MANUAL OF CLINICAL PR
IN INTERNAL MEDICINE
WITH ANNOTATED KEY REFERENCES

MANUAL OF CLINICAL PROBLEMS
IN INTERNAL MEDICINE
WITH ANNOTATED KEY REFERENCES

FOURTH EDITION

EDITED BY

JERRY L. SPIVAK, M.D., F.A.C.P.
Professor of Medicine,
Director, Division of Hematology,
Johns Hopkins University School of Medicine,
Baltimore, Maryland

H. VERDAIN BARNES, M.D., F.A.C.P.
Chairman, Department of Medicine,
Professor of Medicine and Pediatrics,
Wright State University School of Medicine,
Dayton, Ohio

Little, Brown and Company
Boston/Toronto/London

To our wives Wendy and Joyce

And children Laura and Adam; and Bradlee, Brendie, Brannon, and Shari

CONTENTS

V. DISEASES OF THE GASTROINTESTINAL TRACT

VII. INFECTIOUS DISEASES

PREFACE

The goal of the first edition of the *Manual of Clinical Problems in Internal Medicine* was to identify the pathophysiology, diagnosis, complications, and general management of clinical disorders likely to be encountered on a medical ward through a critical evaluation of the existing literature. It was felt to be especially important that clinical myths or practices based on anecdotal or questionable evidence be exposed while emphasizing differential diagnosis and the pitfalls encountered in therapy. Specific drugs and their administration were already well covered elsewhere and were not to be emphasized in this volume, although their side effects were.

In the intervening years and through two subsequent editions, there have been profound changes in the way medicine is practiced and in the diseases encountered. Computed axial tomography is now a routine procedure, and magnetic resonance imaging promises to be also. Interventional radiology and cardiology play an integral role in patient management. Successful organ transplantation now encompasses not only the kidney but also the bone marrow, both autologous and allogeneic, the heart, lungs, liver, and pancreas, and has spawned a new spectrum of clinical problems related to the requisite immunosuppressive therapy. Some of the drugs employed, such as cyclosporine and antilymphocyte globulin, have even found a useful role in patients with bone marrow failure or marrow cell aplasia who are not eligible for marrow transplantation.

Recombinant DNA technology has led to the introduction of a new class of drugs, the biologic response modifiers, such as alpha interferon and interleukin 2, both used successfully in cancer chemotherapy, and the hematopoietic growth factors, erythropoietin, granulocyte colony–stimulating factor, and granulocyte macrophage colony–stimulating factor, which can influence bone marrow function in a positive and physiologic manner.

Through recombinant DNA technology, the molecular biology of normal and neoplastic cell proliferation is being clarified. Indeed, at the time of the first edition, the Philadelphia chromosome was just being employed widely as a marker for chronic myelogenous leukemia. Now we understand its molecular basis, and the bcr rearrangement as well as immunoglobin gene and T-cell receptor rearrangements and restriction fragment length polymorphisms have important diagnostic roles.

Biology is never static and new diseases have been encountered since this book first appeared. Foremost among these, of course, is the acquired immunodeficiency syndrome caused by the human immunodeficiency virus (HIV-1), which is occurring in the setting of a resurgence of sexually transmitted diseases and intravenous drug abuse. Cocaine, in its various forms, has supplanted heroin and introduced a different spectrum of side effects. The organism causing antibiotic-associated colitis, *Clostridium difficile,* has been identified, as has the agent causing red cell aplasia in immunosuppressed patients, parovirus B19. Coronary artery disease is now more common on our wards than valvular heart disease, but at the same time there has been a reappearance of historically important illnesses, such as acute rheumatic fever and diphtheria. Clinical pharmacology has fortunately kept pace with these challenges and important new antiarrhythmics, antibiotics, antiviral agents, and thrombolytic drugs have been developed.

As we noted in the preface to the last edition, "the need to have access to the appropriate literature has grown more urgent while that literature has grown in size." This manual was designed to meet that need in the past, and in its most extensive revision to date, we hope that it will continue to do so. To this end, we have not only added new chapters to encompass the problems currently encountered on the medical ward but also have enlisted the expertise of our colleagues as authors. The expanded material has been most concentrated in the sections dealing with cardiology, rheumatology, infectious disease, and medical emergencies. In addition, we have used computer-associated literature searches to ensure completeness. For example, in Chapter 12, Upper Gastrointestinal Tract Hemorrhage, more than 500 references were retrieved and reviewed; other chapters were treated in the same fashion. Selecting references was not an easy task but accessibility as well as informational content was always a major consideration.

We believe this volume will continue to meet the needs of a new generation of physicians, as it has in the past. As before, we encourage your comments and opinions.

J. L. S.
H. V. B.

CONTRIBUTING AUTHORS

Martin D. Abeloff, M.D.
Professor of Oncology, Johns Hopkins University School of Medicine; Associate Director, Oncology Center, Johns Hopkins Hospital, Baltimore, Maryland

Stephen C. Achuff, M.D.
Associate Professor of Medicine, Johns Hopkins University School of Medicine; Director of Clinical Cardiology, Johns Hopkins Hospital, Baltimore, Maryland

H. Verdain Barnes, M.D., F.A.C.P.
Chairman, Department of Medicine, Professor of Medicine and Pediatrics, Wright State University School of Medicine, Dayton, Ohio

John G. Bartlett, M.D.
Professor of Medicine, Chief, Division of Infectious Diseases, Johns Hopkins University School of Medicine, Baltimore, Maryland

Michael A. Baumann, M.D.
Associate Professor of Medicine, Division of Hematology/Oncology, Wright State University School of Medicine, Dayton, Ohio

Theodore M. Bayless, M.D.
Professor of Medicine, Johns Hopkins University School of Medicine; Attending Physician, Division of Gastroenterology, Johns Hopkins Hospital, Baltimore, Maryland

David W. Buchholz, M.D.
Assistant Professor of Neurology, Johns Hopkins University School of Medicine; Director, Ambulatory Services, Clinical Neurosciences, Johns Hopkins Hospital, Baltimore, Maryland

Gina A. Dallabetta, M.D.
Assistant Professor of Epidemiology, Johns Hopkins University School of Public Health, Baltimore, Maryland

Alice Faryna, M.D.
Formerly Associate Professor of Medicine, Chief, Division of Rheumatology, Wright State University School of Medicine, Dayton, Ohio

Luis F. Gimenez, M.D.
Assistant Professor of Medicine, Johns Hopkins University School of Medicine; Attending Physician, Renal Division, Johns Hopkins Hospital, Baltimore, Maryland

Kim Goldenberg, M.D.
Professor of Medicine, Chief, Division of General Internal Medicine, Associate Dean for Students and Curriculum, Wright State University School of Medicine, Dayton, Ohio

Thomas Guarnieri, M.D.
Associate Professor of Medicine, Johns Hopkins University School of Medicine; Director, Cardiac Arrhythmia Service, Division of Cardiology, Johns Hopkins Hospital, Baltimore, Maryland

Alan D. Guerci, M.D.
Associate Professor of Medicine, Johns Hopkins University School of Medicine; Director, Coronary Care Unit, Division of Cardiology, Johns Hopkins Hospital, Baltimore, Maryland

David B. Hellmann, M.D.
Associate Professor of Medicine, Johns Hopkins University School of Medicine; Deputy Director, Department of Medicine, Attending Physician, Division of Rheumatology, Johns Hopkins Hospital, Baltimore, Maryland

H. Franklin Herlong, M.D.
Associate Professor of Medicine, Johns Hopkins University School of Medicine; Attending Physician, Division of Gastroenterology, Johns Hopkins Hospital, Baltimore, Maryland

Steven M. Holland, M.D.
Assistant Professor of Medicine, Johns Hopkins University School of Medicine, Baltimore; Guest Researcher, National Institutes of Health, Bethesda, Maryland

Judith E. Karp, M.D.
Associate Professor of Oncology, Johns Hopkins University School of Medicine; Attending Physician, Adult Leukemia Service, Johns Hopkins Hospital, Baltimore, Maryland

Edward J. Levine, M.D.
Fellow, Division of Gastroenterology, Department of Medicine, Johns Hopkins University School of Medicine, Baltimore, Maryland

James P. McGee, Ph.D.
Director of Psychology, Sheppard Pratt Hospital, Baltimore, Maryland

John R. Michael, M.D.
Associate Professor of Medicine, University of Utah School of Medicine; Director, Medical Intensive Care Unit, University Hospital, Salt Lake City, Utah

Charles B. Payne, Jr., M.D.
Professor of Medicine, Chief, Division of General Medicine/Critical Care, Wright State University School of Medicine; Chief, Medical Chest Section, Assistant Chief, Department of Medicine, Veterans Administration Medical Center, Dayton, Ohio

Michelle Petri, M.D.
Assistant Professor of Medicine, Johns Hopkins University School of Medicine; Attending Physician, Division of Rheumatology, Johns Hopkins Hospital, Baltimore, Maryland

James K. Porterfield, M.D.
Assistant Professor of Medicine, Johns Hopkins University School of Medicine; Attending Physician, Division of Cardiology, Johns Hopkins Hospital, Baltimore, Maryland

Thomas C. Quinn, M.D.
Associate Professor of Medicine, Johns Hopkins University School of Medicine; Attending Physician, Division of Infectious Disease, Johns Hopkins Hospital, Baltimore, Maryland

Mohammad G. Saklayen, M.D.
Assistant Professor of Medicine, Wright State University School of Medicine; Chief, Hemodialysis Unit, Veterans Administration Medical Center, Dayton, Ohio

Jerry L. Spivak, M.D., F.A.C.P.
Professor of Medicine, Director, Division of Hematology, Johns Hopkins University School of Medicine, Baltimore, Maryland

Peter B. Terry, M.D.
Associate Professor of Medicine, Johns Hopkins University School of Medicine; Clinic Director, Asthma and Allergy Center, Johns Hopkins Hospital, Baltimore, Maryland

Thomas A. Traill, B.M., B.Ch., M.R.C.P.
Associate Professor of Medicine, Johns Hopkins University School of Medicine; Attending Physician, Division of Cardiology, Johns Hopkins Hospital, Baltimore, Maryland

Alan Watson, M.D.
Associate Professor of Medicine, Johns Hopkins University School of Medicine; Attending Physician, Division of Nephrology, Johns Hopkins Hospital, Baltimore, Maryland

I. MEDICAL EMERGENCIES

Notice

The indications and dosages of all drugs in this book have been recommended in the medical literature and conform to the practices of the general medical community. The medications described do not necessarily have specific approval by the Food and Drug Administration for use in the diseases and dosages for which they are recommended. The package insert for each drug should be consulted for use and dosage as approved by the FDA. Because standards for usage change, it is advisable to keep abreast of revised recommendations, particularly those concerning new drugs.

1. CARDIAC ARREST AND RESUSCITATION
Alan D. Guerci

Cardiac arrest may be defined as the sudden cessation of effective cardiac activity. Cardiac arrest is not synonymous with death but will ordinarily result in death unless specific measures are taken. In untreated arrest, permanent damage to the cerebral cortex begins within 5 minutes and is total and complete in 10 minutes.

Most cardiac arrests are the result of advanced heart disease and, in particular, advanced atherosclerotic coronary artery disease. Pulmonary embolism, aortic dissection, and intracranial hemorrhage are less common causes of cardiac arrest in previously healthy persons. Obviously, cardiac arrest may occur in the advanced stages of any serious systemic illness.

In an outpatient setting, asphyxiation, usually due to sedative-hypnotic overdose, smoke inhalation, or drowning, and the ingestion of medications or illicit drugs with direct cardiac activity must also be considered. Among hospitalized patients, iatrogenic factors are not infrequent causes of cardiac arrest. Cardioactive drugs and catheters account for most of these cases. Catheters and pacemaker wires can induce complete heart block or atrial or ventricular tachyarrhythmias and may also perforate the heart and great vessels. Severe electrolyte derangements, especially hyperkalemia and hypokalemia, are also common causes of inpatient cardiac arrest.

Like most good medical practice, successful resuscitative efforts are dependent on considerable amounts of physical effort and attention to detail as well as the mastery of a specific fund of knowledge. The American Heart Association's ABCs of basic life support, *A* for airway, *B* for breathing, and *C* for chest compression, remain an invaluable guide to resuscitation, for effective ventilation is not possible without a properly positioned and unobstructed airway, and neither ventilation nor chest compression is ordinarily of value without the other. Proper positioning of the airway requires extension of the neck in order to raise the base of the tongue off the posterior pharyngeal wall. This can usually be achieved by pushing on the forehead with one hand while lifting the chin with the other. Alternatively, the neck may be extended by pushing on the forehead with one hand and lifting the back of the neck with the other. In cases of suspected cervical spine trauma, it may be possible to open the upper airway simply by raising the mandible. This procedure requires two hands and considerable force but, when performed properly, results in little or no movement of the neck. Breathing may be accomplished by mouth-to-mouth ventilation, bag-and-mask techniques, or endotracheal intubation. Effective mouth-to-mouth ventilation requires pinching-off of the nostrils. Proficiency with bag-and-mask techniques can usually be developed with relatively little practice. The greatest difficulty encountered with this technique involves the establishment of a tight seal around the bridge of the nose. Endotracheal intubation should not be attempted by unskilled persons. Whereas improper use of bag-and-mask techniques will result in hypoventilation, inadvertent intubation of the esophagus will result in no ventilation.

Resistance to airflow generally means airway obstruction, and prompt corrective action is required. The Heimlich maneuver is preferred for conscious victims of upper airway obstruction who cannot move enough air past the obstruction to cough vigorously. Rescuers should never place their hands in the mouth of a conscious victim of airway obstruction. If loss of consciousness supervenes, the obstructing object may be dislodged with vigorous chest compressions and abdominal thrusts. Abdominal thrusts are performed by placing the heel of one hand just below the xiphoid, the second hand over the first, and driving in a cephalad and posterior direction. It is likely that this maneuver does not raise intrathoracic pressure, the motive force for expulsion of a foreign object, as high as vigorous chest compression, and the technique should probably be avoided entirely in pregnant women. Although vigorous back blows were once recommended in this situation, it is not known whether back blows dislodge foreign objects obstructing the airway more often than they cause impaction of foreign objects. When chest compressions and abdominal thrusts fail, cricothyroidotomy may be performed.

It is not known whether external chest compression generates blood flow by direct

3

compression of the heart or a generalized increase in intrathoracic pressure. Animal data provide conflicting evidence on this point, and although human data favor the latter hypothesis, published studies are limited in size and scope. What is clear is that effective external chest compression requires vigorous compression and maintenance of this compression for approximately 50 percent of each compression-release cycle. Whether blood flow in a particular patient is due to direct compression of the left ventricle or increased intrathoracic pressure, or both, more forceful chest compression will provide increased vital organ blood flow. Since cerebral blood flow during cardiopulmonary resuscitation (CPR) is usually not sufficient to maintain consciousness, and myocardial blood flow is usually not sufficient to prevent progressively worsening ischemia and acidosis, the factor which sets an upper limit on the force of chest compression is chest wall trauma. It is probably true that if a bone or a joint in the rib cage has not been damaged, then CPR was not performed with adequate vigor. Proper compression duration (50%) and more or less maximal cardiac output can be achieved by compressing the chest at a rate of 80 to 100 per minute. The discomfort and potential for serious chest wall injury inherent in CPR mandate withholding application of this technique in conscious patients, no matter how low the blood pressure. The recommended sequence of ventilation and chest compressions is two ventilations for each 15 chest compressions in single-rescuer CPR and one ventilation for every 5 chest compressions in two-rescuer CPR.

The cardiac rhythms causing cardiac arrest fall into three categories: ventricular tachyarrhythmias, asystole and profound bradyarrhythmias, and electromechanical dissociation. Because myocardial perfusion is usually inadequate during CPR and because most cardiac arrests are due to ventricular tachyarrhythmias, defibrillation occupies a central position in the treatment of cardiac arrest. Defibrillation is the treatment of first choice in monitored arrests due to ventricular fibrillation or ventricular tachycardia, and blind defibrillation should be employed whenever more than a minute or two is required to record the actual arrhythmia responsible for the arrest. The recommended energy levels are 200 joules for the first countershock, 300 joules for the second countershock, and 400 joules for all subsequent countershocks. Countershocks should probably be delivered in pairs, as the first countershock seems to lower transthoracic impedance. The general strategy for the treatment of ventricular fibrillation and ventricular tachycardia with loss of consciousness involves administration of drugs and the performance of CPR for periods of time sufficient to permit drug effect, alternating with countershocks.

In the case of ventricular tachyarrhythmias causing cardiac arrest, if the initial set of countershocks does not restore organized electrical activity, countershock alone must be regarded as inadequate and drug therapy must be initiated. Epinephrine, lidocaine, and bretylium are the drugs of choice in this situation. In high doses (1 mg every 5 minutes) epinephrine causes intense peripheral vasoconstriction and maximizes cerebral and myocardial perfusion. The usual approach to ventricular tachyarrhythmias refractory to initial countershocks, therefore, is to administer 1 mg of epinephrine, continue CPR for 2 to 5 minutes, and repeat the countershocks. If the ventricular tachyarrhythmia persists, lidocaine may be given in a dose of 1 mg/kg followed by 0.5 mg/kg at 8-minute intervals up to a total of 3 mg/kg. Available data indicate that adherence to this protocol will provide therapeutic lidocaine levels for 35 to 40 minutes. Because hepatic blood flow is negligible during CPR, lidocaine metabolism can be disregarded and lidocaine infusions are not necessary. Since the above regimen will provide therapeutic lidocaine levels beginning within a minute or two of the initial dose, it may be argued that a patient who remains in ventricular fibrillation or ventricular tachycardia 5 or more minutes after the initial dose has failed lidocaine therapy. Since time is limited, it may be appropriate to administer bretylium in addition to ongoing administration of lidocaine in such cases. One ampule (500 mg) of bretylium is an appropriate dose and may be repeated in 5 to 10 minutes. Because bretylium is absorbed by cardiac myocytes for several hours after intravenous administration, and because antiarrhythmic effectiveness is proportional to the intramyocardial level, the effectiveness of bretylium will increase rather than decrease over time. Bretylium should not be given to patients with known or suspected digitalis toxicity, as animal models of this situation are characterized by refractory ventricular fibrillation, probably due to the initial bretylium-induced norepinephrine release acting in concert with digitalis-induced increases in intracellular sodium and calcium. Intravenous beta blockade may be of value in cases in which myocardial ischemia is thought to have been the cause of the ventricular tachyarrhythmia. Procainamide is of lesser value in cardiac arrest because a full hour may be required to achieve a loading dose.

Whereas the emphasis in the treatment of ventricular tachyarrhythmias causing cardiac arrest is placed on stopping the heart, with the expectation that the heart's own intrinsic pacemaker cells will take over at rates compatible with life, the emphasis of treatment for bradyarrhythmias causing cardiac arrest is to increase the ventricular rate in the hope that effective contractile activity will accompany the faster rate. Epinephrine is the drug of choice for this purpose. In doses of 1 mg every 5 minutes, epinephrine maximizes coronary and cerebral perfusion for as long as the patient needs CPR and also fully saturates cardiac beta-adrenergic receptors. This means that chronotropic, dromotropic, and inotropic stimulation is maximal. Isoproterenol was once recommended for this purpose but is now understood to be contraindicated in any person who needs CPR to support his or her circulation. A potent vasodilator, isoproterenol reduces aortic pressure during CPR and actually abolishes coronary blood flow. Indeed, in animal models, the administration of isoproterenol for cardiac standstill is uniformly lethal, whereas the administration of high doses of epinephrine, which also fully stimulates heart rate and contractility, is associated with resuscitation rates approaching 100 percent. Atropine, which in doses of 0.5 mg is ordinarily very useful when sinus bradycardia, second-degree heart block, or slow junctional rhythms lead to circulatory compromise, is of little value in asystole or complete heart block causing full cardiac arrest. The one exception to this rule is complete heart block complicating acute inferior myocardial infarction, in which atropine is often effective in restoring atrioventricular (AV) nodal conduction. The dose of atropine for bradyarrhythmias causing full cardiac arrest is 1 mg.

Electromechanical dissociation is defined as a state of normal or relatively normal electrical activity with minimally effective or ineffective contractile activity. Thus, if myocardial disease is the cause, the underlying disease is ordinarily so severe as to militate against successful resuscitation. Alternatively, a number of treatable nonmyocardial disorders may also cause electromechanical dissociation. These include hypovolemia, tension pneumothorax, pericardial tamponade, and profound acidosis. Massive pulmonary embolism may also cause electromechanical dissociation, but is less easily corrected.

Treatment of electromechanical dissociation is based on consideration of thoracentesis, pericardiocentesis or volume infusion, and repeated administration of epinephrine. Correction of acidosis with sodium bicarbonate may also be advisable.

Standard pharmacologic therapy must be modified for two causes of cardiac arrest. Ordinarily of no value in resuscitation, calcium may be lifesaving in hyperkalemic arrests. The role of sodium bicarbonate in cardiac arrest is, in general, uncertain, but sodium bicarbonate is a partial antagonist for tricyclic antidepressants and is therefore indicated in known or suspected tricyclic overdose.

The outcome of resuscitative efforts is, in general, determined by the severity of underlying disease and the elapsed time between arrest and the initiation of resuscitative efforts. Although the majority of patients will not survive, results are not hopeless. Rates of survival to hospital discharge in excess of 60 percent have been reported for out-of-hospital arrest victims receiving CPR within 4 minutes and advanced cardiac life support within 8 minutes of collapse. Forty-nine percent of those surviving to discharge were alive 4 years later, compared to 80 percent 4-year survival among age-adjusted controls. For inpatient arrests, survival to discharge is usually around 15 percent. Up to 80 percent of short-term survivors are alive at 6 months.

Decisions to withhold resuscitative efforts ought to be made in consultation with patients and their families. Discussions of resuscitative status can be positive and constructive, emphasizing consideration of all possible outcomes of the patient's illness and the support which will be provided to the patient, and allowing the patient to participate in choosing the level of care which he or she will receive. A policy requiring discussion of resuscitative status also contains the seeds of conflict, for it is inevitable that resuscitation will be requested for some patients with no reasonable chance of recovery.

Nevertheless, such a policy appears to be the best safeguard of the patient's rights. Unreasonable demands can usually be satisfied with information about prognosis and the efforts of social workers, psychiatrists, and clergy, and resolution of these issues in hospital conference rooms is preferred over resolution in courtrooms.

1. McIntyre, K. M., and Lewis, A. J. (eds.) *Textbook of Advanced Cardiac Life Support.* Dallas: American Heart Association, 1983.
   Comprehensive review of the pathophysiology and treatment of cardiac arrest.
2. Standards and guidelines for cardiopulmonary resuscitation and emergency cardiac care. *J.A.M.A.* 255:2841, 1986.
   Updated recommendations.
3. Proceedings of the 1985 national conference on standards and guidelines for cardiopulmonary resuscitation and emergency cardiac care. *Circulation* 74 (Suppl. 4): 1986.
   Detailed discussions of several controversial issues in resuscitation.
4. Kouwenhoven, W. B., Jude, J. R., and Knickerbocker, G. G. Closed-chest cardiac massage. *J.A.M.A.* 73:1064, 1960.
   Original report from the developers of external chest compression.
5. Rudikoff, M. T., Maughan, W. L., Effron, M., et al. Mechanisms of blood flow during cardiopulmonary resuscitation. *Circulation* 61:258, 1980.
   Blood flow due to increased intrathoracic pressure described.
6. Niemann, J. T., Rosborough, J. R., Hausknecht, M., et al. Pressure synchronized cineangiography during experimental cardiopulmonary resuscitation. *Circulation* 64:985, 1981.
   More on blood flow due to increased intrathoracic pressure.
7. Chandra, N., Guerci, A., Weisfeldt, M. L., et al. Contrasts between intrathoracic pressures during external chest compression and cardiac massage. *Crit. Care Med.* 9:789, 1981.
   More on blood flow due to increased intrathoracic pressure.
8. Maier, G. W., Tyson, G. S., Olsen, C. O., et al. The physiology of external cardiac massage: High impulse cardiopulmonary resuscitation. *Circulation* 70:86, 1984.
   Evidence of direct cardiac compression in a canine model of CPR.
9. Halperin, H., Tsitlik, J. E., Guerci, A. D., et al. Determinants of blood flow to vital organs during cardiopulmonary resuscitation in dogs. *Circulation* 73:539, 1986.
   Analysis which permits mechanistic inferences derived from the effect of compression rate and duration on blood pressure and flow.
10. MacKenzie, G. J., Taylor, S. H., MacDonald, A. H., et al. Hemodynamic effects of external cardiac compression. *Lancet* 1:1342, 1964.
    Left and right heart pressures are similar during CPR in humans.
11. Thomsen, J. E., Stenlund, R. R., and Rowe, G. G. Intracardiac pressure during closed chest massage. *J.A.M.A.* 205:46, 1968.
    As above, this evidence favors the intrathoracic pressure hypothesis for blood flow.
12. Taylor, G. J., Tucker, W. M., Greene, H. L., et al. Importance of prolonged compression during cardiopulmonary resuscitation. *N. Engl. J. Med.* 296:1515, 1977.
    Blood flow in humans is dependent on duration of chest compression, not compression rate.
13. Werner, J. A., Greene, H. L., Janko, C. L., et al. Visualization of cardiac valve motion during external chest compression using two-dimensional echocardiography. *Circulation* 63:1417, 1981.
    The mitral valve is open during CPR in humans, consistent with the heart-as-conduit concept.
14. Pearson, J. W., and Redding, J. S. Influence of peripheral vascular tone on cardiac resuscitation. *Anesth. Analg.* 44:746, 1965.
    Pioneering study of drug therapy for cardiac arrest; observations remain relevant.
15. Redding, J. S., and Pearson, J. W. Resuscitation from ventricular fibrillation. *J.A.M.A.* 203:93, 1968.
    As above, with focus on ventricular fibrillation (VF).
16. Michael, J. R., Guerci, A. D., Koehler, R. D., et al. Mechanisms by which epinephrine

augments cerebral and myocardial perfusion during cardiopulmonary resuscitation in dogs. *Circulation* 69:822, 1984.
Explanation of the benefit of epinephrine during CPR.

17. Chow, M. S. S., Ronfeld, R. A., Ruffett, D., et al. Lidocaine pharmacokinetics during cardiac arrest and external cardiopulmonary resuscitation. *Am. Heart J.* 102:799, 1982.
Rationale for lidocaine loading regimen during CPR.

18. Haynes, R. E., Chinn, T. L., Copass, M. K., et al. Comparison of bretylium tosylate and lidocaine in resuscitation of patients from out-of-hospital ventricular fibrillation. A randomized clinical trial. *Am. J. Cardiol.* 48:353, 1981.
Lidocaine and bretylium are equally effective in out-of-hospital VF.

19. Bishop, R. L., and Weisfeldt, M. L. Sodium bicarbonate administration during cardiac arrest: Effect on arterial pH, pCO_2 and osmolality. *J.A.M.A.* 235:506, 1976.
Sodium bicarbonate raises PCO_2 as well as pH . . .

20. Cingolani, H. E., Faulkner, S. L., Matiazzi, A. R., et al. Depression of human myocardial contractility with "respiratory" and "metabolic" acidosis. *Surgery* 77:427, 1975.
. . . and PCO_2 is a rapid-acting, potent negative inotrope.

21. Guerci, D. A., Chandra, N., Johnson, E., et al. Failure of sodium bicarbonate to improve resuscitation from ventricular fibrillation in dogs. *Circulation* 74 (Suppl. 4):75, 1986.
Results as described in title, with review of the sodium bicarbonate issue.

22. Weaver, W. D., Cobb, L. A., Copass, M. K., et al. Ventricular defibrillation: A comparative trial using 175-J and 320-J shocks. *N. Engl. J. Med.* 207:1101, 1982.
175 joules is an appropriate energy level for initial countershock.

23. Thompson, R. G., Hallstrom, A. P., and Cobb, L. A. Bystander initiated cardiopulmonary resuscitation in the management of ventricular fibrillation. *Ann. Intern. Med.* 90:737, 1979.
Bystander initiation of CPR reduces mortality and improves neurologic status.

24. Eisenberg, M. S., Copass, M. K., Hallstrom, A., et al. Management of out-of-hospital cardiac arrest: Failure of basic emergency medical technician services. *J.A.M.A.* 243:1049, 1980.
Prompt defibrillation increases survival.

25. Eisenberg, M., Hallstrom, A., and Berger, L.,: The ACLS score: Predicting survival from out-of-hospital cardiac arrest. *J.A.M.A.* 246:50, 1981.
Resuscitation rate of nearly 70% is possible for out-of-hospital VF.

26. Bedell, S. E., Delbanco, T. L., Cook, E. F., et al. Survival after cardiopulmonary resuscitation. *N. Engl. J. Med.* 309:569, 1983.
Short- and long-term outcome from in-hospital arrest.

27. Fox, M., and Lipton, H. L. The decision to perform cardiopulmonary resuscitation. *N. Engl. J. Med.* 309:607, 1983.
Introduction to the ethics of withholding treatment.

28. Taffet, G. E., Teasdale, T. A., and Luchi, R. J. In-hospital cardiopulmonary resuscitation. *J.A.M.A.* 260:2069, 1988.
Cancer, sepsis, polypharmacy, and age are predictive of a poor outcome.

2. DISSECTING ANEURYSM OF THE AORTA

Jerry L. Spivak

Dissecting aneurysm is the most common acute disease of the aorta. Dissection can occur at any age but occurs most often between the fifth and seventh decades, and predominantly in men. Factors predisposing to aortic dissection include hypertension, giant cell arteritis, Marfan's syndrome (but not homocystinuria), Ehlers-Danlos syndrome, idiopathic kyphoscoliosis, coarctation of the aorta, Turner's syndrome, aortic hypoplasia, bicuspid aortic valves, pregnancy, trauma, and cardiac surgery. To date, dissection has not been reported in patients taking oral contraceptives. Syphilitic aortitis does not protect against dissection, nor does hypothyroidism predispose to it.

Dissecting aneurysms can be divided into two types depending on whether there is involvement of the ascending aorta. Type A dissections (De Bakey types I and II), the more common, involve the ascending aorta, the aortic arch, or both. Type B dissections (De Bakey type III) are limited to the aorta distal to the origin of the left subclavian artery. Dissections extend antegrade or retrograde, usually in an asymmetric fashion, from the site of the initial intimal tear. Involvement of aortic branches is not uncommon, but it is usually limited to those arteries with more elastic tissue than muscular tissue. They include the iliac, innominate, and subclavian arteries.

The factors responsible for aortic dissection are not totally understood. Defective connective tissue is likely in Marfan's or the Ehlers-Danlos syndrome, coarctation, bicuspid valves, aortic hypoplasia, idiopathic kyphoscoliosis, and possibly pregnancy. On the other hand, many normal aortas show medial degeneration, and it is not clear whether the medial degeneration found in patients with dissections is the cause of the process or a result of it. Because intimal tears are not always found, dissection has been thought to result from an intramural hematoma in some patients. It is unlikely, however, that the vasa vasorum could generate the necessary pressure relative to the aorta to produce such a hematoma. Hypertension is also not an invariable feature, and the aorta can withstand intramural pressures well above those associated with dissection. Atherosclerosis may play a more significant role than is generally accepted, particularly in type B dissections. The process produces damage to the media as well as the intima, and a ruptured plaque can provide the necessary channel for the dissection. In addition, atherosclerosis-induced rigidity and dilatation of the aorta can result in pressure changes (Laplace's law) that may favor dissection. The importance of rigidity is reflected by the area of location of intimal tears, all of which are at points of fixation of the aorta.

Propagation of the dissection seems to be aided by the pulsatile nature of aortic blood flow, suppression of which is the major objective in the medical management of the process. Propagation is also aided by the anatomy of the aortic wall, with its lamellation and vasa vasorum. Most commonly, the dissection occurs in the area between the outer third of the media and the adventitia. As a consequence, there is little support for the false channel, and the result is often rupture into the pericardium, mediastinum, or pleural space. Spontaneous reentry can occur, but that does not protect against rupture of the false lumen.

The onset of aortic dissection is usually abrupt, with the development of severe pain in the chest or abdomen. Although pain limited to the back is distinctive for type B dissection, there is otherwise no relationship between the location of the pain and the intimal tear, nor is there any feature of pain besides its severity that might distinguish a dissection from the other diseases that must be considered in the differential diagnosis. Those diseases include acute myocardial infarction, pancreatitis, pericarditis, perforated peptic ulcer, leaking aortic aneurysm, vertebral collapse, esophageal rupture, and acute cholecystitis. Because of the nonspecific nature of its presentation, aortic dissection must be considered in every acute thoracic and abdominal syndrome. Factors suggesting dissection are chest or abdominal pain associated with loss of one or more peripheral pulses, pericardial tamponade, hemothorax, and neurologic signs. The neurologic signs include sudden coma or syncope, hemiplegia, extraocular paralyses, Horner's syndrome, vocal cord paralysis, neuropathy, and seizures. Either the right or both cerebral hemispheres can be involved, but not the left one alone. The neurologic signs are the result of either hypotension (pericardial tamponade) or arterial occlusion by the dissection. Differences in blood pressure between the extremities or loss of a pulse are important physical signs, as is the development of aortic insufficiency. An uncommon but helpful sign is a prominent pulsation at either sternoclavicular joint. The ECG is helpful only to exclude an acute myocardial infarction but abnormalities suggesting myocardial injury are seen in 20 percent of dissections. A plain chest x ray is never considered diagnostic since aortic widening due to dissection cannot be distinguished from mediastinal fat, hematoma, tumor, or aortitis; aortography is the procedure of choice for the diagnosis and classification of an acute aortic dissection. The procedure is not without risk, and noninvasive procedures such as computed tomography (CT) scanning, two-dimensional echocardiography, and magnetic resonance imaging (MRI) may prove useful in the evaluation of chronic dissections or where another diagnosis, such as acute myocardial infarction, is likely. They may also be useful in following treated patients.

Studies of the natural history of aortic dissection have indicated that 3 percent of patients die immediately, 21 percent within 1 day, 60 percent in 2 weeks, and 90 percent in 3 months. Factors predisposing to a high mortality include the presence of underlying pulmonary or renal disease, severe neurologic involvement, and type A dissection. Type B dissections and failure to opacify the false lumen at aortography are associated with a good prognosis.

There has been considerable debate over the type of management, medical or surgical, for patients with aortic dissection. The problem has not been clarified by the tendency to administer either type of therapy only to good-risk patients. Although the use of drugs that reduce blood pressure and myocardial contractility has been a significant advance in the management of dissections, there has been a tendency for medically treated patients with type B dissections to subsequently develop saccular aortic aneurysms or progressive dissection. In addition, drug therapy is not without hazards, such as acute tubular necrosis, peptic ulcer, myocardial infarction, cerebrovascular accident, postural hypotension, and congestive heart failure. At present, patients with acute ascending aortic dissections (type A) should be treated by surgery. Patients with a leaking aneurysm (pericardial or pleural hemorrhage), aortic insufficiency, occlusion of a major vessel, congestive heart failure, or progression of the dissection with medical therapy, or patients in whom the false channel opacifies should also undergo surgical correction. Medical therapy is indicated for stable type B dissections, particularly those in which the false lumen does not opacify. Whether or not patients with stable type B dissections who are treated medically should have elective surgery at a later date is unclear, but recent data indicate that progressive dissection occurs in a high percentage of type B lesions initially treated medically.

1. DeSanctis, R. W., Doroghazi, R. M., Austen, W. G., et al. Aortic dissection. *N. Engl. J. Med.* 317:1060, 1987.
   A comprehensive review. (See also Lancet *2:827, 1988.)*
2. Hirst, A. E. N., Johns, V. J., Jr., and Kime, S. W., Jr. Dissecting aneurysm of the aorta: A review of 505 cases. *Medicine* (Baltimore) 37:217, 1958.
   A classic article.
3. Wheat, M. W., Jr. Acute dissecting aneurysms of the aorta: Diagnosis and treatment (1979). *Am. Heart J.* 99:373, 1980.
   Excellent review of the subject.
4. Vecht, R. J., Besterman, E. M. M., Bromley, L. L., et al. Acute dissection of the aorta: Long term review and management. *Lancet* 1:109, 1980.
   Surgery for type A dissections; medical therapy for type B.
5. Dalen, J. E., Pape, L. A., Cohn, L. H., et al. Dissection of the aorta: Pathogenesis, diagnosis and treatment. *Prog. Cardiovasc. Dis.* 23:237, 1980.
   Experience with 69 patients.
6. Leonard, J. L., and Hasleton, P. S. Dissecting aortic aneurysms: A clinicopathological study. *Q. J. Med.* 48:55, 1979.
   Cystic medial necrosis, fibrosis, or medionecrosis do not necessarily predispose to aortic dissection. (See also Am. J. Cardiol. *53:849, 1984.)*
7. Williams, G. M., Gott, V. L., Brawley, R. K., et al. Aortic disease associated with pregnancy. *J. Vasc. Surg.* 8:470, 1988.
   Pregnancy is a risk factor for aortic dissection.
8. Gerber, O., Heyer, E. J., and Vieux, U. Painless dissections of the aorta presenting as acute neurologic syndromes. *Stroke* 17:644, 1986.
   Something to remember. (See also Am. J. Med. *84:765, 1988 and* Ann. Emerg. Med. *17:840, 1988).*
9. Pyeritz, R. E., and McKusick, V. A. The Marfan syndrome. *N. Engl. J. Med.* 300:772, 1979.

Propranolol recommended prophylactically to retard aortic dilatation. (See also N. Engl. J. Med. 305:988, 1981 for a discussion of the collagen abnormality.)

10. Gott, V. L., Pyeritz, R. E., and Magovern, G. J., Jr. Surgical treatment of aneurysms of the ascending aorta in the Marfan syndrome. Results of composite-graft repair in 50 patients. *N. Engl. J. Med.* 314:1070, 1986.
    Surgical intervention recommended when aortic dilatation reaches 6 cm.

11. Lin, A. E., Lippe, B. M., Geffner, M. E., et al. Aortic dilation, dissection, and rupture in patients with Turner syndrome. *J. Pediatr.* 109:820, 1986.
    Another risk factor for aortic dissection.

12. Shuford, W. H., Sybers, R. G., and Weens, H. S. Problems in the aortographic diagnosis of dissecting aneurysm of the aorta. *N. Engl. J. Med.* 280:225, 1969.
    Opacification of true and false lumens can simulate a normal aorta. CT scanning may be helpful here.

13. Hayaski, K., Meaney, T. F., Zelch, J. V., et al. Aortographic analysis of aortic dissection. *Am. J. Roentgenol. Radium Ther. Nucl. Med.* 122:769, 1974.
    Detailed review.

14. Eagle, K. A., Quertermous, T., Kritzer, G. A., et al. Spectrum of conditions initially suggesting acute aortic dissection but with negative aortograms. *Am. J. Cardiol.* 57:322, 1986.
    The differential diagnosis of aortic dissection.

15. Kersting-Sommerhoff, B. A., Higgins, C. B., White, R. D., et al. Aortic dissection: sensitivity and specificity of MR imaging. *Radiology* 166:651, 1988.
    MRI is highly sensitive and specific. (See also J. Comput. Assist. Tomogr. 11:975, 1987.)

16. Goldman, A. P., Kotler, M. N., Scanlon, M. H., et al. The complementary role of magnetic resonance imaging, Doppler echocardiography, and computed tomography in the diagnosis of dissecting thoracic aneurysms. *Am. Heart J.* 111:970, 1986.
    Use of noninvasive tests evaluated. (See also J. Comput. Assist. Tomogr. 10:211, 1985).

17. Jagannath, A. S., Sos, T. A., Lockhart, S. H., et al. Aortic dissection: a statistical analysis of the usefulness of plain chest radiographic findings. *Am. J. Roentgenol.* 147:1123, 1986.
    Interpretation of chest x rays is too subjective.

18. Saner, H. E., Gobel, F. L., Nicoloff, D. M., et al. Aortic dissection presenting as pericarditis. *Chest* 91:71, 1987.
    This can be a silent complication revealed only by CT scanning. (See Chest 93:652, 1988.)

19. Pressler, V., and McNamara, J. J. Thoracic aortic aneurysm. *J. Thorac. Cardiovasc. Surg.* 79:489, 1980.
    Dissecting and arteriosclerotic aneurysms compared.

20. Schlatmann, T. J. M., and Becker, A. E. Histologic changes in the normal aging aorta: Implications for dissecting aortic aneurysm. *Am. J. Cardiol.* 39:13, 1977.
    This article and its companion (Am. J. Cardiol. 39:21, 1977) challenge the concept that cystic medionecrosis is a unique pathologic entity. (See also Circulation 28:1071, 1963 and Arch. Pathol. Lab. Med. 106:175, 1982.)

21. Miller, D. C., Stinson, E. B., Oyer, P. E., et al. Operative treatment of aortic dissections. *J. Thorac. Cardiovasc. Surg.* 78:365, 1979.
    Immediate surgery advocated for dissections involving the ascending aorta.

22. Haverich, A., Miller, D. C., Scott, W. G., et al. Acute and chronic aortic dissections—determinants of long-term outcome for operative survivors. *Circulation* 72:1111, 1985.
    See also J. Am. Coll. Cardiol. 3:1026, 1984.

23. Guthaner, D. F., Miller, D. C., Silverman, J. F., et al. Fate of the false lumen following surgical repair of aortic dissections: An angiographic study. *Radiology* 133:1, 1979.
    The false lumen may be the only perfusion channel in some aortic branches.

24. McFarland, J., Willerson, J. T., Dinsmore, R. E., et al. Medical treatment of dissecting aortic aneurysms. *N. Engl. J. Med.* 286:115, 1972.
    Absence of opacification of the false channel is a good prognostic sign.

25. Dalen, J. E., Alpert, J. S., Cohn, L. H., et al. Dissection of the thoracic aorta. *Am. J. Cardiol.* 34:803, 1974.
    High incidence of progression of dissection in medically treated patients with a distal (type B) lesion.
26. Chase, T. N., Rosman, N. P., and Price, D. C. The cerebral syndromes associated with dissecting aneurysm of the aorta: A clinicopathological study. *Brain* 91:173, 1968.
    Cerebral dysfunction due to vascular obstruction may obscure the presence of a dissection.
27. Bieger, R., Vreeken, J., Stibbe, J., et al. Arterial aneurysm as a cause of consumption coagulopathy. *N. Engl. J. Med.* 285:152, 1971.
    Localized clot formation with consumption of coagulation factors.

3. HYPERTENSIVE CRISIS

H. Verdain Barnes

Hypertensive crisis is characterized by severe progressive functional impairment of the kidneys, eyes, and brain of patients with a sustained or sudden rise in diastolic blood pressure, usually to levels greater than 120 mm Hg. The incidence ranges from 1 to 7 percent among known hypertensives, but on rare occasions the condition arises de novo. Crisis is seen most often in the 40- to 60-year age group in the setting of known hypertension of 2 to 10 years' duration. Predisposing factors in the development of hypertensive crisis have been difficult to define. Two factors, however, have emerged, namely, severe hypertension at initial diagnosis prior to crisis, and interruption or withdrawal of antihypertensive therapy. Sudden withdrawal of clonidine and nifedipine may result in a hypertensive crisis. The most common associated diseases are essential hypertension, chronic pyelonephritis, and acute glomerulonephritis. In patients under age 30, the last two conditions predominate. Other associated diseases and circumstances include polyarteritis nodosa, other systemic necrotizing vasculitis, systemic lupus erythematosus, scleroderma, unilateral renal artery stenosis, thrombosis or embolism, toxemia of pregnancy, postirradiation of the renal area, congenitally small kidneys, hydronephrosis, nephrocalcinosis, renal tuberculosis, hyperadrenocorticism, pheochromocytoma, primary aldosteronism, renin-secreting tumor of the kidney, and excessive ingestion of ephedrine, amphetamines, or foods rich in tyramine by patients being treated with monoamine oxidase inhibitors.

Renal, eye, or central nervous system changes may dominate the clinical picture, but changes in all three are usually seen during the course of the illness. Blood pressure levels are usually sustained but may show wide fluctuations. An isolated diastolic blood pressure reading of less or greater than 120 mm Hg neither excludes nor confirms the diagnosis and must always be interpreted in the light of the presenting history and physical findings.

Early ocular changes may include soft exudates, hemorrhages, and/or papilledema. Papilledema is an invariable component of the syndrome if the process has progressed slowly; however, in the patient with rapidly progressive disease, papilledema may be absent. Papilledema is usually accompanied by a neuroretinitis, but can be seen alone. Varying degrees of blindness are present, and usually resolve with appropriate therapy. It should be noted, however, that the eye changes may continue to progress for a week or more after adequate blood pressure control has been achieved. The underlying pathology is that of fibrinoid necrosis of the arterioles with plasma leakage into surrounding areas, resulting in "cotton-wool" exudates and flame-shaped hemorrhages from capillary rupture. The papilledema arises from focal or generalized cerebral edema. Blindness is the result of neuroretinitis and/or severe obliterative arterial spasm.

Hypertensive encephalopathy may be sudden or gradual in onset and is usually preceded or accompanied by a severe headache. The neurologic manifestations are variable and commonly result in seizures and coma. The primary underlying pathology is multiple small thrombi in the brain with associated focal or generalized cerebral edema. This process is set in motion by the cerebral vasoconstriction accompanying high arterial blood pressure. Cerebral vasoconstriction is relatively less than in peripheral vessels, resulting in an increased cerebral capillary pressure and edema. Hypertensive encephalopathy can be mimicked by acute pulmonary edema in patients with hypertensive vascular disease and by acute anxiety producing a transient rise in blood pressure. The neuropsychiatric presentations of these three conditions may be indistinguishable. Hypertensive encephalopathy can be seen in some patients with toxemia of pregnancy and in children and adolescents with acute nephritis when blood pressures are around 149/90 mm Hg, since for these age groups such a reading may represent a 30- to 50-mm Hg rise in diastolic pressure.

Some degree of renal failure is invariably present and may dominate the clinical picture. The pathology is that of fibrinoid necrosis and endarteritis of the preglomerular arterioles and interlobular arteries of the kidney. The result is ischemia and necrosis of glomeruli and renal failure. In addition, the distinctive pathology of an underlying disease, such as chronic pyelonephritis, may be seen. Hypertensive crisis can present as acute oliguric renal failure with or without associated encephalopathy. Only about 40 percent of the patients have papilledema, but an additional 50 percent have hemorrhages and/or exudates. Hypertensive crisis must be kept in mind when the diagnosis of acute renal failure due to acute vasculitis, glomerulonephritis, or tubular necrosis is considered. Progressive uremia accounts for 30 to 60 percent of the deaths in malignant hypertension. It is clear that these patients benefit from having their diastolic blood pressure lowered to the 90- to 100-mm Hg range. The reduction in blood pressure benefits the ischemic kidney and often results in a significant return of function, although a general worsening of renal function is often seen with the initial lowering of the blood pressure. Renal function, however, will in most patients improve in subsequent weeks and months.

Finally, the other notable clinical features seen in hypertensive crisis are severe headache (more commonly seen in younger patients), weight loss, and elevated sedimentation rate. Uncommon but important findings are microangiopathic hemolytic anemia and aortic dissection.

1. Kincaid-Smith, P., McMichael, J., and Murphy, E. A. The clinical course and pathology of hypertension with papilloedema (malignant hypertension). *Q. J. Med.* 27:117, 1958.
   An excellent review of the natural history and clinical characteristics of malignant hypertension.
2. Dollery, C. T., Ramalho, P. S., Patterson, J. W., et al. Retinal microemboli: Experimental production of "cotton wool" spots. *Lancet* 1:1303, 1965.
   Occlusion of arterioles with focal necrosis and leakage of plasma results in typical exudates.
3. Adams, R. D. Observations on brain embolism with special reference to the mechanism of hemorrhage infarction. *J. Clin. Invest.* 29:795, 1950.
   In hypertensive encephalopathy multiple small thrombi are found in the cerebral vessels, helping to account for an often bizarre neurologic picture.
4. Finnerty, F. A., Jr. Hypertensive encephalopathy. *Am. J. Med.* 52:672, 1972.
   Hypertensive encephalopathy can be mimicked by acute pulmonary edema and acute anxiety.
5. Wilson, C., and Byron, F. B. Renal changes in malignant hypertension: Experimental evidence. *Lancet* 1:136, 1939.
   Fibrinoid necrosis and endarteritis fibrosa are the primary pathologic findings in the kidney.
6. Sevitt, L. H., Evans, D. J., and Wrong, O. M. Acute oliguric renal failure due to accelerated (malignant) hypertension. *Q. J. Med.* 40:127, 1971.
   Acute renal failure without an obvious precipitating cause may dominate the picture in hypertensive crisis.
7. Mroczek, W. J., Davidov, M., Gavnlovich, L., et al. The value of aggressive therapy in the hypertensive patient with azotemia. *Circulation* 40:893, 1969.

Acutely as the blood pressure was lowered, these patients showed an increase in serum creatinine and BUN by 17% and 19% respectively, but by 3 to 6 months there was an average decrease to below pretreatment levels—24 mg/dl in the BUN and 2.8 mg/dl in serum creatinine.

8. Breckenridge, A., Dollery, C. T., and Parry, E. H. O. Prognosis of treated hypertension. *Q. J. Med.* 39:411, 1970.
   Uremia is the leading cause of death in patients with hypertension, followed in order by cerebrovascular accidents and myocardial infarction.

9. Glazener, F. S., Morgan, W. A., Simpson, J. M., et al. Pargyline, cheese, and acute hypertension. *J.A.M.A.* 188:754, 1964.

10. Lee, M. R. Renin-secreting kidney tumors: Rare but remediable cause of serious hypertension. *Lancet* 2:254, 1971.

11. Dalakos, T. G., Streeten, D. H. P., Jones, D., et al. "Malignant" hypertension resulting from atheromatous embolization predominantly of one kidney. *Am. J. Med.* 57:135, 1974.

12. Kanada, S. A., Kanada, D. J., and Hutchinson, R. A. Angina-like syndrome with diazoxide therapy for hypertensive crisis. *Ann. Intern. Med.* 84:696, 1976.

13. Slotkoff, L. M. Prostaglandin A in hypertensive crisis. *Ann. Intern. Med.* 81:345, 1974.
    Articles 12 and 13 discuss therapeutic modalities.

14. Matas, B. R. The optic fundus and hypertension. *Med. Clin. North Am.* 61:547, 1977.

15. Cuneo, R. A., and Caronna, J. J. The neurologic complications of hypertension. *Med. Clin. North Am.* 61:565, 1977.
    Articles 14 and 15 offer concise reviews of these two areas.

16. Strauss, F. G., Franklin, S. S., Lewin, A. J., et al. Withdrawal of antihypertensive therapy: Hypertensive crisis in renovascular hypertension. *J.A.M.A.* 238:1734, 1977.
    Clonidine hydrochloride withdrawal can precipitate hypertensive crisis and those with renovascular disease may be unusually susceptible.

17. Elkik, F., Cornol, P., Idatte, J.-M., et al. Renal segmental infarction: A cause of reversible malignant hypertension. *J. Hypertension* 2:149, 1984.
    An entity to keep in mind in young adults with sudden-onset hypertensive crisis which can be treated medically until remission.

4. PULMONARY EDEMA
John R. Michael

Pulmonary edema develops because of either an increase in pulmonary capillary pressure (cardiogenic) or an increase in the permeability of the pulmonary microvessels (noncardiogenic). Cardiogenic pulmonary edema may occur as a result of systemic hypertension, or myocardial, pericardial, or valvular heart disease. Many disorders can cause noncardiogenic pulmonary edema (also called the adult respiratory distress syndrome or ARDS) by increasing the permeability of the pulmonary vessels. A helpful mnemonic for conditions that cause ARDS is "SHOOT CALL PATH" which stands for sepsis especially gram-negative; hematologic disorders such as disseminated intravascular coagulopathy or thrombotic thrombocytopenic purpura; overdoses with heroin or similar compounds; other infections; trauma, especially associated with long-bone fractures; chemical inhalation of toxic gases or smoke; all other miscellaneous conditions; hemorrhagic pancreatitis; aspiration of gastric contents, freshwater, or saltwater; transfusion of 5 to 10 units of blood over 24 hours; and head injuries or intracranial events, such as subarachnoid hemorrhage.

Patients with cardiogenic pulmonary edema can usually be distinguished from patients with noncardiogenic pulmonary edema, although prospective studies suggest that approximately 10 to 20 percent of patients may have a mixed picture. An enlarged heart or bilateral pleural effusions suggest cardiogenic pulmonary edema, although patients with tight mitral stenosis, left atrial myxoma, or recent myocardial infarctions may have cardiogenic pulmonary edema with a normal-sized heart. The most helpful features that distinguish cardiogenic from noncardiogenic edema are the pulmonary capillary wedge pressure and the concentration of protein in the pulmonary edema fluid. Patients with cardiogenic edema will usually have a wedge pressure exceeding 20 to 25 mm Hg; whereas patients with noncardiogenic pulmonary edema will generally have a wedge pressure less than 15 to 18 mm Hg. Patients with noncardiogenic pulmonary edema will have pulmonary edema fluid with a high concentration of protein because of the increase in the permeability to protein. This can be quantified by determining the ratio of alveolar to plasma protein. In patients with noncardiogenic edema this ratio is usually 0.8 to 1.0; whereas in cardiogenic edema this ratio is generally less than 0.5. Patients with severe cardiogenic edema often have a combined metabolic and respiratory acidosis in addition to severe hypoxemia; whereas patients with noncardiogenic pulmonary edema rarely have respiratory acidosis.

The treatment of cardiogenic pulmonary edema should focus on reducing pulmonary venous pressure. This can usually be accomplished by using morphine, nitrates, diuretics, and oxygen. Morphine is useful in the treatment of cardiogenic pulmonary edema, but should not be used in patients who are unconscious, hypotensive, or have depressed respiration. Diuretics are particularly helpful in patients who are salt and water overloaded. One should remember, however, that many patients with cardiogenic edema are not salt and water overloaded. These patients develop pulmonary edema because sudden left ventricular failure leads to a rapid shift of intravascular volume into the lungs. In a patient with cardiogenic pulmonary edema who does not have peripheral edema, overdiuresis may lead to hypotension. Thus, the convention that all patients with cardiogenic pulmonary edema need diuresis may be incorrect. It is preferable to give sublingual nitrates because of their rapid absorption. Transdermal nitrates should not be used in hypotensive patients. Patients with cardiogenic pulmonary edema who are in extremis should be intubated. The positive intrathoracic pressure resulting from mechanical ventilation reduces venous return, afterloads the left ventricle, and shifts edema fluid from alveoli to the perivascular space. All of these effects improve cardiogenic pulmonary edema.

In treating these patients one should quickly identify conditions that may require additional therapy, such as mitral stenosis, tachyarrhythmias or bradyarrhythmias, myocardial ischemia, or prosthetic heart valves. Mitral stenosis should be considered in all patients, but especially young or middle-aged patients without a prior cardiac history who present with a normal-sized heart and atrial fibrillation. Because in mitral stenosis the increased pulmonary venous pressure is due to obstructed flow across the mitral valve rather than volume overload, measures that reduce venous return such as morphine, diuretics, and nitrates may dramatically reduce cardiac output and arterial blood pressure. In a patient with mitral stenosis and a rapid ventricular rate, the rate should be slowed in order to allow more time for filling of the left ventricle. Verapamil or digoxin are the drugs of choice. Patients with myocardial ischemia may develop mitral regurgitation because of papillary muscle rupture or dysfunction or a ventricular septal defect. Prosthetic valves may become infected, clotted, or unseated, leading to heart failure. In contrast to the excellent prognosis in patients with cardiogenic pulmonary edema, in patients with noncardiogenic pulmonary edema the mortality rate exceeds 50 percent. The first goal of therapy in ARDS is to treat or correct the underlying disorder that has led to an increase in pulmonary vascular permeability. Although the primary defect leading to the development of pulmonary edema is an increase in vascular permeability, there is no therapy that reduces the increase in permeability. The amount of edema, however, can be reduced by keeping the pulmonary wedge pressure as low as possible without significantly reducing cardiac output. Because of the severe lung injury these patients usually require treatment with high concentrations of oxygen and positive end-expiratory pressure (PEEP). PEEP improves PaO_2 primarily by increasing lung volume and by shifting fluid out of alveoli into the perivascular and interstitial space. The major cause of death in ARDS is not respiratory failure but infection, which most often arises in the abdomen or lungs. A multicenter controlled clinical trial indicates that steroid therapy does not improve survival in ARDS.

1. Robin, E. D., Cross, C. E., and Zelis, R. Pulmonary edema. *N. Engl. J. Med.* 288:239, 1973.
   An exhaustive review.
2. Staub, N. C. Pulmonary edema. *Chest* 74:559, 1978.
   Physiologic approach to the pathogenesis.
3. Fein, A., Grossman, R. F., Jones, J. G., et al. The value of edema fluid protein measurement in patients with pulmonary edema. *Am. J. Med.* 67:32, 1979.
   Protein measurements employed to separate overperfusion from increased permeability pulmonary edema.
4. Trapnell, D. H. The differential diagnosis of linear shadows in chest radiographs. *Radiol. Clin. North Am.* 11:77, 1973.
   Kerley lines represent interlobular septa, not lymphatics.
5. Chait, A. Interstitial pulmonary edema. *Circulation* 45:1323, 1972.
   The "silent" stage of pulmonary edema.
6. Hublitz, U., and Shapiro, J. Atypical pulmonary patterns of congestive heart failure in chronic lung disease. *Radiology* 93:995, 1969.
   Altered distribution of edema fluid is related to underlying anatomic and functional defects.
7. Finlayson, J. K., Luria, M. N., Stanfield, C. A., et al. Hemodynamic studies in acute pulmonary edema. *Ann. Intern. Med.* 54:244, 1961.
   One of the few studies of hemodynamic changes during the acute event in patients with cardiac disease.
8. Trapnell, D. H., and Thurston, J. G. B. Unilateral pulmonary oedema after pleural aspiration. *Lancet* 1:1367, 1970.
   Rapid expansion of collapsed lung resulting in pulmonary edema.
9. Mahajan, V. K., Simon, M., and Huber, G. L. Reexpansion pulmonary edema. *Chest* 75:192, 1979.
   Prolonged duration of collapse and application of excess negative pressure are two important factors.
10. Ciongoli, A. K., and Poser, C. M. Pulmonary edema secondary to subarachnoid hemorrhage. *Neurology* 22:867, 1972.
    The complication may mask the primary event.
11. Huff, R. W., and Fred, H. C. Postictal pulmonary edema. *Arch. Intern. Med.* 117:824, 1966.
    Edema is predominantly in the upper lobes.
12. Carilli, A. D., Ramamurty, M. V., Chang, Y. S., et al. Noncardiogenic pulmonary edema following blood transfusion. *Chest* 74:310, 1978.
    Pulmonary edema due to increased microvascular permeability.
13. Zelis, R., Mansour, E. J., Capone, R. J., et al. The cardiovascular effects of morphine. *J. Clin. Invest.* 54:1247, 1974.
    Morphine produces venous and arteriolar dilatation by reduction in alpha-adrenergic tone.
14. Dikshit, K., Vyden, J. K., Forrester, J. S., et al. Renal and extrarenal hemodynamic effects of furosemide in congestive heart failure after acute myocardial infarction. *N. Engl. J. Med.* 288:1087, 1973.
    Relief of pulmonary congestion by furosemide is not related to its diuretic properties.
15. Figueras, J., and Weil, M. H. Blood volume prior to and following treatment of acute cardiogenic pulmonary edema. *Circulation* 57:349, 1978.
    Blood volume falls during acute cardiogenic pulmonary edema and expands with reversal of the pulmonary edema.
16. Figueras, J., and Weil, M. H. Hypovolemia and hypotension complicating management of acute cardiogenic pulmonary edema. *Am. J. Cardiol.* 44:1349, 1979.
    Volume expansion advocated in cardiogenic pulmonary edema complicated by hypotension.
17. Ayres, S. M. Ventilatory management in acute pulmonary edema. *Am. J. Med.* 54:558, 1973.
    Good advice.

18. Bussmann, W. D., and Schupp, D. Effect of sublingual nitroglycerin in emergency treatment of severe pulmonary edema. *Am. J. Cardiol.* 41:931, 1978.
   Rapid decrease in left ventricular filling pressure and relief of symptoms and sublingual nitroglycerin.
19. Aberman, A., and Fulop, M. The metabolic and respiratory acidosis of acute pulmonary edema. *Ann. Intern. Med.* 76:173, 1972.
   Acidosis was present in 80% of patients and hypercapnea in 20%.
20. Habak, P. A., Mark, A. C., Kiosckos, J. M., et al. Effectiveness of congesting cuffs ("rotating tourniquets") in patients with left heart failure. *Circulation* 50:366, 1974.
   The use of tourniquets produces less pooling in heart failure than in absence of that condition.
21. Heffner, J. E., and Salin, S. A. Salicylate-induced pulmonary edema: clinical features and prognosis. *Ann. Intern. Med.* 95:405, 1981.
   This diagnosis may be missed especially in the elderly.
22. Narins, R. G., and Chusid, P. Diuretic use in critical care. [Review] *Am. J. Cardiol.* 57:26A, 1986.
   Rational use of diuretics.
23. Matthay, M. A. Pathophysiology of pulmonary edema. [Review] *Clin. Chest Med.* 6:301, 1985.
   Good discussion.
24. O'Quin, R., and Marini, J. J. Pulmonary artery occlusion pressure: clinical physiology, measurement, and interpretation. *Am. Rev. Respir. Dis.* 128:319, 1983.
   Excellent discussion of the wedge pressure.
25. Colice, G. L., Matthay, M. A., Bass, E., et al. Neurogenic pulmonary edema. *Am. Rev. Respir. Dis.* 130:941, 1984.
   Excellent review of this condition.
26. Shaw, T. J., and Caterine, J. M. Recurrent re-expansion pulmonary edema. *Chest* 86:784, 1984.
   Nice description of this entity.
27. Montgomery, A. B., Stager, M. A., Carrico, C. J., et al. Causes of mortality in patients with the adult respiratory distress syndrome. *Am. Rev. Respir. Dis.* 132:485, 1985.
   Infection is the major cause of death rather than respiratory failure.
28. Bell, R. C., Coalson, J. J., Smith, J. D., et al. Multiple organ system failure and infection in adult respiratory distress syndrome. *Ann. Intern. Med.* 99:293, 1983.
   The multiorgan failure predisposes these patients to infection.
29. Pepe, P. E., Hudson, L. D., and Carrico, C. J. Early application of positive end-expiratory pressure in patients at risk for adult respiratory distress syndrome. *N. Engl. J. Med.* 311:281, 1984.
   PEEP is not protective.

5. PULMONARY EMBOLISM
H. Verdain Barnes

Pulmonary embolism can be defined as the occlusion of one or more vessels in the pulmonary arterial tree by matter from a source extrinsic to the lung. The process is almost invariably acute but may on occasion be chronic. The obstruction is usually by a clot from the distal venous system, but it can result from fat, amniotic fluid, air, or particulate matter from intravenous injection. Depending on the size and number of emboli, the clinical features may range from mild tachycardia and anxiety to shock and sudden death. Pulmonary emboli are a major cause of death in hospitalized patients. It has been estimated that at least 50,000 deaths per year are due to pulmonary emboli with only about 50 to 75 percent suspected ante mortem.

A number of inherited and acquired factors are associated with an increased risk of venous thromboembolism. The inherited risks include antithrombin III, protein C and protein S deficiency states, plus dysfibrinogenemia and abnormalities of plasminogen and its activation. The acquired risk factors are systemic lupus erythematosus; nephrotic syndrome; paroxysmal nocturnal hemoglobinuria; cancer (particularly lung, pancreas, breast, prostate, colon, and stomach); stasis states (congestive heart failure, cardiomyopathy, constrictive pericarditis, myocardial infarction, and immobilization); sepsis; polycythemia rubra vera; inflammatory bowel disease; significant obesity; sickle cell disease or trait; dysproteinemias; pregnancy; birth control with oral contraceptives; the early postpartum period; and after major surgery, especially pelvic, lower-extremity, and portacaval procedures. Major fractures of the pelvis and lower extremities are a common background for thromboembolism and fat emboli. The potential of thromboembolism occurring in association with any of these conditions is enhanced by increasing age. Approximately 90 percent of pulmonary emboli occur in patients over age 50 years.

The clinical presentation is quite varied. It can easily be confused with acute myocardial infarction, pneumonia, congestive heart failure (with or without pulmonary edema), chronic obstructive pulmonary disease, and/or bronchial asthma. Typical clinical manifestations and their approximate percentages include dyspnea (84%), pleuritic chest pain (74%), apprehension (59%), cough (53%), tachypnea (90%), pulmonary crackles (58%), and an increased pulmonary second heart sound (53%). Less frequent features are hemoptysis (30%), syncope (14%), nonpleuritic chest pain, often anginalike (14%), fever (57%), tachycardia (44%), diaphoresis (36%), gallop (34%), and cyanosis (19%). Clear evidence of thrombophlebitis is present in fewer than 50 percent of patients. Additional clues to be sought on physical examination include cyanosis, hypotension, right-sided congestive heart failure with or without hepatomegaly, increased dullness to the right of the sternum on percussion, distended neck veins with a prominent A wave, pulmonary systolic murmur and thrill in association with an accentuated pulmonary second heart sound, and wheezing. Wheezing, which is common and often prominent in these patients, is typically localized to the involved side and occasionally to the site of the embolus.

The current gold standard for laboratory diagnosis is pulmonary angiography. Arteriography is the most accurate but carries some morbidity and mortality. The angiographic abnormalities are (1) intraluminal filling defects, (2) discrete arterial cutoffs, (3) oligemic areas, and (4) total absence of arteries in the involved area. The first two, when clearly present, are diagnostic; the last two may be hard to interpret without a comparison study before or after since they can also be seen in focal emphysema and bronchiectasis. With angiography there are no false-positives when intraluminal filling defects and/or discrete arterial cutoffs are present; however, false-negatives can occur when the emboli are in the smaller-than-second-order arteries. The following constellation of findings derived from discriminant analysis appears to predict the results of arteriography in about 82 percent of patients: age less than 65 years, cancer, leg pain, substernal chest pain, tachycardia greater than 90 per minute or an increase of more than 20 beats per minute over baseline, new S3 or S4 gallop, and a positive lung scan.

The routine scintillation lung scan is easily performed; however, false-positive and false-negative results are seen. Segmental filling defects can also be seen in chronic obstructive pulmonary disease, asthma, pneumonia, lung cysts, bronchiectasis, and atelectasis. An unequivocally normal lung scan, however, makes the diagnosis unlikely. The combination of a perfusion and ventilation scan offers greater accuracy. In acute pulmonary embolism the area of decreased perfusion usually has essentially normal ventilation, whereas in other lung diseases, particularly pneumonia and chronic obstructive lung disease, there are abnormalities in both the ventilation and the perfusion scan.

Hypoxemia is usually present in acute pulmonary embolism. The cause is multifactorial, but recent evidence supports the theory that bronchoconstriction and pneumoconstriction are the primary components. Constriction of the bronchi, bronchioles, alveolar ducts, and alveoli occurs primarily as a result of serotonin release by platelet aggregates on the surface of the thrombus. This leads to ventilation-perfusion mismatching and increased arteriovenous mixing. Additional factors include decreased diffusing capacity, anatomic right-to-left shunting, and atelectasis. Patients with a normal heart and otherwise normal lungs can usually compensate by increasing their inspiratory capacity, whereas patients with significant heart and/or lung disease cannot. Consequently, when patients are breathing room air, a PO_2 of less than 80 mm Hg is common with pulmonary embolism. If the lungs are otherwise normal, there is an accompanying decrease in PCO_2 and an increase in pH due to hyperventilation. This arterial blood gas pattern is not specific for pulmonary embolism; it can also be seen in left ventricular heart failure and acute myocardial infarction. The combination of a normal lung scan and a normal PO_2, however, makes the diagnosis of embolism unlikely.

A variety of other studies can be used to support the diagnosis, but none are diagnostic. Routine chest x ray reveals nonspecific changes of pulmonary infiltrate and/or pleural effusion in two-thirds of patients, but in the remainder it is normal. The ECG changes most commonly seen are atrial arrhythmias, prominent P waves, staircase ST wave ascent, an S in lead I and a Q in lead III, right bundle branch block, right axis deviation, ischemia, a Q in lead V_1, T wave inversion, and first-degree heart block.

The search for a source of thrombophlebitis is facilitated by venography, isotope-labeled fibrinogen scanning, plethysmography, and/or ultrasound flow detection with a Doppler device. The Doppler evaluation is readily available, is noninvasive, and has a greater than 90 percent correlation with venography. About 25 percent of pulmonary embolism patients with a negative clinical examination for thrombophlebitis will have an abnormal Doppler test, a fact that is clinically useful even though false-positives do occur. Combined plethysmography and Doppler flow studies have been shown to predict venogram results with a sensitivity of 96 percent and specificity of 93 percent; however, none of these modalities are optimal in detecting calf thrombophlebitis and, more importantly, do not exclude pulmonary embolism.

Patients with massive pulmonary emboli usually die within the first few hours, whereas those with smaller emboli generally live. Varying periods of time are required for resolution. The rate of resolution depends on age, clot size, and number of clots. About two-thirds of patients show complete or almost complete resolution within 6 months. Some 20 percent show resolution within about 5 weeks. In most patients the pulmonary artery pressure returns to or approaches normal in 1 to 3 weeks. Emboli have a predilection for the lower lung fields, and a single embolus is the exception rather than the rule.

1. Soloff, L. A., and Rodman, T. Acute pulmonary embolism: I. Review. *Am. Heart J.* 74:710, 1967.
   A well-done article with an emphasis on predisposing factors and pathophysiology.
2. Stein, J. M., and Pruitt, B. A. Suppurative thrombophlebitis. *N. Engl. J. Med.* 282:1452, 1970.
   Another cause of pulmonary embolism; seen in heroin addicts and patients with venous cannulas.
3. Olazabal, F., Roman-Irizarry, L. A., Oms, J. D., et al. Pulmonary emboli masquerading as asthma. *N. Engl. J. Med.* 278:999, 1968.
   Wheezing may be a prominent clue.
4. Thomas, D. P., Gurewich, V., and Ashford, T. P. Platelet adherence to thromboemboli in relation to the pathogenesis and treatment of pulmonary embolism. *N. Engl. J. Med.* 274:953, 1966.
   Serotonin release from the clot produces bronchospasm.
5. Dalen, J. E., Mathin, V. S., and Evans, H. Pulmonary angiography in experimental pulmonary embolism. *Am. Heart J.* 72:509, 1966.
   Angiography provides the most objective evidence of pulmonary emboli, but false-negatives occur if emboli are in the smaller arteries.
6. Szucs, M. M., Jr., Brooks, H. L., Banas, J. S., Jr., et al. Diagnostic sensitivity of laboratory findings in acute pulmonary embolism. *Ann. Intern. Med.* 74:161, 1971.
   A valuable study defining the correlation of various tests for pulmonary emboli. A normal PO_2 and negative lung scan together make the diagnosis of acute pulmonary emboli unlikely.
7. Wilson, J. E., III, Pierce, A. R., Johnson, R. L., et al. Hypoxemia in pulmonary embolism: A clinical study. *J. Clin. Invest.* 50:481, 1971.

Hypoxemia due to anatomic right-to-left shunting is usually associated with localized atelectasis.

8. Tow, D. E., and Wagner, H. N., Jr. Recovery of pulmonary arterial blood flow in patients with pulmonary embolism. *N. Engl. J. Med.* 276:1053, 1967.
   Most emboli are to the lower lung fields. Four months or longer is required for resolution in the majority of patients.
9. Dalen, J. E., Banas, J. S., Jr., Brooks, H. L., et al. Resolution rate of acute embolism in man. *N. Engl. J. Med.* 280:1194, 1969.
   In 1 to 3 weeks, the right heart pressures return to normal or almost normal.
10. Tilkian, A. G., Schroeder, J. S., and Robin, E. D. Chronic thromboembolic occlusion of main pulmonary artery or primary branches. *Am. J. Med.* 60:563, 1976.
    A rare but recognizable entity.
11. Bell, W. R., Simon, T. L., and DeMets, D. L. The clinical features of submassive and massive pulmonary emboli. *Am. J. Med.* 62:355, 1977.
    An effective clinical comparison of two quantitative types of pulmonary emboli.
12. Stein, P. D., Willis, P. W., III, and DeMets, D. L. History and physical examination in acute pulmonary embolism in patients without preexisting cardiac or pulmonary disease. *Am. J. Cardiol.* 47:218, 1981.
    Tachypnea (respiratory rate >20/min) or dyspnea occurred in 96% and one of those and/or clinical evidence of deep venous thrombosis occurred in 99% (N-215).
13. Murray, H. W., Ellis, G. C., Blumenthal, D. S., et al. Fever and thromboembolism. *Am. J. Med.* 67:233, 1979.
    About 57% of their patients had a fever due solely to their pulmonary embolism, one >40°C.
14. Wilson, J. E., III, Bynum, L. J., and Parkey, R. W. Heparin therapy in venous thromboembolism. *Am. J. Med.* 70:808, 1981.
    A convincing article showing fewer embolic recurrences in those treated with intermittent as compared to continuous heparin.
15. Bell, W. R. Pulmonary embolism: Progress and problems. *Am. J. Med.* 72:181, 1982.
    Good advice from an expert.
16. Fulkerson, W. J., Coleman, C., Ravin, C. E., et al. Diagnosis of pulmonary embolism. *Arch. Intern. Med.* 146:961, 1986.
    A critical discussion of clinical and laboratory features.
17. Libby, L. S., King, T. E., LaForce, F. M., et al. Pulmonary cavitation following pulmonary infarction. *Medicine* 64:342, 1985.
    A diagnostic consideration in cavitary lung disease.
18. Hoellerich, V. L., and Wigton, R. S. Diagnosing pulmonary embolism using clinical findings. *Arch. Intern. Med.* 146:1699, 1986.
    An effective use of discriminant analysis.
19. Hull, R. D., Hirsh, J., Carter, C. J., et al. Pulmonary angiography, ventilation lung scanning and venography for clinically suspected pulmonary embolism with abnormal perfusion lung scan. *Ann. Intern. Med.* 98:891, 1983.
    A scholarly review of these diagnostic modalities.
20. Schiff, M. J., Feinberg, A. W., and Naidich, J. B. Noninvasive venous examinations as a screening test for pulmonary embolism. *Arch. Intern. Med.* 147:505, 1987.
21. Thaler, E., and Lechner, K. Antithrombin III deficiency and thromboembolism. *Clin. Haematol.* 10:369, 1981.
22. Broekmans, A. W. Hereditary protein C deficiency. *Haemostasis* 15:233, 1985.
23. Engesser, L., Broekmans, A. W., Briet, E., et al. Hereditary protein S deficiency: Clinical manifestations. *Ann. Intern. Med.* 106:677, 1987.
    These articles (21–23) describe the inherited risk factors for thromboembolism.
24. Sharma, G. V. R. K., McIntyre, K. M., Sharma, S., et al. Clinical and hemodynamic correlates in pulmonary embolism. *Clin. Chest Med.* 5:421, 1984.
    An up-to-date review comparing patients with and without underlying cardiopulmonary disease.
25. Petitti, D. B., Strom, B. L., and Melmon, K. L. Duration of warfarin anticoagulant therapy and the probabilities of recurrent thromboembolism and hemorrhage. *Am. J. Med.* 81:255, 1986.
    A large study showing the problems encountered in long-term anticoagulant therapy.

6. SEPTIC SHOCK
H. Verdain Barnes

Septic shock is a dynamic syndrome of inadequate tissue perfusion and metabolic dysfunction. In about two-thirds of patients it results from a gram-negative infection and in the rest from gram-positive infection. Twenty-five percent of all patients having a gram-negative bacteremia develop the complete syndrome. Several epidemiologic observations are important. The syndrome occurs most often in men over age 40 years, while in the under-40 age group, females with obstetric or gynecologic problems predominate. The majority of patients have one or more of the following underlying conditions: diabetes mellitus, cirrhosis, alcoholism, leukemia, lymphoma, metastatic carcinoma, urinary or biliary tract disease, extensive burns, and prior surgery or manipulation of the genitourinary or gastrointestinal tracts. The potential for septic shock in any one of these conditions is enhanced when associated with irradiation, corticosteroid, or antimetabolite therapy. The most common gram-negative organisms are *Escherichia coli, Klebsiella-Aerobacter, Proteus* species, *Pseudomonas,* paracolon, *Bacteroides, Salmonella,* and *Mina herellea* species. The most frequent gram-positive organisms are staphylococci, streptococci, pneumococci, and clostridia.

The pathophysiology of septic shock is multifactorial. For gram-negative organisms a major factor is the release of endotoxin, a lipopolysaccharide, as well as the lysis of leukocytes with the release of serotonin, histamine, kinins, lysosomal enzymes, and superoxide radicals into the circulation. The initial systemic changes are in large measure related to the interference with cell function due to the action of the endotoxin. This appears to be primarily initiated by an activation of the classic and/or alternative pathways of the complement system. The overall result is a decrease in peripheral vascular resistance; increase in central venous pressure; increase in pulmonary vascular resistance; increase in ventilatory insufflation pressure; diversion of all metabolism toward gluconeogenesis, ketone body formation, and reduced energy producing oxidative metabolism; decreased oxygen consumption; increased tissue permeability; and hyperkinetic hemodynamic changes. There is a rise in cardiac output that is usually not adequate to compensate for the fall in vascular resistance. The net result is pooling of blood in the body's microvascular beds, ineffective cardiac output, hypotension, and tissue anoxia. If this persists, there is inadequate perfusion of the brain, kidney, lungs, and heart and an overproduction of lactic acid. It appears that a higher initial heart rate and cardiac index are the only significant hemodynamic differences between gram-positive and gram-negative septic shock.

Recognition of the fully developed syndrome rarely presents a clinical problem; however, atypical or early manifestations of septic shock may cause considerable difficulty. Its potential should be considered in any elderly patient who has unexplained mental changes, drop in blood pressure, hyperventilation, and/or a high fever. In the early stages of the syndrome, "warm shock" is often present. This includes mild hypotension, full pulse pressure, warm dry skin, and only minimal decrease in urinary output. At that juncture, there is a respiratory alkalosis with a low PCO_2 and an elevated arterial pH. With time, untreated as well as some treated patients develop "cold shock." In this stage, hypotension becomes more profound and the patient is characteristically pale, cold, clammy, and peripherally cyanotic, with a weak, thready pulse and a marked decrease in urinary output. A metabolic acidosis supervenes with a low PCO_2 and arterial pH. The central venous pressure drops. There is usually a leukocytosis with a shift to the left, decreased platelets, and often an initial hematocrit elevation. The serum urea nitrogen and creatinine increase, as does the blood lactate level. Blood cultures are usually, but not invariably, positive. A Gram's stain of the peripheral blood or buffy coat may be positive and help differentiate between a gram-positive and a gram-negative bacteremia. About 90 percent of patients have fever and about 35 percent present with a sudden onset of chills, nausea, vomiting, and/or diarrhea. All patients suspected of having septic shock should have careful central venous pressure and urinary output monitoring.

The differential diagnosis includes pulmonary embolism, myocardial infarction, aortic dissection, occult hemorrhage, cerebrovascular accident, and occasionally pericardial disease with tamponade. If a well-equipped intensive care unit is available, a hemodynamic evaluation may be useful. In septic shock, the cardiac output is high or normal and the vascular resistance and filling pressure low, whereas in myocardial infarction, the cardiac output is low and vascular resistance normal or high, and in hemorrhage the cardiac output is low and vascular resistance high. In patients with septic shock, a thorough, aggressive, and rapid evaluation and early institution of specific therapy are the keys to survival.

A serious illness, toxic shock syndrome, has been delineated. It occurs most often in otherwise healthy menstruating females who are using tampons, but can occur in men with localized infections. The inciting organism is primarily *Staphylococcus aureus* soft tissue infection with and without demonstrable bacteremia. The clinical manifestations are variable, but most have fevers above 100.5°F (38°C), hypotension or syncope, skin rash with ultimate desquamation, and mucous membrane hyperemia. Gastrointestinal and central nervous system signs and symptoms and myalgias are common. The differential diagnosis includes leptospirosis, Rocky Mountain spotted fever, measles, and mucocutaneous lymph node syndrome. Significant mortality and morbidity occur, particularly if a timely diagnosis is not made.

1. Waisbren, B. A. Bacteremia due to gram-negative bacilli other than the salmonella: Clinical and therapeutic study. *Arch. Intern. Med.* 88:467, 1951.
   The initial description of the syndrome. The most common portal of entry was the genitourinary tract.
2. McHenry, M. C., Martin, W. J., and Wellman, W. E. Bacteremia due to gram-negative bacilli: Review of 113 cases encountered in five-year period of 1955–1959. *Ann. Intern. Med.* 56:207, 1962.
   About 60% of the persons reviewed were over age 60, with men predominating. Escherichia coli was the most common organism, accounting for about 25% of cases.
3. Weil, M. H., Shubin, H., and Biddle, M. Shock caused by gram-negative micro-organisms. *Ann. Intern. Med.* 60:384, 1964.
   24% of these authors' gram-negative bacteremic patients developed shock.
4. Guenter, C. A., and Hindshaw, L. B. Comparison of septic shock due to gram-negative and gram-positive organisms. *Proc. Soc. Exp. Biol. Med.* 134:780, 1970.
   Gram-positive organisms can also produce septic shock.
5. Winslow, E. J., Loeb, H. S., Rahimtoola, S. H., et al. Hemodynamic studies and results of therapy in 50 patients with bacteremic shock. *Am. J. Med.* 54:421, 1973.
   The primary difference between gram-negative and gram-positive shock is a higher heart rate and cardiac index in gram-positive patients.
6. Blain, C. M., Anderson, T. O., Pietras, R. J., et al. Immediate hemodynamic effects of gram-negative vs gram-positive bacteremia in man. *Arch. Intern. Med.* 126:260, 1970.
   Both types of bacteremia showed a decrease in vascular resistance and an increase in cardiac output.
7. Nishijima, H., Weil, M. H., Shubin, H., et al. Hemodynamic and metabolic studies on shock associated with gram negative bacteremia. *Medicine* 52:287, 1973.
   Survival is more likely in those who maintain a high cardiac output. The cardiac index has potential prognostic value.
8. Maki, D. G., Rhame, F. S., Mackel, M. S., et al. Nationwide epidemic of septicemia caused by contaminated intravenous products. *Am. J. Med.* 60:471, 1976.
   An important potential cause of septicemia. In this epidemic septicemia was due to Enterobacter cloacae or Escherichia agglomerans.
9. Gerlin, L.-E., Davidson, I., Haglund, U., et al. Septic shock. *Surg. Clin. North Am.* 60:161, 1980.
10. Siegel, J. H., Cerra, F. B., Coleman, B., et al. Physiological and metabolic correlations in human sepsis. *Surgery* 86:163, 1979.
    These (articles 9 and 10) provide up-to-date comprehensive reviews of the pathophysiology of sepsis and shock.
11. Rector, W. G., Jr. Fever, shock and chills in gram-negative bacteremia: Clinical correlations in 100 cases. *Johns Hopkins Med. J.* 149:175, 1981.

A useful clinical analysis—shock developed in this series only in the presence of a serious underlying disease or postinstrumentation.
12. Tofte, R. W., and Williams, D. N. Toxic shock syndrome. *Ann. Intern. Med.* 94:149, 1981.
  An important, recently described illness that predominates in menstruating females using tampons. Clinicians should keep this in mind.
13. Micheles, T. C. Mucocutaneous lymph node syndrome: Differentiation from toxic shock syndrome. *Am. J. Med.* 80:724, 1986.
  Adult Kawaksaki syndrome is in the differential diagnosis.
14. Schumer, W. Pathophysiology and treatment of septic shock. *Am. J. Med.* 2:74, 1984.
  A brief well-organized review.
15. Corrin, B. Lung pathology in septic shock. *J. Clin. Pathol.* 33:891, 1980.
  Features include congestive atelectasis, impaired surfactant secretion, platelet aggregation, fibrin deposition, and alveolar epithelium necrosis.

7. INFECTIOUS AIRWAY OBSTRUCTION: LUDWIG'S ANGINA; ACUTE INFECTIOUS EPIGLOTTITIS
Jerry L. Spivak

The anatomy of the upper airway makes it vulnerable to obstruction, which may be produced by trauma (endotracheal intubation, bronchoscopy), tumor, foreign body, laryngospasm occurring with tetanus or hypocalcemic tetany, soft tissue hemorrhage, and edema resulting from allergic reactions, vasculitis, or C1 esterase inhibitor deficiency. Occasionally infection may produce acute upper airway obstruction. In adults (as opposed to children), diphtheria is rare, a tendency to subglottic edema is not present, and infectious processes resulting in airway obstruction usually involve the oropharynx, not the glottis.

Infectious airway obstruction involving the oropharynx is a feature of two unusual syndromes—Ludwig's angina and acute infectious epiglottitis. Both conditions are uncommon, and both are potentially lethal if not recognized and managed correctly. Ludwig's angina is a cellulitis of the submaxillary space of the submandibular area. The submaxillary space is formed by the deep cervical fascia, the mylohyoid muscle, and the hyoid bone. Infection in the submaxillary space may be the result of oral lacerations, mandibular fractures, or even oral cancers, but most commonly it occurs with infection of the second and third molars. Those molars are situated behind the insertion of the mylohyoid muscle in potential communication with the submaxillary space. The first molar is anterior to the mylohyoid and communicates with the sublingual space. In addition, the mandibular bone in the area of the second and third molars is relatively thin, providing an accessible route for periapical or periodontal abscesses to reach the submaxillary space. Occasionally infections of the submaxillary gland or suppuration from the submaxillary nodes may empty into the submaxillary space. Characteristically the infection takes the form of a phlegmonous cellulitis, beginning with unilateral involvement but soon spreading contralaterally, along fascial planes into the neck, and eventually entering the sublingual space as well. The results are edema of the floor of the mouth, which pushes the tongue posteriorly, and cervical swelling (the familiar bull neck), with respiratory embarassment and dysphagia. There is no adenopathy or loculation of pus, and involvement of the tonsils and pharynx is minimal. Rarely the infection may spread by continuity to the retropharyngeal space and superior mediastinum.

The principal threat to the patient with Ludwig's angina is not sepsis but airway obstruction. Absence of stridor is no guarantee of a patent airway since the vocal cords are not involved, and obstruction of the airway by the tongue or by supraglottic or cervical swelling may occur with little warning. Soft tissue x rays can provide an indication of the degree of tracheal compromise, but it is difficult to estimate the degree of supraglottic involvement, and manipulations in the supraglottic area may precipitate airway obstruction. Consequently, early intubation or tracheostomy is the treatment of choice in the patient with full-blown Ludwig's angina. Aerobic and anaerobic gram-positive and gram-negative organisms have been implicated in Ludwig's angina, and broad antibiotic coverage should be given initially until culture results are available. Surgical drainage may be necessary in some patients. The most important treatment, however, is prophylactic; patients with abscesses of the posterior molars should receive antibiotic therapy as well as surgical drainage.

Acute infectious epiglottitis is an uncommon condition in adults. It may be produced by a variety of gram-positive organisms, but the most common offender is *Haemophilus influenzae* type B. Infection with that organism is also uncommon in adults since immunity to it is usually acquired in childhood. Ampicillin-resistant *H. influenzae* has been identified in some patients and *Streptococcus pneumoniae* has been cultured from a number of patients. In general, throat cultures are less reliable than blood cultures and antibiotic coverage should be broad.

The symptoms of acute infectious epiglottitis in the adult are chills, choking, drooling, dysphagia, and sore throat. The symptoms may be present for several days before respiratory difficulty or stridor occurs. Hoarseness is not present since the infection does not involve the vocal cords. Fever, often high, is common, and the patient may appear toxic out of proportion to signs or symptoms.

Physical examination may reveal little evidence of pharyngitis, in contrast to the patient's symptoms. Occasionally cervical swelling or adenopathy may be present. The nature of the problem can be determined only by indirect laryngoscopy, which reveals edema and inflammation of the epiglottic and supraglottic tissues. In contrast to Ludwig's angina, abscesses are not uncommon. A brisk neutrophilic leukocytosis is usual, and bacteremia is common. Respiratory obstruction is indicated by dyspnea, cyanosis, stridor, flaring alae, accessory respiratory muscle activity, and suprasternal and intercostal retraction. Respiratory arrest follows within hours.

Recognition of the illness is the key to avoiding catastrophe. In adults, unlike children, symptoms are usually present for several days before respiratory obstruction occurs. Most of the patients seen in clinical practice who complain of pharyngitis have evident pharyngeal inflammation. Consequently, the physician should be alert for the patient whose complaints of sore throat are out of proportion to what can be seen on direct examination, particularly if tender tonsillar nodes are not present. Laryngoscopy should settle the issue, but an overenthusiastic examination can precipitate obstruction. Lateral neck x rays are usually but not always diagnostic, but definitive therapy should not be delayed to obtain them. Patients with infectious epiglottitis should be hospitalized. Signs or symptoms of respiratory distress demand immediate intubation or tracheostomy. If the airway is not compromised, the patient can be put under careful observation. Since intubation or tracheostomy is lifesaving in infectious epiglottitis, the physician must not be too conservative in this regard. Antibiotic therapy should cover both gram-positive organisms and *H. influenzae*, including strains resistant to ampicillin. There has been no controlled experience with the use of corticosteroids in adults.

1. Chow, A. W., Roser, S. M., and Brady, F. A. Orofacial odontogenic infections. *Ann. Intern. Med.* 88:392, 1978.
   Comprehensive review of pathophysiology and treatment. (See also Laryngoscope *97:271, 1987.)*
2. Moreland, L. W., Corey, J., and McKenzie, R. Ludwig's angina. *Arch. Intern. Med.* 148:461, 1988.
   Comprehensive review. (See also J.A.M.A. 243:1171, 1980.)
3. Meyers, B. R., Lawson, W., and Hirschman, S. Z. Ludwig's angina. *Am. J. Med.* 53:257, 1972.
   A case with all the classic features, including sudden respiratory arrest.
4. Lindner, H. H. The anatomy of the fasciae of the face and neck with particular reference to the spread and treatment of intraoral infections (Ludwig's) that have progressed into adjacent fascial spaces. *Ann. Surg.* 204:705, 1986.
   Review of the anatomy of the submandibular and cervical spaces. (See also Laryngoscope *80:409, 1970.)*

5. Snow, N., Lucas, A. E., Grau, M., et al. Purulent mediastinal abscess secondary to Ludwig's angina. *Arch. Otolaryngol.* 109:53, 1983.
   A potential complication of Ludwig's angina. (See also J. Otolaryngol. *12:50, 1983.)*
6. Allen, D., Loughnan, T. E., and Ord, R. A. A re-evaluation of the role of tracheostomy in Ludwig's angina. *J. Oral. Maxillofac. Surg.* 43:436, 1985.
   Intubation employed instead of tracheostomy.
7. Mayosmith, M. F., Hirsch, P. J., Wodzinski, S. F., et al. Acute epiglottitis in adults. *N. Engl. J. Med.* 314:1133, 1986.
   Early airway control and protection against ampicillin-resistant H. influenzae *are recommended.*
8. Khilanani, U., and Khatib, R. Acute epiglottitis in adults. *Am. J. Med. Sci.* 287:65, 1984.
   Comprehensive review.
9. Gorfinkel, J. H., Brown, R., and Kabins, S. A. Acute infectious epiglottitis in adults. *Ann. Intern. Med.* 70:289, 1969.
   A fatal illness if it is not recognized (See also Arch. Otolaryngol. *80:110, 1964.)*
10. Johnstone, J. M., and Lawy, H. S. Acute epiglottitis in adults due to infection with *Haemophilus influenzae* type B. *Lancet* 2:134, 1967.
    Cervical swelling may occur with epiglottitis.
11. Matteson, A. R. Acute epiglottitis. *Arch. Otolaryngol.* 76:465, 1962.
    Prostration and symptoms of pharyngitis out of proportion to physical findings should suggest epiglottic inflammation.
12. Bass, J. W., Steele, R. W., and Wiebe, R. A. Acute epiglottitis. *J.A.M.A.* 229:671, 1974.
    A review of 97 patients.
13. Shapiro, J., Eavey, R. D., and Baker, A. S. Adult supraglottitis. *J.A.M.A.* 259:563, 1988.
    A condition which is not usually life-threatening nor due to H. influenzae.
14. Schabel, S. I., Katzberg, R. W., and Burgener, F. A. Acute inflammation of epiglottic and supraglottic structures in adults. *Radiology* 122:601, 1977.
    Radiographic findings are reviewed.
15. Ossoff, R. H., and Wolff, A. P. Acute epiglottitis in adults. *J.A.M.A.* 244:2639, 1980.
    Use of steroids advocated.
16. Ward, C. F., Benumof, J. L., and Shapiro, H. M. Management of adult acute epiglottitis by tracheal intubation. *Chest* 71:93, 1977.
    Endotracheal intubation may be as effective as tracheostomy.
17. Bougas, T. P., and Cook, C. D. Pressure-flow characteristics of needles suggested for transtracheal resuscitation. *N. Engl. J. Med.* 262:511, 1960.
    Large-bore needles are not adequate for effective ventilation.
18. Rivera, M., Hadlock, F. P., and O'Meara, M. E. Pulmonary edema secondary to acute epiglottis. *AJR* 132:991, 1979.
    Upper airway obstruction from any cause can produce pulmonary edema.
19. Walsh, T. J., and Gray, W. C. *Candida* epiglottitis in immunocompromised patients. *Chest* 91:482, 1987.
    An unusual cause of epiglottitis.

8. HEMOPTYSIS
John R. Michael

The major causes of hemoptysis are pulmonary *infections,* such as bronchitis, bronchiectasis, pneumonia, tuberculosis, lung abscess, or fungal masses (fungus balls); *tumors,* usually bronchogenic cancer or bronchial adenomas; pulmonary *vascular disease* such as pulmonary emboli, arteriovenous malformations, Wegener's granulomatosis, Goodpasture's syndrome, idiopathic pulmonary hemosiderosis, or rupture of the pulmonary artery during the placement of a Swan-Ganz catheter; and *mitral stenosis*. Bronchiectasis, lung cancer, and tuberculosis are the most common causes; in 15 percent of cases, however, the cause of hemoptysis is unidentified. Rare causes to consider are a broncholith, aortic dissection, and hemoptysis and pneumothorax associated with menses (catamenial hemoptysis). Hemoptysis is more common in patients with inactive rather than active tuberculosis. Bleeding in these patients usually comes from an area of bronchiectasis and arises from the bronchial circulation. Although hemoptysis may occur in patients with pulmonary emboli, the bleeding is rarely massive and does not represent a contraindication to heparin therapy. Fungus balls develop in preexisting lung cavities as in patients with sarcoidosis or bullous emphysema. The fungal mass often moves around inside the cavity and this feature can be helpful in the diagnosis. The fungus has colonized the cavity and only rarely has the organism actually invaded lung tissue. Pulmonary hemorrhage can also arise from rupture of the pulmonary artery by a Swan-Ganz catheter. The rupture is believed to occur when inflation of the balloon causes a tear in the pulmonary artery. Elderly patients and patients with pulmonary hypertension appear to be at increased risk for this complication which occurs in approximately one out of every 1000 or 2000 catheterizations. Such a rupture is fatal in 50 percent of patients.

The appropriate management of hemoptysis depends on the situation. Coughing up small specks of blood is common in patients with acute bronchitis, pneumonia, or bronchiectasis. This by itself rarely warrants evaluation. However, in the patient who coughs up larger amounts of blood or persistently brings up blood, evaluation is indicated. The initial evaluation should be directed toward determining the rate, site, and cause of the bleeding. In a patient with a history of coughing up blood it is important to consider the possibility that the blood is coming from the nasopharynx, throat, or gastrointestinal tract rather than from the lungs. Blood from the lungs is often frothy, and hemosiderin-laden macrophages in the sputum are another indication of intrapulmonary bleeding. The two most helpful diagnostic studies are the chest radiograph and fiberoptic bronchoscopy. Bronchoscopy may lead to a pathologic diagnosis, identify an intrabronchial lesion that is not seen on the chest radiograph, or determine whether the bleeding is coming from the right or left lung. Patients with hemoptysis who do not have a radiographic lesion should generally undergo bronchoscopy. A normal chest radiograph and bronchoscopic examination virtually eliminate lung cancer as the cause for the hemoptysis.

Massive or life-threatening hemoptysis (sometimes called pulmonary hemorrhage) occurs most commonly in patients with tuberculosis, lung abscess, bronchiectasis, lung cancer, and fungus balls. Although the definition is arbitrary, massive hemoptysis is generally defined as more than 200 ml in a few hours or 400 to 600 ml over 24 hours. Managing a patient with massive hemoptysis requires the wisdom of King Solomon. The majority of patients will stop bleeding with conservative therapy, but a rare patient will die from uncontrolled hemorrhage. Many patients with significant hemoptysis appear to have acute bronchitis superimposed on their underlying lung condition and therapy with broad-spectrum antibiotics can lead to a rapid decrease in the amount of bleeding. It is also generally recommended that patients receive cough suppressants. Coagulation studies should be checked and any abnormalities corrected. Controversy exists about when a patient with massive hemoptysis should be bronchoscoped. Many chest physicians believe the bronchoscopy may cause more bleeding by stimulating coughing. These physicians recommend that bronchoscopy be delayed until the bleeding has stopped or slowed markedly. Other physicians would prefer to bronchoscope the patient while he is bleeding in the hopes that the bronchoscopist can identify the source and determine whether the bleeding is coming from the right or left lung. It is probably desirable to not bronchoscope during the acute bleeding because it is often extremely difficult to see anything but blood.

In the patient with massive hemoptysis whose bleeding has slowed or stopped, there are three basic approaches: watchful waiting, surgery, or embolization of the bronchial arteries. Many patients with massive hemoptysis are poor surgical candidates because of their lung disease which may involve the pleura, making the surgical removal difficult and bloody. Embolization is helpful in patients who are not good surgical candidates and who are bleeding from the bronchial circulation. In these patients embolization of the feeding vessel may stop the bleeding. The bleeding site cannot usually be seen during arteriography because the rate of bleeding is not rapid enough, but an abnormal vascular pattern is often found. An absolute contraindication to embolization of a bronchial artery is if this vessel also supplies the spinal cord. In this situation embolization can lead to severe spinal cord injury.

Because the patient with massive hemoptysis does not die from blood loss but from asphyxiation, several techniques have been used in an attempt to isolate the bleeding lung from the nonbleeding lung. The most common is to insert an endotracheal tube that can separate the right from the left lung. Although the bleeding most frequently comes from the bronchial circulation, in the patient who is bleeding from the pulmonary circulation it may be helpful to block the pulmonary artery on the bleeding side by inflating the balloon on a Swan-Ganz catheter.

1. Crocco, J. A., Rooney, J. J., Fankushen, D. S., et al. Massive hemoptysis. *Arch. Intern. Med.* 121:495, 1968.
   Early surgery advocated when blood loss exceeds 600 ml in 16 hours.
2. Stinghe, R. A., and Manguilea, V. G. Hemoptysis of bronchial origin occurring in patients with arrested tuberculosis. *Am. Rev. Respir. Dis.* 101:84, 1970.
   Posttuberculosis bronchiectasis resulting in hemorrhage.
3. Finley, T. N., Aronow, A., Cosentino, A. M., et al. Occult pulmonary hemorrhage in anticoagulated patients. *Am. Rev. Respir. Dis.* 112:23, 1975.
   Dyspnea, acute anemia, alveolar infiltrates without hemoptysis, and hemosiderin-laden alveolar macrophages suggest the presence of pulmonary hemorrhage.
4. Schwartz, R., Myerson, R. M., Lawrence, T., et al. Mitral stenosis, massive pulmonary hemorrhage and emergency valve replacement. *N. Engl. J. Med.* 275:755, 1966.
   Elevated left atrial pressure and bronchial varices are relieved by surgery.
5. Saw, E. C., Gottlieb, L. S., Yakoyama, T., et al. Flexible fiberoptic bronchoscopy and endobronchial tamponade in the management of massive hemoptysis. *Chest* 70:589, 1976.
   Immediate bronchoscopy is indicated in patients with massive hemoptysis.
6. Barbash, G. I., Solomon, A., Reider-Grosswasser, I., et al. Aortic dissection presenting with hemoptysis: diagnostic confirmation of dissection and leak by computerized tomography. *Heart Lung* 12:633, 1983.
   Aortic dissection may cause hemoptysis.
7. Israel, R. H., and Poe, R. H. Hemoptysis. *Clin. Chest Med.* 8:197, 1987.
   General review.
8. Gong, H. Jr., and Salvatierra, C. Clinical efficacy of early and delayed fiberoptic bronchoscopy in patients with hemoptysis. *Am. Rev. Respir. Dis.* 124:221, 1981.
   Retrospective study suggests that early bronchoscopy does not lead to improved outcome.
9. Uflacker, R., Kaemmerer, A., Picon, P. D., et al. Bronchial artery embolization in the management of hemoptysis: technical aspects and long-term results. *Radiology* 157:637, 1985.
   Description of the use of bronchial artery embolization.
10. Haponik, E. F., Britt, E. J., Smith, P. L., et al. Computed chest tomography in the evaluation of hemoptysis. Impact on diagnosis and treatment. *Chest* 91:80, 1987.
    Evaluates the role of chest computed tomography.
11. Noseworthy, T. W., and Anderson, B. J. Massive hemoptysis. [Review] *Can. Med. Assoc. J.* 135:1097, 1986.
12. Conlan, A. A. Massive hemoptysis—diagnostic and therapeutic implications. [Review] *Surg. Annu.* 17:337, 1985.
    Extensive experience with massive hemoptysis.
13. Leatherman, J. W., Davies, S. F., and Hoidal, J. R. Alveolar hemorrhage syndromes: diffuse microvascular lung hemorrhage in immune and idiopathic disorders. [Review] *Medicine* (Baltimore) 63:343, 1984.
    Excellent discussion of these conditions.
14. Howard, W. J., Rosario, E. J., and Calhoon, S. L. Hemoptysis. Causes and a practical management approach. *Postgrad. Med.* 77:53, 1985.
    Practical review.

15. Adelman, M., Haponik, E. F., Bleecker, E. R., et al. Cryptogenic hemoptysis. Clinical features, bronchoscopic findings, and natural history in 67 patients. *Ann. Intern. Med.* 102:829, 1985.
Natural history of patients with hemoptysis and a normal chest radiograph.

16. Elliot, D. L., Barker, A. F., and Dixon, L. M. Catamenial hemoptysis. New methods of diagnosis and therapy. *Chest* 87:687, 1985.
Rare cause of hemoptysis.

9. RESPIRATORY FAILURE
Peter B. Terry

Respiratory failure can usefully be defined as hypoxemic failure (PO_2 <55 mm Hg) or hypercarbic failure (PCO_2 >50 mm Hg). Hypoxemic failure implies that the lungs are being adequately ventilated but that alveolar oxygen is not transferred into the pulmonary capillary bed because of intrinsic lung disease. In contrast, hypercarbic failure implies failure of one or more components of the respiratory system to effectively move air in and out of the lungs. There are exceptions to these physiologic definitions such as the patient who is breathing a low inspired oxygen concentration (hypoxic failure not due to intrinsic lung disease), and some patients may have both forms of failure. These definitions do not imply acuteness or chronicity nor do they imply anything about the patient's clinical status. For example a patient with severe emphysema may be ambulatory with a PCO_2 of 60 mm Hg.

Hypoxemic failure results from poor matching of ventilation and perfusion in the lung due to (1) poor ventilation of alveoli because of airways disease (asthma, bronchitis), (2) alveolar collapse (atelectasis, adult respiratory distress syndrome), (3) alveoli filled with fluid or pus (pneumonia, pulmonary edema). Hypoxemic failure also occurs in association with hypercarbic failure in emphysema patients when inadequate ventilation of alveoli leads to an elevated alveolar PCO_2 which in turns lowers the inspired oxygen concentration in alveoli and consequently in the blood. Hypoxemic respiratory failure occurs most commonly in patients with pneumonia, adult respiratory distress syndrome, and in association with hypercarbic failure due to bronchitis and emphysema.

Hypercarbic respiratory failure may be due to failure of (1) the respiratory centers (heroin overdose), (2) the phrenic nerves (Guillain-Barré syndrome), (3) the neuromuscular junctions (myasthenia gravis), (4) diaphragms (emphysema, glycogen storage disease).

Patients with respiratory failure present a considerable challenge to the physician since they are often as much at risk from therapy as from their disease. Management is based upon an understanding of the above-mentioned pathophysiologic processes.

Hypoxemic failure due to an alveolar filling process such as pneumonia is treated with appropriate antibiotics and supplemental oxygen when the arterial oxygen falls below 60 mm Hg. Antipyretic agents may reduce the consumption of oxygen and in turn increase the arterial PO_2. There is no good evidence that postural drainage and percussion are helpful in patients with pneumonia and otherwise normal lungs.

Hypoxemic failure can occur in patients with previously normal lungs after trauma, burns, sepsis, fractures, pancreatitis, aspiration, viral pneumonia, cardiopulmonary bypass, drug intoxication, or shock. This syndrome is known as the adult respiratory distress syndrome (ARDS) and results from alveolar collapse and increased capillary permeability. ARDS is managed by treating the underlying process leading to this condition (e.g., antibiotics for septic shock) and by using supplemental oxygen to maintain the arterial PO_2 at 60 mm Hg. When the inspired oxygen concentration needed to maintain this PO_2 exceeds 50 percent, then intubation should be considered so that assisted ventilation can be used. The use of assisted ventilation may itself decrease the work of breathing and raise the arterial PO_2. If the arterial PO_2 remains below 60 mm Hg, then consideration should be given to using positive end-expiratory pressure (PEEP) to open the collapsed alveoli and improve the arterial PO_2. Careful attention to fluid balance, cardiac output, and avoidance of alkalosis is important. In some cases of severe hypoxemia not responsive to the above measures, oxygen consumption can be reduced (thus leading to an increased mixed venous oxygen and an increased arterial oxygen concentration) by paralyzing the patient.

Acute hypercarbic failure due to sudden failure of the respiratory centers, phrenic nerves, neuromuscular junctions, or diaphragms can be corrected with medicines if available (naloxone [Narcan] for heroin overdose, pyridostigmine [Mestinon] for myasthenia gravis), or if unavailable or unsuccessful, with general measures which support ventilation (intubation and mechanical ventilation). The hypoxemia which accompanies acute hypercarbic failure can be easily corrected by either improving ventilation or by having the patient inspire a low concentration of supplemental oxygen. If altered mental status accompanies the acute hypercarbic failure, as in drug intoxication, ancillary measures such as proper positioning to prevent aspiration are important.

Chronic hypercarbic respiratory failure is most commonly seen with severe emphysema and bronchitis. The severe airways obstruction leads to hypercarbia and hypoxemia because of respiratory muscle fatigue secondary to the increased work of breathing. Treatment in this instance is directed at correcting the concomitant hypoxemia (low-flow oxygen), reducing the work of breathing (bronchodilators for bronchospasm), strengthening the diaphragm (improved nutrition and diaphragmatic exercises), delaying diaphragmatic fatigue (theophylline preparations), and treating the precipitating cause of the respiratory failure (antibiotics for infection). Care must be taken not to further suppress respiration by giving excessive oxygen (an arterial PO_2 of 60–65 mm Hg is adequate) or by using sedatives.

Low-flow oxygen can be administered in stepwise concentrations of 24 to 28 percent by Venturi mask. Repeat arterial blood gases are necessary to document that the arterial PO_2 is rising to an acceptable range (60–65 mm Hg) without suppressing ventilation to the degree that the arterial PCO_2 rise is associated with acidosis (pH <7.30), or causing end-organ dysfunction (e.g., altered mental status, arrhythmias).

1. West, J. B. Ventilation-perfusion relationships. *Am. Rev. Respir. Dis* 116:919, 1977. *State of the art review. (See also N. Engl. J. Med. 316:1336, 1987.)*
2. Roussos, C. Function and fatigue of respiratory muscles. *Chest* 88:124S, 1985. *Comprehensive review of respiratory muscle failure physiology.*
3. Leitch, A. G. The hypoxic drive to breathing in man. *Lancet* 1:428, 1981. *The response to hypoxia is genetically determined and can be enhanced with medroxyprogesterone.*
4. Butler, J. Clinical problems of disordered respiratory control. *Am. Rev. Respir. Dis.* 110:695, 1974. *A brief review of neurogenic disorders of respiration. (See also Arch. Intern. Med. 140:29, 1980.)*
5. Schwartz, W. B., de Strihou, C. V. P., and Kassirer, J. P. Role of anions in metabolic alkalosis and potassium deficiency. *N. Engl. J. Med.* 279, 1968. *The importance of hypochloremia is stressed.*
6. Newman, J. H., Neff, T. A., and Ziporin, P. Acute respiratory failure associated with hypophosphatemia. *N. Engl. J. Med.* 296:110, 1977. *Neuromuscular impairment caused by a low serum phosphate level.*
7. Hugh-Jones, P., and Whimster, W. The etiology and management of disabling emphysema. *Am. Rev. Respir. Dis.* 117:343, 1978. *Comprehensive review.*
8. Snider, G. L. The pathogenesis of emphysema: Twenty years of progress. *Am. Rev. Respir. Dis.* 124:321, 1981. *Examination of the elastase-antielastase hypothesis.*
9. Fishman, A. P. Chronic cor pulmonale. *Am. Rev. Respir. Dis.* 114:775, 1976. *A comprehensive review.*
10. Brackett, N. C., Wingo, C. F., Muren, O., et al. Acid-base response to chronic hypercapnia in man. *N. Engl. J. Med.* 280:124, 1969.

Use of significance bands to detect mixed acid-base disturbances in the presence of carbon dioxide retention. Note also the accompanying editorial.

11. Block, A. J., and Ball, W. C., Jr. Acute respiratory failure. *Ann. Intern. Med.* 65:957, 1966.
Effectiveness of a volume-cycled respirator and lack of toxicity from rapid reduction of the PCO_2.

12. Douglas, N. J., Leggett, R. J. E., Calverley. P. M. A., et al. Transient hypoxemia during sleep in chronic bronchitis and emphysema. *Lancet* 1:1, 1979.
Nocturnal hypoxemia may be responsible for secondary polycythemia and pulmonary hypertension.

13. Miller, P. D., and Berns, A. S. Acute metabolic alkalosis perpetuating hypercapnia: Role for acetazolamide in chronic obstructive pulmonary disease. *J.A.M.A.* 238:2400, 1977.
Diuretic-induced metabolic acidosis causes hypoventilation and hypercapnia.

14. Stevens, P. M., Austen, K. F., and Knowles, J. H. Prognostic significance of papilledema in course of respiratory insufficiency. *J.A.M.A.* 183:161, 1963.
Papilledema is a complication of carbon dioxide retention.

15. George, R. B., Herbert, S. J., Shames, J. M., et al. Pneumothorax complicating pulmonary emphysema. *J.A.M.A.* 234:389, 1975.
A cause of dyspnea that is easily overlooked.

16. Hudson, L. D., Kent, T. L., et al. Arrhythmias associated with acute respiratory failure in patients with chronic airway obstruction. *Chest* 63:661, 1973.
The incidence of arrhythmias will be underestimated unless continuous monitoring is performed. (See Am. Rev. Respir. Dis. *108:879, 1973.)*

17. Shine, K. I., Kastor, J. A., and Yurchak, P. M. Multifocal atrial tachycardia. *N. Engl. J. Med.* 279:344, 1968.
Chaotic atrial activity is commonly precipitated by bronchodilators in patients with obstructive lung disease.

18. McNicol, M. W., and Campbell, E. J. M. Severity of respiratory failure. *Lancet* 1:336, 1965.
A PCO_2 greater than 80 mm Hg is usually due to uncontrolled oxygen administration.

19. Campbell, E. J. M. The management of acute respiratory failure in chronic bronchitis and emphysema. *Am. Rev. Respir. Dis.* 96:626, 1967.
Rationale for the use of the Venturi mask.

20. Mithoefer, J. C., Keighley, J. F., and Karetzky, M. Response of the arterial PO_2 to oxygen administration in chronic pulmonary disease. *Ann. Intern. Med.* 74:328, 1971.
Guidelines for the selection of the appropriate inspired oxygen concentration for the correction of hypoxia.

21. Rosen, R. L. Acute respiratory failure and chronic obstructive lung disease. *Med. Clin. North Ame.* 70:895, 1986.
Thorough review of the topic.

22. Bartlett, R. H., Morris, A. H., Fairley, H. B., et al. A prospective study of acute hypoxic respiratory failure. *Chest* 89:684, 1986.
A 40% mortality rate occurs with only lung disease.

23. Epstein, R. L. Constituents of sputum: A simple method. *Ann. Intern. Med.* 77:259, 1972.
A useful review.

24. Stauffer, J. L., Olson, D. E., and Petty, T. L. Complications and consequences of endotracheal intubation and tracheotomy. *Am. J. Med.* 70:65, 1981.
Adverse effects are common; tracheotomy was associated with more side effects than endotracheal intubation.

25. Zwillich, C. W., Pierson, D. J., Creagh, C. E., et al. Complications of assisted ventilation. *Am. J. Med.* 57:161, 1974.
Intubation of the right mainstem bronchus, endotracheal tube malfunction, and alveolar hypoventilation were the most serious complications.

26. Sladen, A., Laver, M. D., and Pontoppidan, H. Pulmonary complications and water retention in prolonged mechanical ventilation. *N. Engl. J. Med.* 279:448, 1968.

27. Jardin, F., Farcot, J. C., Boisante, L., et al. Influence of positive end expiratory pressure on left ventricular performance. *N. Engl. J. Med.* 304:387, 1981.
Decreased cardiac output with PEEP is due to restriction of left ventricular filling by displacement of the interventricular septum. (See also the accompanying editorial on p. 421.)
28. Powell, J. R., Vozeh, S., Hopewell P., et al. Theophylline disposition in acutely ill hospitalized patients. *Am. Rev. Respir. Dis.* 118:229, 1978.
Theophylline disposition varies in patients with different diseases. Recommendations concerning theophylline administration are provided.
29. Hasting, P. R., Shillman, J. J., Bushnell, L. S., et al. Antacid titration in the prevention of acute gastrointestinal bleeding. *N. Engl. J. Med.* 298:1041, 1978.
Antacids reduce gastrointestinal hemorrhage associated with a stress such as respiratory failure.
30. Albert, R. K., Martin, T. R., and Lewis, S. W. Controlled clinical trial of methylprednisolone in patients with chronic bronchitis and acute respiratory insufficiency. *Ann. Intern. Med.* 92:753, 1980.
Methylprednisolone improved airflow in patients with chronic bronchitis and acute respiratory insufficiency. (See also Chest 73:389, 1978.)
31. Hedley-Whyte, J., and Winter, P. M. Oxygen therapy. *Clin. Pharmacol. Ther.* 8:696, 1967.
A thorough review.
32. Frank, L., and Massaro, D. Oxygen toxicity. *Am. J. Med.* 69:117, 1980.
Comprehensive review.
33. Hill, N. S. Clinical applications of body ventilators. *Chest* 90:897, 1986.
Alternative kinds of ventilators work well in selected patients.
34. Gillespie, D. J., Marsh, H. M. M., Divertie, M. B., et al. Clinical outcome of respiratory failure in patients requiring prolonged (>24 hours) mechanical ventilation. *Chest* 90:364, 1986.
Mortality increases with the number of organs involved.
35. Shelhamer, J. H., Natanson, C., and Parillo, J. E. Positive end expiratory pressure in adults. *J.A.M.A.* 251:2692, 1984.
Practical approach to use of PEEP.
36. Tobin, M. J., Perez, W., Guenther, S. M., et al. The pattern of breathing during successful and unsuccessful trials of weaning from mechanical ventilation. *Am. Rev. Respir. Dis.* 134:1111, 1986.
Weaning failures are associated with rapid shallow breathing.
37. Bergofsky, E. H. Respiratory failure in disorders of the thoracic cage. *Am. Rev. Respir. Dis.* 119:643, 1979.
State-of-the-art review.
38. Miller, A., and Granada, M. In-hospital mortality in the Pickwickian syndrome. *Am. J. Med.* 56:144, 1974.
Sudden unexplained death is common.
39. Sundarrajan, E. V., Davenport, J. The Guillain-Barré syndrome: pulmonary-neurologic correlations. *Medicine* 64:333, 1985.
40. Pingleton, S. K. Complications of acute respiratory failure. *Am. Rev. Respir. Dis.* 137:1463, 1988.
A comprehensive review.

1C. STATUS ASTHMATICUS
H. Verdain Barnes

Status asthmaticus is a medical emergency with a mortality as high as 30 percent in patients with recurrent episodes. Prompt diagnosis and treatment are essential. Asthma is characterized by diffuse tracheobronchial narrowing. The pathophysiology of bronchial smooth muscle contraction and the associated inflammation in asthma is multi-factorial and not fully understood. Major components in the process include airway epithelial cells, mast cells, secretory cells of the respiratory system, neutrophils, eosinophils, smooth muscle cells, and the parasympathetic nervous system. The airway epithelial cells and mast cells are critical to the initiation of this overall process. The airway epithelial cells when stimulated appear to generate and release several lipoxygenase metabolites of arachidonic acid leading to a migration of neutrophils into the area with a release of prostaglandins and/or thromboxane. The mast cell's central role in beginning bronchospasm and subsequent inflammation is in response to immunologic and nonimmunologic stimuli. The major immunologic activators are antigens and IgE. The numerous nonimmunologic mediators include vasoactive and spasmogenic substances such as histamine and adenosine; chemoattracting substances including specific neutrophil, basophil, and eosinophil chemotactic factors; and enzymes and proteoglycans such as some acid hydrolases, proteases, and heparin. It is the interactions of these components and mediators which produce the primary clinical features of bronchospastic disease.

Constriction of the tracheobronchial tree leads to a general decrease in ventilatory capacity, with nonuniform alveolar ventilation, accentuated changes in regional ventilation-perfusion ratios, and arterial hypoxemia. Microscopically the asthmatic lung shows some thickening of the bronchial smooth muscle and the alveolar basement membrane, an increase in the size and number of goblet cells and submucosal mucous glands, decreased numbers of normal ciliated columnar cells, and conglomerations of desquamated epithelial cells, eosinophils, and inspissated mucus plugging the lumen of the bronchi.

In status asthmaticus there is a marked accentuation of these processes and changes, together with a resistance to the simpler modes of therapy. Clinically the patients almost invariably have some degree of dyspnea, varying patterns of inspiratory and expiratory wheezing, and tachycardia. Other common findings include retraction of the sternocleidomastoid muscles, pulsus paradoxus, thoracic hyperinflation, dehydration, cyanosis, and a mental state ranging from agitation to somnolence. Sternocleidomastoid retraction and pulsus paradoxus have a high correlation with severity of the impairment of the patient's pulmonary function and therefore should be routinely evaluated. Arterial blood gas determinations are essential for optimum management of these patients. There is always some degree of hypoxia. In most patients there is initially mild hypoxemia, mild hypocapnia, and modest respiratory alkalosis. The presence of moderate hypoxia along with a normal arterial PCO_2 and pH may herald the onset of a rapid decline to marked hypoxia, hypercapnia, and respiratory acidosis. Since there are no clinical clues to the crossover from respiratory alkalosis to the development of serious respiratory acidosis, serial arterial blood gas determinations are usually required.

In evaluating the patient presenting with acute bronchial asthma the index of Fischl et al. may prove useful in predicting the potential for immediate relapse and/or the need for hospitalization. The presenting factors used include a pulse rate 120 or more per minute; respiratory rate 30 or more per minute; pulsus paradoxicus 18 or more mm Hg; peak expiratory flow rate 120 or more liters/minute; and moderate to severe dyspnea, accessory muscle use, or wheezing. Each presenting parameter that is found is assigned a numerical value of 1 (index score ranges from 0–7). An index of 4 or more indicates a 95 percent risk of immediate relapse and a similar level of confidence of the need for hospital admission.

The principles of management are (1) relieve bronchoconstriction and maintain a patent airway, (2) maintain adequate ventilation, oxygenation, and hydration, and (3) correct any acid-base imbalance. Those objectives can be accomplished by the judicious use of bronchodilators, fluids, corticosteroids, antibiotics, mechanical ventilators, endotracheal intubation, alkalinizing agents, and mucolytic agents. Excessive utilization of some nebulized bronchodilators and mucolytic agents may result in increased bronchoconstriction.

The complications of status asthmaticus arise from the underlying pathophysiology and/or inappropriate therapy. Mucus plugging, atelectasis, and increased right-to-left shunting, pneumomediastinum, tension pneumothorax, massive pulmonary collapse, arterial air embolism, respiratory fatigue, circulatory collapse due to uncorrected hypovolemia, cardiac arrhythmias due to overuse of bronchodilators, and/or uncorrected hypoxemia and respiratory acidosis are of primary concern. Death from asthma is usually from cardiac arrest and can occur suddenly outside the hospital at night, particularly in patients with large diurnal variations in airflow obstruction or in the setting of a prolonged attack, exhaustion, respiratory muscle fatigue, raising PCO_2, and, in some, associated hypokalemia.

When managing these patients, physicians should keep in mind the leading causes of therapeutic failure—untreated bronchopulmonary infection, oversedation, insufficient use of bronchodilators, occasionally an overdose of nebulized sympathomimetic aerosols, and respiratory fatigue. Adequately treated patients initially respond by loss of respiratory muscle contraction followed by resolution of wheezing and dyspnea. At a much slower rate the other features of decreased ventilatory capacity resolve. It may take a week or more for the 1-second forced expiratory volume (FEV_1) to return to baseline, and several weeks may be required for the arterial oxygen tension to return to baseline. Although the patients may have no symptoms during their recovery phase, these residual abnormalities may serve as a basis for another attack. Consequently, the patient recovering from status asthmaticus should be watched carefully until he has returned to a baseline state.

1. McFadden, E. R., Kiser, R., and DeGroot, W. J. Acute bronchial asthma: Relations between clinical and physiologic manifestations. *N. Engl. J. Med.* 288:221, 1973.
   Correlates sternocleidomastoid retraction with the severity of pulmonary function impairment.
2. McFadden, E. R., and Harold, L. A. Arterial blood gas tension in asthma. *N. Engl. J. Med.* 278:1027, 1968.
   With severe degrees of bronchial obstruction, hypoxia is invariably present and carbon dioxide retention may occur.
3. Rees, H. A., Millar, J. S., and Donald, K. W. A study of the clinical course and arterial blood gas tensions of patients in status asthmaticus. *Q. J. Med.* 37:541, 1968.
   FEV_1 is not a reliable guide to hypoxemia. When present, severe hypercapnia is usually indicative of a fatal outcome.
4. Weiss, E. B., and Faling, L. J. Clinical significance of Pa CO_2 during status asthmaticus, the crossover point. *Ann. Allergy* 26:545, 1968.
   Watch for the crossover from early mild hypoxemia, hypocapnia, and respiratory alkalosis to increased hypoxia, normocapnia, and normalized pH as heralding more severe decompensation.
5. Mitenko, P. A., and Ogilvie, R. I. Rational intravenous doses of theophylline. *N. Engl. J. Med.* 289:600, 1973.
   A safe and effective dose regimen is described.
6. Karetzky, M. S. Asthma mortality: An analysis of one year's experience, review of the literature and assessment of current modes of therapy. *Medicine* 54:471, 1975.
   Intermittent positive-pressure breathing therapy may be a major contributor to asthma mortality, and if it is used it should be administered with small doses of nebulized bronchodilators and oxygen and careful monitoring of arterial blood gases. A well-referenced article.
7. El-Shaboury, A. H. Adrenal failure complicating status asthmaticus in steroid-treated patients. *Br. Med. J.* 2:1478, 1966.
   An important potential problem to keep in mind.
8. Fischl, M. A., Pitchenick, A., and Gardner, L. B. An index predicting relapse and need for hospitalization in patients with acute bronchial asthma. *N. Engl. J. Med.* 305:783, 1981.
   A useful clinical index and treatment protocol are provided.
9. Rossing, T. H., Fanta, C. H., Goldstein, J. R., et al. Emergency therapy of asthma: Comparison of acute effects of parenteral and inhaled sympathomimetics and infused aminophylline. *Am. Rev. Respir. Dis.* 122:365, 1980.
   This study demonstrates that epinephrine subcutaneously (3 doses 20 minutes apart 1:1000 0.3 cc subcutaneously) is the most effective, followed by inhaled isoproterenol.
10. Benatar, S. R. Fatal asthma. *N. Engl. J. Med.* 314:423, 1986.
    A concise review of the causes of death in asthma.

11. Wasserman, S. I. Mediators of immediate hypersensitivity. *J. Allergy Clin. Immunol.* 72:101, 1983.
   A comprehensive review of the current understanding of the mediators involved in asthma.
12. Li, J. T. C., and Reed, C. E. Nocturnal asthma and the timing of treatment. *Am. J. Med.* 79 (Suppl. 6A):10, 1985.
   Asthma deaths occur more frequently at night.
13. Lazarus, S. C. Role of inflammation and inflammatory mediators in airways disease. *Am. J. Med.* 81 (Suppl. 5A):2, 1986.
   Inflammation is an important component of the process.
14. Marney, S. R., Jr. Asthma: Recent developments in treatment. *South. Med. J.* 78:1084, 1985.
   A concise up-to-date review of asthma therapy.

11. CARBON MONOXIDE POISONING
Jerry L. Spivak

Carbon monoxide intoxication, both accidental and intentional, continues to be a major cause of illness and death. Improperly adjusted or vented gas appliances and fires account for most accidental intoxications with the gas, and exposure to automobile exhaust fumes remains a popular method of suicide. Carbon monoxide is an odorless and colorless gas whose toxicity is due to its ability to produce hypoxia in a manner that defeats the mechanisms designed to maintain adequate tissue oxygenation.

Humans require 4 cc of oxygen per kg/minute for basal metabolic processes; since oxygen stores amount to only 20 cc/kg, a constant supply of oxygen is required. A decrease in oxygen supply or an increase in oxygen demand results in immediate compensatory changes in cardiac output, ventilation, distribution of blood flow, and hemoglobin-oxygen affinity. A continuing imbalance results in an erythropoietin-mediated increase in the red blood cell mass. Changes in ventilation and cardiac output are relatively inefficient in increasing oxygenation since they require a further increase in oxygen consumption. In addition, pathologic processes affecting the heart and lungs or lack of conditioning may impair the efficiency of these responses. Changes in hemoglobin-oxygen affinity, however, provide a very efficient mechanism for increasing oxygenation. Under normal circumstances, the shape of the hemoglobin-oxygen dissociation curve provides for maximum oxygen saturation over a wide range of alveolar oxygen tensions, and maximum oxygen release with only small changes in tissue oxygen tension. The shape of the dissociation curve can also be modified to either increase or decrease oxygen release at a given oxygen tension. Thus, a decrease in pH or an increase in temperature shifts the curve to the right and increases oxygen release while alkalosis or hypothermia shifts the curve to the left. In addition to pH and temperature, a major determinant of hemoglobin-oxygen affinity is the organic phosphate compound, 2,3-diphosphoglycerate (2,3-DPG), which has an increased affinity for deoxyhemoglobin. A rise in red cell 2,3-DPG results in a decrease in the affinity of hemoglobin for oxygen and a shift to the right in the hemoglobin-oxygen dissociation curve. The resultant increase in oxygen delivery minimizes the need for a large increase in cardiac output to improve oxygenation. An increase in red cell 2,3-DPG occurs with anemia or hypoxia or when there is an increase in oxygen utilization as in hyperthyroidism. Prolonged acidosis, alkalosis, and certain disorders of the glycolytic cycle decrease red cell 2,3-DPG.

In carbon monoxide poisoning, the mechanisms for improving oxygen transport are profoundly impaired. Carbon monoxide has an affinity for hemoglobin 240 times greater than that of oxygen. The affinity is due not to a greater rate of association, but rather to a slower rate of dissociation of carbon monoxide from the hemoglobin molecule. As a corollary, the affinity of carbon monoxide for myoglobin, a compound that binds tightly to oxygen, is 14 times less than its affinity for hemoglobin. Carbon monoxide also binds to other heme compounds in the respiratory chain and thus affects oxygen utilization at multiple points during cell metabolism. The formation of carboxyhemoglobin results in a reduction in the amount of oxyhemoglobin. The effect is more profound than that produced by a comparable degree of anemia since the oxygen-hemoglobin dissociation curve is also shifted to the left. In addition, carboxyhemoglobin has a reduced affinity for 2,3-DPG and at high levels of carbon monoxide, 2,3-DPG production may be suppressed. Thus carbon monoxide is responsible for both hypoxia and suppression of adaptive mechanisms. The effect of the gas is further magnified by any abnormalities in ventilation producing a venous admixture effect or by right-to-left shunts. In such situations, carbon monoxide–induced alterations in the oxygen-hemoglobin dissociation curve accentuate the shunt effect on arterial oxygenation. Finally, as tissue oxygen tension falls, more carbon monoxide is bound to myoglobin and cytochrome oxidase, further impairing cellular respiration.

Clinically, carbon monoxide intoxication may take the form of chronic sublethal poisoning, with alterations in mental and physical performance, particularly in patients with cardiorespiratory compromise. A long-term effect on atherogenesis has also been postulated. Acutely, the poison may rapidly produce coma and death, but recovery may occur with or without neurologic residua. The symptoms of intoxication vary with the type of exposure and the clinical status of the victim. At blood levels of 20 to 30 percent, headache, nausea, and vomiting may occur. At higher levels, vertigo, tachypnea, and tachycardia ensue, followed by seizures and coma. Prior elevation of the blood carbon monoxide concentration from cigarette smoking or environmental exposure may accelerate the process. Hyperventilation or increased metabolic demands also accelerate toxicity. There is no correlation between symptoms and the blood carboxyhemoglobin level. Characteristically, the two tissues most sensitive to oxygen lack, the brain and myocardium, are the most affected. Coma, seizures, and diffuse and fluctuating neurologic deficits may be seen. Cerebral edema may develop. Myocardial damage can be immediate or delayed, with ischemia, infarction, arrhythmias, and conduction defects occurring. Depression of myocardial function also serves to impair oxygen transport elsewhere, continuing the pathologic cycle. Increases in serum transaminase levels cannot always be attributed to cardiac damage since skeletal muscle necrosis and myoglobinuria with acute renal failure can occur with carbon monoxide poisoning (as it can with other intoxicants causing coma and hypoxia). Erythematous and vesicular skin lesions may be seen at pressure areas and should suggest the possibility of underlying muscle damage. These lesions can also occur elsewhere and may not be evident until several days after exposure. The skin lesions show sweat gland necrosis on biopsy. The characteristic pink- or cherry-colored skin is not commonly observed. Adverse signs include congestive heart failure, leukocytosis, fever, metabolic acidosis, and coma. Delayed postanoxic encephalopathy may occur; in this syndrome initial recovery from coma is followed after an interval of 2 to 10 days by relapse with a multifocal neurologic syndrome often terminating fatally. Less profound late neurologic deterioration can also occur in survivors who do not develop this syndrome.

The treatment of carbon monoxide poisoning is removal from the toxic environment, rapid reduction of carbon monoxide levels by ventilation with 100 percent oxygen, and surveillance for cardiac or skeletal muscle necrosis and cerebral edema. Hyperbaric oxygen is the quickest method of lowering carbon monoxide levels. The use of 5% carbon dioxide with 95% oxygen has no place since ventilation is usually maximal. If ventilation is impaired in the comatose patient, intubation and administration of 100% oxygen are more prudent. Fever with the concomitant elevation of metabolic rate should be avoided; hypothermia with careful observation of myocardial function may be useful. Cerebral edema can be treated in this fashion as well or with steroids.

---

1. Dolan, M. C. Carbon monoxide poisoning. *Can. Med. Assoc. J.* 131:392, 1985.
   Concise review. (See also Brit. Med. J. *296:77, 1988.)*
2. Heckerling, P. S., Leikin, J. B., and Maturen, A. Occult carbon monoxide poisoning: Validation of a prediction model. *Am. J. Med.* 84:251, 1988.
   An attempt to improve recognition of this disorder. (See also Ann. Intern. Med. *107:174, 1987.)*

3. Coburn, R. F. Biologic effects of carbon monoxide. *Ann. N.Y. Acad. Sci.* 174:1, 1970.
   Comprehensive symposium on the effects of carbon monoxide.
4. Goldsmith, J. R., and Landaw, S. A. Carbon monoxide and human health. *Science* 162:1352, 1968.
   An important review.
5. Bartlett, D. Pathophysiology of exposure to low concentrations of carbon monoxide. *Arch. Environ. Health* 16:719, 1968.
   Quantitative comparison of carbon monoxide and other hypoxic influences.
6. McBay, A. J. Carbon monoxide poisoning. *N. Engl. J. Med.* 272:252, 1965.
   Epidemiology of carbon monoxide intoxication. (See also J.A.M.A. 261:1177, 1989.)
7. Meigs, J. W., and Hughes, J. P. N. Acute carbon monoxide poisoning. *Arch. Ind. Hyg. Occup. Med.* 6:344, 1952.
   Detailed observations of 105 patients.
8. Thomas, H. M., III, Lefrak, S. S., Irwin, R. S., et al. The oxyhemoglobin dissociation curve in health and disease. *Am. J. Med.* 57:331, 1974.
   Interaction of hemoglobin and 2,3-DPG.
9. Finch, C. A., and Lenfant, C. Oxygen transport in man. *N. Engl. J. Med.* 286:407, 1972.
   Biochemical adaptation to hypoxia.
10. Mitchell, J. H., and Blomquist, G. Maximal oxygen uptake. *N. Engl. J. Med.* 284:1018, 1971.
    Mechanisms responsible for meeting oxygen demands and their limitations.
11. Anderson, R. F., Allensworth, D. C., and De Groot, W. J. Myocardial toxicity from carbon monoxide poisoning. *Ann. Intern. Med.* 67:1172, 1967.
    Ischemia, infarction, arrhythmias, and conduction defects occur, occasionally with a delayed onset.(See also Am. J. Med. 38:316, 1965 and Angiology 37:671, 1986.)
12. Buehler, J. H., Berns, A. S., Webster, J. R., et al. Lactic acidosis from carboxyhemoglobinemia after smoke inhalation. *Ann. Intern. Med.* 82:803, 1975.
    A manifestation of tissue hypoxia.
13. Larkin, J. M., Brahos, G. J., and Moylan, J. A. Treatment of carbon monoxide poisoning: Prognostic factors. *J. Trauma* 16:111, 1976.
    Metabolic acidosis carries a poor prognosis.
14. Garland, H., and Pearce, J. Neurological complications of carbon monoxide poisoning. *Q. J. Med.* 36:445, 1967.
    Cortical blindness, parietal failure, psychosis, and seizures.
15. Plum, F., Posner, J. B., and Hain, R. F. Delayed neurological deterioration after anoxia. *Arch. Intern. Med.* 110:18, 1962.
    Apparent recovery from coma followed by relapse with a multifocal neurologic deficit and a poor prognosis.
16. Leavell, W. W., Farley, C. H., and McIntyre, J. S. Cutaneous changes in a patient with carbon monoxide poisoning. *Arch. Dermatol.* 99:429, 1969.
    Erythema, vesicles, and sweat gland necrosis often occur after the initial insult. (See also Ann. Emerg. Med. 14:603, 1985 and Br. J. Dermatol. 119:45, 1988.)
17. Wilson, E. F., Rich, T. H., and Messman, H. C. The hazardous hibachi. *J.A.M.A.* 221:404, 1972.
    Lethal accumulation of carbon monoxide when ventilation is inadequate.
18. Craig, T. V., Hunt, W., and Atkinson, R. Hypothermia: Its use in severe carbon monoxide poisoning. *N. Engl. J. Med.* 261:854, 1959.
    Use of hypothermia to prevent anoxic damage.
19. Smith, J. S., and Brandon, S. Morbidity from acute carbon monoxide poisoning at three year follow up. *Br. Med. J.* 1:318, 1973.
    Level of consciousness on admission correlates with subsequent development of neuropsychiatric sequelae.
20. Sawada, Y., Takahashi, M., Ohashi, N., et al. Computerized tomography as an indication of long-term outcome after acute carbon monoxide poisoning. *Lancet* 1:783, 1980.
    Computed tomography abnormalities in the globus pallidus indicate a poor prognosis.

21. Horowitz, A. L., Kaplan, R., and Sarpel, G. Carbon monoxide toxicity: MR imaging in the brain. *Radiology* 162:787, 1987.
    MRI is a useful technique for evaluating cerebral damage.
22. Hebbel, R. P., Eaton, J. W., Modler, S., et al. Extreme but asymptomatic carboxyhemoglobinemia and chronic lung disease. *J.A.M.A.* 239:2584, 1978.
    Extreme elevation of carboxyhemoglobin due to inhalation of cigar smoke.
23. Stewart, R. D., and Hake, C. L. Paint remover hazard. *J.A.M.A.* 235:398, 1976.
    Methylene chloride in paint removers is metabolized to carbon monoxide.
24. Caravati, E.M., Adams, C.J., Joyce, S.M., et al. Fetal toxicity associated with maternal carbon monoxide poisoning. *Ann. Emerg. Med.* 17:714, 1988.
    Fetal mortality is substantial.
25. Kelly, J. S., and Sophocleus, G. J. Retinal hemorrhages in subacute carbon monoxide poisoning. *J.A.M.A.* 239:1515, 1978.
    Retinal hemorrhages may be a clue to the presence of carbon monoxide intoxication.
26. Myers, R. A. M., Snyder, S. K., Linberg, S., et al. Value of hyperbaric oxygen in suspected carbon monoxide poisoning. *J.A.M.A.* 246:2478, 1981.
    Hyperbaric oxygen recommended for severe carbon monoxide poisoning. (See also Ann. Emerg. Med. 14:1233, 1985.)

12. UPPER GASTROINTESTINAL TRACT HEMORRHAGE (EXCLUDING VARICES)

Jerry L. Spivak

In managing the patient with upper gastrointestinal tract hemorrhage, attention should be directed to four factors: (1) the extent of blood loss, (2) the rate of blood loss, (3) the location of bleeding, and (4) the cause of the hemorrhage. Evaluation and therapy are best conducted by a multidisciplinary approach with the internist, endoscopist, radiologist, and surgeon collaborating.

The extent of blood loss can be roughly gauged by determination of the hemoglobin, blood pressure, and BUN. A hemoglobin less than 11 gm/dl, a systolic blood pressure less than 100 mm Hg, and a BUN greater than 40 mg/dl suggest loss of at least a liter of blood. Obviously the measurements are crude guides that can be influenced by prior iron deficiency and by underlying cardiac or renal disease. Other clues are pallor of the palmar creases, which suggests at least a 50 percent decrease in red cell mass (hemoglobin < 7 gm/dl) and a history of hematemesis. Hematemesis is usually associated with at least a 25 percent fall in red blood cell volume. The pulse rate reflects in part the adrenergic response to stress and may be misleading, as may the hematocrit, which takes more than 30 hours to equilibrate and the degree of hemodilution is influenced by whether there is hematemesis, or melena with subsequent absorption of water and protein. The BUN is influenced by the latter as well. Historical inquiry about prior bleeding is important since many patients come to the hospital only after the second episode of hemorrhage.

The rate of blood loss is best determined by insertion of a nasogastric tube and lavage of the stomach. It is characteristic of duodenal ulcers to bleed intermittently, a phenomenon described as stutter bleeding, with bursts of hemorrhage of approximately 30 minutes in duration. Blood that is not refluxed into the stomach cannot be measured, but most patients with melena alone have not been found to be bleeding briskly.

Evaluation of the location and cause of bleeding begins with the history and physical examination. The history should include inquiry into previous bleeding episodes, the circumstances surrounding the present episode particularly with reference to vomiting and retching, and inquiry about the use of antacids, aspirin, steroids, nonsteroidal anti-inflammatory agents (NSAIDs), anticoagulants, and alcohol. Up to 50 percent of patients with upper gastrointestinal hemorrhage have a recent history of salicylate ingestion. A history of a bleeding tendency should also be sought. Physical examination should include a search for the stigmata of cirrhosis, mucocutaneous lesions such as telangiectasia, café au lait spots, aortic valve murmurs, and connective tissue abnormalities, such as pseudoxanthoma elasticum. However, it must be remembered that the history and physical examination can be misleading since 40 percent of patients with peptic ulcer or esophageal varices are found to be bleeding from another lesion. In large series, the causes of upper gastrointestinal hemorrhage include duodenal ulcer, esophageal varices, gastric ulcer, gastritis, esophagitis, Mallory-Weiss syndrome, gastric carcinoma, unusual lesions (telangiectasia, Peutz-Jeghers syndrome, etc.), and anastomotic ulcers. In approximately 10 percent of patients, no cause for bleeding is found.

When the patient's blood volume has been replenished and the vital signs are stable, diagnostic studies can be considered. Endoscopy is superior to x-ray studies in identifying bleeding lesions. Barium contrast x rays offer no assurance that an identified lesion is actually bleeding, cannot be used in the diagnosis of gastritis, are inferior for the identification of varices, and obscure the intestinal tract for both endoscopy and angiography for at least 8 hours. One pitfall in endoscopy is being misled by lesions produced during gastric lavage. If a lesion cannot be identified by endoscopy, then either a barium study or angiography should be performed. The latter is preferred if bleeding is continuing, particularly if there is rapid blood loss per rectum without evidence of a bleeding site. In such a situation the cause is usually either a duodenal ulcer or diverticular hemorrhage.

It should be emphasized that the routine use of endoscopy as a diagnostic procedure in patients with gastrointestinal bleeding is by no means established. Although a vigorous diagnostic approach to gastrointestinal tract hemorrhage has been advocated for many years, recent studies suggest that endoscopy was not beneficial in patients whose bleeding ceased during hospitalization in response to conservative medical therapy. Patients with alcoholic cirrhosis may prove to be an exception since such patients, if they stop bleeding, are likely to rebleed and in them hemorrhage can occur from a variety of causes, each of which requires a different form of therapy. Consequently, patients with liver disease may represent a subgroup in whom emergency endoscopy may play an important role in determining treatment. Rebleeding in patients with peptic ulcer is most likely to occur when there is a visible vessel in the ulcer crater. However, rebleeding in such a situation is not inevitable.

Additional diagnostic studies performed at the time of initial evaluation should include liver function tests, coagulation studies (prothrombin time, partial thromboplastin time, fibrinogen and platelet count), a smear for red cell morphology, a creatinine determination, and an ECG. Normal liver function tests exclude portal hypertension due to intrahepatic disease as a cause of hemorrhage, and normal coagulation studies rule out a hemorrhagic diathesis. Identification of a hemorrhagic diathesis is of great therapeutic importance but does not exclude an anatomic basis for gastrointestinal hemorrhage. Although a site of bleeding is rarely identified in von Willebrand's disease, peptic ulcer disease is the most common cause of upper gastrointestinal bleeding in classical hemophilia and bleeding in an anticoagulated patient may be due to an occult carcinoma. A reduced platelet count is not uncommon in alcoholics. Red cell morphology may reveal macrocytosis, microcytosis, or the fragmentation seen with disseminated intravascular coagulation (DIC) or metastatic tumor. The serum creatinine is a better guide to renal function than the BUN owing to resorption of protein from the gut. The ECG may indicate the presence of subendocardial ischemia, a not uncommon finding with hypovolemia and the attendant release of catecholamines.

Although determination of the site and cause of bleeding is important in the definitive treatment of gastrointestinal tract hemorrhage, the single most important initial therapeutic maneuver is adequate volume replacement. This is one of the few situations in which use of whole blood is indicated. The most common cause of death in patients with upper gastrointestinal tract hemorrhage, whether treated medically or surgically, is inadequate blood replacement and most fatalities occur during the first hospitalization for bleeding. The patient with a duodenal ulcer must be approached with the assumption that the bleeding that precipitated admission is probably the second episode of hemorrhage and that if the hemoglobin is less than 9 gm/dl, rebleeding will occur. In addition, patients with hematemesis have a 20 percent incidence of rebleeding within the first 48 hours of hospitalization. Thus blood replacement must be vigorous. If a catheter can be placed safely, observation of the central venous pressure may be the best way to monitor replacement therapy in the older patient.

If bleeding is not controlled by gastric lavage and blood replacement, other measures must be considered. These measures include administration of vasopressin, embolization, endoscopic cautery, and surgery. Selective arterial vasoconstrictive therapy is probably the method of choice when intervention is necessary for the initial management of gastritis and the Mallory-Weiss syndrome. Results with peptic ulcer bleeding have been less satisfactory. Surgery is indicated in patients requiring more than 6 units of blood, in those with bleeding gastric ulcers (recurrent bleeding is 3 times more common than with duodenal ulcers), in patients over age 50, in patients with unusual blood types, and in patients whose hemorrhage is associated with continuing pain or obstruction. It should be remembered, however, that although surgery is an effective immediate means for the mechanical control of hemorrhage, it provides no guarantee against future bleeding. Embolization or endoscopic cautery may also be useful in selected situations.

1. Gostout, C. J. Acute gastrointestinal bleeding—a common problem revisited. *Mayo Clin. Proc.* 63:596, 1988.
   A useful, concise review which summarizes the results of endoscopic cautery (See also Am. J. Med. *83:(suppl 6A):41, 1987.)*
2. Bordley, D. R., Mushlin, A. I., Dolan, J. G., et al. Early clinical signs identify low-risk patients with acute upper gastrointestinal hemorrhage. *J.A.M.A.* 253:3282, 1985.
   Low-risk patients are younger without multiorgan failure, hypotension, or active bleeding.
3. Larson, G., Schmidt, T., Gott, J., et al. Upper gastrointestinal bleeding: predictors of outcome. *Surgery* 100:765, 1986.
   Age, multiorgan failure, and extent and rate of hemorrhage were important. (See also Am. J. Med. Sci. *294:26, 1987 and Br. J. Surg. 73:985, 1986.)*
4. Snook, J. A., Holdstock, G. E., and Bamforth, J. Value of a simple biochemical ratio in distinguishing upper and lower sites of gastrointestinal haemorrhage. *Lancet* 1:1064, 1986.
   If the plasma urea-creatinine ratio is 100 or greater, upper gastrointestinal hemorrhage is likely.
5. Sutton, F. M. Upper gastrointestinal bleeding in patients with esophageal varices. What is the most common source? *Am. J. Med.* 83:273, 1987.
   Esophageal varices.
6. Wilcox, C. M., and Truss, C. D. Gastrointestinal bleeding in patients receiving long-term anticoagulant therapy. *Am. J. Med.* 84:683, 1988.
   The bleeding is usually due to an underlying lesion. (See also Am. J. Med. *83:269, 1987.)*
7. Peterson, W. L., Barnett, C. C., Smith, H. J., et al. Routine early endoscopy in upper-gastrointestinal-tract bleeding: A randomized, controlled trial. *N. Engl. J. Med.* 304:925, 1981.
   Endoscopy was not found to influence prognosis when upper gastrointestinal bleeding responded to conservative therapy. (See also the accompanying editorial on p. 967.)
8. Mailer, C., Goldberg, A., Harden, R. M., et al. Diagnosis of upper gastrointestinal bleeding. *Br. Med. J.* 2:784, 1965.
   A hemoglobin less than 11 gm/dl or a systolic blood pressure less than 100 mm Hg suggests that more than 1 liter of blood has been lost.
9. Northfield, T. C., and Smith, T. Hematemesis as an index of blood loss. *Lancet* 1:990, 1971.
   Hematemesis signifies at least a 25 percent loss of red cell volume.

10. Graham, D. Y., and Schwartz, J. T. The spectrum of the Mallory-Weiss tear. *Medicine* 57:307, 1977.
   Comprehensive review; in most cases bleeding stops spontaneously.
11. Sheedy, P. F., II, Fulton, R. E., and Atwell, D. T. Angiographic evaluation of patients with chronic gastrointestinal bleeding. *AJR* 123:338, 1975.
   The occult site of hemorrhage was identified by angiography in 45 percent of cases; most often it was an arteriovenous malformation.
12. Northfield, T. C. Factors predisposing to recurrent haemorrhage of acute gastrointestinal bleeding. *Br. Med. J.* 1:26, 1971.
   Most recurrent bleeding occurs within 48 hours after the patient's admission to the hospital.
13. Borland, J. L., Sr., Hancock, W. R., and Borland, J. L., Jr. Recurrent upper gastrointestinal hemorrhage in peptic ulcer. *Gastroenterology* 52:631, 1967.
   30% recurrence rate after the initial hemorrhage.
14. Storey, D. W., Brown, S. G., Swain, C. P., et al. Endoscopic prediction of recurrent bleeding in peptic ulcer. *N. Engl. J. Med.* 305:915, 1981.
   Rebleeding occurs predominantly when there is a visible vessel in the ulcer crater. (See also N. Engl. J. Med. 300:1411, 1979.)
15. Fleischer, D. Endoscopic therapy of upper gastrointestinal bleeding in humans. *Gastroenterology* 90:217, 1986.
   The role of endoscopic therapy is not definitively established. (See also N. Engl. J. Med. 316:1652, 1987.)
16. Collins, R., and Langman, M. Treatment with histamine H2 antagonists in acute upper gastrointestinal hemorrhage. Implications of randomized trials. *N. Engl. J. Med.* 313:660, 1985.
   These agents may reduce the rebleeding rate in patients with gastric ulcers.
17. Fisher, R. D., Ebert, P. A., and Zuidema, G. D. Peptic ulcer disease. *Arch. Surg.* 92:909, 1966.
   Mortality in emergency surgery for gastrointestinal tract hemorrhage is reduced by preoperative correction of hypovolemia. (See also Ann. Surg. 164:840, 1966.)
18. Cannon, L. A., Heiselman, D., Gardner, W., et al. Prophylaxis of upper gastrointestinal tract bleeding in mechanically ventilated patients. *Arch. Intern. Med.* 147:2101, 1987.
   Cimetidine, sulcralfate, and antacids were effective but renal failure was more common with antacid therapy.
19. Levy, M., Miller, D. R., Kaufman, D. W., et al. Major upper gastrointestinal tract bleeding. *Arch. Intern. Med.* 148:281, 1988.
   Aspirin increases the risk as do NSAIDs. (See Ann. Intern. Med. 109:359, 1988 and Arch. Intern. Med. 147:85, 1987.)
20. Bjarnason, I., Zanelli, G., Prouse, P., et al. Blood and protein loss via small-intestinal inflammation induced by non-steroidal anti-inflammatory drugs. *Lancet* 2:711, 1987.
   Mechanism for gastrointestinal hemorrhage with NSAIDs.
21. Hubert, J. P., Jr., Kiernan, P. D., Welch, J. S., et al. The surgical management of bleeding stress ulcers. *Ann. Surg.* 191:672, 1980.
   Extensive resection advocated if medical therapy is unsuccessful.
22. Franco, D., Durandy, Y., Deporte, A., et al. Upper gastrointestinal haemorrhage in hepatic cirrhosis: Causes and relation to hepatic failure and stress. *Lancet* 1:218, 1977.
   Stress-induced subepithelial erosions predominate as the cause of upper gastrointestinal tract bleeding with severe hepatic failure. (See also Gastroenterology 93:1054, 1987 and 94:1254, 1988.)
23. Lau, W. Y., Fan, S. T., Wong, S. H., et al. Preoperative and intraoperative localization of gastrointestinal bleeding of obscure origin. *Gut* 28:869, 1987.
   Use of multiple diagnostic approaches was required. (See also Br. Med. J. 296:3, 1988.)
24. Clark, R. A., Colley, D. P., and Eggers, F. M. Acute arterial gastrointestinal hemorrhage: Efficacy of transcatheter control. *AJR* 136:1185, 1981.

Embolization should not be employed as the primary therapy in gastrointestinal hemorrhage.

25. Keller, F. S., Rosch, J., Baur, G. M., et al. Percutaneous angiographic embolization: A procedure of increasing usefulness. *Am. J. Surg.* 142:5, 1981.
    Results of 152 embolizations reviewed.

26. Hussey, K. P. Vasopressin therapy for upper gastrointestinal tract hemorrhage. Has its efficacy been proven? *Arch. Intern. Med.* 145:1263, 1985.
    The exact role of vasopressin is still undefined. (See also Ann. Intern. Med. *96:565, 1982.)*

27. Waltman, A. C., Greenfield, A. J., Novelline, R. A., et al. Pyloroduodenal bleeding and intraarterial vasopressin: Clinical results. *AJR* 133:643, 1979.
    Intraarterial vasopressin alone is not effective in controlling duodenal hemorrhage.

28. Briley, C. A., Jr., Jackson, D. C., Johnsrude, I. S., et al. Acute gastrointestinal hemorrhage of small-bowel origin. *Radiology* 136:317, 1980.
    Causes of hemorrhage included vascular malformations, fistulas, tumors, ulcers, and granulomatous inflammation.

29. Smith, R., Copely, D. J., and Bolen, F. H. 99mTc RBC scintigraphy: correlation of gastrointestinal bleeding rates with scintigraphic findings. *Am. J. Roentgenol.* 148:869, 1987.
    A useful diagnostic technique.

30. Harris, S. K., Bone, R. C., and Ruth, W. E. Gastrointestinal hemorrhage in patients in a respiratory intensive care unit. *Chest* 72:301, 1977.
    Hemorrhage occurs more often with acute respiratory failure than with chronic obstructive disease.

31. Adamson, J. W., and Hillman, R. S. Blood volume and plasma protein replacement following acute blood loss in normal man. *J.A.M.A.* 205:60, 1968.
    The hematocrit is a poor index of acute blood loss.

32. Bredgaard-Sorensen, M., Christiansen, L. A., Malmstrom, J., et al. Central hemodynamics in acute gastrointestinal bleeding. *Surgery* 145:685, 1977.
    In patients without heart failure, pulmonary artery pressure was the best measure of hypovolemia; with heart failure, the central venous pressure was more useful.

33. Luk, G. D., Bynum, T. E., and Hendrix, T. R. Gastric aspiration in localization of gastrointestinal hemorrhage. *J.A.M.A.* 241:576, 1979.
    Gastric aspiration is a reliable method of distinguishing upper gastrointestinal bleeding from lower. (For the use of labeled red cells, see J.A.M.A. 247:789, 1982.)

34. Spechler, S. J., and Schimmel, E. M. Gastrointestinal tract bleeding of unknown origin. *Arch. Intern. Med.* 142:236, 1982.
    A useful review.

35. Zuckerman, G. R., Cornette, G. L., Clouse, R. E., et al. Upper gastrointestinal bleeding in patients with chronic renal failure. *Ann Intern. Med.* 102:588, 1985.
    Angiodysplasia was the most common lesion.

36. Bronner, M. H., Pate, M. B., Cunningham, J. T., et al. Estrogen-progesterone therapy for bleeding gastrointestinal telangiectasias in chronic renal failure. An uncontrolled trial. *Ann. Intern. Med.* 105:371, 1986.
    An interesting therapeutic approach. (See also Am. J. Gastroenterol. *83:556, 1988.)*

37. Imperiale, T. F., and Ransohoff, D. F. Aortic stenosis, idiopathic gastrointestinal bleeding, and angiodysplasia: Is there an association? *Gastroenterology* 95:1670, 1988.
    A definitive association has not been demonstrated.

38. Vase, P., and Grove, O. Gastrointestinal lesions in hereditary hemorrhagic telangiectasia. *Gastroenterology* 91:1079, 1983.
    A difficult therapeutic problem.

39. Pointner, R., Schwab, G., Konigsrainer, A., et al. Endoscopic treatment of Dieulafoy's disease. *Gastroenterology* 94:563, 1988.
    An unusual cause of hemorrhage which is amenable to endoscopic cautery.

40. Simon, J. B. Occult blood screening for colorectal carcinoma: a critical review. *Gastroenterology* 88:820, 1985.
    An excellent summary of the literature.

41. Barer, D., Ogilvie, A., Henry, D., et al. Cimetidine and tranexamic acid in the treatment of acute upper-gastrointestinal-tract bleeding. *N. Engl. J. Med.* 308:1571, 1983.
    Both were effective in reducing mortality.
42. Shuman, R. B., Schuster, D. P., and Zuckerman, G. R. Prophylactic therapy for stress ulcer bleeding: a reappraisal. *Ann. Intern. Med.* 106:562, 1987.
    Cimetidine is equivalent to antacids in preventing stress ulcer bleeding.

13. ESOPHAGEAL VARICEAL HEMORRHAGE
H. Franklin Herlong

Esophageal variceal hemorrhage is the most serious consequence of chronic liver disease. While only about 25 percent of patients with varices ever bleed from them, once patients do bleed most will rebleed within 6 months. The mortality from a variceal hemorrhage depends on the stage of the underlying liver disease. Approximately half of patients with decompensated cirrhosis, manifested by jaundice and coagulopathy, die as a direct result of the hemorrhage, whereas only about 10 percent of patients with well-compensated liver disease die because of the bleed.

Varices develop when resistance to blood flow through the liver causes portal blood to reroute to the systemic circulation through collateral vessels. Varices may develop when there is obstruction of hepatic blood flow in the hepatic veins (Budd-Chiari syndrome, venoocclusive disease), the hepatic sinusoids (cirrhosis, granulomatous hepatitis), or the portal veins (schistosomiasis, portal vein thrombosis). Patients who bleed from varices secondary to a portal vein thrombosis who have intact hepatocellular function have an excellent prognosis. Isolated gastric varices with no esophageal varices are most often caused by a splenic vein thrombosis.

Variceal hemorrhage is rare when the portal pressure is less than 12 mm Hg (normal portal pressure = 5 mm Hg) but the risk of hemorrhage correlates poorly with the degree of portal hypertension as measured by the wedged hepatic venous pressure. There is a better correlation between the risk of hemorrhage and the size of the esophageal varices. These observations suggest that transmural pressure, which is influenced to a greater degree by the radius of the varix than the portal pressure, is the most important factor in predicting whether a varix will bleed.

Precipitating factors for hemorrhage have been difficult to identify. Esophagitis caused by gastroesophageal reflux does not appear to increase the risk of bleeding. Similarly, the presence of ascites does not increase the risk of hemorrhage. In some reports, the use of nonsteroidal anti-inflammatory agents has been associated with esophageal variceal hemorrhage.

Variceal hemorrhage often causes hematemesis, but may also present as melena. When the bleeding is brisk, hematochezia may be the presenting symptom. Rarely, subclinical variceal bleeding may cause occult iron-deficiency anemia.

Esophageal variceal hemorrhage is diagnosed most reliably by endoscopy. Barium studies play no role in the diagnosis of esophageal variceal bleeding. Endoscopy should be performed as soon as the patient is hemodynamically stable. Prompt restoration of circulating blood volume is essential in managing patients with variceal bleeding. Prolonged arterial hypotension dramatically impairs hepatic function since the regenerating nodules in the cirrhotic liver are virtually entirely dependent on hepatic arterial flow. The adequacy of intravenous volume support is best assessed by measuring the central venous pressure. Maintaining the central venous pressure between 5 and 8 cm of water confirms an adequate filling pressure of the right heart. Further elevation of the central venous pressure will unnecessarily expand the plasma volume, increase portal blood flow, and may exacerbate bleeding. Blood loss should be replaced by packed red blood cells, and fresh frozen plasma if the prothrombin time is prolonged.

Therapy for esophageal variceal hemorrhage is directed at controlling the acute bleed and reducing the risk of subsequent rebleeding. Endoscopic sclerotherapy and vasopressin infusion are the two modalities most commonly used to control acute bleeding. Sclerotherapy is usually performed at the time of the initial diagnostic endoscopy if a varix is the source of the bleeding. Esophageal varices are considered to be responsible for the hemorrhage if blood is seen coming from the varix or no other diagnostic finding is identified in the esophagus, stomach, or duodenum which would explain the bleed.

Several sclerosing agents including sodium morrhuate and sodium tetradecyl sulfate and ethanolamine oleate have been used. As yet, no single agent has clearly proved superior. The sclerosant induces inflammation of the intima of the varix with formation of a thrombus. After the thrombosis occludes the varix, developing fibrosis tissue results in eventual obliteration of the varix. Intravariceal and paravariceal injections have been used to treat bleeding esophageal varices. While both appear to be efficacious, intravariceal injection results in better thrombosis and is usually the preferred technique.

Fifteen percent of patients who undergo sclerotherapy develop clinically significant complications. Esophageal ulceration with secondary stricture formation is the most common. Most patients develop chest pain during the first 24 hours after sclerotherapy which usually resolves with no therapy. Pleural effusion, pericarditis, or aspiration pneumonitis occurs in fewer than 10 percent of patients. Sclerotherapy is repeated at intervals of 1 to 2 weeks until the varices in the distal esophagus are completely obliterated. If variceal obliteration is successful, rebleeding is rare.

In the acutely bleeding patient, vasopressin is often used as an adjunct to endoscopic sclerotherapy. Vasopressin is administered through a large peripheral vein at a dose of 0.4 unit/minute. Directly infusing vasopressin into the superior mesenteric artery offers no advantage over peripheral infusion. The dose of vasopressin is tapered by 0.1 unit every 12 hours, if no further bleeding occurs. Predictable hemodynamic effects which occur during vasopressin infusion include increased systemic vascular resistance and blood pressure, accompanied by a reflex bradycardia. Since vasopressin may cause vasoconstriction of the coronary arteries, the drug must be used with great caution in patients at risk for ischemic heart disease. The drug should not be used in patients with clinically apparent cardiac ischemia or in individuals who have had a recent myocardial infarction. Vasopressin may cause retention of free water and hyponatremia.

Nitroglycerin has been used as an adjunct to vasopressin therapy. This potent venous dilator can reduce the undesirable side effects of vasopressin in addition to reducing portal pressure. It increases cardiac output by reducing afterload, while its vasodilator properties reduce directly portal blood flow and pressure. If the combination of sclerotherapy and pharmacologic therapy fails to control bleeding, a Sengstaken-Blakemore tube may be used. Numerous complications limit the effectiveness of esophageal tamponade. The tube may obstruct the upper airway or cause pressure necrosis of the gastric fundus and distal esophagus. It should not be left in place for more than 24 hours.

For patients who continue to bleed despite vasopressin therapy, sclerotherapy, and Sengstaken-Blakemore tube, emergency shunt surgery may be the only alternative. Since the mortality is so high in decompensated cirrhotic patients, surgery should be avoided if at all possible.

Once the acute bleed has been controlled, therapy is directed at prevention of recurrent variceal hemorrhage. Several controlled trials have been published evaluating the efficacy of beta blockade in preventing bleeding. The results remain controversial. In most studies, patients with decompensated cirrhosis have little benefit from propranolol. In well-compensated Child's class A cirrhotic patients, propranolol may reduce the incidence of bleeding. Repeated endoscopic sclerotherapy appears to be the most satisfactory modality to control recurrent variceal bleeding. As mentioned previously, when sclerotherapy leads to esophageal variceal obliteration, hemorrhage is usually controlled.

The role of portosystemic shunts in preventing recurrent bleeding remains controversial. Several controlled trials have compared distal splenorenal shunts with endoscopic sclerotherapy. Both approaches are about equally efficacious in controlling bleeding. Since sclerotherapy is technically much easier, portosystemic shunts are reserved for those patients who have recurrent bleeding despite sclerotherapy.

Many centers consider hepatic transplantation an alternative to shunt therapy. For patients who have recurrent variceal hemorrhage this approach is recommended if they are appropriate candidates for hepatic transplantation.

One would like to identify effective prophylactic therapy to prevent the initial hemorrhage in a patient with esophageal varices. Several approaches have been used to prevent the first variceal bleed. Prophylactic portosystemic shunts reduce the prevalence of the frequency of hemorrhage, but do not change overall mortality. Postshunt encephalopathy is common. Several controlled trials have been performed to evaluate endoscopic sclerotherapy in patients with varices who have never bled. Most have shown a reduction in hemorrhage and several have reported an apparent reduction in mortality. It also appears that prophylactic therapy with beta-adrenergic blockers may reduce the risk of bleeding. Patients with large varices discovered prior to the first hemorrhage are candidates for beta-adrenergic blockade and sclerotherapy.

1. Italian Liver Cirrhosis Project: Reliability of endoscopy in the assessment of variceal features. *J. Hepatology* 4:93, 1987.
   Criteria to standardize the endoscopic description of features of the esophageal varices are presented.
2. Garcia-Tsao, G., Groszmann, R. J., Fisher, R., et al. Portal pressure, presence of esophageal varices and variceal bleeding. *J. Hepatology* 5:419, 1985.
   The risk of variceal bleeding was shown to correlate with the size of varices more than portal pressure suggesting transmural pressure was the most important factor in determining the risk of hemorrhage.
3. Arsene, D., Bruley des Varannes, S., Galmiche, J. T., et al. Gastroesophageal reflux and alcoholic cirrhosis. A reappraisal. *J. Hepatology* 4:250, 1987.
   25% of patients with cirrhosis had evidence of gastroesophageal reflux with no episodes present in controls. However, there was no difference in incidence of reflux in patients who had bled from varices compared with those who had not.
4. Graham, D. Y., and Smith, J. L. The course of patients with variceal hemorrhage. *Gastroenterology* 80:800, 1981.
   The risk of rebleeding was greatest during the first 6 months to 1 year after a bleed from esophageal varices.
5. Sutton, N., and Sutton, F. M. Upper gastrointestinal bleeding in patients with esophageal varices. What is the most common source? *Am. J. Med.* 83:273, 1987.
   The study evaluated the sources of bleeding in patients known to have varices. In 65% of the patients, only varices were found, 15% had varices and erosions in the stomach and duodenum, 8% had gastric ulcer, 3% had a duodenal ulcer, esophagitis was present in 4%, and a Mallory-Weiss tear was present in 3%.
6. Gimson, A. F. S., Westaby, D., and Hegarty, J. A randomized trial of vasopressin and vasopressin plus nitroglycerin in the control of acute variceal hemorrhage. *Hepatology* 6:410, 1986.
7. Tsai, Y. T., Lay, C. S., Lai, K. H., et al. Controlled trial of vasopressin and nitroglycerine versus vasopressin alone in the treatment of esophageal varices. *Hepatology* 6:406, 1986.
   These two studies confirm that nitroglycerin negates the negative hemodynamic effects of vasopressin while further reducing portal pressure.
8. Conn, H. O., Lindenmuth, W. W., May, C. J., et al. Prophylactic portocaval anastomosis. A tale of two studies. *Medicine* 51:27, 1972.
9. Resnick, R. H., Chalmers, T. C., Ishihara, A. M., et al. A controlled study of the prophylactic portocaval shunt. *Ann. Intern. Med.* 70:675, 1969.
10. Jackson, F. C., Perrin, E. B., Smith, A. G., et al. A clinical investigation of the portocaval shunt. *Am. J. Surg.* 115:22, 1968.
    The above studies all confirm that prophylactic portosystemic shunts reduce the incidence of hemorrhage from varices, but in no study was there an improvement in mortality.
11. LeBrec, D., Poynard, T., Bernuau, J., et al. A randomized controlled study of propranolol for prevention of recurrent gastrointestinal bleeding in patients with cirrhosis: A final report. *Hepatology* 4:355, 1984.
    This paper was the first report suggesting that propranolol effectively prevented re-

current bleeding in patients with cirrhosis. While some patients had bled from varices, many had bled from acute gastric erosions.

12. Poynard, T., Lebrec, D., Hillon, P., et al. Propranolol for prevention of recurrent gastrointestinal bleeding in patients with cirrhosis. *Hepatology* 7:447, 1987.
    This prospective study evaluated factors associated with rebleeding.

13. Pascal, J. P., and Cales, P. Multi-center study group: Propanolol in the prevention of first upper gastrointestinal tract hemorrhage in patients with cirrhosis of the liver and esophageal varices. *N. Engl. J. Med.* 317:856, 1987.
    In this study, 27% of patients in the placebo group bled from varices compared with 17% in the propranolol group. There was also a suggestion of improved survival in the group receiving propranolol.

14. Italian Multi-Center Project for Propranolol in Prevention of Bleeding: Propranolol for prophylaxis of bleeding in cirrhotic patients with large varices: A multi-center randomized trial. *Hepatology* 8:1, 1988.

15. Ideo, J., Bellati, G., Fesce, E., et al. Nadolol for preventing the first gastrointestinal bleeding. *Hepatology* 8:6, 1988.
    The two above articles published in the same issue confirmed a beneficial effect of propranolol on bleeding episodes. In these two studies, mortality was not significantly improved.

16. Sarin, S. K., Nanda, R., Sachded, G., et al. Intravariceal versus paravariceal sclerotherapy: A prospective controlled randomized trial. *Gut* 28:657, 1987.
    In this study, bleeding was controlled in 90% of patients by intravariceal injection, while only 19% of patients were controlled who received paravariceal injection.

17. Teres, J., Bordas, J. M., Bravo, D., et al. Sclerotherapy versus splenorenal shunt in the elective treatment of variceal hemorrhage: A randomized controlled trial. *Hepatology* 7:430, 1987.
    In this study survival was similar in the sclerotherapy and distal splenorenal shunt groups. Hemorrhage occurred in about 50% of patients in the sclerotherapy group, while only 26% of the patients who bled received a shunt. More patients in the distal splenorenal shunt group developed encephalopathy. In some, this encephalopathy was severe and recurrent.

18. Rikkers, L. F., Burnett, D. A., Volentine, G. D., et al. Shunt surgery versus endoscopic sclerotherapy for long-term treatment of variceal bleeding: Early results of a randomized trial. *Ann. Surg.* 206:261, 1987.
    In this study, 60% of patients who received sclerotherapy rebled, whereas only 19% of the patients who had a shunt rebled. The shunt group required 28 transfusions, whereas 228 transfusions were given to the sclerotherapy group.
    The following randomized trials have investigated prophylactic sclerotherapy.

19. Paquet, K. J. Prophylactic endoscopic sclerosing treatment of esophageal wall varices: A prospective controlled randomized trial. *Endoscopy* 14:4, 1982.

20. Witzel, L., Wolbergs, E., and Merki, H. Prophylactic endoscopic sclerotherapy of esophageal varices—A prospective randomized trial. *Lancet* 1:773, 1985.
    In both of the above studies, prophylactic sclerotherapy significantly reduced hemorrhage compared to no therapy. There was also a significant reduction in mortality.

21. Santangelo, W. C., Dueno, M. J., Estes, B. L., et al. Prophylactic sclerotherapy of large esophageal varices. *N. Engl. J. Med.* 318:814, 1988.
    In this study the prevalence of variceal bleeding was greater in the sclerotherapy group. There was no significant difference in mortality between the two groups.

14. HYPOGLYCEMIA
H. Verdain Barnes

Hypoglycemia is a state in which the rate of glucose removal from the blood exceeds sufficient replacement to maintain normoglycemia. The exact glucose level required to remain asymptomatic varies according to (1) the rapidity of the fall, (2) individual and sex variations, and (3) age. From the clinical and pathophysiologic perspectives, cerebral hypoglycemia is essentially identical to cerebral anoxia. Central nervous system tissues have diminished oxygen utilization despite adequate arterial oxygen saturation. Macroscopically the brain shows hemorrhages and edema, and microscopically pyknotic nuclei and vacuolar changes. To some degree, all cells can use ketones and/or free fatty acids for energy in the absence of adequate glucose, but brain cells and erythrocytes have far less adaptability than other tissues. To maintain optimum integrity and function, brain cells require about 100 gm and erythrocytes 14 gm of glucose per day.

The primary glucoregulatory organs are the liver, pancreas, adrenals, and pituitary. In hypoglycemia the liver responds with increased glycogenolysis and gluconeogenesis. These three glands secrete at least five important hormones that work to prevent hypoglycemia. The pancreas releases glucagon, an activator of a hepatic phosphorylase that stimulates glycogenolysis and enhances gluconeogenesis. The pituitary releases growth hormone and adrenocorticotropic hormone (ACTH). Growth hormone enhances lipolysis and inhibits glucose utilization by muscle. ACTH stimulates the adrenal cortex to release cortisol, which has a catabolic action on proteins, induces increments in other hormones that stimulate gluconeogenesis, and helps to diminish the muscle uptake of glucose. In hypoglycemia there is a release of epinephrine from the adrenal medulla. Epinephrine, an insulin antagonist, inhibits the uptake of glucose by muscle and partially inhibits the release of insulin from the pancreas. It also activates a hepatic phosphorylase, which induces glycogenolysis, and fat cell lipase, which stimulates lipolysis. The result is an increased availability of free fatty acids, an additional energy source, and glycerol, a gluconeogenic precursor. When one or more of these homeostatic factors is lost, impaired, or overpowered, there is a potential for symptomatic hypoglycemia. The differential diagnosis is long. Comprehensive and detailed discussions of potential causes are found in the first three references.

The clinical presentation of hypoglycemia is variable, depending on the individual, the cause, and the level of the blood glucose. Typically the first manifestations are parasympathetic, including hunger, nausea, eructation, and occasionally bradycardia and mild hypotension. Then a cerebral response generally occurs. The patient may exhibit less spontaneous conversation and mentation, lethargy, lassitude, and frequent yawning. The sympathetic response is usually next, with an increase in pulse rate and blood pressure, with an accompanying diaphoresis and hyperventilation. Finally, seizures and/or coma supervene if the process is not interrupted by an increase in blood glucose levels. Although there is no absolute correlation of signs and symptoms with the level of blood glucose, the parasympathetic response usually begins when the true glucose level drops rapidly to below 70 mg/dl, the cerebral response when the level is below 50 mg/dl, the sympathetic response when the level is below 35 mg/dl, and coma and/or seizures when the level is below 20 mg/dl. The onset of signs and symptoms in fasting or reactive hypoglycemia may be insidious, with lower levels of blood sugar than would be expected from the clinical presentation. On the other hand, signs and symptoms of excess endogenous or exogenous insulin are often acute in onset and may progress rapidly to coma, with the patient having little or no forewarning. The elderly patient, however, may develop profound signs and symptoms with only modest falls in blood glucose, whereas younger persons, especially women, may have true glucose levels well below 40 mg/dl without hypoglycemia signs or symptoms.

When fasting hypoglycemia is suspected, the diagnosis should be confirmed with an 18- to 24-hour fast and/or by a low blood sugar at the onset of signs and symptoms. When reactive hypoglycemia is suspected, a 5-hour oral glucose tolerance test may be useful. Caution is needed when a dumping syndrome is suspected since profound hypoglycemia may occur rapidly after an oral glucose load. Currently, a fingerstick blood sugar using Dextrostix or Chemstrip bG offers relatively accurate estimates in emergencies and for home monitoring. However, if the diagnosis is not easily established but the physician's suspicion is high, more sophisticated tests should be used.

1. Arky, R. A. Pathophysiology and therapy of the fasting hypoglycemias. *D.M.* February, 1968.

2. Eastman, R. C., Rittmaster, R. S., and Kahn, C. R. Hypoglycemia. In P. O. Kohler (eds.), *Clinical Endocrinology*. New York: John Wiley & Sons, 1986. P. 465.
   References 1 and 2 provide the best available in-depth general discussions of hypoglycemia.
3. Merimee, T. J., and Tyson, J. E. Stabilization of plasma glucose during fasting: normal variations in two separate studies. *N. Engl. J. Med.* 291:1275, 1974.
   After a 24-hour fast in women true glucose levels must fall below 35 mg/dl to be significant. Sex standards are needed to judge fasting glucose levels.
4. Strauch, B. S., Felig, P., Baxter, J. D., et al. Hypothermia in hypoglycemia. *J.A.M.A.* 210:345, 1969.
5. Ramos, E., Zorilla, E., and Hadley, W. B. Fever as a manifestation of hypoglycemia. *J.A.M.A.* 205:590, 1968.
   It can happen either way (4, 5).
6. Arky, R. A., and Arons, D. L. Hypoglycemia in diabetes mellitus. *Med. Clin. North Am.* 55:919, 1971.
   A well-referenced article with tables listing causes of hypoglycemia including drugs.
7. Madison, L. L., Lochner, A., and Wulff, J. Ethanol-induced hypoglycemia II: Mechanism of suppression of hepatic gluconeogenesis. *Diabetes* 16:252, 1967.
   This syndrome is characterized by an increased $NADH_2/NAD$ ratio.
8. MacCuish, A. C., Munro, J. F., and Duncan, L. J. P. Treatment of hypoglycemic coma with glucagon, intravenous dextrose and mannitol infusion in 100 diabetics. *Lancet* 2:946, 1970.
   The discussion is probably applicable to all types of hypoglycemia. Consciousness may not return for hours or days after the blood glucose has returned to nonhypoglycemic levels.
9. Frerichs, H., and Creutzfeldt, W. Hypoglycemia 1: Insulin secreting tumors. *Clin. Endocrinol. Metabol.* 5:747, 1976.
10. Marks, V. Hypoglycemia 2: Other causes. *Clin. Endocrinol. Metabol.* 5:769, 1976.
    Articles 9 and 10 are well-referenced reviews.
11. Miller, S. I., Wallace, R. J., Jr., Musher, D. M., et al. Hypoglycemia as a manifestation of sepsis. *Am. J. Med.* 68:649, 1980.
    The most frequent organisms were Streptococcus pneumoniae *and* Haemophilus influenzae *type b. An important entity to keep in mind both in the diagnosis of sepsis and in monitoring patients with sepsis, particularly in the alcoholic.*
12. Boden, G., Reichard, G. A., Jr. Hoeldtke, R. D., et al. Severe insulin induced hypoglycemia associated with deficiencies in the release of counterregulatory hormone. *N. Engl. J. Med.* 305:1200, 1981.
    This can occur in diabetics, after complete sympathectomy, adrenalectomy, or in normal subjects whose responses are blocked by adrenergic blockers.
13. Rizza, R. A., Cryer, P. E., Heymond, M. W., et al. Adrenergic mechanisms for the effects of epinephrine on glucose production and clearance in man. *J. Clin. Invest.* 65:682, 1980.
    Propranolol blocked the epinephrine increase in glucose released by the liver and reduced glucose clearance from the blood as well as the adrenergic clinical manifestations of hypoglycemia.
14. Gordon, P., Hendricks, C. M., Kahn, C. R., et al. Hypoglycemia associated with non-islet-cell tumor and insulin-like growth factors. *N. Engl. J. Med.* 305:1452, 1981.
    Insulin-like growth factor (NSILAs) was most often found with hemangiopericytoma, fibrosarcoma, leiomyosarcoma, malignant pheochromocytoma, adrenocortical carcinoma, and hepatoma.
15. Anderson, N., and Lokich, J. J. Mesenchymal tumors associated with hypoglycemia: Case reports and review of the literature. *Cancer* 44:785, 1979.
    About 50% were retroperitoneal.
16. Jordan, R. M., Kammer, H., and Riddle, M. R. Sulfonylurea-induced factitious hypoglycemia: A growing problem. *Arch. Intern. Med.* 137:390, 1977.
    A problem to keep in mind, C peptide levels don't help with this diagnosis, but blood levels of the sulfonylurea agents do.
17. Scarlett, J. A., Mako, M. E., Rubenstein, A. H., et al. Factitious hypoglycemia. *N. Engl. J. Med.* 297:1029, 1977.

C peptide and free insulin levels are useful in diagnosis including in insulin-treated diabetics.

18. Hoeldtke, R. D., Boden, G., Shuman, C. R., et al. Reduced epinephrine secretion and hypoglycemia unawareness in diabetic autonomic neuropathy. *Ann. Intern. Med.* 96:459, 1982.
   Beware of delayed, diminished, or absent epinephrine-mediated responses to hypoglycemia in diabetics.
19. Hogan, M. J., Service, F. J., Starbrough, F. W., et al. Oral glucose tolerance test compared with a mixed meal in the diagnosis of reactive hypoglycemia: A caveat on stimulation. *Mayo Clin. Proc.* 58:491, 1983.
   Postprandial hypoglycemia (reactive hypoglycemia) is rare after a mixed meal stimulus.
20. Sklenar, J., Wilkin, T. J., Diaz, J. L., et al. Spontaneous hypoglycemia associated with autoimmunity specific to human insulin. *Diabetes Care* 10:152, 1987.
21. Stuart, C. A., Prince, M. J., Peters, E. J., et al. Insulin receptor proliferation: A mechanism for tumor associated hypoglycemia. *J. Clin. Endocrinol. Metab.* 63:879, 1986.
   Two articles (20, 21) report rare causes of hypoglycemia.
22. Fischer, K. F., Lees, J. A., and Newman, J. H. Hypoglycemia in hospitalized patients: Causes and outcomes. *N. Engl. J. Med.*315:1245, 1986.
   A relatively common problem in hospitalized patients, particularly those with renal failure.
23. DeFeo, P., Perriello, G., DeCosmo, S., et al. Comparison of glucose counterregulation during short-term and prolonged hypoglycemia in normal humans. *Diabetes* 35:563, 1986.
   In the short term the primary factors are increased glucose production, insulin suppression, and increased glucagon secretion, while in the long term there is suppression of glucose utilization plus increased glucose production.
24. Boyle, P. J., Schwartz, N. S., Shah, S. D., et al. Plasma glucose concentrations at the onset of hypoglycemic symptoms in patients with poorly controlled diabetes and in nondiabetics. *N. Engl. J. Med.* 318:1487, 1988.
   Poorly controlled diabetics have hypoglycemic symptoms at higher glucose levels than normals.
25. Service, F. J. Hypoglycemia. *Endocrinol. Metab. Clin. North Am.* 17:601, 1988.
   A concise review of diagnostic methods.

15. DIABETIC KETOACIDOSIS
H. Verdain Barnes

Ketoacidosis can develop in any patient with diabetes mellitus, and it can be a rare complication in the nondiabetic patient receiving intravenous diazoxide, high-dose diphenylhydantoin (Dilantin), or high-dose glucocorticoids.

The factors precipitating ketoacidosis in the diabetic are variable. The most common include (1) omission of insulin or oral hypoglycemic, (2) longstanding lack of control, (3) acute infection, (4) acute cardiovascular events, and (5) acute emotional upheaval. The person with insulinopenic juvenile-onset diabetes is the most prone to develop ketoacidosis.

Severe (relative to absolute) insulin deficiency is prerequisite to the development of severe diabetic ketoacidosis. In addition, plasma glucagon is usually elevated. Lipolysis is increased by insulin deficiency, resulting in an elevation of plasma-free fatty acids. The liver is unable to handle the increased free fatty acid load in the absence of insulin. The result is the production and release of the strong acids acetoacetic and β-hydroxybutyrate in about a 1:3 ratio. The ensuing ketonuria and ketonemia lead to a decrease in arterial pH and serum bicarbonate concentration. The effect of insulin deficiency on protein metabolism is increased catabolism leading to aminoacidemia and nitrogen loss. Aminoacidemia enhances gluconeogenesis, thus augmenting the hyperglycemia. The effect of insulin deficiency on carbohydrate metabolism is a decrease in the peripheral utilization of glucose. Hyperglycemia results from an overproduction of glucose and the decrease in the ability of cells to use the glucose. The result is glucosuria and an osmotic diuresis, which is accompanied by an obligatory loss of free water, sodium, potassium, phosphorus, and magnesium. In summary, major insulin deficiency ultimately leads to (1) acidosis; (2) dehydration, hypovolemia and hyperosmolarity; (3) total body depletion of sodium, potassium, phosphorus, and magnesium; (4) lipolysis; and (5) negative nitrogen balance. All these parameters must be considered in the therapy of diabetic ketoacidosis.

The complications of diabetic ketoacidosis (DKA) can be divided into those related to therapy and those related to the disease. Those related to therapy include hypoglycemia, hypokalemia, and cerebral edema. All three complications can in most cases be avoided by careful observation and attention to detail while the ketoacidosis is progressively corrected avoiding sudden rapid changes in glucose, electrolytes, and osmolarity. Cerebral edema is almost always fatal. Current evidence suggests that brain edema occurs as a result of the accumulation of nonglucose metabolites within the brain. These osmotically active substances (idiogenic osmoles) are most likely to occur with a rapid lowering of plasma glucose levels to below 250 mg/dl.

The degree of acidosis deserves attention in therapy. When the arterial pH is less than 7.0, there is a relative impairment of cardiovascular and respiratory function and an increased potential for the development of life-threatening arrhythmias and/or cardiorespiratory arrest. Nonetheless, it is still controversial whether bicarbonate therapy is indicated, even when the pH drops below 7.0, or if used, at what level of pH it should be initiated and how much should be given.

The most frequent complications unrelated to therapy are hypotension, shock, vascular thrombosis, and renal failure. Hypotension and shock are usually related to dehydration and hypovolemia, and usually respond promptly to appropriate therapeutic measures for ketoacidosis. If hypotension and shock persist despite these measures, another cause should be sought. In the older diabetic, congestive heart failure and/or acute myocardial infarction are not uncommon. Arterial thrombosis is a relatively common and a potential cause of death in patients with DKA. Any artery can be involved, but the most common are the carotid, coronary, mesenteric, iliac, and renal. The onset is usually hours or days after initial presentation. Oliguria and progressive azotemia, despite adequate therapy, are most often related to underlying chronic renal disease, acute urinary tract infection, obstructive uropathy, and/or varying degrees and severity of acute tubular necrosis. This situation, however, should not be confused with the transient "functional nephropathy" that occurs not uncommonly in patients with ketoacidosis.

1. Schade, D. S., and Eaton, R. P. Diabetic ketoacidosis—Pathogenesis, prevention and therapy. *Clin. Endocrinol. Metab.* 12:321, 1983.
   A concise well-referenced review.
2. Atchley, D. W., Loeb, R. F., Richards, D. W., Jr., et al. On diabetic acidosis: A detailed study of electrolyte balances following the withdrawal and reestablishment of insulin therapy. *J. Clin. Invest.* 12:297, 1933.
3. Butler, A. M., Talbot, N. B., Burnett, C. H., et al. Metabolic studies in diabetic coma. *Trans. Assoc. Am. Phys.* 60:102, 1947.
4. Seldin, D. W., and Tarail, R. The metabolism of glucose and electrolytes in diabetic acidosis. *J. Clin. Invest.* 29:552, 1950.
5. Nabarro, J. D. N., Spencer, A. G., and Stowers, J. M. Metabolic studies in severe diabetic ketosis. *Q. J. Med.* 21:225, 1952.
   References 2 to 5 are classic references on the metabolic changes during ketoacidosis and the time required for full recovery.
6. Dillon, E. S., Riggs, H. E., and Dyer, W. W. Cerebral lesions in uncomplicated fatal diabetic acidosis. *Am. J. Med. Sci.* 192:360, 1936.
   The pathologic findings in the brain are discussed.

7. Opie, L. H. Cardiac metabolism: The effect of some physiologic, pharmacologic and pathologic influences. *Am. Heart J.* 69:401, 1965.
   The effects on the cardiovascular and respiratory system of a pH <7.1.

8. Watkins, P. J., Smith, J. S., Fitzgerald, M. G., et al. Lactic acidosis in diabetes. *Br. Med. J.* 1:744, 1969.
   Lactic acid may on rare occasions be a significant contributor to the acidosis.

9. Trever, R. W., and Cluff, L. E. The problem of increasing azotemia during management of diabetic acidosis. *Am. J. Med.* 24:368, 1958.
   Acute tubular necrosis may be the answer.

10. Morris, L. R., and Kitabchi, A. E. Efficacy of low-dose insulin therapy in severely obtunded patients in diabetic ketoacidosis. *Diabetes Care* 3:53, 1980.

11. Burghen, G. A., Etteldorf, J. N., Fisher, J. N., et al. Comparison of high-dose and low-dose insulin continuous intravenous infusion in the treatment of diabetic ketoacidosis in children. *Diabetes Care* 3:15, 1980.
   Articles 10 and 11 document the ease and effectiveness of low-dose intravenous or intramuscular insulin in the treatment of ketoacidosis. The advantages are numerous, the two most important being the rarity of rapid electrolyte shifts and, if properly monitored, the avoidance of hypoglycemia.

12. Guisado, R., and Arieff, A. I. Neurologic manifestations of diabetic comas: Correlation with biochemical alterations in the brain. *Metabolism* 24:665, 1975.
   A good review that includes a discussion of hyperosmolar nonketotic coma.

13. Arieff, A. I., and Carroll, H. J. Cerebral edema and depression of sensorium in nonketotic hyperosmolar coma. *Diabetes* 23:565, 1974.
   Decreased sensorium is highly correlated with plasma osmolality and occurs when blood glucose falls below 250 mg/dl.

14. Knight, A. H., Williams, D. N., Ellis, G., et al. Significance of hyperamylasaemia and abdominal pain in diabetic ketoacidosis. *Br. Med. J.* 3:128, 1973.
   Elevated amylase levels in DKA may or may not indicate acute pancreatitis.

15. Fulop, M., and Hoberman, H. D. Alcoholic ketosis. *Diabetes* 24:785, 1975.
   An important entity to recognize. Therapy is critically discussed.

16. Molitch, M. E., Radman, E., Hirsch, C. A., et al. Spurious serum creatinine elevations in ketoacidosis. *Ann. Intern. Med.* 93:280, 1980.
   The marked elevations in acetoacetate in DKA interfere with the automated determinations.

17. Owen, O. E., Licht, J. H., and Sapir, D. G. Renal function and effects of partial rehydration during diabetic ketoacidosis. *Diabetes* 30;510, 1981.
   The early fall in plasma glucose is primarily related to renal glucose excretion.

18. Miles, J. M., Rizza, R. A., Haymond, M. W., et al. Effects of acute insulin deficiency on glucose and ketone body turnover in man: Evidence for the primary overproduction of glucose and ketone bodies in the genesis of diabetic ketoacidosis. *Diabetes* 29:926, 1980.
   Only a rise in glucagon was coincident with the overproduction of glucose and ketone bodies.

19. Owen, O. E., Trapp, V. E., Reichard, G. A., et al. Effects of therapy on the nature and quantity of fuels oxidized during diabetic ketoacidosis. *Diabetes* 29:365, 1980.
   The predominant initial effect of insulin appears to be the promotion of fuel storage rather than glucose and ketone oxidation.

20. Clements, R. S., Jr., and Vourganti, B. Fatal diabetic ketoacidosis: Major causes and approaches to their prevention. *Diabetes Care* 1:314, 1978.
   The culprits are infection, arterial thrombosis, shock, and cerebral edema.

21. Adrogue, H. J., Wilson, H., Boyd, A. E. III, et al. Plasma acid-base patterns in diabetic ketoacidosis. *N. Engl. J. Med.* 307:1603, 1982.
   DKA patients presenting with hyperchloremic acidosis may respond more slowly than those with pure anion gap acidosis.

22. Paulson, W. D. Anion gap–bicarbonate relation in diabetic ketoacidosis. *Am. J. Med.* 81:995, 1986.
   You cannot depend on the anion gap in assessing for mixed acid-base disorders in DKA.

23. Morris, L. R., Murphy, M. B., and Kitabchi, A. E. Bicarbonate therapy for organic acidosis: The case for its continued use. *Ann. Intern. Med.* 105:836, 1986.
24. Narins, R. G., and Cohen, J. J. Bicarbonate therapy for organic acidosis: The case for its continued use. *Ann. Intern. Med.* 106:615, 1987.
    Some (23) say no, others (24) say yes.
25. Kebler, R., McDonald, F. D., and Cadnapaphornchai, P. Dynamic changes in serum phosphorus levels in diabetic ketoacidosis. *Am. J. Med.* 79:571, 1985.
    Hyperphosphatemia is initially present in over 90% but falls dramatically during the first 12 hours of therapy.
26. Adrogue, H. J., Lederer, E. D., Suki, W. N., et al. Determinants of plasma potassium levels in diabetic ketoacidosis. *Medicine* 65:163, 1986.
    A comprehensive well-referenced review.
27. Foley, R. J. Inhaled industrial acetylene: A diabetic ketoacidosis mimic. *J.A.M.A.* 254:1066, 1985.
    Something to add to the differential diagnosis.

16. HYPEROSMOLAR HYPERGLYCEMIC NONKETOTIC SYNDROME

H. Verdain Barnes

The hyperosmolar hyperglycemic nonketotic syndrome (HHNS) is a medical emergency that can occur at any age, although the median age is in the sixties. Only about 25 percent of the patients present in coma, although all progress to coma if left untreated. The initiating event is the development of hyperosmolarity as a result of hyperglycemia and/or hypernatremia. A variety of precipitating causes have been reported. The most common is untreated or uncontrolled type II diabetes mellitus. Less common causes or associations include high-dose corticosteroid therapy, intravenous diphenylhydantoin, immunosuppressive agents, thiazide diuretics, glycerol therapy for cerebral edema, propranolol, ethacrynic acid, mafenide burn ointment, diazoxide, gram-negative pneumonia, pancreatitis, acute pyelonephritis, hepatitis, acute myocardial infarction, subdural hematoma, arterial thrombosis, gastrointestinal tract hemorrhage, pemphigus, systemic lupus erythematosus, eczematoid dermatitis, status epilepticus, peritoneal dialysis with high glucose or sorbital dialysate, or uncontrolled insulin-dependent diabetes mellitus.

When initially seen, most patients have had polyuria and polydipsia for days to weeks and are therefore markedly dehydrated, with dry mucous membranes and doughy skin. The mentally alert patients usually complain of extreme thirst, weakness, and fatigue. Neurologic manifestations may dominate. The mental status may range from mild confusion to hallucinations to coma. Focal neurologic and motor function abnormalities may include hemisensory defects, hemiparesis, homonymous hemianopsia, coarse flapping of the upper extremities, unilateral or bilateral hyperreflexia, to areflexia, tremors, fasciculations, nuchal rigidity, and opisthotonus. About 15 percent of patients have seizures, of which the majority are focal. Orthostatic hypotension and tachycardia are common. Any patient who presents with marked dehydration with or without coma should have a quick estimation of blood or urine sugar to screen for the possibility of HHNS.

Hematologic and chemical laboratory values are in accordance with the hyperglycemia and dehydration. Glucose levels range from 600 to 2800 mg/dl, with the average being just over 1000. Urine usually shows 4-plus glucosuria and no ketones although an occasional patient has small to moderate amounts of ketones in the urine. The white blood cell count, hematocrit, and hemoglobin are usually elevated, reflecting dehydration. Serum urea nitrogen and proteins are elevated. The sodium is usually elevated, but it can be normal or low. Sodium when elevated is primarily a manifestation of dehydration; however, there is a tendency toward real sodium excess due to increased aldosterone levels and decreased glomerular filtration rate. Serum potassium values can be decreased or normal. The rise in glucocorticoids with stress probably contributes to the sodium and potassium abnormalities. The bicarbonate level is normal or only slightly decreased. The effective osmotic pressure across the cell is usually between 330 and 460 mOsm, and it can be estimated by the following formula:

Plasma osmolarity (mOsm/L)

$$= 2 \times \text{serum sodium (mEq/liter)} + \frac{\text{serum glucose (mg/dl)}}{18} + \frac{\text{BUN (mg/dl)}}{2.8}$$

The hyperglycemia in HHNS syndrome is related to an increased glucose load and a lack of appropriate amounts of insulin or peripheral insulin action. The increased glucose load appears to be primarily the result of stress-induced glycogenolysis. Some patients, however, also have a history of an increased intake of glucose. Insulin levels are routinely low but typically no different from those in patients who develop ketoacidosis. Why the patients with HHNS do not develop ketoacidosis is not easily explained. The most popular explanation hypothesizes that the amount of insulin present is sufficient to inhibit lipid mobilization and insulinize the liver, but insufficient to promote effective glucose transport into the cell. Several studies support that hypothesis, finding that many patients have comparatively low human growth hormone and free fatty acid levels; however, other workers have found the levels to be no different from those in patients with ketoacidosis. The question at the moment remains unresolved.

Therapy should be tailored to the findings of the individual patient. The average total body water deficit is about 24 percent. The fluid lost usually contains about 60 mEq/liter of sodium and potassium. To avoid cerebral edema, lower the glucose cautiously, keeping the blood level above 250 mg/dl, and reverse the hyperosmolarity slowly. To avoid hypoglycemia, if insulin is used start with small doses, since some of these patients are exquisitely sensitive to insulin, and glucose levels may drop precipitously. The patient should be carefully observed for the following complications: seizures, hypotension, cardiac arrhythmias, myocardial infarction, acute tubular necrosis, arterial or venous thrombosis, and lactic acidosis. The mortality continues to be 35 to 50 percent.

1. McCurdy, D. K. Hyperosmolar hyperglycemic nonketotic diabetic coma. *Med. Clin. North Am.* 54:683, 1970.
   A good review of the syndrome and its therapy. Hyperosmolarity is not an absolute criterion for diagnosis.
2. Gerich, J. E., Martin, M. M., and Recant, L. Clinical and metabolic characteristics of hyperosmolar nonketotic coma. *Diabetes* 20:228, 1971.
   The average duration of symptoms before therapy was 12 days. Average water deficit was 8.2 liters.
3. Brockman, W., Cordova, L. J., and Davis, P. J. Hyperglycemic nonketotic coma in insulin-dependent diabetes mellitus. *Johns Hopkins Med. J.* 127:119, 1970.
   Uncommon.
4. Seltzer, H. S., and Allen, E. W. Hyperglycemia and inhibition of insulin secretion during administration of diazoxide and trichlormethiazide in man. *Diabetes* 18:19, 1969.
5. Halmos, P. B. Hyperosmolar non-ketoacidotic diabetic coma in a patient with necrotizing pancreatitis. *Br. Med. J.* 2:685, 1966.
6. Goldberg, E. M., and Sanbar, S. S. Hyperglycemic, nonketotic coma following administration of Dilantin (diphenylhydantoin). *Diabetes* 18:101, 1969.
7. Spenney, J. G., Eure, C. A., and Kreisberg, R. A. Hyperglycemia, hyperosmolar, nonketoacidotic diabetes: A complication of steroid and immunosuppressive therapy. *Diabetes* 18:107, 1969.
8. Fernandez, J. P., McGinn, J. T., and Hoffman, R. S. Cerebral edema from blood-brain glucose: Differences in complicating peritoneal dialysis. *N.Y. State J. Med.* 68:677, 1968.
9. Monteleone, J. A., and Keefe, D. M. Transient hyperglycemia and aketotic hyperosmolar acidosis with heat stroke. *Pediatrics* 41:737, 1969.
10. Oakes, D. D., Schreibman, P. H., Hoffman, R. S., et al. Hyperglycemic nonketotic coma in the patient with burns. *Metabolism* 18:103, 1969.
11. Manzano, F., and Kozak, G. P. Acute quadriplegia in diabetic hyperosmotic coma with hypokalemia. *J.A.M.A.* 207:2278, 1969.

12. Sears, E. S. Nonketotic hyperosmolar hyperglycemia during glycerol therapy for cerebral edema. *Neurology* 26:89, 1976.
    Articles 4–12 document some circumstances associated with the syndrome.
13. Zierler, K. L., and Rabinowitz, D. Role of insulin and growth hormone based on forearm metabolism in man. *Medicine* 42:385, 1963.
    Only 10% of the insulin required for glucose transport is needed to inhibit lipolysis.
14. Arieff, A. I., and Carroll, H. J. Nonketotic hyperosmolar coma with hyperglycemia. *Medicine* 51:73, 1972.
    In this series, all patients with coma had a plasma osmolarity of 350 mOsm/kg, a blood glucose level above 600 mg/dl, and a less than 2 + Acetest at 1:1 dilution of plasma.
15. Keller, U., and Berger, W. Prevention of hypophosphatemia by phosphate infusion during treatment of diabetic ketoacidosis and hyperosmolar coma. *Diabetes* 29:87, 1980.
    The HHNS patients had normal 2,3-diphosphoglycerate levels; phosphorus falls with therapy; phosphorus replacement did not seem to change the patient's course.
16. Khardori, R., and Soler, N. G. *Hyperosmolar hyperglycemia nonketotic syndrome: Report of 22 cases and brief review. Am. J. Med.* 77:899, 1984.
    Hyperosmolality was not related to outcome.
17. West, M. L., Marsden, P. A., Singer, G. G., et al. Quantitative analysis of glucose loss during acute therapy for hyperglycemic hyperosmolar syndrome. *Diabetes Care* 9:465, 1986.
    Insulin is not needed in some patients. A good brief review of selective aspects of pathophysiology.

17. HYPERCALCEMIA

H. Verdain Barnes

Hypercalcemia can be an insidious or acute life-threatening manifestation of a variety of diseases. Its clinical features include anorexia, constipation, nausea, vomiting, polydipsia, polyuria, dry mouth, dry nose, dysesthesia, myalgia, bone pain, decreasing memory, apathy and—with very high levels of calcium—stupor, coma, and cardiac arrest. The renal effects include decreased glomerular filtration rate and concentrating ability, potassium wasting, and occasionally nephrolithiasis and/or nephrocalcinosis. When longstanding or severe, these changes can result in increased serum creatinine, urea nitrogen, and uric acid levels. In hypercalcemia the ECG typically shows a shortened Q–T interval that is inversely proportional to the level of serum calcium. The EEG may show slowing of the postcentral rhythm, lambda waves, high voltage, bilateral synchronous frontal delta activity, and excess theta activity. The ECG and EEG findings are not specific.

The diagnosis is made by determining the level of serum calcium. To interpret the value obtained, the level of serum protein must be known. About 0.8 mg of calcium is bound to 1.0 gm of serum albumin and globulin. Therefore, essentially 50 percent of the serum calcium is bound to protein. Some laboratories provide determinations of unbound or ionized calcium which can eliminate problems caused by the presence of protein abnormalities. In most settings, more than one calcium determination is needed to confirm the diagnosis. Spurious elevations in calcium can occur after prolonged venous stasis and/or exposure of the sample of cork stoppers. A false lowering can occur when serum or plasma is allowed to stand without separating the erythrocytes, which absorb calcium. Once the diagnosis of hypercalcemia has been established, determinations of serum phosphorus, chloride, bicarbonate, alkaline phosphatase, magnesium, and urinary calcium may be useful.

Diseases of diverse causes can have associated hypercalcemia. Adenomas or hyperplasia of the parathyroid gland(s) produce excess parathyroid hormone (PTH), resulting in hypercalcemic primary hyperparathyroidism (discussed on pp. 216–219).

Hypercalcemia is associated with a wide variety of clinical disorders ranging from malignancy to granulomatous diseases to the factitious. Malignancy-associated hypercalcemia, however, is by far the most common. Among the malignancies reported are carcinoma of the lung, kidney, bladder, uterus, vulva, ovary, liver, stomach, pancreas, colon, rectum, esophagus, penis, prostate, and parotid; leiomyoblastoma; rhabdomyosarcoma; Hodgkin's disease; B cell and T cell non-Hodgkin's lymphomas; reticulum cell sarcoma; Burkitt's lymphoma; multiple myeloma; acute myeloblastic leukemia; and chronic lymphocytic leukemia. In these patients the common mechanism in the development of hypercalcemia is increased bone reabsorption. There appears to be a heterogeneous group of factors responsible. The most obvious and probably most frequent is tumor growth in bone, either metastatic or primary, which produces local osteolysis. Next are a variety of humoral factors produced by the malignant process remote from bone such as parathyroid hormone–like peptides, 1,25-dihydroxyvitamin D_3, 1,24(R)-dihydroxyvitamin D_3–like bone-resorbing lipid, osteoclast-activating factor, some transforming growth factors, and prostaglandins E and A, which are known to stimulate bone reabsorption.

Hypercalcemia is also seen in association with a variety of nonmalignancy disorders such as the milk-alkali syndrome; neuroleptic malignant syndrome; sarcoidosis; tuberculosis; disseminated coccidioidomycosis, candidiasis, and histoplasmosis; chronic berylliosis; eosinophilic granuloma; immobilization with major fractures, Paget's disease, and the Landry-Guillain Barré syndrome; disseminated cytomegalovirus infection; silicone-induced granulomas; advanced chronic liver disease; plasma cell granuloma; pheochromocytoma; absorptive hypercalcemia; rhabdomyolysis; idiopathic hypercalcemia of infancy; bronchial carcinoid; hyperthyroidism; hypothyroidism; hypoadrenocorticism; diuretic phase of acute renal failure; and vitamin D intoxication. Here again the final common pathway is increased bone reabsorption. For most the factors responsible are not fully defined or unknown. However, for sarcoidosis, and perhaps other granulomas, the humoral mechanism appears to be the synthesis of 1,25-hydroxyvitamin D_3 by the alveolar macrophages in the sarcoid lung.

Clinically, it appears that high levels of fasting calcium excretion, normal or low immunoreactive PTH levels, low 1,25-dihydroxyvitamin D concentrations, and, in some, low urinary levels of nephrogenic cyclic AMP may help separate cancer-associated hypercalcemia from that of primary hyperparathyroidism.

Patients with familial hypocalciuric hypercalcemia can be differentiated from typical primary hyperparathyroidism by their lower levels of calcium excretion and higher levels of serum magnesium, which are directly proportional to the degree of hypercalcemia. Abnormal vitamin D metabolism is found in infants having idiopathic hypercalcemia with and without supravalvular aortic stenosis. Excess calcium intake from milk or calcium-containing antacids may result in calcium elevation. Paget's disease of bone rarely produces hypercalcemia and only in association with immobilization. A variety of other nonneoplastic associations have been reported, with the underlying pathophysiology undetermined or incompletely understood. These include thiazide therapy, postdiuretic phase of acute renal failure, postrenal transplant, sarcoidosis, and tuberculosis. Several endocrinopathies other than primary hyperparathyroidism may have associated hypercalcemia such as adrenocortical insufficiency, usually following adrenalectomy, (rarely) Addison's disease, hypothyroidism, and hyperthyroidism.

In primary hyperparathyroidism, the plasma chloride is usually increased and the phosphorus and bicarbonate decreased by the renal tubular effects of PTH. In hypercalcemia due to tumors, the plasma phosphorus and chloride levels are usually normal or low and the bicarbonate level is normal or increased. Plasma phosphorus is routinely elevated in vitamin D intoxication and occasionally in multiple myeloma, lymphoma, leukemia, and the idiopathic hypercalcemia of infancy, while plasma chlorides are decreased and bicarbonate increased. In all other types of hypercalcemia, the plasma phosphorus is variable but usually normal, whereas the chloride is decreased and the bicarbonate increased. These changes are due to the effects of excess calcium on the renal tubule. A nomogram for first-order discriminate function has been generated using the plasma phosphorus, chloride, alkaline phosphatase, bicarbonate, and urea nitrogen. Using this nomogram primary hyperparathyroidism was successfully separated from other causes of hypercalcemia about 90 percent of the time in a small series of patients. A serum chloride-phosphate ratio greater than 33 appears to be equally effective. Serum alkaline phosphatase is usually markedly elevated in Paget's disease of the bone and with immobilization following major fractures, whereas in other forms of hypercalcemia it is normal or modestly increased. Blood urea nitrogen is routinely increased in vitamin D intoxication, milk-alkali syndrome, multiple myeloma, and idiopathic hypercalcemia of infancy and occasionally increased in lymphoma, leukemia, and glucocorticoid insufficiency.

1. Howard, J. E., and Thomas, W. C., Jr. Clinical disorders of calcium homeostasis. *Medicine* 42:25, 1963.
   A superb general review of calcium homeostasis as understood in the 1960s.
2. Lafferty, F. W. Pseudohyperparathyroidism. *Medicine* 45:247, 1966.
   Rapid progression of hypercalcemia favors an underlying tumor. Plasma chloride is usually less than 102 mEq/liter.
3. Rawson, A. J., and Sunderman, F. W. Studies in serum electrolytes. XV. calcium-binding property of serum proteins. *J. Clin. Invest.* 27:82, 1948.
   Approximately 50% of calcium is bound to albumin and globulin.
4. Smith, F. E., Reinstein, H., and Braverman, L. E. Cork stoppers and hypercalcemia. *N. Engl. J. Med.* 272:787, 1965.
   Beware of venous stasis and cork stoppers, because they can produce false elevations in serum calcium.
5. Bronsky, D., Dubin, A., Kushner, D. S., et al. Calcium and electrocardiogram. *Am. J. Cardiol.* 7:840, 1961.
   Inverse relationship between the duration of the Q–T interval and the serum calcium level.
6. Robertson, R. P., Baylink, D. J., Marini, J. J., et al. Elevated prostaglandins and suppressed parathyroid hormone associated with hypercalcemia and renal cell carcinoma. *J. Clin. Endocrinol. Metabol.* 41:164, 1975.
7. Mundy, G. R., Raisz, L. G., Cooper, R. A., et al. Evidence for the secretion of an osteoclast stimulating factor in myeloma. *N. Engl. J. Med.* 291:1041, 1974.
8. Norrby, K., and Vikrot, O. Hypercalcemia in chronic lymphocytic leukemia. *Scand. J. Haematol.* 15:132, 1975.
9. Griboff, S. I. Hypercalcemia secondary to bone metastases from carcinoma of the breast. *J. Clin. Endocrinol. Metab.* 14:378, 1954.
10. Winters, J. L., Kleinschmidt, A. G., Jr., Frensilli, J. J., et al. Hypercalcemia complicating immobilization in the treatment of fractures: A case report. *J. Bone Joint Surg.* 48:1182, 1966.
11. Segal, A. J., Miller, M., and Moses, A. M. Hypercalcemia during the diuretic phase of acute renal failure. *Ann. Intern. Med.* 68:1066, 1968.
12. Schwartz, G. H., David, D. S., Riggio, R. R., et al. Hypercalcemia after renal transplantation. *Am. J. Med.* 49:42, 1970.
13. Garcia, R. E., Friedman, W. F., Kaback, M. M., et al. Idiopathic hypercalcemia and supravalvular aortic stenosis. *N. Engl. J. Med.* 271:117, 1964.
14. Stote, R. M., Smith, L. H., Wilson, D. M., et al. Hydrochlorothiazide effects on serum calcium and immunoreactive parathyroid hormone. *Ann. Intern. Med.* 77:587, 1972.
15. Meier, D. A., Arnstein, R. A., and Hamburger, J. I. Symptomatic thyrotoxic hypercalcemia. *Mich. Med.* 73:19, 1974.
16. Smith, R. E. Hand-mirror-cell variant of B-cell lymphoma with hypercalcemia. *Arch. Intern. Med.* 146:2273, 1986.
17. Maislos, M., Sobel, R., and Shany, S. Leiomyoblastoma associated with intractable hypercalcemia and elevated 1,25-dihydroxycholecalciferol levels. *Arch. Intern. Med.* 145:565, 1985.

18. Murray, J. J., and Heim, C. R. Hypercalcemia in disseminated histoplasmosis: Aggravated by vitamin D. *Am. J. Med.* 78:881, 1985.
19. Zaloga, G. P., Chernow, B., and Eil, C. Hypercalcemia and disseminated cytomegalovirus infection in the acquired immunodeficiency syndrome. *Ann. Intern. Med.* 102:331, 1985.
20. Wang, R. T., Aftergood, D. E., and Carlson, H. E. Hypercalcemia in the neuroleptic malignant syndrome. *Arch. Intern. Med.* 145:143, 1985.
21. Kapsner, P., Langsdorf, L., Marcus, R., et al. Milk-alkali syndrome in patients treated with calcium carbonate after cardiac transplantation. *Arch. Intern. Med.* 146:1965, 1986.
22. Dodd, R. C., Winkler, C. F., Williams, M. E., et al. Calcitriol levels in hypercalcemic patients with adult T-cell lymphoma. *Arch. Intern. Med.* 146:1971, 1986.
23. Helikson, M. A., Havey, A. D., Zerwekh, J. E., et al. Plasma-cell granuloma producing calcitriol and hypercalcemia. *Ann. Intern. Med.* 105:379, 1986.
24. Meythaler, J. M., Korkor, A. B., Nanda, T., et al. Immobilization hypercalcemia associated with Landry-Guillain-Barré syndrome. *Arch. Intern. Med.* 146:1567, 1986.
25. Frame, B., and Parfitt, A. M. Corticosteroid-responsive hypercalcemia with elevated serum 1-alpha, 25-dihydroxyvitamin D. *Ann. Intern. Med.* 93:449, 1980.
26. Gerhardt, A., Greenberg, A., Reilly, J. J., Jr., et al. Hypercalcemia: A complication of advanced chronic liver disease. *Arch. Intern. Med.* 147:274, 1987.
27. Akwal, M., Bishop, J. E., Telfer, N., et al. Hypocalcemia and hypercalcemia in patients with rhabdomyolysis with and without acute renal failure. *J. Clin. Endocrinol. Metab.* 63:137, 1986.
28. Jurney, T. H. Hypercalcemia in a patient with eosinophilic granuloma. *Am. J. Med.* 76:527, 1984.
29. Kozeny, G. A., Barbato, A. L., Bansal, V. K., et al. Hypercalcemia associated with silicone-induced granulomas. *N. Engl. J. Med.* 311:1103, 1984.
    Articles 6–29 illustrate the many disease associations with hypercalcemia and discuss the potential etiologic factors involved.
30. Palmer, F. J., Nelson, J. C., and Bacchus, H. Chloride-phosphate ratio in hypercalcemia. *Ann. Intern. Med.* 80:200, 1974.
    The ratio was greater than 33:1 in 96% of patients with primary hyperparathyroidism.
31. Frame, B., Jackson, G. M., Keerckoper, M. Acute severe hypercalcemia a la Münchausen. *Am. J. Med.* 70:316, 1981.
    No question Os-Cal 500 raises your serum calcium.
32. Skrabanek, P., McPartlin, J., and Powell, D. Tumor hypercalcemia and "ectopic hyperparathyroidism." *Medicine* 59:262, 1980.
    A well-done critical review that justly concludes that there is no clear demonstration that any tumor has produced ectopic PTH.
33. Mundy, G. R., Ibbotson, K. J., D'Souza, S. M., et al. The hypercalcemia of cancer: Clinical implications and pathogenic mechanisms. *N. Engl. J. Med.* 310:1718, 1984.
    A concise well-referenced review.
34. Shigeno, C., Yamamoto, I., Dokoh, S., et al. Identification of 1,24(R)-dihydroxyvitamin D3–like bone-resorbing lipid in a patient with cancer-associated hypercalcemia. *J. Clin. Endocrinol. Metab.* 61:761, 1985.
35. Adams, J. S., Singer F. R., Gacad, M. A., et al. Isolation and structural identification of 1,25-dihydroxyvitamin D_3 produced by cultured alveolar macrophages in sarcoidosis. *J. Clin. Endocrinol. Metab.* 60:960, 1985.
    Articles 34 and 35 detail recent advances in understanding the pathophysiologic factors that may be operative in selected patients with hypercalcemia.
36. Orwall, E. S. The milk-alkali syndrome: Current concepts. *Ann. Intern. Med.* 97:242, 1982.
    A concise review of this complex syndrome about which much is still unknown.
37. Mundy, G. R., Wilkinson, R., and Heath, D. A. Comparative study of available medical therapy for hypercalcemia of malignancy. *Am. J. Med.* 74:421, 1983.
38. Singer, F. R., and Fernandez, M. Therapy of hypercalcemia of malignancy. *Am. J. Med.* 82(suppl 2A):34, 1987.

Articles 37 and 38 bring you up-to-date on the therapy of malignancy-related hyper-calcemia.

39. Klee, G. G., Kao, P. C., and Heath H., III. Hypercalcemia. *Endocrinol. Metab. Clin. North Am.* 17:573, 1988.
Concise review with emphasis on diagnostic testing. No one test is diagnostic for etiology.

18. THYROID STORM
H. Verdain Barnes

Thyroid storm is a rare complication of hyperthyroidism. In the pre-iodine era, thyroid storm commonly occurred after subtotal thyroidectomy for thyrotoxicosis and accounted for about 70 percent of postoperative deaths. The incidence has declined dramatically due to preoperative preparation with iodine and/or a thioamide. Today, thyroid crisis arises most often with nonthyroidal stress in an untreated or partially treated hyperthyroid patient. On a rare occasion thyroid storm occurs after radioiodine therapy for thyrotoxicosis.

The underlying pathophysiology of thyroid storm is not clear. There is some support for the hypothesis that the primary event during thyroid surgery and after radioiodine therapy is the sudden release of stored thyroxine and triiodothyronine into the circulation. There is no direct evidence of such release when the stress is nonthyroidal. Consideration must also be given to the possibilities of a sudden change in thyroid hormone binding in serum, a sudden release of thyroid hormone from peripheral stores, and/or a sudden increase in circulating catecholamines.

The following stresses have been reported to precipitate thyroid crisis: infection, septicemia, trauma, nonthyroid surgery, severe fright, eclampsia, dehydration, pulmonary embolism, parturition, rapid iodine withdrawal, congestive heart failure, and diabetic ketoacidosis. The most common precipitating factor is infection although in a significant number of patients there may be no immediately obvious precipitating event. Thyroid storm occurs primarily in patients with toxic diffuse goiter (Graves' disease), but it can be seen in toxic nodular goiter.

Clinically the onset is usually abrupt, with the principal features being those of hypermetabolism and/or adrenergic excess. The cardiovascular, central nervous, and gastrointestinal systems are predominantly affected. A key to diagnosis is a temperature greater than 37.7°C (100°F) and a disproportionate increase in heart rate. Arrhythmias are common, and high output congestive heart failure may occur even in the absence of underlying heart disease. Central nervous system manifestations vary in severity. Tremor and agitation are the most common initial manifestations. Progression to overt psychosis or apathy, stupor, and coma may occur. Coma may dominate the clinical picture and be misleading in patients with apathetic hyperthyroidism. Gastrointestinal tract signs and symptoms are typically present. Diarrhea is classic, but it may be absent or less prominent than crampy abdominal pain and/or nausea and vomiting. Marked weight loss, dyspnea, palpitations, wide pulse pressure, and stare are often present. Muscle wasting, weakness, tender hepatomegaly, and jaundice may be prominent. The skin is usually fine, smooth, warm, flushed, and excessively moist. Since all of these signs and symptoms are accentuations of many of the features common to thyrotoxicosis, it should be recognized that without an alteration in mental function and temperature regulation a clinical diagnosis of thyroid storm cannot be made with certainty.

Thyroid function tests are useful to establish a diagnosis of hyperthyroidism, but do not confirm or rule out the diagnosis of thyroid storm. In storm, serum total and free thyroxine and triiodothyronine are typically, but not invariably, elevated, but are not distinctly different from those levels seen in patients without thyroid storm. The laboratory feature with the greatest potential for enhancing the probability of thyroid storm is a higher level of free thyroxine in comparison to the level of total thyroxine that is seen in nonstorm patients.

Hypocholesterolemia and hyperglycemia are common and hypercalcemia has been reported. Plasma cortisol is normal in uncomplicated hyperthyroidism since the increased production rate is offset by accelerated peripheral metabolism. Cortisol levels, however, have not been carefully monitored in thyroid storm.

Patients with uncontrolled thyrotoxicosis who develop a marked accentuation of their hypermetabolic state should be considered to have incipient thyroid storm and should be so treated. Therapy should include (1) diagnosis and treatment of the precipitating cause, (2) blockade of thyroid hormone production, (3) blockade of thyroid hormone release from the thyroid, (4) blockade of abnormal central nervous system thermoregulation; (5) when needed, blockade of excessive adrenergic system function; (6) supportive measures to ensure adequate blood pressure, plasma cortisol, and blood sugar levels, and (7) control of hyperthermia if present. The blockade of hormone production can be accomplished with a thioamide; propylthiouracil is preferred because of its rapid inhibition of peripheral deiodination of thyroxine to triiodothyronine. Blockade of hormone release from the thyroid is best accomplished with iodine, which blocks proteolysis by 70 to 80 percent. Adrenergic blockade can be accomplished with reserpine, guanethidine, or propranolol. Propranolol is the drug of choice unless it is contraindicated because of bronchospasm or complete heart block. Most authors agree that glucocorticoids should be given, because with the already increased production of cortisol there may be an inadequate reserve for the additional stress. Early therapy before the complete picture of thyroid storm has developed may be lifesaving.

1. Ingbar, S. H. Thyrotoxic storm. *N. Engl. J. Med.* 274:1252, 1966.
   A good general discussion.
2. Mazzaferri, E. L., and Skillman, T. G. Thyroid storm: A review of 22 episodes with special emphasis on the use of guanethidine. *Arch. Intern. Med.* 124:684, 1969.
   A careful review of 20 cases. No laboratory findings were diagnostic of thyroid storm.
3. Mackin, J. F., Canary, J. J., and Pittman, C. S. Thyroid storm and its management. *N. Engl. J. Med.* 291:1396, 1974.
   An excellent review of the subject, including the specifics of therapy.
4. Thomas, F. B., Mazzaferri, E. L., and Skillman, T. G. Apathetic thyrotoxicosis: A distinctive clinical and laboratory entity. *Ann. Intern. Med.* 72:679, 1970.
   Beware of thyroid storm in this setting.
5. Aach, R., and Kissane, J. Thyroid storm shortly after ^{131}I therapy of a toxic multinodular goiter. *Am. J. Med.* 52:786, 1972.
   Another precipitating circumstance.
6. Stoffe, S. S., Jiang, N. S., Gorman, C. A., et al. Plasma catecholamines in hypothyroidism and hyperthyroidism. *J. Clin. Endocrinol. Metabol.* 36:587, 1973.
   The mean plasma value is low in uncomplicated hyperthyroidism. Values are unknown in thyroid storm.
7. Levey, G. S. Catecholamine sensitivity, thyroid hormone, and the heart. *Am. J. Med.* 50:413, 1971.
   Thyroid hormone also has a direct inotropic and chronotropic effect on the heart.
8. Gallagher, T. F., Hellman, L., Finkelstein, J., et al. Hyperthyroidism and cortisol secretion in man. *J. Clin. Endocrinol. Metabol.* 34:919, 1972.
   Peripheral metabolism of cortisol is increased, with a resultant increase in production rate.
9. Ashkar, F. S., Katims, R. B., Smoak, W. M., III, et al. Thyroid storm treatment with blood exchange and plasmapheresis. *J.A.M.A.* 214:1275, 1970.
   A radical but apparently effective mode of therapy that merits consideration when other therapy fails.
10. Wartofsky, L. W., Ransil, B. J., and Ingbar, S. H. Inhibition by iodine of the release of thyroxine from the thyroid glands of patients with thyrotoxicosis. *J. Clin. Invest.* 49:78, 1970.
   A rapid decrease is seen, with the nadir in about 4 days.

11. Brooks, M. H., Waldstein, S. S., Bronsky, D., et al. Serum triiodothyronine concentration in thyroid storm. *J. Clin. Endocrinol. Metab.* 40:339, 1975.
    Total triiodothyronine levels are usually increased.
12. Oppenheimer, J. H., Schwartz, H. L., and Surks, M. L. Propylthiouracil inhibits conversion of L-thyroxine to L-triiodothyronine. *J. Clin. Invest.* 51:2493, 1972.
    In thyroid storm propylthiouracil appears to be the drug of choice since it blocks peripheral conversion.
13. Brooks, M. H., and Waldstein, S. S. Free thyroxine concentrations in thyroid storm. *Ann. Intern. Med.* 93:694, 1980.
    Those with storm consistently had a high free thyroxine.
14. Eriksson, M., Rubenfeld, S., Garber, A. J., et al. Propranolol does not prevent thryoid storm. *N. Engl. J. Med.* 296:263, 1977.
    Something to keep in mind.
15. Ahmad, N., and Cohen, M.P. Thyroid storm with normal triiodothyronine level during diabetic ketoacidosis. *J.A.M.A.* 245:2516, 1981.
    Worthy of note.
16. Nicoloff, J.T. Thyroid storm and myxedema coma. *Med. Clin. North Am.* 69:1005, 1985.
    An up-to-date review of the key pathophysiologic features of thyroid storm and the principles of therapy.

19. MYXEDEMA COMA

H. Verdain Barnes

Myxedema coma, a rare complication of untreated hypothyroidism, is a medical emergency. It can occur at any age and in either sex, but it is most common in women over age 50 years. The typical features of hypothyroidism are invariably present. The vast majority of patients who develop coma have a precipitating cause, most commonly infection. Pneumonia leads the list, followed by infections ranging from mastoiditis to pyelonephritis. Other precipitating factors include myocardial infarction, congestive heart failure, cold exposure, alcohol, and drugs. Hypothyroid patients are hypersensitive to sedatives, narcotics, and tranquilizers. This is due, at least in part, to diminished drug metabolism and clearance in myxedema.

Coma in myxedema can occur spontaneously without hypoventilation, but is almost invariably associated with depressed pulmonary ventilation. The respiratory rate can be less than four per minute. As carbon dioxide retention increases, varying degrees of respiratory acidosis supervene. Carbon dioxide narcosis is a predominant factor in at least one-third of patients. Coma as a result of hypoglycemia occurs most often in secondary hypothyroidism but can occur in primary disease. Hypothermia is common, except in the presence of infection, in which case the temperature may be normal or modestly elevated. About 15 percent of patients have temperatures of 29.4°C (85°F) or less. The development of hypothermia in myxedema is a warning sign of impending progressive central nervous system depression, stupor, and coma. Hyponatremia and hypochloremia are present in about 50 percent of patients. The potential causes are (1) a reduction in effective blood volume reaching the distal diluting segment of the nephron and a diminished ability to excrete water, (2) an inappropriate excess of antidiuretic hormone, and/or (3) glucocorticoid deficiency and some degree of associated hyperkalemia. These conditions may be seen alone or in combination. Hypotension is not uncommon and presents a particular problem since hypothyroid patients are relatively insensitive to vasopressor agents. In primary hypothyroidism, hypoadrenocorticism is rare, but in secondary hypothyroidism, it is not infrequent. Since the differentiation of primary and secondary hypothyroidism usually requires days, the therapeutic regimen for the patient should include the administration of glucocorticoids. Complications (in addition to those already noted) are gastrointestinal tract bleeding, megacolon, and psychosis.

The basics of therapy can be summarized in order of importance. First, a patent airway and ventilation must be maintained, a task that frequently requires intubation or tracheostomy and mechanical ventilation. Second, hypoglycemia must be corrected. Third, any treatable precipitating cause should be vigorously treated. Fourth, thyroxine or triiodothyronine should be administered. There is no general agreement as to the most effective route and dosage of thyroid hormone. Finally pharmacologic doses of glucocorticoids should be given. Several cautions should be noted: (1) Fluids and electrolytes must be administered slowly and monitored carefully to avoid cardiovascular overload; (2) simultaneous administration of thyroid hormone and vasopressors may result in serious arrhythmias; (3) effort should be made to prevent progressive hypothermia, but aggressive warming should be avoided since it inappropriately increases body metabolism and oxygen consumption; and (4) smaller doses than usual of cardiac glycosides are required to treat congestive heart failure in myxedema.

Mortality is 20 to 80 percent in most series, regardless of the therapeutic approach. Death is usually due to peripheral vascular collapse.

1. Royce, P. C. Severely impaired consciousness in myxedema: A review. *Am. J. Med. Sci.* 261:46, 1971.
   An excellent review.
2. Perlmutter, M., and Cohn, H. Myxedema crisis of pituitary or thyroid origin. *Am. J. Med.* 36:883, 1964.
   The distinction between primary and secondary hypothyroidism is not necessary in this setting.
3. Edwards, G. A. Myxedema crisis. *Med. Sci.* 16:56, 1965.
   Coma in myxedema can be spontaneous or secondary to carbon dioxide retention hypoglycemia or induced by sedatives or narcotics.
4. Forlster, C. F. Coma in myxedema: Report of a case and review of the world literature. *Arch. Intern. Med.* 111:734, 1963.
   50% of patients have low serum sodium and about 15% have a temperature less than 29.4°C (85°F).
5. Catz, B., and Russell, S. Myxedema, shock, and coma: Seven survival cases. *Arch. Intern. Med.* 108:129, 1961.
   Infection is the most common precipitating cause.
6. Derubertis, F. R., Jr., Michelis, M. F., and Bloom, M. E. Impaired water excretion in myxedema. *Am. J. Med.* 51:41, 1971.
   The inability to handle a water load is probably due to a decrease in the effective blood volume reaching the nephron.
7. Pettinger, W. A., Talner, L., and Ferris, T. F. Inappropriate secretion of antidiuretic hormone due to myxedema. *N. Engl. J. Med.* 272:362, 1965.
   Inappropriate antidiuretic hormone may also be a problem.
8. Brewster, W. R., Isaacs, J. P., Osgood, P., et al. The hemodynamic and metabolic interrelationships in the activity of epinephrine, norepinephrine, and the thyroid hormones. *Circulation* 13:1, 1956.
   Thyroid hormone and catecholamines are synergistic.
9. Means, J. H., Hertz, S., and Lerman, J. The pituitary type of myxedema. *Trans. Assoc. Am. Physicians* 55:32, 1940.
   Adrenal insufficiency may complicate the course of these patients.
10. Nickerson, J. F., Hill, S. R., Jr., McNeil, J. H., et al. Fatal myxedema with and without coma. *Ann. Intern. Med.* 53:475, 1960.
    Watch for hypoglycemia, particularly in secondary hypothyroidism.
11. Browning, T. B., Atkins, R. W., and Weiner, H. Cerebral metabolic disturbances in hypothyroidism. *Arch. Intern. Med.* 93:938, 1954.
    Diffuse EEG changes are seen in these patients, but they are not pathognomonic.
12. Zwillich, C. Z., Pierson, D. J., Hofeldt, F. D., et al. Ventilatory control in myxedema and hypothyroidism. *N. Engl. J. Med.* 292:662, 1975.
    Hypoxic ventilatory drive is significantly depressed in both.

13. Santos, A. D., Miller, R. P., Matthew, P. K., et al. Echocardiographic characterization of the reversible cardiomyopathy of hypothyroidism. *Am. J. Med.* 68:675, 1980.
    About 90% of their patients had assymetric septal hypertrophy, a consideration in therapy.
14. Valente, W. A., Goldiner, W. H., Hamilton, B. P., et al. Thyroid hormone levels after acute L-thyroxine loading in hypothyroidism. *J. Clin. Endocrinol. Metab.* 53:527, 1981.
    Beware—large doses of L-thyroxine contain enough contamination with L-triiodothyronine (T_3) to acutely raise circulating T_3 levels significantly.
15. Lizarralde, G., Baldwin, J. G., McCulley, H. G., Jr., et al. Myxedema coma and normal serum thyroxine. *South Med. J.* 71:860, 1978.
    An interesting and logical possibility, but their case is not airtight.
16. Nicoloff, J. T. Thyroid storm and myxedema coma. *Med. Clin. North Am.* 69:1005, 1985.
    An up-to-date review of selected pathophysiologic features and the principles of therapy.
17. Bastenie, P. A., Bonnyns, M., and Vanhaelst, L. Natural history of primary myxedema. *Am. J. Med.* 79:91, 1985.
    A concise well-referenced review of the clinical course of hypothyroidism.

20. SALICYLATE INTOXICATION: WITH A NOTE ON ACETAMINOPHEN
Jerry L. Spivak

The antipyretic, anti-inflammatory, and analgesic effects of acetylsalicylic acid (ASA) make it one of the most useful therapeutic agents and at the same time one of the most abused. Although the metabolism of ASA is well understood, its mechanism of action is not. The antipyretic and analgesic activities result from a direct effect of the drug on the central nervous system, whereas the anti-inflammatory activity appears to be mediated peripherally, by protein acetylation and inhibition of prostaglandin synthesis. ASA is an organic acid ester and is poorly soluble in water in the nonionized form. Because of its low pK, it exists largely in the nonionized form in gastric juice, and although that form is lipid-soluble, its low water solubility reduces the amount available for mucosal penetration. In contrast, buffered or effervescent ASA, although poorly lipid-soluble, is more effectively absorbed because of its greater solubility in gastric juice. It is for this reason that ASA is also absorbed in the small intestine. Once absorbed, ASA is deacetylated to salicylic acid, which binds to plasma proteins and is either hydroxylated, conjugated, or excreted unchanged. With increasing doses of ASA, the conjugation mechanism becomes saturated and the rate of elimination of the drug becomes independent of its plasma concentration. Consequently, in patients on maintenance therapy, small increments in dose can result in large increases in plasma salicylate level and sudden toxicity. In addition, small changes in urine pH can produce large changes in serum salicylate levels. ASA toxicity can be idiosyncratic as well as dose-related. Idiosyncratic toxicity results in skin rash, angioedema, rhinitis, polyposis, and asthma, usually in patients without a history of atopy.

Occult gastrointestinal bleeding is a side effect of ASA ingestion. With the dose of ASA used for mild analgesia the average daily blood loss is 5 ml. Major gastrointestinal hemorrhage is usually associated with regular and heavy ASA consumption. ASA-induced bleeding is the result of both local injury to the mucosa, producing increased permeability to hydrogen ions, and an effect on platelet function, resulting in defective platelet plug formation. Impaired synthesis of the vitamin K–dependent clotting factors requires a suicidal dose of ASA. At plasma levels that are therapeutic for rheumatic inflammation, ASA causes headache, tinnitus, hearing loss, nausea, and vomiting. The exact level for these toxic symptoms varies from patient to patient owing to differences in plasma protein concentration and renal function. In general, severe toxicity is usually seen with ingestion of ASA for suicidal purposes, but because of the mechanism of ASA biotransformation and excretion, patients on maintenance salicylate therapy are also at risk. The toxicity of ASA at high plasma concentrations is due to its effect on respiration and metabolic processes. ASA stimulates respiration, both by a direct effect on the respiratory center and also by increasing carbon dioxide production. Hyperventilation initially is inappropriate for the magnitude of carbon dioxide production, and respiratory alkalosis occurs, with an attendant loss of bicarbonate due to buffering by hemoglobin and body tissues. Renal compensation causes increased potassium excretion. Alkalosis is helpful since it maintains salicylic acid in its ionized form, preventing tissue uptake and enhancing urinary excretion. On the other hand, ASA increases oxygen consumption by uncoupling oxidative phosphorylation, while alkalosis increases the affinity of hemoglobin for oxygen. If toxic levels of salicylate persist, a metabolic acidosis develops. This is the result of accumulation of organic acids resulting from salicylate-induced inhibition of the tricarboxylic acid cycle and from ketone formation in the presence of reduced buffering capacity. In addition, high salicylate levels eventually result in depression of respiration, resulting in an increase in the PCO_2. The acid-base disturbance is further complicated by fluid loss resulting from both hyperventilation and sweating. The latter is due to increased heat production resulting from uncoupled oxidative phosphorylation in muscle. Increased heat production may outstrip heat loss, resulting in hyperthermia. Acidosis potentiates tissue uptake of salicylates, and patients with salicylate-induced acidosis are usually in coma. Recent experimental evidence indicates that salicylates lower brain glucose, and this phenomenon may be involved in the central nervous system disturbances seen in salicylate intoxication. The possibility that other drugs were ingested simultaneously must also be considered, particularly when significant respiratory acidosis is present.

The clinical presentation of the patient with severe salicylate toxicity is similar to that of the patient with diabetic ketoacidosis, including hyperglycemia, ketonuria, and a positive urine reaction with Benedict's reagent. The ferric chloride test or Phenistix can be used to determine the presence of salicylic acid in the urine. Hypouricemia is also a clue to salicylate ingestion.

In the patient with salicylate intoxication, prompt reduction of plasma salicylate levels is mandatory. Since salicylates cause pylorospasm and remain in the gut for prolonged periods, gastric lavage is a useful maneuver to prevent continued absorption of the drug. Activated charcoal is also useful in preventing ASA absorption. In the comatose patient or when renal function is impaired, hemodialysis is the method of choice since continued toxicity can result in sudden cardiovascular collapse. In the less urgent situation, peritoneal dialysis with 5% albumin, osmotic diuresis, or alkaline diuresis is satisfactory. Oxygen should be administered to all patients, and glucose as well if hyperglycemia is not present. Dehydration is usually hypertonic, and diuresis will not be initiated until volume depletion is corrected. Hypokalemia may be manifested by arrhythmias, areflexia, and muscle weakness; if hypokalemia is not corrected, attempting alkalinization is dangerous and ineffective. Hyperpyrexia must be reversed quickly; vitamin K_1 may be required to correct hypoprothrombinemia. Since ASA is a carbonic anhydrase inhibitor, acetazolamide (Diamox) should not be used to alkalinize the urine. Salicylate intoxication can result in neurogenic pulmonary edema; therefore, fluid therapy should be monitored carefully. Correction of salicylate-induced acidosis does not result in immediate compensatory changes in respiration. Consequently, overvigorous alkalinization can lead to severe alkalosis.

Recognition that ASA has a number of side effects has led to the increased use of acetaminophen (Paracetamol), a drug that is equipotent to aspirin with respect to antipyretic activity and analgesia. Acetaminophen also appears to have some anti-inflammatory activity although not in arthritic conditions. Acetaminophen is metabolized by the liver to a toxic arylating agent, a process that is stimulated by phenobarbital and probably ethanol. Conjugation with glutathione detoxifies the toxic metabolite. With excessive ingestion of acetaminophen, intracellular glutathione stores become depleted, and centrolobular hepatic necrosis, pancreatic, cardiac, and renal damage result. Hepatocellular damage by acetaminophen is predictable and can be produced by ingestion of 10 gm of the drug. Hepatic damage is signified by marked elevations in serum transaminase levels, an increase in alkaline phosphatase, and a prolonged prothrombin time.

The increase in serum bilirubin is not marked. Death usually ensues within 4 to 18 days in untreated patients. If recovery occurs, normal liver morphology is usually restored within 3 months. Acetaminophen is rapidly absorbed and little is left in the stomach after 60 minutes. Therefore gastric lavage or the use of activated charcoal must be prompt if they are to be effective. Hemodialysis removes at best only 10 percent of the drug and the most effective therapy is treatment with nucleophilic agents such as cysteine, cysteamine, methionine, and N-acetylcysteine. Therapy must be instituted within 8 hours to prevent tissue damage. Recent studies have indicated that intravenous administration of N-acetylcysteine is the most effective method of preventing tissue damage due to acetaminophen, but the compound must be administered within 8 hours of drug ingestion to be completely effective.

1. Cooper, S. A. Comparative analgesic efficacies of aspirin and acetaminophen. *Arch. Intern. Med.* 141:282, 1981.
   Part of an important symposium on aspirin and acetaminophen.
2. Levy, G., and Tsuchiya, T. Salicylate accumulation kinetics in man. *N. Engl. J. Med.* 287:430, 1972.
   Small increases in dose can result in large increases in body salicylate levels.
3. Miller, R. R., and Jick, H. Acute toxicity of aspirin in hospitalized medical patients. *Am. J. Med. Sci.* 274:271, 1977.
   Adverse reactions, most commonly gastrointestinal disturbances, occurred in 5% of patients, with females predominating.
4. Davison, C. Salicylate metabolism in man. *Ann. N.Y. Acad. Sci.* 179:249, 1971.
   Paradoxically, buffered aspirin is absorbed more rapidly and effectively than plain aspirin, and is excreted more rapidly in the urine.
5. Anderson, R. J., Potts, D. E., and Gabow, P. A. Unrecognized adult salicylate intoxication. *Ann. Intern. Med.* 85:745, 1976.
   Misdiagnosis due to failure to recognize the cardiopulmonary manifestations of salicylate toxicity.
6. Hill, J. B. Salicylate intoxication. *N. Engl. J. Med.* 288:1110, 1973.
   Death is presumably due to central nervous system dysfunction.
7. Heffner, J. E., and Sahn, S. A. Salicylate-induced pulmonary edema. *Ann. Intern. Med.* 95:405, 1981.
   Salicylate levels were greater than 40 mg/dl and proteinuria was present. (See also Am. J. Med. 66:1046, 1979.)
8. Robin, E. D., Davis, R. P., and Rees, S. B. Salicylate intoxication with special reference to the development of hypokalemia. *Am. J. Med.* 26:869, 1959.
   Salicylate-induced respiratory alkalosis results in hypokalemia.
9. Proudfoot, A. J., and Brown, S. S. Acidemia and salicylate poisoning in adults. *Br. Med. J.* 2:547, 1969.
   Acidosis promotes intracellular accumulation of salicylates.
10. Arbus, G. S., Herbert, L. A., Levesque, P. R., et al. Application of the "significance band" for acute respiratory alkalosis. *N. Engl. J. Med.* 280:117, 1969.
    An approach to the evaluation of complex acid-base disturbances.
11. Gabow, P. A., Anderson, R. J., Potts, D., et al. Acid-base disturbances in the salicylate-intoxicated adult. *Arch. Intern. Med.* 138:1481, 1978.
    Respiratory acidosis is often a consequence of ingestion of other drugs in addition to salicylates.
12. Arena, F. P., Dugowson, C., and Saudek, C. D. Salicylate-induced hypoglycemia and ketoacidosis in a nondiabetic adult. *Arch. Intern. Med.* 138:1153, 1978.
    An unusual complication of salicylate ingestion in an adult.
13. Myers, E. N., Bernstein, J. M., and Fostiropoulous, G. Salicylate ototoxicity. *N. Engl. J. Med.* 273:587, 1965.
    Reversible sensorineural hearing loss.
14. Zimmerman, H. J. Aspirin-induced hepatic injury. *Ann. Intern. Med.* 80:103, 1974.
    High blood levels of ASA are associated with hepatocellular damage.
15. Lawson, A. A. H., Proudfoot, A. J., Brown, S. S., et al. Forced diuresis in the treatment of acute salicylate poisoning in adults. *Q. J. Med.* 38:31, 1969.

Use of potassium supplements to prevent hypokalemia during bicarbonate adminis-tration.
16. Beveridge, G. W., Forshall, W., Munro, J. F., et al. Acute salicylate poisoning in adults. *Lancet* 1:1406, 1964.
Effectiveness of hemodialysis and alkaline diuresis compared.
17. Graham, D. Y., and Smith, J. L. Aspirin and the stomach. *Ann. Intern. Med.* 104:390, 1986.
Comprehensive review of a complex topic.
18. Roth, S. H., and Bennett, R. E. Nonsteroidal anti-inflammatory drug gastropathy. Recognition and response. *Arch. Intern. Med.* 147:2093, 1987.
Salicylates are not the only offenders.
19. O'Laughlin, J. C., Silvoso, G. R., and Ivey, K. J. Healing of aspirin-associated peptic ulcer diseases despite continued salicylate ingestion. *Arch. Intern. Med.* 141:781, 1981.
Evidence for the development of mucosal resistance.
20. Muther, R. S., Potter, D. M., and Bennett, W. M. Aspirin-induced depression of glomerular filtration rate in normal humans: Role of sodium balance. *Ann. Intern. Med.* 94:317, 1981.
Aspirin depresses glomerular filtration in the presence of salt depletion.
21. Weiss, H. J., Aledort, L. M., and Kochwa, S. The effect of salicylates on the hemostatic properties of platelets in man. *J. Clin. Invest.* 47:2169, 1968.
Aspirin irreversibly impairs platelet aggregation and prolongs the bleeding time.
22. Suarez, M., and Krieger, B. P. Bronchoalveolar lavage in recurrent aspirin-induced adult respiratory distress syndrome. *Chest* 90:452, 1986.
An unusual complication mediated by leukocytes.
23. Filippone, G. A., Fish, S. S., Lacouture, P. G., et al. Reversible adsorption (desorption) of aspirin from activated charcoal. *Arch. Intern. Med.* 147:1390, 1987.
Emesis may be preferable.
24. Berkowitz, J. M., Rogenes, P. R., Sharp, J. T., et al. Ranitidine protects against gastroduodenal mucosal damage associated with chronic aspirin therapy. *Arch. Intern. Med.* 147:2137, 1987.
Cimetidine and sucralfate are also protective. (See Am. J. Med. *84:35, 1988 and 83:83, 1987.)*
25. Szczeklik, A. Adverse reactions to aspirin and nonsteroidal anti-inflammatory drugs. *Ann. Allergy* 59:113, 1987.
A useful review.
26. Black, M. Acetaminophen hepatotoxicity. *Gastroenterology* 78:382, 1980.
Comprehensive review.
27. Ameer, B., and Greenblatt, D. J. Acetaminophen. *Ann. Intern. Med.* 87:202, 1977.
Slow onset of clinical manifestations of intoxication may delay initiation of therapy, which should be started within 8 hours after drug ingestion.
28. Seeff, L. B., Cuccherini, B. A., Zimmerman, H. J., et al. Acetaminophen hepatotoxicity in alcoholics. A therapeutic misadventure. *Ann. Intern. Med.* 104:399, 1986.
Ethanol potentiates the hepatic toxicity of acetaminophen. (See also Dig. Dis. Sci. *31:103, 1986 and* Ann. Intern. Med. *104:427, 1986.)*
29. Caldarola, V., Hassett, J. M., Hall, A. H., et al. Hemorrhagic pancreatitis associated with acetaminophen overdose. *Am. J. Gastroenterol.* 81:579, 1981.
An uncommon complication.
30. Prescott, L. F., Illingworth, R. N., Critchley, J. A. J. H., et al. Intravenous *N*-acetylcysteine: The treatment of choice for paracetamol poisoning. *Br. Med. J.* 2:1097, 1979.
N-acetylcysteine, if given within 8 hours after drug ingestion, blocks the toxic effects of acetominophen.
31. Levy, G., and Giacomini, K. M. Rational aspirin dosage regimens. *Clin. Pharmacol. Ther.* 23:247, 1978.
Good advice.
32. Gault, M. H., Rudwal, T. C., Engles, W. D., et al. Syndrome associated with the abuse of analgesics. *Ann. Intern. Med.* 68:906, 1968.

Anemia, renal papillary necrosis, peptic ulceration, headache, and underlying personality disorders associated with mixed analgesic abuse. (See also Ann. Intern. Med. 90:432, 1979.)

21. SEDATIVE INTOXICATION
Jerry L. Spivak

In this era of polypharmacy, barbiturates are among the drugs of choice for committing suicide. Although usually a single agent is involved, it is not uncommon for mixtures of different barbiturates or combinations of barbiturates and other intoxicants, such as meprobamate, glutethimide, and alcohol, to be ingested simultaneously. The central nervous system effects of all barbiturates are similar, the various analogues differing only in their speed of onset and duration of action. The latter properties are a function of the length of the alkyl side chains on the barbituric acid skeleton. Compounds with long alkyl side chains, such as secobarbital and pentobarbital, are lipid-soluble, have a rapid onset and short duration of action, and are metabolized by the liver, while a compound such as phenobarbital, with an aromatic substitution, has reduced lipid solubility, a longer duration of action, and is eliminated by the kidneys. The duration of action is an important determinant of the quantity of drug required for death to occur. In general, most deaths due to short-acting barbiturates occur with ingestion of 3 gm or more of the particular agent; prognostically a blood level of 3.5 mg/dl is considered potentially lethal. For phenobarbital, the corresponding values are 5 to 10 gm and 8 mg/dl. These values are not absolute and are affected by age, underlying disease, duration of intoxication before therapy, drug tolerance, and development of secondary complications, such as hypotension and aspiration.

Initial management of the patient with sedative intoxication is no different from that for any other comatose patient. Immediate attention must be given to maintenance of a patent airway, adequate oxygenation, and support of the circulation. Classification of the degree of central nervous system depression is helpful in determining the severity of intoxication and in following the clinical course. Nervous system depression occurs in a rostral-caudal pattern, and initially there are delirium, ataxia, and nystagmus followed by stupor and coma, with spasticity, decerebration, and flaccidity. The response to noxious stimuli is impaired before the loss of deep tendon reflexes, and the pupillary light reflex is preserved until the late stages of intoxication. Pupillary dilatation may, however, be a clue that the intoxication is due to glutethimide. Barbiturates depress respiration and venous tone, and hypercapnia and hypotension are not uncommon. Hypothermia can also occur but in this situation the possibility of hypoglycemia or ingestion of another agent such as an opiate, glutethimide, or ethchlorvynol should also be considered. Seizure activity may be the result of hypoglycemia, hypoxia, or simultaneous amphetamine abuse.

When the patient's vital functions are stable and a cuffed airway is in place, gastric aspiration and lavage should be performed. With the use of mass spectroscopy, rapid identification of ingested intoxicants can be performed on the gastric contents. Alternatively, the blood may be examined for the presence and concentration of drugs, but for the reasons listed above that procedure is of more value for diagnosis than prognosis. Gastric lavage is useful because of the tendency for sedative intoxication to produce ileus and retention of the offending agent, but care must be taken to avoid hypoxia and aspiration. Activated charcoal, given in repeated doses by nasogastric tube without a cathartic, has proved to be an effective agent in enhancing the elimination of a variety of drugs including barbiturates. Removal of barbiturates from the blood can also be accelerated by forced diuresis, peritoneal dialysis, or hemodialysis. Hemodialysis is the most effective method of removing all barbiturates; forced diuresis is equal to or more efficient than peritoneal dialysis. Barbiturates are weak organic acids, but only phenobarbital has a pK (7.2) low enough for therapy with alkali to promote excretion by increasing the ratio of ionized to nonionized drug. Hemodialysis is indicated in patients with impaired hepatic, renal, or cardiovascular function; underlying disease; coma; secondary complications such as infection or aspiration; or known ingestion of a fatal quantity of drug. Otherwise, aggressive diuretic and fluid therapy suffices to promote excretion of both long- and short-acting barbiturates. It should be recognized, however, that hypovolemia must be corrected before any diuresis can occur. If hypovolemia is corrected, the use of osmotic agents such as mannitol is not usually necessary. The role of resin hemoperfusion is unestablished but is unlikely to be important in the treatment of sedative-hypnotic intoxications.

Attention to avoiding the complications ensuing from the comatose state is probably the most important aspect of the therapy of sedative intoxication. Positioning the patient on the side with the head slightly dependent, turning frequently, and using a cuffed endotracheal airway should prevent aspiration. Hyperventilation and overly vigorous alkali therapy must be avoided since alkalosis impairs tissue oxygen delivery and results in hypokalemia. Sudden cessation of mechanical ventilation in an alkalotic patient may result in apnea. The importance of meticulous supportive care is accentuated by the fact that a lethal dose of barbiturate is much greater than that required to depress respiration or cause hypotension. The management of these patients does not end when they awake since elimination of the systemic toxin is not correlated with either elimination of the desire to attempt suicide or protection from an abstinence reaction. Careful observation is required during the rehabilitation period.

1. Goldberg, M. J., Spector, R., Park, G. D., et al. An approach to the management of the poisoned patient. *Arch. Intern. Med.* 146:1381, 1986.
   A comprehensive review (See also Med. Clin. North Am. *67:1279, 1983.)*
2. Brett, A. S., Rothschild, N., Gray, R., et al. Predicting the clinical course in intentional drug overdose. Implications for use of the intensive care unit. *Arch. Intern. Med.* 147:133, 1987.
   High-risk and low-risk patients.
3. Khantzian, E. J., and McKenna, G. J. Acute toxic and withdrawal reactions associated with drug use and abuse. *Ann. Intern. Med.* 90:361, 1979.
   Comprehensive review of both overdose and abstinence reactions.
4. Arena, J. Poisoning: General treatment and prevention. *J.A.M.A.* 232:1272, 233:358, 900, 1975.
   An extensive review, with many useful tables.
5. Sabin, T. D. The differential diagnosis of coma. *N. Engl. J. Med.* 290:1062, 1974.
   A brief review. (See also Med. Clin. North Am. *65:15, 1981.)*
6. Jay, S. J., Johanson, W. G., Jr., and Pierce, A. K. Respiratory complications of overdose with sedative drugs. *Am. Rev. Respir. Dis.* 112:591, 1975.
   Hypotension and aspiration carry a poor prognosis.
7. Ross, J. F., Hewitt, W. L., Wahl, G. W., et al. The management of the presuicidal, suicidal and postsuicidal patient. *Ann. Intern. Med.* 75:441, 1971.
   Discussion of the psychopathology of the suicidal patient.
8. Mandy, S., and Ackerman, A. B. Characteristic traumatic skin lesions in drug-induced coma. *J.A.M.A.* 213:253, 1970.
   Erythematous and bullous skin lesions at sites of trauma and pressure.
9. Bird, T. D., and Plum, F. Recovery from barbiturate overdose coma with a prolonged isoelectric electroencephalogram. *Neurology* 18:456, 1968.
   In the presence of barbiturate intoxication, an isoelectric EEG cannot be considered a sign of cerebral death.
10. Linton, A. L., and Ledingham, I. M. Severe hypothermia with barbiturate intoxication. *Lancet* 1:24, 1966.
    Drug intoxication should always be considered in the differential diagnosis of hypothermia.
11. Henderson, L. W., and Merrill, J. P. Treatment of barbiturate intoxication. *Ann. Intern. Med.* 64:876, 1966.
    Critical review advocating conservative therapy.
12. Park, G. D., Spector, R., Goldberg, M. J., et al. Expanded role of charcoal therapy in the poisoned and overdosed patients. *Arch. Intern. Med.* 146:969, 1986.

13. Shubin, H., and Weil, M. The mechanism of shock following suicidal doses of barbiturates, narcotics and tranquilizer drugs with observations on the effects of treatment. *Am. J. Med.* 38:853, 1965.
Hypotension is best treated with volume expansion, not vasopressors.
14. Morgan, A. G., Bennett, J. M., and Polak, A. Mannitol retention during diuretic treatment of barbiturate and salicylate overdosage. *Q. J. Med.* 37:589, 1968.
Mannitol retention is usual and may result in cell dehydration and pulmonary edema.
15. McCarron, M. M., Schulze, B. W., Walberg, C. B., et al. Short-acting barbiturate overdosage. Correlation of intoxication score with serum barbiturate concentration. *J.A.M.A.* 248:55, 1982.
A technique for correlating clinical status with the blood barbiturate level.
16. Linton, A. C., Luke, R. G., and Briggs, J. D. Methods of forced diuresis and its application in barbiturate poisoning. *Lancet* 2:377, 1967.
Forced diuresis without osmotic agents is effective in drug removal.
17. Bloomer, H. A. A critical evaluation of diuresis in the treatment of barbiturate intoxication. *J. Lab. Clin. Med.* 67:989, 1966.
Alkalinization does not promote the excretion of short-acting barbiturates.
18. Setter, J. G., Maher, J. F., and Schreiner, G. E. Barbiturate intoxication. *Arch. Intern. Med.* 117:224, 1966.
Hemodialysis found to be effective for both long- and short-acting barbiturates.
19. Berman, L. B., and Vogelsang, P. Removal rates for barbiturates using two types of peritoneal dialysis. *N. Engl. J. Med.* 270:77, 1964.
Use of albumin to improve efficiency of dialysis.
20. Barley, D. N., and Jaslow, P. I. Barbital overdose and abuse. *Am. J. Clin. Pathol.* 64:291, 1975.
A serum barbiturate level greater than 20 mg/dl in a living patient suggests barbital abuse.
21. Maher, J. F., Schreiner, G. E., and Westervelt, F. B. Acute glutethimide intoxication. *Am. J. Med.* 33:70, 1962.
The clinical features are reviewed. (See J. Toxicology 23:557, 1985 for a review of combined glutethimide-codeine intoxication.)
22. Chazan, J. A., and Cohen, J. J. Glutethimide intoxication. *Arch. Intern. Med.* 128:215, 1971.
Hemodialysis was not found to improve survival.
23. Hansen, A. R., Kennedy, K. A., and Ambre, J. J. Glutethimide poisoning. *N. Engl. J. Med.* 292:250, 1975.
Severity of intoxication may not be due to the drug itself but rather to accumulation of a metabolite.
24. Bowyer, K., and Glasser, S. P. Chloral hydrate overdose and cardiac arrhythmias. *Chest* 77:232, 1980.
Propranolol was effective in correcting ventricular arrhythmias associated with chloral hydrate intoxication.
25. Teehan, B. P., Maher, J. F., Carey, J. J. H., et al. Acute ethchlorvynol (Placidyl) intoxication. *Ann. Intern. Med.* 72:875, 1970.
Prolonged coma, respiratory depression and hypothermia; hemodialysis is effective in removing the drug.
26. Lorch, J. A., and Garella, S. Hemoperfusion to treat intoxications. *Ann. Intern. Med.* 91:301, 1979.
Hemoperfusion is not effective for many drugs and has not been proved to be more effective than conventional therapy for sedative-hypnotic intoxication. (See also Clin. Pharmacol. Ther. 27:236, 1980.)
27. Vale, J. A., Meredith, T. J., and Proudfoot, A. T. Syrup of ipecacuanha: Is it really useful? *Br. Med. J.* 22:293, 1986.
A vote against ipecac.
28. Levy, G. Gastrointestinal clearance of drugs with activated charcoal. *N. Engl. J. Med.* 307:676, 1982.
Brief review. (See also Lancet 1:1013, 1987 and Q. J. Med. 235:997, 1986.)

22. HEAT STROKE
Jerry L. Spivak

Body temperature is maintained within a narrow range by the hypothalamic regulatory centers responsible for heat conservation and dissipation. Dissipation of heat occurs by radiation, convection, and conduction from the surface of the body, by evaporation from the skin and the lungs, by warming of inspired air, and by excretion of urine and feces. The efficiency of radiation and convection depends on an adequate circulatory system and a gradient between body and ambient temperature. When the ambient temperature reaches 95°F (35°C), these mechanisms become inefficient and evaporation becomes the major pathway for heat exchange. The effectiveness of evaporation, however, varies inversely with the degree of ambient humidity. Tolerance to heat can be increased by the process of acclimatization. With acclimatization the rate of sweating is increased, sodium excretion in sweat and urine is decreased, and blood volume and cardiac output are increased. The degree of acclimatization is proportional to the imposed heat stress. Age conditions the degree to which heat adaptation can take place. Older individuals have reduced sweat gland activity and generally have an inadequate circulatory response to an imposed heat load. Heat toxicity results when homeostatic mechanisms are inadequate to compensate for the heat load, a problem that can occur in acclimatized as well as unacclimatized persons.

Disorders resulting from heat exposure include heat cramps due to salt depletion, heat exhaustion due to either salt or volume depletion, and heat stroke. In heat exhaustion due to salt depletion, hyperpyrexia generally does not occur, while in the heat stroke syndrome temperatures of 106°F (41°C) are usually seen. Heat exhaustion due to salt depletion usually does not lead to heat stroke since it prevents the degree of muscular activity that would cause hyperpyrexia. In heat stroke, heat dissipation mechanisms are overwhelmed but heat production continues unabated resulting in widespread tissue damage and often death. Factors predisposing to heat stroke include an elevated ambient temperature and humidity; lack of acclimatization; obesity; old age; strenuous exercise; dehydration; fever; cardiovascular or central nervous system disease (hypothalamic disease, autonomic neuropathy); delirium tremens; diabetes mellitus; skin disease (miliaria, scleroderma); alcohol ingestion; phenothiazine, diuretic, anticholinergic, or antihistamine therapy; amphetamine abuse; anesthesia (malignant hyperthermia); concomitant therapy with narcotics or tricyclic antidepressants and a monoamine oxidase inhibitor; and neuroleptic drugs (the neuroleptic malignant syndrome).

Clinically two settings for heat stroke are common. In younger individuals, the setting is one of strenuous exercise in a warm and humid environment. The onset of symptoms is sudden with confusion, weakness, or collapse. Sweating is usually observed. Initially, the temperature may only be mildly elevated but it continues to rise. In older individuals heat stroke usually occurs after a prolonged period of unusually hot weather. The victims usually live in poorly ventilated dwellings and on the higher floors, are often overclothed, frequently have impaired mobility, occasionally have deficient thirst mechanisms, and may be taking diuretics, tranquilizers, or abusing ethanol. Prodromal symptoms of anorexia, nausea, vomiting, and weakness may be present for several days before collapse. Anhidrosis is common in this group, but its role in the pathogenesis of the heat stroke is unknown. Decreased sweating can occur with hypothalamic lesions but in epidemic heat stroke hypothalamic damage is likely to be the result of the hyperthermia rather than the cause of it.

When first seen, patients with heat stroke may be either irrational or comatose. Seizures are not uncommon and hypotension may be present. Hypokalemia is not infrequent in patients with exertional heat stroke and hypocalcemia and hypophosphatemia are frequently found. Metabolic acidosis, alone or in combination with a respiratory alkalosis, is the most common acid-base disturbance. Serum aminotransferase and creatine kinase (CK) levels are usually elevated reflecting liver and muscle injury; urinalysis may reveal myoglobin. ECG abnormalities are generally limited to nonspecific

ST–T wave changes and prolongation of the Q–T interval. Coagulation studies may reveal abnormalities compatible with intravascular coagulation.

The diagnosis of heat stroke is usually evident but the physician must consider the possibility that the hyperpyrexia is due to meningitis, intracranial hemorrhage, typhoid fever, Rocky Mountain spotted fever, adrenal insufficiency, thyroid storm, delirium tremens, malaria, pyogenic infections, or drug abuse. As the rectal temperature rises above 105°F (40.5°C) with failure of heat-dissipating mechanisms, the body becomes poikilothermic. Temperatures above 107°F (41.6°C) are usually incompatible with life; lower temperatures can be fatal in the presence of an underlying disease.

The principal objective in treating the patient with heat stroke is reduction of the body temperature and the attendant increased oxygen requirements by rapid (within 1 hour) lowering of the rectal temperature to 102°F (38.8°C). Since the rectal temperature lags behind the core temperature, the latter will be even lower. Vigorous cooling is mandatory if the body temperature is above 106°F (41°C). Hypotension may respond to cooling alone but many patients require substantial volume replacement, particularly elderly individuals who have had prolonged heat exposure. The use of chlorpromazine to prevent shivering and vasoconstriction is not recommended. Steroids are also not helpful, and aspirin should be avoided. Seizures, azotemia, hyperkalemia, temperatures greater than 106°F (41.1°C), and evidence of severe tissue damage (such as prolonged coma or renal failure) are poor prognostic signs. Acute renal failure is an indication for early dialysis. After initial cooling, the body temperature will continue to fall but it may rise again and it is usually labile for several days. If anhidrosis is present, the return of sweating may be delayed.

1. Knochel, J. P. Environmental head injury. *Arch. Intern. Med.* 133:841, 1974.
   A comprehensive review. (See also Adv. Intern. Med. *28:115, 1983.)*
2. Hart, G. R., Anderson, R. J., and Crumpler, C. P. Epidemic classical heat stroke: Clinical characteristics and course of 28 patients. *Medicine* 61:188, 1982.
   Exertional and epidemic heat stroke compared.
3. Clowes, G. H. A., Jr., and O'Donnell, T. F., Jr. Heat stroke. *N. Engl. J. Med.* 291:564, 1974.
   Pathophysiology and management reviewed.
4. O'Donnell, T. F., and Clowes, G. H. A. The circulatory abnormalities of heat stroke. *N. Engl. J. Med.* 287:734, 1972.
   Hyperdynamic circulatory pattern with elevated pulmonary vascular resistance.
5. Sprung, C. L. Hemodynamic alterations of heatstroke in the elderly. *Chest* 75:362, 1979.
   Elderly individuals generally develop an inadequate circulatory response to heat stress.
6. Costrini, A. M., Pitt, H. A., Gustafson, A. B., et al. Cardiovascular and metabolic manifestations of heatstroke and severe heat exhaustion. *Am. J. Med.* 66:296, 1979.
   Myocardial damage was rare: dehydration was common.
7. Levine, J. A. Heat stroke in the aged. *Am. J. Med.* 47:251, 1969.
   A high-risk group of persons in whom heat stroke often presents with anhidrosis and infection.
8. Schrier, R. W., Hano, J., and Keller, H. I. Renal, metabolic and circulatory responses to heat and exercise. *Ann. Intern. Med.* 73:213, 1970.
   An integrated hypothesis for heat- or exercise-induced renal failure.
9. Schrier, R. W., Henderson, H. S., Fisher, C. C., et al. Nephropathy associated with heat stress and exercise. *Ann. Intern. Med.* 67:356, 1967.
   The functional abnormalities are more striking than the histologic abnormalities.
10. Knochel, J. P., and Caskey, J. H. The mechanism of hypophosphatemia in acute heat stroke. *J.A.M.A.* 238:425, 1977.
    Hypophosphatemia occurs as a consequence of respiratory alkalosis.
11. Knochel, J. P., and Vertel, R. M. Salt loading as a possible factor in the production of potassium depletion, rhabdomyolysis and heat injury. *Lancet* 1:659, 1967.
    Possible association between potassium loss and muscle injury in heat stroke.

12. Knochel, J. P., Dotin, L. N., and Hamburger, R. J. Heat stress, exercise, and muscle injury: Effects on urate metabolism and renal function. *Ann. Intern. Med.* 81:321, 1974.
    Hyperuricemia associated with muscle injury.
13. Sprung, C. L., Portocarrero, C. J., Fernaine, A. V., et al. The metabolic and respiratory alterations of heat stroke. *Arch. Intern. Med.* 140:665, 1980.
    Metabolic acidosis or a mixed metabolic acidosis and a respiratory acidosis are the most common acid-base disturbances.
14. Bradley, A. F., Stupfel, M., and Severinghaus, J. W. Effect of temperature on PCO_2 and PO_2 of blood in vitro. *J. Appl. Physiol.* 9:201, 1956.
    A 1°C rise in temperature elevates PO_2 by 6% and the PCO_2 by 4.4%.
15. Vertel, R. M., and Knochel, J. P. Acute renal failure due to heat injury. *Am. J. Med.* 43:435, 1967.
    A complication of heat stroke frequently associated with myoglobinuria.
16. Nolph, K. D., Whitcomb, M. E., and Schrier, R. W. Mechanisms for inefficient peritoneal dialysis in acute renal failure associated with heat stress and exercise. *Ann. Intern. Med.* 71:317, 1969.
    Increased catabolism and defective peritoneal permeability may necessitate the use of hemodialysis.
17. Kew, M., Bersohn, I., Seftel, H., et al. Liver damage in heatstroke. *Am. J. Med.* 49:192, 1970.
    Abnormal liver function tests are common; severe damage is unusual.
18. Weber, M. D., and Blakely, J. A. The hemorrhagic diathesis of heatstroke. *Lancet* 1:1190, 1969.
    Defibrinogenation is presumably due to intravascular coagulation.
19. Yaqub, B. A. Neurologic manifestations of heatstroke at the Mecca pilgrimage. *Neurology* 37:1004, 1987.
    Neurologic dysfunction can be global. (See also Neurology 20:336, 1970.)
20. Knochel, J. P. Dog days and siriasis. *J.A.M.A.* 233:513, 1975.
    Seven ways to kill a football player.
21. Leithead, C. S., Leithead, L. A., and Lee, F. D. Salt-deficiency heat exhaustion. *Ann. Trop. Med. Parasitol.* 52:456, 1958.
    Hyperpyrexia does not usually occur in this syndrome.
22. Shapiro, Y., Magazanik, A., Udassin, R., et al. Heat intolerance in former heatstroke patients. *Ann. Intern. Med.* 90:913, 1979.
    Persistent defect in thermoregulation with impaired heat loss.
23. Willner, J. H., Wood, D. S., Cerri, C., et al. Increased myophosphorylase A in malignant hyperthermia. *N. Engl. J. Med.* 303:138, 1980.
    Muscle phosphorylase A levels suggested as a diagnostic test for malignant hyperthermia.
24. Ginsberg, M. D., Hertzman, M., and Schmidt-Nowara, W. W. Amphetamine intoxication with coagulopathy, hyperthermia and reversible renal failure. *Ann. Intern. Med.* 73:81, 1970.
    Hyperpyrexia is a common feature of amphetamine poisoning.
25. Wyndham, C. H. Heatstroke and hyperthermia in marathon runners. *Ann. N.Y. Acad. Sci.* 301:128, 1977.
    A hazard of exertion that is magnified by heat and humidity. (See also Ann N.Y. Acad. Sci. 301:262, 1977.)
26. Shkolnik, A., Taylor, C. R., Finch, V., et al. Why do Bedouins wear black robes in hot deserts? *Nature* 283:373, 1980.
    Black robes are no warmer than white ones.
27. Bernheim, H. A., Block, L. H., and Atkins, E. Fever: Pathogenesis, pathophysiology, and purpose. *Ann. Intern. Med.* 91:261, 1979.
    Comprehensive review.
28. Rodbard, D. The role of regional body temperature in the pathogenesis of disease. *N. Engl. J. Med.* 305:808, 1981.
    Interesting observations.
29. Graham, B. S., Lichtenstein, M. J., Hinson, J. M., et al. Nonexertional heatstroke.

Physiologic management and cooling in 14 patients. *Arch. Intern. Med.* 146:87, 1986. *A simple, effective technique.*

30. Guze, B. H., and Baxter, C. R., Jr. Current concepts: neuroleptic malignant syndrome. *N. Engl. J. Med.* 313:163, 1985.
    Excellent, concise review. (See also Arch. Intern. Med. *142:601, 1982 and 145:143, 1985 and* Lancet *1:545, 1984.)*
31. Kilbourne, E. M., Choi, K., Jones, S., et al. Risk factors for heatstroke. *J.A.M.A.* 247:3332, 1982.
    Alcoholism, tranquilizers, anticholinergics, and living on an upper floor.

23. HYPOTHERMIA
Jerry L. Spivak

Hypothermia is defined as a temperature of 96°F (35.5°C) or less. Conditions causing hypothermia include hypoglycemia; myxedema; hypopituitarism; adrenal insufficiency; uremia; starvation; cerebrovascular accidents; diabetic ketoacidosis; drug intoxication (sedatives, ethanol, opiates, phenothiazines); bacterial sepsis; Wernicke's encephalopathy; hypothalamic lesions; exfoliative dermatitis; and intentional, iatrogenic (cold blood, cold operating suites, gastric lavage, hypothermia blankets, peritoneal dialysis, and antipyretics), or accidental exposure to cold. Accidental exposure occurs most often in alcoholic or senile individuals who are unable to protect themselves from their environment.

The normal physiologic responses to cold exposure are vasoconstriction, tachycardia, shivering, and diuresis. As the body cools, a predictable sequence of events occurs. When the temperature falls below 90°F (32.2°C), shivering ceases, muscular rigidity ensues, and judgment and consciousness become impaired. Further cooling produces bradycardia and ECG changes that include prolongation of the P–R, QRS, and Q–T intervals and the development of an abnormal terminal deflection of the QRS complex known as the J wave. Although considered diagnostic for hypothermia, J waves have been observed in normal individuals and in normothermic patients with subarachnoid hemorrhage or other central nervous system problems or with myocardial ischemia. Cooling also causes a reduction in blood pressure and respiratory activity. Below 85°F (29.5°C) atrial fibrillation occurs. Continued cooling results in a loss of atrial activity and the appearance of idioventricular rhythms and ventricular fibrillation. Metabolic activity decreases in direct proportion to the temperature depression. Renal blood flow and glomerular filtration are reduced but since renal tubular function is also depressed, urine production continues until 81°F (27°C). Below 79°F (26°C) ventricular fibrillation can occur spontaneously. Hypothermia causes a shift in intravascular fluid resulting in hypovolemia and hemoconcentration. Reversible thrombocytopenia has also been described. Metabolic acidosis is usually present and arterial PO_2 and PCO_2 measurements will be spuriously high unless corrected for the current body temperature. The median lethal temperature (LT_{50}) for man as determined in contravention of the Geneva Convention is 81°F (27°C).

Hypothermia, particularly in the elderly, has a high mortality. Its complications include infection, frostbite, gastrointestinal tract hemorrhage, pancreatitis, vascular accidents, and cardiac arrest. It is noteworthy that standard clinical thermometers are usually calibrated only as low as 95°F (35°C). Consequently not only may the diagnosis of hypothermia initially be overlooked but its severity initially underestimated. Biochemical abnormalities associated with hypothermia include elevations in serum transaminase levels and hyperglycemia. Hypothermia also increases the affinity of hemoglobin for oxygen and because most biochemical reactions undergo a twofold reduction for every 10°C (18°F) decrease in temperature, production of 2,3-diphosphoglycerate, which would tend to correct the shift in hemoglobin-oxygen affinity, is prevented.

When treating a hypothermic patient, the initial objectives are to stop further heat loss and initiate rewarming. The method for rewarming and the rate of rewarming depend on the clinical situation. A patient who has not lost heat production mechanisms such as shivering can be rewarmed passively without danger. On the other hand, elderly patients or those who suffer from physical exhaustion, such as immersion victims or hikers, should be rewarmed actively. This approach should be employed regardless of the possibility of an underlying disease such as hypothyroidism. The most important fact to consider in the treatment of a hypothermic patient is that the heart is the target organ. A patient whose temperture is 86°F (30°C) or less is in danger of spontaneous ventricular fibrillation. Furthermore, when such patients develop ventricular fibrillation, the arrhythmia is refractory to therapy until the body temperature is elevated. In addition, in such patients simple manipulation such as intratracheal intubation can trigger ventricular fibrillation. Consequently, manipulation should be kept to a minimum until the patient's body temperature has reached a safe level. Thus, active rewarming is mandatory since not only is the patient at risk of a fatal cardiac arrest, but the means for treating the patient are restricted as long as the temperature remains low. Once, however, the temperature is above the critical level for spontaneous ventricular arrhythmias, rewarming can proceed at a slower pace.

There is substantial controversy in the literature over the method that should be used for rewarming. The need for rapid rewarming under certain situations has been discussed above. The best method for this has not been established. Advocates can be found for core rewarming and external rewarming. Since the clinical status of the patients described and the causes of hypothermia vary in different published series, it is difficult to make valid comparisons of the different methods employed. Many published articles contain caveats concerning possible adverse effects on blood pressure produced by peripheral vasodilation and by the shunting of cold blood to the core when external rewarming is employed. Published data to substantiate these hypothetical effects are almost nonexistent. To the contrary, however, the large body of data derived from the sordid and sadistic experiments at Dachau provide ample evidence that rapid external rewarming is superior to all other forms of resuscitation for hypothermia. Thus, while there is theoretically much to be said for core rewarming techniques, rapid external rewarming by immersing the patient in a bath of hot water is probably just as effective and removes the hazards of invasive manipulation as well as any attendant delays to set up such procedures as peritoneal dialysis or cardiac bypass. With respect to rewarming immersion victims, it should be remembered that the body temperature in these patients continues to drop after removal from the hypothermic environment. In such a situation passive rewarming will be ineffective. During the course of rewarming arrhythmias may occur but they should resolve spontaneously when a normal body temperature is achieved.

1. Reuler, J. B. Hypothermia: Pathophysiology: Clinical settings, and management. *Ann. Intern. Med.* 89:519, 1978.
   In-depth review. (See also Adv. Intern. Med. 27:127, 1982.)
2. Hagnauer, A. H. Lethal hypothermic temperatures in dog and man. *Ann. N.Y. Acad. Sci.* 80:315, 1952.
   LT_{50} *is 81°F (27°C).*
3. Severinghaus, J. W. Respiration and hypothermia. *Ann. N.Y. Acad. Sci.* 80:384, 1959.
   Spurious elevation of the PO_2 and PCO_2 if not corrected for temperature.
4. Collins, K. J., Dore, C., Exton-Smith, A. N. Accidental hypothermia and impaired temperature homeostasis in the elderly. *Br. Med. J.* 1:353, 1977.
   Loss of cutaneous vasoconstriction, reduction in peripheral blood flow, and shivering with aging.
5. Frienkel, N., Metzger, B. E., Harris, E., et al. The hypothermia of hypoglycemia. *N. Engl. J. Med.* 287;841, 1972.
   A central nervous system effect of intracellular glucose deprivation.
6. Whittle, J. L., and Bates, J. H. Thermoregulatory failure secondary to acute illness. *Arch. Intern. Med.* 139:418, 1979.
   The method of correction of hypothermia should be matched to the clinical situation.

7. Duguid, H., Simpson, R. G., and Stowers, J. M. Accidental hypothermia. *Lancet* 2:1213, 1961.
   Visceral infarctions, gastric erosions, and pancreatitis found at autopsy.
8. Weyman, A. E., Greenbaum, D. M., and Grace, W. J. Accidental hypothermia in an alcoholic population. *Am. J. Med.* 56:13, 1974.
   Mortality was found to be related to the presence of underlying disease rather than the degree of hypothermia.
9. Gale, E. A. M., and Tattersall, R. B. Hypothermia: A complication of diabetic ketoacidosis. *Br. Med. J.* 1:1387, 1978.
   Hypothermia was commonly observed in patients with untreated severe ketoacidosis.
10. Philip, G., and Smith, J. F. Hypothermia and Wernicke's encephalopathy. *Lancet* 2:122, 1973.
    Posterior hypothalamic damage resulting in hypothermia.
11. Fox, R. H., Davies, T. W., Marsh, F. P., et al. Hypothermia in a young man with an anterior hypothalamic lesion. *Lancet* 2:185, 1970.
    Recurrent hypothermia.
12. Clements, S. D., Jr., and Hurst, W. Diagnostic value of electrocardiographic abnormalities observed in subjects accidentally exposed to cold. *Am. J. Cardiol.* 29:729, 1972.
    Bradycardia, atrial fibrillation, and J waves.
13. Maclean, D., Griffiths, P. D., and Emslie-Smith, D. Serum enzymes in relation to electrocardiographic changes in accidental hypothermia. *Lancet* 2:1266, 1968.
    Elevation of serum levels of muscle enzymes reflects alterations in membrane permeability, not histologic damage.
14. Maclean, D., Griffiths, P. D., Browning, M. C. K., et al. Metabolic aspects of spontaneous rewarming in accidental hypothermia and hypothermic myxoedema. *Q. J. Med.* 43:371, 1974.
    Mechanisms of adaptation are reviewed.
15. Woolf, P. D., Hollander, C. S., Mitsuma, T., et al. Accidental hypothermia: Endocrine function during recovery. *J. Clin. Endocrinol. Metab.* 34:460, 1972.
    The hypothalamic-pituitary-thyroid axis is intact.
16. Sprunt, J. G., Maclean, D., and Browning, M. C. K. Plasma corticosteroid levels in accidental hypothermia. *Lancet* 1:324, 1970.
    Corticosteroid levels are usually elevated.
17. Lewin, S., Brettman, L. R., and Holzman, R. S. Infections in hypothermic patients. *Arch. Intern. Med.* 141:920, 1981.
    A high incidence of infection was found in hypothermic alcoholics.
18. Niazi, S. A., and Lewis, F. J. Profound hypothermia in man. *Ann. Surg.* 147:264, 1958.
    Survival after 45 minutes at 48°F (9°C) with no cardiac activity.
19. Laufman, H. Profound accidental hypothermia. *J.A.M.A.* 147:1201, 1951.
    An interesting and well-studied case with a core temperature of 64.4°F (18°C).
20. Meriwether, W. D., and Goodman, R. M. Accidental hypothermia with survival after rapid rewarming. *Am. J. Med.* 53:505, 1972.
    Rapid rewarming is advocated. (See also J. Trauma 27:89, 1987.)
21. Lash, R. F., Burdette, J. A., and Ozdel, T. Accidental profound hypothermia and barbiturate intoxication. *J.A.M.A.* 201:269, 1967.
    Core rewarming by peritoneal dialysis.
22. Fernandez, J. P., O'Rourke, R. A., and Ewy, G. A. Rapid active external rewarming in accidental hypothermia. *J.A.M.A.* 212:153, 1970.
    External rewarming advocated.
23. Reuler, J. B., and Parker, R. A. Peritoneal dialysis in the management of hypothermia. *J.A.M.A.* 240:2289, 1978.
    Core rewarming by peritoneal dialysis advocated.
24. Southwick, F. S., and Dalglish, P. H., Jr. Recovery after prolonged asystolic cardiac arrest in profound hypothermia. *J.A.M.A.* 243:1250, 1980.
    Patients who are hypothermic should not be pronounced dead until they are warm and dead.

25. Fischbech, K. H., and Simon, R. P. Neurological manifestations of accidental hypothermia. *Ann. Neurol.* 10:384, 1981.
    Concise review.
26. MacMillan, A. L., Corbett, J. L., Johnson, R. H., et al. Temperature regulation in survivors of accidental hypothermia of the elderly. *Lancet* 2:165, 1967.
    Both the production and conservation of heat are impaired.
27. Pugh, L. G.-C. E. Tolerance to extreme cold at altitude in a Nepalese pilgrim. *J. Appl. Physiol.* 18:1234, 1963.
    Interesting case report.
28. Washburn, B. Frostbite. *N. Engl. J. Med.* 266:974, 1962.
    Excellent review stressing rapid rewarming.
29. Gagge, A. P., and Herrington, L. P. Physiological effects of heat and cold. *Annu. Rev. Physiol.* 9:409, 1947.
    Review of the Dachau experience.
30. Swain, J. A. Hypothermia and blood pH. *Arch. Intern. Med.* 148:1643, 1988.
    Suggestion that pH should be allowed to remain above 7.4.
31. Steinman, A. M. Cardiopulmonary resuscitation and hypothermia. *Circulation* 74 (pt. 2):IV29, 1986.
    The theoretical possibility of inducing ventricular fibrillation is outweighed by the benefits of cardiopulmonary resuscitation if cardiac arrest is suspected.

II. DISEASES OF THE CARDIOVASCULAR SYSTEM

Pathogenesis of low voltage, electrical alternans, injury current, and T wave changes. (See also Circulation 48:1268, 1973.)

12. Charles, M. A., Bensinger, T. A., and Glasser, S. P. Atrial injury current in pericarditis. *Arch. Intern. Med.* 131:657, 1973.
    An easily overlooked diagnostic aid.

13. Spodick, D. H. Differential characteristics of the electrocardiogram in early repolarization and acute pericarditis. *N. Engl. J. Med.* 295:523, 1976.
    Absence of RS–T deviations in the limb leads favors early repolarization.

14. Klacsmann, P. G., Bulkley, B. H., and Hutchins, G. M. The changed spectrum of purulent pericarditis. *Am. J. Med.* 63:666, 1977.
    An important review; staphylococci and gram-negative organisms are the major pathogens; aseptic pericarditis and surgery are important antecedents.

15. Berk, S. L., Rice, P. A., Reynholds, C. A., et al. Pneumococcal pericarditis: A persisting problem in contemporary diagnosis. *Am. J. Med.* 70:247, 1981.
    The development of cardiomegaly and S–T segment elevations are important clues to the presence of pericardial involvement. (See also Arch. Intern. Med. 146:1174, 1986.)

16. Nelson, D. P., Rensimer, E. R., and Raffin, T. A. *Legionella pneumophila* pericarditis without pneumonia. *Arch. Intern. Med.* 145:926, 1985.
    An unusual complication.

17. Rubin, R. H., and Moellering, R. C., Jr. Clinical, microbiologic, and therapeutic aspects of purulent pericarditis. *Am. J. Med.* 59:68, 1975.
    There was a high incidence of fungal pericarditis in this series.

18. Morse, J. R., Oretski, M. I., and Hudson, J. A. Pericarditis as a complication of meningococcal meningitis. *Ann. Intern. Med.* 74:212, 1971.
    A complication that is being reported with increasing frequency. (See also N. Engl. J. Med. 290:143, 1974.)

19. Kumar, S., and Lesch, M. Pericarditis in renal disease. *Prog. Cardiovasc. Dis.* 22:357, 1980.
    Comprehensive review of a complex problem.

20. Seifert, F. C., Miller, D. C., Oesterle, S. N., et al. Surgical treatment of constrictive pericarditis: analysis of outcome and diagnostic error. *Circulation* 72:II264, 1985.
    Differentiating between pericardial constriction and restrictive myocardiopathy is a problem. (See also Radiology 156:753, 1985.)

21. Kumpe, D. A., Jaffe, R. B., Waldmann, T. A., et al. Constrictive pericarditis and protein losing enteropathy. *Am. J. Roentgenol. Radium Ther. Nucl. Med.* 124:365, 1975.
    The presence of pericardial disease is overshadowed by the gastrointestinal tract complications.

22. Nicholson, W. J., Cobbs, B. W., Jr., Franck, R. H., et al. Early diastolic sound of constrictive pericarditis. *Am. J. Cardiol.* 45:378, 1980.
    Squatting employed to accentuate the knock of constrictive pericarditis.

23. Nishimura, R. A., Connolly, D. C., Parkin, T. W., et al. Constrictive pericarditis: assessment of current diagnostic procedures. *Mayo Clin. Proc.* 60:397, 1985.
    A useful, brief review of various diagnostic tests. (See also Lancet 2:372, 1987.)

24. Bush, C. A., Stang, J. M., Wooley, C. F., et al. Occult constrictive pericardial disease. *Circulation* 56:924, 1977.
    Rapid volume expansion employed to unmask the presence of pericardial constriction.

25. Kutcher, M. A., King, S. B., III, Alimurung, B. N., et al. Constrictive pericarditis as a complication of cardiac surgery: recognition of an entity. *Am. J. Cardiol.* 50:742, 1982.
    This can occur early or late. (See also Am. J. Cardiol. 43:657, 1979.)

26. Solano, F. X., Jr., Young, E., Talamo, T. S., et al. Constrictive pericarditis mimicking Budd-Chiari syndrome. *Am. J. Med.* 80:113, 1986.
    It is important to consider the pericardium in patients with hepatomegaly, ascites or protein-losing enteropathy. The ascitic fluid protein may be high.

27. Saner, H. E., Gobel, F. L., Nicholoff, D. M., et al. Aortic dissection presenting as pericarditis. *Chest* 91:71, 1987.
    Something to remember.

28. Hara, K. S., Ballard, D. J., Ilstrup, D.C., et al. Rheumatoid Pericarditis: Clinical features and survival. *Medicine* 69:81, 1990.
Pericardiectomy may be necessary.

29. Thompson, D. G., Lennard-Jones, J. E., Sevorbrid, E. T., et al. Pericarditis and inflammatory bowel disease. *Q. J. Med.* 48:93, 1979.
An uncommon complication usually occurring when the bowel disease is active. An association of pericarditis with celiac sprue has also been described (Lancet 1:1021, 1981).

30. Weiss, J., and Spodick, D. Association of left pleural effusion with pericardial disease. *N. Engl. J. Med.* 308:696, 1983.
High incidence of left-sided pleural effusions in constrictive pericarditis (See also Arch. Intern. Med. 149:201, 1989.)

31. Singh, S., Wann, S., Schuchard, G. H., et al. Right ventricular and right atrial collapse in patients with pericardial tamponade—a combined echocardiographic and hemodynamic study. *Circulation* 70:966, 1984.
Right atrial collapse occurs earlier than right ventricular collapse in the course of tamponade and both can be used to detect the development of cardiac tamponade.

32. Isner, J. M., Carter, B. L., Bankoff, M. S., et al. Computed tomography in the diagnosis of pericardial heart disease. *Ann. Intern. Med.* 97:473, 1982.
Computed tomography scanning is a valuable adjunct to echocardiography particularly for evaluation of pericardial thickening.

25. ACUTE MYOCARDIAL INFARCTION
Alan D. Guerci

More than 1 million acute myocardial infarctions occur each year in the United States. In the industrialized West, the acute and chronic manifestations of myocardial infarction account for more deaths than any other single disease entity. Full discussion of the pathophysiology and treatment of acute myocardial infarction is beyond the scope of this text, and this chapter will focus on diagnostic and therapeutic problems related to the patient's presentation.

The majority of myocardial infarctions are caused by thrombosis of severely atherosclerosed coronary arteries. Coronary spasm is an unusual cause of acute myocardial infarction, and coronary artery embolism, congenital anomalies of the coronary circulation, and inflammatory arteritides are rare causes of myocardial infarction. Necrosis is determined by the duration and intensity of ischemia. Available data suggest that most myocardial infarctions are complete in 4 to 6 hours.

Patients with acute myocardial infarction typically complain of squeezing or crushing retrosternal discomfort, often with radiation to the neck, jaw, or left arm. Radiation to the right arm or back is less common. In some cases the discomfort is epigastric and may be mistaken for indigestion. Still other patients present not with pain but with symptoms of disordered electrical or mechanical activity such as syncope or shortness of breath.

Electrocardiography remains the single most useful diagnostic test in the initial phase of myocardial infarction. Although fallible, electrocardiography usually offers insight into the location, size, age, and consequently, the prognosis of an infarct.

ST segment elevation is the ECG hallmark of acute, transmural ischemia involving the anterior, inferior, and lateral walls of the left ventricle. When viewed from above, the ST segment elevations of infarction often have a convex shape, as opposed to the concave upward appearance of the ST segment elevations of pericarditis and early repolarization. In some cases hyperacute T waves, defined as greater than 1.0-mV-high T waves, may be the earliest and only ECG evidence of infarction. Deep (usually more than 0.2 mV), horizontal, or slowly upsloping ST segment depressions in the precordial leads may be the only evidence of transmural ischemia involving the posterior wall of the left ventricle. These ST segment depressions are actually the reciprocal representation of ST elevations, as may be appreciated by turning the ECG over and viewing it against a source of light. The development of Q waves and loss of R waves occur in parallel and indicate necrosis. Like the infarction itself, these ECG processes are ordinarily complete in 4 to 6 hours. Indeed, when chest pain and ST segment elevations persist for more than 3 or 4 hours without R wave loss or the development of Q waves, it is appropriate to consider the possibility of preservation of myocardium due to abundant collateral blood flow to the ischemic region or nonischemic causes of ST segment elevation.

The ECG expression of subendocardial infarction is less precise. Deep (>0.2 mV), symmetric T wave inversions and persistent ST segment depressions are considered typical, but many cases are manifested by nonspecific ST and T wave abnormalities or no abnormality at all. Thus, while the ECG is useful in guiding therapy, it is of less value in triage. Coronary-prone individuals with a history of typical ischemic myocardial pain lasting more than 20 or 30 minutes should be admitted for observation even if their ECGs are normal.

The differential diagnosis of acute myocardial infarction includes aortic dissection, pulmonary embolism, pericarditis, and a variety of disorders involving the chest wall and upper gastrointestinal tract. The pain of aortic dissection ordinarily radiates to the back and is usually described in terms more severe than that of myocardial infarction. Although the dissection may involve the aortic root, occlude a coronary artery, and cause an acute myocardial infarction, most aortic dissections do not cause infarction and, in addition, do not cause changes in the ECG. This latter feature may be a useful point in differential diagnosis.

Like myocardial infarction, pulmonary embolism may cause severe chest pain and shortness of breath. Pulmonary embolism may also cause T wave inversions or minor nonspecific ST and T wave abnormalities, which lack diagnostic utility. Alternatively, the ECG may be normal or minimally abnormal in massive pulmonary embolism. Excluding acute ischemic mitral regurgitation, this is not true of myocardial infarction causing hemodynamic compromise, that is, although the ECG may be normal in small myocardial infarctions, it is grossly abnormal when the infarct is large enough to cause hypotension or respiratory distress.

The pain of pericarditis is almost pleuritic, whereas that of the initial phase of myocardial infarction is rarely, if ever, pleuritic. Several other clinical and ECG features of pericarditis are also distinctive. The PR segment may be depressed, and ST segment elevations are often present in all of the left ventricular leads. ST segment elevations may be widespread in acute myocardial infarction as well, but extensive ST elevations are the result of massive infarction, and some hemodynamic compromise would ordinarily accompany such cases. Thus, normal heart rate, blood pressure, and lung examination in the face of widespread ST segment elevations (e.g., I, II, AVL, AVF, and V_3–V_6) suggest pericarditis. Normal ventricular wall motion in regions with ST segment elevation as, for example, might readily be demonstrated with echocardiography, would also support the diagnosis of pericarditis, for ischemia severe enough to cause ST segment elevation invariably abolishes contraction.

Esophageal spasm may cause pain which is indistinguishable from that of acute myocardial infarction but does not cause ST segment or T wave abnormalities. Cholecystitis and pancreatitis more commonly cause confusion, for both may cause minor, nonspecific ST–T wave abnormalities or even T wave inversions, and the pain of acute myocardial infarction may be epigastric. Physical examination, that is, demonstration of right upper quadrant or epigastric tenderness, is usually sufficient to establish the correct diagnosis.

A number of diseases of the chest wall, ranging from muscle spasm and rib fractures to herpes zoster radiculitis, may cause aching or nondescript discomfort similar to that of acute myocardial infarction. Again, careful physical examination usually distinguishes these cases from myocardial infarction.

Treatment of acute myocardial infarction consists of measures applicable to all patients and measures which must be individualized according to the ECG and the patient's overall condition. In the absence of a specific contraindication, oxygen, lidocaine, and narcotic analgesics should probably be administered to all patients, whereas nitroglycerin, thrombolytic agents, calcium antagonists, beta blockers, heparin, and intravenous fluids must be given more selectively.

The principal justification for routine administration of oxygen is that approximately 10 percent of patients with Killip I infarcts have a PaO_2 of 55 to 60 mm Hg. While this partial pressure will ordinarily provide adequate hemoglobin saturation, any deterioration in the left ventricular function of such patients will result in serious deficits in oxygen delivery. Routine measurement of arterial blood gas tensions, on the other hand, has never been shown to favorably affect outcome, should not substitute for clinical judgment, and is not indicated.

Lidocaine dramatically reduces the incidence of primary ventricular fibrillation (ventricular fibrillation occurring in hemodynamically stable patients). It is usually given for 12 to 24 hours.

Whereas it may be impossible to abolish the pain of myocardial infarction without serious respiratory depression, substantial relief can be provided with opiates. This is an important goal of therapy and can usually be achieved in 20 to 45 minutes with 8 to 20 mg of morphine given intravenously in 2- to 5-mg increments. Morphine also causes vasodilation and should not be given to hypotensive patients. Nalbuphine, a potent synthetic narcotic with mild vasoconstricting properties, may be given in such cases.

A small percentage of transmural infarcts are due to coronary spasm, with or without underlying atherosclerotic disease. Nitroglycerin may be effective in such cases, and should be administered immediately to all patients with transmural infarcts and systolic blood pressures greater than 100 mm Hg. The preferred dose and route is 0.4 mg sublingually.

If chest pain and ST segment elevations persist after one or two sublingual nitroglycerin tablets, it must be assumed that the infarct-related artery is occluded by thrombus. The focus of therapy should be shifted to thrombolytic therapy or primary angioplasty. Streptokinase, 1.5 million units given intravenously over 1 hour, has been shown to reduce mortality by 20 percent when given within 6 hours of the onset of myocardial infarction. Benefit is concentrated among patients treated within 1 hour of symptom onset and those with anterior infarctions. Tissue plasminogen activator, a nonantigenic agent with significantly greater thrombolytic efficacy than streptokinase, has not been studied in terms of mortality, but has been shown to improve left ventricular function in two placebo-controlled trials. Benefit is significant for patients with inferior infarctions as well as those with anterior infarctions, but more studies are needed.

Beta blockers have been shown to ameliorate several indirect indices of myocardial injury when administered at a mean of 3.4 hours after symptom onset. Administration at means of 8 to 11 hours into the course of a myocardial infarction is ineffective. Moreover, the strategy of treatment with beta blockers is limited by the fact that patients with the greatest need for intervention, those with large infarcts, will not tolerate beta blockade.

Although individual studies of nitroglycerin and nitroprusside in acute myocardial infarction have, for the most part, been inconclusive, pooled data indicate a reduction in mortality when these agents are given for at least 48 or more hours.

Right ventricular infarction is diagnosed on the basis of inferior ST segment elevations, hypotension, and the absence of pulmonary congestion. Treatment is based on elevation of right ventricular preload with volume. Infusion of as much as 5 to 10 liters of normal saline may be necessary.

Subendocardial infarction poses a number of problems in pathophysiology and treatment. It is likely that many subendocardial infarctions are due to subtotal occlusion or transient total occlusion of vessels with moderate to abundant distal collateral flow. Thus, therapy is directed at maintaining vessel patency with nitrates, calcium antagonists, and heparin. Early catheterization is appropriate in many patients, particularly those with evidence of widespread ischemia.

Treatment of heart failure due to myocardial infarction is similar to the treatment of heart failure from other causes, with the exception that digitalis glycosides are usually withheld for several days when the stability of atrioventricular nodal function is uncertain. Preload, afterload, and contractility may all be manipulated in an effort to relieve lung congestion, optimize ventricular filling, and maintain tissue perfusion.

As in the case of heart failure, treatment of rhythm disturbances due to acute myocardial infarction is generally similar to treatment of arrhythmias from any cause. The exception to this rule concerns conduction disturbances. New left bundle branch block, bifascicular block, and alternating bundle branch block are associated with 15 to 40 percent risk of progression to complete heart block. Prophylactic, temporary transvenous pacing for 48 to 72 hours is the usual treatment for these conduction disturbances.

Emergency coronary angioplasty is a rapidly evolving therapy with as yet incompletely defined indications in acute myocardial infarction. References discussing angioplasty and other topics in acute myocardial infarction can be found in the bibliography.

1. Guerci, A. D., and Weisfeldt, M. L. Acute Myocardial Infarction. In A. M. Harvey (ed.), *Principles and Practice of Medicine* (22nd ed.) New York: Appleton, Century, Crofts, 1988. P. 99.

2. DeWood, M. A., Spores, J., Notske, R., et al. Prevalence of total coronary occlusion during the early hours of acute myocardial infarction. *N. Engl. J. Med.* 303:897, 1980.
   Role of coronary thrombosis in transmural infarction.

3. DeWood, M. A., Stifter, W. F., Simpson, C. S., et al. Coronary arteriographic findings soon after non-Q wave myocardial infarction. *N. Engl. J. Med.* 303:417, 1986.
   Coronary anatomy in subendocardial infarction.

4. Maseri, A., L'Abbate, A., Baroldi, G., et al. Coronary vasospasm as a possible cause of myocardial infarction: A conclusion derived from the study of "preinfarction angina." *N. Engl. J. Med.* 299:1271, 1978.
   As entitled.

5. Rivas, F., Cobb, F. R., Bache, R. J., et al. Relationship between blood flow to ischemic regions and extent of myocardial infarction. *Circ. Res.* 38:439, 1976.
   Important study in experimental infarction; approximately 40% of normal flow is necessary to maintain viability.

6. Vatner, S. F. Correlation between acute reductions in myocardial blood flow and function in conscious dogs. *Circ. Res.* 47:201, 1980.
   Regional function is very sensitive to reductions in blood flow.

7. Gruppo Italiano per lo Studio della Streptochinasi nell'Infarto Miocardico (GISSI). Effectiveness of intravenous thrombolytic treatment in acute myocardial infarction. *Lancet* 1:397, 1986.
   Landmark study of streptokinase in myocardial infarction; benefit is concentrated in patients treated early and patients with anterior infarcts.

8. Guerci, A. D., Gerstenblith, G., Brinker, J. A., et al. A randomized placebo-controlled, double-blinded trial of intravenous tissue plasminogen activator [tPA] for acute myocardial infarction with subsequent randomization to elective coronary angioplasty. *N. Engl. J. Med.* 317:1613, 1987.
   When administered within 4.5 hours of symptom onset, tPA improves left ventricular function.

9. Simoons, M. L., Serruys, P. W., van den Brand, M., et al. Improved survival after early thrombolysis in acute myocardial infarction. *Lancet* 2:578, 1985.
   Aggressive revascularization strategy, consisting of streptokinase and emergency angioplasty, reduces mortality.

10. O'Neill, W., Timmis, G. C., Bourdillon, P., et al. A prospective randomized clinical trial of intracoronary streptokinase versus coronary angioplasty for acute myocardial infarction. *N. Engl. J. Med.* 314:812, 1986.
    Primary angioplasty is associated with high patency rates and improved left ventricular function.

11. Kennedy, J. W., Ritchie, J. L., Davis, K. B., et al. The western Washington randomized trial of intracoronary streptokinase in acute myocardial infarction: A 12-month follow-up report. *N. Engl. J. Med.* 312:1073, 1985.
    Benefit of intracoronary streptokinase is maintained over ensuing year.

12. Anderson, J. L., Marshall, H. W., Bray, B. E., et al. A randomized trial of intravenous and intracoronary streptokinase in patients with acute myocardial infarction. *Circulation* 70:606, 1984.

Intracoronary administration of streptokinase yields high patency rates but delays in initiation of therapy may negate benefit.

13. International Collaborative Study Group. Reduction of infarct size with the early use of timolol in acute myocardial infarction. *N. Engl. J. Med.* 310:9, 1984.
When administered within 4 hours of symptoms timolol reduces several indirect indices of infarct size.

14. Roberts, R., Croft, C., Gold, H. K., et al. Effect of propranolol on myocardial infarct size in a randomized blinded multicenter trial. *N. Engl. J. Med.* 311:218, 1984.
No benefit when beta blockers are given 8 hours after symptom onset.

15. Lie, K. I., Wellens, H. J., Capelle, F. J., et al. Lidocaine in the prevention of primary ventricular fibrillation. *N. Engl. J. Med.* 291:1324, 1974.
Lidocaine sharply reduces the incidence of ventricular fibrillation.

16. Yusuf, S., and Collins, R. IV nitroglycerin and nitroprusside therapy in acute myocardial infarction reduces mortality: Evidence of randomized controlled trials (abstracted). *Circulation* 72 (suppl 3):224, 1985.
Pooling of studies reveals vasodilator-associated reduction of mortality.

17. VA Cooperative Trial. Anticoagulants in acute myocardial infarction. *J.A.M.A.* 225:724, 1973.
Anticoagulation for 1 month reduces the incidence of stroke. This study does not answer questions of duration of therapy or patient selection.

18. Report of the Sixty Plus Reinfarction Study Research Group. A double-blinded trial to assess long-term or anticoagulant therapy in elderly patients after myocardial infarction. *Lancet* 2:889, 1980.
Elderly patients benefit from prolonged anticoagulation.

19. Hindman, M. C., Wagner, G. S., Jaro, M., et al. The clinical significance of bundle branch block complicating acute myocardial infarction. 2. Indications for temporary and permanent pacemaker insertion. *Circulation* 58:689, 1978.
As entitled. Classic study.

20. Killip, T., and Kimball, J. T. Treatment of myocardial infarction in a coronary care unit. A two-year experience with 250 patients. *Am. J. Cardiol.* 201:457, 1967.
Another classic. This study relates clinical features to prognosis.

21. Forrester, J. S., Diamond, G., Chatterjee, K., et al. Medical therapy of acute myocardial infarction by application of hemodynamic subsets. *N. Engl. J. Med.* 295:1356,1404, 1976.
As entitled. A third classic.

22. Multicenter Postinfarction Research Group. Risk stratification and survival after myocardial infarction. *N. Engl. J. Med.* 309:331, 1983.
Fine study of an important problem, left ventricular (LV) function is the major determinant of survival after infarction.

23. Sanz, G., Castaner, G., Betriu, A., et al. Determinants of prognosis in survivors of myocardial infarction. *N. Engl. J. Med.* 306:1065, 1982.
As above. LV function and, to a lesser extent, coronary anatomy, determine prognosis.

24. Moss, A. J., David, H. T., DeCamilla, J., et al. Ventricular ectopic beats and their relation to sudden and non-sudden cardiac death after myocardial infarction. *Circulation* 60:998, 1979.
Premature ventricular contractions correlate with LV function but also appear to be an independent risk factor for late cardiac death.

25. DeBusk, R. F., Blomqvist, G. G., et al. Identification and treatment of low risk patients after acute myocardial infarction and coronary artery bypass graft surgery. *N. Engl. J. Med.* 314:161, 1986.
Consensus statement by leaders in risk stratification.

26. Turner, J. D., Rogers, W. J., Mantle, J. A., et al. Coronary angiography soon after myocardial infarction. *Chest* 77:58, 1980.
Majority of infarct survivors have multivessel coronary disease.

27. Schuster, E. H., and Bulkley, B. H. Early post-infarction angina. Ischemia at a distance and ischemia in the infarct zone. *N. Engl. J. Med.* 305:1101, 1981.
Biased sample (i.e., patients in a referral center); nevertheless, postinfarction angina treated medically has a devastating (50%) 1-year mortality rate.

28. Baumgartner, W. A., Borkon, A. M., Gardner, T. J., et al. Operative intervention for post-infarction angina. *Ann. Thorac. Surg.* 38:265, 1984.
   Surgical mortality is 5 to 8%.
29. DeFeyter, P. J., Serruys, P. W., Simoons, M., et al. Coronary angioplasty for early post-infarction unstable angina. *Circulation* 74:1365, 1986.
   Mortality rate of 2% when angioplasty is applied to a selected subset of patients with postinfarct angina.
30. Norwegian Multicenter Study Group. Timolol induced reduction in mortality and reinfarction in patients surviving acute myocardial infarction. *N. Engl. J. Med.* 304:802, 1981.
   Beta blockers reduce incidence of sudden cardiac death by approximately 33%.
31. Furburg, C. D., Hawkins, C. M., and Lichstein, E. Effect of propranolol in postinfarction patients with mechanical or electrical complications. *Circulation* 69:761, 1984.
   Benefit of long-term therapy is concentrated in patients with complicated infarcts.
32. Folts, J. D., Crowell, E. B., and Rowe, G. G. Platelet aggregation in partially obstructed vessels and its elimination with aspirin. *Circulation* 54:365, 1976.
   Pathophysiologic and therapeutic intrigue.
33. Canner, P. L. Aspirin in coronary heart disease: Comparison of six clinical trials. *Isr. J. Med. Sci.* 19:413, 1983.
   Aspirin reduces mortality by approximately 10%.
34. Geft, P. L., Shah, P. K., Rodriguez, L., et al. ST elevation in leads V1 to V5 may be caused by right coronary occlusion and acute right ventricular infarction. *Am. J. Cardiol.* 53:991, 1984.
   Diagnostic approach and introduction to literature on right ventricular infarction.
35. Schroeder, J. S., Lamb, I. H., and Harrison, D. C. Patients admitted to the coronary care unit for chest pain: High risk subgroup for subsequent cardiovascular death.
   Patients with transient ST-T wave changes and normal creatine kinase levels have 1-year cardiac mortality rate similar to infarct survivors.

26. ACUTE RHEUMATIC FEVER IN ADULTS
Jerry L. Spivak

Acute rheumatic fever is primarily a disease of children and adolescents, but its occurrence in adults is not uncommon. In one epidemiologic study, 18 percent of all patients hospitalized for acute rheumatic fever were over age 20 years. The frequency and morbidity of rheumatic fever in adults are greatest in the third decade, but this disease can occur at any age and without regard to a history of prior attacks or the presence of underlying rheumatic heart disease.

The diagnosis is easily overlooked because of the similarity of the clinical features of acute rheumatic fever to other illnesses that are encountered more frequently—systemic lupus erythematosus; serum sickness; rheumatoid arthritis; viral myopericarditis; sarcoidosis; bacterial endocarditis; viral or gonococcal arthritis; postinfectious arthritis associated with *Yersinia, Salmonella,* or *Shigella;* and cardiac failure in patients with established rheumatic heart disease. The problem is further compounded in the adults because the presentation of the disease is different in children. Chorea, subcutaneous nodules, and erythema marginatum are not seen, while arthralgias and polyarthritis of both a migratory, additive, and symmetric nature are more common than carditis. Lower-extremity, large-joint involvement, and tenosynovitis are frequently observed. Joint fluid is somewhat turbid, and the leukocyte count is usually over 10,000 per cu mm, of which 50 percent or more are neutrophils. The mucin clot is good, and the glucose level is normal. In addition to the acute and transient polyarthritis, chronic joint deformities have been described (under the term *Jaccoud's arthritis*). A particular problem in recognizing acute rheumatic activity occurs in patients with established rheumatic heart disease. In such patients fever, leukocytosis, and atrial arrhythmias may indicate the presence of endocarditis or pulmonary embolism with infarction as well as acute rheumatic fever. The diagnosis of acute rheumatic fever is established first by considering the possibility and then by determining the antistreptolysin O titer and performing a throat culture. Minimal signs of pharyngitis and the absence of clinical symptoms are no guarantee that a streptococcal infection is not present; neither is a negative throat culture in a patient taking penicillin prophylactically.

Therapy for the episode should include a course of antibiotics to eradicate the streptococcus, and anti-inflammatory agents to suppress inflammation. Salicylates are generally effective if adequate blood levels are obtained, but when severe exudative manifestations are present, steroids are more efficient. Bed rest, particularly if signs of carditis are present, seems prudent. Since the treatment of acute rheumatic fever is palliative and not curative, every effort should be directed at preventing the illness. To that end, monthly injections of benthazine penicillin G are the most effective prophylactic measure. Recent data suggest that shortening this interval to 3 weeks may be more effective (*J. Pediatr.* 108:299, 1986). For adults, the issue is more problematic. Individuals who develop acute rheumatic fever but not carditis, will not develop carditis with subsequent attacks. Thus, for these patients lifelong prophylaxis seems pointless. For those with a history of carditis, lifelong prophylaxis seems appropriate. Penicillin prophylaxis, however, does not constitute protection against bacterial endocarditis.

1. Veasy, L. G., Wiedmeier, S. E., Orsmon, G. S., et al. Resurgence of acute rheumatic fever in the intermountain area of the United States. *N. Engl. J. Med.* 316:421, 1987. *Acute rheumatic fever is now appearing in new population groups.*

2. Wee, A. S. T., and Goodwin, J. F. Acute rheumatic fever and carditis in older adults. *Lancet* 2:239, 1966. *Polyarthritis, atrial arrhythmias, and an elevated erythrocyte sedimentation rate were frequent features. (For ventricular arrhythmias, see* Cereb. Intern. Med. *145:1904, 1985.)*

3. Adatto, I. J., Poske, R. M., Ponget, J. M., et al. Rheumatic fever in the adult. *J.A.M.A.* 194:1043, 1965. *Polyarthritis was found to be the most common manifestation.*

4. Barnert, A. L., Terry, E. E., and Persellin, R. H. Acute rheumatic fever in adults. *J.A.M.A.* 232:925, 1975. *Arthritis involving the large joints was common; carditis was rare and transient.*

5. McDonald, E. C., and Weisman, M. H. Articular manifestations of rheumatic fever in adults. *Ann. Intern. Med.* 89:917, 1978. *Addictive symmetric, lower-extremity, large-joint polyarthritis, and tenosynovitis.*

6. Persellin, R. H. Acute rheumatic fever: Changing manifestations. *Ann. Intern. Med.* 89:1002, 1978. *Acute rheumatic fever must be distinguished from the postinfectious polyarthritis associated with certain enteric pathogens such as* Yersinia, Shigella, *and* Salmonella. *(See also* Ann. Intern. Med. *81:458, 1974.)*

7. Elster, S. K., Pader, E., and Horn, H. Fever in patients with rheumatic heart disease. *Arch. Intern. Med.* 112:476, 1963. *Fever may be the only clinical manifestation of acute rheumatic fever.*

8. Davis, E. Criteria of rheumatic fever. *Lancet* 1:1043, 1970. *Improvements suggested. (See also* Circulation 32:664, 1965.)

9. Ward, C. A reappraisal of the clinical features in acute and chronic rheumatic heart disease: Etiological implications. *Am. Heart J.* 98:298, 1979. *Suggestion that acquired valvular heart disease is not always due to acute rheumatic fever.*

10. Feinstein, A. R., and Stern, E. K. Clinical effects of recurrent attacks of acute rheumatic fever. *J. Chronic Dis.* 20:13, 1967.

Recurrent rheumatic fever seldom damages previously unaffected hearts. (see also J. Chronic. Dis. 39:361, 1986.)

11. Spagnuolo, M., Pasternack, B., and Taranta, A. Risk of rheumatic fever recurrences after streptococcal infections. *N. Engl. J. Med.* 285:641, 1971.
    Recurrence rate is influenced by the severity of the infection, residual heart disease, recent acute rheumatic fever, and a young age.

12. Feinstein, A. R., and Levitt, M. The role of tonsils in predisposing to streptococcal infections and recurrences of rheumatic fever. *N. Engl. J. Med.* 282:285, 1970.
    If prophylaxis is poor, large tonsils are associated with reinfection and relapse.

13. Kaplan, E. L., Bisno, A., Derrick, W., et al. Prevention of rheumatic fever. *Circulation* 55:223, 1977.
    Guidelines from the American Heart Association; benzathine penicillin is the antibiotic of choice. (and Circulation 70:1118A, 1984.)

14. Mortimer, E. A., Jr., and Rammelkamp, C. H. Prophylaxis of rheumatic fever. *Circulation* 14:1144, 1976.
    Chance of exposure is important in determining the need for continuous prophylaxis in the adult.

15. Johnson, E. E., Stollerman, G. H., and Grossman, B. J. Rheumatic recurrences in patients not receiving continuous prophylaxis. *J.A.M.A.* 190:407, 1964.
    The recurrence rate in adults is lower than in children, but recurrence still occurs and continuous prophylaxis is advised.

16. Griffith, G. C., and Taranta, A. Should adults with rheumatic heart disease be kept on continuous penicillin prophylaxis? *Am. J. Cardiol.* 18:627, 1966.
    Yes.

17. Thompkins, D. G., Boxerbaum, B., and Liebman, J. Long-term prognosis of rheumatic fever patients receiving regular intramuscular benzathine penicillin. *Circulation* 45:543, 1972.
    Reduced incidence of valvular stenosis with penicillin prophylaxis.

18. Spencer, W. H., III, Thornsberry, C., Moody, M. D., et al. Rheumatic fever, chemoprophylaxis and penicillin-resistant gingival organisms. *Ann. Intern. Med.* 73:683, 1970.
    Benzathine penicillin G prophylaxis results in the lowest number of resistant organisms.

19. Ben-Dov, I., Berry, E. M., and Kopolovic, J. Poststreptococcal nephritis and acute rheumatic fever in two adults. *Arch. Intern. Med.* 145:338, 1985.
    An unusual occurrence. (See also N. Engl. J. Med. 282:561, 1970.)

20. Zvaifler, N. J. Chronic postrheumatic fever (Jaccoud's) arthritis: *N. Engl. J. Med.* 267:10, 1962.
    Ulnar deviation, periarticular swelling, and flexion deformity of the metatarsophalangeal joints.

21. Ignaczak, T., Espinoza, L. R., Kantor, O. S., et al. Jaccoud arthritis. *Arch. Intern. Med.* 135:577, 1975.
    Evidence that the entity is a variant of rheumatoid arthritis and not a result of acute rheumatic fever.

22. Combined Rheumatic Fever Study Group. A comparison of short-term intensive prednisone and acetylsalicylic acid therapy in the treatment of acute rheumatic fever. *N. Engl. J. Med.* 272:63, 1965.
    Steroids are not superior to aspirin in preventing residual heart disease, but they are effective in controlling acute inflammatory manifestations.

23. Gibney, R., Reineck, J., Bannayan, G. A., et al. Renal lesions in acute rheumatic fever. *Ann. Intern. Med.* 94:322, 1981.
    Renal lesions are uncommon, variable in histology, and transient. (See also Arch. Intern. Med. 127:245, 1971.)

24. Svartman, M., Potter, E. V., Poon-King, T., et al. Immunoglobulins and complement components in synovial fluid of patients with acute rheumatic fever. *J. Clin. Invest.* 56:111, 1975.
    The arthritis of rheumatic fever may be due to immune complexes (as may the pericarditis. Arthritis Rheum. 25:1054, 1982).

25. Ayoub, E. M., Barrett, D. J., Maclaren, N. K., et al. Association of class II human histocompatibility leukocyte antigens with rheumatic fever. *J. Clin. Invest.* 77:2019, 1986.
   Genetic basis for rheumatic fever suggested. (See also Nature *278:173, 1979.)*
26. Pantell, R. H. Cost-effectiveness of pharyngitis management and prevention of rheumatic fever. *Ann. Intern. Med.* 86:497, 1977.
   This article and the accompanying editorial (p. 494) provide a rational approach to the problem.
27. Massell, B. F. Prophylaxis of streptococcal infections and rheumatic fever: A comparison of orally administered clindamycin and penicillin. *J.A.M.A.* 241:1589, 1979.
   Oral clindamycin was as effective as penicillin in this study.
28. Doyle, E. F., Spagnuolo, M., Taranta, A., et al. The risk of bacterial endocarditis during antirheumatic prophylaxis. *J.A.M.A.* 201:807, 1967.
   The risk of endocarditis is not increased but it is not reduced either; blood cultures should be obtained in patients with arthritis and fever.
29. Stollerman, G. H. Streptococcal immunology: Protection versus injury. *Ann. Intern. Med.* 88:422, 1978.
   Strains of streptococci differ in their ability to cause acute rheumatic fever. (See also Circulation *71:1077, 1985.)*
30. Bisno, A. Primary prevention of acute rheumatic fever: Quo vadis. *J. Lab. Clin. Med.* 98:323, 1981.
   Concise review of the treatment of pharyngitis in the setting of a declining incidence of acute rheumatic fever.

27. ANGINA PECTORIS
Thomas A. Traill

Angina pectoris is a symptom, often difficult to describe, caused by temporary imbalance between myocardial oxygen supply and demand. Although its most common cause is coronary atherosclerosis, the term should not be used as though it was a synonym for coronary vascular stenosis; there are several nonvascular diseases that cause angina, in particular aortic stenosis, hypertrophic cardiomyopathy, and, less commonly, severe pulmonary hypertension.

In patients with coronary artery disease and angina pectoris, the most fundamental issue in determining prognosis and management is whether the imbalance between supply and demand is the result of temporary increase in myocardial oxygen demand, or decrease in supply. The former causes the common pattern of "stable" exertional angina. It usually has as its underlying pathophysiology fixed arteriosclerotic narrowing of one or more major coronary vessels, the stenosis reducing the lumen by 70 percent or more. "Supply-side" angina is caused by temporary, reversible reduction in caliber or occlusion of a coronary artery, by coronary artery spasm, thrombosis, or both, usually in the presence of underlying coronary arteriosclerosis. Since coronary occlusion may lead to infarction if sufficiently protracted, supply-side angina has a much more ominous prognosis than demand angina and requires prompt treatment. The clinical syndromes that imply such interruption in supply have acquired a number of names, including unstable angina, preinfarction angina, and rest angina. "Crescendo angina" means exertional angina with a rapidly falling threshold, and since it also implies that there is a rapidly changing coronary supply, its clinical significance is the same as other presentations of supply-side or unstable angina.

The diagnosis of angina is clinical, based on interpretation of the patient's history. Because of its limited specificity and sensitivity for coronary artery disease, stress testing has its main value not so much for diagnosis as for assessing severity and potential risk. Thus, most new patients with demand angina due to arteriosclerotic coronary artery disease undergo stress testing not to "confirm" the diagnosis but to help decide on a plan of action. The signs on stress testing that indicate the existence of a left main coronary artery stenosis or other life-threatening disease are a fall in blood pressure during exercise, very pronounced (> 4 mm) or widespread (more than one vascular distribution) ST segment shift, or a positive test at a low level of oxygen demand, in the sense either of heart rate less than 140 per minute or less than 6 minutes on the treadmill. There is no role for stress testing in the patient with supply-side or unstable angina; it is both dangerous and, since it does not reproduce the pathophysiologic circumstances of ischemia, very insensitive.

Many patients with angina pectoris undergo cardiac catheterization. In general, angiography should be reserved for when clinical circumstances or the results of stress testing indicate that the patient may require a revascularization procedure, either bypass surgery or percutaneous transluminal coronary angioplasty (PTCA). Thus, the indications for coronary angiography include angina refractory to medical treatment, or intolerance of medical treatment; unstable or crescendo angina; angina following a myocardial infarction (which carries the ominous message that there is still additional myocardium in jeopardy); angina with an early, strongly, or hypotensive-positive stress test; and angina and cardiac syncope. Additional, less clear-cut indications are diagnostic angiography in some patients whose histories are difficult to interpret; angiography for prognosis in the young patient with newly discovered coronary disease; angiography to check coronary anatomy in patients who require heart surgery for other conditions.

It is seldom possible to decide on the overall approach to treatment of coronary artery disease simply on the results of coronary angiography. Only in the case of left main coronary artery stenosis has it been possible to show that surgery is superior to medical treatment irrespective of other nonangiographic variables. In this case PTCA is contraindicated. In other patients the decision to operate should require both an unfavorable clinical situation—unstable, worsening, or refractory angina, or an early positive stress test—and coronary artery anatomy that is at the same time severe and surgically remediable. There should be tight proximal stenosis, usually of more than one vessel, combined with adequate distal run-off. The potential for coronary artery bypass to improve prognosis is greater when left ventricular function is impaired. Therefore, in the patient with extensive coronary artery disease and previous ischemic myocardial damage, it may be appropriate to operate even in the absence of profound limitation by symptoms. In patients with less extensive disease, often involving only one vessel, PTCA may be recommended, with results in some cases approaching those of surgical bypass.

Unstable phases of coronary artery disease involve activation of blood platelets, leading to coronary spasm and thrombosis. Unless there is a hematologic contraindication, or a potential bleeding site in the gastrointestinal tract or elsewhere, patients with symptomatic coronary disease should be treated with aspirin. In unstable angina heparin or thrombolytic agents may be required for prevention or lysis of coronary thrombus; aspirin is also effective in this situation, but is often avoided for fear of bleeding complications if the patient requires surgery.

Three classes of vasoactive drugs are used in the medical treatment of patients with angina pectoris, namely beta-adrenergic blocking agents, nitrate compounds, and a less homogeneous group of drugs which act on the calcium channel, referred to as calcium channel blockers. Of course each type of agent has a distinct pharmacologic mechanism of action which suits it for use in its own particular pathophysiologic circumstance; there is therefore no single algorithm in treatment of angina, nor any one agent that is the "first line" of therapy for all patients. When we attempt to optimize therapy we do not simply add drugs in increasing dosage to the limit of tolerance; we make as precise an appraisal as possible of the mechanisms governing symptoms in a particular patient and thereby choose the most closely applicable treatment.

Beta-adrenergic blocking agents act by limiting the rise in heart rate and blood pressure during exercise or other "stress," and thereby improve exercise tolerance in demand angina. They represent the logical treatment for the patient with normal left ventricular function and stable exertional angina. Except in patients with hypertrophic cardiomyopathy, beta blockers do not influence oxygen supply, so that the threshold for chest pain defined by the rate-pressure product is not increased, but treatment allows this threshold level of rate-pressure product to be reached at a higher workload. By virtue of their negative chronotropic and inotropic effect they may also be used to reduce myocardial oxygen consumption at rest, and thus have a role in the treatment of unstable supply-side angina. The theoretical possibility of aggravating arterial spasm by the vasoconstrictive effect of beta-2 blockade seems in practice not to be a problem, and can in any case be overcome by using a cardioselective beta-1–blocking agent. In the intensive care unit short-acting drugs such as propranolol and metoprolol are used so that dosage levels can be rapidly adjusted. Esmolol administered intravenously has an even more rapid onset and offset of action and may be used as a continuous infusion to allow the most precise adjustment of dose. In outpatients nadolol and atenolol are generally preferred because they can be given once daily and seem to have fewer and less severe side effects. The dosages of these two water-soluble drugs should be reduced in patients with renal failure.

Sublingual nitroglycerin usually terminates an episode of angina, the mode of action depending on the circumstances. In stable demand-side angina nitroglycerin lowers oxygen demand by virtue of abruptly lowering systemic arterial pressure. Its coronary vasodilator effect does not act at the site of fixed arteriosclerotic narrowing and is thus irrelevant. As with beta-blocking therapy, any enhancement of exercise performance following prophylactic nitroglycerin is attributable not to an increase in rate-pressure product at the onset of pain, but to an increased workload when that threshold level of oxygen demand is reached. In contrast, in the patient whose supply-side, unstable angina is due to coronary spasm, nitroglycerin has its effect directly on the coronary artery. Even though it will not dilate a fixed stenosis, it is highly effective at abolishing a transient narrowing or increase in narrowing due to spasm. Patients with impaired left ventricular function may benefit from a third mechanism of action of nitrates, namely, their venodilator property. In this respect they act in a fashion comparable to rapid venesection, lowering the ventricular filling pressures. In the patient with ventricular dysfunction whose subendocardial perfusion is compromised by a high diastolic intracavitary pressure, they thereby improve subendocardial ischemia.

The phenomena of tachyphylaxis and nitrate tolerance make it impossible to extrapolate directly from the acute effects of nitroglycerin to the actions of longer-acting nitrate compounds. A single dose of isosorbide dinitrate, for example, may provide a hypotensive effect that lasts for several hours, thereby improving exercise tolerance long enough to complete some specific task or activity. However, the same dose taken regularly 4 times per day quickly becomes ineffective, hence the absence of a role for nitrates in the chronic treatment of hypertension. One possible way round this is to leave an untreated period of 12 hours or more daily, but in general long-acting nitrates have only a very limited role in treatment of stable angina in the presence of normal ventricular function. In contrast, continuous administration of nitrates by infusion or transdermally may be invaluable in the patient for whom prevention of coronary artery spasm is the aim of therapy, and may therefore be the first choice of treatment for a patient with unstable angina. The venodilator effects of nitrates seems to be less subject to tachyphylaxis than the arterial effect, so that in patients with left ventricular dysfunction chronic nitrate treatment, whether transcutaneous or oral, may be of long-term benefit in maintaining subendocardial perfusion. A particular circumstance where such treatment should be considered is the patient with angina decubitus, a symptom whose significance is comparable to that of paroxysmal nocturnal dyspnea, in whom additional diuretic therapy leads only to dehydration, while nitrates given at night successfully counteract the effect of recumbency on ventricular filling.

Of the three calcium channel blockers in general use, nifedipine is the most potent vasodilator, and hence the most effective for treatment of coronary spasm. It thus has its role almost exclusively in the treatment of supply-side unstable angina. Its side effects naturally include hypotension, and the resulting refex tachycardia may occasionally lead to problems by increasing oxygen demand. It has no role in treatment of stable angina and should be used cautiously in patients with impaired left ventricular function because of some negative inotropic effect.

Verapamil is a much less potent vasodilator than nifedipine, but has a much more depressant effect on heart rate and inotropic state. It has no role in treatment of unstable angina, but may on occasion be used for demand angina as a substitute for beta-blocking agents in patients who have asthma, Raynaud's phenomenon, or some other contraindication to beta blockade. The drug has its chief value as an antiarrhythmic agent rather than in the treatment of ischemia.

The clinical effects of diltiazem lie somewhere in between those of nifedipine and verapamil. The drug does seem to be effective for patients with coronary artery spasm, and can be used in unstable angina; it is not such a powerful vasodilator as nifedipine and tends therefore to be better tolerated. It also has some effect on heart rate and blunts the reflex response to vasodilation as well as reducing the heart rate response to exercise so that it may also be of some value in patients with demand angina.

In summary, management strategy in patients with angina depends on a detailed appraisal of the pathophysiologic mechanisms at work, and of the patient's prognosis. When clinical findings indicate that the patient is at high risk, or when medical therapy is ineffective, then coronary angiography and a revascularization procedure may be required. Otherwise, drug treatment should be offered, the choice of medications depending on the particular clinical circumstances.

1. Fowler, N. O. Angina pectoris: clinical diagnosis. *Circulation* 46:1079, 1972.
   Clues and pitfalls in clinical evaluation of chest pain.
2. Robinson, B. F. Relation of heart rate and systolic blood pressure to the onset of pain in angina pectoris. *Circulation* 35:1073, 1967.
   Defines threshold for demand angina in terms of rate-pressure product.
3. Lange, R. L., Reid, M. S., Tresch D. D., et al. Nonatheromatous ischemic heart disease following withdrawal from industrial nitroglycerin exposure. *Circulation* 46:666, 1972.
   First demonstration of coronary spasm in patients.
4. Maseri, A., Chierchia, S., and L'Abbate, A. Pathogenetic mechanisms underlying the clinical events associated with atherosclerotic heart disease. *Circulation* 62 (Suppl. 5):V-3, 1980.
   Pathogenetic mechanisms—particularly coronary spasm—in unstable angina, reviewed by the group who demonstrated them in patients.
5. Sherman, C. T., Litvack, F., Grundfest, W., et al. Coronary angioscopy in unstable angina pectoris. *N. Engl. J. Med.* 315:913, 1986.
   Direct visualization of thrombosis in unstable angina.
6. McNeer, J. F., Margolis, J. R., Lee, K. L., et al. The role of the exercise test in the evaluation of patients for ischemic heart disease. *Circulation* 57:64, 1978.
   Stress tests predict the extent of coronary artery disease, and also have independent predictive value for prognosis.
7. Goldschlager, N., Selzer, A., and Cohn, K. Treadmill stress tests as indicators of presence and severity of coronary artery disease. *Ann. Intern. Med.* 85:277, 1976.
   Criteria for strong positivity.
8. Thompson, P. T., and Kelemen, M. H. Hypotension accompanying the onset of exertional angina. *Circulation* 52:28, 1975.
   Predicts left main narrowing or coronary disease of comparable severity.
9. Friesinger, G. C. The reasonable workup before recommending medical or surgical therapy: an overall strategy. *Circulation* 65 (Suppl. 2):II–21, 1982.
   Indications for coronary angiography.
10. Lewis, H. D., Davis, J. W., Archibald, D. G., et al. Protective effects of aspirin against acute myocardial infarction and death in men with unstable angina. *N. Engl. J. Med.* 309:396, 1983.
    Aspirin reduced likelihood of myocardial infarction in unstable angina.
11. Telford, A. M., and Wilson, C. Trial of heparin versus atenolol in prevention of myocardial infarction in intermediate coronary syndrome. *Lancet* 1:1225, 1981.
    Heparin improves outcome in unstable angina.
12. Mandelkorn, J. B., Wolf, N. M., Singh, S., et al. Intracoronary thrombus in non-transmural myocardial infarction and in unstable angina pectoris. *Am. J. Cardiol.* 52:1, 1983.
    Coronary thrombosis doesn't always cause transmural infarction—hence the thrombolytic treatment of unstable angina.
13. Brunton, T. L. On the use of nitrite of amyl in angina pectoris. *Lancet* 2:97, 1867.

First use of vasodilators in angina; their efficacy predicted from the temporary improvement in some patients following venesection.

14. Robinson, B. F. Mode of action of nitroglycerin in angina pectoris. *Br. Heart J.* 30:295, 1968.
    In stable demand angina, effects of trinitroglycerin (TNG) accounted for by arterial hypotension.
15. Ganz, W., and Marcus, H. S. Failure of intracoronary nitroglycerin to alleviate pacing-induced angina. *Circulation* 46:880, 1972.
    Implying that coronary vasodilation is not the mechanism for pain relief in demand angina.
16. Feldman, R. L., Pepine, C. J., and Conti, C. R. Magnitude of dilatation of large and small coronary arteries by nitroglycerin. *Circulation* 64:324, 1981.
    Least dilatation by TNG in the narrowest stenoses.
17. Thadani, U., Fung, H.-L. Darke. A. C., et al. Oral isosorbide dinitrate in angina pectoris: comparison of duration of action and dose-response relation during acute and sustained therapy. *Am. J. Cardiol.* 49:411, 1982.
    Arterial vasodilator effect of isosorbide dinitrate not sustained in chronic therapy.
18. Leier, C. V., Huss, P., Magovern, R. D., et al. Improved exercise capacity and differing arterial and venous tolerance during chronic isosorbide dinitrate therapy for congestive heart failure. *Circulation* 67:817, 1983.
    Sustained effect of isosorbide dinitrate on ventricular filling pressure during chronic treatment, even after developing arterial tolerance.
19. Gerber, J. G., and Nies, A. S. Beta-adrenergic blocking drugs. *Ann. Rev. Med.* 36:145, 1985.
    General review of beta-blocking drugs.
20. Braunwald, E. Mechanism of action of calcium-channel-blocking agents. *N. Engl. J. Med.* 307:1618, 1982.
    Helpful account of calcium channels for the clinician.
21. Henry, P. D. Comparative pharmacology of calcium antagonists: nifedipine, verapamil and diltiazem. *Am. J. Cardiol.* 46:1047, 1980.
    Pharmacokinetics of nifedipine, diltiazem, and verapamil.
22. Gerstenblith, G., Ouyang, P., Achuff, S. C., et al. Nifedipine in unstable angina: a double-blind, randomized trial. *N. Engl. J. Med.* 306:885, 1982.
    Nifedipine in patients with pure supply-side unstable angina.

28. AORTIC STENOSIS
H. Verdain Barnes

Aortic stenosis (AS) is a frequent cause of functionally significant cardiac disease and death. It can be subvalvular, valvular, or supravalvular. For practical purposes, *subvalvular* aortic stenosis can be divided into membranous and muscular types. Membranous obstruction to left ventricular outflow is produced by a ring of fibrous tissue below the aortic ring that may be due to incomplete atrophy of the bulbus cordis. The muscular variety of subaortic stenosis is the more common type. It is called *hypertrophic cardiomyopathy.* In hypertropic cardiomyopathy the obstruction to left ventricular outflow is secondary to an asymmetric thickening of the anterior myocardium with predominant involvement of the ventricular septum. The impedance to systolic flow is a consequence of reduced compliance and impaired left ventricular function.

The clinical differences between the two types of subvalvular aortic stenosis are important to diagnosis and therapy. The characteristics of hypertrophic cardiomyopathy *not* seen in the membranous type are (1) onset of murmur in late childhood or adult life, (2) a positive family history, (3) postexercise syncope or angina, (4) increasing symptoms after nitroglycerin and occasionally digitalis, (5) brisk upstroke of the carotid pulse, (6) maximum murmur and thrill along the left sternal edge to the apex, (7) almost invariably an increase in murmur intensity during Valsalva maneuver and frequently a decrease on squatting, (8) right ventricular enlargement, (9) presence of atrial fibrillation (in about 10 percent of patients), (10) Q waves in standard and left precordial leads of the electrocardiogram and delta waves in some, (11) decrease in systemic arterial pulse pressure in the postventricular contraction period, (12) increase in outflow pressure gradient during Valsalva maneuver, and (13) clinical improvement with beta-adrenergic blockade. In hypertrophic cardiomyopathy the most common complaints are those of dyspnea on exertion, increased fatigability, syncope, and angina. Sudden death occurs in up to 5 percent of patients.

Valvular aortic stenosis is congenital or acquired. In recent studies from 33 to 43 percent of surgical cases were for a congenitally abnormal valve while the cases due to postinflammatory disease ranged from 18 to 33 percent and those due to degenerative calcification from 23 to 46 percent. In congenital AS the valve can have a single cusp and commissure, two cusps and commissures, or a fusion of the three cusps. The bicuspid variety is present in more than 50 percent of these patients. In unicuspid disease, the murmur is present at birth or in infancy; in bicuspid disease, the stenosis may have its onset from infancy to middle age. With the unicuspid valve, there is about a 90 percent incidence of associated aortic insufficiency whereas with the bicuspid valve, aortic insufficiency is uncommon. Differentiation between unicuspid and bicuspid disease cannot be made by physical examination. The differentiation can be made with an angiogram since the leaflets of the bicuspid valve are dome-shaped during systole, the ejection jet is central, and the sinuses of Valsalva reflect bicuspid anatomy during diastole.

In *congenital* AS, the majority of patients do well during the first three decades of life. Hemodynamic changes, however, are often progressive during these asymptomatic decades. Consequently all patients should be closely followed. Sudden death accounts for about 50 percent of the deaths in children and one-third of the deaths in adults. The incidence of sudden death is about 0.4 percent per year during the first three decades in untreated patients; thereafter, it increases with age. Bacterial endocarditis occurs in approximately 1 percent of patients per year.

The most common variety of acquired valvular AS is the degenerative calcific variety, which occurs primarily in the elderly. Calcific AS can occur on a congenitally bicuspid valve or a normal valve. In many patients, calcific AS produces no significant hemodynamic changes, and the patients remain asymptomatic. Calcification is located at the base of the aortic cusps, and increases with age. In the elderly, the classic findings of AS are often modified or absent. Most older patients have a moderately loud (low grade in about 10%) rather than a loud murmur, rarely have an inaudible second heart sound or a narrow pulse pressure, and do not have chest x-ray evidence of a markedly enlarged heart. On the other hand, ECG evidence of left ventricular hypertrophy is characteristic in this age group. A long asymptomatic period is common and the complications of angina and syncope often develop prior to dyspnea or overt congestive heart failure. Over half of these patients will have at least one of these complications at the time of presentation. Two unusual but major complications are hemolytic anemia and gastrointestinal bleeding. In the unoperated patient death usually occurs within 2 years after the onset of congestive heart failure, within 3 years after the onset of syncope, and within 5 years after angina begins.

Supravalvular aortic stenosis is a rare congenital abnormality that is inherited as an autosomal dominant. It may or may not be associated with hypercalcemia in infancy. Those patients who have both AS and hypercalcemia have mental retardation and an "elfin" facies. Three pathologic types of supravalvular AS have been described—focal hourglass, hypoplastic ascending aorta, and membranous.

1. Cohen, J., Effat, H., Goodwin, J. F., et al. Hypertrophic obstructive cardiomyopathy. *Br. Heart J.* 26:16, 1964.
   Discusses membranous and muscular subvalvular aortic stenosis.
2. Frank, S., and Braunwald, E. Idiopathic hypertrophic subaortic stenosis. *Circulation* 37:759, 1968.
   Sudden death occurred in about 5% of patients, atrial fibrillation in 8%, and symptomatic pulmonary hypertension in about 30%.

3. Mason, D. T., Braunwald, E., and Ross, J., Jr. Effects of changes in body position on the severity of obstruction to left ventricular outflow in idiopathic hypertrophic subaortic stenosis. *Circulation* 33:374, 1966.
Decreased venous return results in an increase in the signs and symptoms of IHSS.

4. Reeve, R. Clues to the bedside diagnosis of mild idiopathic subaortic stenosis. *J.A.M.A.* 195:131, 1966.
Valsalva maneuver can be helpful at the bedside, producing an increase in the intensity and duration of the murmur.

5. Stefadouros, M. A., Mucha, E., and Frank M. J. Paradoxic response to the murmur of idiopathic hypertrophic subaortic stenosis to the Valsalva maneuver. *Am. J. Cardiol.* 37:89, 1976.
Beware—an occasional patient's murmur attenuates with Valsalva maneuver.

6. Bulkley, B. H., Weisfeldt, M. L., and Hutchins, G. M. Isometric cardiac contraction. *N. Engl. J. Med.* 295:135, 1977.
The unusual septal architecture in IHSS may result from a small systolic ventricular cavity and late systolic isometric contraction.

7. Simon, A. L., Ross, J., Jr., and Gault, J. H. Angiographic anatomy of the left ventricle and mitral valve in idiopathic hypertrophic subaortic stenosis. *Circulation* 36:852, 1968.
The angiographic findings in IHSS are discussed in detail.

8. Roberts W. C. Anatomically isolated aortic valve disease. *Am. J. Med.* 49:151, 1970.
Isolated valvular AS is rarely the result of rheumatic valvular disease.

9. Campbell, M. The natural history of congenital aortic stenosis. *Br. Heart J.* 30:514, 1968.
Most patients do well during the first three decades. Sudden death occurred in 0.4% of the patients per year.

10. Simon, A. L., and Reis, R. E. The angiographic features of bicuspid and unicommissural aortic stenosis. *Am. J. Cardiol.* 28:353, 1971.
The criteria for an angiographic distinction between unicuspid and bicuspid disease are presented.

11. Falcone, M. W., Roberts, W. C., Morrow, A. G., et al. Congenital aortic stenosis resulting from unicommissural valve: Clinical and anatomic features in 21 adult patients. *Circulation* 44:272, 1971.
88% of the patients with unicuspid disease had associated aortic insufficiency.

12. Friedman, W. F., Modlinger, J., and Morgan, J. R. Serial hemodynamic observations in asymptomatic children with valvar aortic stenosis. *Circulation* 43:91, 1971.
The disease may be hemodynamically progressive in the asymptomatic patient.

13. Marsh, G. W., and Lewis, S. M. Cardiac haemolytic anaemia. *Semin. Hematol.* 6:133, 1969.
Hemolytic anemia can be seen in the patients prior to surgery. A good general review.

14. Galloway, S. J., Casarella, W. J., and Shimkin, P. M. Vascular malformations of the right colon as a cause of bleeding in patients with aortic stenosis. *Radiology* 113:11, 1974.
A possible explanation of this perplexing problem in some AS patients.

15. Ross, J., Jr., Fisher, D., Behrendt, D. M., et al. Obstruction to left ventricular outflow: Current concepts of management and operative treatment. *Ann. Intern. Med.* 69:1255, 1968.
A discussion of the natural history of AS before and after the onset of symptoms and complications.

16. Adelman, A. G., Wigle, E. D., Ranganathan, N., et al. The clinical course in muscular subaortic stenosis. *Ann. Intern. Med.* 77:515, 1972.
68% of patients had a murmur as the first evidence of disease. 93% developed class II symptoms within 10 years.

17. Ross, J., Jr. Left ventricular function and the timing of surgery in valvular heart disease. *Ann. Intern. Med.* 94:498, 1981.
A useful discussion of this perplexing problem. In AS the primary indicator appears to be the development of significant clinical symptoms.

18. Carabello, B. A., Green, L. H., Grossman, W., et al. Hemodynamic determinants of

prognosis of aortic valve replacement in critical aortic stenosis and advanced congestive heart failure. *Circulation* 62:42, 1980.
*When the reduction in ejection fraction is not related to increased afterload, the sur-
gical prognosis is very poor.*

19. Mills, P., Leech, G., Davis, M., et al. Natural history of a nonstenotic bicuspid aortic valve. *Br. Heart J.* 40:951, 1978.
    The prognosis is generally good. Only two of 41 patients developed enough stenosis in an 11-year follow-up to require surgery, but three patients had infective endocarditis.

20. Strickberger, S. A., Schulman, S. P., and Hutchins, G. M. Association of Paget's disease of bone with calcific aortic valve disease. *Am. J. Med.* 82:953, 1987.
    The more advanced the Paget's the greater the calcification.

21. Passik, C. S., Ackermann, D. M., Pluth, J. R., et al. Temporal changes in the causes of aortic stenosis: A surgical pathologic study of 646 cases. *Mayo Clin. Proc.* 62:119, 1987.
    During the 5-year study period there was a decrease in rheumatic (postinflammatory) and bicuspid valve disease and an increase in degenerative calcific disease.

22. Lombard, J. T., and Selzer, A. Valvular aortic stenosis: A clinical and hemodynamic profile of patients. *Ann. Intern. Med.* 106:292, 1987.
    The classic findings of AS may not be present in the elderly.

23. Hoagland, P. M., Cook, E. F., Wynne, J., et al. Value of noninvasive testing in adults with suspected aortic stenosis. *Am. J. Med.* 80:1041, 1986.

24. Johnson, G. R., Myers, G. S., Lees, R. S., et al. Evaluation of aortic stenosis by spectral analysis of the murmur. *Am. Coll. Cardiol.* 6:55, 1985.
    It may be possible to effectively evaluate patients noninvasively (articles 23, 24). More data are needed.

25. Selzer, A. Changing aspects of the natural history of valvular aortic stenosis. *N. Engl. J. Med.* 317:91, 1987.
    Current well-referenced review.

26. Schneider, J. F., Wilson, M., and Gallant, T. E. Percutaneous balloon aortic valvuloplasty for aortic stenosis in elderly patients at high risk for surgery. *Ann. Intern. Med.* 106:696, 1987.
    In selected patients, at least short-term improvement can be achieved.

29. ATRIAL MYXOMA
Jerry L. Spivak

Myxoma is the most common primary cardiac tumor. It can arise in any chamber of the heart, but it is found most often in the left atrium, where it arises from the septum near the fossa ovalis. The tumor is usually pedunculated rather than sessile, is rarely multiple, may be gelatinous or firm in consistency and rarely, bilateral in location. Myxomas can occur at any age, but they usually present in the fifth decade, most commonly in females, and tumor growth may be rapid.

The clinical presentation is variable, depending on the location, size, and consistency of the tumor. By virtue of its location, the tumor is likely to obstruct the flow of venous blood in and out of the atrium. In addition, large mobile tumors may disrupt the continuity of the valvular apparatus, resulting in regurgitation as well as stenosis. If trauma from a mobile tumor is sufficient, valvular damage and chordal rupture can occur. Obstructive tumors in the right atrium can mimic constrictive pericarditis, tricuspid stenosis, tricuspid insufficiency, Ebstein's anomaly, carcinoid, and right ventricular failure.

Such tumors have also been associated with right-to-left shunts at the atrial level, clubbing, cyanosis, erythrocytosis, and vena caval obstruction. Since these features may also occur in cirrhosis and with hepatoma—a tumor known to invade the vena cava and occasionally the right atrium—the diagnosis is not easy. A left atrial myxoma can produce pulmonary hypertension by obstructing either or both pulmonary venous or atrioventricular flow. Postural dyspnea can result from either type of obstruction. Tumor growth usually exceeds any compensatory atrial enlargement, further compounding the problem. It is of interest that pulmonary hypertension resulting from an atrial myxoma is much more severe than would be expected for the duration and degree of obstruction. Pulmonary hypertension is not, however, a feature peculiar to left-sided myxomas and can occur with right-sided tumors as a consequence of embolic phenomena. Embolic events are not uncommonly the first sign of the presence of these tumors. Hemiplegia in a young adult or emboli in the absence of heart failure or atrial fibrillation should arouse suspicion that the source is an atrial myxoma. The diagnosis has also been suggested by the discovery of myxomatous tissue on careful sectioning of an arterial embolus. Constitutional signs may be a prominent part of the clinical picture. They include fever, arthralgias, weight loss, clubbing, anemia, hyperglobulinemia, and an elevated erythrocyte sedimentation rate. The anemia is not uncommonly hemolytic, and although a positive Coombs' test has been reported, hemolysis is more often due to trauma by the tumor or turbulent flow. In some cases thrombocytopenia has also been found, suggesting that in these patients disseminated intravascular coagulation (DIC) with resultant microangiopathy is the mechanism for hemolysis. A low erythrocyte sedimentation rate in one such case supports this conclusion.

Recently, a unique familial syndrome has been recognized in which cardiac myxomas occur in association with pigmented microcutaneous and ocular lesions (lentigines), skin myxomas, Cushing's syndrome, mammary fibroadenomas, testicular tumors, and pituitary adenomas. The syndrome appears to be inherited in a dominant mode and the cutaneous manifestations may precede the development of the cardiac lesions. In contrast to "sporadic" or nonfamilial myxomas, cardiac myxomas which develop as part of the familial syndrome occur at an earlier age, are more often multiple, occasionally ventricular in location, and are more likely to recur. Cytogenetic studies have documented the clonal origin of these tumors.

The possibility of an atrial myxoma should be considered in any patient with unexplained dyspnea, pulmonary edema, isolated tricuspid valve disease, refractory and rapidly progressive right or left heart failure (particularly when it develops in a setting of good health), myocardial infarction at a young age, progressive pulmonary hypertension, mitral stenosis without left atrial enlargement or atrial fibrillation, "culture-negative" bacterial endocarditis, and when there are cutaneous lesions or an endocrinopathy. Rheumatic fever, mitral stenosis, infectious endocarditis, cardiac calcification, mitral regurgitation, and atrial fibrillation have all occurred in patients with myxomas and cannot be used to exclude the diagnosis. Most patients with myxomas have cardiac murmurs and occasionally friction rubs. The tumors can mimic mitral stenosis or regurgitation although S1 is usually split and the S2–OS interval is long. The ECG and chest x ray are usually of no diagnostic help. Contrary to popular belief, syncope occurs in less than 25 percent of patients with atrial myxomas, and postural changes are not always present.

With the development of echocardiography and newer techniques such as magnetic resonance imaging (MRI), safe noninvasive diagnostic techniques are available for identifying the presence of cardiac tumors. Echocardiography should be performed in all the clinical situations listed above, as well as in every patient with suspected mitral or tricuspid stenosis. Atrial myxoma is a curable cause of mitral or tricuspid stenosis, but if left undiagnosed can result in the death of the patient, often as a sudden event. In addition, transseptal cardiac catheterization can be fatal in patients with an atrial myxoma. If echocardiography is not available, a cardiac blood pool scan may provide evidence of an intracardiac filling defect. Removal of the tumor usually results in complete reversal of cardiac and constitutional symptoms. The picture at the 5- to 10-year follow-up is excellent but both recurrences and metastases including arterial wall invasion with aneurysm formation have been documented. Recent studies have documented the epithelial origin of certain myxomas.

portant to be aware that a wide fixed split of the second heart sound may not be present, and splitting may be normal or near normal. The first heart sound may be split. Diagnosis is usually uncomplicated in older children or young adults, but is frequently missed in infants or small children and may be missed in middle-aged adults. In the older adult it may be misdiagnosed as mitral stenosis and insufficiency. Since the defect is surgically correctable, it is important to thoroughly evaluate those patients with findings compatible with but not diagnostic of ASD.

It is often impossible to distinguish the various types of ASD by auscultation. The ostium primum variety, however, should be suspected in the presence of a holosystolic murmur medial to the apex of the heart. The ECG is often helpful. In the primum defect, 90 percent of patients show left axis deviation, whereas in the other types there is usually right axis deviation, incomplete right bundle branch block, and an RSR in V_1. The chest x ray usually shows mild cardiomegaly, an enlarged pulmonary artery segment, and increased vascular markings in the peripheral lung fields. The ECG and chest x ray, however, may be normal if the left-to-right shunt is small. When ASD is suspected, its presence can be confirmed by right heart catheterization. Before catheterization, consideration should be given to documenting the diagnosis by contrast two-dimensional echocardiography and scintigraphy, useful noninvasive diagnostic tools.

In caring for ASD patients, one should appreciate the natural history of the disease and the results of surgical correction. According to most series, young adult patients are usually asymptomatic and well. Dyspnea on exertion is the most common symptom, but it is usually not disabling in the young adult. Eighty-six percent of patients experience no change in their status until their mid-fifties to sixties. In the older age group, progressive disability is most often associated with atrial fibrillation or flutter. The single most important complication and risk factor is pulmonary hypertension, which occurs in about 14 percent of young adult patients. Pulmonary hypertension may be abrupt in onset and progress rapidly over a 2- to 3-year period. Its presence can lead to shunt reversal and cyanosis, apparently a key factor in operative morbidity and mortality. The exact cause of the pulmonary hypertension is unknown; however, current data support the concept of a hyperreactive vasculature, resulting in a state of chronic pulmonary hypercirculation and changes in the intima of the vessels. Congestive heart failure is uncommon, occurring in only 4 percent of patients with ASD. Atrial arrhythmias are common, and they increase in incidence with age. Stroke due to cerebral embolization may be the presenting manifestation in undiagnosed, or a complication in diagnosed, patients. It can occur with or without an associated atrial arrhythmia. In the absence of an arrhythmia, it appears to be due to paradoxical embolism.

In general, life expectancy is decreased. In one series, 87 percent of patients without pulmonary vascular changes were alive after 10 years as compared to 25 percent of those with pulmonary vascular disease. Surgery may produce a significant fall in pulmonary artery systolic pressure without any demonstrable change in established pulmonary vascular resistance. Operative mortality and morbidity are significantly increased when the pulmonary artery systolic pressure is greater than 75 mm Hg. Since there is currently no way to predict when and who will develop pulmonary hypertension and pulmonary vascular disease, surgical repair should be considered in all ASD patients, regardless of their age or the size of the defect and shunt. This is particularly true in uncomplicated secundum ASD, in which operative mortality is less than 1 percent in most centers. The surgical mortality in primum defect repair is somewhat higher. On occasion surgical repair may be successful in patients who already have moderate pulmonary hypertension and/or congestive heart failure.

1. Craig, R. J., and Selzer, A. Natural history and prognosis of atrial septal defect. Circulation 37:805, 1968.
   The best series concerning the natural history of ASD.
2. Sudarshan, K., and Luisada, A. A. The second heart sound in atrial septal defect. Am. J. Cardiol. 28:168, 1971.
   The split second sound is due to a dilated pulmonary artery.
3. Edwards, J. E. Functional pathology of the pulmonary vascular tree in congenital cardiac disease. Circulation 15:164, 1957.
   Pulmonary arterial changes are primarily intimal.

4. Kimball, K. G., and McIlroy, M. B. Pulmonary hypertension in patients with congenital heart disease. *Am. J. Med.* 41:883, 1966.
   Pulmonary arterial hypertension and vascular changes increase the operative risk.
5. Dalen, J. E., Haynes, F. W., and Dexter, L. Life expectancy with atrial septal defect. *J.A.M.A.* 200:442, 1967.
   Life expectancy is clearly related to the presence or absence of increased pulmonary vascular resistance.
6. Saksena, F. B., and Aldridge, H. E. Atrial septal defect in the older patient: A clinical and hemodynamic study in patients operated on after age 35. *Circulation* 42:1009, 1970.
   Surgical correction can be beneficial in patients with moderate pulmonary hypertension and/or congestive heart failure.
7. Andersen, M., Lyngborg, K., Moller, I., et al. The natural history of small atrial septal defects: Long-term follow-up with serial heart catheterizations. *Am. Heart J.* 92:302, 1976.
   No clinical deterioration was seen during a mean follow-up of 11.6 years, but of the 26 patients, 4 showed a significant increase in left-to-right shunt, of whom 3 were from the 10 patients whose defects were first diagnosed as adults.
8. Popio, I. A., Gorlin, R., Teichholz, L. E., et al. Abnormalities of left ventricular function and geometry in adults with an atrial septal defect. *Am. J. Cardiol.* 36:302, 1975.
   Patients with an ostium secundum defect showed a subnormal left ventricular volume, and the majority of these showed an abnormal sequence of septum contraction.
9. Losay, J., Rosenthal, A., Castaneda, A. R., et al. Repair of atrial septal defect primum: Results, course and prognosis. *J. Thorac. Cardiovasc. Surg.* 75:248, 1978.
   A study of 92 patients supporting the need for early repair.
10. Forfang, K., Simonsen, S., Andersen, A., et al. Atrial septal defect of secundum type in the middle aged. *Am. Heart J.* 94:44, 1977.
    Repair in patients over age 40 resulted in about 23% of the preoperative functional class III and IV patients becoming class I.
11. Betrinick, E. H., and Schiller, N. B. The complementary roles of M mode echocardiography and scintigraphy in the evaluation of adults with suspected left-to-right shunts. *Circulation* 62:1070, 1980.
    A sensitive, noninvasive duo for diagnosing ASD.
12. Winer, H. E., and Kronzon, I. Absence of paradoxical pulse in patients with cardiac tamponade and atrial septal defects. *Am. Heart J.* 44:378, 1979.
13. Radtke, W. E., Smith, H. C., Fulton, R. E., et al. Misdiagnosis of atrial septal defect in patients with hereditary telangiectasia (Osler-Rendu-Weber disease) and hepatic arteriovenous fistulas. *Am. Heart J.* 95:235, 1978.
    Pearls (12, 13) to keep in mind.
14. Harvey, J. R., Teague, S. M., Anderson, J. L., et al. Clinically silent atrial septal defects with evidence of cerebral embolization. *Ann. Intern. Med.* 105:695, 1986.
    ASD should be suspected in younger patients with an embolic stroke.

31. CARDIAC ARRHYTHMIAS
Thomas Guarnieri

The approach to the patient with a cardiac arrhythmia is quite variable, ranging from emotional support to emergent cardiopulmonary resuscitation and cardioversion. The modalities for the treatment of cardiac arrhythmias have expanded remarkably in the last decade and range from a variety of antiarrhythmic drugs to sophisticated devices and/or surgical techniques for correction. There are three principles in the approach to the management of a patient with a cardiac arrhythmia: (1) an *exact* definition of the cardiac arrhythmia; (2) placement of the arrhythmia in the overall perspective of the physiologic and pathologic status of the cardiovascular system, that is, is there significant heart disease present?; and (3) deciding what type of treatment, if any, is appropriate.

In the last decade a significant amount of information has evolved documenting the mechanisms of cardiac arrhythmia in man. The mechanisms are grouped as disturbances of automaticity, conduction, or both. Reentry is probably the most frequent mechanism of cardiac arrhythmia. It has been proved that reentry is the mechanism of the atrioventricular (AV) reciprocating tachycardia seen in the Wolff-Parkinson-White syndrome (WPW). WPW has served as a model for understanding cardiac arrhythmia for the last decade, as all principles of reentry are present, and can be easily understood. It is probable, though not proved, that reentry is the cause for most forms of ventricular tachycardia (VT), paroxysmal supraventricular tachycardia (PSVT), and atrial flutter. Abnormal automaticity is a mechanism of cardiac arrhythmia most frequently seen in either drug-induced arrhythmias or in incessant atrial tachycardia of childhood (ectopic tachycardia). In the last several years a third mechanism of tachycardia, called triggering, has emerged. This mechanism is thought to occur from incomplete repolarization of the cardiac cell or de novo depolarization of the cardiac cell, which is dependent on the previous beat, hence the term "triggering." This mechanism of arrhythmia is probably present in digitalis overdose, or some forms of disorganized ventricular tachycardia, especially torsade des pointes.

Defining the cardiac arrhythmia can seldom be done on the basis of the history and physical examination. Some clues on the physical examination can be helpful, including flutter waves in the jugular venous wave form, or varying first heart sound with a regular rhythm (suggestive of AV dissociation). Other than these clues the history and physical examination are frequently nonspecific in the patient with cardiac arrhythmia, and in fact can be misleading during the evaluation of a patient with a wide complex QRS tachycardia (see below). The recording of a 12-lead ECG during the cardiac arrhythmia is the single most important piece of information that can be gathered for the definition of the arrhythmia. Frequently, mistakes in the definition of a cardiac arrhythmia (the wide QRS complex tachycardia) are made by examining only a single channel or a monitored lead recording. Every effort must be made on the 12-lead ECG to determine the AV relationship during the tachycardia. Additional leads are frequently helpful for determining the relationship between the atria and the ventricles during the tachycardia, including Lewis surface leads or esophageal recording.

One particular example in the problem of the differential diagnosis of a cardiac arrhythmia is the so-called wide QRS complex tachycardia. In older literature this problem is called differentiating ventricular tachycardia from supraventricular tachycardia (SVT) with aberrancy (SVT with bundle branch block). It is clear that the patient presenting to the emergency room with a wide QRS complex tachycardia is frequently mismanaged. Overwhelmingly, the mistake in the emergency room stems from the assumption that a wide QRS complex tachycardia cannot be ventricular tachycardia because the "patient looks so good" or had normal blood pressure during the arrhythmia. This assumption has led to significant and dangerous errors, as many individuals with sustained ventricular tachycardia walk into the emergency room. As a first and important principle it should be remembered that most episodes of wide QRS complex tachycardia presenting to an emergency room are ventricular tachycardia and should be regarded as such. Once this assumption is made, the treatment modalities which then can be employed will rarely make the arrhythmia worse. Conversely the misdiagnosis of the wide QRS complex tachycardia as supraventricular can frequently lead to the misuse of intravenous verapamil or beta blockers, which can be disastrous to an individual with ventricular tachycardia.

Once the arrhythmia is defined, then it must be put into perspective. The most common example of this analysis is the management of the asymptomatic patient with frequent or complex ventricular ectopy in the setting of a normal heart. In individuals with complex ventricular ectopy or unsustained ventricular tachycardia who have normal cardiac function (demonstrated by history, physical examination, chest x ray, echocardiogram, and exercise test) there is little evidence that suppressing the arrhythmia will have any benefit. In fact, the antiarrhythmic drugs which would be used under these circumstances frequently are more dangerous than the arrhythmias themselves. Management in this case should be conservative. On the other hand, one of the most difficult dilemmas is the treatment of frequent or complex ectopy in asymptomatic individuals after myocardial infarction or with evidence of substantial heart disease. To date a satisfactory method for deciding which patient requires treatment has not been established. Evaluation and therapy in these types of individuals must be individualized and unfortunately is frequently empiric.

After defining the cardiac arrhythmia and placing the arrhythmia in perspective the decision must be made as to what type of management to employ. Far too often nonpharmacologic management of cardiac arrhythmia is ignored. It cannot be overemphasized that careful attention to management of factors which can precipitate cardiac arrhythmia need attention. For example, it is clear in the patient with recurrent atrial fibrillation and flutter that abstinence from alcohol or caffeine may be the only treatment necessary to prevent the recurrence of arrhythmia or to diminish its frequency. On a more serious note, it should be stated that very close attention must be paid to the interaction between the aggressive management of heart failure (diuretics) and the maintenance of a normal serum potassium in those individuals with congestive heart failure and ventricular arrhythmias. The maintenance of a normal serum potassium remains one of the major, but overlooked, cornerstones of arrhythmia management in these individuals.

If simple measures are unsuccessful, or not warranted, the choice of antiarrhythmic drug is first decided by attacking the "weak link" of the tachycardia. In those tachycardias which use the AV node as a link (PSVT or atrial fibrillation), agents which directly increase the effective refractory period of the AV node are still the most useful, including digoxin, calcium channel blockers, or beta blockers. Rhythms located primarily in the atria, especially atrial flutter or fibrillation, can be managed with either type Ia (quinidinelike) agents or type Ic (flecainide or encainide) agents. Type Ic agents have the advantage of slightly increasing the effective refractory period of the AV node in addition to increasing the effective refractory period of the atrium. This means that at the least these agents will not accelerate conduction through the AV node, similar to the well-known quinidinelike effect of type Ia agents.

When treating ventricular tachycardia the choices become even more difficult and the approach is often limited by the interaction between proved efficacy and intolerable side effects. The efficacy of the drug can be assayed either through Holter monitoring or through provocative testing (electrophysiologic testing), but side effects are generally idiosyncratic. In individuals with significant heart disease who have had serious episodes of ventricular tachycardia or survive cardiac arrest, there is a clear tendency away from using drugs as primary management. In these individuals (aborted sudden death) impressive survival results have been obtained either through direct surgical excision of the tachycardia site or by the use of implantable defibrillators to cardiovert the rhythm. The development of implantable defibrillators is currently in a nascent stage, and it is clear that over the next 5 to 10 years the engineering and modifications necessary to make these devices more useful and widespread will emerge. It is quite possible that within the next 5 years that for individuals who survived an episode of out-of-hospital cardiac arrest or very significant ventricular tachycardia, antiarrhythmic devices will supplant antiarrhythmic drugs as a therapy of first choice.

1. Alpert, J. S., Haffajee, C. I., Young, M. D., et al. Chemistry, pharmacology, antirhythmic efficacy and adverse effects of tocainide hydrochloride, an orally active structured analog of lidocaine. *Pharmacotherapy* 3:316, 1983.
   Extensive review of tocainide.
2. Bigger, J. T. Symposium on flecainide acetate. *Am. J. Cardiol.* 53:1B, 1984.
   The use of flecainide, pre-CAST study.
3. Cox, J. L. The status of surgery for cardiac arrhythmias. *Circulation* 71:413, 1985.
   Critically details the application of surgical techniques; surgery is not the last resort.
4. Echt, D. S., Armstrong, K., Schmidt, P., et al. Clinical experience, complications, and survival in 70 patients with the automatic implantable cardioverter/defibrillator [AICD]. *Circulation* 71:289, 1985.
   The original Stanford experience with the AICD.
5. Gallagher, J. J., Pritchett, E. L. C., Sealy, W. C., et al. The preexcitation syndromes.

Prog. Cardiovasc. Dis. 20:285, 1978.
Duke surgical experience in WPW.
 6. Grant, A. O., Starmer, C. F., and Strauss, H. C. Antiarrhythmic drug action blockade
of the inward sodium current. *Circ. Res.* 55:427, 1984.
Basic mechanisms of antiarrhythmic drugs.
 7. Hammill, S. C., and Pritchett, E. L. C. Simplified esophageal electrocardiography
using bipolar recording leads. *Ann. Intern. Med.* 95:14, 1981.
"How to" approach for esophageal electrocardiography.
 8. Josephson, M. E., Harkin, A. H., and Horowitz, L. N. Endocardial excision: a new
surgical technique for the treatment of recurrent ventricular tachycardia. *Circulation* 60:1430, 1979.
World's largest experience with surgical treatment of VT.
 9. Knochel, J. P. The cardiovascular effects of alcohol. *Ann. Intern. Med.* 98:849, 1983.
Review of the multiple effects of ethanol on cardiac excitation.
10. Mirowski, M., Reid, P. R., Mower, M. M., et al. Termination of malignant ventricular
arrhythmias with implanted automatic defibrillators in human beings. *N. Engl. J.
Med.* 303:322, 1980.
Original report of the AICD.
11. Smith, W. M., and Gallagher, J. J. Les torsades des pointes: an unusual ventricular
arrhythmia. *Ann. Intern. Med.* 93:578, 1980.
Torsade as a drug intoxication rhythm.
12. Spear, J. F., and Moore, E. N. Mechanism of cardiac arrhythmias. *Annu. Rev. Physiol.* 44:485, 1982.
Review of basic mechanism of arrhythmia.
13. Stewart, R. B., Bardy, G. H., and Greene, H. The wide complex tachycardia: misdiagnosis and outcome after emergent therapy. *Ann. Intern. Med.* 104:766, 1986.
*Important reference on the approach to patients with tachycardia in the emergency
room.*
14. Sun, J., Ruey, J., Shapiro, W. A., et al. Effects of verapamil on ventricular tachycardias possibly caused by reentry automaticity and triggered activity. *J. Clin. Invest.*
72:350, 1983.
Speculation on whether some cardiac arrhythmias in humans are "triggered."
15. Wellens, H. J. J., Barr F. W. H. M., and Lie, K. I. The value of the electrocardiogram
in the differential diagnosis of a tachycardia with a widened QRS complex. *Am. J.
Med.* 64:27, 1978.
*First report of correlation of surface ECG and intracardiac ECG to differentiate VT
from SVT with aberrancy.*
16. Wellens, H. J. J. Wolff-Parkinson-White syndrome. *Mod. Concepts Cardiovasc. Dis.*
52:53, 1987.
Practical approach to WPW.
17. Wilbur, D. J., Garan, H., Finklestein, D., et al. Out of hospital cardiac arrest: the use
of electrophysiologic testing in the prediction of the long-term outcome. *N. Engl. J.
Med.* 318:19, 1988.
*One of the largest series of the use of electrophysiologic testing to prevent recurrent
cardiac arrest.*
18. Zipes, D. P., Prystowski, E. N., Heger, J. J., et al. Amiodarone: electrophysiologic
actions, pharmacokinetics, and clinical effects. *J. Am. Coll. Cardiol.* 3:1059, 1984.
Review of the pharmacology of amiodarone.

32. CARDIOMYOPATHY
James K. Porterfield

The cardiomyopathies comprise a group of disorders of varying etiology and pathophysiology in which the major feature is involvement of the heart muscle itself. Cardiomyopathies are divided into three broad categories based on the underlying pathophysiology: (1) *dilated,* or "congestive," characterized by ventricular dilatation and contractile dysfunction; (2) *hypertrophic,* characterized by an inappropriate increase in ventricular muscle mass, often with asymmetric involvement of the septum, and preserved systolic function; and (3) *restrictive,* marked by impaired diastolic filling due to noncompliance of the endocardium or myocardium. The differences between these three types of cardiomyopathy are not absolute and it may be particularly difficult to distinguish between the hypertrophic and restrictive forms. Our ability to diagnose and accurately categorize the cardiomyopathies has been aided by recent technologic advances, particularly the widespread use of echocardiography and endomyocardial biopsy, through which samples can be obtained for histologic analysis.

Dilated cardiomyopathy (DCM) is a syndrome characterized by cardiac enlargement and contractile dysfunction. Symptoms are those of heart failure, primarily dyspnea due to pulmonary venous congestion, along with weakness and fatigue due to diminished cardiac output. Chest pain, when present, suggests associated coronary artery disease. Characteristic physical signs include narrow pulse pressure and pulses alternans. The apical impulse is enlarged and laterally displaced. A presystolic gallop (S4) is usually present and a ventricular gallop (S3) can be heard during periods of cardiac decompensation. A holosystolic blowing murmur is commonly noted, due to dilatation of the mitral valve annulus with resultant failure of leaflet coaptation. If right heart failure develops, the systolic murmur may be due to tricuspid regurgitation, as evidenced by prominent V waves in the jugular pulse and an enlarged, pulsatile liver. The development of pulmonary hypertension with right heart failure and tricuspid regurgitation are late signs and are associated with a particularly poor prognosis. The etiology of DCM is likely multifactorial and may represent a "final common pathway" for myocardial injury due to a variety of toxic, metabolic, and infectious insults. Viral myocarditis is often cited as the initiating event leading to DCM, possibly through an autoimmune mechanism. Although there are well-documented cases of progression from myocarditis to DCM, the percentage of individuals with histologic evidence of myocarditis on biopsy has varied widely in several clinical series. In most patients with DCM there is little clinical evidence to suggest a preceding viral infection. Thus, the role of *routine* endomyocardial biopsy in DCM to detect myocarditis and other potentially reversible causes remains controversial. Other established causes of DCM include excessive chronic alcohol ingestion, endocrine disorders (i.e., hyperthyroidism, pheochromocytoma), and selenium deficiency.

The diagnosis of DCM is generally easily made with noninvasive studies. Chest radiography shows cardiomegaly and, with left ventricular failure, pulmonary vascular redistribution. The ECG generally shows sinus tachycardia and intraventricular conduction delay. Both atrial and ventricular tachyarrhythmias are common; indeed, arrhythmias are second in frequency to heart failure as clinical manifestations of DCM. Echocardiography and radionuclide ventriculography are extremely useful techniques for assessing ventricular size and function. The former technique also allows assessment of concomitant valvular or pericardial disease. Cardiac catheterization is performed primarily to evalute ventricular filling pressures and coronary anatomy. Specific therapy for DCM is generally not possible except when a potentially reversible cause, such as myocarditis, is found. Management therefore is directed at controlling symptoms of heart failure and consists of sodium restriction, diuretics, digitalis, nitrates, and vasodilator therapy. Beta blocker therapy has also been employed by some investigators in view of evidence that activation of the sympathetic nervous system may have deleterious effects on the cardiovascular system in these patients, but this therapy has yet to be widely employed. Because of the frequency of embolic events, anticoagulant therapy is recommended for patients with DCM, even in the absence of direct evidence of intracavitary thrombus formation. In appropriate patients, cardiac transplantation has been very successfully employed as treatment for DCM.

Hypertrophic cardiomyopathy (HCM) was first described in detail by Teare in 1958.[13] The most characteristic anatomic feature is inappropriate myocardial hypertrophy, often involving the intraventricular septum out of proportion to the left ventricular (LV) free wall. Soon after the discovery of HCM, reports appeared describing a dynamic pressure gradient in the subaortic area, prompting the descriptive term "idiopathic hyper-trophic subaortic stenosis" (IHSS). Subsequent studies have shown that many patients do not have LV outflow obstruction and therefore HCM is considered to be the more appropriate term. The most characteristic pathophysiologic abnormality in HCM is di-astolic dysfunction. Abnormal diastolic relaxation results in impaired LV filling and el-evated LV end-diastolic pressure. This elevation in LV filling pressure results in dyspnea which is the most common symptom in HCM. In over half the patients, HCM appears to be genetically transmitted as an autosomal dominant trait with a high degree of pene-trance. Sporadic cases are presumably due to new mutations. The underlying defect leading to the myocardial hypertrophy in HCM remains obscure. The concept of a dy-namic outflow gradient due to systolic anterior motion (SAM) of the mitral valve against the septum has been a source of considerable controversy. Despite the presence of an outflow gradient, it is unlikely that blood flow is actually obstructed in HCM in view of the characteristic finding of rapid ventricular emptying and high ejection fraction. Im-paired diastolic filling is now felt to be the major pathophysiologic abnormality account-ing for the symptoms associated with HCM. The clinical picture ranges from the asymp-tomatic individual who has inappropriate ventricular hypertrophy on echocardiogram to the patient with incapacitating symptoms. Although symptomatic HCM is most com-monly a disease of young adulthood, it occurs more often than previously suspected in elderly patients. It occurs with equal frequency in men and women. The most common symptom is dyspnea which is due to the elevated LV filling pressure. Angina pectoris, syncope, and palpitations are also commonly seen in HCM, while overt heart failure occurs less often. Syncope and sudden death may result from inadequate cardiac output with exertion or from malignant cardiac arrhythmias. The association of sudden cardiac death in these patients with competitive sports and severe exertion necessitates the proscription of these activities.

The physical examination in HCM is noteworthy for a LV with prominent pre-systolic apical impulse. The jugular pulse may show a sharp A wave due to right ven-tricular noncompliance. The carotid pulse is characteristically bifid. The most promi-nent physical sign is a systolic murmur which reflects both outflow tract turbulence and concomitant mitral regurgitation. Thus, the murmur is often more holosystolic and blowing at the apex and midsystolic and harsher along the left sternal border. Unlike valvular aortic stenosis, the systolic murmur of HCM is accentuated by maneuvers which diminish venous return to the heart, such as the Valsalva maneuver or standing. The ECG in HCM commonly exhibits ST segment and T wave abnormalities as well as tall mid-precordial R waves consistent with LV hypertrophy. Prominent, abnormal Q waves in the inferior or lateral leads occur in 20 to 50 percent of patients. The echocar-diogram is the single most useful study in diagnosing HCM. The cardinal feature of echocardiogram is myocardial hypertrophy. The classic pattern of asymmetric septal hy-pertrophy (ASH) occurs in over half of HCM patients although a variety of hypertrophic patterns have been described. The second feature of HCM is narrowing of the LV outflow tract due to anterior motion of the mitral valve during systole (SAM), although this is not pathognomonic of HCM. Doppler ultrasound demonstrates mitral regurgitation and marked deceleration of aortic blood flow coincident with SAM. Cardiac catheterization often demonstrates an intracavitary gradient between the body of the left ventricle and a subaortic chamber from which it is separated by the thickened septum and the ante-rior leaflet to the mitral valve. Care must be taken to avoid artifactual outflow gradients due to catheter entrapment in the hypertrophied trabeculae. Ventriculography typically shows vigorous systolic contraction, often with virtual cavity obliteration. The medical management of patients with HCM is aimed at decreasing the ventricular contractility and increasing ventricular compliance. Beta blockers and calcium antagonists, partic-ularly verapamil, have been shown to reduce LV outflow gradient and improve diastolic filling. Disopyramide has recently been shown to produce symptomatic improvement through its negative inotropic effect. Both supraventricular and ventricular arrhyth-mias can be suppressed with amiodarone. Antibiotic prophylaxis to prevent infective endocarditis is indicated. Septal myotomy-myectomy, with or without concomitant mi-tral valve replacement, has been shown to produce symptomatic improvement in the medically refractory patient.

Restrictive cardiomyopathy is the least common type of cardiomyopathy in Western countries. It is characterized by excessively rigid ventricular walls which impede diastolic filling. Contractile function is generally well preserved. The causes of restrictive cardiomyopathy are numerous and include amyloidosis, hemochromatosis, endomyocardial fibrosis, and neoplastic infiltration. The clinical manifestations include diminished exercise tolerance, weakness, and dyspnea. Common physical signs include elevated central venous pressure with peripheral edema, hepatomegaly, and ascites. Restrictive cardiomyopathy may be very difficult to distinguish from constrictive pericarditis as they have similar hemodynamic and clinical features. Differentiation is crucial in view of the potential for surgical treatment of constrictive pericarditis and can generally be achieved through computed tomography (CT) scanning, magnetic resonance imaging, and endomyocardial biopsy, although exploratory thoracotomy may be rarely needed. The medical treatment of restrictive cardiomyopathy varies widely depending on the underlying cause, which can in many cases be determined by endomyocardial biopsy.

1. Wynne, J., and Braunwald, E. The Cardiomyopathies and Myocarditides. In E. Braunwald (ed.), *Heart Disease* (3rd ed.). Philadelphia: Saunders, 1988.
   Comprehensive review of all of the cardiomyopathies.
2. Mason, J. W. Endomyocardial biopsy: the balance of success and failure. *Circulation* 71:185, 1985.
   Excellent discussion of the role of endomyocardial biopsy in managing patients with cardiomyopathy.
3. Johnson, R. A., and Palacios, I. Dilated cardiomyopathies of the adult. *N. Engl. J. Med.* 307:1051 and 1119, 1982.
   Good general review of DCM.
4. Parrillo, J. E., Aretz, H. T., Palacios, I., et al. The results of transvenous endomyocardial biopsy can frequently be used to diagnose myocardial diseases in patients with idiopathic heart failure. Endomyocardial biopsies in 100 consecutive patients revealed a substantial incidence of myocarditis. *Circulation* 69:93, 1984.
   Authors found a high incidence of myocarditis in patients with DCM.
5. Fenoglio, J. J., Jr., Ursell, P. C., Kellogg, C. F., et al. Diagnosis and classification of myocarditis by endomyocardial biopsy. *N. Engl. J. Med.* 308:12, 1983.
   Good discussion of criteria for diagnosis of myocarditis.
6. Dee, G. W., Jr., Palacios, I. F., Fallon, J. T., et al. Active myocarditis in the spectrum of acute dilated cardiomyopathies. Clinical features, histologic correlates, and clinical outcome. *N. Engl. J. Med.* 312:885, 1985.
   Review of the experience with DCM and myocarditis at the Massachusetts General Hospital.
7. Anderson, J. L., Carlquist, J. F., and Hammond, E. H. Deficient natural killer cell activity in patients with idiopathic dilated cardiomyopathy. *Lancet* 2:1124, 1982.
   Authors suggest a possible role of immune disorder in DCM.
8. Katz, A. M., Freston, J. W., Messineo, F. C., et al. Membrane damage and the pathogenesis of cardiomyopathies. *J. Mol. Cell. Cardiol.* 17:11, 1985.
   Interesting discussion of pathogenesis of DCM.
9. Pasternac, A., Noble, J., Steulens, Y., et al. Pathophysiology of chest pain in patients with cardiomyopathies and normal coronary arteries. *Circulation* 65:778, 1982.
   Author suggests that subendocardial ischemia may be present in DCM in the absence of coronary artery disease.
10. Huang, S. K., Messer, J. V., and Denes, P. Significance of ventricular tachycardia in idiopathic dilated cardiomyopathy: Observations in 35 patients. *Am. J. Cardiol.* 51:507, 1983.
    Relationship between ventricular arrhythmias and risk of sudden cardiac death in patients with DCM has been difficult to establish.
11. Cohn, J. N., Archibald, D. G., Ziesche, S., et al. Effect of vasodilator therapy on mortality in chronic congestive heart failure. Results of Veterans Administration cooperative study. *N. Engl. J. Med.* 314:1547, 1986.
    Study suggests that long-term therapy with hydralazine and nitrates can reduce mortality in DCM.

12. Engelmeier, R. S., O'Connell, J. B., Walsh, R., et al. Improvement in symptoms and exercise tolerance by metoprolol in patients with dilated cardiomyopathy: A double-blind, randomized, placebo-controlled trial. *Circulation* 72:536, 1985.
    Authors found beneficial effect of metoprolol on symptoms and exercise tolerance in patients with DCM.
13. Teare, R. D. Asymmetrical hypertrophy of the heart in young adults. *Br. Heart J.* 20:1, 1958.
    Classic paper describing clinical features of HCM.
14. Morrow, A. G., and Braunwald, E. Functional aortic stenosis: A malformation characterized by resistance to left ventricular outflow without anatomic obstruction. *Circulation* 20:181, 1959.
    Original report of subaortic outflow obstruction in patients with HCM.
15. Epstein, S. E., Henry, W. L., Clark, C. E., et al. Asymmetric septal hypertrophy. *Ann. Intern. Med.* 81:650, 1974.
    Authors propose criteria for defining HCM based on septal–free wall thickness ratio.
16. Maron, B. J., Gottdiener, J. S., Roberts, W. C., et al. Left ventricular outflow tract obstruction due to systolic anterior motion of the anterior mitral leaflet in patients with concentric left ventricular hypertrophy. *Circulation* 57:527, 1978.
    Suggests that the gradient in HCM is due to narrowing of the LV outflow tract by SAM.
17. Come, P. C., Bulkley, B. H., Goodman, Z. D., et al. Hypercontractile cardiac states simulating hypertrophic cardiomyopathy. *Circulation* 55:901, 1977.
    SAM can occur in conditions other than HCM.
18. Topol, E. J., Traill, T. A., and Fortuin, N. J. Hypertensive hypertrophic cardiomyopathy of the elderly. *N. Engl. J. Med.* 312:277, 1985.
    HCM in elderly patients may present as congestive heart failure. Therapy with diuretics and nitrates can be hazardous.
19. Henry, W. L., Clark, C. E., Roberts, W. C., et al. Differences in the distribution of myocardial abnormalities in patients with obstructive and nonobstructive asymmetric septal hypertrophy (ASH). Echocardiographic and gross anatomic findings. *Circulation* 50:447, 1974.
    Authors noted myocardial fiber disarray as an important histopathologic characteristic of HCM.
20. Maron, B. J. Myocardial disorganization in hypertrophic cardiomyopathy. Another point of view. *Br. Heart J.* 50:1, 1983.
    Further analysis of myocardial fiber disarray in HCM.
21. Fiorito, S., Autore, C., Fragola, P. V., et al. HLA-DR3 antigen linkage in patients with hypertrophic obstructive cardiomyopathy. *Am. Heart J.* 111:91, 1986.
    HCM may be linked to the HLA system.
22. Pearce, P. C., Hawkey, C., Symons, C., et al. Role of calcium in the induction of cardiac hypertrophy and myofibrillar disarray. Experimental studies of a possible cause of hypertrophic cardiomyopathy. *Br. Heart J.* 54:420, 1985.
    Study suggests that HCM may be due to abnormal handling of calcium by the myocardium.
23. Maron, B. J., Bonow, R. O., Cannon, R. W., III, et al. Hypertrophic cardiomyopathy: Interrelations of clinical manifestations, pathophysiology and therapy. *N. Engl. J. Med.* 316:780, 844, 1987.
    Good general review of HCM.
24. Criley, J. M., and Siegel, R. J. Has "obstruction" hindered our understanding of hypertrophic cardiomyopathy? *Circulation* 72:1148, 1985.
    Emphasizes the importance of diastolic properties in HCM.
25. Maron, B. J., Roberts, W. C., Edwards, J. E., et al. Sudden death in patients with hypertrophic cardiomyopathy: Characterization of 26 patients without functional limitation. *Am. J. Cardiol.* 41:803, 1978.
    Sudden death may occur in previously asymptomatic patients.
26. Spicer, R. L., Rocchini, A. P., Crowley, D. C., et al. Hemodynamic effects of verapamil in children and adolescents with hypertrophic cardiomyopathy. *Circulation* 67:413, 1983.

Verapamil can decrease the LV outflow gradient by depressing myocardial contractility.

27. Beahrs, M. M., Tajik, A. J., Seward, J. B., et al. Hypertrophic obstructive cardiomyopathy: Ten- to 21-year followup after partial septal myectomy. *Am. J. Cardiol.* 51:1160, 1983.
    Summary of Mayo Clinic experience with surgical treatment of HCM.
28. Maron, B. J., Epstein, S. E., and Roberts, W. C. Causes of sudden death in competitive athletes. *J. Am. Coll. Cardiol.* 7:204, 1986.
    Unsuspected HCM is the most common autopsy finding in young athletes who die suddenly.
29. Benotti, J. R., and Grossman, W. Restrictive cardiomyopathy. *Annu. Rev. Med.* 35:113, 1984.
    Good general review of restrictive cardiomyopathy.
30. Janos, G. G., Arjunan, K., Meyer, R. A., et al. Differentiation of constrictive pericarditis and restrictive cardiomyopathy using digitized echocardiography. *J. Am. Coll. Cardiol.* 1:541, 1983.
    Echocardiography may be useful in distinguishing between restrictive and constrictive processes.
31. Hodkinson, H. M., and Pomerance, A. The clinical signifiance of senile cardiac amyloidosis: A prospective clinicopathological study. *Q.J. Med.* 46:381, 1977.
    Cardiac involvement in senile amyloidosis ranges from asymptomatic deposits to extreme infiltration leading to heart failure.

33. CONGENITAL HEART DISEASE IN ADULTS
Thomas A. Traill

Congenital anomalies in adult patients do not cover the whole range of congenital heart disease. Seriously symptomatic but correctable defects are usually repaired in childhood, so that those left in adults are largely asymptomatic and undetected, hemodynamically trivial, or for some reason uncorrectable. There are only a few patients who require surgical repair of lesions that have gone undiscovered in childhood, or in whom correction has been delayed; in the majority of cases, the decisions to be made pertain to medical management or to such questions as fitness for employment, pregnancy, or insurance.

Lesions that should be repaired if they escape detection until adult life include atrial septal defect, coarctation of the aorta, persistent ductus arteriosus, and the rarer obstructive lesions such as congenital mitral stenosis. Surgical repair of atrial septal defect and other left-to-right shunts at atrial level in middle-aged and elderly patients, when they have reached the inevitable stage of being symptomatic, is particularly rewarding. These are often patients with severe right heart enlargement, fluid retention, dyspnea, and arrhythmias, in whom the first impression may be that they are unlikely to be much improved by anything; however, the results of surgery are gratifying, even in the presence of moderate pulmonary hypertension. Timing of surgery in congenital aortic valve disease is no different from that of acquired aortic valve disease, except that in a few children and teenagers surgery may be deferred at a time of rapid growth so that the final prosthetic replacement may be of adult size. Young people wear out tissue valves faster than old people, so mechanical prostheses should be recommended, unless pregnancy is planned or there exist other contraindications to anticoagulants.

Very few adults with congenital ventricular septal defect (VSD) require surgical attention. If a ventricular septal defect is large enough to cause heart failure or pulmonary vascular disease, it invariably does so in the first few years of life. By the time a patient is fully grown he either has Eisenmenger's syndrome or his lesion is small enough that it can safely be ignored. There are three exceptions to this, namely, recurrent endocarditis; development of aortic regurgitation due to prolapse of the right coronary cusp through the septal defect; and in a few cases progressive left ventricular dilatation due to the volume load imposed by the shunt. Significant pulmonic stenosis rarely escapes detection until adult life because the murmur is so loud. In general the prognosis is predicted by the transvalvular gradient; when the gradient exceeds about 50 mm Hg, the patient should be referred for balloon valvuloplasty or surgical commissurotomy.

Cyanotic congenital heart disease in adult patients is most commonly the result of the Eisenmenger reaction complicating a large VSD or other similar defect. Patients with Eisenmenger's syndrome are of course not suitable for corrective surgery. A few in the late stages of the disease can be treated by heart and lung transplantation but the majority are managed medically, with attention paid to the hematocrit, treatment of arrhythmias, and eventually fluid retention and dyspnea. They are at formidable risk for any major surgery and, like other cyanotic patients, they should be advised against pregnancy.

The cyanotic patient who does not have pulmonary hypertension necessarily has reduced pulmonary blood flow as the result of obstruction at or below the level of the pulmonary valve. From the practical point of view, the immediate diagnostic question in such a patient is whether there is a "complete set of parts" for corrective surgery, or whether the patient has only a single ventricle or great artery. In the former case, typified by tetralogy of Fallot, surgery will often be recommended after appropriate studies have defined the detailed diagnosis and hence the risk of operation. Management of the more complicated lesions has to be worked out case by case. In a few, "physiologic correction" may be achieved by a Fontan procedure, in which the systemic venous return is rerouted to the pulmonary arteries via the right atrium, with no ventricular pump interposed. Such surgery seems to work best in younger patients, and of course requires that the pulmonary vascular resistance and left atrial pressure both be very low.

1. Campbell, M., Neill, C., and Suzman, S. The prognosis of atrial septal defect. *Br. Med. J.* 1:1375, 1957.
   In time all patients with sizeable atrial septal defects seem to become symptomatic.
2. St. John Sutton, M. G., Tajik, A. J., McGoon, D. C., et al. Atrial septal defect in patients ages 60 years or older: operative results and long-term postoperative follow-up. *Circulation* 64:402, 1981.
   Low risk and excellent long-term benefit from ASD repair in the elderly.
3. Weidman, W. H., Blount, S. G., DuShane, J. W., et al. Clinical course in ventricular septal defect. *Circulation* 56 (Suppl. 1):I-56, 1977.
   Natural history study: same issue contains results for pulmonic stenosis, and other acyanotic lesions.
4. Presbitero, P., Demarie, D., Villani, M., et al. Long term results (15–30 years) of surgical repair of aortic coarctation. *Br. Heart J.* 57:462, 1987.
5. Wood, P. The Eisenmenger syndrome. *Br. Med. J.* 2:701, 709, 1958.
   The first, largest, and best-described series of patients with the syndrome.
6. Editorial. Tetralogy of Fallot in adults. *Lancet* 1:74, 1980.
   Bleak outlook for patients not operated upon contrasts with good results of surgery, even for patients in their thirties and older.
7. Driscoll, D., Danielson, G., Puga, F., et al. Exercise tolerance and cardiorespiratory response to exercise after the Fontan operation for tricuspid atresia or functional single ventricle. *J. Am. Coll. Cardiol.* 7:1087, 1986.
   One of several uncontrolled studies attesting to the benefits of the Fontan type of repair.

34. CONGESTIVE HEART FAILURE
Stephen C. Achuff

Congestive heart failure is a clinical syndrome rather than a disease entity. Recognition of this distinction is critical to assessing prognosis and instituting appropriate therapy.

While the congestive and low cardiac output symptoms and signs of dyspnea, fluid retention, and fatigue are easily diagnosed, all too often clinicians leap to the conclusion that a failing pump is the crux of the problem. Drugs such as digoxin, diuretics, and vasodilators should not be prescribed without a systematic evaluation of pathophysiology and etiology. It is important to ascertain whether the syndrome is due primarily to left ventricular systolic or diastolic dysfunction, as these are treated entirely differently. One should consider the possibility of a reversible cause for heart failure such as hyperthyroidism, thiamine deficiency, pheochromocytoma, or myocarditis. Correctable mechanical problems such as constrictive pericarditis, atrial septal defect, ventricular aneurysm, and various valvular lesions may also be discovered after appropriate investigation. In addition to a meticulous history and physical examination, noninvasive studies, either echocardiography or radionuclide ventriculography, are mandatory before embarking on therapy. In some cases endomyocardial biopsy and cardiac catheterization are necessary to establish or rule out specific etiologies.

When heart failure is due to impaired systolic function the long-term prognosis is extremely poor. Community-based studies indicate a 5-year survival under 50 percent while referral centers dealing with refractory cases report figures of 20 percent or less for the same time period. Death is often sudden and presumably due to arrhythmias; indeed, the most important prognostic factor in most studies is the presence or absence of frequent and complex ventricular ectopy. Recent attention has focused on the contribution of the body's own compensatory mechanisms in heart failure, such as activation of the renin-angiotensin-aldosterone and sympathetic nervous systems, to this propensity towards fatal arrhythmias. While therapy with conventional antiarrhythmic drugs has not been shown to improve survival, newer agents that alter various components of the neurohormonal milieu appear more promising. Other causes of morbidity and mortality in patients with congestive heart failure such as systemic and pulmonary emboli (especially with atrial fibrillation) and refractory failure itself may be more amenable to treatment with standard medications.

Assuming the etiologic basis for congestive heart failure cannot be corrected, the physician must resort to supportive therapy. Nonpharmacologic approaches may be of particular value in some patients (e.g., salt restriction, reduction of excessive physical and emotional activity). However, most patients will require some form of medication, usually combinations of drugs. Traditionally, diuretics have been first-line therapy and this is still entirely appropriate, assuming precautions are taken to avoid electrolyte imbalance and excessive fluid loss. It is also important to match the power of the diuretic with the magnitude of the heart failure. Patients with mild degrees of fluid retention will benefit from a relatively weak agent such as a thiazide, whereas refractory patients may require a more potent loop diuretic (bumetanide, furosemide, ethacrynic acid) perhaps in combination with a drug that acts in a different portion of the nephron like the distal tubule (metolazone, spironolactone). Symptomatic relief from congestive symptoms can usually be obtained with judicious use of diuretics, although improvement in long-term survival has not been demonstrated. The other traditional therapy is with digitalis and, while considerable doubts have been raised concerning its efficacy, recent studies establish its appropriate use in treating congestive heart failure. Patients in normal sinus rhythm (the benefit in atrial fibrillation is obvious) have been shown clearly to achieve improved hemodynamic and symptomatic status with digoxin as compared with placebo. However, because digoxin has only a modest inotropic effect other agents are being actively sought. Among those tested to date are oral catecholamines (L-dopa, pirbuterol, salbutamol) and phosphodiesterase inhibitors (amrinone, milrinone), but thus far none has proved clearly efficacious and safe.

Vasodilator drugs have been used successfully to lower systemic vascular resistance and filling pressures of the heart since the late 1960s. Two key determinants of cardiac performance, preload and afterload, are elevated to detrimental levels in heart failure; lowering them through arteriolar and venous dilators, respectively, improves symptoms and signs of congestion as well as increases the cardiac output. Combination isosorbide dinitrate and hydralazine has been shown to improve survival compared with placebo or prazosin in patients already on diuretics and digoxin. Likewise the angiotensin-converting enzyme (ACE) inhibitors captopril, enalapril, and lisinopril have a sustained beneficial effect on hemodynamics and symptoms and one of these (enalapril) also on survival. The principal caution with this latter class of drugs is that they may exacerbate renal insufficiency. Current practice is to begin one of the ACE-inhibitors if diuretics and digoxin no longer control symptoms of heart failure.

When heart failure becomes refractory to oral pharmacotherapy there are few remaining options. Some patients can be hospitalized and brought back to stable hemodynamic status with careful use of intravenous diuretics and inotropic drugs. A few of these may even benefit from out-patient intermittent or continuous (via infusion pump) dobutamine or dopamine. For the remaining group of patients with end-stage congestive heart failure and a limited prognosis the question of cardiac transplantation may arise. This is no longer considered experimental therapy and for carefully selected patients, generally those under 60 years old who are nondiabetic and in reasonably good condition apart from their heart disease, transplantation is a realistic and promising option. Current results indicate an 80 to 90 percent 1-year survival and projected 60 to 70 percent 5-year survival after surgery.

1. Parmley, W. W. Pathophysiology and current therapy of congestive heart failure. *J. Am. Coll. Cardiol.* 13:771, 1989.
   Superb review of the entire topic by a master clinician.
2. Maron, B. J., Bonow, R. O., Cannon, R. O., et al. Hypertrophic cardiomyopathy: Interrelations of clinical manifestations, pathophysiology and therapy. *N. Engl. J. Med.* 316:780, 844, 1987.
   Comprehensive current review of this disorder.
3. Criley, J. M., and Siegel, R. J. Has "obstruction" hindered our understanding of hypertrophic cardiomyopathy? *Circulation* 72:1148, 1985.
   Emphasizes the crucial role of impaired diastolic filling as opposed to obstruction to left ventricular emptying.
4. Topol, E. J., Traill, T. A., and Fortuin, N. J. Hypertensive hypertrophic cardiomyopathy of elderly. *N. Engl. J. Med.* 312:277, 1985.
   Affectionately known as "little old lady's heart," this disorder is actually quite common and is another example of heart failure with preserved systolic function.
5. Benotti, J. R., Grossman, W., and Cohn, P. F. The clinical profile of restrictive cardiomyopathy. *Circulation* 61:1206, 1980.
   Reduced ventricular diastolic compliance ("stiff heart") is the common pathophysiologic feature. Examples include amyloidosis and hemochromatosis.
6. Mason, J. W. Endomyocardial biopsy: The balance of success and failure. *Circulation* 71:185, 1985.
   When is a biopsy appropriate? What can be learned that is helpful clinically?
7. Dec, G. W., Palacios, I. F., Fallon, J. T., et al. Active myocarditis in the spectrum of acute dilated cardiomyopathies—clinical features, histologic correlates, and clinical outcome. *N. Engl. J. Med.* 312:885, 1985.
   Highlights the importance of considering myocarditis with the first presentation of otherwise unexplained congestive heart failure.
8. Johnson, R. A., and Palacios, I. F. Dilated cardiomyopathies of the adult. *N. Engl. J. Med.* 307:1051, 1119, 1982.
   Landmark comprehensive review.
9. McKee, P. A., Castelli, W. P., McNamara, P. M., et al. The natural history of congestive heart failure: The Framingham study. *N. Engl. J. Med.* 285:1441, 1971.
   A background history of hypertension was present in 75% of cases.
10. Fuster, V., Gersh, B. J., Giuliani, E. R., et al. The natural history of idiopathic dilated cardiomyopathy. *Am. J. Cardiol.* 47:525, 1981.
    Long-term follow-up of patients referred to the Mayo Clinic.
11. Massie, B. M., and Conway, M. Survival of patients with congestive heart failure: Past, present, and future prospects. *Circulation* 75(Suppl. IV):IV-11, 1987.
    Reviews studies of prognosis and examines various factors that indicate high risk.
12. Chakko, C. S., and Gheorghiade, M. Ventricular arrhythmias in severe heart failure: Incidence, significance, and effectiveness of antiarrhythmic therapy. *Am. Heart J.* 109:497, 1985.

One of numerous studies showing the presence of ventricular ectopy to be a bad prognostic sign. Also emphasizes lack of efficacy of conventional antiarrhythmic drugs.

13. Packer, M., Lee, W. H., Kessler, P. D., et al. Role of neurohormonal mechanisms in determining survival in patients with severe chronic heart failure. *Circulation* 75(Suppl. IV):IV-98, 1987.
   Good review of current understanding of biochemical pathophysiology. Provides rationale for using some of the newer agents.

14. Dargie, H. J., Cleland, J. G. F., Leckie, B. J., et al. Relation of arrhythmias and electrolyte abnormalities to survival in patients with severe chronic heart failure. *Circulation* 75(Suppl. IV):IV-98, 1987.
   Similar to preceding but emphasizes electrolyte abnormalities which are potentially treatable.

15. Lee, W. H., and Packer, M. Prognostic importance of serum sodium concentration and its modification by converting-enzyme inhibitors in patients with severe chronic heart failure. *Circulation* 73:257, 1986.
   Unfavorable prognosis for hyponatremic patients is related to marked elevation of plasma renin activity and may be modified by ACE-inhibition.

16. Cohn, J. N., Levine, T. B., Olivari, M. T., et al. Plasma norepinephrine as a guide to prognosis in patients with chronic congestive heart failure. *N. Engl. J. Med.* 311:819, 1984.
   A single venous blood sample showing increased plasma norepinephrine may provide a better guide to prognosis than other commonly measured parameters.

17. Lapeyre, A. C., Steele, P. M., Kazmier, F. J., et al. Low incidence of systemic embolism in left ventricular aneurysm—a comparison with idiopathic dilated cardiomyopathy. *J. Am. Coll. Cardiol.* 1:704, 1983.
   Patients with dilated cardiomyopathy are at high risk of embolism and should be treated with chronic warfarin anticoagulation.

18. Packer, M. Therapeutic options in the management of chronic heart failure. Is there a drug of first choice? *Circulation* 79:198, 1989.
   Thoughtful editorial in light of recent enthusiasm for new drugs.

19. Gheorghiade, M., St. Clair, J., St. Clair, C., et al. Hemodynamic effects of intravenous digoxin in patients with severe heart failure initially treated with diuretics and vasodilators. *J. Am. Coll. Cardiol.* 9:849, 1987.
   Intravenous digoxin improved cardiac function even when diuretics and vasodilators appeared clinically successful.

20. Lee, D. C., Johnson, R. A., and Bingham, J. B. Heart failure in out-patients: A randomized trial of digoxin vs. placebo. *N. Engl. J. Med.* 306:699, 1982.
   Presence of an S3 gallop had the strongest correlation with a favorable response to digoxin.

21. Cohn, J. N., Archibald, D. G., Ziesche, S., et al. Effect of vasodilator therapy on mortality in chronic congestive heart failure. *N. Engl. J. Med.* 314:1547, 1986.
   Veterans Administration cooperative study showing the benefit of combined hydralazine and isosorbide dinitrate.

22. The CONSENSUS Trial Study Group. Effects of enalapril on mortality in severe congestive heart failure. *N. Engl. J. Med.* 316:1429, 1987.
   The addition of the ACE inhibitor enalapril to conventional therapy reduced mortality and improved symptoms in patients followed long-term.

23. The Captopril-Digoxin Multicenter Research Group. Comparative effects of therapy with captopril and digoxin in patients with mild to moderate heart failure. *J.A.M.A.* 259:539, 1988.
   Patients already on maintenance diuretics benefit from captopril and digoxin alone or in combination.

24. Roth, A., Kulick, D., Freidenberger, L., et al. Early tolerance to hemodynamic effects of high dose transdermal nitroglycerin in responders with severe chronic heart failure. *J. Am. Coll. Cardiol.* 9:858, 1987.
   Cutaneous nitrates are attractive for their simplicity and convenience but long-term efficacy is unlikely.

25. DiBianco, R., Shabetai, R., Kostuk, W., et al. A comparison of oral milrinone, digoxin,

and their combination in the treatment of patients with chronic heart failure. *N. Engl. J. Med.* 320:677, 1989.
While milrinone improved symptoms it was no better than digoxin and had more problems in terms of increased ventricular arrhythmias.

26. Packer, M., Lee, W. H., Medina, N., et al. Functional renal insufficiency during long-term therapy with captopril and enalapril in severe chronic heart failure. *Ann. Intern. Med.* 106:346, 1987.
Deterioration of renal function after ACE inhibitor therapy is usually transient and is ameliorated by sodium repletion.

27. Swedberg, K., Hjalmarson, A., Waagstein, F., et al. Beneficial effects of long-term beta-blockade in congestive cardiomyopathy. *Br. Heart J.* 44:117, 1980.
Symptomatic improvement and lower than expected mortality—a provocative study but this form of therapy is not to be recommended casually.

28. Applefeld, M. M., Newman, K. A., Sutton, F. J., et al. Outpatient dobutamine and dopamine infusions in the management of chronic heart failure: Clinical experience in 21 patients. *Am. Heart J.* 114:589, 1987.
An effective form of therapy for selected patients refractory to more conventional treatment or who are awaiting heart transplant.

29. Baumgartner, W. A. Role of cardiac transplantation in the management of congestive heart failure. *Am. J. Med.* 80(Suppl. 2B):51, 1986.
Brief review that hits all the highlights of current practice of this ultimate form of therapy for CHF.

30. Copeland, J. G., Emery, R. W., Levinson, M. M., et al. Selection of patients for cardiac transplantation. *Circulation* 75:2, 1987.
Details criteria for selecting who will and who will not be likely to benefit from transplantation.

35. MITRAL STENOSIS
H. Verdain Barnes

Mitral stenosis (MS) is the most common and important cause of apical diastolic murmurs. It is the only cardiac valvular disease that is predominantly rheumatic in origin and accounts for about 50 percent of all rheumatic valve disease. Nonetheless, only about 50 percent of all patients with MS have a clear-cut history of acute rheumatic fever. It has a 4:1 predilection for females over males.

Pathologically there are three main types of *rheumatic* stenosis. The commissural type exhibits fusion of the commissures with little involvement of the chordae and/or cusps. The chordae type exhibits fusion and thickening of the chordae, resulting in shortened and decreased mobility of the valve leaflets. In the third type the leaflets or cusps become stiff and rigid and ultimately calcify. These types may be pure or in combination. There are four anatomic types of *congenital* mitral stenosis. About one-half are of the typical type characterized by short chordae, obliteration of the interchordal spaces, and reduction of the interpapillary distance. Next in frequency is the hypoplastic type, which is usually associated with the hypoplastic left heart syndrome. Next is the type caused by a stenosing supramitral ring; finally there is the parachute mitral valve with a single papillary muscle. Common associated malformations include endocardial sclerosis, marked endocardial fibroelastosis, hypoplasia of the aortic isthmus, aortic valve stenosis or atresia, and coarctation of the aorta, in descending order of frequency. The parachute type of stenosis has the best prognosis of the congenital forms of stenosis.

The resultant stenosis of each pathologic type is characterized by varying degrees of obstruction to left ventricular filling. The greater the obstruction, the more pronounced are the associated features of decreased cardiac output and increased left atrial size and pressure. The increase in left atrial pressure causes a rise in pulmonary artery pressure and results in varying levels of increased pulmonary capillary pressure. These changes set the stage for the clinical findings and natural history of the disease.

The murmur in MS is produced by the flow of blood from the atrium to the ventricle during diastole in the presence of a significant left atrial to left ventricular pressure gradient. The murmur occurs well after the second sound and is, therefore, termed a *middiastolic murmur.* Initially with mild stenosis, the murmur may be short with no presystolic component, and is characteristically low-pitched and rumbling. As stenosis advances, left ventricular filling becomes slower and the murmur prolonged. As this progresses, a murmur develops at the time of left atrial contraction into the unfilled ventricle. This presystolic murmur is crescendo in character and ends at the first heart sound. This component of the murmur is obviously absent in the presence of atrial fibrillation. An opening snap is frequently heard along the left sternal border in the fourth intercostal space. Recent studies have identified the opening snap as the point at which the valve is maximally open and there is a rapid cessation of movement of the anterior leaflet. At this point, mechanical energy is converted to acoustic energy. In the presence of major mitral valve calcification, an opening snap may not be audible due to decreased valve mobility. A major consideration in listening for the murmur of MS is that the apex area is not only the point of maximum intensity but may be the only place the murmur is heard. The murmur area may be small and well-defined and is frequently audible only when the patient is in the supine or left lateral position. In tight mitral stenosis, the murmur may be less prominent and the findings may be primarily those of pulmonary hypertension.

The natural history of rheumatic MS is not clear, but in general there is a stage of development, a stage of fully developed asymptomatic MS, and a stage of symptomatic MS. The average latent period is about 19 years. The period from onset of symptoms to total disability averages about 7 years in untreated patients. Most patients become symptomatic in the fourth or fifth decade of life. Symptoms develop gradually or abruptly in about equal frequency. The onset of symptoms is frequently associated with development of paroxysmal or persistent atrial fibrillation, which occurs in at least 40 percent of patients. The complications of MS are (1) systemic embolization in 9 to 25 percent of patients with the most common site being the cerebral hemispheres, (2) hemoptysis in 17 percent, with a rare instance of pulmonary apoplexy, (3) pulmonary hypertension, (4) increased incidence of respiratory infections, which may precipitate pulmonary edema, (5) occasional occurrence of angina pectoris, (6) a rare instance of bacterial endocarditis, and (7) impaired pulmonary function.

The long-term prognosis in untreated patients with MS is variable, but one longitudinal study shows that about 40 percent die within 10 years and 80 percent within 20 years of diagnosis. At 10 years, approximately 40 percent of the patients showed no change, with the remaining 20 percent showing progression. By 20 years only 13 percent showed no progression. In another study dealing with already symptomatic patients, by 11 years approximately 70 percent were dead with only 11 percent unchanged, and by 18 years 83 percent were dead, with a mere 3 percent showing no progression.

Surgical correction is possible by a variety of procedures and may well extend life in symptomatic patients. Therapy should be individually tailored and carefully considered in view of the natural history.

1. Wood, P. An appreciation of mitral stenosis. *Br. Med. J.* 1:1051, 1954.
   A classic review of the disease, with an emphasis on its natural history.
2. Roberts, W. C., and Perloff, J. K. Mitral valvular disease: A clinicopathologic survey of the conditions causing the mitral valve to function abnormally. *Ann. Intern. Med.* 77:939, 1972.
   This review has an emphasis on pathology.
3. Selzer, A., and Cohn, K. E. Natural history of mitral stenosis: A review. *Circulation* 45:878, 1972.
   A compilation of what is known about the natural history of MS and a provocative discussion of therapy.

4. Dubin, A. A., March, H. W., Cohn, K., et al. Longitudinal hemodynamic and clinical study of mitral stenosis. *Circulation* 44:381, 1971.
   Valve involvement can be progressive, which may be related to the chronic trauma from altered flow through the valve.

5. Friedman, N. J. Echocardiographic studies of mitral valve motion: Genesis of the opening snap in mitral stenosis. *Am. Heart J.* 80:177, 1970.
   The sudden cessation of motion of the anterior leaflet producing the opening snap in MS can be documented by echocardiographic techniques.

6. Selzer, A. Effects of atrial fibrillation upon the circulation in patients with mitral stenosis. *Am. Heart J.* 59:518, 1960.
   Atrial fibrillation produces a lower resting cardiac output and is the most common antecedent moving the patient from an asymptomatic to a symptomatic state.

7. Casella, L., Abelmann, W. H., and Ellis, L. B. Patients with stenosis and systemic emboli. *Arch. Intern. Med.* 114:773, 1964.
   Most emboli find their way to the cerebral circulation.

8. Ramsey, H. W., DeLa Torre, A., Bartley, T. D., et al. Intractable hemoptysis in mitral stenosis treated by emergency mitral commissurotomy. *Ann. Intern. Med.* 67:588, 1967.
   Emergency commissurotomy may be lifesaving.

9. Heller, S. J., and Carleton, R. A. Abnormal left ventricular contraction in patients with mitral stenosis. *Circulation* 42:1099, 1970.
   The immobile mitral valve ring, valve leaflets, chordae tendineae, and capillary muscles restrict the motion of the adjacent left ventricle.

10. Rowe, J. C., Blawd, E. F., Sprague, H. B., et al. The course of mitral stenosis without surgery: Ten and twenty year perspectives. *Ann. Intern. Med.* 52:741, 1960.

11. Olesen, K. H. The natural history of 271 patients with mitral stenosis under medical treatment. *Br. Heart J.* 24:349, 1962.
    Articles 10 and 11 are the best longitudinal studies of the natural history of medically treated mitral stenosis.

12. Coulshed, N., Epstein, E. J., McKendrick, C. S., et al. Systemic embolism in mitral disease. *Br. Heart J.* 32:26, 1970.
    Only patients without atrial fibrillation have fewer emboli after valve surgery.

13. Henry, W. L., Griffith, J. M., Michaelis, L. L., et al. Measurement of mitral orifice area in patients with mitral valve disease by real-time, two dimensional echocardiography. *Circulation* 51:827, 1975.
    An important advance in noninvasive evaluation of mitral valve disease.

14. Ruchman, R. N., and VanPraagh, R. Anatomic types of congenital mitral stenosis: Report of 49 autopsy cases with consideration of diagnosis and surgical implications. *Am. J. Cardiol.* 42:592, 1978.
    Four anatomic types and their prognosis are described.

15. Ahmed, S. S., Regan, T. J., Fiore, J. J., et al. The state of the left ventricular myocardium in mitral stenosis. *Am. Heart J.* 94:28, 1977.

16. Thompson, M. E., Shaver, J. A., and Leon, D. F. Effect of tachycardia on atrial transport in mitral stenosis. *Am. Heart J.* 94:297, 1977.

17. Marco, J. D., Standeven, J. D., Barnes, H. B. Pulmonary and left atrial hemodynamics in mitral stenosis. *Am. Heart J.* 94:73, 1977.
    These articles (15–17) illuminate some of the pathophysiologic concomitants of this disease.

18. Cortese, D. A. Pulmonary function in mitral stenosis. *Mayo Clin. Proc.* 53:321, 1978.
    There is a significant impact of increased atrial pressure on the pulmonary function.

19. Bonchek, L. I. Indications for surgery of the mitral valve. *Am. J. Cardiol.* 46:155, 1980.
    A concise discussion of a controversial area.

20. Rahko, P. S., Salerni, R., Reddy, P. S., et al. Extent of mitral calcific deposits determined by cineangiography in mitral stenosis and their effect on valve motion, hemodynamics, and clinical signs. *Am. J. Cardiol.* 58:121, 1986.
    An opening snap may not be audible in patients with significant valve calcification.

36. MITRAL VALVE PROLAPSE

H. Verdain Barnes

Mitral valve prolapse (also referred to as a floppy or billowing mitral valve, Reid-Barlow syndrome, or click-late systolic murmur syndrome) is among the most common abnormalities of the heart. The clinical spectrum ranges from a nonejection click and no murmur or mitral insufficiency to severe mitral regurgitation with a holosystolic murmur and no click. The precise incidence is not known, but from the combined data of the reported studies of 100 or more female patients the condition appears to be found in about 4 percent of the general female population. Consequently, an understanding of the ubiquitous mitral valve prolapse (MVP) complex is important.

The underlying histopathology is variable ranging from myxomatous degeneration to typical postinflammatory changes. The components involved include the mitral valve leaflets and annulus, chordae tendineae, and left ventricular myocardium. The valve leaflets may or may not be redundant, but all have mitral leaflet displacement during systole. One or more of the scallops of the posterior leaflet may be affected alone or in combination with the anterior leaflet. Isolated anterior leaflet ballooning is rare. The chordae are usually thin, elongated, and attenuated, but in some thickening occurs. The anulus of the valve may be moderately or severely dilated—on occasion up to two-thirds greater in circumference than normal. Many patients show segmental dyskinesis of the left ventricle during systole. This dyskinesis may include excessive posteromedial or midventricular contraction, a reduction in the long axis of the ventricle, posterior akinesis, and left ventricular cavity obliteration. In patients with isolated MVP and little or no mitral insufficiency, hemodynamics are normal as determined by angiography.

Most patients with MVP are asymptomatic, although a significant number are clearly symptomatic, often for years before diagnosis. MVP has been diagnosed from childhood to old age, but is most often first discovered during the third through the fifth decades of life. Females predominate among younger patients, but both sexes are about equally involved in patients beyond middle age. A familial history is uncommon in most studies, but when present, an autosomal dominant pattern of inheritance is usually found.

Symptomatic patients most commonly complain of fatigue and dyspnea. Palpitations occur in up to 50 percent and chest pain is reported by about one-third. Some patients report decreased functional capacity, primarily exercise intolerance. Documented arrhythmias are not uncommon, particularly in those with recurrent palpitations; however, Holter monitor arrhythmias often do not correlate with the patient's report of palpitations. Induced arrhythmias occur in close to 75 percent of patients during exercise testing. Chest pain, when present, may range from annoying discomfort to disabling pain. It is usually a sharp, short-lived precordial discomfort that is unrelated to exertion or emotional stress and does not respond to nitroglycerin. On occasion, however, it is clinically indistinguishable from classic angina pectoris. Of those complaining of recurrent lightheadedness, dizziness, or syncope, a significant number have their symptoms associated with orthostatic hypotension.

In suspected MVP, the physical examination should focus on the patient's physical appearance and cardiac evaluation. The patient often has an asthenic body habitus, often with a loss of the normal thoracic kyphosis, scoliosis, pectus excavatum, and/or a narrow anterior-posterior chest diameter and long arm span. Palpation of the precordium may reveal (1) an interruption of the normal outward systolic movement of the chest with an unequivocal midsystolic retraction coincident with the auscultatory click or (2) a bifid point of maximal impulse in the left lateral decubitus position. On auscultation, systole may be silent, but with repeated examination all but about 10 percent have a distinct snapping or clicking sound and/or a systolic murmur. These so-called clicks may be single or multiple, and typically occur in midsystole although they may occur early or late in systole. On occasion, the patient may have a burst of definite systolic "crackles." The typical murmur is usually crescendo, beginning at the time of the click or shortly after the click and ending at or just beyond A2. About 10 percent of patients have an apical holosystolic murmur and no audible click. A smaller percentage of patients have an intermittent systolic "honk," which is easily audible to both the patient and physician. When present, this high-frequency musical sound is accompanied by an easily palpable thrill. When MVP is suspected, it is critical to listen to the heart with the patient in the left lateral decubitus, sitting, leaning forward, and standing positions, because these positions accentuate chordae and leaflet displacement by decreasing left ventricular volume. Sitting, standing, or Valsalva maneuver tends to move the click earlier in systole with an associated lengthening of the systolic murmur and on occasion the honk will appear. In contrast, rapid squatting and isometric exercise move the click in the opposite direction and shorten the murmur although it may become louder.

The initial laboratory evaluation of suspect patients should include a chest x ray, ECG, and echocardiogram. The more common and important ECG findings which may be associated include (1) ST and T wave abnormalities in leads II, III, aVF, and V_{4-6}, (2) prolongation of the Q–T interval, (3) single or multifocal premature ventricular or apical contractions, (4) ventricular or supraventricular tachycardia, (5) first-, second-, or third-degree heart block, and/or (6) the Lown-Ganong-Levine or Wolff-Parkinson-White syndrome. Echocardiography, an important noninvasive technique, can usually define the late systolic displacement of one or both mitral valve leaflets. Suggestive but nonspecific echographic findings include (1) minimal systolic mitral leaflet sagging with a decrease in anterior leaflet motion, (2) multiple parallel mitral leaflet echoes, and (3) excessive motion of the leaflets that brings them in contact with the intraventricular septum during diastole. Meticulous echographic technique and stringent diagnostic criteria are necessary to minimize false-positive and false-negative interpretations. In selected patients, left ventricular and occasionally right ventricular and coronary angiograms are required for complete evaluation.

The diagnostic criteria for MVP are not universally agreed upon which has led to a proposal of major and minor criteria by Perloff and his colleagues.[26] These criteria include auscultatory, two-dimensional echocardiography, and combination findings to help differentiate pathologic MVP from a potentially normal superior displacement of the mitral valve during systole. Further use and evaluation are needed to establish the usefulness of these criteria.

The conditions reported to be associated with MVP include Marfan's syndrome, trauma, rheumatic valvulitis, myotonic dystrophy, atrial septal defect, hypertrophic cardiomyopathy, cardiomyopathy, periarteritis nodosa, systemic lupus erythematosus, ischemic heart disease, Ehlers-Danlos syndrome, psoriatic arthritis, and Ebstein's anomaly.

Coronary artery disease is not more frequent than expected for the general population and no significant correlation between MVP and the distribution of coronary artery lesions has been found. There is, however, evidence for an increased incidence of MVP in patients with severe coronary atherosclerosis as well as in patients with atypical precordial chest pain and normal coronary arteriogram. There are six well-documented potential complications of MVP: progressive mitral insufficiency requiring surgical intervention (approx. 7.2%), sudden death (approx. 2.5%), infective endocarditis (approx. 1.3%), cerebral embolic event (approx. 0.8%), ruptured chordae tendineae, and recurrent syncope. The most likely subset of MVP patients to experience these complications are those with redundant mitral leaflets and a left ventricular dimension during diastole of greater than 60 mm.

1. Devereaux, R. B., Perloff, J. K., Reichek, N., et al. Mitral valve prolapse. *Circulation* 54:3, 1976.
   A superb overall review article that is extraordinarily complete and lucid.
2. Procacci, P. N., Savran, S. V., Schreiter, S. L., et al. Prevalence of clinical mitral-valve prolapse in 1169 young women. *N. Engl. J. Med.* 294:1086, 1976.
   In this large series of asymptomatic young women, 6.3% were found to have MVP, with a combined female study incidence in 2792 subjects of 4.2%.
3. Barlow, J. B., Bosman, C. K., Pocock, W. A., et al. Late systolic murmurs and nonejection (mid-late) systolic clicks: An analysis of 90 patients. *Br. Heart J.* 30:203, 1968.
   The chordae tendineae are usually thin, elongated, and attenuated.

4. Scameardonis, G., Yang, S. S., Maranhao, V., et al. Left ventricular abnormalities in prolapsed mitral leaflet syndrome. *Circulation* 48:287, 1973.
   Left-sided ventricular dyskinesis occurs in this syndrome.
5. Brown, O. R., Kloster, F. E., and DeMots, H. Incidence of mitral valve prolapse in the asymptomatic normal. *Circulation* 52(Suppl. 2):77, 1975.
   The majority are asymptomatic.
6. Barlow, J. B., and Pocock, W. A. The problem of non-ejection systolic clicks and associated mitral systolic murmurs: Emphasis on the bellowing mitral leaflet syndrome. *Am. Heart J.* 90:636, 1975.
   When a familial history is present, an autosomal dominant inheritance is suggested.
7. Gooch, A. S., Vicencio, F., Maranaho, V., et al. Arrhythmias in left ventricular asynergy in the prolapsing mitral leaflet syndrome. *Am. J. Cardiol.* 29:611, 1972.
   The authors found arrhythmias in about 75% of their subjects during exercise testing.
8. BonTenvo, C. P., Ronan, J. A., deLeon, A. C., et al. Radiographic appearance of the thorax and systolic-click, late systolic murmur syndrome. *Am. J. Cardiol.* 36:27, 1975.
   In these patients, there is often a loss of normal thoracic kyphosis, scoliosis, or pectus excavatium.
9. Winkle, R. A., Lopes, M. G., and Fitzgerald, J. W. Arrhythmias in patients with mitral valve prolapse. *Circulation* 52:23, 1975.
   A wide variety of ECG abnormalities are seen. The most common are ST/T abnormalities that occur in at least one-third of patients.
10. Verani, M. S., Carroll, R. J., and Falsetti, H. L. Mitral valve prolapse in coronary artery disease. *Am. J. Cardiol.* 37:1, 1976.
    In this study no significant correlation was found between the MVP and the distribution of coronary artery disease.
11. Goodman, D., Kimbiris, D., and Lenhart, J. W. Chordae tendineae rupture complicating the systolic click-late systolic syndrome. *Am. J. Cardiol.* 33:681, 1974.
    Spontaneous rupture of the chordae is a well-documented complication of MVP that results in a sudden augmentation of mitral insufficiency.
12. Winters, S. J., Schreiner, B., Griggs, R. C., et al. Familial mitral valve prolapse and myotonic dystrophy. *Ann. Intern. Med.* 85:19, 1976.
    In this kindred, about 25% had evidence of both disorders.
13. Leichtman, D., Nelson, R., Gobel, R. L., et al. Bradycardia with mitral valve prolapse: A potential mechanism of sudden death. *Ann. Intern. Med.* 85:453, 1976.
    Another potential mechanism of sudden death.
14. Barnett, H. J. M., Boughner, D. R., Taylor, D. W., et al. Further evidence relating to mitral valve prolapse to cerebral ischemic events. *N. Engl. J. Med.* 302:139, 1980.
15. Steele, P., Weily, H., Rainwater, J., et al. Platelet survival time and thromboembolism in patients with mitral valve prolapse. *Circulation* 60:43, 1979.
    These articles (14, 15) discuss cerebral ischemic events in MVP and a possible etiology, particularly those with myxomatous degeneration of the valve.
16. Schutte, J. E., Gaffney, F. A., Blend, L., et al. Distinctive anthropometric characteristics of women with mitral valve prolapse. *Am. J. Med.* 71:533, 1981.
    MVP patients in these families tended to have a decreased anterior-posterior chest diameter and longer arm span.
17. Santos, A. D., Mathew, P. K., Hilal, A., et al. Orthostatic hypotension: A commonly unrecognized cause of symptoms in mitral valve prolapse. *Am. J. Med.* 71:746, 1981.
    May cause lightheadedness, dizziness, and/or syncope.
18. Cabin, H. S., and Roberts, W. C. Ebstein's anomaly of the tricuspid valve and prolapse of the mitral valve. *Am. Heart J.* 101:177, 1981.
    Rare, but interesting, syndrome that may include MVP.
19. McKinsey, D. S., Ratts, T. E., and Bisno, A. L. Underlying cardiac lesions in adults with infective endocarditis. *Am. J. Med.* 82:681, 1987.
20. Devereux, R. B., Hawkins, I., Kramer-Fox, R., et al. Complications of mitral valve prolapse: Disproportionate occurrence in men and older patients. *Am. J. Med.* 81:751, 1986.
    Of their endocarditis patients 29% had MVP (article 19), and those at greater risk (article 20).

21. Pines, A., Ehrenfeld, M., Fisman, E. Z., et al. Mitral valve prolapse in psoriatic arthritis. *Arch. Intern. Med.* 146:1371, 1986.
Another disease with an apparent association with MVP.
22. Come, P. C., Riley, M. F., Carl, L. V., et al. Pulsed Doppler echocardiographic evaluation of valvular regurgitation in patients with mitral valve prolapse: Comparison with normal subjects. *J. Am. Coll. Cardiol.* 8:1355, 1986.
Another adjunct to functional diagnosis.
23. Kolibash, A. J., Bush, C. A., Fontana, M. B., et al. Mitral valve prolapse syndrome: Analysis of 62 patients aged 60 years and older. *Am. J. Cardiol.* 52:534, 1983.
An important review of MVP in the elderly.
24. Tomaru, T., Uchida, Y., Mohri, N., et al. Postinflammatory mitral and aortic valve prolapse: A clinical and pathologic study. *Circulation* 76:68, 1987.
In this study population, a substantial number had a postinflammatory histopathology.
25. Nishimura, R. A., McGoon, M. D., Shub, C., et al. Echocardiographically documented mitral valve prolapse: Long-term followup of 237 patients. *N. Engl. J. Med.* 313:1305, 1985.
Redundant valve leaflets and a left ventricular dimension during diastole of ≥60 mm had the greatest predictive value for complications.
26. Perloff, J. K., Child, J. S., and Edwards, J. E. New guidelines for the clinical diagnosis of mitral valve prolapse. *Am. J. Cardiol.* 57:1124, 1986.
Based on "major" and "minor" criteria, this system merits further use and evaluation. A step in the right direction.

37. PERICARDIAL EFFUSION AND PERICARDIOCENTESIS
Jerry L. Spivak

In evaluating the patient with an enlarged cardiac silhouette, the physician must decide whether it is due to myocardial dilatation, pericardial effusion, pericardial thickening, or a combination of these. The history is often of no help since the symptoms of chronic pericarditis are similar to those of myocardiopathy, and acute pericarditis can be difficult to distinguish from acute myocardial infarction or dissecting aneurysm. The findings on physical examination may also not permit distinction between pericardial and myocardial processes. Venous distention, hepatomegaly, and edema are common to both. The presence of a rub does not guarantee that the process is entirely pericardial (acute myocardial infarction, dissecting aneurysm, atrial septal defect, pulmonary embolism, thyroid storm, and atrial myxoma), nor does the absence of a friction rub exclude pericardial disease. Atrial fibrillation, cardiac murmurs, and gallops occur in the presence of pericardial as well as myocardial disease, and with tamponade it is possible on palpation of the radial pulse to confuse a pulsus paradoxus with atrial fibrillation. Friedreich's sign is present in myocardial failure as well as in constrictive pericarditis, and Kussmaul's sign is absent with lax pericardial effusions. In addition, it may be difficult to distinguish between a third-sound gallop and a diastolic knock. Finally, the systemic manifestations of pericardial disease (chronic passive congestion, protein-losing enteropathy, and nephrotic syndrome) are similar to those found in myocardial disease.

Until recently this problem in differential diagnosis was complicated by the need to use invasive techniques (angiocardiography, cardiac catheterization) to distinguish between myocardial dilatation and pericardial effusion. The problem was further compounded when pericardiocentesis was used to determine the presence of fluid since it is precisely when fluid is absent that the complications of pericardiocentesis occur. Echocardiography, cardiac blood pool scanning, and computed tomography (CT) scanning obviate the need for invasive procedures to determine the presence of pericardial fluid. Carbon dioxide contrast radiography is also a safe technique, but it requires a degree of cooperation that may be difficult to obtain in an acutely ill patient.

If the presence of pericardial fluid is suggested by echocardiography, a pericardiocentesis should be performed to determine the cause of the effusion. It should be borne in mind, however, that tumor, fibrosis, epicardial fat, and pleural effusion can mimic pericardial effusion on echocardiography.

If properly performed, pericardiocentesis can be approached with respect for its complications rather than with trepidation. There are several requirements for proper performance: (1) Premedication with atropine to prevent vasovagal reactions. (2) Proper positioning of the patient in the sitting position. Patients with acute pericarditis assume a position of sitting and leaning forward to relieve their pain. Such a position provides relief because the heart recedes posteriorly away from the anterior chest wall. If pericardiocentesis is performed with the patient supine, the operator can expect to encounter myocardium more frequently than fluid. (3) The approach should always be at the apex unless purulent pericarditis is suspected or there is a left pleural effusion, empyema, or pneumonia. The apex is preferred for several reasons. The myocardium is thicker and the coronary vessels are smaller, reducing the chance of laceration, bleeding, and air embolism. In addition, the bulk of the fluid in pericardial effusions accumulates posterolaterally, not anteriorly, and with insertion of the needle at the fifth left intercostal space there is little chance of puncturing the lingula. (4) The anesthesia needle as well as the pericardial aspirating needle must always be attached to an ECG monitor. In addition, the patient must be isolated from ground (turn off the electric bed and remove all other monitors). (5) The venous pressure must be monitored with a catheter proximal to the shoulder since more peripheral readings can be misleading. (6) Sonography, fluorography, or echocardiography can be employed to assist in guiding the needle but they do not exempt the procedure from the other requirements.

Following removal of fluid (no more than 500 ml at one time), further diagnostic information can be obtained by the injection of air. This procedure is safe as long as fluid can be withdrawn and the ECG monitor reveals no injury current. Since air is compressible, it will not impede cardiac activity, but neither will the air impede adhesion formation secondary to pericardial inflammation since it is relatively quickly absorbed. The importance of air contrast lies in the fact that it provides information about heart size and pericardial wall thickness. Such information can spare a patient with a myocardiopathy from unnecessary surgery and speed a patient with pericardial constriction to the operating room. Under normal circumstances the pericardium is distensible, and can hold a considerable amount of fluid if accumulation is slow. In the presence of inflammation, edema, and rapid fluid accumulation, its properties change and a much smaller amount of fluid will cause cardiac embarrassment. Removal of a small quantity of fluid in such instances should lower the venous pressure and bring relief. If it does not, possible explanations include the presence of loculated fluid, myocardial restriction or failure, or pericardial thickening with constriction. Air contrast studies will identify this last condition, in which the risk of tamponade is greatest. Such patients should either have definitive surgery or be watched carefully for signs of recurrent tamponade, which usually develops within 12 hours. The presence of pulsus paradoxus and elevation of the venous pressure, as well as increasing dyspnea, signal the occurrence of tamponade and the need for pericardiectomy. However, it should be noted that demonstration of a normal pericardial thickness does not imply absence of pericardial disease. In neoplastic invasion of the pericardium, involvement can be limited solely to the posterior pericardium, an area that is not visible with the air contrast technique.

1. Holt, J. P. The normal pericardium. *Am. J. Cardiol.* 26:455, 1970.
   Review of the physiology and function of the pericardium.
2. Shabetai, R. The pericardium: An essay on some recent developments. *Am. J. Cardiol.* 42:1036, 1978.
   Review of recently published studies on pericardial physiology and pathology.
3. Conner, L. A. On the diagnosis of pericardial effusion. *Am. Heart J.* 1:421, 1925.
   An excellent discussion of the distribution of pericardial fluid.
4. Ewart, W. Practical aids in the diagnosis of pericardial effusion in connection with the question as to surgical treatment. *Br. Med. J.* 1:717, 1896.
   A classic description of the physical signs of pericardial effusion.

5. Hancock, E. W. On the elastic and rigid forms of constrictive pericarditis. *Am. Heart J.* 100:917, 1980.
   Hemodynamic features of the various forms of cardiac compressive syndromes. (See also Am. J. Cardiol. *45:386, 1980.)*
6. Stein, L., Shubin, H., and Weil, M. H. Recognition and management of pericardial tamponade. *J.A.M.A.* 225:503, 1973.
   A concise review.
7. Tajik, A. J. Echocardiography in pericardial effusion. *Am. J. Med.* 63:29, 1977.
   Comprehensive review. (See also Ann. Intern. Med. *86:434, 1977 and* Arch. Intern. Med. *138:622, 1978.)*
8. Horowitz, M. S., Schultz, C. S., Stinson, E. B., et al. Sensitivity and specificity of echocardiographic diagnosis of pericardial effusion. *Circulation* 50:239, 1974.
   20 ml of fluid is the lower limit of sensitivity.
9. Chen, J. T. T., Petter, R. H., Orgain, E. J., et al. The pitfalls in interpreting artificial pneumopericardium. *Am. J. Roentgenol. Radium Ther. Nucl. Med.* 116:91, 1972.
   Injection of compressible gas results in fluid wave formation and deceptive changes in the cardiac silhouette.
10. Baron, M. G. Pericardial effusion. *Circulation* 44:294, 1971.
    Review of the x-ray diagnosis of pericardial effusion.
11. Tomoda, H., Hoshiai, M., and Furuya, H. Evaluation of pericardial effusion with computed tomography. *Am. Heart J.* 99:701, 1980.
    CT scanning was found to be comparable to echocardiography.
12. Unverferth, D. V., Williams, T. E., and Fulkerson, P. K. Electrocardiographic voltage in pericardial effusion. *Chest* 75:157, 1979.
    A low-voltage ECG per se is not specific for pericardial effusion but a reduction in voltage on serial studies suggests the development of an effusion.
13. Markiewicz, W., Brik, A., and Brook, G. Pericardial rub in pericardial effusion: Lack of correlation with amount of fluid. *Chest* 77:643, 1980.
    The presence of a pericardial rub is not related to the amount of pericardial fluid present.
14. Reddy, P. S., Curtiss, E. I., O'Toole, J. D., et al. Cardiac tamponade: Hemodynamic observations in man. *Circulation* 58:265, 1978.
    Cardiac tamponade can occur in the absence of a paradoxical pulse.
15. Friedman, H. S., Sakurai, H., Choe, S.-S., et al. Pulsus paradoxus: A manifestation of a marked reduction of left ventricular end-diastolic volume in cardiac tamponade. *J. Thorac. Cardiovasc. Surg.* 79:74, 1980.
    Pulsus paradoxus was found to be a late manifestation of cardiac tamponade.
16. Krikorian, J. G., and Hancock, E. W. Pericardiocentesis. *Am. J. Med.* 65:808, 1978.
    An important review of the risks and benefits of pericardiocentesis. (See also Am. J. Cardiol. *44:1110, 1979).*
17. Kelbaek, H., Skagen, K., and Godtfredsen, J. Pericardiocentesis in patients with and without incipient cardiac tamponade due to pericardial effusion. An easy and safe bedside approach. *Acta Med. Scand.* 217:289, 1985.
    The experience at the bedside. (See also Surg. Gynecol. Obstet. *160:414, 1985 for the left subcostal approach.)*
18. Schaffer, A. I. Pericardiocentesis with the aid of a plastic catheter and ECG monitor. *Am. J. Cardiol.* 4:83, 1959.
    ECG monitoring is an absolute necessity.
19. Kerber, R. E., Ridges, J. D., and Harrison, D. C. Electrocardiographic indications of atrial puncture during pericardiocentesis. *N. Engl. J. Med.* 282:1142, 1970.
    Deviation of the P–T$_a$ segment indicates atrial injury.
20. Clarke, D. P., and Cosgrove, D. O. Real-time ultrasound scanning in the planning and guidance of pericardiocentesis. *Clin. Radiol.* 38:119, 1987.
    Use of sonography in pericardiocentesis. (See also Ann. Thorac. Surg. *45:99, 1988 and* Mayo Clin. Proc. *60:344, 1985 for use of echocardiography.)*
21. Alcan, K. E., Zabetakis, P. M., Marino, N. D., et al. Management of acute cardiac tamponade by subxiphoid pericardiotomy. *J.A.M.A.* 247:1143, 1982.

This is currently a popular approach. (See also Surgery *96:738, 1984 and* Arch. Intern. Med. *146:1113, 1986.)*

22. Kessler, K. M., Rodriguez, D., Rahim, A., et al. Echocardiographic observations regarding pericardial effusions associated with cardiac disease. *Chest* 78:736, 1980.
    Congestive heart failure was the most common cause of pericardial effusion in this series. (See also Chest *74:174, 1978.)*

23. Kerber, R. E., and Sherman, B. Echocardiographic evaluation of pericardial effusion in myxedema. *Circulation* 52:823, 1975.
    10% had an effusion but physical examination was not a reliable indication of this, none developed tamponade, and in all the effusion disappeared with thyroid hormone replacement.

24. Thomas, C. S., Carter, J. W., and Lowder, S. C. Pericardial tamponade from central venous catheters. *Arch. Surg.* 98:217, 1969.
    Iatrogenic pericardial effusion.

25. Peters, R. W., Scheinman, M. M., Raskin, S., et al. Unusual complications of epicardial pacemakers. *Am. J. Cardiol.* 45:1088, 1980.
    Cardiac tamponade, recurrent pericarditis, and pericardial constriction.

26. Brawley, R. K., Vasko, J. S., and Morrow, A. G. Cholesterol pericarditis. *Am. J. Med.* 41:235, 1966.
    Cholesterol pericarditis is a result of either chronic pericardial inflammation or hypothyroidism.

27. Ruckdeschel, J. C., Chang, P., Martin, R. G., et al. Radiation-related pericardial effusions in patients with Hodgkin's disease. *Medicine* 54:245, 1975.
    Risk factors predisposing to this complication include mediastinal adenopathy and adjuvant chemotherapy.

28. Tabibian, N., Schwartz, J. T., Smith, J. L., et al. Cardiac tamponade as a result of endoscopic sclerotherapy: report of a case. *Surgery* 102:546, 1987.
    Something to remember.

29. Rutsky, E. A., and Rostand, S. G. Treatment of uremic pericarditis and pericardial effusion. *Am. J. Kidney Dis.* 10:2, 1987.
    Intensive dialysis is the initial therapy of choice. (See also Arch Intern. Med. *143:1673, 1983.)*

30. Galve, E., Garcia-Del-Castillo, H., Evangelista, A., et al. Pericardial effusion in the course of myocardial infarction: incidence, natural history, and clinical relevance. *Circulation* 73:294, 1986.
    The incidence was 28% and most common with anterior infarctions. Heparin is not contraindicated but streptokinase may cause effusions (See Chest *85:494, 1984,* Lancet *1:1015, 1986, and also* J. Am. Coll. Cardiol. *8:517, 1986.)*

31. Thadani, U., Iveson, J. M. I., and Wright, V. Cardiac tamponade, constrictive pericarditis, and pericardial resection in rheumatoid arthritis. *Medicine* 54:261, 1975.
    Corticosteroids were not found to be effective. (See also N. Engl. J. Med. *289:597, 1973 and* Medicine *69:81, 1990.)*

32. Lorell, B., Leinbach, R. C., Pohost, G. M., et al. Right ventricular infarction. *Am. J. Cardiol.* 43:465, 1979.
    Right ventricular infarction can be misdiagnosed as cardiac tamponade.

33. Press, O. W., and Livingston, R. Management of malignant pericardial effusion and tamponade. *J.A.M.A.* 257:1088, 1987.
    An important review.

34. Shepherd, F. A., Morgan, C., Evans, W. K., et al. Medical management of malignant pericardial effusion by tetracycline sclerosis. *Am. J. Cardiol.* 60:1161, 1987.
    An effective procedure which is not without complications. (See also Clin. Oncol. *2:631, 1984.)*

35. Carey, R. W., Sawicka, J. M., and Choi, N. C. Cytologically negative pericardial effusion complicating combined modality therapy for localized small-cell carcinoma of the lung. *J. Clin. Oncol.* 5:818, 1987.
    Not all effusions in cancer patients are due to the malignancy. (See also Cancer *60:263, 1987 and* Cancer *62:1904, 1988.)*

38. POSTMYOCARDIAL INFARCTION SYNDROME (DRESSLER'S SYNDROME)
H. Verdain Barnes

Postmyocardial infarction syndrome was first described by Dressler in 1955. The primary clinical features are fever, pericarditis, pneumonitis, and pleuropericardial pain. The diagnosis cannot be made on the basis of a pericardial friction rub alone, since this sign is also a feature of postmyocardial infarction pericarditis. The incidence of postmyocardial infarction pericarditis ranges from 7 to 42 percent, with only a small percentage of patients ultimately having a classic Dressler's syndrome. The exact incidence of Dressler's syndrome is not clear, but probably does not exceed 4 percent.

The pain in Dressler's syndrome is induced or accentuated by inspiration, when the person is lying flat or in the left lateral position, and is partially or totally relieved by sitting. Pain is rarely, if ever, entirely absent. The pain is characterized as a pressing, squeezing, drawing, and/or sticking sensation. It is primarily in the substernal or precordial areas but occasionally radiates to the neck, jaws, shoulders, arms, or epigastrium. Pain may precede all other manifestations by days to weeks. The presence of a pericardial friction rub can be documented in at least 75 percent of patients at some point during the course of the illness despite the fact that it is usually not loud and is frequently evanescent. In about one-third of patients, however, the rub persists for 7 to 21 days. The rub may occur in the first week after infarction, but more commonly occurs in the second to eleventh weeks. A pericardial effusion can be documented in about two-thirds of patients.

Fever is observed at some point in the course in virtually all patients. Temperatures usually range from 101° (38.3°) to 102°F (38.8°C), but may not exceed 100°F. The fever may run a daily spiking pattern or plateau, but it rarely returns to normal, even during periods when the pleuropericarditis is asymptomatic. Pleuritis with pleural effusion is also a common feature, occurring in about two-thirds of patients. The pleural effusion has the characteristics of an exudate and is bilateral in 50 percent of patients. A patchy or linear pulmonary infiltrate occurs in 25 percent of patients. Several laboratory features are of note: (1) There is usually a leukocytosis ranging from 10,000 to 20,000, with a shift to the left, (2) 20 percent of patients have eosinophilia, and (3) the sedimentation rate is almost invariably elevated. In a few patients, a mild normochromic normocytic anemia develops.

The course of the illness is characterized by remissions and exacerbations. Eighty percent have recurrent episodes, with about 40 percent having three or more episodes. Relapses have been reported over a year after the initial myocardial infarction. The major complications of the syndrome are serious arrhythmias and cardiac tamponade. The most common arrhythmia is supraventricular tachycardia, which occurs in about one-third of patients in some series. Most recent studies have not found any adverse effects from anticoagulants nor have they found postmyocardial infarction pericarditis or Dressler's syndrome to indicate a poorer prognosis. Standard therapy consists of anti-inflammatory agents, salicylates, and/or steroids. Recently, immunosuppressive agents have been reported to be effective, but they are probably unnecessary. The response to anti-inflammatory agents is in most cases dramatic, with relief of the fever and pain within 24 to 36 hours. The syndrome is often misdiagnosed as pulmonary embolism, bacterial pneumonia, congestive heart failure, or late extension of the initial myocardial infarction. A missed diagnosis can result in unwarranted therapy or a prolonged hospital stay.

The cause is probably autoimmune. Antimyocardial antibodies have been demonstrated by direct immunofluorescence and antiglobulin consumption tests in the sera of these patients. In addition, many of the clinical signs and symptoms and the response to steroids and immunosuppressive agents are similar to those of other autoimmune disorders. Pathophysiologically, pericarditis occurs whenever the etiologic process involves the visceral pericardium. The propensity for supraventricular arrhythmias relates to an involvement of the atrial myocardium and specifically the superficially located sinoatrial node.

1. Dressler, W. A complication of myocardial infarction: Resembling idiopathic recurrent benign pericarditis. *Circulation* 12:697, 1955.
   The original abstract describing the syndrome.
2. Dressler, W. The post-myocardial-infarction syndrome. *Arch. Intern. Med.* 103:28, 1959.
   Carefully describes the signs, symptoms, and course of the syndrome.
3. Thadani, U., Chopra, M. P., Cline, P. A., et al. Pericarditis after acute myocardial infarction. *Br. Med. J.* 2:135, 1971.
   Analyzes the incidence and course of postmyocardial infarction pericarditis and Dressler's syndrome in 779 patients with myocardial infarction. Anticoagulants seem to have no adverse effect.
4. Kossowsky, W. A., Epstein, P. J., and Levine, R. S. Post myocardial infarction syndrome: An early complication of acute myocardial infarction. *Chest* 63:35, 1973.
   The syndrome can on rare occasions occur within 4 to 5 days of the infarction.
5. Davies, A. M., and Gery, I. The role of antibodies in heart disease. *Am. Heart J.* 60:669, 1960.
6. Van der Geld, H. Anti-heart antibodies in the postpericardiotomy and the postmyocardial-infarction syndromes. *Lancet* 2:617, 1964.
7. Kaplan, M. H., and Frengley, J. D. Autoimmunity to the heart in cardiac disease. *Am. J. Cardiol.* 24:459, 1969.
   Articles 5–7 discuss the role of autoimmunity and the presence of antiheart antibodies.
8. James, T. N. Pericarditis and the sinus node. *Arch. Intern. Med.* 110:305, 1962.
   Involvement of the sinoatrial node by the inflammatory process probably accounts for the high incidence of supraventricular arrhythmias.
9. McGuinness, J. B., and Taussig, H. B. The postpericardotomy syndrome. *Circulation* 26:500, 1962.
   The presentation and course are similar to those of Dressler's syndrome, and antiheart antibodies are present. The most constant clinical feature is the pleuropericardial friction rub.
10. Domby, W. R., and Whitcomb, M. E. Pleural effusion as a manifestation of Dressler's syndrome in the distant post-infarction period. *Am. Heart J.* 96:243, 1978.
    This occurred 2.5 years after the onset of Dressler's syndrome.

39. PRIMARY PULMONARY HYPERTENSION
Charles B. Payne, Jr.

The presence of sustained mean blood pressures greater than 20 mm Hg in the pulmonary artery without any identifiable cause defines primary pulmonary hypertension. The disease may have more than one etiology. In this discussion, venoocclusive disease and pulmonary hypertension arising from multiple pulmonary embolic episodes are excluded. The disease is uncommon with a frequency cited as being 0.25 to 1.1 percent in unselected right heart catheterizations. The disease occurs in infants as early as 2 months of age and, in infancy, the sex distribution is equal. Women are afflicted at a 5:1 ratio over men in the ages ranging over the childbearing years from 15 to 50 years. Men usually are diagnosed at older ages than women. The disease is usually not diagnosed until symptoms occur, at which time the underlying pathologic process is well established and therapeutic interventions may be of little or doubtful value. Recent advances in basic knowledge of the pathophysiology of the pulmonary vasculature may make earlier diagnosis assume a high priority as new treatments are developed. The prognosis is variable with survival for up to 39 years being recorded. Most patients progress to death from hypoxemia and intractable cor pulmonale or sudden arrhythmias within 2 to 4 years from the onset of symptoms.

A familial form of the disorder is well described. A large variety of factors may be involved in the etiology of primary pulmonary hypertension. There may be a relationship to the syndrome of persistence of the fetal pulmonary circulation. Hereditary factors may play a role in this persistence although a definitive relationship has not yet been established. Although there is still controversy regarding the possibility that the syndrome is produced by "silent showers" of pulmonary microemboli, there is evidence that this mechanism does not account for all of the available facts. These include an incidence of embolic disease greatest in patients over age 50, not young women who are the most frequently seen patients in adult medicine. The presence of vascular webs and recanalization in thromboembolic disease is not found in primary pulmonary hypertension. More detailed evidence is available in the literature. Primary pulmonary hypertension occurs in association with collagen-vascular diseases more frequently than expected by chance. Raynaud's syndrome is reported in 7 to 30 percent of patients with the disorder and other evidence suggests that vasoconstriction may be involved in the etiology. Unexplained antinuclear antibodies have been found in a group of 14 of 17 patients with primary pulmonary hypertension while none were found in pulmonary hypertension secondary to congenital heart disease.

Drug-induced disease has been well described following the use of the appetite suppressant aminorex in Europe from 1967 to 1970. Other factors implicated have included hypoxemia, liver disease, and various "vasoconstrictive factors." The lung has been shown to be an active metabolic organ in a number of conditions such as the carcinoid syndrome when metabolically active compounds are infused directly into the pulmonary vascular bed. There is current interest in the finding of a gradient for thromboxane across the lung. Whether or not it is a cause or an effect of prostaglandin actions on the pulmonary vasculature is being investigated. It may be that therapy based on alterations of metabolic pathways of thromboxane will result.

Initial symptoms are usually those of exertional dyspnea and fatigue. Syncope and right ventricular failure occur as the disease progresses. If increasing pulmonary artery pressure opens the foramen ovale, cyanosis may occur and rarely there may be hoarseness from recurrent laryngeal nerve palsy from the pressure of an aneurysmal dilatation of the pulmonary artery. Physical findings show a prominent A wave of the jugular venous pulse associated with a right ventricular heave and an accentuated pulmonic valve closure sound. Right heart third and fourth sounds are common and a murmur of tricuspid valve incompetence occurs. Occasionally, there may be a Graham-Steele diastolic murmur of pulmonic valve regurgitation. Chest x-ray examination shows prominence of the pulmonary outflow tract together with right ventricular enlargement causing cardiomegaly. Pruning of the vasculature may occur with progress of the disease. The ECG is that of cor pulmonale with right axis deviation, right atrial P wave changes, and right ventricular hypertrophy. The echocardiogram shows right atrial and ventricular enlargement and flattening of the ventricular septum. Characteristic patterns of pulmonary valve echocardiograms are also described.

The diagnosis is one of exclusion. Pulmonary arteriography may be quite hazardous with elevated pulmonary artery pressures. Ventilation-perfusion scans are preferable screening devices to exclude segmental abnormalities compatible with pulmonary embolic disease. If cardiac catheterization is done, the right ventricular end-diastolic pressure is elevated, the systolic pressures in the right ventricle and pulmonary arteries are increased, but the wedge pressure is normal. Cardiac catheterization must be done cautiously and, if indicated, is usually combined with a therapeutic trial of drugs to be used in therapeutic attempts. Occasionally, lung biopsy is required and, if so, an open lung biopsy rather than a transbronchoscopic biopsy is the method of choice. Pulmonary function studies usually show no airflow obstruction but there may be an increased dead space – tidal volume ratio. Arterial blood gas data commonly show mild to moderate chronic hyperventilation (hypocapnea) with reduced oxygenation from increased alveolar-arterial oxygen gradients felt to represent ventilation-perfusion imbalance with a possible component of a diffusion abnormality. The diffusing capacity may be mildly to strikingly reduced.

At this time there is enthusiasm for the use of various vasodilator drugs in the treatment of primary pulmonary hypertension. A variety of agents, usually investigated under strict protocols, have been tried. The effects of these drugs are measured during cardiac catheterization against the administration of oxygen, which is a known vasodilator. Isoproterenol, hydralazine, verapamil, nifedipine, prostaglandin E_1, and others are currently being evaluated. One attempts to avoid reducing the systemic vascular resistance to a greater degree than the pulmonary resistance to avoid hypotension and aggravation of the disease. There is, as yet, no evidence to suggest that long-term use of any agent or combination correlates well with the initial laboratory measurements or prolongs survival. Although the chronic administration of anticoagulants has been a standard therapy, this treatment has never been known to reverse the course of the disease. Rare spontaneous remissions are recorded.

1. Enson, Y. Pulmonary Hypertension and Its Consequences. In G. L. Baum and E. Wolinsky, eds., *Textbook of Pulmonary Diseases* (3rd ed.). Boston: Little, Brown & Co., 1983. P. 1007.
   An overview and classification of disorders of the pulmonary vasculature.
2. Jones, R. C., and Reid, L. M. Structural Basis of Pulmonary Hypertension. In D. Simmons, (eds.), *Current Pulmonology*. Chicago: Year Book Medical Publishers Inc., 1987. Vol. 8, p. 175.
   A beautifully illustrated description of the morphologic changes in the pulmonary vasculature, including those of early primary pulmonary hypertension.
3. Jones, R. C., Langleben, D., and Reid, L. M. Patterns of Remodeling of Pulmonary Circulation in Acute and Subacute Lung Injury. In S. I. Said (ed.), *The Pulmonary Circulation and Acute Lung Injury*. New York: Futura Publishing Co., 1985. P. 137.
   A more mechanistic approach to the morphologic changes resulting from injury to the pulmonary vasculature outlining evidence from both human disease and animal models.
4. Voelkel, N., and Reeves, J. T. Primary Pulmonary Hypertension. In *Lung Biology in Health and Disease*. Vol 14. Moser, K. M. (ed.), *Pulmonary Vascular Diseases*. New York: Marcel Dekker, Inc., 1979. P. 573.
   An authoritative review of the subject combining epidemiologic, pathologic, clinical, and therapeutic information and giving German and English references up to the time of publication.
5. Nanda, N. C., Gramiak, R., Robinson, T. I., et al. Echocardiographic evaluation of pulmonary hypertension. *Circulation* 50:575, 1974.
   The basic descriptive reference outlining the usual findings from the use of this valuable, noninvasive technique in right ventricular overload syndromes.
6. Shah, A., Schwartz H., and Class, R. N. Unusual echocardiographic findings in primary pulmonary hypertension. *Arch. Intern. Med.* 143:820, 1983.
   A case report enlivened by additional findings of echos generated by hypertrophy of the right ventricular musculature.
7. Ross, R. S. Right ventricular hypertension as a cause of precordial pain. *Am. Heart J.* 61:134, 1961.
   One of several articles which estabished pulmonary hypertension and right ventricular hypertrophy as one of the causes of angina pectoris.
8. Zimmerman, D., and Parker, B. M. The pain of pulmonary hypertension: fact or fancy? *J.A.M.A.* 246:2345, 1981.
   Controlled observations of the frequency of chest pain in patients with pulmonary hypertension found it no more common than in those with normal pulmonary artery pressures.
9. Daoud, F. S., Reeves, J. T., and Kelly, D. B. Isoproterenol as a potential pulmonary vasodilator in primary pulmonary hypertension. *Am. J. Cardiol.* 42:817, 1978.
   One of the seminal papers in the attempt to develop a pharmacologic therapy for relief of the vasoconstrictive aspects of primary pulmonary hypertension.
10. Pietro, D. A., LaBresh, K. A., Shulman, R. M., et al. Sustained improvement in primary pulmonary hypertension during six years of treatment with sublingual isoproterenol. *N. Engl. J. Med.* 310:1032, 1984.
    A single case report illustrating that, in some patients, isoproterenol may be effective when compared to the natural history of the disease.

11. Rubin, L. J., and Peter, R. H. Oral hydralazine therapy for primary pulmonary hypertension. *N. Engl. J. Med.* 302:69, 1980.
    Report of the effects of hydralazine in four patients suggesting a possible therapeutic role in some patients based on cardiac catheterization data.
12. Packer, M., Greenberg, B., Massie, B., et al. Deleterious effects of hydralazine in patients with pulmonary hypertension. *N. Engl. J. Med.* 306:1326, 1982.
    If the effects on systemic vascular resistance outweigh those effects on the pulmonary vascular resistance, then patients may deteriorate quickly.
13. Kronzon, I., Cohen, M., and Winer, H. E. Adverse effect of hydralazine in patients with primary pulmonary hypertension. *J.A.M.A.* 247:3112, 1982.
    A further two cases illustrating the problem of all investigators in attempting to study infrequent cases of this disease.
14. Ruskin, J. N., and Hutter, A. M. Primary pulmonary hypertension treated with oral phentolamine. *Ann. Intern. Med.* 90:772, 1979.
    Outlining the results of a trial of another vasoactive drug.
15. Persen, B., and Proctor, R. J. Primary pulmonary hypertension response to indomethacin, terbutaline and isoproterenol. *Chest* 76:601, 1979.
    An example of careful comparison of the acute effects of various agents during the study of primary pulmonary hypertension.
16. Crevey, B. J., Dantzker, D. R., Bower, J. S., et al. Hemodynamic and gas exchange effects of intravenous diltiazem in patients with pulmonary hypertension. *Am. J. Cardiol.* 49:578, 1982.
    In which the calcium channel blockers are discussed and one studied prospectively in five patients, four of whom had primary pulmonary hypertension.
17. Rubin, L. J., Groves, B. M., Reeves, J. T., et al. Prostacyclin induced acute pulmonary vasodilation in primary pulmonary hypertension. *Circulation* 64:181, 1981.
    An abstract illustrating the potent vasodilator effects of prostacyclin (PGI$_2$) which demonstrated that PGI$_2$ can increase cardiac output and reduce pulmonary vascular resistance.
18. Moser, K. M. Idiopathic pulmonary hypertension: therapeutic opportunities and pitfalls. *J.A.M.A.* 247:3119, 1982.
    A thoughtful editorial calling for careful and closely monitored evaluation of the various drugs done prospectively in spite of the urge to "do something."
19. Hyman, A. L., and Kadowitz, P. J. Vasodilator therapy for pulmonary hypertensive disorders. *Chest* 85:145, 1984.
    This editorial reviews the pathophysiology and unpredictability of reported studies, points directions for further research, and ends on an optimistic note.

III. DISEASES OF CONNECTIVE TISSUE

40. GIANT CELL ARTERITIS
H. Verdain Barnes

Giant cell arteritis (GCA) should be considered in patients over age 50 who have a diagnosis of cerebrovascular insufficiency or occlusion, seizures, dementia, meningoencephalitis, arterial aneurysm, aortic arch syndrome, aortic dissection, myocardial failure, myocardial infarction, unilateral renal hypertension, anemia, fever of unknown origin, sudden or gradual loss of vision, unexplained generalized headaches, gangrene of the extremities, nephrotic syndrome, mononeuritis multiplex, ischemic bowel disease, or hypochondriasis. GCA can involve any part of the arterial tree. The process may be limited to small or large segments of a single artery or may involve small or large segments of many vessels. The primary histologic feature is the presence of lymphocytes, plasma cells, histiocytes, monocytes, and/or macrophages within the arterial wall. The lymphocytes appear to be primarily T cells with a predominance of Leu-3a helper/inducer cells. The intima of the vessel shows loose fibrous tissue proliferation, and the elastic tissues are frayed and fragmented. It is the altered elastic tissue that probably incites the foreign body reaction and giant cell formation that are almost invariably present. Immunofluorescent studies of involved artery may show deposits of IgG, IgM, IgA, and/or complement (C3) in at least four staining patterns: cytoplasmic, elastic, nuclear, and/or linear. The exact pathogenesis remains unclear; these findings suggest the possibility of a cell-mediated, a humoral-mediated, or a combination pathogenesis.

The average age of patients with GCA is about 66 years, with a slight predominance in females. The patient's initial complaint is usually nonspecific and frequently not clearly suggestive of arterial occlusive disease. Consequently, the interval between symptoms and diagnosis is usually a matter of months with a range from 1 week to 3 years. Headache is the most common presenting complaint and occurs as a feature at some time in close to 97 percent. Classically it is temporal, continuously boring and sudden in onset, often with radiation to the face, jaws, and occiput with associated scalp tenderness. Unfortunately, these findings are the exception rather than the rule. Most patients experience nondescript headaches that are often described as "tension headaches." Intermittent tender areas and/or nodules of the scalp are not uncommon and should not be discounted because they are not limited to the temporal areas. Physical examination may reveal scalp nodules and tenderness and/or a thick nonpulsatile temporal artery. On the other hand, the examination is not uncommonly normal. Facial artery involvement is seen in half the patients. A typical complaint is claudication of the jaw or tongue with vigorous chewing or talking. True intermittent claudication of the jaw, however, is not pathognomonic. The arteritic process often involves branches of the ophthalmic arteries, posterior ciliary arteries, and in rare instances the retinal arteries or arteries of the occipital cortex. Ocular manifestations are seen in about half the patients. Sudden blindness or progressive loss of vision is not uncommon; it is bilateral in about half. In sudden blindness the initial ophthalmologic examination is usually normal, only to be followed in 24 to 48 hours by papilledema often in association with hemorrhages and/or cotton-wool exudates. Resolution of these changes typically occurs within 10 to 14 days, but total vision rarely returns. Other eye manifestations include blurred vision, amaurosis fugax, scintillating scotomata, transient ophthalmoplegia, iritis, conjunctivitis, and glaucoma.

Fever occurs in over 50 percent of the patients. It is usually persistent and low grade, but on occasion is high and spiking. Associated night sweats are not uncommon. Anorexia, weight loss, and anemia are seen in about 40 percent. Weight loss may be severe. The anemia is normochromic or minimally hypochromic, with hematocrit values usually between 30 and 35 percent. Polymyalgia rheumatica characterized by pain and stiffness in the proximal muscles and a constellation of constitutional signs and symptoms is associated in about 20 percent. In classic GCA, arthralgias of the knees, shoulders, and hips are not uncommon but frank arthritis is rare. GCA, Takayasu's arteritis, and polymyalgia rheumatica represent a spectrum of a common disease process. Other clinical manifestations of GCA include malaise, easy fatigue, dementia, depression, psychosis, memory loss, focal or generalized seizures, hemiparesis, hearing loss, facial pain or edema, vertigo, deep throat pain, polyneuropathy, myositis, intermittent claudication of the arms and legs, pericarditis, and pulmonary infarction. Renal involvement is rare. Definite diagnosis is made by a positive arterial biopsy, but a negative biopsy does not rule out the diagnosis. A markedly elevated sedimentation rate is typical but not invariable. The course of the ESR tends to follow the course of disease activity. The white blood cell count may be normal or elevated, usually with a normal differential cell count or a slight lymphocytosis. Thrombocytosis may be seen. The bone marrow is normal. The alpha globulin fraction of the serum proteins is frequently elevated, as is fibrinogen. In some patients three of the factor VIII–von Willebrand components and plasminogen activator levels have also been reported to be elevated. None of these tests is diagnostic. Angiographic studies may show alternating areas of ectasia and stenosis in involved areas. Arterial biopsy is the diagnostic tool of choice. Several points need emphasis: (1) The temporal and facial arteries are frequently involved whether or not they are clinically abnormal. (2) The artery segment excised should be 5 cm or greater in length and should have multiple histologic sections made since the involvement may be focal. (3) The introduction of steroid therapy need not be deferred until after the biopsy since arterial healing requires weeks to months. If the biopsy is negative but the suspicion of GCA is high, corticosteroids should be given. A dramatic response to high-dose steroids in 12 to 48 hours supports a presumptive diagnosis.

1. Hamilton, C. R., Jr., Shelley, W. M., and Tumulty, P. A. Giant cell arteritis: Including temporal arteritis and polyalgia rheumatica. *Medicine* 50:1, 1971.
   The best general well-referenced review. The protean manifestations of the disease are carefully presented.
2. Hollenhorst, R. W., Brown, J. R., Wagner, H. P., et al. Neurologic aspects of temporal arteritis. *Neurology* 10:490, 1960.
   Describes classic headache. Watch for GCA in patients with cerebrovascular accidents.
3. Harrison, M. J. G., and Bevan, A. T. Early symptoms of temporal arteritis. *Lancet* 2:638, 1967.
   Signs and symptoms had been present from 1–15 months in 78% of patients.
4. Hunder, G. G., Disney, T. F., and Ward, L. E. Polymyalgia rheumatica. *Mayo Clin. Proc.* 44:849, 1969.
   Not infrequently a component of GCA.
5. Fauchald, P., Rygvold, O., and Øystese, B. Temporal arteritis and polmalgia rheumatica. *Ann. Intern. Med.* 77:845, 1972.
   A practical distinction between these two disorders is difficult if not impossible.
6. Soloway, M., Moir, T. W., and Linton, D. S. Takayasu's arteritis. *Am. J. Cardiol.* 25:258, 1970.
   GCA, polymalgia rheumatica, and Takayasu's arteritis appear to be autoimmune disorders.
7. Heptinstall, R. H., Porter, K. A., and Barkley, H. Giant-cell (temporal) arteritis. *J. Pathol. Bacteriol.* 67:507, 1954.
   The coronary arteries, arteries of the occipital cortex, and the brainstem can be involved.
8. Wagener, H. P., and Hollenhorst, R. W. The ocular lesions of the temporal arteritis. *Am. J. Ophthalmol.* 45:617, 1958.
   A useful review.
9. Liang, G. C., Simkim, P. A., and Mannik, M. Immunoglobulins in temporal arteritis. *Ann. Intern. Med.* 81:19, 1974.
   Deposition of IgG, IgA, IgM, and/or C3 documented.
10. Klein, R. G., Hunder, G. G., Stanson, A. W., et al. Large artery involvement in giant cell (temporal) arteritis. *Ann. Intern. Med.* 83:806, 1975.
    About 14% of these authors' patients had involvement of the aorta or its major branches.
11. Klein, R. G., Campbell, R. J., Hunder, G. G., et al. Skip lesions in temporal arteritis. *Mayo Clin. Proc.* 51:504, 1976.
    The lesion may be as short as 330μ in length; multiple histologic sections are a must.

12. Hunder, G. G., Shelps, S. G., Allen, G. L., et al. Daily and alternate day corticosteroid regimens in treatment of giant cell arteritis. *Ann. Intern. Med.* 82:613, 1975.
    An excellent discussion of therapy.
13. Lupi-Herrera, E., Sánchez-Torres, G., Marcushamer, J., et al. Takayasu's arteritis. Clinical study of 107 cases. *Am. Heart J.* 93:94, 1977.
    The four types of anatomic involvement are discussed.
14. Fauci, A. S., Haynes, B. F., and Katz, P. The spectrum of vasculitis: Clinical pathologic, immunologic and therapeutic considerations. *Ann. Intern. Med.* 89:660, 1978.
    A useful review and comparison of GCA and Takayasu's arteritis.
15. Persellin, S. T., Daniels, T. M., Tings, L. J., et al. Factor VIII–von Willebrand factor in giant cell arteritis and polymyalgia rheumatica. *Mayo Clin. Proc.* 60:457, 1985.
    Elevated levels appear to be normal factor VIII–von Willebrand factor.
16. Lipton, R. B., Solomon, S., and Wertenbaker, C. Gradual loss and recovery of vision in temporal arteritis. *Arch. Intern. Med.* 145:2252, 1985.
    A gradual loss of vision over months can occur.
17. Wong, R. L., and Korn, J. H. Temporal arteritis without an elevated erythrocyte sedimentation rate. *Am. J. Med.* 80:959, 1986.
    Headaches, visual symptoms, and temporal artery signs were the most common in those without an elevated ESR.
18. Green, G. M., Lain, D., Sherwin, R. M., et al. Giant cell arteritis of the legs: Clinically isolation of severe disease with gangrene and amputation. *Am. J. Med.* 81:727, 1986.
19. Feigel, D. W., Robbins, D. L., and Leek, J. C. Giant cell arteritis associated with mononeuritis multiplex and complement-activating 19S IgM rheumatoid factor. *Am. J. Med.* 79:495, 1985.
20. Perruguet, J. L., Davis, D. E., and Harrington, T. M. Aortic arch arteritis in the elderly: An important manifestation of giant cell arteritis. *Arch. Intern. Med.* 146:289, 1986.
21. Truong, L., Kopelman, R. G., Williams, G. S., et al. Temporal arteritis and renal disease. *Am. J. Med.* 78:171, 1985.
    These articles (18–21) illustrate the protean manifestations of this disease.
22. Banks, P. M., Cohen, M. D., Ginsburg, W. W., et al. Immunohistologic and cytochemical studies of temporal arteritis. *Arthritis Rheum.* 26:1201, 1983.
    Cell-mediated immunity may be involved in the pathogenesis.
23. Save-Soderbergh, J., Malmvall, B.-E., Anderson, R., et al. Giant cell arteritis as a cause of death. *J.A.M.A.* 255:493, 1986.
    Cerebrovascular accident appeared to cause the most deaths.
24. Gertz, M. A., Kyle, R. A., Griffing, W. L., et al. Jaw claudication in primary systemic amyloidosis. *Medicine* 65:173, 1986.
    Nothing is pathognomonic.

---

41. JUVENILE RHEUMATOID ARTHRITIS
H. Verdain Barnes

Juvenile rheumatoid arthritis (JRA), or Still's disease, is a protean disorder of uncertain etiology. It occurs primarily in children and adolescents, but can occur in adults. The precise incidence of the disease is not known, but it is not rare in children and youth. In most series, misdiagnosis for weeks, months, and occasionally years is common. JRA has three typical presentations: febrile systemic, polyarticular, and pauciarticular.

JRA with a febrile systemic presentation is usually acute in onset. It occurs in about 20 percent of children and adolescents and is characteristic of the adult form. In children and adolescents the other notable findings and approximate incidences are rash (90%), generalized lymphadenopathy (85%), splenomegaly (75%), pericarditis (35%), pneumonitis and/or pleuritis (35%), hepatomegaly (20%), abdominal pain (10%), myocarditis (2%), and iridocyclitis (less than 1%). The joint complaints range from none to arthralgias to florid arthritis. In only about one-third of patients do the joint complaints arise simultaneously with the onset of systemic manifestations. The fever pattern is typically quotidian or double quotidian, with temperature spikes that may reach as high as 40.5°C (105°F). Remittent, relapsing, or periodic patterns may occur, but are rare. The diurnal temperature range may be as wide as 4 to 5°C (7.2–9.0°F); hence in a 24-hour period both high and subnormal temperatures may be seen in the same patient. The classic rash is an evanescent eruption consisting of discrete or confluent macules and/ or papules. It usually involves the face, trunk, and/or extremities, including the palms and soles. Erythema is variable in degree and can often be increased by rubbing or warming. Interestingly, the rash can be elicited or intensified by rubbing or mild trauma—Koebner's phenomenon. Pericarditis when present without associated myocarditis usually runs a benign but recurrent course. Patients with pericarditis are generally asymptomatic, but the diagnosis can usually be made by ECG and/or echocardiography. Pneumonitis and/or pleuritis when present is often asymptomatic. The primary importance of evaluating the patient for pericarditis, pneumonitis, and pleuritis is that these conditions may herald the onset of myocarditis. Myocarditis is a serious manifestation often accompanied by rapid cardiac enlargement and congestive heart failure. Vasculitis and encephalopathy are rare. Typical laboratory findings include a leukocyte count of 20,000 to 30,000, mild anemia, an elevated erythrocyte sedimentation rate (ESR), and negative standard rheumatoid factor and antinuclear antibody (ANA) tests. The differential diagnosis includes systemic lupus erythematosus, infection, polyarteritis, Henoch-Schönlein purpura, leukemia, inflammatory bowel disease, and familial Mediterranean fever. The adult form is similar, except for a lesser frequency of pneumonitis, pleuritis, generalized adenopathy, iridocyclitis, and myocarditis.

The polyarticular presentation occurs in 30 to 50 percent of children and adolescents, with a predominance among females. About 80 percent have symmetric involvement of more than four joints, most commonly the knees, ankles, elbows, cervical spine, hips, and metacarpal phalangeal and proximal interphalangeal joints. Systemic manifestations include a daily low-grade fever (in about 60%), rash and lymphadenopathy (40%), subcutaneous nodules (25%), splenomegaly (22%), and pericarditis, pneumonitis, pleuritis, and hepatomegaly (4%). Myocarditis and iridocyclitis are rare. The laboratory findings are variable, but the majority of patients have a leukocyte count in the 20,000 to 30,000 range, an elevated ESR, and a minimal to moderate anemia. The standard rheumatoid factor is elevated (1:160 or greater) in 25 to 75 percent and antinuclear factor is present in low titers in about 25 percent. An elevated antistreptolysin O (ASO) titer is not uncommon, often confusing the diagnosis with acute rheumatic fever. The immunoglobulins IgG, IgM, and IgA are elevated in about 30 percent, and IgA is decreased in about 4 percent. The differential diagnosis of the polyarticular form includes acute rheumatic fever, serum sickness, viral hepatitis, rubella, systemic lupus erythematosus, dermatomyositis, and drug reactions.

The pauciarticular presentation involves four or fewer joints. This mode of onset occurs in 30 to 50 percent with a female-male ratio of about 3:1. The arthritis is usually insidious in onset, consisting primarily of swelling and stiffness, with minimal to no pain, except with hip involvement where pain is often severe. In descending order of frequency, the joints involved are the knee, hip, ankle, and elbow. The systemic manifestations are low-grade quotidian fever (in about 50% of patients), rash, lymphadenopathy and splenomegaly (20%), and hepatomegaly (10%). Close to 25 percent of these patients have or develop iridocyclitis. Pericarditis, pneumonitis, pleuritis, myocarditis, and subcutaneous nodules are rare. The white blood count is usually normal, and when elevated is rarely more than 18,000. The ESR is elevated in just over 50 percent of patients, and anemia occurs in less than 20 percent. Rheumatoid factor is seldom elevated, but a positive antinuclear factor (ANA) occurs in about one-third of patients. The differential diagnosis includes inflammatory bowel disease, traumatic arthritis, infection (particularly gonococcal), juvenile ankylosing spondylitis, systemic lupus erythematosus, psoriatic arthritis, hemophilia, and Reiter's syndrome.

The principal complications of JRA are myocarditis, iridocyclitis, deforming arthritis, delayed growth and development, amyloidosis, and psychosocial adjustment problems. Iridocyclitis deserves special emphasis. It occurs most frequently in females who have an early age of pauciarticular onset and positive ANA. Early iridocyclitis is often asymptomatic; it may first present with a decrease in vision. An early diagnosis in asymptomatic patients requires a slit-lamp examination. About 45 percent of patients initially complain of a red eye, ocular pain, and/or photophobia. Iridocyclitis may precede arthritic manifestations by as much as 2 to 4 years. Once present, the disease is chronic, with remissions and exacerbations, and demands aggressive steroid therapy. The sequelae of active disease are synechiae, glaucoma, cataracts, band keratopathy, and blindness.

The course of JRA is variable, but in general seems to fall into three categories: (1) termination of active disease within 2 years of onset and no sequelae, (2) recurrent febrile flares, with inactive interludes of weeks to months, (3) chronic arthritis, with varying degrees of joint deformity. Mortality ranges from 2 to 5 percent, with the most common causes of death being secondary amyloidosis in polyarticular disease and myocarditis in the febrile systemic group. Complete remission occurs in about 50 percent of patients, with at least 70 percent regaining normal joint function. An occasional patient with a remission of long duration will have a severe exacerbation and progressive disability as an adult.

1. Still, G. S. On a form of chronic joint disease in children. *Med. Chir. Trans.* 80:47, 1897.
   A classic description of the systemic features of JRA.
2. Calabro, J. J., Holgerson, W. B., Sonpal, G. M., et al. Juvenile rheumatoid arthritis: A general review and report of 100 patients observed for 15 years. *Semin. Arthritis Rheum.* 5:257, 1976.
   A well-written and referenced review.
3. Grossman, B. J., Ozoa, N. F., and Arya, S. C. Problems in juvenile rheumatoid arthritis. *Med. Clin. North Am.* 49:33, 1965.
   In this survey, diagnostic errors were found to occur in about 50% of patients.
4. Calabro, J. J., and Marchesano, J. M. Fever associated with juvenile rheumatoid arthritis. *N. Engl. J. Med.* 276:11, 1967.
   The typical fever pattern is quotidian or double quotidian.
5. Calabro, J. J., and Marchesano, J. M. Rash associated with juvenile rheumatoid arthritis. *J. Pediatr.* 72:611, 1968.
   The characteristics of the rash are discussed, and Koebner's phenomenon is detailed.
6. Lietman, P. F., and Bywaters, E. G. L. Pericarditis in juvenile rheumatoid arthritis. *Pediatrics* 32:855, 1963.
   Pericarditis is usually a benign, recurrent process.
7. Bernstein, B., Takahashi, M., and Hanson, V. Non-invasive techniques in the study of cardiac involvement in juvenile rheumatoid arthritis. *Arthritis Rheum.* 16:535, 1973.
   Currently the most sensitive diagnostic procedure is echocardiography.
8. Rudnicki, R. D., Ruderman, M., Scull, E., et al. Clinical features and serologic abnormalities in juvenile rheumatoid arthritis. *Arthritis Rheum.* 17:1007, 1974.
   A concise review of the serologic findings in JRA as well as its multifaceted clinical features.
9. Torrigiani, G., Roitt, I. M., Lloyd, K. M., et al. Elevated IgG antiglobulins in patients with seronegative rheumatoid arthritis. *Lancet* 1:14, 1970.
   Many seronegative JRA patients have an IgG–anti-IgG rheumatoid factor that is not picked up by routine agglutination tests.
10. Schaller, J., Kupfer, C., and Wedgwood, R. J. Iridocyclitis in juvenile rheumatoid arthritis. *Pediatrics* 44:92, 1969.
    This chronic eye disease may precede the development of arthritis by months to years.
11. Chylack, L. T., Binfang, D. C., Bellows, A. R., et al. Ocular manifestations of juvenile rheumatoid arthritis. *Am. J. Ophthalmol.* 79:1026, 1975.
    In this series the patients most commonly developing iridocyclitis were young women with monoarticular or pauciarticular presentations. 44% had identifiable ocular signs and symptoms at the time of examination.
12. Schaller, J. G., Johnson, G. D., Holborow, E. J., et al. The association of antinuclear

antibodies with the chronic iridocyclitis of juvenile rheumatoid arthritis (Still's disease). *Arthritis Rheum.* 17:409, 1974.
The authors found that 88% of their patients with chronic iridocyclitis had positive tests for antinuclear factor.

13. Bywaters, E. G. L., and Ansell, B. M. Cause of death in juvenile rheumatoid chronic polyarthritis. *J. Rheumatol.* 1:178, 1974.
The most common cause of death in this group is secondary amyloidosis.

14. Schaller, J., and Wedgwood, R. J. Juvenile rheumatoid arthritis: A review. *Pediatrics* 50:940, 1972.
In this series, 26% of patients presented with febrile systemic manifestations, 37% with polyarticular disease, and 37% with pauciarticular disease.

15. Goel, K. M., and Shanks, R. A. Follow-up study of 100 cases of juvenile rheumatoid arthritis. *Ann. Rheum. Dis.* 33:25, 1974.
In this series, prognosis was better in late-onset and monoarticular disease.

16. Jan, J. E., Hill, R. H., and Low, M. D. Cerebral complications in juvenile rheumatoid arthritis. *Can. Med. Assoc. J.* 107:623, 1972.
In this series 7% of the patients were found to have some cerebral complications, of which the most common was toxic encephalopathy.

17. Oen, K., Wilkins, J. A., and Krzekotowska, D. OKT4:OKT8 ratios of circulating T cells and in vitro suppressor cell function of patients with juvenile rheumatoid arthritis (JRA). *J. Rheumatol.* 12:321, 1985.
JRA patients (children and adolescents) had increased OKT4:OKT8 ratios compared to controls.

18. Larson, E. B. Adult Still's disease. *Medicine* 63:82, 1984.

19. Cush, J. J., Medsger, T. A., Jr., Christy, W. C., et al. Adult-onset Still's disease. *Arthritis Rheum.* 30:186, 1987.
These articles (18, 19) define the presentation and course of adult JRA. An entity not to be overlooked.

42. RHEUMATOID ARTHRITIS
Alice Faryna

Rheumatoid arthritis (RA) is a systemic disease characterized by immunologic abnormalities and the manner in which it affects the joints. Its prevalence, when the strictest criteria are applied, is between 0.5 and 1.0 percent of the adult population, with a peak incidence in the fourth decade, although the disease may occur at any age. Females are affected 2 to 3 times as often as men, but this difference is more pronounced in younger adults, and becomes negligible in the elderly.

The etiology is unknown, although evidence of activation of both cellular and humoral limbs of the immune system suggests that exogenous (e.g., bacteria or viruses) or endogenous (e.g., collagen) antigens may initiate the process. Rheumatoid factors (immunoglobulins with specificity for the Fc portion of IgG) are produced as part of the polyclonal activation of B cells by the persistently activated T cells, and are more likely a product of the rheumatoid process rather than its cause. However, complement-activating immune complexes containing rheumatoid factor may well amplify the inflammatory process in the synovium. Genetic factors are thought to play a role in susceptibility of RA, since the HLA type DR4 is found more frequently in RA patients than in controls.

The initial pathologic lesion is an acute inflammatory synovitis, which may be accompanied by joint effusions of inflammatory fluid. The synovial tissue becomes greatly thickened by synovial cell hyperplasia and infiltration of inflammatory cells, which sometimes form aggregates or lymphoid follicles. The majority of cells are T cells. The hypertrophied synovium (pannus) produces immunoglobulins and a variety of inflammatory molecules (lymphokines, collagenases, proteases, complement fragments, prostaglandins, superoxide radicals), which are capable of degrading cartilage and bone. The invasion of bone and cartilage by pannus adds to this destruction. Surprisingly, ankylosis of the joints is rare in RA.

In the majority (two-thirds) of patients, the onset is insidious. About 5 to 10 percent have an abrupt onset, and the remainder an intermediate onset. Malaise and fatigue may precede joint symptoms by months. Joint pain with swelling of joints and tendon sheaths are the hallmarks of the disease, and while any synovial joint may be affected initially, the characteristic pattern of established RA is a symmetric large and small joint polyarthritis with a predilection for the joints of the hands and wrists. The 1987 revised classification criteria of the American Rheumatism Association have been shown to have 93 percent sensitivity and 90 percent specificity when four or more of the following are met: (1) morning stiffness for at least 1 hour for a duration of 6 weeks or more; (2) swelling of at least three joints for 6 weeks or more; (3) swelling of wrist metacarpophalangeal (MP) or proximal interphalangeal (PIP) joints for 6 weeks or more; (4) symmetry of swollen joint areas for 6 weeks or more; (5) typical hand x-ray changes; (6) physician-confirmed subcutaneous nodules; and (7) abnormal amounts of rheumatoid factor in the serum.

Deformities of hands and feet result from tendon sheath swelling or erosions, producing displacement of tendons and subluxation of joints. Prolonged disuse or joint destruction often lead to marked limitation of motion of larger joints such as the knees, hips, and shoulders. The most common deformities are ulnar deviation of the fingers, swanneck or boutonnière deformities of the fingers, and cocked-up toes. Joints rarely affected by RA are the distal interphalangeal joints, and the thoracic and lumbar regions of the spine. Rarely, joint disease may create life-threatening situations. Subluxation of C1 on C2 from erosive disease around the odontoid process may cause cervical cord compression. Fixation of the cricoarytenoid joints in adduction may result in laryngeal stridor and asphyxiation. Other clinical events may result indirectly from the rheumatoid process. A common consequence of thickened synovial tissue and the associated local inflammatory mass are neural entrapment syndromes (30%), most commonly in the carpal tunnel, causing numbness and weakness in the median distribution of the hand. Other areas vulnerable to entrapment are the tarsal tunnel (ankle), the popliteal fossa, and the forearm near the elbow.

Extraarticular manifestations are frequently found. The most common (up to 35%) are subcutaneous nodules, which are usually situated over pressure joints or the extensor tendons of the fingers. Rheumatoid nodules have the histologic appearance of foreign body granulomas, and have been found in deeper structures such as the lungs, heart, sclera, vocal cords, and the lining membranes of the central and peripheral nervous systems. Sjögren's syndrome (diminished secretion of tears and saliva), splenomegaly, and evidence of active or prior pleuritis or pericarditis may be found in 10 to 15 percent of RA patients. Scleritis, necrotizing vasculitis, pulmonary fibrosis, and amyloidosis are rare complications of RA. Felty's syndrome (leukopenia with selective neutropenia and splenomegaly) is also a rare complication, with a poor prognosis because of recurrent gram-positive infections.

There are no laboratory tests which are pathognomonic for RA. The rheumatoid factor is present in 80 percent. Most authorities consider titers below 1:160 as not likely to be significant. Although very high titers of rheumatoid factor appear to be markers of destructive and complicated disease, variations in titer do not correlate with clinical activity. The sedimentation rate and C-reactive protein are usually elevated during periods of activity, but the best clinical marker of activity is the duration of morning stiffness. A normochromic, normocytic anemia is often present in severe RA. Rheumatoid effusions (joint, pleural, pericardial) are characterized by elevated WBC, low glucose, and low complement levels. Serum complement is usually normal. About 25 percent of patients have a positive test for antinuclear antibody (ANA). The earliest radiographic changes in RA are soft tissue swelling around the joints, and periarticular osteopenia, best appreciated in hand films. Uniform joint space narrowing due to loss of cartilage occurs later. Erosions may take years to appear, and typically begin at the periphery of the joint.

The diseases most commonly confused with RA are systemic lupus erythematosus

(SLE), fibrositis, and polymyalgia rheumatica (PMR). Occasionally, elderly patients with hand deformities due to osteoarthritis (OA) will be labeled as RA because of a positive test for rheumatoid factor. It is well to remember that false-positive tests for autoantibodies are more common in the elderly. The OA patients have a shorter duration of morning stiffness, and no evidence of soft tissue swelling. SLE patients can be distinguished by the presence of typical rashes, CNS manifestations, renal disease, or the presence of specific ANAs such as anti-DNA or anti-Sm. Fibrositis patients present with symptoms resembling RA (morning stiffness, widespread symmetric pain), but have no objective joint findings, have normal laboratory tests, and have tenderness localized to specific soft tissue areas rather than over the joints. Patients with PMR complain of pain and stiffness in the shoulder and hip girdle regions. While they may have objective evidence of synovitis in the more peripheral joints, the predilection for the hands and wrists is not seen as often as in RA. A greatly elevated sedimentation rate (80–120 mm) is usually found in PMR.

In 15 to 22 percent of RA patients, the disease has an intermittent course of remissions and relapses, but the majority have a chronic and progressive course if untreated. No more than 10 percent have a spontaneous and long-lasting remission. Most patients will improve with pharmacologic therapy, which should be continued indefinitely, as relapses are common if treatment is discontinued. About 5 percent are unresponsive to all standard therapies, and are candidates for experimental therapies.

1. Kelley, W. N., Harris, E. D., Ruddy, S., et al. (eds.). *Textbook of Rheumatology.* Philadelphia: W.B. Saunders Co., 1989.
   Chapters 51–63 are the best comprehensive reference source.
2. Rodnan, G. P., and Schumacher, H. R. (eds). *Primer on the Rheumatic Diseases.* Atlanta: Arthritis Foundation, 1988.
   The best condensed overview of rheumatic diseases including RA.
3. Arnett, F. C., Edworthy, S., Bloch, D. A., et al. The 1987 revised ARA criteria for rheumatoid arthritis. *Arthritis Rheum.* 30(Suppl.):S17, 1987.
   The lengthy 1958 criteria have been reduced to 7 simplified criteria which have high sensitivity and specificity.
4. Decker, J. L., Malone, D. G., Haraoui, B., et al. Rheumatoid arthritis: Evolving concepts of pathogenesis and treatment. *Ann. Intern. Med.* 101:810, 1984.
   Histologic and immunologic abnormalities suggest a major role for cell-mediated immune mechanisms. The causes of RA may be multiple.
5. Masi, A. T., and Feigenbaum, S. L. Seronegative rheumatoid arthritis, fact or fiction? *Arch. Intern. Med.* 143:2167, 1983.
   A concise summary of other rheumatic disorders to be considered in patients with rheumatoid factor–negative polyarthritis.
6. Aho, K., Palosuo, T., Raunio, J., et al. When does rheumatoid disease start? *Arthritis Rheum.* 28:485, 1985.
   Rheumatoid factor may be present several years before the onset of clinically evident RA. The risk for asymptomatic seropositive persons is 5%.
7. Kaufman, R. L., and Glenn, W. V. Rheumatoid cervical myelopathy: Evaluation by computerized tomography with multiplanar reconstruction. *J. Rheumatol.* 10:42, 1983.
   Cervical disease occurs in a high proportion of RA patients with severe peripheral disease. Computed tomography scans are useful in identifying compressive myelopathy resulting from subluxation.
8. Hurd, E. R. Extraarticular manifestations of rheumatoid arthritis. *Semin. Arthritis Rheum.* 8:151, 1979.
   The most comprehensive literature review of extraarticular RA.
9. Kaye, B. R., Kaye, R. L., and Bobrove, A. Rheumatoid nodules: Review of the spectrum of associated conditions and proposal of a new classification, with a report of four seronegative cases. *Am. J. Med.* 76:279, 1984.
   Rheumatoid nodules occur in a variety of immunologic and infectious diseases. Other nodular conditions may resemble rheumatoid nodules.
10. Nakano, K. K. The entrapment neuropathies. *Muscle Nerve.* 1:264, 1978.
    An excellent description of clinical findings in entrapment syndromes.

11. Cervantes-Perez, P., Toro-Perez, A. H., and Rodriguez-Jurado, P. Pulmonary involvement in rheumatoid arthritis. *J.A.M.A.* 243:1715, 1980.
    A prospective study of 140 hospitalized RA patients which showed that 80% had interstitial disease even though half of those were asymptomatic.
12. Franco, A. E., Levine, H. D., and Hall, A. P. Rheumatoid pericarditis: Report of 17 cases diagnosed clinically. *Ann. Intern. Med.* 77:837, 1972.
    A review of 17 cases recognized clinically, comparing clinical, radiographic, and laboratory features with cases of uncomplicated RA.
13. Thorne, C., and Urowitz, M. B. Long-term outcome in Felty's syndrome. *Ann. Rheum. Dis.* 41:486, 1982.
    A review of 35 cases of Felty's syndrome. Mortality was 36% at 5 years. Splenectomy did not prevent sepsis.
14. Abruzzo, J. L. Rheumatoid arthritis and mortality. *Arthritis Rheum.* 25:1020, 1982.
    Shortened survival has been demonstrated in RA patients who have severe disease. Aggressive treatment may also be a factor. Major causes of death are infection, vasculitis, or amyloidosis.
15. Abramowicz, M. (ed.). Drugs for rheumatoid arthritis. *Med. Lett. Drugs Ther.* 29:21, 1987.
    A concise summary of drugs commonly used in RA, including a list of available nonsteroidal drugs, their dosages, and costs.
16. Bunch, T. W., and O'Duffy, J. D. Disease-modifying drugs for progressive rheumatoid arthritis. *Mayo Clin. Proc.* 55:161, 1980.
    A thorough review of the pharmacology and toxicity of second-line antirheumatic drugs.
17. Abruzzo, J. L. Auranofin: A new drug for rheumatoid arthritis. *Ann. Intern. Med.* 105:274, 1986.
    An editorial review of chrysotherapy. Oral gold has an efficacy approaching that of injectable gold, and has far fewer adverse reactions.
18. Kremer, J. M., and Lee, J. K. The safety and efficacy of the use of methotrexate in long-term therapy for rheumatoid arthritis. *Arthritis Rheum.* 29:822, 1986.
    Methotrexate has the advantages of rapid onset of action and once-weekly dosing. The possibility of late-onset liver damage is of concern.
19. Tanay, A., Field, E. H., Hoppe, R. T., et al. Long-term followup of rheumatoid arthritis patients treated with total lymphoid irradiation. *Arthritis Rheum.* 30:1, 1987.
    Patients with severe and intractable RA often improve after total lymphoid radiation. Complications of this therapy are described. Four of 32 patients have died of causes not directly related to radiation.
20. Pinals, R. S., Masi, A. T., and Larsen, R. A. Preliminary criteria for clinical remission in rheumatoid arthritis. *Arthritis Rheum.* 24:1308, 1981.
    Criteria proposed for evidence of remission of RA include absence of morning stiffness and fatigue, absence of joint/tendon tenderness and swelling, and normal sedimentation rate.
21. Sherrer, Y. S., Bloch, D. A., Mitchell, D. M., et al. The development of disability in rheumatoid arthritis. *Arthritis Rheum.* 29:494, 1986.
    Only 10% of RA patients remain free of disability on long-term follow-up. Older women and early radiographic progression had the worst prognosis.

43. SPONDYLOARTHROPATHIES

Michelle Petri
David B. Hellmann

The spondyloarthropathies are disorders characterized chiefly by inflammatory arthritis of the spine. The members of the spondyloarthropathy family include ankylosing spondylitis, Reiter's syndrome, reactive arthritis, and the arthritis associated with inflammatory bowel disease and psoriasis.

Though each member is clinically distinct, the family has many common features. First, inflammation of the spine usually dominates the clinical picture. Second, the predominant site of inflammation is not the synovium (as in rheumatoid arthritis) but ligaments and tendons, particularly at their bony attachments. This form of inflammation (enthesopathy) explains why the spine, the Achilles tendon, the heel (at the insertion of the plantar fascia) are so frequently and so distinctively involved. Third, all of these disorders are frequently associated with uveitis, especially anterior uveitis. Other extra-articular sites of inflammation can also be seen, including the skin and mucous membranes (psoriasis, keratodermia blennorrhagicum, circinate balanitis), the heart (conduction defects, aortitis, aortic regurgitation), and the lung (apical fibrosis). Fourth, the spondyloarthropathies are seronegative; the serum does not contain autoantibodies such as rheumatoid factors or antinuclear antibodies. Fifth, HLA-B27 is strikingly more prevalent in patients with spondyloarthropathies than in the normal population. How these or other linked genes increase the risk of developing a spondyloarthropathy remains one of the most important enigmas in rheumatology.

The most common spondyloarthropathy is ankylosing spondylitis, a disease that affects one out of every 100 adults. Clinically significant disease is 9 times more common in men than in women. The most prominent early symptom is low back pain that differs from common back strain in that the pain of ankylosing spondylitis (1) begins insidiously (over months), (2) almost always begins before age 40 (often during late adolescence), (3) is aggravated by rest, and (4) is improved with moderate activity. Because the predominant pathology is inflammation at the bony insertions of ligaments and tendons (enthesopathy), patients may also have chest pain, Achilles tendinitis, plantar fascitis with heel pain, and sausage-shaped digits. Uveitis or synovitis of peripheral joints, especially an oligoarthritis of the lower extremities, can also occur. Evidence of restricted motion either by chest expansion or lumbosacral spine motion (the Schober test) may be found on physical examination. Occasionally, maneuvers that stress the sacroiliac joints may be painful.

The diagnosis of ankylosing spondylitis is confirmed by x rays. The earliest changes are erosions and sclerosis of the sacroiliac joints. Radionuclide bone scans or computed tomography may identify early sacroiliitis when plain films are normal. Later in the disease syndesmophytes may be found in the lumbosacral spine. In severe disease, involvement progresses up the spine, leading to a "bamboo spine."

Ninety percent of white patients with ankylosing spondylitis are positive for HLA-B27. However, this test is not diagnostic since the gene is present in 14 percent of the normal white population.

In many patients the disease process stabilizes and does not affect longevity. Yet, approximately 40 percent will develop severe spinal restriction. Other late complications of ankylosing spondylitis can include destruction of peripheral joints (especially hip and shoulder), (fatal) spinal fracture, aortic regurgitation, conduction disturbances, cauda equina syndrome, apical fibrotic lung disease, and renal amyloidosis. Treatment includes physical therapy to preserve extension of the spine and anti-inflammatory agents, especially indomethacin. Phenylbutazone, although effective, is reserved for appropriate patients who fail multiple other nonsteroidal anti-inflammatory drugs.

Another important member of the spondyloarthropathy family is Reiter's syndrome, which was originally described as a triad of conjunctivitis, urethritis, and arthritis that develops days to weeks after dysentery. It is now known that Reiter's can follow a non-gonococcal urethritis, dysentery, or occur idiopathically. The classic triad is not always present, and other features such as mucocutaneous lesions (aphthous ulcers, keratodermia blennorrhagicum, circinate balanitis), Achilles tendinitis, plantar fascitis ("lover's heel"), and dactylitis (sausage-shaped digits) are also characteristic of Reiter's.

Reiter's is second only to gonococcal infection as the most frequent cause of inflammatory arthritis in young men. The disease is less frequently diagnosed in women, but this may be because cervicitis, a counterpart of urethritis, is undetected. The arthritis, the most salient clinical feature, is usually a lower-extremity oligoarthritis. In some, the arthritis is severe and associated with fever and weight loss. Twenty percent will have low back pain from sacroiliitis.

In the absence of the classic extraarticular features, so-called incomplete Reiter's can be difficult to distinguish from gonococcal arthritis. Where there is doubt, appropriate antibiotic treatment is advised; prompt response and positive cultures will provide proof of gonococcal infection.

In Reiter's, as in ankylosing spondylitis, the great majority of patients (>75%) are HLA-B27–positive. Sacroiliitis is seen eventually in 20 to 30 percent but may not be present initially. The earliest x-ray changes in some cases may be reactive heel spurs from plantar fascitis. It often takes months before peripheral joints show the character- istic periosteal new bone "whiskering." The joint fluid is inflammatory and routine cul- tures are negative.

Though Reiter's was originally thought to be a self-limited arthritis of several weeks to months, it is now apparent that most cases produce a chronic waxing and waning course. While life span is not affected, disability may be persistent.

Treatment of Reiter's disease consists mainly of nonsteroidal anti-inflammatory agents. Large knee or other joint effusions may require periodic drainage and intra- articular corticosteroids. In rare cases, antimetabolites, such as methotrexate or aza- thioprine, are necessary.

With the use of careful and sophisticated microbiologic techniques, it has become clear that an (usually sterile) arthritis can develop following diarrhea due to *Shigella, Salmonella, Campylobacter, Clostridium difficile, Yersinia,* or *Giardia*. Many of these cases lack the other features of Reiter's, and have therefore been termed "reactive arthritis." There is, however, tremendous clinical overlap among cases of reactive arthritis, Rei- ter's, and "incomplete Reiter's." The high prevalence of HLA-B27 in all of these groups suggests a shared genetic predisposition to develop an abnormal immune response to certain infections, which, in turn, results in an inflammatory arthritis. It seems likely, then, that each of these conditions is a "reactive arthritis," and that "Reiter's" simply designates a subset with characteristic extraarticular features.

Inflammatory bowel disease is associated with both a spondyloarthropathy (often HLA-B27–associated) and a peripheral arthritis. The spondyloarthropathy progresses independently of the bowel disease. Sacroiliitis, if present, is usually symmetric and syndesmophytes, if found, are marginal and symmetric, as is the case with ankylosing spondylitis.

Psoriatic arthritis most commonly presents with an oligoarticular "skip-hit" pattern or a rheumatoidlike pattern, but it can also present as a spondyloarthropathy (with an increased incidence of HLA-B27). Asymmetric sacroiliitis, as in Reiter's disease, is com- monly found.

1. Carette, S., Graham, D., Little, H., et al. The natural disease course of ankylosing spondylitis. *Arthritis Rheum.* 26:186, 1983.
   Thirty-year follow-up of a large cohort shows that 41% develop severe spine restric- tion, 20% or less have significant disability, and that early peripheral joint disease, particularly of the hip, augurs a poor prognosis.
2. Lehtinen, K. 76 patients with ankylosing spondylitis seen after 30 years of disease. *Scand. J. Rheum.* 12:5, 1983.
   A discussion of the natural history of the disease, including cardiac, renal, and pul- monary complications.
3. McGuigan, L. E., Geczy, A. F., Edmonds, J. P. The immunopathology of ankylosing spondylitis—a review. *Semin. Arthritis Rheum.* 15:81, 1985.
   Review of HLA-B27, immune function, and Klebsiella cross-reactive determinants in ankylosing spondylitis.
4. Geczy, A. F., Alexander, K., and Bashir, H. V. A factor(s) in *Klebsiella* culture filtrates specifically modifies an HLA-B27–associated cell-surface component. *Nature* 283:182, 1980.
   Rabbits immunized with Klebsiella antigens develop antibodies that specifically lyse the lymphocytes of patients with ankylosing spondylitis.
5. Terasaki, P. I., and Yu, D. T. Regarding the ankylosing spondylitis/*Klebsiella*/HLA- B27 problem. *Arthritis Rheum.* 30:353, 1987.
   Editorial discussing the difficulties of confirming the findings in reference 4.

6. Brewerton, D. A., Goddard, D. H., Moore, R. B., et al. The myocardium in ankylosing spondylitis. *Lancet* 1:995, 1987.
   In addition to conduction defects and aortic root abnormalities, some patients have echocardiographic evidence of functional disturbance of the left ventricle, especially during diastole. The long-term clinical ramifications are unknown.
7. Bergfeldt, L. HLA-B27-associated rheumatic diseases with severe cardiac bradyar-rhythmias. *Am. J. Med.* 75:210, 1983.
   13% of patients with severe bradyarrhythmias had a spondyloarthropathy.
8. Bergfeldt, L., Edhag, O., Vedin, L., et al. Ankylosing spondylitis: An important cause of severe disturbances of the cardiac conduction system. *Am. J. Med.* 73:187, 1982.
   Ankylosing spondylitis is 15 times more common in patients requiring pacemakers than in the normal population.
9. Rosenow, E. C., III, Strimline, C. V., Muhm, J. R., et al. Pleuropulmonary manifes-tations of ankylosing spondylitis. *Mayo Clin. Proc.* 52:641, 1977.
   Review of 2080 patients; 1.3% had pleuropulmonary manifestations, most commonly fibrobullous changes in the upper lobes.
10. Fransen, M. J. A. M., VanHerwaarden, C. L. A. A., van de Putstes, L. B. A., et al. Lung function in patients with ankylosing spondylitis. *J. Rheum.* 13:936, 1986.
    Slight restrictive lung disease is common, but usually clinically silent, because nor-mal diaphragmatic function compensates for chest wall restriction.
11. Ryan, L. M., Carrera, G. F., Lightfoot, R. W., Jr., et al. The radiographic diagnosis of sacroiliitis. *Arthritis Rheum.* 26:760, 1983.
    Single posteroanterior view of the sacroiliac joints is 70–80% accurate.
12. Bellamy, N., Park, W., and Rooney, P. J. What do we know about the sacroiliac joint? *Semin. Arthritis Rheum.* 12:282, 1983.
    Extensive review.
13. Resnik, C. S., and Resnick, D. Radiology of disorders of the sacroiliac joints. *J.A.M.A.* 253:2863, 1985.
    A concise description of the differentiation of sacroiliac findings.
14. Russell, A. S., Masksymowych, W., LeClerq, S. Clinical examination of the sacroiliac joints: A prospective study. *Arthritis Rheum.* 24:1575, 1981.
    This study demonstrates the lack of discriminatory function of techniques for sacro-iliac assessment.
15. Jacobs, J. C. Spondyloarthritis and enthesopathy. *Arch. Intern. Med.* 143:103, 1983.
    A discussion of enthesopathy, the pathologic process underlying the spondyloarthrop-athies.
16. Calin, A., and Fries, J. F. Striking prevalence of ankylosing spondylitis in "healthy" W27 positive males and females: a controlled study. *N. Engl. J. Med.* 293:835, 1975.
    In this study a person with HLA-B27 has a 20% chance of developing ankylosing spondylitis, suggesting a prevalence of 10–15 per 1000.
17. Wasner, C., Britton, M. C., Kraines, G., et al. Nonsteroidal anti-inflammatory agents in rheumatoid arthritis and ankylosing spondylitis. *J.A.M.A.* 246:2168, 1981.
    Patients with ankylosing spondylitis preferred naproxen, indomethacin, and fenopro-fen in this study.
18. Hunter, T., and Dubo, H. Spinal fractures complicating ankylosing spondylitis. *Ann. Intern. Med.* 88:546, 1978.
    Minor trauma can produce spinal fracture. The most common site is lower cervical spine.
19. Murray, G. C., and Persellin, R. H. Cervical fracture complicating ankylosing spon-dylitis. *Am. J. Med.* 70:1033, 1981.
    35% of spinal fractures in ankylosing spondylitis are fatal, twice the rate seen in fractures of normal spines.
20. Ginsburg, W., and Cohen, M. C. Peripheral arthritis in ankylosing spondylitis: a review of 209 patients followed up for more than 20 years. *Mayo Clin. Proc.* 58:593, 1983.
    32% of patients had peripheral arthritis, excluding hip and shoulder involvement.
21. Rosenbaum, J. T., and Nozid, R. A. Uveitis: Many diseases, one diagnosis. *Am. J. Med.* 79:545–547, 1985.
    A succinct review of anterior uveitis in systemic diseases.

22. Keat, A. Reiter's syndrome and reactive arthritis in perspective. *N. Engl. J. Med.* 309:1606, 1983.
    Excellent review. Keratodermia blenorrhagicum is not seen with gut-associated arthritis. The only reactive arthritis associated with erythema nodosum is Yersinia arthritis.
23. Winchester, R., Bernstein, D. H., Fischer, H. D., et al. The co-occurrence of Reiter's syndrome and acquired immunodeficiency. *Ann. Intern. Med.* 106:19, 1987.
    Experiment of nature that suggests that cytotoxic T cells, but not helper T cells, are pathogenic in Reiter's.
24. Fox, R., Calin, A., Gerber, R. C., et al. The chronicity of symptoms and disability in Reiter's syndrome. *Ann. Intern. Med.* 91:190, 1979.
    83% of all patients have chronic symptoms: 27% had to change or stop their work. Heel pain was the only clinical predictor of chronicity.
25. Arnett, F. C., McClusky, O. E., Schacter, B. Z., et al. Incomplete Reiter's syndrome: discriminating features and HLA W27 in diagnosis. *Ann. Intern. Med.* 84:8, 1976.
    Incomplete Reiter's syndrome was used to describe patients with reactive arthritis who did not have the classic triad of conjunctivitis, urethritis, and arthritis.
26. Smith, D. L., Bennett, R. M., and Regan, M. G. Reiter's disease in women. *Arthritis Rheum.* 23:335, 1980.
    Cervicitis may be missed in women.
27. Calin, A. A placebo controlled, crossover study of azathioprine in Reiter's syndrome. *Ann. Rheum. Dis.* 45:653, 1986.
    Five of six patients who completed the trial preferred azathioprine to placebo.
28. Noer, H. R. An "experimental" epidemic of Reiter's syndrome. *J.A.M.A.* 198:693, 1966.
29. Keat, A., Thomas, B., Dixey, J., et al. *Chlamydia trachomatis* and reactive arthritis: the missing link. *Lancet* 1:72, 1987.
    Chlamydial elementary bodies were seen in joint material from five patients with reactive arthritis.
30. Ebright, J. R., and Ryan, L. M. Acute erosive reactive arthritis associated with *Campylobacter jejuni*–induced colitis. *Am. J. Med.* 76:321, 1984.
    Most patients reported with Campylobacter-reactive arthritis have had an asymmetric oligoarthritis. True Reiter's disease has been uncommon.
31. Ahvonen, P., Seivers, K., and Aho, K. Arthritis associated with *Yersinia enterocolitica* infection. *Acta Rheum. Scand.* 15:232, 1969.
    The duration of arthritis in cases in which it eventually subsided was 1 week to 5 months. Some patients had erythema nodosum and some had more classic symptoms of Reiter's disease (conjunctivitis, iritis, urethritis).
32. McEwen, C., DiTata, D., Lingg, C., et al. Ankylosing spondylitis and spondylitis accompanying ulcerative colitis, regional enteritis, psoriasis and Reiter's disease.
    Ankylosing spondylitis and spondylitis with inflammatory bowel disease are similar, with symmetric sacroiliitis and bilaterally symmetric syndesmophytes (marginal type). Conversely, in Reiter's and psoriatic spondyloarthropathy unilateral sacroiliitis and syndesmophytes are common.
33. Kammer, G. M., Soter, N. A., Gibson, D. J., et al. Psoriatic arthritis: A clinical, immunologic and HLA study of 100 patients. *Semin. Arthritis Rheum.* 9:75, 1979.
    Psoriatic arthritis occurs in 5% of psoriasis patients. It can be divided into subgroups.
34. Lambert, J. R., and Wright, V. Psoriatic spondylitis: a clinical and radiological description of the spine in psoriatic arthritis. *Q. J. Med.* 46:411, 1977.
    Spondylitis was found in 40% and sacroiliitis in 21% of this series of 130 patients.
35. Aho, K., Ahvonen, P., Lassus, A., et al. HLA-27 reactive arthritis. *Arthritis Rheum.* 17:521, 1974.
36. Bocanegra, T. S., Espinoza, L. R., Bridgefore, P. H., et al. Reactive arthritis induced by parasitic infestation. *Ann. Intern. Med.* 94:207, 1981.
37. Granfors, K., Jalkanen, S., von Essen, R., et al. Yersinia antigens in synovial-fluid cells from patients with reactive arthritis. *N. Engl. J. Med.* 320:216, 1989.
    Synovial fluid from 10 to 15 patients contained Yersinia antigens.

38. Danzi, J. T. Extraintestinal manifestations of idiopathic inflammatory bowel disease. *Arch. Intern. Med.* 148:297, 1988.
    Recent review of the literature.

44. POLYARTERITIS NODOSA
H. Verdain Barnes

Polyarteritis is an uncommon disease of small and middle-sized arteries that occurs primarily in young and middle-aged men. Histologically, fibrinoid necrosis and leukocyte infiltration are seen in and around an involved vessel. Eosinophils are often the predominant cell type. Giant cell formation is rare. Involvement may be focal or diffuse. Aneurysm formation in the parenchyma of involved organs is common. The exact cause is unknown, but current evidence supports a hypersensitivity etiology.

The clinical presentation and course depend on the arteries involved, and thus there is no truly typical onset or symptom complex. The onset and course are usually gradual and chronic, respectively, but can be abrupt and acute. Early in the disease, complaints referable to a single organ system are not uncommon, but as the disease progresses, an involvement of many systems is the rule. The recognized triad of fever, abdominal pain, and hypertension is rare. Frequent early complaints are weakness, myalgia, arthralgia, easy fatigue, headache, anorexia, weight loss, fever, chilliness, drenching sweats, asthma, hepatitis, serous otitis media, and periumbilical or right upper quadrant abdominal pain. Skin manifestations occur in about 25 percent. Cutaneous or subcutaneous nodules may occur along the course of an involved blood vessel. These lesions are often tender and may appear and regress in a matter of a day or so. Other lesions include urticaria, petechiae, hemorrhagic bullae, dermatitis gangrenosa, and a variety of erythematous eruptions. Local or generalized edema can occur. Raynaud's phenomenon and mucosal lesions are rare.

In order of decreasing frequency, the systems or organs involved are the genitourinary, cardiac, peripheral or central nervous, gastrointestinal, pulmonary, and musculoskeletal systems, the eye, and ear. Genitourinary tract involvement is chiefly renal, which occurs in about 80 percent of patients. Renal involvement results in a focal or diffuse glomerulonephritis, infarcts, and aneurysms. About 60 percent have proteinuria and 40 percent hematuria. The most common complications are hypertension (often malignant) and uremia. Hemorrhagic cystitis and testicular pain with or without infarction and atrophy may occur.

The most common cardiac involvement is the myocardium, which may result in tachycardia, ischemia, infarction, arrhythmias (usually supraventricular), and occasionally myocardial failure. The second most common is the pericardium, leading to recurrent pericarditis, which is often hemorrhagic. Tamponade may occur.

Peripheral neuropathy, which occurs in about 50 percent of patients, can be a mono- or polyneuropathy. It is commonly bilateral but asymmetric. Pain is almost invariably present and is often associated with paresthesias and motor nerve involvement. Central nervous system involvement may result in behavior and mentation changes, seizures, hemiplegia, aphasia, and subarachnoid hemorrhage.

Gastrointestinal tract involvement can result in anorexia, nausea, vomiting, watery or bloody diarrhea, or severe pain simulating an acute surgical abdomen. Mesenteric arteritis may lead to thrombosis and/or bowel perforation. Arteritis may involve the gallbladder and result in rupture. Liver involvement can produce jaundice, aneurysms, and infarcts. Polyarteritis accounts for more than 50 percent of all large liver infarcts. Splenomegaly of minimal to moderate degree is seen in about one-third of patients.

Pulmonary and pleural vasculitis can result in hemoptysis and bloody pleural effusion. Thrombosis of the pulmonary artery has been reported. There may be associated lung cavitation and/or pulmonary hypertension. As many as 18 percent of patients have bronchial asthma. Patchy, nodular, and frequently changing densities may be seen on the chest x ray. Hypertrophic pulmonary osteoarthrophy has been reported.

Voluntary muscle is involved in 20 to 25 percent of patients. It is commonly asymptomatic, but muscle pain, tenderness, atrophy, and weakness may occur. Arthralgias are frequent, but joint effusion is rare. Migratory polyarthritis occurred in about 7 percent of the patients in one series, and antedated the other manifestations of the disease.

Ocular changes may be striking. Exudates, hemorrhages, cytoid bodies, papilledema, optic atrophy, retinal detachment, scleritis, iritis, episcleritis, corneal ulcers, extraocular muscle paralyses, and visual field defects may be seen. Finally, about 10 percent have serous otitis media and an occasional patient will have hearing loss.

Two presentations of polyarteritis nodosa are being increasingly recognized. First, there is the localized form, which may involve only the skin or the muscle, run a relatively benign course, and have perhaps some presentations with only renal involvement; this form has a less optimistic prognosis. Second, polyarteritis nodosa may be a component of the polyangiitis overlap syndrome. It has been reported in combination with Churg-Strauss disease, giant cell arteritis, Takayasu's arteritis, Henoch-Schönlein purpura, and Wegener's granulomatosis.

The diagnosis of polyarteritis is often missed initially. Biopsy of a nodule, purpuric area, or painful muscle will usually provide a definitive diagnosis. Biopsy of uninvolved skin, subcutaneous tissue, and muscle will make the diagnosis in only about 13 percent of patients. In one autopsy series, testicular biopsy was positive in 86 percent. About 60 percent of patients have parenchymal aneurysms that are arteriographically demonstrable, a sign that many consider diagnostic. There are no characteristic laboratory values. About 80 percent of patients have leukocytosis with or without a prominent eosinophilia. The urinalysis may show red cells, white cells, oval fat bodies, fatty casts, and proteinuria. The erythrocyte sedimentation rate is often elevated, serum albumin decreased, and globulins increased. Rheumatoid factor, if present, suggests associated rheumatoid arthritis. Recent studies have shown hepatitis B (HB) surface antigen to be present in up to 55 percent of patients and antihepatitis B surface antibody in about 15 percent. The differential diagnosis includes a variety of vasculitides, such as hypersensitivity angiitis, rheumatoid arteritis, allergic granulomatous arteritis, Wegener's granulomatosis, giant cell arteritis, aortic arch arteritis, erythema nodosum, Henoch-Schöenlein purpura, and serum sickness.

Prognosis is guarded. The 5-year survival without therapy is about 13 percent and with therapy nearly 48 percent. The most common cause of death is uremia and hypertension, followed by congestive heart failure with or without associated myocardial infarction.

1. Ross, G. A. The natural history of polyarteritis. *Br. Med. J.* 2:1148, 1957.
   A comprehensive review.
2. James, T. N., and Birk, R. E. Pathology of the cardiac conduction system in polyarteritis nodosa. *Arch. Intern. Med.* 117:561, 1966.
   Structural damage was found in the sinoatrial node. Atrial flutter was the most frequent arrhythmia.
3. Maxeimer, S. R., McDonald, J. R., and Kirklin, J. W. Muscle biopsy in diagnosis of periartertitis nodosa; evaluation. *Surg. Clin. North Am.* 32:1225, 1952.
   In this series, muscle biopsy was positive in only 13% while 30% had the disease at autopsy.
4. Dahl, E. V., Baggenstoss, A. H., and DeWeerd, J. H. Testicular lesions of periarteritis nodosa, with special reference to diagnosis. *Am. J. Med.* 28:222, 1960.
   86% of patients in this series had a diagnostic biopsy.
5. Krimbrell, O. C. Polyarteritis nodosa complicated by bilateral optic neuropathy. *J.A.M.A.* 201:139, 1967.
   A rare complication.
6. Curran, R. E., Steinberg, I., and Hagstrom, W. C. Arteriovenous fistula complicating percutaneous renal biopsy in polyarteritis nodosa. *Am. J. Med.* 43:465, 1967.
   A complication of renal biopsy worth noting.

7. Bron, K. M., and Gajaraj, A. Demonstration of hepatic aneurysms in polyarteritis nodosa by arteriography. *N. Engl. J. Med.* 282:1024, 1970.
   Visceral aneurysms were seen in 60% of patients.
8. Trepo, C. G., Zuckerman, A. J., Bird, R. C., et al. Role of circulating hepatitis B antigen-antibody immune complexes in pathogenesis of vascular and hepatic manifestations in polyarteritis nodosa. *J. Clin. Pathol.* 27:863, 1974.
   A potential pathogenetic mechanism is reported. About 55% of patients had HB surface antigen and about 15% had anti-HB surface antibody.
9. Frohnert, P., and Sheps, S. G. Long-term follow-up study of periarteritis nodosa. *Am. J. Med.* 43:8, 1967.
   13% survival of untreated patients and 48% survival of treated patients.
10. Pettersen, E., and Carlsen, B. H. Hearing impairment as an initial sign of polyarteritis nodosa. *Acta Otolaryngol.* 61:189, 1966.
    Deafness can be the presenting manifestation.
11. Phanuphak, P., and Kohler, P. F. Onset of polyarteritis nodosa during allergic hyposensitization treatment. *Am. J. Med.* 68:479, 1980.
    Vasculitic symptoms began during hyposensitization therapy in 6 of their 20 consecutive patients. They hypothesize that their hyposensitization was indirectly responsible in the majority.
12. Holt, P. J. A., Davies, M. G., Saunders, K. C., et al. Pyoderma gangrenosum: Clinical and laboratory findings in 15 patients with special reference to polyarteritis. *Medicine* 59:114, 1980.
    About half of their patients had polyarteritis.
13. Leavitt, R. Y., and Fauci, A. S. Polyangitis overlap syndrome: Classification and prospective clinical experience. *Am. J. Med.* 81:79, 1986.
    Polyarteritis is a common component in this increasingly recognized syndrome.
14. Ferreiro, J. E., Saldana, M. J., and Azevedo, S. J. Polyarteritis manifesting as calf myositis and fever. *Am. J. Med.* 80:312, 1986.
15. Croker, B. P., Lee, T., and Gunnells, J. C. Clinical and pathologic features of polyarteritis nodosa and its renal-limited variant: Primary crescentic and necrotizing glomerulonephritis. *Hum. Pathol.* 18:38, 1987.
    These articles (14, 15) discuss two of the localized forms of polyarteritis nodosa.

45. CRYOGLOBULINEMIA AND MIXED CONNECTIVE TISSUE DISEASE
David B. Hellmann
Michelle Petri

Cryoglobulins are antibodies that precipitate when cooled and dissolve when rewarmed. Cryoglobulinemia may occur by itself or, more frequently, may be associated with other conditions, chiefly connective tissue diseases and malignancies. Clinically, cryoglobulinemia will manifest itself either as a vasculitis or as a hyperviscosity syndrome. Cryoglobulins should not be confused with cold agglutinins, which are present in various disease states (e.g., mycoplasma pneumonia), and are defined as IgM antibodies that agglutinate red blood cells in the cold. Occasionally in normals and in certain disease states, fibrinogen will precipitate in the cold. Such cryofibrinogens do not dissolve on rewarming, and are therefore readily distinguished from cryoglobulins.

Cryoglobulins can be classified by immunochemical techniques into threee types. Type I cryoglobulins are *monoclonal* immunoglobulins that *do not have rheumatoid factor* activity. Type II cryoglobulins are also *monoclonal* but *do have rheumatoid factor* activity; that is, type II cryoglobulins can bind to the Fc portion of other antibodies. Type III cryoglobulins are *polyclonal* and *have rheumatoid factor* activity.

The immunochemical differences in the types of cryoglobulins result in predictable differences in clinical manifestations. Since types II and III cryoglobulins have rheumatoid factor activity, they can form immune complexes that readily activate complement and produce inflammatory damage to blood vessels (i.e., vasculitis). In contrast, the type 1 cryoglobulins do not have rheumatoid factor activity, do not readily activate complement, and are therefore more likely to produce a hyperviscosity syndrome (visual or central nervous system abnormalities, bleeding disorders, Raynaud's syndrome) than a vasculitis.

The clonal differences in the cryoglobulins help explain which diseases are associated with each type of cryoglobulin. As expected, monoclonal cryoglobulins (types I and III) are most frequently associated with malignancies (especially Waldenström's macroglobulinemia, multiple myeloma, lymphocytic leukemias, and lymphoma). Polyclonal cryoglobulins (type III) frequently occur as a primary disorder or are associated with rheumatic disorders (such as Sjögren's syndrome, systemic lupus erythematosus (SLE), rheumatoid arthritis, polyarteritis), or are associated with infections (such as hepatitis B, syphilis, leprosy, mononucleosis, toxoplasmosis, malaria, acquired immunodeficiency disease, or Lyme disease). Clearly, "cryoglobulinemia" is no more a single disease than "anemia" is. Knowing the rheumatoid factor activity and the clonal nature of the cryoglobulin helps formulate the differential diagnosis and defines the additional tests (e.g., bone marrow biopsy) needed to identify the underlying disease process.

While approximately 50 percent of all cryoglobulins are due to lymphoproliferative diseases and another 25 percent are associated chiefly with autoimmune diseases, 25 percent of all cases have no identifiable cause even after many years of follow-up. Such cases have been called "mixed, essential cryoglobulinemia" or "Meltzer's syndrome." The classic clinical features of this condition are *palpable* purpura (predominantly on the lower extremities), polyarthralgias, renal disease, leg ulcers, and peripheral neuropathy (especially mononeuritis multiplex). Laboratory evidence of liver disease and previous hepatitis B infection are often present. In all of these patients the cryoglobulins have rheumatoid factor activity (i.e., types II and III) and the majority are polyclonal (i.e., type III). Hypocomplementemia is common. Indeed, the combination of a rheumatoid factor and low complement levels in a patient not known to have lupus or rheumatoid arthritis should strongly suggest mixed, essential cryoglobulinemia. The course of these patients is variable. Prognosis is most adversely influenced by the presence of renal disease. Neuropathy may be resistant to therapy. Patients are usually managed symptomatically, with immunosuppressive therapy and plasmapheresis reserved for those with progressive damage to critical organs.

The above discussion indicates that searching for cryoglobulins is appropriate in any patient with unexplained hyperviscosity syndrome or vasculitis (especially when associated with purpura, renal disease, or peripheral neuropathy). The search must be done carefully. Blood must be collected and handled at normal body temperature to prevent precipitation and "loss" of the cryoglobulin from the serum layer when the blood is centrifuged. Careless handling often results in false-negatives. The separated serum is then refrigerated at 4°C (39.2°F) and inspected daily for 1 week. The cryoglobulin nature of any precipitate is verified by showing that the precipitate dissolves on warming and reforms on cooling. Further analysis of the cryoglobulin's rheumatoid factor activity and clonality are essential steps in the diagnostic evaluation.

Patients who have overlapping features of SLE, scleroderma, and polymyositis and who have antibodies to ribonucleoprotein (RNP), a specific nuclear antigen, are said to have mixed connective tissue disease (MCTD).

Recognition of MCTD as an independent disease entity is controversial. Critics point to the hazards of pinning any clinical diagnosis on the presence of a single autoantibody. Fully 30 percent of clinically diagnosed patients with SLE have antibodies to RNP, making some claim that MCTD is simply a subset of SLE. Other skeptics note that with long-term follow-up many patients initially diagnosed as having MCTD do not continue to have overlapping manifestations. It is likely this controversy will end only when the pathogenesis of these autoimmune conditions is understood.

The clinical hallmark of MCTD is the presence of overlapping clinical features. While SLE-like features predominate, these patients frequently have puffy and tight skin over the fingers as in scleroderma, and may have the rash and weakness characteristic of dermatomyositis. Other manifestations of MCTD are similar to those in SLE except that in MCTD renal disease is less frequent.

Laboratory results are similar to those in SLE except that, by definition, antibodies to nuclear RNP are seen in 100 percent of MCTD patients.

Originally it was thought that MCTD patients were exquisitely sensitive to low- to moderate-dose corticosteroids and had little to no increase in mortality. Long-term studies have suggested, however, that the outcome is not always benign; disability or death from pulmonary hypertension occurs in some patients.

The treatment of MCTD depends on the features present, and in most cases is similar to that in SLE.

1. Wintrobe, M. M., and Buell, M. V. Hyperproteinemia, associated with multiple myeloma. *Johns Hopkins Hosp. Bull.* 52:156, 1933.
   The initial description.

2. Lightfoot, R. W. Cryoglobulinemia. In W. N. Kelly, E. D. Harris, S. Ruddy, et al. (eds.), *Textbook of Rheumatology.* Philadelphia: W.B. Saunders Co., 1985. P. 1337.
   Excellent general review with 39 references.

3. Gorevic, P. D., Kassab, H. J., Levo, Y., et al. Mixed cryoglobulinemia: Clinical aspects and long-term follow up of 40 patients. *Am. J. Med.* 69:287, 1980.
   Clinical features: palpable purpura (100%), polyarthralgias (73%), renal disease (55%), hepatic dysfunction (70%), evidence of previous hepatitis B infection (60%), leg ulcers (30%), and neuropathy (12.5%). Three main causes of death: renal disease, systemic vasculitis, and infection.

4. Brouet, J. C., Clauvel, J. P., Danon, F., et al. Biologic and clinical significance of cryoglobulins. *Am. J. Med.* 57:775, 1974.
   Compares the clinical features seen with the three different classes of cryoglobulins. Vasculitis manifestations are more common in types II and III. Overall prevalence: type I 25%, type II 25%, and type III 50%. Immunoproliferative and autoimmune diseases are frequently associated with cryoglobulinemia. 30% of cases are idiopathic even after a mean follow-up of 9 years. Plasmapheresis and chemotherapy produced a clinical remission in 9/10 patients.

5. Ferri, C., Moriconi, L., Gremignai, G., et al. Treatment of the renal involvement in mixed cryoglobulinemia with prolonged plasma exchange. *Nephron* 43:246, 1986.
   Plasmapheresis alone or in combination with corticosteroids but not with cytotoxic agents improved 5/9 patients.

6. Horowitz, J., Klein, M., and Sukenik, S. Cryoglobulinemia and hepatitis B markers in North African Jews with Raynaud's disease. *Arthritis Rheum.* 29:1026, 1986.
   Cryoglobulinemia is commonly (11/20) associated with Raynaud's in this unusual population.

7. Inman, R. D., Hodge, M., Johnston, M. E. A., et al. Arthritis, vasculitis, and cryoglobulinemia associated with relapsing hepatitis A virus infection. *Ann. Intern. Med.* 105:700, 1986.
   Mixed cryoglobulinemia is a rare complication of hepatitis A.

8. Geltner, D., Kohn, R., Gorevic, P., et al. The effect of combination therapy (steroids, immunosuppressives, and plasmapheresis) on 5 mixed cryoglobulinemia patients with renal, neurologic, and vascular involvement. *Arthritis Rheum.* 24:1121, 1981.
   Cutaneous ulcers healed (3/3), renal function improved (4/4), purpura diminished (2/2), but peripheral neuropathy changed little.

9. Singer, R. J., Venning, M. C., Lockwood, C. M., et al. Cryoglobulinemia: clinical features and response to treatment. *Ann. Intern. Med.* 137:251, 1986.
   English series. 1/16 had human T cell lymphotrophic virus type III infection.

10. Duggan, D. B., and Schattner, A. Unusual manifestations of monoclonal gammopathies; autoimmune and idiopathic syndromes. *Am. J. Med.* 864, 1986.

11. Gamble, C. N., and Ruggles, S. W. The immunopathogenesis of glomerulonephritis associated with mixed cryoglobulinemia. *N. Engl. J. Med.* 299:81, 1978.
    Case report of glomerulonephritis due to renal deposition of cryoglobulin.

12. Bombardieri, S., Paoletti, P., Ferri, C., et al. Lung involvement in essential mixed cryoglobulinemia. *Am. J. Med.* 66:629, 1979.
    Italian study showing that while pulmonary symptoms are rare (3/23), pulmonary

function abnormalities (indicative of small airway disease) and chest x-ray abnormalities (suggestive of mild interstitial involvement) are common.

13. Levo, Y., Gorevic, P. D., Kassab, H. J., et al. Liver involvement in the syndrome of mixed cryoglobulinemia. *Ann. Intern. Med.* 87:287, 1977.
    11% had overt hepatic disease, but 77% had hepatomegaly and abnormal liver function tests.

14. Dolin, R. In R. E. Scully, E. J. Mark, and B. U. McNeely (eds.), *Case Records of the Massachusetts General Hospital. N. Engl. J. Med.* 306:657, 1982.
    Type II cryoglobulinemia associated with Kaposi's sarcoma.

15. Letendre, L., and Kyle, R. A. Monoclonal cryoglobulinemia with high thermal insolubility. *Mayo Clin. Proc.* 57:629, 1982.
    Two cases in which severe manifestations occurred despite small amounts of cryoglobulins.

16. Luzar, M. J., Camisa, C., and Neff, J. C. Essential mixed cryoglobulinemia (type II) with pseudoleukocytosis. *Arthritis Rheum.* 27:353, 1984.
    Cryoglobulin crystals can produce pseudoleukocytosis when total white cell counts are performed on Coulter-type particle counters.

17. Weinberger, A., Berliner, S., and Pinkhas, J. Articular manifestations of essential cryoglobulinemia. *Semin. Arthritis Rheum.* 10:224, 1981.
    25% have arthralgias, 25% have arthritis.

18. Germain, M. J., Anderson, R. W., and Keane, W. F. Renal disease in cryoglobulinemia type II: Response to therapy. *Am. J. Nephrol.* 2:221, 1982.
    A case of renal disease responsive to cyclophosphamide and prednisone.

19. Sharp, G. C., Irvin, W. S., Tan, E. M., et al. Mixed connective tissue disease: an apparently distinct rheumatic disease syndrome associated with a specific antibody to an extractable nuclear antigen (ENA). *Am. J. Med.* 52:148, 1972.
    The original report suggesting that patients with antibodies to RNP had overlapping features of lupus, scleroderma, and polymyositis. Renal disease was absent and most manifestations were responsive to prednisone.

20. Sharp, G. C., Irvin, W. S., May, C. M., et al. Association of antibodies to ribonucleoprotein and Sm antigens with mixed connective-tissue disease, systemic lupus erythematosus and other rheumatic diseases. *N. Engl. J. Med.* 295:1149, 1976.
    74% of patients with antibodies to RNP have clinical features of mixed connective tissue disease.

21. Sullivan, W. D., Hurst, D. J., Harmon, C. E., et al. A prospective evaluation emphasizing pulmonary involvement in patients with mixed connective tissue disease. *Medicine* 63:92, 1984.
    Pulmonary involvement in MCTD is common (80%) and often severe. Predominant problem is pulmonary hypertension in the absence of severe interstitial disease.

22. Alpert, M. A., Goldberg, S. H., Bernhard, H., et al. Cardiovascular manifestations of mixed connective tissue disease in adults. *Circulation* 68:1182, 1983.
    Manifestations in 38 patients include pericarditis, pericardial effusion, mitral valve prolapse, intimal hyperplasia of coronary arteritis, myocardial inflammation, and pulmonary hypertension.

23. Prakash, U. B. S., Luthra, H. S., and Divertie, M. B. Intrathoracic manifestations in mixed connective tissue disease. *Mayo Clin. Proc.* 60:813, 1985.
    Pleuropulmonary involvement occurred in 25% of 81 patients.

24. Hosoda, Y., Suzuki, Y., Takano, M., et al. Mixed connective tissue disease with pulmonary hypertension: A clinical and pathological study. *J. Rheumatol.* 14:826, 1987.
    Pathologic changes mimic those of primary pulmonary hypertension.

25. Nimelstein, S. H., Brody, S., McShane, D., et al. Mixed connective tissue disease: A subsequent evaluation of the original 25 patients. *Medicine* 59:239, 1980.
    Argument against recognizing MCTD as a distinct entity: with time, patients generally evolve away from an MCTD picture to that of systemic sclerosis. Course is not benign; 8 of the 22 original patients were dead within 10 years.

26. Ginsburg, W. W., Conn, D. L., Bunch, T. W., et al. Comparison of clinical and serologic markers in systemic lupus erythematosus and overlap syndrome: a review of 247 patients. *J. Rheumatol.* 10:235, 1983.
    The case against anti-RNP as a marker of a distinct entity: a review of 247 patients.

All overlap patients had a high frequency of arthritis and Raynaud's regardless of serologic profile. The presence or absence of RNP and Sm did not distinguish SLE from overlap patients.

27. Munves, E. F., and Schur, P. H. Antibodies to Sm and RNP. *Arthritis Rheum.* 26:848, 1983.
    The case against anti-RNP as a marker of a distinct entity: chart review of 150 patients suggested that antibodies are not disease-specific.

28. Hardin, J. A., Rahn, D. R., Shen, C., et al. Antibodies from patients with connective tissue diseases bind specific subsets of cellular RNA-protein particles. *J. Clin. Invest.* 1982;70:141, 1982.
    One of a series of experiments that has helped define the antigens recognized by some autoantibodies. RNP, Sm, Ro, and La antigens are complexes of molecules of small nuclear or cytoplasmic RNA and protein.

29. Lazaro, M. A., Maldonado Cocco, J. A., Catoggio, L. J., et al. Clinical and serologic characteristics of patients with overlap syndrome: Is mixed connective tissue disease a distinct clinical entity? *Medicine* 68:58, 1989.
    Review of 27 patients indicating that "mixed connective tissue disease" is not a distinct entity.

46. SYSTEMIC SCLEROSIS (SCLERODERMA)

H. Verdain Barnes

Systemic sclerosis (SS) is a chronic disease with protean manifestations. The exact cause is unknown. Several potential pathogenic mechanisms have been proposed. Endothelial cell injury may be a primary factor as suggested by specific endothelial cell cytotoxic activity, increased factor VIII (von Willebrand factor), factor VIII antigen, factor VIII activity, beta-thromboglobulin, and fibrin degeneration products in the sera of SS patients. The factor VIII antigen–factor VIII coagulant ratio has been reported to correlate with the severity of nail bed vascular changes. Recently, increased numbers of mast cells have been reported in the early cutaneous lesions of SS patients. These cells may induce fibroblast overproduction of collagen as well as endothelial cell injury. All of these potential mechanisms are consistent with an autoimmune disease mechanism. Histologic examination of involved areas reveals dense, swollen, hypertrophied collagen with varying degrees of inflammation. The small arterial walls often show "fibrinoid" necrosis with or without vessel occlusion. Changes in the microvasculature include decreased numbers of vessels, and thickening and reduplication of vascular basement membranes. These changes may be limited to the integument and can be localized or generalized. On the other hand, they may be limited to the viscera. During the course of the disease both cutaneous and visceral changes are usually demonstrable. The onset is usually insidious but may be acute. Females predominate 3:1. The peak incidence is in persons between 20 and 50 years of age.

Early in the history of the disease the clinical manifestations are often subtle and nonspecific, including such features as easy fatigability, weakness, weight loss, neurasthenia, impotence, arrhythmias, telangiectases, and/or vague complaints of arthralgias, myalgias, dyspnea on exertion, dyspepsia, or dysphagia. The most common complaint at the time of diagnosis, however, is Raynaud's phenomenon (occurring in about 35% of patients), followed by joint and dermatologic complaints (in 29% and 26% respectively). The remainder have complaints referable to specific organ system involvement. Focal dermatologic involvement, morphea, may begin as a plaquelike area of shiny edematous skin, or as linear sclerotic streaks often following the course of nerves or blood vessels, or as sclerodactylia. The face, hands, and arms are most frequently involved. Localized or generalized edema is on occasion the only change. Hyperpigmentation and telangiectasia are common. Varying degrees of alopecia can be seen, as well as metastatic subcutaneous calcification. Ulcerations in involved areas, particularly the finger tips and toes, may be a major feature. The following disease processes can produce skin changes that to varying degrees mimic scleroderma: scleredema, scleromyxedema, carcinoid, phenylketonuria, porphyria cutanea tarda, acromegaly, congenital porphyria, primary amyloidosis, Werner's syndrome, Rothmund's syndrome, lichen sclerosus et atrophicus, acrodermatitis chronica atrophicans, progeria, and acroosteolysis.

The musculoskeletal system in SS may show the following types of involvement: frank arthritis with or without joint deformity, myositis with and without clear evidence of myopathy, and bone ischemia with reabsorption of the phalanges or heads of the femur, ulna, radius, or mandible. The nervous system rarely shows primary involvement. When present, the most common is a neuropathy involving single or multiple cranial or peripheral nerves or the autonomic nervous system.

Gastrointestinal tract involvement is common. Smooth muscle degeneration and microvascular occlusion in the esophagus, small bowel, or colon can produce a variety of signs and symptoms, including mild to marked dysphagia, reflux esophagitis, small or large bowel obstruction, ulceration, constipation, and/or diarrhea. Complications such as malabsorption, infarction, hemorrhage, or perforation may occur. Radiographic and motility studies are often characteristic. Barrett's metaplasia, particularly in patients with the CREST syndrome (calcinosis, Raynaud's phenomenon, esophageal dysfunction, sclerodactyly, and telangiectasia), with long-standing dysphagia or a very low lower-esophageal sphincter pressure, may be seen. These patients appear to have an increased risk of esophageal stricture and adenocarcinoma. Lung involvement is common. Pulmonary fibrosis and microvascular obstruction can result in pulmonary cysts, emphysema, atelectasis, bronchiectasis, pulmonary hypertension, pleural fibrosis, cor pulmonale, and a partially or totally fixed chest wall. As a result, the patients are prone to recurrent or chronic bronchospasm, lung abscesses, pneumonia, embolism, and some develop alveolar cell carcinoma. Pulmonary function tests usually show a decreased vital capacity, carbon monoxide diffusion capacity, and lung capacity, with a corresponding increase in dead space and venous admixture. The pulmonary arterial pressure is increased, with a decrease in pulmonary blood flow.

The kidney and the heart are frequently involved. Renal involvement occurs in at least 45 percent of patients. Histologically, the kidney usually shows (1) fibrinoid necrosis and mucoid intimal proliferation of the interlobular arteries and arterioles and/or (2) glomerulitis with hypercellular mesangium and lobulated capillary tufts. These changes can be focal or diffuse. Clinical manifestations in focal disease are usually absent, but in those with diffuse disease they may dominate the picture. A rapid onset of malignant hypertension occurs in about one-third of those with hypertension. Rapid progression of uremia is not uncommon. The incidence of myocardial fibrosis, small coronary arteries, and arteriolar lesions is increased in SS. The clinical correlates are ischemic and mechanical myocardial decompensation, conduction defects, arrhythmias, and pericarditis. Valvular lesions are rare. Pericarditis is not uncommon, and in one recent series was found at autopsy in 62 percent. Two clinical patterns of pericarditis may occur. The most common is chronic pericarditis with associated cardiomegaly, pleural effusion, dyspnea, and Raynaud's phenomenon. The second is an acute pericarditis associated with fever, cardiomegaly, pericardial friction rub, chest pain, and dyspnea. The pericardial effusion has the characteristics of an exudate, but differs from that seen in rheumatoid arthritis and systemic lupus erythematosus (SLE), in that no autoantibodies, immune complexes, or complement depletion is seen. Tamponade is unusual. The occurrence of malignant hypertension, uremia, and pericarditis in a patient with scleroderma, however, does not relieve the physician of the responsibility of seeking other more easily treatable causes for these disorders.

During the course of the disease, involvement of the skin is seen in 95 to 98 percent of patients, Raynaud's phenomenon in 35 to 83 percent, involvement of the joints in 29 to 61 percent, of the esophagus in 54 to 74 percent, of the lungs in 29 to 59 percent, of the heart in 22 to 62 percent, of the kidney in 21 to 49 percent, of the muscles in 29 to 41 percent, and of the small or large intestine in 8 to 46 percent.

Diagnosis may be difficult since SS can be confused with other connective tissue diseases, as a component of mixed connective tissue disease (SS, SLE, and polymyositis) or the "overlap syndrome" (i.e., two or more connective tissue diseases). Anticentromere antibody is common in the CREST form of the disease. From 40 to 90 percent have antinuclear antibodies with abnormal DNA binding and antinuclear ribonucleoprotein activity. About 25 percent have a positive rheumatoid factor and up to 22 percent a positive LE cell preparation. The erythrocyte sedimentation rate is frequently elevated. A modest elevation in gamma globulin levels (usually IgG) is found in about 50 percent of patients. Biologic false-positive tests for syphilis can also be seen, and a rare patient has a low serum complement. The significance of these findings is not clear.

The course of the disease can be intermittent or relentless, with slow or rapid progression. About 10 percent of patients die in less than a year after diagnosis, 45 percent in 1 to 3 years, 30 percent in 3 to 10 years; and 15 percent live longer than 10 years. The most common causes of death are renal and cardiac (in 50% and 21% respectively).

1. Tumulty, P. A. Clinical synopsis of scleroderma, simulator of other diseases. *Johns Hopkins Med. J.* 122:236, 1968.
   A concise clinical discussion.
2. D'Angelo, W. S., Fries, J. F., Masi, A. T., et al. Pathologic observations in systemic sclerosis. *Am. J. Med.* 46:428, 1969.
   A good review of pathologic findings in various organ systems. Vascular lesions can exist in organs without clinical evidence of disease.
3. Rodnan, G. P. The natural history of progressive systemic sclerosis (diffuse scleroderma). *Bull. Rheum. Dis.* 13:301, 1963.
   Renal and cardiac involvement were the principal causes of death.
4. Clark, J. A., Winkelmann, R. K., and Ward, L. E. Serologic alterations in scleroderma and sclerodermatomyositis. *Mayo Clin. Proc.* 46:104, 1971.
   ESR was normal in 33% of patients, the rheumatoid factor was present in 35%, and the results of the serologic test for syphilis were positive in 5%.
5. Notman, D. D., Kurata, N., and Tan, E. M. Profiles of antinuclear antibodies in systemic rheumatic diseases. *Ann. Intern. Med.* 83:464, 1975.
   Only abnormal DNA binding and antinuclear ribonucleoprotein antibodies were found in SS.
6. Hassar, M., Case, D. B., Casarella, W. J., et al. Relationship of hypertension and renal failure in scleroderma (progressive systemic sclerosis) to structural and functional abnormalities of renal cortical circulation. *Medicine* 53:1, 1974.
   A good review.
7. Meihoff, W. E., Hirschfield, J. S., and Kern, F., Jr. Small intestinal scleroderma with malabsorption and pneumatosis cystoides intestinalis: Report of three cases. *J.A.M.A.* 204:854, 1968.
   Uncommon complications of importance.
8. Bulkley, B. H., Ridolfi, R. L., Salyer, W. R., et al. Myocardial lesions of progressive systemic sclerosis: A cause of cardiac dysfunction. *Circulation* 53:483, 1976.
   An excellent study of the correlation of pathology and clinical manifestations.
9. McWhorter, J. E., and Leroy, E. C. Pericardial disease in scleroderma (systemic sclerosis). *Am. J. Med.* 57:566, 1974.
   Two clinical patterns are identified.
10. Gladman, D. D., Gordon, D. A., Urowitz, M. B., et al. Pericardial fluid analysis in scleroderma (systemic sclerosis). *Am. J. Med.* 60:1064, 1976.
    An exudate with no detectable autoantibodies or immune complexes.
11. Medsger, T. A., Masi, A. T., Rodnan, G. P., et al. Survival with systemic sclerosis. *Ann. Intern. Med.* 75:369, 1971.
    Seven-year accumulated survival rate of 35%. Poorest prognosis with renal involvement.
12. Leroy, E. C. Increased collagen synthesis by scleroderma skin fibroblasts in vitro. *J. Clin. Invest.* 54:880, 1974.
    Scleroderma fibroblasts synthesize more soluble collagen and at a faster rate than normals.

24. Matthay, R. A., Schwartz, M. I., Petty, T. L., et al. Pulmonary manifestations of systemic lupus erythematosus: review of twelve cases of acute lupus pneumonitis. *Medicine* 54:397, 1975.
   Shock lung–like picture with 50% mortality.
25. Segal, A. M., Calabrese, L. H., Ahmad, M., et al. The pulmonary manifestations of systemic lupus erythematosus. *Semin. Arthritis Rheum.* 14:202, 1985.
26. Perez, H. D., and Dramer, N. Pulmonary hypertension in systemic lupus erythematosus. Report of 4 cases and review of the literature. *Semin. Arthritis Rheum.* 11:177, 1981.
   Present in 10% of patients; unresponsive to hydralazine or prednisone.
27. Perez, H. D., and Goldstein, I. M. Infection and Host Defenses in Systemic Lupus Erythematosus. In E. Franklin (ed.), *Clinical Immunology Update.* New York. Elsevier, 1979. P. 133.
28. Ginzler, A., Diamond, H., Kaplan, D. Computer analysis of factors influencing frequency of infection in systemic lupus erythematosus. *Arthritis Rheum.* 21:37, 1978.
29. Hellmann, D. B., Petri, M., and Whiting-O'Keefe, Q. Fatal infections in systemic lupus erythematosus: The role of opportunistic organisms. *Medicine* 66:341, 1987.
   Many fatal infections are due to occult, opportunistic organisms.
30. Stahl, N. I., Klippel, J. H., and Decker, J. L. Fever in systemic lupus erythematosus. *Am. J. Med.* 67:935, 1979.
   Leukocytosis, neutrophilia, shaking chills, and normal anti-DNA were predictors of infection.
31. Weinstein, A. Drug-induced systemic lupus erythematosus. *Prog. Clin. Immunol.* 4:1, 1980.
32. Johnson, R. T., and Richardson, E. P. The neurological manifestations of systemic lupus erythematosus. *Medicine* 47:337, 1968.
   Classic pathologic study showing small vessel vasculopathy is much more common than true vasculitis.
33. Bluestein, H. G., Williams, G. W., and Steinberg, A. D. Cerebrospinal fluid antibodies to neuronal cells: Association with neuropsychiatric manifestations of systemic lupus erythematosus. *Am. J. Med.* 70:240, 1981.
   Diffuse, but not focal, CNS disease associated with antineuronal antibodies.
34. Feinglass, E. J., Arnett, F. C., Dorsch, C. A., et al. Neuropsychiatric manifestations of systemic lupus erythematosus: Diagnosis, clinical spectrum, and relationship to other features of the disease. *Medicine* 55:323, 1976.
   37% of patients had neuropsychiatric dysfunction, including seizures, long tract signs, cranial neuropathy, and peripheral neuropathy.
35. Bonfa, E., Golombek, S. J., and Kaufman, L. D. Association between lupus psychosis and anti-ribosomal P protein antibodies. *N. Engl. J. Med.* 317:265, 1987.
   90% of patients with psychosis have anti-P. Yet 50% of patients with anti-P do not have CNS disease.
36. Budman, D.R., and Steinberg, A. D. Hematologic aspects of systemic lupus erythematosus. Current concepts. *Ann. Intern. Med.* 86:220, 1977.
37. Arnett, F. C., Reveille, J. D., Wilson, R. W., et al. Systemic lupus erythematosus: current state of the genetic hypothesis. *Semin. Arthritis Rheum.* 14:24, 1984.
   A review of genetic influences in SLE, including HLA, hereditary deficiencies of complement, sex and hormonal influences.
38. Petri, M., Rheinschmidt, M., Whiting-O'Keefe, Q. E., et al. The frequency of lupus anticoagulant in systemic lupus erythematosus. *Ann. Intern. Med.* 106:524, 1987.
39. Lockshin, M. D., Druzin, M. L., Goei, S., et al. Antibody to cardiolipin as a predictor of fetal distress or death in pregnant patients with systemic lupus erythematosus. *N. Engl. J. Med.* 313:152, 1985.
40. Hughes, G. R. V., Harris, E. N., Gharavi, A. E. The anticardiolipin syndrome. *J. Rheumatol.* 13:486, 1986.
41. Felson, D. T., and Anderson, J. J. Across-study evaluation of association between steroid dose and bolus steroids and avascular necrosis of bone. *Lancet* 2:902, 1987.
   A strong correlation was found between daily prednisone dose and avascular necrosis.

42. Zizic, T. M., Marcoux, C., Hunberford, D. S., et al. Corticosteroid therapy associated with ischemic necrosis of bone in systemic lupus erythematosus. *Am. J. Med.* 79:596, 1985.
   52% of patients afflicted; mean daily prednisone dose for the highest single month is a greater risk factor than duration of steroid therapy or total steroid dose.
43. Lockshin, M. D., Reinitz, E., Druzin, M. L., et al. Lupus pregnancy. Case-control prospective study demonstrating absence of lupus exacerbation during or after pregnancy. *Am. J. Med.* 77:893, 1984.
44. Fine, L. G., Barnett, E. V., Danovitch, G. M., et al. Systemic lupus erythematosus in pregnancy (UCLA Conference). *Ann. Intern. Med.* 94:667, 1981.
   Fertility (articles 43, 44) usually normal. Maternal side effects infrequent if disease stable. Fetal wastage common, especially in the presence of renal disease. (See also Medicine *63:362, 1984.)*
45. Jonsson, H., Nived, Ol, and Sturfelt, G. Outcome in systemic lupus erythematosus: a prospective study of patients from a defined population. *Medicine* 68:141, 1989.
   Neuropsychiatric and immunologic abnormalities were associated with a high frequency of relapse.
46. Balow, J. E., Austin III, H. A., Tsokos, G. C., et al. Lupus nephritis. *Ann. Intern. Med.* 106:79, 1987.
   Thorough review of pathophysiology, pathology, and treatment, with emphasis on the role of cytotoxic therapies.
47. McCune, W. J., Golbus, J., Zeldes, W., et al. Clinical and immunologic effects of monthly administration of intravenous cyclophosphamide in severe systemic lupus erythematosus. *N. Engl. J. Med.* 318:1423, 1988.
   Uncontrolled study on 9 patients treated monthly for 6 months suggesting efficacy of cyclophosphamide.
48. Asherson, R. A., Khamashta, M. A., Gil, A., et al. Cerebrovascular disease and antiphospholipid antibodies in systemic lupus erythematosus, lupuslike disease, and the primary antiphospholipid syndrome. *Am. J. Med.* 86:391, 1989.
   Multiple strokes and multiinfarct dementia may be associated with antiphospholipid antibodies in the presence or absence of SLE.
49. Lockshin, M. D. Pregnancy does not cause systemic lupus erythematosus to worsen. *Arthritis Rheum.* 32:665, 1989.
   Worsening of SLE during pregnancy is uncommon; prophylactic increase of prednisone is not warranted.

48. WEGENER'S GRANULOMATOSIS
H. Verdain Barnes

Wegener's granulomatosis (WG), a disease of unknown cause, was first defined as a clinical entity in 1936. The classic anatomic features include (1) necrotizing granulomas in the upper and lower respiratory system, (2) generalized focal necrotizing vasculitis of the arteries and veins, and (3) focal necrosis and fibrin thrombosis in the glomerular tufts. The necrotizing angiitis primarily involves small arteries, arterioles, small veins, and venules, but can involve vessels of any size. Any organ can be involved. In recent years limited forms of the disease have been described. Patients may have isolated involvement of the upper airways or lungs or both, with or without renal involvement.

Clinically the generalized and limited forms of the disease usually have their onset in the fourth and fifth decades. Males and females are affected about equally in generalized WG, whereas females predominate about 3:1 in the limited forms. The majority of patients have been previously healthy, and their history is strikingly devoid of allergy, asthma, and drug exposure. The onset in both forms is most often insidious, but may be acute. The classic triad in generalized WG is (1) intractable rhinitis and sinusitis, (2) nodular pulmonary lesions, and (3) end-stage uremia. About 85 percent of patients have purulent rhinorrhea and sinus opacities on x ray; most of the remainder have persistent pneumonitis. Other early manifestations include nasal obstruction, epistaxis, perforation of the nasal septum, otorrhea, cough, hemoptysis, pleurisy, exophthalmos, chemosis, corneal ulceration, scleritis, episcleritis, uveitis, parotitis, inflammatory polyarthritis, myositis, pericarditis, prostatitis, myocarditis, peripheral neuropathy, dermopathy, and constitutional signs and symptoms. Fever is almost invariably present; it shows no characteristic pattern. Easy fatigability, malaise, and weight loss are common. About 50 percent of the patients will have neuromuscular involvement, of which about 25 percent will have mononeuritis multiplex. Skin lesions are common; the most frequent are dermal nodules, petechiae, vesicular eruptions, hemorrhagic bullae, pyoderma gangrenosum, and papulonecrotic tuberculids. These lesions are usually found on the extremities and buttocks. Biopsy may show unequivocal granulomatous vasculitis. Skin, nasopharyngeal lesions, and pulmonary nodules may precede other manifestations of the disease by weeks to years, especially in the limited form. The course after diagnosis is usually rapidly progressive over a matter of weeks to months in the generalized form. The average time from diagnosis until death is about 5 months in most series, with a range from 2 weeks to 4 years. Without cytotoxic therapy about 80 percent are dead in 1 year and 93 percent by 2 years. About 80 percent die as a result of uremia; the remainder usually succumb to respiratory and/or cardiac failure. Hypertension is uncommon until the terminal stage. Recent reports show a far better prognosis for those treated with immunosuppressive agents, especially in limited disease.

The diagnosis is confirmed by biopsy with the open lung biopsy still being the most productive. Recently, an IgG autoantibody against polymorphonuclear leukocytes and monocytes has been described which may prove useful in diagnosis as well as in monitoring disease activity. The most prominent pulmonary findings on x ray are discrete nodular densities usually greater than 1 cm in diameter and remarkably thin-walled cavities with ragged edges surrounded by parenchymal infiltrates. These findings are multiple in over 70 percent and bilateral in about 60 percent. About 90 percent have lesions predominantly in the lower lobes, but often with adjacent involvement of the inferior aspect of the upper lobes. A rare patient will have only upper lobe involvement, but the apices are almost invariably spared. About one-third will have a radiographically demonstrable cavity. At some point in the disease a mild to moderate anemia is seen in over 90 percent. A leukocytosis is seen in about 70 percent and a mild eosinophilia is not uncommon in generalized WG while rare in the limited forms. Serum globulins are in general normal, but some authors have reported decreased IgM and increased secretory and serum IgA. Recently, circulating immunoglobulin complexes have been demonstrated as have elevations of rheumatoid factor and immunoglobulin (L chain) excretion in the urine. All of these return toward normal when therapy is effective.

The following must be considered in the differential diagnosis: tuberculosis, histoplasmosis, coccidiodomycosis, sarcoidosis, berylliosis, syphilis, blastomycosis, allergic angiitis, Henoch-Schönlein purpura, rheumatoid arthritis, Sjögren's syndrome, systemic sclerosis, systemic lupus erythematosus, polyarteritis nodosa, dermatomyositis, allergic granulomatosis, Leoffler's syndrome, eosinophilic pneumonia, Goodpasture's syndrome, nasopharyngeal neoplasm, metastatic carcinoma, Hodgkin's disease, polymorphic reticulosis, and primary carcinoma of the lung.

1. Fahey, J. L., Leonard, E., Churg, J., et al. Wegener's granulomatosis. *Am. J. Med.* 17:168, 1954.
   Frequently begins with destructive sinusitis, rhinitis, or persistent pneumonitis. A good review.
2. Godman, G. C., and Churg, H. Wegener's granulomatosis: Pathology and review of the literature. *Arch. Pathol.* 58:533, 1954.
   A classic.
3. DeRemee, R. A., McDonald, T. J., Harrison, E. G., et al. Wegener's granulomatosis: Anatomic correlates, a proposed classification. *Mayo Clin. Proc.* 51:777, 1976.
   A useful classification of the disease.

4. Drachman, D. A. Neurological complications of Wegener's granulomatosis. *Arch. Neurol.* 8:145, 1963.
   54% have neurologic manifestations.
5. Cassan, S. M., Divertie, M. B., Hollenhorst, R. W., et al. Pseudotumor of the orbit: Limited Wegener's granulomatosis. *Ann. Intern. Med.* 72:687, 1970.
6. Jordan, J. M., Rowe, W. T., and Allen, N. B. Wegener's granulomatosis involving the breast. *Am. J. Med.* 83:159, 1987.
   Two (5,6) rare presentations to keep in mind.
7. Bischoff, M. E. Noninfectious necrotizing granulomatosis: The pulmonary roentgen signs. *Radiology* 75:752, 1960.
   X-ray findings are reviewed.
8. Israel, H. L., and Patchefsky, A. S. Wegener's granulomatosis of lung: Diagnosis and treatment. *Ann. Intern. Med.* 74:881, 1971.
   Diagnosis is by lung biopsy. The course is variable.
9. Cassan, S. M., Coles, D. T., and Harrison, E. G., Jr. The concept of limited forms of Wegener's granulomatosis. *Am. J. Med.* 49:366, 1970.
   The prognosis and response to steroids appears to be better in the absence of renal involvement.
10. Fauci, A. S., and Wolff, S. M. Wegener's granulomatosis: Studies in 18 patients and a review of the literature. *Medicine* 52:535, 1973.
    Necrotizing granulomatous vasculitis of the upper and lower respiratory tracts, glomerulonephritis, and varying degrees of systemic vasculitis are discussed.
11. McDonald, T. J., DeRemee, R. A., and Weiland, L. H. Wegener's granulomatosis and polymorphic reticulosis: Two diseases or one? *Arch. Otolaryngol.* 107:141, 1981.
    Convincing histologic and clinical differences support these being two diseases.
12. Haynes, B. F., Fishman, M. L., Fauci, A. S., et al. The ocular manifestations of Wegener's granulomatosis: Fifteen years experience and a review of the literature. *Am. J. Med.* 63:131, 1977.
    A good review; 47% have some form of ocular involvement.
13. Lampman, J. H., Queribin, R., and Kondapalli, P. Subglottic stenosis in Wegener's granulomatosis. *Chest* 79:230, 1981.
14. Oimomi, M., Suehiro, I., Mizuno, N., et al. Wegener's granulomatosis with intracerebral granuloma and mammary manifestation: Report of a case. *Arch Intern. Med.* 140:853, 1980.
15. Hensley, M. J., Feldman, N. T., Lazarus, J. M., et al. Diffuse pulmonary hemorrhage and rapidly progressive renal failure: An uncommon presentation of Wegener's granulomatosis. *Am. J. Med.* 66:894, 1979.
    Some (articles 13–15) rare but important presentations and manifestations of this protean disease.
16. Rosenberg, D. M., Weinberger, S. E., Fulmer, J. D., et al. Functional correlates of lung involvement in Wegener's granulomatosis. *Am. J. Med.* 69:387, 1980.
    The most common finding was obstruction to airflow.
17. Hu, C.-H., O'Loughlin, S., and Winkelmann, R. K. Cutaneous manifestations of Wegener granulomatosis. *Arch. Dermatol.* 113:175, 1977.
    A comprehensive review of the skin manifestations.
18. van der Woude, F. J., Rasmussen, N., Lobatto, S., et al. Autoantibodies against neutrophils and monocytes: Tool for diagnosis and marker of disease activity in Wegener's granulomatosis. *Lancet* 1:425, 1985.
    Looks promising but needs further study.
19. Brandwein, S., Esdaile, J., Danoff, D., et al. Wegener's granulomatosis: Clinical features and outcomes in 13 patients. *Arch. Intern. Med.* 143:476, 1983.
    Survival rate was 56% at 1 year in the nine patients treated with a cytotoxic agent.

IV. DISEASES OF THE ENDOCRINE SYSTEM AND METABOLIC DISORDERS

49. ACROMEGALY
H. Verdain Barnes

"For some 15 to 20 years, each day when I looked into the glass to brush my hair or to shave, there was a typical acromegalic literally staring me in the face. Yet, I never recognized the fact." This statement made in 1912 by a physician, Leonard Mark, dramatically demonstrates the insidious onset of this rare disease of excess human growth hormone (HGH).

The etiology of acromegaly is usually an HGH-producing anterior pituitary tumor, but on occasion results from a growth hormone (GH)–producing adenoma of neural origin outside of the pituitary, an ectopic HGH-producing neoplasm, or an ectopic production of growth hormone releasing hormone (GHRH). HGH-producing pituitary adenomas can be classified as densely or sparsely granulated GH cell, mixed GH and prolactin cell, acidophil stem cell, mammosomatotroph cell, and unclassified plurihormonal cell types. Rarely the source is a GH cell carcinoma or GH cell hyperplasia. Ectopic GH cell adenomas may be located in the sphenoid sinus or parapharyngeal areas. Ectopic GH-producing tumors have been reported in the lung, ovary, breast, and pancreas. Ectopic production of GHRH has been reported with hypothalamic hamartomas or choristomas, and ectopic GHRH-producing neoplasms have been found in the pancreas, bronchus, and intestine. Suprasellar extension of the pituitary adenomas is not uncommon.

In most patients the disease presents in the third or fourth decade often with a delay in diagnosis of 10 to 20 years. Virtually all patients have varying degrees of acral enlargement. However, the presenting complaint is more likely to be (1) headaches; (2) visual disturbance; (3) hyperhydrosis; (4) fatigue and lethargy; (5) arthritis or arthralgias; (6) peripheral neuropathy (commonly carpal tunnel syndrome); (7) polyuria, polydipsia, or polyphagia with overt diabetes mellitus; (8) galactorrhea; (9) goiter (occasionally with hyperthyroidism); (10) nephrolithiasis; or (11) cardiovascular decompensation and/or hypertension.

Once the diagnosis is clinically suspected, active disease should be confirmed by the measurement of a basal serum HGH level or fasting somatomedin C level. A very high (>50 ng/ml) basal HGH level is virtually diagnostic as is an elevated insulin-like growth factor I (IGF-I, somatomedin C) level except for the latter during the adolescent growth spurt and normal pregnancy. If the diagnosis is still in doubt then one or more provocative tests should be used (oral glucose tolerance test, thyrotropin releasing hormone (TRH) test, or L-dopa test). Classically, acromegalics are unable to suppress their immunoreactive HGH levels to less than 5 ng/ml at the time of maximum hyperglycemia. Three responses can be seen: (1) a sustained elevation of HGH throughout the test, (2) a minimal depression of HGH, or (3) a paradoxical rise in HGH. In 70 to 80 percent of acromegalies the TRH test shows a paradoxical rise in HGH by 50 to 150 percent above the baseline. In the L-dopa test over 60 percent of acromegalics have a paradoxical suppresion of HGH by greater than 50 percent below the basal level. Once the diagnosis has been established, all patients should have a visual field examination, radiographs of the sella turcica, and a computed tomograph (CT) scan of the head. The plain skull x rays of the sella are normal in 10 to 24 percent of patients, but tomograms of the sella identify abnormalities in the majority of patients. In McLachlan's series,[3] 138 of 140 acromegalics were found to have sellar abnormalities when both the plain film and tomograms were used. Suprasellar extension can usually be documented by CT scan and/or elevated HGH levels in the cerebrospinal fluid. Somatomedin C levels appear to correlate with clinical disease activity as does heel pad thickness.

The natural history of the disease suggests a relatively early death, with approximately 64 percent of patients dying before 60 years. The most common cause of death is cardiovascular disease (in at least one-third of patients). The cardiovascular complications are (1) accelerated arteriosclerotic vascular disease with or without associated diabetes mellitus or hypertension, (2) arrhythmias, and (3) cardiomyopathy. Some (occasionally all) complications regress or stabilize after therapy. Significant visual impairment and progressive cardiovascular disease are complications demanding immediate therapy.

1. Mark, L. P. *Acromegaly: A Personal Experience.* Paris: Baillière, 1912.
   Just for fun.
2. Earll, J. M., Sparks, L. L., and Forsham, P. H. Glucose suppression of serum growth hormone in the diagnosis of acromegaly. *J.A.M.A.* 201:628, 1967.
   The criteria for diagnosis.
3. McLachlan, M. S. F., Wright, A. D., and Doyle, F. H. Plain film and tomographic assessment of the pituitary fossa in 140 acromegalic patients. *Br. J. Radiol.* 43:360, 1970.
   The radiologic criteria for the diagnosis of sellar abnormalities in acromegaly.
4. Kho, K. M., Wright, A. D., and Doyle, F. H. Heel pad thickness in acromegaly. *Br. J. Radiol.* 43:119, 1970.
   Technique and diagnostic criteria for evaluating heel pad thickness.
5. Wright, A. D., Hill, D. M., Lowry, C., et al. Mortality in acromegaly. *Q. J. Med.* 39:1, 1970.
   Deaths in 194 acromegalic patients: cardiovascular disease (38.5%), malignancy (18%), respiratory disease (18%), and miscellaneous disorders (25.5%).
6. Mastaglia, F. L., Barwick, D. D., and Hall, R. Myopathy in acromegaly. *Lancet* 2:907, 1970.
   Pathophysiology may be related to increased protein synthesis secondary to HGH effect on myocardial ribosomes.
7. Frohman, L. A., Szabo, M., and Berelowitz, M. Partial purification and characterization of a peptide with growth hormone–releasing activity from extrapituitary tumors in patients with acromegaly. *J. Clin. Invest.* 65:43, 1980.
   Found in extracts of carcinoid and islet cell tumors.
8. Savage, D. D., Henry, W. L., Eastman, R. C., et al. Echocardiographic assessment of cardiac anatomy and function in acromegalic patients. *Am. J. Med.* 67:823, 1979.
   80% had abnormal echocardiograms by this noninvasive technique.
9. Corenblum, B., LeBlanc, F. E., and Watanabe, M. Acromegaly with an adenomatous pharyngeal pituitary. *J.A.M.A.* 243:1456, 1980.
   Embryology can be important.
10. Scheithauer, B. W., Kovacs, K., Randall, R. V., et al. Pathology of excessive production of growth hormone. *Clin. Endocrinol. Metab.* 15:655, 1986.
    A well-done and well-referenced review.
11. Melmed, S., Braunstein, G. D., Horvath, E., et al. Pathophysiology of acromegaly. *Endocr. Rev.* 4:271, 1983.
    An effective method of histologic classification is presented as well as a comprehensive theory of tumorigenesis.
12. Melmed, S., Braunstein, G. D., Chang, J., et al. Pituitary tumors secreting growth hormone and prolactin. *Ann. Intern. Med.* 105:238, 1986.
    A concise review including the differential diagnosis.
13. Daughaday, W. H., Starkey, R. H., Saltman, S., et al. Characterization of serum growth hormone (GH) and insulin-like growth factor I in active acromegaly with minimal elevation of serum GH. *J. Clinic Endocrinol. Metab.* 65:617, 1987.
    IGF-I (somatomedin C) was distinctly elevated in these two patients who appeared to have an increased sensitivity to GH. Diagnosis is not always easy.
14. Verde, G. G., Santi, I., Chiodinid, P., et al. Serum type III procollagen propeptide levels in acromegaly. *J. Clin. Endocrinol. Metab.* 63:1406, 1986.
    Levels were elevated in acromegalics and may prove useful in diagnosis, but more study is needed.
15. Dinn, J. J., and Dinn, E. I. Natural history of acromegalic peripheral neuropathy. *Q. J. Med.* 224:833, 1985.
    The basic lesion is demylination with hypertrophy of the Schwann cell system and small-diameter fibers. If the acromegaly is untreated the course appears to be progressive.
16. Melmed, S., Ezrin, C., Kovacs, K., et al. Acromegaly due to secretion of growth hormone by an ectopic pancreatic islet-cell tumor. *N. Engl. J. Med.* 312:9, 1985.
17. Boizel, R., Halimi, S., Labat, F., et al. Acromegaly due to a growth hormone-releasing hormone–secreting bronchial carcinoid tumor: Further information on the abnormal

responsiveness of the somatotroph cells and their recovery after successful treatment. *J. Clin. Endocrinol. Metab.* 64:304, 1987.

18. Roth, K. A., Wilson, D. M., Eberwine, J., et al. Acromegaly and pheochromocytoma: A multiple endocrine syndrome caused by a plurihormonal adrenal medullary tumor. *J. Clin. Endocrinol. Metab.* 63:1421, 1986.
    The three articles (16–18) illustrate three different ectopic etiologies for acromegaly.

19. Reubi, J. C., Heitz, P. U., and Landolt, A. M. Visualization of somatostatin receptors and correlation with immunoreactive growth hormone and prolactin in human pituitary adenomas: Evidence for different tumor subclasses.
    Based on somatostatin receptor density, there may be subclasses of GH-producing adenomas.

20. Bjerre, P., Lindholm, J., and Videbaek, H. The spontaneous course of pituitary adenomas and occurrence of an empty sella in untreated acromegaly. *J. Clin. Endocrinol. Metab.* 63:287, 1986.
    Partial or complete disappearance of GH-secreting pituitary adenomas may be more frequent than recognized, but normalization of serum GH is rare.

21. Abboud, C. F., and Laws, E. R., Jr. Diagnosis of pituitary tumors. *Endocrinol. Metab. Clin. North Am.* 17:241, 1988.
    A concise discussion of the laboratory evaluation of acromegaly.

50. ANOREXIA NERVOSA AND BULIMIA NERVOSA

James P. McGee
Jerry L. Spivak

The primary characteristic of *anorexia nervosa* is a pathologic refusal to eat and a failure to maintain body weight over a minimal normal weight for age and height. The weight loss is *not* caused by an organic disorder and it leads to a body weight at least 15 percent below what is appropriate.

Anorexic patients display a morbid fear of gaining weight or becoming obese even while they are both malnourished and emaciated, and a distorted body image marked by gross misperception of body size, weight, and shape is usually present. True loss of appetite is quite rare in these patients and, if seen at all, appears only at an advanced stage of the illness. Most anorexics experience persistent and intense feelings of hunger but refuse to eat in spite of that. Ninety-five percent of anorexia patients are adolescent or young adult females with the onset of the disorder frequently coinciding with puberty. It rarely occurs after age 35 and older patients usually give a history of similar symptoms at a younger age. In those rare instances of anorexia nervosa in a male, the symptom picture and mode of presentation is often remarkably similar to that found in female patients.

The typical course for both male and female patients is a single episode followed by return to normal weight. Some patients, however, have episodic bouts of the disorder which alternate with periods of remission. The mortality rate among anorexic patients has been reported to be anywhere from 5 to 22 percent, including deaths that are either the direct consequence of starvation or from suicide by some other method.

Weight loss of a profound and distressing degree to all but the patient is the most striking feature of anorexia nervosa. Self-imposed restriction of total food intake frequently accompanied by excessive exercising accounts for the weight loss though binge eating followed by self-induced vomiting, laxative, and diuretic abuse may also be present (see bulimia nervosa below).

The typical anorexic patient is a lean, possibly emaciated-looking, shy, and immature young white female from a social background that is middle class or above. Psychosexual development is usually delayed and in older patients there is a notable lack of interest in, or fear of, sex. Perfectionism, scholastic overachievement, lowered sense of self-esteem, excessive sensitivity to criticism and rejection, and social-interpersonal anxiety are also usually present. There may have been a period of mild overweight to obesity before the onset of the illness and weight gain may be fearfully and subconsciously equated with independence, psychosexual maturity, and/or pregnancy. Preoccupation with food selection and preparation, compulsive recipe collecting, and rigidly scheduled eating routines are common and the patient may hoard, conceal, ritualistically cut or dice food, or throw food away. Many of these patients prepare elaborate meals for others while simultaneously limiting themselves to a narrow selection of low calorie or dietetic foods. Other compulsive behaviors such as repeated hand washing may be present and may justify the additional diagnosis of obsessive-compulsive disorder.

Examination frequently reveals hypothermia, bradycardia, and hypotension. There is amenorrhea; however, cessation of menses frequently precedes weight loss and menstruation may not resume even after normal body weight is restored. If the patient is a laxative abuser, rectal prolapse may be present and some anorexics who purge with repeated enemas have been known to produce bowel tearing and even perforation.

Secondary sexual characteristics including pubic and axillary hair are preserved even in the presence of marked weight loss. Hypertrichosis or flossy neonatal-like lanugo hair is often present. The relaxation time of the deep tendon reflexes may be prolonged. The presence of dehydration, muscle weakness and atrophy, pedal edema, and signs of vitamin lack are dependent on the degree and duration of starvation. The latter may be conditioned by the tendency of some patients to eat surreptitiously. In contrast to true protein and calorie malnutrition, most patients with anorexia nervosa have a diet that is more depleted in carbohydrates than protein. Vomiting or laxative and diuretic abuse may lead to hypokalemia, hypochloremia, and a mixed alkalosis. This is compounded by dehydration and a failure of renal conservation of water that appears to respond to exogenous vasopressin. Hypokalemia undoubtedly contributes to polyuria in some patients. Mild metabolic acidosis with ketonuria, hyperuricemia, and asymptomatic hypoglycemia may be present. Carotenemia is also common; the serum cholesterol level may be normal or elevated. Anemia and neutropenia are generally associated with a hypocellular bone marrow. Bone marrow neutrophil reserves, however, are generally adequate. Urine output is low, bowel movements are infrequent, and thirst is minimal. In spite of a wasted appearance, however, many patients are energetic and hyperactivity is not uncommon.

Hypothalamic dysfunction is a fundamental feature of anorexia nervosa and appears to correlate best with the degree of weight loss. Estradiol, luteinizing hormone (LH), and follicle-stimulating hormone (FSH) levels in the plasma are reduced; thyrotropic-stimulating hormone (TSH) levels are normal while thyroxine (T_4) levels are at the lower limits of normal. The serum triiodothyronine (T_3) level is low; reverse T_3 levels, however, are high. In contrast to hypopituitarism, growth hormone levels are elevated. Serum cortisol levels may be normal or high. In approximately 50 percent of patients, the normal diurnal variation is lost, presumably due to a prolonged half-life of plasma cortisol.

Anorexic patients produce false-positive results to a challenge dose of oral dexamethasone as given in the dexamethasone suppression test (DST), a test which has achieved some popularity in the psychiatric diagnosis of certain types of endogenous depression.

Low levels of urinary 17-hydroxysteroids and 17-ketosteroids reflect a reduced rate of steroid degradation. Serum prolactin levels are normal. Hypothermia and a decreased ability to maintain a normal body temperature when exposed to heat or cold are not uncommon. Bradycardia and hypotension appear to correlate with reduced levels of norepinephrine and urine catecholamine metabolites. The response of the pituitary to hypothalamic releasing factors may be either normal or blunted. With refeeding both the pituitary response and plasma hormone levels normalize. The possibility of an occult cerebral neoplasm should, of course, always be considered, particularly in patients presenting with atypical manifestations.

Concerning differential diagnosis, loss of appetite is common in depressive disorders and in many physical illnesses. However, unlike in anorexia, these patients do not show the characteristic disturbance of body image or phobic aversion to weight gain. In schizophrenia, bizarre and ritualized eating behaviors are not unusual but true anorexia is rarely present. In bulimia nervosa (see below) fear of obesity and weight instability also appear but weight remains above the minimal normal weight for height.

The precise etiology of anorexia nervosa remains unknown. Pedigree research reveals an increased incidence of anorexia among female siblings and mothers of proband cases. Major depression, manic-depressive illness, and alcoholism are also reported to be more common among first-degree relatives of people with anorexia nervosa. Stressful life situations frequently precede the onset of the illness and in male anorexics a traumatic homosexual experience is a common triggering event.

The treatment of patients with anorexia nervosa is a difficult proposition involving both medical and psychological aspects. Most anorexic patients stridently deny or minimize the severity of their illness, and passive, manipulative, or direct stubborn resistance to therapy is typical. Even in a closely monitored hospital setting these patients are known to continue patterns of food restriction, binge eating, self-induced vomiting, and laxative abuse. Ironically, the psychic impairment seen in these patients including depression, irritability, concreteness, cognitive rigidity, erratic behavior, and compulsivity, may, at least partially, be the result of an organic brain syndrome due to the malnourished state. Patiently attentive nursing care and a rigorously supervised refeeding program is essential. Judicious use of positive reinforcement contingent on treatment compliance and weight gain can be helpful. It is important to evaluate all patients for signs of vitamin lack that may be reflected by muscle tenderness, peripheral neuropathy, bruising, or bleeding. Adequate replacement of vitamins must accompany refeeding since an acute imbalance between vitamin and caloric intake may produce the symptoms of a vitamin-deficient state. Administration of glucose should be continuous to avoid reactive hypoglycemia, and potassium supplementation should be included if urine production flow is sufficient. The administration of glucose or protein can result in the development of edema, presumably because of improved medullary sodium transport and decreased sodium excretion. Supplemental magnesium may be required. Abnormalities in bone marrow function do not require specific therapy; they respond to refeeding alone. It must be emphasized that refeeding has little impact on the underlying mental disorder. When weight loss is severe and there is resistance to voluntary feeding, nutrition must be effected by a parenteral route or by nasogastric tube. Tube feeding, however, is not without risks; they include aspiration, diarrhea, dehydration, and hypernatremia. The risk of tube feeding is compounded because these patients have delayed gastric emptying. The use of chlorpromazine and insulin to reduce anorexia and promote hunger has been advocated. However, hypotension, hypokalemia, and hypoglycemia can result from these agents and they are not recommended. Cyproheptadine has also been employed to promote weight gain but without notable success. Tricyclic antidepressants and monoamine oxidase inhibitors (MAOIs) may benefit patients who remain depressed after weight has been restored and stabilized and some clinicians enthusiastically endorse the use of antidepressants for the control of symptoms of binge eating and purging.

While most patients with anorexia nervosa do not suffer from severe or recurrent infections, it should be remembered that malnourished, leukopenic patients do not tolerate infections once they become established, and develop metabolic acidosis under minimal stress. In the early literature on anorexia nervosa, tuberculosis was a frequent occurrence. Overwhelming sepsis in the absence of fever has also been described in these patients.

While refeeding corrects most of the observed metabolic abnormalities, a successful functional outcome depends on effective psychologic interventions. Individual psychotherapy is almost always a requirement and psychotherapy groups and self-help programs composed of other eating disorder patients can also be of benefit. Parents and/or spouses usually participate in family therapy. Favorable outcome is associated with less denial and immaturity in the patients, the presence of physical hyperactivity, stable family background, and early recognition and treatment. Poor prognostic features include long duration of illness, older age of onset, cycles of binging and vomiting, and poor social and family relationships.

Finally, there is an increased frequency of both anorexia and bulimia among amateur and professional dancers and among some athletes such as marathon runners and gymnasts where weight requirements are stringent.

Current classification systems identify *bulimia nervosa* as a separate diagnostic entity though it clearly shares features common to anorexia nervosa. Criteria for the diagnosis of bulimia nervosa include recurrent episodes of binge eating, followed by self-induced purging through vomiting and/or laxative, cathartic, or diuretic abuse. The disorder is about 10 times more common among females and onset is typically during adolescence and before age 25. Unlike anorexia, weight is usually maintained in bulimia though there may be frequent fluctuations within the normal range due to alternating binges, purging, and fasting. Bulimics experience a subjective sense of loss of control during eating binges and a binge is typically followed by a period of depression, remorse, and self-deprecation. Episodes of strict dieting or fasting accompanied by vigorous exercising are common and there must be, on average, a minimum of two binge eating episodes per week for at least 3 months for the diagnosis to apply. Like anorexic patients, bulimics show obsessive mental preoccupation with their body shape and weight.

When a bulimic patient embarks on an eating binge she may consume as many as 24,000 calories in a single episode. The food is typically bolted down in huge portions, the eating is done in secret, and sweet, easily swallowed foods are preferred. Abdominal pain and distention, sleep from exhaustion, or interruption by others causes binge eating to stop. Purposeful vomiting reduces physical discomfort in order to permit continued gorging or to terminate the binge. Sometimes the vomiting becomes an end in itself so that the patient eats in order to vomit. Though the eating binge may be experienced as pleasurable, it is almost always followed by a psychic letdown or mood "crash."

The course of bulimia is frequently chronic with weekly or more frequent episodes of binging and purging occurring for years at a time. There may be periods of spontaneous remission to normalized eating habits but these are usually followed by a return to the binge-purge pattern. In the most severe cases, periods of normal eating are completely absent. Obesity and depressive illness are more common among first-degree relatives of bulimic patients and adolescent obesity may be a predisposing factor to the development of the condition. Some bulimics are prone to substance abuse involving sedatives, amphetamines, cocaine, or alcohol.

Metabolic disturbances similar to those found in anorexic patients are sometimes present. Vomiting produces painless bilateral swelling of the parotid glands, and erosion of the tooth enamel, particularly of anterior teeth, occurs owing to exposure to gastric fluids. If the patient induces vomiting by inserting fingers in her throat, there may be noticeable scarring on the knuckles and repeated vomiting can produce esophageal tears or gastric rupture. Electrolyte imbalance and dehydration raises the potential for cardiac arrhythmias and even sudden cardiac arrest.

Concerning differential diagnosis, severe weight loss, a central feature of anorexia, is absent in bulimia nervosa. Abnormal eating patterns are common to neurologic diseases such as CNS tumor, Kleine-Levin syndrome, and Klüver-Bucy syndrome, but a true bulimic pattern is rarely present. Overeating and food regurgitation is found among some regressed schizophrenic patients but they almost never have bulimia nervosa.

Bulimic patients tend to be less resistant to therapeutic intervention than their anorexic counterparts but they nonetheless remain a particularly challenging group of individuals to treat. Once the binge-purge pattern of eating behavior becomes established it takes on many of the characteristics of a compulsion and it is thus extremely difficult to change. In some cases, particularly where depression is a prominent feature, tricyclic antidepressants or MAOIs may be of benefit.

1. Frisch, R. E., and McArthur, J. W. Menstrual cycles: Fatness as a determinant of minimum weight for height necessary for their maintenance or onset. *Science* 185:949, 1974.
   Approximately 17% of body weight must be fat for menses to occur.
2. Vigersky, R. A., Andersen, A. E., Thompson, R. H., et al. Hypothalamic dysfunction in secondary amenorrhea associated with simple weight loss. *N. Engl. J. Med.* 297:1141, 1977.
   Simple weight loss produces changes in hypothalamic function, which are qualitatively similar to those found in anorexia nervosa.
3. Hsu, L. K. G., Crisp, A. H., and Harding, B. Outcome of anorexia nervosa. *Lancet* 1:61, 1979.

4. American Psychiatric Association. *Diagnostic and Statistical Manual of Mental Disorders* (3rd ed. rev.). Washington, D.C.: American Psychiatric Press, 1987.
   Current diagnostic criteria for anorexia and bulimia.
5. Drossman, D. A., Ontjes, D. A., and Heizer, W. D. Anorexia nervosa. *Gastroenterology* 77:1115, 1979.
   A global review of the disease.
6. Schwabe, A. D., Lippe, B. M., Chang, R. J., et al. Anorexia nervosa. *Ann. Intern. Med.* 94:371, 1981.
   Clinical data from 36 patients.
7. Warren M. P., and Vande Wiele, R. L. Clinical and metabolic features of anorexia nervosa. *Am. J. Obstet. Gynecol.* 117:435, 1973.
   A thorough and thoughtful review.
8. Mecklenburg, R. S., Loriaux, D. C., Thompson, R. H., et al. Hypothalamic dysfunction in patients with anorexia nervosa. *Medicine* 53:147, 1974.
   Impaired thermoregulation is thought to be due to hypothalamic dysfunction.
9. Boyar, R. M., Katz, J., Finkelstein, J. W., et al. Anorexia nervosa *N. Engl. J. Med.* 291:861, 1974.
   LH secretory activity correlates with body weight.
10. Boyar, R. M., Hellman, L. D., Roffwarg, H., et al. Cortisol secretion and metabolism in anorexia nervosa. *N. Engl. J. Med.* 296:190, 1977.
    Elevated plasma cortisol levels with reduced T_3 levels are due to the state of undernutrition.
11. Avery, D. H. Dexamethasone suppression test as a marker for depression. *Resident Staff Physician,* 9:63, 1983.
    Anorexia produces false-positive DST results.
12. Leslie, R. D. G., Issacs, A. J., Gomez, J., et al. Hypothalamopituitary-thyroid function in anorexia nervosa: Influence of weight gain, *Br. Med. J.* 2:526, 1978.
    T_3 is low but increases with weight gain; T_4 shows less change with weight gain.
13. Hay, G. G., and Leonard, J. C. Anorexia nervosa in males. *Lancet* 2:574, 1979.
    Exclusion of organic disorders causing cachexia must be pursued before considering this diagnosis in a male.
14. Kron, L., Katz, J. L., Gorzynsky, G., et al. Anorexia nervosa and gonadal dysgenesis. *Arch. Gen. Psychiatry* 34:332, 1977.
    A relationship whose occurrence appears to be more than coincidental.
15. Gottdiener, J. S., Gross, H. A., Henry, W. L., et al. Effects of self-induced starvation on cardiac size and function in anorexia nervosa. *Circulation* 48:425, 1978.
    Reduction in cardiac size without alteration in ventricular function.
16. White, J. H., Kelly, P., and Dorman, K. Clinical picture of atypical anorexia nervosa associated with hypothalamic tumor. *Am. J. Psychiatry* 134:323, 1977.
    One of several reports of a hypothalamic tumor presenting as anorexia nervosa.
17. Fowler, P. B. S., Banim, S. O., and Ikran, H. Prolonged ankle reflex in anorexia nervosa. *Lancet* 2:307, 1972.
    An example of delayed relaxation not due to hypothyroidism.
18. Bowers, T. K. and Eckert, E. Leukopenia in anorexia nervosa. *Arch. Intern. Med.* 138:1520, 1978.
    Marrow neutrophil reserves are normal.
19. Mant, M. J., and Faragher, B. S. The haematology of anorexia nervosa. *Br. J. Haematol.* 23:737, 1972.
    Hypoplasia, gelatinous transformation of ground substance, and spiculated red cells.
20. Cornblee, P. J., Moir, R. C., and Wolf, P. L. A histochemical study of bone marrow hypophasis in anorexia nervosa. *Virchows Arch. (Pathol. Anat.)* 374:239, 1977.
    Serious fat atrophy without an increase in ground substance.
21. Levin, P. A., Falko, J. M., Dixon, K., et al. Benign parotid enlargement in bulimia. *Ann. Intern. Med.* 93:827, 1980.
    An interesting clinical observation.
22. Russell, G. F., and Bruce, J. T. Impaired water diuresis in patients with anorexia nervosa. *Am. J. Med.* 40:38, 1986.

Delayed and decreased response to water loading is due to a decrease in glomerular filtration rate.

23. Saudek, C. D., and Felig, P. The metabolic events of starvation. *Am. J. Med.* 60:117, 1976.
    A brief review of compensatory mechanisms.

24. Spencer, H., Lewin, I., Samachson, J., et al. Changes in metabolism in obese persons during starvation. *Am. J. Med.* 40:27, 1966.
    During the period of metabolic acidosis, hypercalciuria is marked and hyperuricemia occurs.

25. Klahr, S., Tripathy, K., and Lotero, H. Renal regulation of acid-base balance in malnourished man. *Am. J. Med.* 48:325, 1970.
    Starvation causes an impaired renal response to an acid load.

26. Barrett, P. V. D. Hyperbilirubinemia of fasting. *J.A.M.A.* 217:1349, 1971.
    Fasting results in a slight increase in direct bilirubin.

27. Doekel, R. C., Jr., Zwillich, C. W., Scoggin, C. H., et al. Clinical semi-starvation: Depressin of hypoxic ventilatory response. *N. Engl. J. Med.* 295:358, 1976.
    Another adverse effect of the starved state.

28. Cahill, G. F. Starvation in man. *N. Engl. J. Med.* 282:668, 1970.
    Review of the metabolic changes preventing excessive protein catabolism during starvation.

29. Weinsier, R. L. Fasing: A review with emphasis on the electrolytes. *Am J. Med.* 50:233, 1971.
    Carbohydrate ingestion reverses sodium loss during fasting, causing refeeding edema.

30. Drenick, E. J., Joven, C. B., and Swenseid, M. E. Occurrence of acute Wernicke's encephalopathy during prolonged starvation for the treatment of obesity. *N. Engl. J. Med.* 274:937, 1966.
    Latent thiamine deficiency unmasked by refeeding with glucose.

31. Heymsfield, S. B., Bethel, R. A., Ansley, J. D., et al. Enteral hyperalimentation: An alternative to central venous hyperalimentation. *Ann. Intern. Med.* 90:63, 1979.
    Hyperalimentation by the enteric route is safer and more physiologic than by venous access.

32. McGee, K. T., McGee, J. P. Behavioral treatment of eating disorders. *Occup. Ther. Men. Health.* 6:1, 1986.
    Behavioral therapy useful with anorexic patients.

33. Anderson, A. E., *Practical Comprehensive Treatment of Anorexia Nervosa and Bulimia.* Baltimore: Johns Hopkins Press, 1985.
    Describes multimodal treatment approach.

34. Geracrote, T. D., Jr., and Liddle, R. A. Impaired cholecystokenin secretion in bulimia nervosa. *N. Engl. J. Med.* 319:683, 1988.
    Defective satiety in bulimia related to impaired secretion of cholecystokinin. (See also N. Engl. J. Med. 319:716, 1988.)

51. CONGENITAL ADRENAL HYPERPLASIA
H. Verdain Barnes

The known inborn errors of adrenal steroidogenesis result from a partial or complete absence of a specific, occasionally more than one, enzyme necessary in steroid biosynthesis. Genetic transmission is as in autosomal recessive disorders. The defect is typically present in the gonads as well as the adrenals.

1. The 20,22-desmolase defect prevents the conversion of cholesterol to pregnenolone, the first step in steroid biosynthesis. Cortisol, aldosterone, and androgens are absent,

leading to salt loss, glucocorticoid deficiency, and death. Genetic males have feminized external genitalia, and females have normal genital development.

2. The microsomal 3-β-hydroxysteroid dehydrogenase enzyme required to convert pregnenolone to progesterone is deficient or absent. There is a classic and nonclassic form of this disorder with the latter probably involving two isoenzymes. In the classic form the primary hormones in excess are 17-hydroxypregnenolone and dehydroepiandrosterone (DHEA) while aldosterone, cortisol, and testosterone are decreased. Salt wasting and glucocorticoid deficiency are severe. In the nonclassic form 17-hydroxypregnenolone and DHEA are usually increased and no steroid is decreased. Since in the classic form, there are two weak androgens (Δ-5-pregnenolone and DHEA) in excess which are converted by the liver to androstenedione and testosterone, there is some masculinization of genetic females and incomplete masculinization of genetic males. In the nonclassic form pubertal or postpubertal hirsutism in women may be the primary clinical feature.

3. The 17-α-hydroxylase defect results in impaired synthesis of cortisol and testosterone. Aldosterone synthesis is possible but diminished or absent due to the excess of deoxycorticosterone (DOC) that arises from the excess progesterone synthesized in the presence of this enzyme block. The disorder is characterized by increased levels of plasma corticosterone, ACTH, and DOC and decreased levels of cortisol, aldosterone, renin, and testosterone. The genetic female has normal external genitalia, and the male presents as a normal phenotypic female or (rarely) as an incompletely masculinized male. Since deficiencies may be minimal to moderate, patients may present as adolescents or young adults with a lack of secondary sexual development, including lack of sexual hair in both sexes and primary amenorrhea in the female. DOC excess results in salt retention, increased vascular volume, and hypertension. Serum electrolyte levels may mimic those of primary aldosteronism, but urine aldosterone is low or absent. The 17,20-lyase deficiency produces a decrease in DHEA, testosterone, and androstenedione, which typically leads to ambiguous genitalia in males.

4. The 21-hydroxylase defect is the most common, accounting for at least 60 percent of all cases of congenital adrenal hyperplasia. There are at least four forms of this disorder of which one is a combination of 21- and 11-hydroxylase deficiency. The salt-wasting form has an increase in 17-hydroxyprogesterone (17-OHP) and androstenedione and a decrease in aldosterone and cortisol. The simple virilizing form exhibits the same except aldosterone is essentially normal. The nonclassic form is the same except both cortisol and aldosterone are normal. This form is typically associated with HLA-B14, DR1 and is among the most common of the known autosomal recessive diseases. In the salt-wasting and simple virilizing forms the genetic female may exhibit partial to complete masculinization of the external genitalia, and the male has varying degrees of macrogenitosomia. In the male the size of the penis and prostate are disproportionate to testicular size. A rare male has large nodular testes resulting from overstimulated adrenal rest tissue within the gonads. These otherwise normal testes may be mistakenly considered to have bilateral tumors. Hyperpigmentation of the hands, elbows, axillary folds, scrotum, penis, clitoris, labia, and areolae mammae is common. If untreated, these patients are typically taller than their peers in childhood, becoming shorter than their peers in adolescence or as adults due to premature epiphyseal closure by androgen excess. Recently, late-onset 21-hydroxylase deficiency has become more clearly defined. There appear to be several phenotypes: androgen excess similar to patients with polycystic ovary disease, but no consistent elevation in the luteinizing hormone (LH)–follicle-stimulating hormone (FSH) ratio; isolated hirsutism; and a cryptic form with no clinical evidence of androgen excess. An important entity to keep in mind when evaluating the hirsute female with menstrual problems.

5. Deficiency of the mitochondrial enzyme 11-β-hydroxylase occurs in about 10 percent of patients with congenital adrenal hyperplasia. This disorder has classic and nonclassic forms. In the former, hypertension is present accompanied by an increase in DOC and 11-deoxycortisol and a decrease in cortisol plus, on occasion, aldosterone. The other clinical manifestations are the same as in the 21-hydroxylase deficiency. The serum electrolyte levels mimic those of primary aldosteronism, but urinary aldosterone is low or absent, as it is in the 17-α-hydroxylase defect. In the nonclassic form, 11-deoxycortisol is increased, DOC may be slightly increased or normal, while cortisol and aldosterone

are normal. As noted above, this defect may occur in combination with 21-hydroxylase deficiency.

6. The rare 18-oxidase defect prevents aldosterone synthesis. The production and metabolism of other steroids are unimpaired. The only clinical feature is salt loss. In this disorder, 18-hydroxycorticosterone is increased and aldosterone is decreased or absent.

Adolescents or young adults who have a lack of secondary sexual hair, infantile external genitalia, and hypertension should be screened for a possible 17-hydroxylase defect; those who are short, with masculinization, hirsutism, with or without ambiguous genitalia or hypertension, should be screened for the 11- and/or 21-hydroxylase defects. A buccal smear should be done and if the result is equivocal, a chromosome analysis performed. Therapy for these patients consists of adequate doses of glucocorticoids. In patients with the 17-hydroxylase defect, appropriate male or female hormone therapy is also required. Psychologic counseling should be provided for all these patients, especially those requiring corrective surgical procedures.

1. Hamilton, W. Congenital adrenal hyperplasia. *J. Clin. Endocrinol. Metab.* 1:503, 1972.
   A comprehensive review with an emphasis on pathophysiology and treatment.
2. Fore, W. W., Bledsoe, T., Weber, D. M., et al. Cortisol production by testicular tumors in adrenogenital syndrome. *Arch. Intern. Med.* 130:59, 1972.
   What appear to be testicular tumors may be adrenal rests or testicular interstitial cells; both respond to cortisol therapy.
3. Wilkins, L., Lewis, R. A., and Klein, R. The suppression of androgen secretion by cortisone in a case of congenital hyperplasia. *Bull. Johns Hopkins Hosp.* 81:249, 1950.
   A classic study of therapy in these patients by the father of pediatric endocrinology.
4. Money, J., Hampson, J. G., and Hampson, J. L. Hermaphroditism: Recommendations concerning assignment of sex, changes of sex, and psychological management. *Bull. Johns Hopkins Hosp.* 97:284, 1955.
   A good discussion of an approach to the psychologic management of these patients.
5. Jones, H. W., Jr., and Wilkins, L. Gynecological operations in ninety-four patients with intersexuality. *Am. J. Obstet. Gynecol.* 82:1142, 1961.
   A discussion of the surgical procedures that may be required.
6. Mckenna, T. J., Jennings, A. S., Liddle, G. W., et al. Pregnenolone, 17-OH-pregnenolone, and testosterone in plasma of patients with congenital adrenal hyperplasia. *J. Clin. Endocrinol. Metab.* 42:918, 1976.
   Control is not easily achieved.
7. Newmark, S., Dluky, R., Williams, G., et al. Partial 11 and 21 hydroxylase deficiencies in hirsute women. *Am. J. Obstet. Gynecol.* 127:594, 1977.
   The so-called acquired adrenal hyperplasia.
8. Kuhnle, U., Chow, D., Rapaport, R., et al. The 21-hydroxylase activity in the glomerulosa and fasciculata of the adrenal cortex in congenital adrenal hyperplasia. *J. Clin. Endocrinol. Metab.* 52:534, 1981.
   In the salt- and non–salt-losing varieties there is a zona fasciculata defect, but only the salt-losing patient has a zona glomerulosa defect.
9. Kirkland, R. T., Keenan, B. S., Holcombe, J. H., et al. Effect of therapy on mature height in congenital adrenal hyperplasia. *J. Clin. Ednocrinol. Metab.* 47:1320, 1978.
   The earlier the patient is effectively treated the greater the potential for achieving an average adult height.
10. White, P. C., New, M. I., and DuPont, B. Congenital adrenal hyperplasia (Pt. I and II). *N. Engl. J. Med.* 316:1519 and 1580, 1987.
    An up-to-date review including a concise review of steroidogenesis.
11. New, M. I., and Speicer, P. W. Genetics of adrenal steroid 21-hydroxylase deficiency. *Endocr. Rev.* 7:331, 1986.
12. Speicer, P. W., New, M. I., and White P. C. Molecular genetic analysis of nonclassic steroid 21-hydroxylase deficiency associated with HLA-B14, DR1. *N. Engl. J. Med.* 319:19, 1988.
    These two articles (11, 12) define the current understanding of this deficiency.

. Hurwitz, A., Brautbar, C., Milwidsky, A., et al. Combined 21- and HB-hydroxylase deficiency in familial congenital adrenal hyperplasia. *J. Clin. Endocrinol. Metab.* 60:631, 1985.
   The clinical manifestations are quite variable.
14. Pang, S., Lerner, A. J., Stoner, E., et al. Late-onset adrenal steroid 3-beta-hydroxysteroid dehydrogenase deficiency: I. A cause of hirsutism in pubertal and postpubertal women. *J. Clin. Endocrinol. Metab.* 60:428, 1985.
   Another potential cause of hirsutism.
. Cravioto, M. A. C., Ulloa-Aguirre, A., Bermudez, J. A., et al. A new inherited variant of the 3-beta-hydroxysteroid dehydrogenase-isomerase deficiency syndrome: Evidence for the existence of two isoenzymes. *J. Clin. Endocrinol. Metab.* 62:360, 1986.
   These isoenzymes may have different genetic foci.
16. Dewailly, D., Vantyghem-Handiquet, M.-C., Sainsard, C., et al. Clinical and biological phenotypes in late-onset 21-hydroxylase deficiency. *J. Clin. Endocrinol. Metab.* 63:418, 1986.
   There may be several different phenotypes.
/. Georgitis, W. T. Clinically silent congenital adrenal hyperplasia masquerading as ectopic adrenocorticotropic hormone syndrome. *Am. J. Med.* 80:703, 1986.
   A really late onset with bilateral adrenal enlargement on computed tomography scan.
18. Zerah, M., Pang, S., and New, M. I. Morning salivary 17-hydroxyprogesterone as a useful screening test for nonclassical 21-hydroxylase deficiency. *J. Clin. Endocrinol. Metab.* 65:227, 1987.
19. Baskins, H. J. Screening for late-onset congenital adrenal hyperplasia in hirsutism and amenorrhea. *Arch. Intern. Med.* 147:847, 1987.
   These articles (18, 19) discuss two methods of screening for late-onset 21-hydroxylase deficiency.

52. DIABETES INSIPIDUS

. Verdain Barnes

Diabetes insipidus (DI) is a disease produced by a partial or complete lack of antidiuretic hormone (ADH), endogenous arginine vasopressin. The result is an inability of the kidney to concentrate urine in spite of increased serum solute concentration. The clinical manifestations are polyuria, polydipsia, and an intense thirst, particularly for cold fluids. About 50% of cases are idiopathic. The most common idiopathic type is sporadic and can occur at any age beyond infancy. A second type is a rare familial form involving both sexes and having its onset in infancy. In both types, there is a decrease in the number of neurons in the paraventricular and supraoptic nuclei of the hypothalamus.

The remaining cases of DI are due to a variety of secondary causes that can be categorized into trauma, infection, vascular, neoplastic, and miscellaneous. The head trauma most likely to produce DI is that resulting in a basilar skull fracture or rupture of the pituitary stalk. The acute infectious causes include measles, mumps, basilar meningitis, encephalitis, diphtheria, and scarlet fever. DI may also result from chronic infections, such as tuberculosis, brucellosis, syphilis, and actinomycosis. Any disease process capable of producing intracranial vasculitis, thrombosis, hemorrhage, or aneurysm can, if appropriately placed, result in ADH deficiency. Any primary or secondary tumor in the pituitary-hypothalamic area has the potential of producing DI. Of the primary tumors, craniopharyngioma is the most common. Juvenile astrocytomas, meningiomas, and pinealomas follow in frequency. DI may follow pituitary, hypothalamic, or pituitary stalk surgery. Other known associations include histiocytosis X, sarcoidosis, Sheehan's syndrome, sickle cell disease, amyloidosis, lymphoma, and leukemia.

ADH deficiency must be differentiated from the other causes of polyuria, polydipsia, and thirst. These causes include hereditary and acquired nephrogenic DI, compulsive water drinking, and diabetes mellitus. In hereditary nephrogenic DI, there is an X-linked deficiency in renal cyclic 3'5'-adenosine monophosphate production resulting in renal tubular insensitivity to ADH. In sickle cell disease or trait the renal tubule is also insensitive to ADH. Acquired nephrogenic DI includes hypokalemic and hypercalcemic nephropathy and drug-induced renal tubular insensitivity to ADH that may be associated with demeclocycline or lithium therapy. Compulsive water drinking is psychogenic in origin. Chronic renal disease with polyuria and diabetes mellitus are the result of an excess osmotic load per nephron.

Compulsive water drinking (psychogenic polydipsia) is the most difficult to differentiate. Both the compulsive water drinker and the patient with ADH deficiency will frequently drink over 5 liters per day. Both generally show a normal response to exogenous vasopressin though occasionally the patient with psychogenic polydipsia does not. Generally, after 8 hours of water deprivation, the compulsive water drinker responds normally by maintaining a normal serum osmolarity and increasing urine osmolarity, whereas the patient with DI does not. However, a partial response toward normal may be seen in partial DI. In nephrogenic DI there is no response to exogenous vasopressin and minimal response to water deprivation.

The therapy of DI usually consists of exogenous vasopressin and/or chlorpropamide, the latter being effective only when some vasopressin is present. Natriuretic agents are effective in nephrogenic DI and to some degree in DI. A note of caution should be raised regarding therapy in patients who develop DI after intracranial surgery or trauma. The course is usually triphasic with immediate polyuria and polydipsia for 2 to 5 days, followed by a period of 2 to 6 days of antidiuresis, after which permanent DI may or may not recur. Consequently, in the immediate postoperative or trauma period control should be achieved with a short-acting rather than a long-acting vasopressin preparation to avoid renal shutdown during the period of antidiuresis.

1. Thomas, W. C. Diabetes insipidus. *J. Clin. Endocrinol.* 17:565, 1957.
   A variety of causes are discussed, including sarcoidosis, birth injuries, and eosinophilic granuloma. The patient prefers cold beverages.
2. Schwartz, W. B., and Relman, A. S. Effects of electrolyte disorders on renal structure and function. *N. Engl. J. Med.* 276:383, 452, 1967.
   Hypokalemic and hypercalcemic nephropathy impairs the kidney's ability to concentrate the urine.
3. Miller, M., Dalakos, T., Moses, A. M., et al. Recognition of partial defects in antidiuretic hormone secretion. *Ann. Intern. Med.* 73:721, 1970.
   A combination of dehydration and vasopressin is used to identify patients with partial ADH deficiency.
4. Miller, V. I., and Campbell, W. G., Jr. Diabetes insipidus as a complication of leukemia: Case report and review of the literature. *Cancer* 28:666, 1971.
   Leukemic infiltrates are the most common pathogenetic mechanism, followed by vascular thrombosis.
5. Bode, H. H., Harley, B. M., and Crawford, J. D. Restoration of normal drinking behavior by chlorpropamide in patients with hypodipsia and diabetes insipidus. *Am. J. Med.* 51:304, 1971.
   A difficult therapeutic problem resulting from damage to the hypothalamic thirst center and neighboring vasopressin nuclei.
6. Fichman, M. P., and Brooker, G. Deficient renal cyclic adenosine 3'5' monophosphate production in nephrogenic diabetes insipidus. *J. Clin. Endocrinol. Metab.* 35:35, 1972.
   The probable pathogenetic mechanism. A nicely done study.
7. Singer, I., and Rotenberg, D. Demeclocycline-induced nephrogenic diabetes insipidus. *Ann. Intern. Med.* 79:679, 1973.
8. Singer, I., Rotenberg, D., and Puschett, J. B. Lithium-induced nephrogenic diabetes insipidus: In vivo and in vitro studies. *J. Clin. Invest.* 51:1081, 1972.
   Articles 7 and 8 document drug-induced renal tubular insensitivity to ADH.
9. Berndt, W. O., Miller, M., Kettyle, W. Potentiation of the anti-diuretic effect of vasopressin by chlorpropamide. *Endocrinology* 86:1028, 1970.
10. Delzant, G., Sebaom, J., and Krivitzky, A. Use of carbamoyldebenzoazepine (Tegretol) in treatment of diabetes insipidus. *Ann. Endocrinol.* 32:540, 1971.

11. Decourt, M. J. Value of clofibrate in a case of diabetes insipidus. *Ann. Endocrinol.* 32:284, 1971.
12. Robinson, A. G. DDAVP in the treatment of central diabetes insipidus. *N. Engl. J. Med.* 294:507, 1976.
    These articles (9–12) discuss the usefulness and mechanism of action of various agents in therapy. Desmopressin (DDAVP) is the current treatment of choice.
13. Sridhar, C. B., Calvert, G. D., and Ibbertson, H. K. Syndrome of hypernatremia, hypodipsia and partial diabetes insipidus: New interpretation. *J. Clin. Endocrinol. Metabol.* 38:890, 1974.
    Essential hypernatremia is another entity to keep in mind.
14. Gossain, V. V., Sugawara, M., and Hagen, G. A. Co-existent diabetes mellitus and diabetes insipidus, a familial disease. *J. Clin. Endocrinol. Metabol.* 41:1020, 1975.
    Just to keep us on our toes.
15. Hays, R. M. Antidiuretic hormone. *N. Engl. J. Med.* 295:659, 1976.
    An excellent discussion.
16. Dorfman, S. G., Ruark, G. W., Agus, S., et al. Transient diabetes with elevated serum osmolarity associated with "benign" febrile illness. *Arch. Intern. Med.* 137:1479, 1977.
    An interesting, well-studied case of a disorder not previously reported in the United States.
17. Manelfe, C., and Louvet, J.-P. Computed tomography (CT) in diabetes insipidus. *J. Comput. Assist. Tomogr.* 3:309, 1979.
    Nine of these patients with idiopathic DI had an abnormal CT. Eight had small isodense masses in the chiasmatic cistern that disappeared after vasopressin therapy.
18. Zebre, R. L., and Robertson, G. L. A comparison of plasma vasopressin measurements with a standard indirect test in the differential diagnosis of polyuria. *N. Engl. J. Med.* 305:1539, 1981.
    The vasopressin assay significantly improves diagnosis.
19. Durr, J. A., Hoggard, J. G., Hunt, J. M., et al. Diabetes insipidus in pregnancy associated with abnormally high circulating vasopressinase activity. *N. Engl. J. Med.* 316:1070, 1987.
    A rare but interesting cause of DI.
20. Baylis, P. H. Posterior pituitary function in health and disease. *Clin. Endocrinol. Metab.* 12:747, 1983.
21. Robinson, A. G. Disorders of antidiuretic hormone secretion. *Clin. Endocrinol. Metab.* 14:55, 1985.
    Two (20, 21) well-referenced recent reviews of ADH disorders including diagnosis.

53. ENDOCRINE EXOPHTHALMOS

H. Verdain Barnes

Endocrine exophthalmos is most common in dysthyroid disease but can be seen with Cushing's syndrome and acromegaly. Dysthyroid disease accounts for over 90 percent of all exophthalmos and over 95 percent of endocrine exophthalmos. The pathologic findings of exophthalmos are well-known, but the pathogenesis is less clear. Most current evidence suggests an autoimmune process. The pathologic changes include (1) essentially a doubling of the fat content of the extraocular muscles; (2) focal accumulations of mast cells, plasma cells, lymphocytes; (3) thickened connective tissue septa; (4) newly formed collagen containing hydrophilic hyaluronic acid; and (5) increased mucopolysaccharides. Degenerative changes and edema are seen in the extraocular muscles. Ultimately, varying degrees of fibrosis occurs. In Graves' disease, these changes may be secondary to an increased secretory activity of the orbital fibroblasts.

A variety of biochemical presentations of dysthyroid exophthalmos have been described. The vast majority of patients have Graves' disease with an elevated total serum thyroxine (T_4) and triiodothyronine (T_3), free thyroxine index (FTI), radioiodine uptake (RAIU), nonsuppression by T_3 suppression test, and no response to thyrotropin releasing hormone (TRH). These patients may or may not have low titers of thyroid antibodies. In Graves' disease about 50 percent of the patients have the onset of exophthalmos after they are hyperthyroid, and about 12 percent months and occasionally years before their hyperthyroidism. Some thyrotoxic patients will have "T_3 toxicosis" in which case the total serum T_3 is elevated while the T_4, FTI, and usually the RAIU are normal. A small number of patients have euthyroid Graves' ophthalmopathy. They usually have a normal total serum T_4, T_3, FTI, and a normal or low RAIU, although an occasional patient will be hypothyroid with low values. They may have nonsuppression by T_3 suppression test and no response to TRH stimulation, or one test may be abnormal and the other normal. They may or may not have elevated titers of antithyroid antibodies. Rarely, exophthalmos occurs in patients with chronic lymphocytic thyroiditis (Hashimoto's struma) with a normal or low total and free serum T_4, normal or low radioiodine uptake, normal T_3 suppression test, and very high titers of thyroid antibodies.

Endocrine exophthalmos may have a noninfiltrative as well as a distinctive infiltrative component. The noninfiltrative component consists of upper lid retraction resulting from excessive sympathetic stimulation of Müller's superior palpebral muscle. This is a direct result of excess thyroid hormone and can be seen with any cause of hyperthyroidism. The infiltrative component includes venous engorgement, varying degrees of proptosis, and extraocular muscle involvement. A convenient clinical classification can be remembered by Werner's mnemonic NO SPECS:

Class 0   No signs or symptoms
Class 1   Only the signs of upper lid retraction and stare with or without associated lid
           lag and exophthalmos
Class 2   Soft tissue involvement
Class 3   Proptosis
Class 4   Extraocular muscle involvement
Class 5   Corneal involvement
Class 6   Sight loss; optic nerve involvement

The complications of proptosis include lagophthalmos, exposure keratitis, corneal ulceration, and stretching or compression of the optic nerve. Lagophthalmos of 2 mm or greater predisposes the patient to exposure of the cornea during sleep, which, if untreated, may lead to keratitis and ulceration. Optic nerve involvement due to pressure may result in decreased visual acuity and peripheral vision, and finally papilledema. The complications of extraocular muscle involvement are varying degrees of muscle paralysis most often involving the inferior and lateral recti. Inferior rectus muscle involvement results in a limitation of upward gaze whereas lateral rectus muscle involvement causes limited convergence. With time, some patients develop a fixed strabismus due to fibrosis and shortening of the extraocular muscles. The complications of chronic venous engorgement are chemosis, orbital pain, and occasionally glaucoma or subconjunctival hemorrhage. The typical clinical expressions of chemosis are conjunctival edema, excess lacrimation, photophobia, and a foreign body sensation in the eye. Periorbital edema is common and primarily involves the upper lid with a sparing of the tarsal border in contrast to the predominant lower lid and total tarsal edema seen in hypothyroidism.

The workup of a patient with bilateral exophthalmos should be designed in accordance with the clinical picture. If there is no suspicion of hyperthyroidism, hyperadrenocorticism, or excess growth hormone, the evaluation should typically consist of (1) a thorough eye examination by an ophthalmologist, including orbital computed tomography (CT), and (2) determination of total and free serum T_4, total serum T_3, thyroid antibodies, a TRH stimulation test, and if normal perhaps a radioiodine uptake and T_3 suppression test. Unilateral exophthalmos occurs in about 16 percent of the patients with dysthyroid disease. Most of these patients, however, have bilateral exophthalmos with a unilateral prominence. In true unilateral exophthalmos 80 percent of the cases are about equally distributed among dysthyroid disease, hemangiomas, lymphomas, and pseudotumor cerebri.

If all thyroid function tests are normal, the nonendocrine causes must be considered. For bilateral proptosis, the causes are lithium therapy, hepatic cirrhosis, pseudotumor cerebri, Wegener's granulomatosis, Sjögren's syndrome, arteriovenous malformations, and metastatic tumors from the breast or lung. For unilateral proptosis, primary orbital neoplasm and myositis as well as metastatic disease should be considered.

There is no ideal therapy. Two points, however, are clear. First, hyperthyroidism, if present, should be controlled. Special care should be taken not to overtreat since hypothyroxemia may be associated with worsening of the infiltrative component of the disease. Second, steroids, immunosuppression, or surgical decompression are in order if there is a fixed strabismus and/or optic nerve involvement with decreasing vision. In these patients most authors favor an initial trial with high-dose steroids unless contraindicated. When the disease is less severe, supportive local therapy should not be overlooked since it can be rewarding to the distraught patient. Finally, in choosing the therapy for hyperthyroidism, consideration should be given to the possibility of a significant increase in exophthalmos after partial ablative therapy with radioiodine or subtotal thyroidectomy.

1. Riley, F. C. Orbital pathology in Graves' disease. *Mayo Clin. Proc.* 47:975, 1972.
   Micropolysaccharides, connective tissue, water, mast cells, and lymphocytes are increased.
2. Werner, S. C. Classification of the eye changes of Graves' disease. *J. Clin. Endocrinol. Metab.* 44:203, 1977.
   A useful mneumonic is given.
3. Hamburger, J. I., and Sugar, S. What the internist should know about the ophthalmopathy of Graves' disease. *Arch. Intern. Med.* 129:131, 1972.
   A superb and comprehensive clinical article that should be read by all.
4. Solomon, D. H., Chopra, I. J., Chopra, U., et al. Identification of subgroups of euthyroid Graves' ophthalmopathy. *N. Engl. J. Med.* 296:181, 1977.
   This is probably a heterogeneous group of patients; some had no demonstrable thyroid pathology.
5. Wyse, E. P., McConahey, W. M., Woolner, L. B., et al. Ophthalmopathy without hyperthyroidism in patients with histologic Hashimoto's thyroiditis. *J. Clin. Endocrinol. Metab.* 28:1623, 1968.
   Rarely, chronic lymphocytic thyroiditis may be the only demonstrable thyroid pathology.
6. Hales, I. B., and Rundle, F. F. Ocular changes in Graves' disease. A long-term follow-up study. *Q. J. Med.* 29:113, 1960.
   The long-term prognosis is not good.
7. Rundle, F. F., and Wilson, C. W. Development and course of exophthalmos and ophthalmoplegia in Graves' disease with special reference to the effect of thyroidectomy. *Clin. Sci.* 5:177, 1945.
   Static and dynamic phases occur in the natural history of exophthalmos.
8. Day, R. M., and Carroll, F. D. Optic nerve involvement associated with thyroid dysfunction. *Arch. Ophthalmol.* 67:289, 1962.
   A dreaded complication that can occur with minimal proptosis.
9. Barbosa, J., Wong, E., and Doe, R. P. Ophthalmopathy of Graves' disease: Outcome after treatment with radioactive iodine, surgery, or antithyroid drugs. *Arch. Intern. Med.* 130:111, 1972.
   An appropriate therapeutic caution to be considered before treating patients with toxic diffuse goiter and eye disease.
10. Tmai, H., Nakagawa, T., Ohsako, N., et al. Changes in thyroid functions in patients with euthyroid Graves' disease. *J. Clin. Endocrinol. Metab.* 50:108, 1980.
    The instability and variations in thyroid function tests are emphasized.
11. deJuan, E., Jr., Hurley, D. P., and Sapira, J. D. Racial differences in normal values of proptosis. *Arch. Intern. Med.* 140:1230, 1980.
    They found the upper limits of normal in white females to be 19 mm, for white males 21 mm, for black females 23 mm, and for black males 24 mm. Between eye difference should be at least 2 mm for whites and 3 mm for blacks before diagnosing unilateral exophthalmos.

12. Trokel, S. L., and Hilal. Recognition and differential diagnosis of enlarged extraocular muscles in computed tomography. *Am. J. Ophthalmol.* 87:503, 1979.
    Enlargement is usually Graves' disease but can be seen in arteriovenous malformations, carotid cavernous fistulas, acute orbital myositis, and orbital tumors.
13. Jacobson, D. H., and Gorman, C. A. Endocrine ophthalamopathy: Current ideas concerning etiology, pathogenesis and treatment. *Endocr. Rev.* 5:200, 1984.
    The most comprehensive, well-referenced, current review of the subject.
14. Ahmann, A., Baker, J. R., Weetman, A. P., et al. Antibodies to porcine eye muscle in patients with Graves' ophthalamopathy: Identification of serum immunoglobulins directed against unique determinants by immunoblotting and enzyme-linked immunosorbent assay. *J. Clin. Endocrinol. Metab.* 64:454, 1987.
    Antigenic differences between eye and skeletal muscle may provide the specificity for the eye muscle disease in Graves'.
15. Rotella, C. M., Zonefrati, R., Toccafondi, R., et al. Ability of monoclonal antibodies to the thyrotropin receptor to increase collagen synthesis in human fibroblasts: An assay which appears to measure exophthalmogenic immunoglobins in Graves' sera. *J. Clin. Endocrinol. Metab.* 62:357, 1986.
    More evidence for an autoimmune etiology.
16. Sebastin, P. A. Euthyroid Graves' disease: Report of a case observed over a 12-year period. *Am. J. Med.* 80:1197, 1986.
    An unusual case which clinically supports the distinction between Graves' and euthyroid Graves' ophthalmopathy.
17. Mengistu, M., Laryea, E., Miller, A., et al. Clinical significance of a new autoantibody against a human eye muscle soluble antigen, detected by immunofluorescence. *Clin. Exp. Immunol.* 65:19, 1986.
    A potentially useful clinical marker found in a majority of patients with Graves' and euthyroid Graves' disease.
18. Bahn, R. S., Garrity, J. A., Bartley, G. B., et al. Diagnostic evaluation of Graves' ophthalmopathy. *Endocrinol. Metab. Clin. North Am.* 17:527, 1988.
    A concise review including differential diagnosis.

54. GALACTORRHEA
H. Verdain Barnes

Normally the human female breast does not secrete except in late pregnancy and in the first few weeks post partum or during nursing. At other times breast secretion in the female and in the male at any time is abnormal. Breast secretions may be clear, bloody, or opalescent; only opalescent secretions can properly be called galactorrhea. Unfortunately the character of the discharge does not indicate the underlying cause, although a bloody secretion is more likely to result from an intramammary lesion, of which carcinomas and ductal papillomas are the most common. A wide variety of causes of galactorrhea have been reported and must be considered in the differential diagnosis. They can be categorized as physiologic, intracranial, intramammary, neurothoracic, neuropsychiatric, genital-gonadal, drug-induced, hormon-induced, or idiopathic. In all but the intramammary causes, excess prolactin appears to play a pathogenic role. Prolactin, an anterior pituitary hormone, is heterogeneous in size ranging from the predominant single-chain low-molecular-weight (22,000-dalton) to a high-molecular-weight variant ($\geq$100,000-dalton) protein. Its production and release are controlled by prolactin-inhibiting factor (PIF), a tonic inhibitor secreted from the median eminence of the hypothalamus. When the control system is changed or a tumor produces prolactin, elevated levels of prolactin may be found in the serum and lactation may occur. About 30 to 40 percent of patients with elevated serum prolactin have galactorrhea. The physiologic causes of hyperprolactinemia can be divided into those that typically result in galactorrhea (pregnancy and lactation) and those that do not (sleep, exercise, coitus, stress, and chest wall stimulation).

The intracranial causes of galactorrhea involving the hypothalamic-pituitary area are pituitary tumors producing prolactin alone or in association with Cushing's disease, acromegaly, craniopharyngioma, pineal psammosarcoma, pituitary angiosarcoma, encephalitis, pituitary stalk section, pseudotumor cerebri, basal meningitis, postencephalitis parkinsonism, idiopathic, posttraumatic, or postpartum hypopituitarism, pseudocyesis, empty-sella syndrome, and postpneumoencephalography.

The intramammary causes of breast discharges or (less commonly) galactorrhea can be divided into malignant and benign. The malignant lesions are adenocarcinoma, adenofibrosarcoma, fibrosarcoma, liposarcoma, Paget's disease of the breast, and malignant melanoma. There may or may not be a palpable breast mass at the time of presentation. About 1 to 5 percent of these patients have a discharge. About 10 percent of all patients with benign breast disease have a spontaneous or expressible discharge. The most common lesion is fibrocystic disease, but the lesion most frequently presenting with a discharge is an intraductal papilloma. Other benign breast diseases that may have secretions include papillary cystadenoma, sclerosing adenosis, duct ectasia, galactoceles, fat necrosis, acute mastitis, breast abscess, tuberculosis of the breast, and eczema of the nipple.

The neurothoracic causes of galactorrhea result from a neuroendocrine reflex, which begins with an impulse generated from the breast and nipple. The stimulatory impulse is transmitted via the peripheral nerves of the chest wall to the spinal cord to the hypothalamus. Prolactin is then generated and released. The most common cause is mechanical manipulation of the breast or suckling. Stimulation may also arise from chest wall trauma, thoracoplasty, mastectomy, mammoplasty, burns of the chest wall, herpes zoster, tabes dorsalis, and syringomyelia. The genital-gonadal causes of galactorrhea include partial ovarian resection, corpus luteum cysts, ovarian carcinoma, dermoids, hysterectomy, uterine myomata, menopause, and chorioepithelioma of the testes. Galactorrhea has also been reported in hypothyroidism, hyperthyroidism, Addison's disease, and hypernephroma.

The most common cause of galactorrhea is drug therapy with reserpine, chlorpromazine hydrochloride, trifluoperazine dihydrochloride, prochlorperazine, meprobamate, thioridazine hydrochloride, fluphenazine, imipramine hydrochloride, heroin, α-methyldopa, testosterone, estrogens, progesterones, or combinations of the last two for contraception. The breast discharge usually occurs at higher dose levels and after several months of therapy; however, the breast discharge may appear after the withdrawal of contraceptive therapy and is accompanied by amenorrhea. All these drugs interfere with the hypothalamic-pituitary axis and may result in hyperprolactinemia.

Patients with galactorrhea should have a careful evaluation. Emphasis should be placed on drug, sexual, neurologic, and endocrine aspects of the history. A careful physical examination is mandatory. If the cause is not established, computed tomograms of the head should be performed, the endocrine status evaluated, visual fields examined, and consideration given to discharge cytology and mammography. Determination of prolactin levels by radioimmunoassay is important. Patients with idiopathic galactorrhea have normal prolactin levels.

1. Barnes, A. B. Diagnosis and treatment of abnormal breast secretions. *N. Engl. J. Med.* 275:1184, 1966.
   A superb, general review of breast discharges.
2. Atkins, H., and Wolff, B. Discharges from the nipple. *Br. J. Surg.* 51:602, 1964.
   In this series, 41% had fibroadenomas and 8% had carcinoma of the breast.
3. Hooper, J. H., Jr., Welch, V. C., and Shackelford, R. T. Abnormal lactation associated with tranquilizing drug therapy. *J.A.M.A.* 178:506, 1961.
4. Pettinger, W. A., Horwitz, D., and Sjoerdsma, A. Lactation due to methyldopa. *Br. Med. J.* 1:1460, 1963.
5. Klein, J. J., Segal, R. L., and Warner, R. R. Galactorrhea due to imipramine. *N. Engl. J. Med.* 271:510, 1964.

6. Salkin, D., and Davis, E. W. Lactation following thoracoplasty and pneumonectomy. *J. Thorac. Surg.* 18:580, 1949.

7. Gambrell, R. D., Jr., Greenblatt, R. B., and Mahesh, V. B. Post-pill and pill-related amenorrhea-galactorrhea. *Am. J. Obstet. Gynecol.* 110:838, 1971.

8. Gluskin, L. E., Strasberg, B., and Shah, J. H. Verapamil-induced hyperprolactinemia and galactorrhea. *Ann. Intern. Med.* 95:66, 1981.

9. Boyd, A. E., III, Spare, S., Bower, B., et al. Neurogenic galactorrhea-amenorrhea. *J. Clin. Endocrinol. Metab.* 47:1374, 1978.

10. Dobbs, M. E. Amenorrhea-galactorrhea syndrome caused by a benign pituitary cyst: Case report. *Fertil. Steril.* 33:451, 1980.

11. Gomez, F., DeLaCueva, R., Wanters, J.-P., et al. Endocrine abnormalities in patients undergoing long term hemodialysis. The role of prolactin. *Am. J. Med.* 68:522, 1980.
   Articles 3–11 discuss some causes of hyperprolactinemia and/or galactorrhea.

12. Franks, S., Murray, M. A. F., Jequier, A. M., et al. Incidence and significance of hyperprolactinemia in women with amenorrhea. *Clin. Endocrinol.* 4:597, 1975.
   30–40% of patients with elevated serum prolactin had galactorrhea.

13. Tolis, G., Somma, M., Van Campenhout, J., et al. Prolactin secretion in 65 patients with galactorrhea. *Am. J. Obstet. Gynecol.* 118:91, 1974.
   A wide variety of causes were evaluated. "Idiopathic" patients had normal prolactin levels.

14. Zacur, H. A., Chapanis, N. P., Lake, C. R., et al. Galactorrhea-amenorrhea: Psychological interaction with neuroendocrine function. *Am. J. Obstet. Gynecol.* 125:859, 1976.
   Prolactin declined with psychiatric intervention.

15. Pelosi, M. A., Sarna, J. C., Caterini, H., et al. Galactorrhea-amenorrhea syndrome associated with heroin addiction. *Am. J. Obstet. Gynecol.* 118:966, 1974.
   The syndrome occurred in long-term heroin abusers.

16. Kleinberg, D. L., Noel, G. L., and Frantz, A. G. Galactorrhea: A study of 235 cases, including 48 with pituitary tumors. *N. Engl. J. Med.* 296:589, 1977.
   The largest group were women with idiopathic galactorrhea without amenorrhea, and of these 86% had normal prolactin levels.

17. Turksoy, R. N., Faber, M., and Mitchell, G. W., Jr. Diagnostic and therapeutic modalities in women with galactorrhea. *Obstet. Gynecol.* 56:323, 1980.

18. Speroff, L., Levin, R. M., Haning, R. V., Jr., et al. A practical approach for the evaluation of women with polytomography or elevated prolactin levels. *Am. J. Obstet. Gynecol.* 135:896, 1979.
   An approach to diagnosis.

19. March, C. M., Mishell, D. R., Jr., Keltzky, O. A., et al. Galactorrhea and pituitary tumors in post pill and non-post pill secondary amenorrhea. *Am. J. Obstet. Gynecol.* 134:45, 1979.
   Galactorrhea occurred in 65% of their postpill amenorrhea patients.

20. Schlechte, J., Sherman, B., Halmi, N., et al. Prolactin-secreting pituitary tumors in amenorrheic women: A comprehensive study. *Endocr. Rev.* 1:295, 1980.
   An excellent review including therapy.

21. DeMeirleu, K. L., Baeyens, L., L'Hermite-Baleriaux, M., et al. Exercise-induced prolactin release is related to anaerobiosis. *J. Clin. Endocrinol. Metab.* 60:1250, 1985.
   Sufficient exercise to produce anaerobic metabolism was required to significantly raise the prolactin level.

22. Petraglia, F., DeLeo, V., Nappi, C., et al. Differences in the opioid control of luteinizing hormone secretion between pathological and iatrogenic hyperplactinemic states. *J. Clin. Endocrinol. Metab.* 64:508, 1987.
   Opioid modulation of luteinizing hormone secretion appeared to be related to the cause of hyperprolactinemia.

23. Melmed, S., Braustein, G. D., Change, R. J., et al. Pituitary tumors secreting growth hormone and prolactin. *Ann. Intern. Med.* 105:238, 1986.
   A concise review.

24. Martin, T. L., Kim, M., and Malarkey, W. B. The natural history of idiopathic hyperprolactinemia. *J. Clin. Endocrinol. Metab.* 60:855, 1985.

Idiopathic hyperprolactinemia is a relatively common disorder. On a 5-plus–year follow-up, 34% had a normal prolactin level, 17% an increase, and only 1 of the 41 had a prolactinoma.

25. Jackson, R. D., Wortsman, J., and Malarkey, W. B. Characterization of a large molecular weight prolactin in women with idiopathic hyperprolactinemia and normal menses. *J. Clin. Endocrinol. Metab.* 61:258, 1985.
    "Big prolactin" may not intefere with normal menstruation.
26. Sisam, D. A., Sheehan, J. P., and Schumacher, O. P. Lack of demonstrable tumor growth in progressive hyperprolactinemia. *Am. J. Med.* 80:279, 1986.
    Increasing prolactin levels did not signal tumor growth as is usually the case.
27. Bevan, J. S., Burke, C. W., Esiri, M. M., et al. Misinterpretation of prolactin levels leading to management errors in patients with sellar enlargement. *Am. J. Med.* 82:29, 1987.
    Only serum prolactin levels above 8000 mU/liter signaled a prolactinoma, while at all lower elevations the cause was unpredictable.
28. Jackson, R. D., Wortsman, J., and Malarkey, W. B. Macroprolactinemia presenting like a pituitary tumor. *Am. J. Med.* 78:347, 1985.
    "Big prolactin" may lead to very high levels of prolactin by standard radioimmunoassay.
29. Vance, M. L., and Thorner, M. O. Prolactinomas. *Endocrinol. Metab. Clin. North Am.* 16:731, 1987.
30. Abboud, C. F., and Laws, E. R., Jr. Diagnosis of pituitary tumors. *Endocrinol. Metab. Clin. North Am.* 17:241, 1988.
    Two up-to-date reviews (articles 29, 30).

55. GRAVES' DISEASE
H. Verdain Barnes

Graves' disease (GD) is the most common form of hyperthyroidism in the United States, accounting for about 90 percent of all cases. This autoimmune disease only appears to result in clinical disease in a susceptible host, that is, controlled by two genes of the HLA complex and the immunoglobulin allotype (Gm). Substantial evidence suggests an association in whites with HLA-B8-DR3, with HLA-DRw6 in American blacks, HLA-Bw35 in Japanese, and HLA-Bw46 in Chinese. The primary defect appears to be in suppressor T lymphocyte function which in the thyroid may be due to a decrease in $CD4^+$ $2H4^+$ cells. The result is the production of immunoglobulins against the thyroid-stimulating hormone (TSH) receptor, principally human thyroid-stimulating antibody (TSab), and the production of anti-idiotype antibodies which may modulate the clinical expression of the disease. This results in an excess production and release of thyroxine (T_4) and triiodothyronine (T_3) and clinical thyrotoxicosis.

The incidence of GD in the general population is unknown. The predominance of females over males ranges from 4.4 to 8.1:1. The peak ages of presentation are the third and fourth decades for adults and the adolescent years. The classic clinical presentation offers no problem in diagnosis; however, subtle forms of the disease and/or predominant involvement of a single organ system may initially direct the physician away from the thyroid.

Apathetic hyperthyroidism occurs most often in patients over age 50 years, but on rare occasions is seen in children. The primary presenting features are (1) depression, marked lethargy, or apathy, (2) cardiovascular dysfunction, usually with associated atrial fibrillation, (3) placid apathetic facies, (4) pronounced weakness and weight loss, (5) normal-sized or only modestly enlarged thyroid, and (6) blepharoptosis. The first and second features are typical. The remaining components may occur in varying combinations.

The neuromuscular manifestations may dominate the clinical picture. Thyrotoxic myopathy is proximal in about two-thirds of patients and both proximal and distal in the remainder. The associated weakness is usually disproportionately greater than the observable muscle wasting. The extent of the weakness can vary from annoying to totally incapacitating. The electromyogram reveals a decrease in the duration of motor unit potentials and an increase in polyphasic motor unit potentials. Serum creatinine phosphokinase levels are usually normal or low. Some patients have hypokalemic periodic paralysis characterized by episodic attacks of weakness often brought on by exposure to cold, exercise, high carbohydrate meals, or excess sodium intake. Serum potassium levels fall during attacks but not invariably to levels outside the normal range. In contradistinction to other forms of periodic paralysis, men are more often affected than women and 75 percent of patients reported have been Oriental. Attacks are cured by establishing a euthyroid state. Finally, about 1 percent of patients with GD develop myasthenia gravis.

Cardiovascular system problems may predominate. The most common is an arrhythmia, but occasionally high output heart failure occurs in an otherwise normal heart. The most common arrhythmias are first-degree heart block, atrial fibrillation, and premature ventricular contractions. A rare patient will have complete heart block, Wolff-Parkinson-White syndrome, or paroxysmal ventricular tachycardia. These patients are relatively insensitive to the digitalis glycosides and may become toxic to digitalis before the desired effect is achieved. This insensitivity is multifactorial. Hyperthyroid heart muscle exhibits less enhancement of contractility, and less prolongation of the atrioventricular node refractory period with digitalis. In addition serum levels of digitalis are lower for a given dose due to an increased distribution space for the drug.

GD may present as a primary psychopathy. The most common psychiatric manifestations are hyperactivity, tension, anxiety, and marked emotional lability. Depression may predominate, but agitation and extreme restlessness are more common. Occasional patients have a frank toxic psychosis with visual and auditory hallucinations, disorientation, and confusion. Those patients who develop an overt psychosis almost invariably have an underlying psychiatric condition.

Finally, the presentation may be dominated by an infiltrative ophthalmopathy (see Endocrine Exophthalmos) or thyrotoxic crisis (see Thyroid Storm). Myxedema circumscripta, onycholysis, and acropachy are rare but distinctive features when present.

1. Wall, J. R. (ed.). Autoimmune thyroid disease. *Endocrinol. Metab. Clin. North Am.* 16:229, 1987.
   This entire volume offers an up-to-date, comprehensive discussion of autoimmune thyroid disease.
2. Davis, P. J., and Davis, F. B. Hyperthyroidism in patients over the age of 60 years. *Medicine* 53:161, 1974.
   A careful study of older patients. Anorexia and cardiovascular symptoms are the most common in this age group.
3. Engel, A. G. Thyroid function and periodic paralysis. *Am. J. Med.* 30:327, 1961.
   In 95% of patients the thyrotoxic periodic paralysis is sporadic and cure is obtained by achieving a euthryoid state.
4. Gorman, C. A. Unusual manifestations of Graves' disease. *Mayo Clin. Proc.* 47:926, 1972.
   Pretibial myxedema, onycholysis, acropachy, gynecomastia, vitiligo, osteoporosis, hypercalcemia, anemia, and choreoathetosis are discussed.
5. Verbrycke, J. R., Jr. Masked gastrointestinal hyperthyroidism: Report of 34 cases. *J.A.M.A.* 97:513, 1931.
   Diarrhea, abdominal pain, or nausea and vomiting may dominate the clinical picture.
6. Dunlap, H. F., and Moersch, F. P. Psychic manifestations associated with hyperthyroidism. *Am. J. Psychiatry* 91:1215, 1935.
   A classic worth reading.
7. McNicol, G. P. Thyrotoxicosis associated with pernicious anemia. *Am. J. Med. Sci.* 241:336, 1961.
   The incidence of pernicious anemia is increased in GD.

8. Hollander, C. S., Mitsuma, T., Nehei, N., et al. Clinical and laboratory observations in cases of triiodothyronine toxicosis confirmed by radioimmunoassay. *Lancet* 1:609, 1972.
   About 75% have GD. The free and total serum T_4 levels are normal, and the radioiodine uptake is normal or slightly increased, but nonsuppressible by exogenous T_3.

9. Horvath, F., Jr., Teague, P., Gaffney, E. F., et al. Thyroid antigen associated immune complex glomerulonephritis in Graves' disease. *Am. J. Med.* 67:901, 1979.
   The first reported case.

10. Burman, K. D., and Baker, J. R., Jr. Immune mechanisms in Graves' disease. *Endocr. Rev.* 6:183, 1985.
    A comprehensive well-referenced review.

11. Farid, N. R., and Beau, J. C. The human major histocompatibility complex and endocrine disease. *Endocr. Rev.* 2:50, 1981.

12. Sridama, V., Hara, Y., Faushet, R., et al. HLA immunogenetic heterogeneity in black American patients with Graves' disease. *Arch. Intern. Med.* 147:229, 1987.

13. Tamai, H., Uno, H., Hirota, Y., et al. Immunogenetics of Hashimoto's and Graves' diseases. *J. Clin. Endocrinol. Metab.* 60:62, 1985.
    These articles (11–13) discuss the current immunogenetic foundation of Graves' disease as it relates to the HLA complex.

14. Ishikawa, N., Eguchi, K., Otsubo, T., et al. Reduction in the suppressor-inducer T-cell subset and increase in the helper T cell subset in thyroid tissue from patients with Graves' disease. *J. Clin. Endocrinol. Metab.* 65:17, 1987.
    The decrease in suppressor T cell function may be due to the decrease in CD4$^+$ 2H4$^+$ cells.

15. Ueki, Y., Eguchi, K., Fukuda, T., et al. Dysfunction of suppressor T cells in thyroid glands from patients with Graves' disease. *J. Clin. Endocrinol. Metab.* 65:922, 1987.
    The decreased function of the suppressor T cells may result in an increased production of autoantibodies.

16. Raines, K. B., Baker, J. R., Jr., Lukes, Y. G., et al. Antithyrotropin autoibodies in the sera of Graves' disease patients. *J. Clin. Endocrinol. Metab.* 61:217, 1985.
    Anti-idiotype antibodies may regulate the clinical activity of Graves' disease.

17. Zakarija, M., McKenzie, J. M., and Hoffman, W. H. Prediction and therapy of intrauterine and late-onset neonatal hyperthyroidism. *J. Clin. Endocrinol. Metab.* 62:368, 1986.
    A rare but important form of autoimmune hyperthyroidism.

18. Tibaldi, J. M., Barzel, U. S., Albin, J., et al. Thyrotoxicosis in the very old. *Am. J. Med.* 81:619, 1986.
    Twenty-one cases of GD and only three had a palpable goiter. Often, very subtle clinical manifestations were found.

19. Tamai, H., Hirota, Y., Kasagi, K., et al. The mechanism of spontaneous hypothyroidism in patients with Graves' disease after antithyroid drug treatment. *J. Clin. Endocrinol. Metab.* 64:718, 1987.
    Diffuse focal destructive thyroiditis is a prime mechanism.

20. Garrel, D. R., Delimas, P. D., Malaval, L., et al. Serum bone Gla protein: A marker of bone turnover in hyperthyroidism. *J. Clin. Endocrinol. Metab.* 62:1052, 1986.
    Serum bone Gla protein was distinctly elevated in two-thirds of these patients.

21. Culp, K. S., and Piziak, V. K. Thyrotoxicosis presenting with secretory diarrhea. *Ann. Intern. Med.* 1005:216, 1986.

22. Beard, L., Kumar, A., and Estep, H. L. Bilateral carpal tunnel syndrome caused by Graves' disease. *Arch. Intern. Med.* 145:345, 1985.

23. Tucker, W. S., Jr., Niblack, G. D., McLean, R. H., et al. Serositis with autoimmune endocrinopathy: Clinical and immunogenetic features. *Medicine* 66:138, 1987.
    Some rare presentations of Graves' disease (articles 21–23).

24. Chen, J. J. S., and Lademson, P. W. Discordant hypothyroxemia and hypertriiodothyroninemia in the treated patients with hyperthyroid Graves' disease. *J. Clin. Endocrinol. Metab.* 63:102, 1986.
    Thyroid hormone levels may not correlate with the clinical thyrometabolic status. Beware!

25. Cobb, W. E., Lamberton, R. P., and Jackson, I. M. D. Use of a rapid sensitive immu-

noradiometric assay for thyrotropin to distinguish normal from hyperthyroid subjects. *Clin. Chem.* 30:1558, 1984.
The immunoradiometric TSH assay may now be the test of choice for diagnosis.
26. Morris, J. C., III, Hay, I. D., Nelson, R. E., et al. Clinical utility of thyrotropin-receptor antibody assays: Comparison of radioreceptor and bioassay methods. *Mayo Clin. Proc.* 63:707, 1988.
Both assays are useful in the diagnosis of Graves' disease.

56. HYPERCORTISOLISM (CUSHING'S SYNDROME)
H. Verdain Barnes

Hypercortisolism (Cushing's syndrome) is characterized by glucocorticoid excess. This syndrome can result from an overproduction of adrenocorticotropin (ACTH) by the pituitary (Cushing's disease), an excess central production of corticotropin releasing factor (CRF), an ectopic production of ACTH and/or CRF, an overproduction of cortisol by adrenal adenomas and carcinomas which require no ACTH stimulation, or the cause may be iatrogenic or factitious.

Cushing's disease still accounts for a high percentage of hypercortisolism. The usual lesion is a basophilic adenoma of the anterior pituitary; however, on occasion, it will be a chromophobe adenoma. Pituitary carcinoma is rare. In 80 percent, the adenoma is so small that no visual field defect or abnormality on routine x rays of the sella turcica is seen. These tumors may function autonomously and/or perhaps have an abnormally high set point for cortisol in the negative feedback system. The adrenal responds to excess stimulation with bilateral hyperplasia of the zona fasciculata and reticularis. Females show a 4:1 predominance over males. The clinical features are protean. The most common are weakness (about 90%), thin skin (about 84%), obesity (about 79% are centripetal with moon face, buffalo hump and/or supraclavicular adiposity), easy bruising and hypertension (about 77%), menstrual disorders and hirsutism (about 67%), impotence and striae (about 53%), edema and osteopenia (about 48%), and neuropsychiatric symptoms (31–70%). Proximal myopathy with varying degrees of weakness, as well as glucose intolerance with polyuria, polydipsia, and polyphagia, are common. A wide variety of occasional signs and symptoms have been reported, including painful obesity, acne, poor wound healing, pathologic fractures, renal stones, exophthalmos, insomnia, and galactorrhea. Hypokalemic alkalosis is most common with ectopic ACTH secretion. Leukocytosis with a relative lymphopenia is often present, and occasionally polycythemia or hypercalcemia is found.

The following tumors have been reported to produce a polypeptide similar or identical to pituitary ACTH: small-cell carcinoma of the bronchus, thymoma, islet cell tumors of the pancreas, carcinoid-type bronchial adenoma, hypernephroma, neuroblastoma, craniopharyngioma, seminoma, pheochromocytoma, medullary thyroid carcinoma, and carcinoma of the breast, ovary, colon, prostate, parotid, and esophagus. The most common is oat-cell carcinoma of the lung with ectopic ACTH production, occurring in about 2 percent. Clinically, the ectopic ACTH syndrome often presents with marked hypokalemia alkalosis, muscle wasting and weakness, marked hyperpigmentation, and little else in the way of typical features. Hyperpigmentation is of the type seen in Addison's disease and is due to the production of β-melanocyte-stimulating hormone (β-MSH) by the tumor.

Excess CRF production has been reported in hypothalamic gangliogliomas, prostate cancer, and medullary thyroid carcinoma. Combined ectopic production of ACTH and CRF have been reported with the latter having a paracrine function. The culprit neoplasms include small-cell lung cancer, colon carcinoma, nephroblastoma, medullary thyroid carcinoma, and bronchial carcinoid.

Adrenal adenomas account for about 10 percent of the cases of Cushing's syndrome while adrenal carcinoma is much rarer. Adenomas and carcinomas often present with virilization that is disproportionate to the other signs and symptoms of hypercortisolism. The development of a male hair pattern, acne, seborrhea, and deep voice results from a disproportionate increase in androgen production by these tumors, especially in adrenal carcinoma. The prognosis for adenomas is excellent, whereas male adrenal carcinoma patients rarely survive longer than 28 months and females longer than 45 months. These tumors are found more frequently on the left but may be bilateral. The remaining normal adrenal cortical tissue becomes atrophic. Ectopic adrenal rests, most often superior to the adrenal gland or near the gonads, may rarely produce hypercortisolism.

The patient who is suspected of having hypercortisolism should have a careful assessment. The screening test of choice is a pair of 24-hour urine assays for urinary free cortisol (UFC), which in the absence of renal dysfunction provides screening that is as good as or better than the overnight low-dose dexamethasone suppression test (DST). Euadrenal obese patients, who may have modest elevations of 17-hydroxysteroids and 17-ketosteroids, have normal UFC levels. If the UFC level is suspicious or is clearly elevated, a careful evaluation by other tests will be needed. A high (8-mg) single-dose overnight DST has recently been reported to have a diagnostic accuracy of 93 percent, that is, equally as reliable as the 2-day DST. An ovine CRF stimulation test shows an increase in plasma ACTH and cortisol in over 95 percent of patients with a pituitary adenoma, no increase in an already elevated ACTH and no cortisol response in patients with ectopic ACTH production, and a low or undetectable basal ACTH level with no response to stimulation and no increase in cortisol in patients with an adrenal neoplasm. In addition, an overnight metyrapone suppression test outperforms the old standard high-dose DST. The 8 A.M. 11-deoxycortisol level is typically above 14 μg/dl in Cushing's disease and less than 6 μg/dl in patients with an adrenal neoplasm. Due to the variability in cortisol production and release in Cushing's syndrome, testing for a loss of the normal diurnal variation is no longer recommended. In adrenal carcinoma no response is seen to the 2- or 8-mg DST, metyrapone, or exogenous ACTH. The urinary 17-ketosteroid values, however, are high, frequently exceeding 40 mg/day. The use of simultaneous venous ACTH sampling from the periphery and the inferior petrosal sinus may be the most reliable diagnostic procedure for separating pituitary from ectopic Cushing's. Once the diagnosis of Cushing's is made, radiographic evaluation by computed tomography (CT) should be performed. There are several causes of pseudo- and unintended iatrogenic Cushing's which should be considered in the differential diagnosis. A very rare patient will have an inherited autosomal dominant partial insensitivity to cortisol with an associated increase in cortisol and often adrenal androgen production. A more common problem is in the alcohol abuser whose elevated ACTH and cortisol resolves with alcohol withdrawal. Unintended iatrogenic Cushing's has been reported with dexamethasone therapy using every-3-week high-dose intramuscular injections, skin creams, or nose drops.

Finally, factitious Cushing's has been described in patients taking larger glucocorticoid doses than prescribed as well as a rare patient who surreptitiously takes a glucocorticoid.

1. Cushing, H. The basophil adenomas of the pituitary body and their clinical manifestations. *Bull. Johns Hopkins Hosp.* 1:137, 1932.
   The classic description.
2. Plotz, C. M., Knowlton, A. I., and Ragan, C. The natural history of Cushing's syndrome. *Am. J. Med.* 13:597, 1952.
   An excellent review of the natural history.
3. O'Riordan, J. L., Blanshard, G. P., Moxham, A., et al. Corticotrophin-secreting carcinomas. *Q. J. Med.* 35:137, 1966.
   Severe hypokalemic alkalosis may be the tip-off of ectopic ACTH.
4. Butler, P. W., and Besser, G. M. Pituitary-adrenal function in severe depressive illness. *Lancet* 1:1234, 1968.
   The differential diagnosis may not be easy to make; these patients can have increased cortisol, absent diurnal variation, and nonsuppression with dexamethasone. Features disappear with successful therapy of depression.

5. Howard, J. E., and Migeon, C. J. Cushing's syndrome produced by normal replacement doses of cortisone in a patient with defective mechanism for steroid degradation. *Am. J. Med. Sci.* 235:387, 1958.
   Hypothyroidism is the example. Beware!
6. Hajjar, R. A., Hickey, R. C., and Samaan, N. A. Adrenal cortical carcinoma: Study of 32 patients. *Cancer* 35:549, 1975.
   Prognosis is poor, with 28 months overall survival for men and 45 months for women.
7. Nelson, D. H., Meakin, J. W., and Thorn, G. W. ACTH-producing pituitary tumors following adrenalectomy for Cushing's syndrome. *Ann. Intern. Med.* 52:560, 1960.
   Nelson's syndrome.
8. May, P., Stein, E. J., Ryter, R. J., et al. Cushing's syndrome from percutaneous absorption of triamcinolone cream. *Arch. Intern. Med.* 136:612, 1976.
   Another iatrogenic cause of hypercortisolism.
9. Ganguly, A., Stanchfield, J. B., Roberts, T. S., et al. Cushing's syndrome in a patient with an empty sella turcica and a microadenoma of the adenohypophysis. *Am. J. Med.* 60:306, 1976.
10. Visser, J. W., Boeijinga, J. K., and Meer, C. D. Functioning black adenoma of the adrenal cortex: Clinicopathologic entity. *J. Clin. Pathol.* 27:955, 1974.
    Two (9,10) interesting but rare causes of hypercortisolism.
11. Aron, D. C., Tyrrell, J. B., Fitzgerald, P. A., et al. Cushing's syndrome: Problems in diagnosis. *Medicine* 60:25, 1981.
    Problems in diagnosis are not uncommon; drug interference, obesity, alcoholism, and depression are among those discussed.
12. Zadik, Z., DeLacerda, L., DeCarmargo, L. A. H., et al. A comparative study of urinary 17-hydroxycorticosteroids, urinary free cortisol and the integrated concentration of plasma cortisol. *J. Clin. Endocrinol. Metab.* 51:1099, 1980.
13. Findling, J. W., Aron, D. C., Tyrrell, J. B., et al. Selective venous sampling for ACTH in Cushing's syndrome: Differentiation between Cushing's disease and the ectopic ACTH syndrome. *Ann. Intern. Med.* 94:647, 1981.
    Two (articles 12 and 13) advances in diagnostic testing.
14. Krakoff, L. R., and Elijovich, F. Cushing's syndrome and exogenous glucocorticoid hypertension. *Clin. Endocrinol. Metab.* 10:479, 1981.
    A concise, up-to-date review.
15. Cook, D. M., and Meikle, A. W. Factitious Cushing's syndrome. *J. Clin. Endocrinol. Metab.* 61:385, 1985.
16. Kimmerle, R., and Rlooa, A. R. Iatrogenic Cushing's syndrome due to nasal drops. *Am. J. Med.* 79:535, 1985.
17. Hughes, J. M., Hickens, M., Booze, G. W., et al. Cushing's syndrome from the therapeutic use of intramuscular dexamethasone acetate. *Arch. Intern. Med.* 146:1848, 1986.
18. Kapcala, L. P. Alcohol-induced pseudo-Cushing's syndrome mimicking Cushing's disease in a patient with an adrenal mass. *Am. J. Med.* 82:849, 1987.
19. Lamberts, S. W. J., Poldermans, D., Zweens, M., et al. Familial cortisol resistance: Differential diagnostic and therapeutic aspects. *J. Clin. Endocrinol. Metab.* 63:1328, 1986.
    These entities (15–19) should be considered in the differential diagnosis of Cushing's.
20. Carney, J. A., Gordon, H., Carpenter, P. C., et al. The complex of myxomas, spotty pigmentation and endocrine overactivity. *Medicine* 64:270, 1985.
    Over a quarter of these patients had Cushing's.
21. Findling, J. W., and Tyrrell, J. B. Occult ectopic secretion of corticotropin. *Arch. Intern. Med.* 146:929, 1986.
    Clinically apparent disease followed the establishment of chemical disease by 2 to 12 months.
22. Lenkowski, P., Mendlewicz, J., Kerkhofs, M., et al. 24-hour profiles of adrenocorticotropin, cortisol, and growth hormone in major depressive illness: Effect of antidepressant treatment. *J. Clin. Endocrinol. Metab.* 65:141, 1987.
    The abnormalities found appear to be due to the state of the depression rather than a trait of the depression.

23. Kuchel, O., Bolte, E., Chretien, M., et al. Cyclical edema and hypokalemia due to occult episodic hypercorticism. *J. Clin. Endocrinol. Metab.* 64:170, 1987.
Not all of these women were diuretic users or abusers.

24. Vagnucci, A. H., and Evans, E. Cushing's disease with intermittent hypercortisolism. *Am. J. Med.* 80:83, 1986.
Diagnosis is not always easy.

25. Tyrrell, J. B., Findling, J. W., Aron, D. C., et al. An overnight high-dose dexamethasone suppression test for rapid differential diagnosis of Cushing's syndrome. *Ann. Intern. Med.* 104:180, 1986.
The diagnostic accuracy of this test was 93%.

26. Sindler, B. H., Griffing, G. T., and Melby, J. C. The superiority of the metyrapone test versus the high-dose dexamethasone test in the differential diagnosis of Cushing's syndrome. *Am. J. Med.* 74:657, 1983.
Metyrapone proved more effective than the old standard high-dose DST.

27. Nieman, L. K., Chrousos, G. P., Oldfield, E. H., et al. The ovine corticotropin-releasing hormone stimulation test and the dexamethasone suppression test in the differential diagnosis of Cushing's syndrome. *Ann. Intern. Med.* 105:862, 1986.
Cushing's disease patients (96%) responded to CRF while none of the ectopic ACTH patients did.

28. Guerin, C. K., Wahner, H. W., Gorman, C. A., et al. Computed tomographic scanning versus radioisotope imaging in adrenocortical diagnosis. *Am. J. Med.* 75:653, 1983.
CT is the current imaging test of choice.

29. Howlett, T. A., Raes, L. H., and Besser, G. M. Cushing's syndrome. *Clin. Endocrinol. Metab.* 14:911, 1985.
A comprehensive well-referenced review.

30. Aron, D. C., Findling, J. W., and Tyrrell, J. B. Cushing's disease. *Endocrinol. Metab. Clin.* 16:705, 1987.
A concise review including current therapy.

31. Larsen, J. L., Cathey, W. J., and Odell, W. D. Primary adrenocortical nodular dysplasia, a distinct subtype of Cushing's syndrome: Case report and review of the literature. *Am. J. Med.* 80:976, 1986.
This rare bilateral process can be distinguished from other forms of nodular adrenal disease.

32. Lee, P. D. K., Winter, R. J., and Green, O. C. Virilizing adrenocortical tumors in childhood: Eight cases and a review of the literature. *Pediatrics* 76:437, 1985.
A good review of this problem in the pediatric age group.

33. Melmed, S., and Rushakoff, R. J. Ectopic pituitary and hypothalamic hormone syndromes. *Endocrinol. Metab. Clin.* 16:805, 1987.
A concise, well-referenced, up-to-date discussion.

34. Cauter, E. V., and Refetoff, S. Evidence for two subtypes of Cushing's disease based on the analysis of episodic cortisol secretion. *N. Engl. J. Med.* 312:1343, 1985.
Some appear to depend on CRF and some appear to be independent of CRF.

35. Carpenter, P. C. Diagnostic evaluation of Cushing's syndrome. *Endocrinol. Metab. Clin. North Am.* 17:445, 1988.
A concise review of current methods for diagnosis.

57. HYPERLIPOPROTEINEMIAS

H. Verdain Barnes

The clinical and chemical presentations of the hyperlipoproteinemias are protean. The current nomenclature with which the practicing physician should be familiar are chylomicron-large macromolecular lipid complex (about 90% triglycerides)—formed in the intestine to carry the cholesterol and triglycerides from food; very low-density lipo-proteins (VLDL)—produced by the liver to carry endogenously produced cholesterol and triglycerides; intermediate-density lipoproteins (IDL)—formed by the action of lipoprotein lipase on VLDL molecules (relatively richer in cholesterol than VLDL); low-density lipoproteins (LDL)—formed by the further hydrolysis of IDL; and high-density lipoproteins (HDL)—formed in the intestine and liver where cholesterol, cholesterol ester, phospholipids, apoproteins, and some triglycerides are transferred to HDL during lipolysis of the larger lipoproteins. IDL contains two apoproteins, E and B-100, and LDL contains only B-100. These apoproteins are critical in the removal of LDL and IDL from the blood. LDL carries about 65 percent of the cholesterol present in blood and when elevated appears to produce the greatest risk factor for human atherosclerotic vascular disease, whereas high HDL levels appear to provide some protective effect. The Frederickson system of classification defines the various phenotypes for these disorders.[1]

Type I, familial hyperchylomicronemia, is typically juvenile in onset and may be associated with abdominal pain, hepatosplenomegaly, and eruptive xanthomas. The etiology is due to an absence of lipoprotein lipase and its apoprotein activator C-II. The result is a marked elevation in triglycerides, elevated chylomicrons, and a normal cholesterol. Some of the known secondary causes include uncontrolled insulin-dependent diabetes mellitus, systemic lupus erythematosus, lymphoma, and dysglobulinemia.

Type II has two subtypes, a and b, which also have subsets. Type IIa has a homozygous and heterozygous familial subset, that is, familial hypercholesterolemia, a familial combined subset and a polygenetic subset of which the latter is by far the most common hyperlipoproteinemia (85–90%). In each the onset can occur at virtually any age, and there may be associated planar, tendinous, or tuberous xanthomas in both the familial and combined subsets. Relatives are commonly affected in each subset. There is a relative increase in severity as well as an earlier age of onset of clinical atherosclerotic vascular disease. In each there is an elevation in LDL and cholesterol with normal triglycerides.

The type IIb subtype has two subsets, familial hypercholesterolemia and familial combined hyperlipidemia, in which there is an elevation in LDL, VLDL, cholesterol, and triglycerides. The onset in each is typically in adult life with an accompanying relative increase in severity as well as an earlier onset of atherosclerosis. Some documented secondary causes of type IIa include the nephrotic syndrome, hypothyroidism, and acute intermittent porphyria, and of type IIb, obstructive liver disease and multiple myeloma as well as porphyria.

Type III, familial dysbetalipoproteinemia, is typically adult in onset with an increase in atherosclerotic vascular disease and tuberoeruptive and/or palmar xanthomas. In these patients there is an increase in IDL, cholesterol, and triglycerides with a normal LDL. The pathophysiology relates to a deficiency or absence in apoprotein E-III. Some of the known secondary causes of type III are dysgammaglobulinemia and hypothyroidism.

Type IV disease is relatively common and includes two subsets: familial triglyceridemia and familial combined hyperlipidemia. The onset is typically in adult life and may be associated with hyperglycemia, hyperuricemia, obesity, and hypertension. Blood lipids include elevated VLDL and triglyceride levels with a normal cholesterol. A variety of secondary causes have been reported ranging from diabetes mellitus (types I and II) to estrogen therapy to alcoholism to Niemann-Pick disease.

Type V disease also includes two subsets: familial type V and familial hypertriglyceridemia. The clinical features include an adult onset, abdominal pain with or without pancreatitis, eruptive xanthomas, lipemia retinalis, obesity, and diabetes mellitus. In these patients the triglyceride level is markedly elevated in association with increased levels of chylomicrons, cholesterol, and VLDL with a decrease in LDL. The secondary causes are multiple ranging from insulin-dependent diabetes mellitus to multiple myeloma to nephrotic syndrome to alcohol abuse.

The typical laboratory directly measures serum cholesterol, HDL, and triglyceride levels in a lipoprotein profile and calculates the VLDL and LDL. HDL can be determined by several methods, but those that do not precipitate out all other lipoproteins before the assay are generally inaccurate. The prediction of risk for coronary atherosclerosis is complex with no universally agreed upon method. In some studies, the HDL–total cholesterol ratio, an HDL percent of total cholesterol less than 22 percent, and plasma apoprotein A-I and A-II levels, have proved to be the most accurate predictors. Current relative degrees of risk for cholesterol alone are low risk (cholesterol < 200 mg/dl), intermediate risk (cholesterol levels 200–239 mg/dl), and high risk (≥ 240 mg/dl) (National Cholesterol Education Program Guidelines).

1. Fredrickson, D. S., Levy, R. I., and Lees, R. S. Fat transport in lipoproteins: An integrated approach to mechanisms and disorders. *N. Engl. J. Med.* 276:32, 94, 148, 215, 273, 1967.
   This classic series of articles provides a basic classification of the hyperlipoproteinemias.
2. Motulsky, A. G. The genetic hyperlipidemias. *N. Engl. J. Med.* 294:823, 1976.
   The current categorization of the genetic hyperlipidemias. A concise review.
3. Cameron, J. L., Crisler, C., Margolis, S., et al. Acute pancreatitis with hyperlipemia. *Surgery* 70:53, 1971.
   Serum amylase may not be increased in the presence of acute pancreatitis. It was not in 14 of 19 patients in this series.
4. Stone, N. J., Levy, R. I., Fredrickson, D. S., et al. Coronary artery disease in 116 kindred with familial type II hyperlipoproteinemia. *Circulation* 94:476, 1974.
   There was a clearly increased incidence of coronary artery disease in this well-studied kindred.
5. Swanson, J. O., Pierpont, G., and Adicoff, A. Serum high density lipoprotein cholesterol correlates with presence but not severity of coronary artery disease. *Am. J. Med.* 71:235, 1981.
6. Gordon, T., Castelli, W. P., Hjortland, M. C., et al. High-density lipoprotein as a protective factor against coronary heart disease: The Framingham study. *Am. J. Med.* 62:707, 1977.
   Low HDL levels seem to have a strong correlation with coronary artery disease and perhaps high levels a negative correlation (articles 5, 6).
7. Hazzard, W. R., O'Donnell, T. F., and Lee, Y. L. Broad-beta disease (type III hyperlipoproteinemia) in a large kindred. *Ann. Intern. Med.* 82:141, 1975.
8. Fredrickson, D. S., Morganroth, J., and Levy, R. I. Type III hyperlipoproteinemia: An analysis of two contemporary definitions. *Ann. Intern. Med.* 82:150, 1975.
9. Morganroth, J., Levy, R. I., and Fredrickson, D. S. The biochemical, clinical, and genetic features of type III hyperlipoproteinemia. *Ann. Intern. Med.* 82:158, 1975.
   Articles 7–9 define type III disease.
10. Carlson, L. A., and Bottiger, L. E. Ischaemic heart disease in relation to fasting values of plasma triglycerides and cholesterol. *Lancet* 1:865, 1972.
    In a 9-year follow-up study of a large general population, elevated fasting triglycerides proved to be as great a risk factor in ischemic heart disease as hypercholesterolemia.
11. Falsetti, H. L., Schnatz, J. D., Green, D. G., et al. Serum lipids and glucose tolerance in angiographically proven coronary artery disease. *Chest* 58:111, 1970.
    In this series 27% of patients had type IV disease.
12. Blacket, R. B., Woodhill, J. M., Leelarthaepin, B., et al. Type IV hyperlipidemia and weight gain after maturity. *Lancet* 2:517, 1975.
    Maturity-onset weight gain is associated with an increased frequency of type IV disease.
13. Buckingham, R. B., Bole, G. G., and Bassett, D. R. Polyarthritis associated with type IV hyperlipoproteinemia. *Arch. Intern. Med.* 135:286, 1975.
    A new asymmetric, oligoarticular arthritis is reported.
14. Wiedeman, E., Rose, H. G., and Schwartz, E. Plasma lipoproteins, glucose tolerance and insulin response in primary gout. *Am. J. Med.* 53:299, 1972.
    A direct relationship is proposed between primary gout and type IV disease.
15. Schaefer, E. I., and Levy, R. I. Pathogenesis and management of lipoprotein disorders. *N. Engl. J. Med.* 312:1300, 1985.
    A concise well-referenced up-to-date review.

16. Brown, M. S., and Goldstein, J. L. A receptor-mediated pathway for cholesterol ho-
    meostasis. *Science* 232:34, 1986.
    *LDL is removed by a receptor-mediated system which recognizes apoprotein B-100 or
    E.*
17. Concensus Conference: Lowering blood cholesterol to prevent heart disease. *J.A.M.A.*
    253:2080, 1985.
    *Patients with cholesterol values equal to or greater than 240 mg/dl are considered at
    high risk for coronary artery disease.*
18. Levy, R. I., Brensike, J. F., Epstein, S. E., et al. The influence of changes in lipid
    values induced by cholestyramine and diet on progression of coronary artery disease:
    Results of the NHLBI type II coronary intervention study. *Circulation* 69:325, 1984.
19. Arntzenius, A. C., Kromhout, D., Barth, J. D., et al. Diet, lipoproteins and the pro-
    gression of coronary atherosclerosis: The Leiden intervention trial. *N. Engl. J. Med.*
    312:805, 1985.
    *HDL–total cholesterol ratio was the best predictor of disease progression (articles 18,
    19).*
20. Anderson, K. M., Castelli, W. P., and Levy, D. Cholesterol and mortality: 30 years of
    follow-up from the Framingham study. *J.A.M.A.* 257:2176, 1987.
    *HDL percent of total cholesterol appeared to be an effective predictor of the risk for
    coronary artery disease.*
21. Freedman, D. S., Srinivasan, S. R., Shear, C. L., et al. The relation of apolipoproteins
    A-I and B in children to parental myocardial infarction. *N. Engl. J. Med.* 315:721,
    1986.
22. Kattke, B. A., Zinsmeister, A. R., Holmes, D. R., Jr., et al. Apolipoproteins and cor-
    onary artery disease. *Mayo Clin. Proc.* 61:313, 1986.
    *The apoproteins A-I, A-II, and B may be among the most sensitive indicators of cor-
    onary artery disease (articles 21, 22).*
23. Lipid Research Clinics Program: The lipid research clinics coronary primary preven-
    tion trial results. 1. Reduction in incidence of coronary heart disease. *J.A.M.A.*
    251:351, 1984.
    *Lowering LDL appears to reduce coronary artery disease mortality and morbidity in
    high-risk men.*
24. McManus, B. M. Reference ranges and ideal patient values for blood cholesterol: Can
    there be reconciliation? *Arch. Pathol. Lab. Med.* 110:469, 1986.
    A potentially useful algorithm for assessing coronary artery disease risk is detailed.
25. Knopp, R. H., Walden, C. E., Heiss, G., et al. Prevalence and clinical correlates of
    beta-migrating very-low-density lipoprotein: Lipid research clinics program preva-
    lence study. *Am. J. Med.* 81:493, 1986.
    The vast majority (93%) with beta-VLDL had some type of lipoprotein abnormality.
26. Bergman, M., Gidez, L. I., and Eder, H. A. High-density lipoprotein subclasses in
    diabetes. *Am. J. Med.* 81:488, 1986.
    The change is primarily in subclass 2.
27. Brewer H. B., Zech, L. A., Gregg, R. E., et al. Type III hyperlipoproteinemia: Diag-
    nosis, molecular defects, pathology and treatment. *Ann. Intern. Med.* 98:623, 1983.
    *Three defects predispose to type III disease: deficient apolipoprotein E, structural
    defect in E, or liver receptor defect.*
28. Taylor, W. C., Pass, T. M., Shepard, D. S., et al. Cholesterol reduction and life expec-
    tancy: A model incorporating multiple risk factors. *Ann. Intern. Med.* 106:605, 1987.
    *This model calculates the increase in life expectancy in high-risk patients on dietary
    therapy (range 18 days–1 year).*
29. Graber, M. L., Quigg, R. J., Stempsey, W. E., et al. Spurious hyperchloremia and
    decreased anion gap in hyperlipidemia. *Ann. Intern. Med.* 98:607, 1983.
    Worth noting along with pseudohyponatremia.
30. Peters, W. L., and Goroll, A. H. The evaluation and treatment of hypercholesterol-
    emia in primary care practice. *J. Gen. Intern. Med.* 1:183, 1986.
31. Gotto, A. M., Jr. Cholesterol: New approaches to screening, management. *Diagnosis*
    10:40, 1988.
    Two concise up-to-date reviews.

32. Grundy, S. M. HMG-CoA reductase inhibitors for treatment of hypercholesterolemia. *N. Engl. J. Med.* 319:24, 1988.
   A new class of drugs for treating hypercholesterolemia; the initial results are promising.
33. Gotto, A. M., Jr., Jones, P. H., and Scott, L. W. The diagnosis and management of hyperlipidemia. D.M., 1986.
   This monograph provides a detailed and comprehensive review of the hyperlipidemias.

58. HYPERTHYROIDISM
H. Verdain Barnes

An excess in circulating thyroid hormone may occur under a variety of circumstances. Graves' disease is clearly the most common (see Chapter 55). Next in frequency is toxic nodular goiter, which may be either multinodular (Plummer's disease) or uninodular. The more unusual causes of hyperthyroidism include jodbasedow, autonomous thyroid-stimulating hormone production by a pituitary tumor, toxic struma ovarii, thyrotoxicosis factitia, functional metastatic thyroid carcinoma, hyperthyroidism due to acute or chronic thyroiditis, tumors producing a thyroid-stimulating substance, and thyrotropin induced due to selective pituitary resistance to thyroid hormone. In general, both the serum thyroxine (T_4) and triiodothyronine (T_3) are elevated. However, in recent years, it has been recognized that a small number of hyperthyroid patients may in the course of their disease have only an elevated serum level of T_3 (T_3 toxicosis) or T_4 (T_4 toxicosis). To document hyperthyroidism in the presence of an excess of only T_3 or T_4, thyroid gland autonomy and/or hypothalamic-pituitary nonresponsiveness must be abnormal on a T_3 suppression test and/or thyrotropin releasing hormone (TRH) stimulation test. T_3 toxicosis is more likely to occur in patients with relative or absolute iodine deficiency while T_4 toxicosis is most likely in those who are elderly or those with severe acute or chronic nonthyroid disease or iodine excess.

Toxic nodular goiter differs from Graves' disease in several respects. It is less common, occurs primarily in the 40- to 65-year age group, and is only rarely if ever associated with infiltrative ophthalmopathy, localized myxedema, onycholysis, or a thyroid bruit. Toxic nodular goiter frequently arises insidiously in a long-standing nontoxic nodular goiter. Estimates of the incidence of hyperthyroidism in nontoxic nodular goiter range from 5 to 13 percent. The signs and symptoms of hypermetabolism are often predominantly cardiovascular. Heart failure and atrial arrhythmias in the older population should routinely raise the suspicion of hyperthyroidism. Nervousness and excitability occur in about 70 percent, palpitations in 55 percent, heat intolerance in 40 percent, and weight loss in 25 percent. Some present with the typical features of apathetic thyrotoxicosis. The incidence of a toxic adenoma in patients with toxic nodular goiter is about 4 percent. The diagnosis of toxic nodular goiter requires an abnormal thyroid scan as well as an elevated serum T_4 and/or T_3. The scan should show an area or areas of increased uptake that are not suppressible by the conventional T_3 suppression test. Jodbasedow is hyperthyroidism induced by an exogenous iodide load. Typically these patients live in an area of iodine deficiency, have long-standing multinodular goiters, and become thyrotoxic after therapy with large doses of iodide. Other cases, however, have been reported in patients from areas not deficient in iodine and some occur after therapy with small doses of iodide. The serum T_4 and/or T_3 is typically elevated and the radioiodine uptake (RAIU) is usually normal or low, depending on the dose of exogenous iodide.

Autonomous production of thyroid-stimulating hormone (TSH) by a pituitary tumor is rare. Serum T_4 and/or T_3, RAIU, and radioimmunoassayable TSH are elevated. Excess TSH may also be the underlying cause of hyperthyroidism in acromegaly. Hyperthyroidism occurs in 4 to 32 percent of patients with struma ovarii. A palpable ovarian mass is almost invariably found, and about two-thirds of patients also have an enlarged thyroid. The tumor is malignant in about 20 percent. These patients typically have an elevated T_4 and/or T_3 with a normal, low, or no radioiodine thyroid uptake in the neck. Radioiodine scanning of the pelvis usually shows an area of increased uptake. Thyrotoxicosis factitia can be self-induced or iatrogenic. When the offending drug is pure T_4 or combination T_4 and T_3, the serum T_4 and T_3 levels are elevated. On the other hand, if pure T_3 is taken, the serum T_4 will be low and only the T_3 will be elevated. The RAIU is low or absent due to suppression by the excess thyroid hormone. An accelerated rate of turnover of labeled T_4 in the presence of an elevated serum T_4, a low protein-bound iodine 131, and a normal response to TSH stimulation may help confirm the diagnosis when it is not evident from the history. To be ruled out when hyperthyroidism is seen with a low RAIU are struma ovarii, acute nonsuppurative thyroiditis, and jodbasedow. On rare occasions thyrotoxicosis can arise from functional metastatic follicular thyroid carcinoma. Functional metastatic foci can usually be demonstrated by radioiodine scanning.

Acute nonsuppurative thyroiditis and chronic lymphocytic thyroiditis can have associated hyperthyroidism (see chapter on thyroiditis). A variety of autoimmune diseases have been associated with thyrotoxicosis including idiopathic adrenal insufficiency, systemic lupus erythematosus, pernicious anemia, and myasthenia gravis. Other diseases include sarcoidosis and Albright's syndrome.

Finally, choriocarcinoma, embryonal cell carcinoma of the testes, and hydatidiform mole may produce a TSH-like substance that occasionally produces hyperthyroidism. The distinctive feature in these patients is an excess of a biologically active TSH in the serum and tumor that is not measured using the human TSH radioimmunoassay. Hyperthyroidism typically disappears within about 6 weeks after a successful removal of the tumor.

1. Plummer, H. S. Function of the thyroid gland containing adenomatous tissue. *Trans. Assoc. Am. Physicians* 43:159, 1928.
   A classic article.
2. Ferriman, D., Hennebry, T. M., and Tassopoulos, C. N. True thyroid adenoma. *Q. J. Med.* 41:127, 1972.
   438 consecutive patients with goiters were analyzed, and overt hyperthyroidism occurred in about 5%. Clinical characteristics and diagnosis are discussed.
3. Morton, W. M., and Runyan, J. W., Jr. The hyperfunctioning thyroid nodule. *South. Med. J.* 62:1036, 1969.
   Exophthalmos, localized myxedema, onycholysis, and thyroid bruit rarely if ever occur in nodular toxic goiter.
4. Hamilton, C. R., Jr., and Maloof, F. Unusual types of hyperthyroidism. *Medicine* 52:195, 1973.
   A careful, well-referenced review.
5. Hamilton, C. R., Jr., and Maloof, F. Acromegaly and toxic goiter. *J. Clin. Endocrinol. Metab.* 35:659, 1972.
   Excess TSH may well be the cause in these patients.
6. Vagenakis, A. G., Maloof, F., Wang, C. A., et al. Iodide-induced hyperthyroidism in Boston. *N. Engl. J. Med.* 287:523, 1972.
   Four of 8 goiter patients prospectively treated with iodide developed thyrotoxicosis.
7. Kempers, R. D., Dockerty, M. B., Hoffman, D. L., et al. Struma ovarii ascitic, hyperthyroid, and asymptomatic syndromes. *Ann. Intern. Med.* 72:883, 1970.
   Eight of 25 had hyperthyroidism, and 5 of 8 had an associated goiter.
8. Gorman, C. A., Wahner, H. W., and Tauxe, W. N. Metabolic malingerers: Patients who deliberately induce or perpetuate a hypermetabolic or hypometabolic state. *Am. J. Med.* 48:708, 1970.
   Thyroid radioiodine uptake is low or absent and the gland responds normally to TSH.
9. Cohen, J. D., and Utiger, R. D. Metastatic choriocarcinoma associated with hyperthyroidism. *J. Clin. Endocrinol. Metab.* 30:423, 1970.
10. Higgins, H. P., Hershman, J. M., Kenimer, J. G., et al. The thyrotoxicosis of hydatidiform mole. *Ann. Intern. Med.* 83:307, 1975.
11. Steigbigel, N. H., Oppeheim, J. J., Fishman, L. M., et al. Metastatic embryonal car-

cinoma of the testes associated with elevated TSH-like activity and hyperthyroidism. *N. Engl. J. Med.* 271:345, 1964.
The TSH-like substance in all three instances (9–11) is biologically active but not immunoreactive to human TSH.

12. Sterling, K., Refetoff, S., and Selenkow, H. A. T3-thyrotoxicosis. *J.A.M.A.* 213:571, 1970.
Isolated T_3 elevations can be seen in toxic diffuse and nodular goiter.

13. Miller, J. M., and Block, M. A. Functional autonomy in multinodular goiter. *J.A.M.A.* 214:535, 1970.
Three apparent stages in the development of hyperthyroidism in multinodular goiter.

14. Marsden, P., and McKerron, C. G. Serum triiodothyronine concentration in diagnosis of hyperthyroidism. *Clin. Endocrinol.* 4:189, 1975.
With a good immunoassay, total T_3 is a must test.

15. Kenimer, J. G., Hershman, J. M., and Higgins, P. M. Thyrotropin in hydatidiform moles is human chorionic gonadotropin. *J. Clin. Endocrinol. Metab.* 40:482, 1975.
The human chorionic gonadotropin levels in molar pregnancy are apparently high enough to produce hyperthyroidism.

16. Hamburger, J. I. Evolution of toxicity in solitary nontoxic autonomously functioning thyroid nodules. *J. Clin. Endocrinol. Metab.* 50:1089, 1980.
Toxicity developed in 14 of 159 (8.8%) untreated patients during a 1- to 6-year follow-up with a 20% chance of becoming toxic if the nodule was ≥ 3 cm in diameter.

17. Sobrinko, L. G., Limbert, E. S., and Santos, M. A. Thyroxine toxicosis in patients with iodine induced thyrotoxicosis. *J. Clin. Endocrinol. Metab.* 45:25, 1977.
T_4 toxicosis was more likely to occur in those patients with iodine excess.

18. Woolf, P. D. Transient painless thyroiditis with hyperthyroidism: A variant of lymphocytic thyroiditis? *Endocr. Rev.* 1:411, 1980.
This type of hyperthyroidism is being increasingly recognized and must be included in the differential diagnosis.

19. Weintraub, B. D., Gershengorn, M. C., Kourides, I. A., et al. Inappropriate secretion of thyroid-stimulating hormone. *Ann. Intern. Med.* 95:339, 1981.
An excellent discussion. Some hyperthyroid patients have tumors of the pituitary thyrotropic cells or some degree of pituitary and peripheral resistance to thyroid hormone action.

20. Grubeck-Lobenstein, B., Derfler, K., Kassol, H., et al. Immunological features of non-immunogenic hyperthyroidism. *J. Clin. Endocrinol. Metab.* 60:150, 1985.
DR^+-T lymphocyte infiltration of the thyroid gland of patients with toxic nodular goiter (solitary) was found.

21. Kraiem, Z., Glaser, B., Yigla, M., et al. Toxic multinodular goiter: A variant of autoimmune hyperthyroidism. *J. Clin. Endocrinol. Metab.* 65:659, 1987.
Two subgroups were identified: one with evidence for an autoimmune process and the other without, potential Graves' disease and toxic adenoma variants, respectively.

22. Lukert, B. P., Higgins, J. A., and Stroskoff, M. M. Serum osteocalcin is increased in patients with hyperthyroidism and decreased in patients receiving glucocorticoids. *J. Clin. Endocrinol. Metab.* 62:1056, 1986.

23. Toh, S. H., Claunch, B. C., and Brown, P. H. Effect of hyperthyroidism and its treatment on bone mineral content. *Arch. Intern. Med.* 145:883, 1985.
Bone demineralization is seen in thyrotoxicosis (articles 22, 23).

24. Blank, M. S., and Tucci, J. R. A case of thyroxine thyrotoxicosis. *Arch. Intern. Med.* 147:863, 1987.
Seen in a 57-year-old patient with no predisposing factors.

25. Cogan, E., and Abramows, M. Transient hyperthyroxemia in symptomatic hyponatremic patients. *Arch. Intern. Med.* 146:545, 1986.
Beware. Interpret initial T_4 values in these patients with caution.

26. Ross, D. S., Neer, R. M., Ridgeway, E. C., et al. Subclinical hyperthyroidism and reduced bone density as a possible result of prolonged suppression of the pituitary-thyroid axis with L thyroxine. *Am. J. Med.* 83:1167, 1987.
Look for more information in this area; patients should probably receive the lowest dose needed for an effective clinical response.

59. HYPERURICEMIA
H. Verdain Barnes

Hyperuricemia is a biochemical abnormality that is being recognized more often since the advent of multichannel analyzers. In adolescents and adults, uric acid levels are generally lower in women than in men. If an accurate enzymatic spectrophotometric method is used, the normal range is 6.9 to 7.5 mg/dl for men and 5.7 to 6.6 mg/dl for women. Elevated levels of uric acid may occur as a result of increased production or decreased renal clearance.

Primary idiopathic hyperuricemia is a polygenetic disorder of unexplained pathogenesis. Two groups can be defined. Seventy to 80 percent are overproducers and/or underexcretors of uric acid. The 24-hour urinary excretion is normal if less than 600 mg/day on a low purine diet. Several specific enzyme defects in purine metabolism result in overproduction. The most common is glucose-6-phosphatase deficiency in type I glycogen storage disease (von Gierke's disease). In this disorder, there is both overproduction and underexcretion of uric acid. Inheritance is autosomal recessive. Less common varieties of excess production are (1) hypoxanthine guanine phosphoribosyltransferase deficiency (Lesch-Nyhan syndrome), (2) glutathione reductase variant with increased enzyme activity, and (3) glutamine–phosphoribosylpyrophosphate amidotransferase feedback resistance. For these three varieties, inheritance is X-linked, autosomal recessive, and unknown, respectively. Secondary causes of excess uric acid production may arise from increased de novo synthesis or from increased nucleic acid turnover. The former cause is rare but may be seen with excess fructose or 2-ethylamino-1,3,4,-thiadiazole intake. Increased nucleic acid turnover, however, is commonly encountered in myeloproliferative and lymphoproliferative disorders, infectious mononucleosis, chronic hemolytic anemias, multiple myeloma, secondary polycythemia, pernicious anemia, psoriasis, and after tumor therapy with drugs or radiation.

Decreased renal excretion of uric acid can result in hyperuricemia. This occurs by a variety of mechanisms: (1) reduced functional renal mass, as in chronic renal disease; (2) decreased renal perfusion, as in hypothyroidism and hypoadrenocorticism; (3) decreased tubular secretion of uric acid in (a) lactic acidemic states, such as acute alcoholism, toxemia of pregnancy, sarcoidosis, and chronic beryllium intoxication, (b) β-hydroxybutyrate and acetoacetate acidemia, such as diabetic ketoacidosis and starvation, (c) drug therapy with pyrazinamide and low-dose salicylates, or (d) lead poisoning, and (4) increased tubular reabsorption of uric acid, such as that associated with diuretic therapy, particularly the thiazides and their derivatives, and in conditions such as the hepatorenal syndrome. Hyperuricemia is also commonly seen in obesity, hyperlipoproteinemia types III, IV, and V, Down's syndrome, primary hyperparathyroidism, plus essential and renovascular hypertension.

The most striking complication of hyperuricemia is gouty arthritis. Primary gouty arthritis occurs mainly in men, with postmenopausal women accounting for only 3 to 7 percent in most series. In males, the incidence typically correlates with serum uric acid levels: 0.6 percent incidence when serum uric acid levels are less than 6 mg/dl, 1.9 percent with 6.0 to 6.9 mg/dl, 16.7 percent with 7.0 to 7.9 mg/dl, 25 percent with 8.0 to 8.9 mg/dl, and 90 percent with 9.0 mg/dl or more. In the two most common forms of secondary hyperuricemia, namely, chronic renal disease and hematologic disorders, the incidence of gouty arthritis is 0.4 and 5.0 percent, respectively.

The other complication of note is nephrolithiasis. In patients with gouty arthritis, about 22 percent with primary and 4.2 percent with secondary hyperuricemia have a stone history. In about 40 percent, urolithiasis precedes gouty arthritis by months or years. The pathophysiologic conditions required for uric acid stone formation appear to be an increased urine uric acid concentration and a persistently acid urine. It should be recognized, however, that uric acid kidney stones can occur in the absence of hyperuricemia. The two most common situations are idiopathic and after ileostomy or small bowel bypass surgery.

The discovery of asymptomatic hyperuricemia by multichannel testing must be viewed with skepticism until proved by a more reliable method. Current evidence suggests that long-standing asymptomatic hyperuricemia does not produce clinically significant azotemia, even after 40 years, unless the levels are persistently over 10 mg/dl in women and 13 mg/dl in men. Nephrolithiasis appears to also be uncommon, occurring in about one out of every 295 asymptomatic hyperuricemic patients per year. Consequently, therapy with allopurinol should probably be reserved for patients who have had a stone, tophaceous gout, gouty arthritis, gouty nephropathy, or asymptomatic patients excreting 1100 mg of uric acid or more in the urine each day.

1. Paulus, H. E., Coutts, A., Calabro, J. J., et al. Clinical significance of hyperuricemia in routinely screened hospital men. *J.A.M.A.* 211:277, 1970.
   13.2% of patients had elevated uric acid levels and of these 70% were secondary.
2. Talbott, J. H. Gout and blood dyscrasias. *Medicine* 38:173, 1959.
   Still a good review.
3. Lynch, E. C. Uric acid metabolism in proliferative diseases of the marrow. *Arch. Intern. Med.* 109:639, 1962.
   Here males and females are equal in incidence: 5% developed gouty arthritis.
4. Barlow, K. A. Hyperlipidemia in primary gout. *Metabolism* 17:289, 1968.
   Hypertriglyceridemia is common.
5. Demartini, F. E., Wheaton, E. A., Healey, L. A., et al. Effect of chlorothiazide on the renal excretion of uric acid. *Am. J. Med.* 32:572, 1962.
   75% of patients on diuretics substantially increase their uric acid levels.
6. Yu, T., and Gutman, A. B. Uric acid nephrolithiasis in gout-predisposing factors. *Ann. Intern. Med.* 67:1133, 1967.
   22% of primary gout patients and 42% of the secondary hyperuricemia patients had urolithiasis.
7. Hall, A. P., Barry, P. E., Dawber, T. R., et al. Epidemiology of gout and hyperuricemia. *Am. J. Med.* 42:27, 1967.
   90% of the males with serum uric acids above 9 mg/dl develop gouty arthritis.
8. Smyth, C. J. Disorders associated with hyperuricemia. *Arthritis Rheum.* 18:713, 1975.
   An excellent review and a listing of 39 causes of secondary hyperuricemia.
9. Fessel, W. J. Renal outcomes of gout and hyperuricemia. *Am. J. Med.* 67:74, 1979.
   No asymptomatic hyperuricemic patient developed azotemia and only 1 out of 295 developed a uric acid renal stone each year.
10. Kelley, W. N. Approach to the Patient with Hyperuricemia. In W. N. Kelley, et al. (eds.), *Textbook of Rheumatology.* Philadelphia: W. B. Saunders Co., 1985. P. 489.
    A comprehensive discussion and review.
11. Dykman, D., Simon, E. E., and Avioli, L. V. (eds). Hyperuricemia and uric acid nephropathy. *Arch. Intern. Med.* 147:1341, 1987.
    A concise review and a therapy algorithm for primary hyperuricemia.

60. HYPOADRENOCORTISOLISM (ADDISON'S DISEASE)
H. Verdain Barnes

Adrenal corticol insufficiency may result from adrenal failure (primary), hypothalamic or pituitary failure (secondary). Varying degrees of hypoadrenalism may occur; consequently, the disease should not be considered an all-or-none phenomenon. The earliest manifestation may be nothing more than an increasing severity of minor illness, such as excessive fever or a prolonged duration of the common cold. Other early general signs and symptoms may include increased fatigue, anorexia, recurrent nausea with or without vomiting, constipation often alternating with diarrhea, intermittent abdominal pain, weight loss, malaise, irritability, sleeplessness, orthostatic dizziness, and varying degrees of weakness. As the disease progresses, these manifestations become more pronounced and episodes of syncope, hypotension, and hypoglycemia develop.

The causes of primary adrenal insufficiency are autoimmune, infectious, congenital, chemical, ischemic, hemorrhagic, or infiltrative. In most current series the autoimmune variety accounts for approximately 75 percent. Histologically, there is a loss of the usual three-layered structure of the cortex with patches of parenchyma surrounded by lymphocytic infiltration and fibrosis. The medulla is not involved or only slightly so. From 48 to 63 percent have immunofluorescent antibodies to a particulate adrenal cell cytoplasmic antigen that apparently arises from the zona fasciculata. The autoimmune disease can be sporadic or part of a polyglandular syndrome. Of the latter there appears to be two types. Type I Addison's polyglandular disease usually has its onset in childhood and has associated hypoparathyroidism in 76 percent, chronic cutaneous mucocutaneous candidiasis in 73 percent, alopecia in 32 percent, malabsorption syndrome in 22 percent, gonad failure in 17 percent, chronic active hepatitis and pernicious anemia in 13 percent, and autoimmune thyroid disease in 11 percent. Type II tends to have its onset in middle age and has associated autoimmune thyroid disease in 69 percent, insulin-dependent diabetes in 52 percent, vitiligo in 4.5 percent, and gonad failure in 3.6 percent. The pathogenesis is not clear, but type I has been postulated to be related to a suppressor T cell defect and type II multifactorial related to the HLA-B8 or Dw3 haplotypes. These associated findings can occur before, with, or after the clinical appearance of adrenal cortical insufficiency. A variety of other disorders have been reported in patients with Addison's disease. Those occurring in over 1 percent are asthma, short stature, seizures, disseminated sclerosis, spastic paraplegia, jejunal diverticulosis, alopecia totalis, and rheumatoid arthritis. Types I and II Addison's disease associated with other diseases have a slight female predominance at all ages.

Tuberculous adrenocortical insufficiency currently accounts for about 21 percent. Less common causes of infectious adrenal gland destruction include histoplasmosis, coccidioidomycosis, cryptococcosis, and septicemia, usually meningococcal or staphylococcal. In this setting, the entire adrenal gland exhibits hemorrhage and necrosis. Congenital enzyme defects are discussed in the section on congenital adrenal hyperplasia. Drugs that can produce adrenal insufficiency by interfering with biosynthesis include metyrapone, amphenone, aminoglutethimide, ketoconazole, and σ-para DDD. Ischemic causes are rare, but embolization and thrombosis do occur. Infiltrative causes include sarcoidosis, metastatic cancer, amyloid, Hodgkin's or non-Hodgkin's lymphomas, and hemochromatosis. Hemorrhage as a cause may occur with anticoagulant therapy, and postoperatively, usually following abdominal surgery, or in association with an adrenal neoplasm, the most common being pheochromocytoma. Miscellaneous causes include irradiation therapy, posttraumatic adrenal vein thrombosis, and bilateral surgical adrenalectomy.

Secondary hypoadrenalism can result from a variety of causes. The most common is postpartum pituitary hemorrhage (Sheehan's syndrome). About 96 percent of these patients at some point develop cortisol insufficiency. The majority have a normal response to adrenocorticotropin hormone (ACTH) stimulation. Next in frequency are the neoplasms involving the hypothalamus and/or pituitary. These include chromophobe adenomas, most commonly in adults or craniopharyngiomas in children, as well as primary or metastatic third ventricle tumors and optic gliomas. Other intracranial causes are trauma, encephalitis, meningitis, stalk section, surgical hypophysectomy, autoimmune hypophysitis, and pituitary apoplexy. In these patients the zona glomerulosa is characteristically unaffected; hence the renin-angiotensin-aldosterone system is intact.

The most common iatrogenic cause of adrenal cortical insufficiency is the administration of pharmacologic doses of corticosteroids for the control of other disease processes. This results in varying degrees of disuse atrophy of the adrenal and pituitary. In general, doses up to 7.5 mg of prednisolone per day (i.e., a replacement dose for most adults) have no demonstrable atrophic effect on the pituitary or adrenal glands. Doses above this level provide varying degrees of suppression of these glands and their axis with the most profound effects seen with doses above 20 mg a day given for months or years. In most individuals the adrenal gland response to ACTH stimulation returns much quicker than the hypothalamic-pituitary-adrenal axis, which may require as much as a year to return to normal after exogenous steroids have been tapered below replacement levels or discontinued. In regard to the feedback axis, alternate-day therapy appears to offer the least suppression. Some authors have suggested that depot tetracosactrin does not significantly disturb this axis in doses of 0.5 mg intramuscularly twice weekly, but further confirmation is needed. It must be noted that patients receiving pharmacologic doses of glucocorticoids may develop acute insufficiency during times of stress despite their already high dose; therefore, doses should be doubled at these times.

Some clinical features can help differentiate primary from secondary hypoadrenalism. Hyperpigmentation is seen in about 94 percent of patients with primary hypoadrenalism and in essentially none of those with secondary disease. This progressive increase in pigmentation is due to the increase in β-melanocyte-stimulating hormone, which accompanies excess ACTH production and release. Areas prone to pigmentation are new scars, palmar creases, knuckles, elbows, knees, areolae, and perianal and mucosal areas. The skin has a dirty appearance, and the mucosal surfaces may have bluish-black patches. Areas of vitiligo are not uncommon in patients with hypoadrenalism of autoimmune origin. Salt craving may be seen in primary Addison's disease, but is rare in secondary. Hypotension is seen in 94 percent of patients and is common to both forms, as are the other typical signs and symptoms. Two unusual manifestations of both are hyperkalemic paralysis or ectopic calcification, which often involves the pinna of the ear and may or may not be accompanied by hypercalcemia. Chemically, primary disease can usually be differentiated from secondary by ACTH and, perhaps, corticotropin releasing hormone (CRH) stimulation testing. An effective screening test is the 30- to 60-minute alpha-1-24-adrenocorticotropin (Cortrosyn) stimulation test. A doubling of a low baseline cortisol level suggests secondary disease, whereas a lesser rise in cortisol suggests adrenal gland disease, but final confirmation requires a lack of response to daily ACTH stimulation for 3 to 4 days. A substantial rise in plasma aldosterone 30 minutes after intramuscular injection of Cortrosyn strongly supports the diagnosis of secondary adrenal insufficiency. In patients presenting with weakness, anorexia, weight loss, and hyperpigmentation, other key diseases in the differential diagnosis are malabsorption, Peutz-Jeghers syndrome, cirrhosis, aleukemic leukemia, hemochromatosis, chronic renal disease with or without salt loss, hyperthyroidism, ectopic ACTH syndrome, anorexia nervosa, acanthosis nigricans, scleroderma, dermatomyositis, polyostotic fibrous dysplasia, neurofibromatosis, inappropriate antidiuretic hormone secretion, arsenic or silver poisoning, and drug therapy with quinacrine (Atabrine) or busulfan.

Acute adrenal insufficiency is a medical emergency characterized by varying degrees of hypotension, nausea and vomiting, hyperthermia, hyponatremia, hyperkalemia, hypoglycemia, and prostration. The clinical suspicion of hypoadrenocorticism should always be confirmed by appropriate laboratory studies. It should be remembered that the total eosinophil count and serum sodium, potassium, and urea nitrogen levels will be normal in 25 to 50 percent and are thus only useful if abnormal.

1. Addison, T. Disease of the suprarenal capsules. *Lon. Med. Gaz.* 43:517, 1855.
   The original description, including discussions of tuberculosis, metastatic disease, and idiopathic causes.
2. Dluhy, R. G., Himathongkam, T., and Greenfield, M. Rapid ACTH test with plasma aldosterone levels: Improved diagnostic discrimination. *Ann. Intern. Med.* 80:693, 1974.
   Patients with secondary adrenal insufficiency show a substantial rise in plasma aldosterone.
3. Wuepper, K. D., Wegienka, L. C., and Fudenberg, H. H. Immunologic aspects of adrenocortical insufficiency. *Am. J. Med.* 46:206, 1969.
   IgG adrenal antibodies were regularly found in idiopathic Addison's disease when studies were made within 1 year of diagnosis.
4. Carpenter, C. C. J., Solomon, N., Silverberg, S. G., et al. Schmidt's syndrome: A review of the literature and a report of fifteen new cases including ten instances of coexistent diabetes mellitus. *Medicine* 43:153, 1964.
   A not uncommon duo and trio.
5. Neufeld, M., MacLaren, N. K., and Blizzard, R. M. Two types of autoimmune Addison's disease associated with different polyglandular autoimmune (PGA) syndromes. *Medicine* 60:355, 1981.
   Types I and II are defined and their clinical courses and importance detailed.

6. Clark, O. H., Hall, A. D., and Schambelan, M. Clinical manifestations of adrenal hemorrhage. *Am. J. Surg.* 128:219, 1974.
   Sudden onset and continuous upper abdominal pain were characteristic in this series. Of particular note is that 35% of patients had their adrenal hemorrhage 1–33 days postoperatively.

7. McDonald, F. D., Myers, R., and Pardo, R. Adrenal hemorrhage during anticoagulant therapy. *J.A.M.A.* 198:1052, 1966.
   Back pain was a common symptom in addition to the classic features of adrenal crisis.

8. Haddock, L., Vega, L. A., Oguilo, F., et al. Adrenocortical, thyroidal, and human growth hormone reserve in Sheehan's syndrome. *Johns Hopkins Med. J.* 131:80, 1972.
   96% of patients had evidence of adrenocortical dysfunction, and isolated ACTH deficiency was not seen.

9. James, U. H. T. The investigation of pituitary-adrenal function: Effects of corticosteroid and corticotropin therapy. *Pharmacol. Clin.* 2:182, 1970.
   Up to 1 year is required for return of pituitary-adrenal axis.

10. Axelrod, L. Glucocorticoid therapy. *Medicine* 56:39, 1976.
    A review that should be read by all who prescribe steroids.

11. Besser, G. M., Cullen, D. R., Irvine, W. J., et al. Immunoreactive corticotropin level in adrenocortical insufficiency. *Br. Med. J.* 1:374, 1971.
    ACTH levels are high in primary adrenal insufficiency and low-normal or low in secondary adrenal insufficiency.

12. Speckart, P. F., Nicoloff, J. T., and Bethune, J. C. Screening for adrenocortical insufficiency with cosyntropin (synthetic ACTH). *Arch. Intern. Med.* 128:761, 1971.
    A useful screening test for primary Addison's disease.

13. Strott, C. A., West, C. D., Nakagawa, K., et al. Plasma 11-deoxycorticosteroid and ACTH response to metyrapone. *J. Clin. Endocrinol. Metab.* 29:6, 1969.
    A useful test for ACTH reserve, but adrenal crisis can be precipitated in primary disease.

14. Schaison, G., Sebaoum, J., Pelzant, G., et al. Mineralocorticoid function in 10 cases of Addison's disease. *Ann. Endocrinol.* 31:609, 1970.
    40% of patients had normal mineralocorticoid function.

15. Lanes, R., Plotnick, L. P., Bynum, T. E., et al. Glucocorticoid and partial mineralocorticoid deficiency associated with achalasia. *J. Clin. Endocrinol. Metab.* 50:268, 1980.
    A rare new syndrome that is probably due to ACTH unresponsiveness.

16. Dolman, L. I., Nolan, G., and Jubiz, W. Metyrapone test with adrenocorticotropic levels: Separating primary from secondary adrenal insufficiency. *J.A.M.A.* 241:1251, 1979.
    A potentially useful initial screening test.

17. Burke, C. W. Adrenocortical insufficiency. *Clin. Endocrinol. Metab.* 14:947, 1985.
    A concise up-to-date review.

18. Jensen, M. D., Handwerger, B. S., Scheithauer, B. W., et al. Lymphocytic hypophysitis with isolated corticotropin deficiency. *Ann. Intern. Med.* 105:200, 1986.
    Is most often seen in association with other endocrine autoimmune processes or post partum.

19. Shea, T. C., Spark, R., Kane, B., et al. Non-Hodgkin's lymphoma limited to the adrenal gland with adrenal insufficiency. *Am. J. Med.* 78:711, 1985.

20. Best, T. R., Jenkins, J. K., Murphy, F. Y., et al. Persistent adrenal insufficiency secondary to low-dose ketoconazole therapy. *Am. J. Med.* 82:676, 1987.
    Two (articles 19, 20) newly recognized causes of hypoadrenocorticism.

21. Chrousos, G. P., Schuermeyer, T. H., Doppman, J., et al. Clinical applications of corticotropin-releasing factor. *Ann. Intern. Med.* 102:344, 1985.
    A corticotropin releasing factor test may be useful in identifying adrenal, pituitary, and hypothalamic etiologies.

22. Vita, J. A., Silverberg, S. J., Goland, R. S., et al. Clinical clues to the causes of Addison's disease. *Am. J. Med.* 78:461, 1985.

Early tuberculous and carcinomatous causes tended to have enlarged adrenals on computed tomography.

23. Yamaji, T., Ishibashi, M., Takaku, F., et al. Serum dehydroepiandrosterone sulfate concentrations in secondary adrenal insufficiency. *J. Clin. Endocrinol. Metab.* 65:448, 1987.
    Decreased levels appear to suggest ACTH deficiency.

24. Stryker, T. D., and Molitch, M. E. Reversible hyperthyrotropinemia, hyperthyroxemia and hyperprolactinemia due to adrenal insufficiency. *Am. J. Med.* 79:271, 1985.
    Cortisol may in part modulate the pituitary-thyroid axis and prolactin release.

25. MacLaren, N. K., and Riley, W. J. Inherited susceptibility to autoimmune Addison's disease is linked to human leukocyte antigens-DR$_3$ and/or DR$_4$, except when associated with type I autoimmune polyglandular syndrome. *J. Clin. Endocrinol. Metab.* 62:455, 1986.
    Another HLA association.

61. HYPOPARATHYROIDISM

H. Verdain Barnes

Hypoparathyroidism (HPT) is an uncommon endocrine disorder that may be transient or permanent, partial or essentially complete. Clinically HPT can be categorized as acquired (parathyroid gland removal or destruction), functional, and idiopathic. The most frequently encountered is parathyroid hormone (PTH) deficiency due to parathyroid gland removal or damage during thyroid, parathyroid, or other extensive neck surgery. In the hands of a capable and experienced neck surgeon, severe, permanent HPT is uncommon. Mild, transient HPT or diminished parathyroid reserve after neck surgery, however, is relatively common. The clinical significance is not clear although some authors have suggested that personality and mentation dysfunction, basal ganglia calcification, and cataracts occur more frequently in these patients. Rare causes of parathyroid gland destruction include external neck irradiation, radioiodine therapy, hemochromatosis, and metastatic disease from breast carcinoma, leukemia, melanoma, lung carcinoma, sarcomas, and lymphomas. The parathyroid glands are congenitally absent in DiGeorge's syndrome and several other bronchial dysembryogenetic syndromes.

The most common form of functional HPT is severe hypomagnesemia, a relative and reversible disorder. Prolonged or pronounced hypomagnesemia results in a decreased production and release of PTH and increases the bone's resistance to the physiologic actions of PTH. The net movement of calcium from the extracellular fluid into bone is increased. When hypomagnesemia occurs in other types of HPT, the patient's vitamin D requirements tend to increase.

Idiopathic familial hypoparathyroidism is a heterogeneous group of disorders in which deficient PTH production or action results in hyperphosphatemia and hypocalcemia. Type I disease has an autosomal dominant inheritance, with a defective structural gene for PTH and a nonlinked mutation form. Type II disease is an autosomal recessive disorder with a linked and nonlinked form. Type III is an X-linked disease which typically becomes clinically apparent in neonatal life. It can be recessive or dominant with variable penetrance. The autosomal dominant form is the most common and is often associated with autoimmune hypoadrenocorticism, pernicious anemia, hypogonadism, and moniliasis. Idiopathic hypoparathyroidism can also occur in a sporadic form without autoimmune-associated diseases. The cause of parathyroid gland destruction is not known.

Another major category of HPT is the spectrum of disorders labeled as pseudohypoparathyroidism. In these disorders there is an end-organ resistance to PTH. Type I pseu-dohypoparathyroidism (PHPT) is the most common. This X-linked dominant disorder with variable penetrance is characterized by hypocalcemia and a variety of associated somatic anomalies. These, in descending order of frequency, are round face, short neck, metacarpal brachydactyly, subcutaneous calcifications, mental retardation, basal gan-glia calcification, short stature, stocky body build, metatarsal brachydactyly, cataracts, thickened calvarium, and increased or decreased bone density on x ray. In these patients there is an insensitivity of the kidney to exogenous PTH, that is, an impaired ability to generate cyclic AMP, and an increase in renal tubular phosphate reabsorption. In ad-dition, there is an apparent defect in the ability of PTH to mobilize calcium from bone, while in most the bone remodeling action of PTH remains intact. Finally, in some pa-tients there may be a biodefective PTH molecule. Type II pseudohypoparathryoidism (PHPT) is heterogeneous in clinical presentation except for the presence of hypocal-cemia. These patients exhibit a normal renal response to the production of cyclic AMP by exogenous PTH, but are hyperphosphatemic. These patients have elevated levels of circulating immunoreactive PTH. A variety of other rare potential expressions have been reported: (1) PHPT with somatic abnormalities, skeletal response to PTH with osteitis fibrosa, and renal resistance to PTH, (2) PHPT with the same features as (1) but without somatic abnormalities, and (3) somatic abnormalities and possible skeletal re-sistance and renal responsiveness to exogenous hormone. These variations probably rep-resent a continuum of disorders of end-organ unresponsiveness rather than individual diseases.

Finally, HPT resulting from biologically defective circulating PTH has been docu-mented in PHPT characterized by normal or elevated immunoreaction PTH levels, hy-pocalcemia, normal somatic features, and normal response to exogenous hormone. De-ficient 25-hydroxyvitamin D or 1,25-dihydroxyvitamin D_3 and resistant states to 1,25-dihydroxyvitamin D_3 can produce HPT as can glucocorticoid and mithramycin therapy. The full spectrum of HPT merits consideration in the differential diagnosis of hypocal-cemia.

1. Nusynowitz, M. L., Frame, B., and Kolb, F. O. The spectrum of the hypoparathyroid states: A classification based on physiologic principles. *Medicine* 55:105, 1976.
   A careful delineation and classification of the hypoparathyroid states based on defi-cient or excessive amounts of PTH.

2. Woodhouse, N. J. Y. Hypocalcemia and hypoparathyroidism. *Clin. Endocrinol. Me-tab.* 3:323, 1974.
   A concise discussion of the common causes of chronic hypocalcemia and their clinical features.

3. Davis, R. H., Fourman, P., and Smith, J. W. G. Problems of parathyroid insufficiency after thyroidectomy. *Lancet* 2:1432, 1961.
   The authors suggest that personality and mentation changes, basal ganglia calcifi-cation, and cataracts are more common in persons with mild or partial postoperative HPT.

4. Horowitz, C. A., Myers, L. W. P., and Foote, F. W. Secondary malignant tumors of the parathyroid glands: Report of two cases with associated hypoparathyroidism. *Am. J. Med.* 52:797, 1972.

5. MacDonald, R. A., and Mallory, G. K. Hemochromatosis and hemociderosis: Study of 211 autopsied cases. *Arch. Intern. Med.* 105:686, 1960.

6. Townsend, J. D. Hypoparathyroidism following radioactive iodine therapy for in-tractable angina pectoris. *Ann. Intern. Med.* 55:662, 1961.
   Articles 4–6 discuss some of the rarer causes of parathyroid gland destruction.

7. Anast, C. S., Winnacker, J. L., Forte, L. R., et al. Impaired release of parathyroid hormone in magnesium deficiency. *J. Clin. Endocrinol. Metab.* 42:707, 1976.
   Elucidates the mechanisms of the effect of hypomagnesemia on calcium homeostasis.

8. Rosler, A., and Rabinowitz, D. Magnesium-induced reversal of vitamin D resistance in hypoparathyroidism. *Lancet* 1:803, 1973.
   Magnesium deficiency may produce an increase in the vitamin D requirement in the therapy of HPT.

9. Drezner, N., Neelon, F. A., and Lebovitz, H. E. Pseudohypoparathyroidism type II:

A possible defect in the reception of the cyclic AMP signal. *N. Engl. J. Med.* 289:1056, 1973.
The initial discussion of a rare disorder.

10. Kolb, F. O., and Steinbach, H. L. Pseudohypoparathyroidism with secondary hyperparathyroidism and osteitis fibrosa. *J. Clin. Endocrinol.* 22:59, 1972.
   These patients have renal resistance and skeletal responsiveness to PTH.

11. Hirano, K., Ishibashi, A., and Yoshino, Y. Cutaneous manifestations in idiopathic hypoparathyroidism. *Arch. Dermatol.* 109:242, 1974.
   The article provides a good discussion of the dermatologic changes seen in this disorder.

12. Juan, D. Hypocalcemia: Differential diagnosis and mechanisms. *Arch. Intern. Med.* 139:1166, 1979.
   A concise, well-done review.

13. Farfel, Z., Brickman, A. S., Kaslow, H. R., et al. Defect of receptor-cyclase coupling protein in pseudohypoparathyroidism. *N. Engl. J. Med.* 303:237, 1980.
   Reduced N protein activity was seen in 50% of their type I PHPT patients.

14. Ahn, T. G., Antonarakis, S. E., Kronenberg, H. M., et al. Familial isolated hypoparathyroidism: A molecular genetic analysis of 8 families with 23 affected persons. *Medicine* 65:73, 1986.
   Autosomal dominant and recessive as well as an X-linked type are defined.

15. Farfel, Z., and Friedman, E. Mental deficiency in pseudohypoparathyroidism type I is associated with Ns-protein deficiency. *Ann. Intern. Med.* 105:197, 1986.
   Reduced Ns protein, cyclic AMP, or both may have a pathophysiologic role in the mental function of some of these patients.

16. Breslau, N. A., Moses, A. M., and Pak, C. Y. C. Evidence for bone remodeling but lack of calcium mobilization response to parathyroid hormone in pseudohypoparathyroidism. *J. Clin. Endocrinol. Metab.* 57:638, 1983.
   Most patients have intact bone remodeling but cannot mobilize calcium from the bone.

17. Rao, D. S., Parfitt, A. M., Kleerekoper, M., et al. Dissociation between the effects of endogenous parathyroid hormone on adenosine 3'5'-monophosphate generation and phosphate reabsorption in hypocalcemia due to vitamin D depletion: An acquired disorder resembling pseudohypoparathyroidism type II. *J. Clin. Endocrinol. Metab.* 61:285, 1985.
   Vitamin D deficiency must be excluded to diagnose PHPT type II.

18. Mitchell, J., and Goltzman, D. Examination of circulating parathyroid hormone in pseudohypoparathyroidism. *J. Clin. Endocrinol. Metab.* 61:328, 1985.
   Defective PTH release and/or metabolism may have a pathophysiologic role in many of these patients.

19. Levine, M. A. Laboratory investigation of disorders of the parathyroid glands. *Clin. Endocrinol. Metab.* 14:257, 1985.
   A concise discussion.

20. Nolten, W. E., Chesney, R. W., Dabbagh, S., et al. Moderate hypocalcemia due to normal serum 1,25-dihydroxyvitamin D levels in an asymptomatic kindred with familial hypoparathyroidism. *Am. J. Med.* 82:1157, 1987.
   Yet another clinical presentation.

62. HYPOTHYROIDISM

H. Verdain Barnes

Hypothyroidism is a systemic disorder resulting from a lack of thyroid hormone due to dysfunction of (1) the thyroid (primary hypothyroidism), or (2) the pituitary or the hypothalamus (secondary hypothyroidism). Primary hypothyroidism is the most common. It can be divided into inherited and acquired. The inherited causes include thyroid agenesis, a hypofunctioning ectopic thyroid, a thyroid-stimulating hormone (TSH)–unresponsive gland, peripheral and/or pituitary resistance to thyroid hormone, thyroid-binding globulin excess or deficiency, iodide transport defect, iodide organification defect without or with Pendred's syndrome, coupling defect, thyroglobulin defect, and deiodination defect. In the main, these disorders are diagnosed in early infancy or childhood, although partial enzyme defects may not become manifest until adolescence or rarely not until adult life.

In the United States, the most common form of acquired hypothyroidism is autoimmune, including primary myxedema and chronic lymphocytic thyroiditis, Hashimoto's disease. Other causes include iodine excess, iodine deficiency, antithyroid drugs, lithium therapy, partial thyroidectomy or radioactive iodine therapy for toxic diffuse goiter, Graves' disease, nontoxic nodular goiter, colloid goiter, and rarely external neck irradiation, granulomatous diseases, and primary or metastatic carcinoma. Secondary hypothyroidism due to pituitary dysfunction may be idiopathic or arise from vascular insufficiency such as Sheehan's syndrome, vascular thrombosis, pituitary tumor, or following head trauma or pituitary-hypothalamic surgery. Secondary hypothyroidism due to hypothalamic dysfunction may be idiopathic or result from hypothalamic injury by a neoplasm or surgery. The differentiation of primary from secondary hypothyroidism can be made by measuring circulating TSH using a sensitive immunoradiometric, fluorometric, chemiluminometric, or enzymometric assay; the thyroid's response to TSH administration; and pituitary's response to thyrotropin releasing hormone (TRH). In primary hypothyroidism, the serum TSH is elevated and there is an exaggerated response to TRH and no thyroid gland response to exogenous TSH stimulation. In secondary hypothyroidism of both types, the serum TSH level is normal or low, but the thyroid gland responds to TSH stimulation. In pituitary failure, there is no response to TRH, whereas in hypothalamic failure there is a response although repeated stimulation may be required.

The clinical manifestations of hypothyroidism are protean and the onset is most often insidious. The most common constitutional manifestations are weakness, fatigue, lethargy, sleepiness, decreased memory, cold intolerance, and modest weight gain with little or no increase in appetite. Common cardiorespiratory complaints include dyspnea, palpitations, and precordial pain. The cutaneous manifestations most frequently seen include dry and coarse skin; edema of the hands, face, and eyelids; alopecia of the lateral third of the eyebrows and, to some extent, of the scalp; pallor or a yellowish discoloration of the skin; malar flush; hypohydrosis; and thick tongue. Myxedematous involvement of the throat may result in a deepening of the voice, and eighth cranial nerve involvement can produce deafness. Arthritis and carpal tunnel syndrome are the most common musculoskeletal problems. Gastrointestinal tract features are dominated by complaints of distention, flatulence, and constipation. The neuropsychiatric manifestations range from cerebellar ataxia to dementia to myxedema coma. Anemia is common. It can be physiologic, due to decreased oxygen demand or secondary to iron, vitamin B_{12}, folic acid, or pyridoxine deficiency. In acquired primary hypothyroidism, achlorhydria occurs in about 50 percent of patients, and frank pernicious anemia in 10 to 15 percent.

The earliest signs and symptoms of hypothyroidism frequently date back several months to years prior to diagnosis. The patients may present with a single-system problem predominating. The cardiovascular system and dominate, with findings of congestive heart failure associated with hypertension, bradycardia, pericardial effusion, and cardiomyopathy. A rare patient presents with cardiac tamponade. Respiratory problems may predominate, with dyspnea, which may be associated with pleural effusion and obstructive sleep apnea. Some patients complain primarily of arthralgias or arthritis, with symptoms ranging from those suggestive of rheumatism to frank rheumatoid arthritis to polymyositis. Constipation may be the leading complaint and myxedema magacolon can occur. Patients may be essentially asymptomatic but found to have hyperlipidemia, particularly type IV. Finally, the primary involvement may be of the central nervous system, with a psychiatric presentation ranging from presenile seizures to psychosis. All patients with the findings described should have a thyroid screen unless another cause is obvious.

When the diagnosis is suspected, a serum thyroxine value should be obtained unless there is a suspicion of serum protein abnormalities, in which case a "free" thyroxine by equilibrium dialysis or its equivalent should be obtained. The workup is not complete without a determination of serum TSH by a sensitive assay. If secondary hypothyroidism is suspected, then a TSH stimulation or TRH stimulation test should be performed. When a diagnosis of secondary hypothyroidism is made, it is mandatory that at least the pituitary-adrenal axis be evaluated prior to therapy since diminished or absent pituitary or adrenal reserve may result in adrenal crisis during thyroid hormone replacement. Therapy should be initiated with low doses of thyroid hormone with a slow, progressive increase until full replacement is achieved as determined by TSH levels in patients with thyroid gland failure.

1. Meinas, F. W., Gorman, C. A., Devine, K. D., et al. Lingual thyroid. *Ann. Intern. Med.* 79:205, 1973.
   Hypothyroidism was frequently associated with throat discomfort, dysphonia, and hemoptysis in these patients.
2. Maenpaa, J. Congenital hypothyroidism. *Arch. Dis. Child.* 47:914, 1972.
   In this study from Finland, the cause was athyrosis (in 30% of patients), ectopic thyroid (in 36%), dyshormonogenesis (in 28%), and hypoplastic thyroid (in 5%).
3. Crowley, W. F., Ridgway, C., Bough, E. W., et al. Noninvasive evaluation of cardiac function in hypothyroidism. *N. Engl. J. Med.* 296:1, 1977.
   The preejection period was prolonged and the left ventricular ejection period shortened in a majority of patients. All abnormalities reversed with adequate thyroid hormone replacement.
4. Kerber, R. E., and Sherman, B. Echocardiographic evaluation of pericardial effusion in myxedema: Incidence and biochemical and clinical correlations. *Circulation* 52:823, 1975.
   Effusion was documented in close to 50% of patients.
5. Ritter, F. N. The effects of hypothyroidism upon the ear, nose, and throat. *Laryngoscope* 67:1427, 1967.
   Varying degrees of deafness are common.
6. Tudhope, G. E., and Wilson, G. M. Deficiency of vitamin B_{12} in hypothyroidism. *Lancet* 1:703, 1962.
   About 10% of patients with acquired primary hypothyroidism have pernicious anemia.
7. Burrell, M., Cronan, J., Megna, D., et al. Myxedema megacolon. *Gastrointest. Radiol.* 5:181, 1980.
   Localized transverse ridging of the colon and megacolon suggests hypothyroidism.
8. Tudhope, G. E., and Wilson, G. M. Anemia in hypothyroidism. *Q. J. Med.* 29:513, 1960.
   The physiologic anemia of hypothyroidism is mild unless complicated by iron or vitamin deficiency.
9. Edson, J. R., Fecher, D. R., and Doe, R. P. Low platelet adhesiveness and other hemostatic abnormalities in hypothyroidism. *Ann. Intern. Med.* 82:342, 1975.
   In addition to low platelet adhesiveness in 75% of patients, a majority also had low levels of factors VII, VIII, IX, and XI.
10. Watanakuna, C., Hodges, R. E., and Evans, T. C. Myxedema: A study of 400 cases. *Arch. Intern. Med.* 116:183, 1965.
    About 4% of patients had secondary hypothyroidism.
11. Nelson, J. C., Johnson, D. E., and Odell, W. D. Serum TSH levels and the thyroidal response to TSH stimulation in patients with thyroid disease. *Ann. Intern. Med.* 76:47, 1972.
    Patients with primary hypothyroidism have elevated TSH levels and little or no response to exogenous TSH stimulation.
12. Luby, E. D., Schwartz, D., and Rosenbaum, H. Lithium carbonate-induced myxedema. *J.A.M.A.* 218:1298, 1971.
    A recently documented iatrogenic cause of hypothyroidism.
13. Bronsky, D., Kiamko, R. T., and Waldstein, S. S. Posttherapeutic myxedema. *Arch. Intern. Med.* 121:113, 1968.
    Iodine 131 therapy and subtotal thyroidectomy for toxic diffuse goiter are the most common causes of iatrogenic hypothyroidism.

14. Royce, P. C. Severely impaired consciousness in myxedema: A review. *Am. J. Med. Sci.* 261:46, 1971.
   Hypoxia, hypercarbia, hyponatremia, and hypopituitarism often provide the pathophysiologic background for myxedema coma.

15. Zwillich, C. W., Pierson, D. J., Hofeldt, F. D., et al. Ventilatory control in myxedema and hypothyroidism. *N. Engl. J. Med.* 292:662, 1975.
   Hypoxic ventilatory drive is depressed in both disorders.

16. Dorwart, B. B., and Schumacher, H. R. Joint effusions, chondrocalcinosis and other rheumatic manifestations of hypothyroidism. *Am. J. Med.* 59:780, 1975.

17. Hochberg, M. C., Koppes, G. M., Edwards, C. Q., et al. Hypothyroidism presenting as a polymyositis-like syndrome. *Arthritis Rheum.* 19:1363, 1976.
   The rheumatologic manifestations may be dramatic and are eminently treatable (16, 17).

18. Wood, L. C., and Ingbar, S. H. Hypothyroidism as a late sequela in patients with Graves' disease treated with antithyroid agents. *J. Clin. Invest.* 64:1429, 1979.
   Graves' disease patients must be followed for life.

19. Klein, I., Parker, M., Shebert, R., et al. Hypothyroidism presenting as muscle stiffness and pseudohypertrophy: Hoffmann's syndrome. *Am. J. Med.* 70:891, 1981.
   It occurs in adults as well as children.

20. Orr, W. C., Males, J. L., and Imes, N. K. Myxedema and obstructive sleep apnea. *Am. J. Med.* 70:1061, 1981.
   A potentially lethal consequence of hypothyroidism to keep in mind.

21. Sawers, J. S. A., Toft, A. D., Irvine, W. J., et al. Transient hypothyroidism after ^{131}I treatment of thyrotoxicosis. *J. Clin. Endocrinol. Metab.* 50:226, 1980.
   Be careful not to treat these patients too quickly with thyroid hormone.

22. Josephson, A. M., and Mackenzie, T. B. Thyroid-induced mania in hypothyroid patients. *Br. J. Psychiatry* 137:222, 1980.
   Preexisting psychiatric symptoms were typically exacerbated between 4 and 7 days into thyroid hormone therapy and usually resolved within a week or two.

23. Konish, J., Iida, Y., Kasagi, K., et al. Primary myxedema with thyrotropin-binding inhibitor immunoglobulins: Clinical and laboratory findings in 15 patients. *Ann. Intern. Med.* 103:26, 1985.
   About 20% of their total patients (N = 43) had inhibiting immunoglobulins.

24. Arikawa, K., Ichikawa, Y., Yoshida, T., et al. Blocking type antithyrotropin receptor antibody in patients with nongoiterous hypothyroidism: Its incidence and characteristics of action. *J. Clin. Endocrinol. Metab.* 60:953, 1985.
   Inhibitory effect may be on the adenylate cyclase system by preventing the TSH molecule from engaging its receptor.

25. Bastenie, P. A., Bonnyns, M., and Vanhaelst, L. Natural history of primary myxedema. *Am. J. Med.* 79:91, 1985.
   A protracted asymptomatic course is common.

26. Tajiri, J., Higashi, K., Morita, M., et al. Studies of hypothyroidism in patients with high iodine uptake. *J. Clin. Endocrinol. Metab.* 63:412, 1986.
   Iodine restriction alone often reverses the hypothyroidism.

27. Gharib, H., and Abboud, C. F. Primary idiopathic hypothalamic hypothyroidism: Report of four cases. *Am. J. Med.* 83:171, 1987.
   In two patients the hypothyroidism appeared to be transient.

28. Robuschi, G., Safran, M., Braverman, L. E., et al. Hypothyroidism in the elderly. *Endocr. Rev.* 8:142, 1987.

29. Livingston, E. H., Hershman, J. M., Sawin, C. T., et al. Prevalence of thyroid disease and abnormal thyroid tests in older hospitalized and ambulatory persons. *J. Am. Geriatr. Soc.* 35:109, 1987.
   Two articles (27, 28) discussing this increasing population's potential for hypothyroidism.

30. Hawthorne, G. C., Campbell, N. P. S., Geddes, J. S., et al. Amiodarone-induced hypothyroidism a common complication of prolonged therapy: A report of eight cases. *Arch. Intern. Med.* 145:1016, 1985.
   An increasingly common cause of iatrogenic hypothyroidism due to the high iodide content of this antiarrhythmic agent.

31. Gow, S. M., Caldwell, G., Toft, A. D., et al. Relationship between pituitary and other target organ responsiveness in hypothyroid patients receiving thyroxine replacement. *J. Clin. Endocrinol. Metab.* 64:364, 1987.
32. Sawin, C. T., Surks, M. I., London, M., et al. Oral thyroxine: Variation in biologic action and tablet content. *Ann. Intern. Med.* 100:641, 1984.
33. Fish, L. H., Schwartz, H. L., Cavanaugh, J., et al. Replacement dose, metabolism, and bioavailability of levothyroxine in the treatment of hypothyroidism. *N. Engl. J. Med.* 316:764, 1987.
34. Hennessey, J. V., Evaul, J. E., Tseng, Y.-C., et al. L-thyroxine dosage: A reevaluation of therapy with contemporary preparations. *Ann. Intern. Med.* 105:11, 1986.
   These articles (31–34) focus on the current state of the art in assessment and dosing.
35. Tachman, M. L., and Guthrie, G. P., Jr. Hypothyroidism: Diversity of presentation. *Endocr. Rev.* 5:456, 1984.
36. Poretsky, L., Garber, J., and Kleefield, J. Primary amenorrhea and pseudoprolactinoma in a patient with primary hypothyroidism. *Am. J. Med.* 81:180, 1986.
37. Zaloga, G. P., Eil, C., and O'Brian, J. T. Reversible hypocalciuric hypercalcemia associated with hypothyroidism. *Am. J. Med.* 77:1101, 1984.
   These articles (35–37) cover some of the multiple clinical presentations of hypothyroidism.
38. Becker, C. Hypothyroidism and atherosclerotic heart disease: Pathogenesis, medical management, and the role of coronary artery bypass surgery. *Endocr. Rev.* 6:432, 1985.
   A concise, timely review of coronary artery disease in hypothyroidism.
39. Caron, P. J., Neiman, L. K., Rose, S. R., et al. Deficient nocturnal surge of thyrotropin in central hypothyroidism. *J. Clin. Endocrinol. Metab.* 62:960, 1986.
   A potentially useful test in differential diagnosis of hypothyroidism.
40. Lever, E. G., Medeiros-Neto, G. A., and DeGroot, L. J. Inherited disorders of thyroid metabolism. *Endocr. Rev.* 4:213, 1983.
   A concise, but comprehensive review.
41. Hamblin, P. S., Dyer, S. A., Mohr, V. S., et al. Relationship between thyrotropin and thyroxine changes during recovery from severe hypothyroxemia of critical illness. *J. Clin. Endocrinol. Metab.* 62:717, 1986.
   In the euthyroid sick syndrome, when you draw the specimen may determine what you see.
42. Sawin, C. T., Castelli, W. P., Hershman, J. M., et al. The aging thyroid: Thyroid deficiency in the Framingham study. *Arch. Intern. Med.* 145:1386, 1985.
   The prevalence in this study population was 4.4%, about 2:1 female to male.

63. INSULINOMA

H. Verdain Barnes

Neoplasms of the pancreatic islets can produce a variety of hormones and syndromes. With current histochemical methods and electron microscopy, at least four cell types can be identified—A-like cells, B-like cells, G-like cells, and EC-like cells, which produce glucagon, insulin, gastrin, and serotonin, respectively. About 50 percent of all islet tumors are functional, and in addition to the hormones just mentioned they may also manufacture and release gastric inhibitory polypeptide, secretin, melanocyte-stimulating hormone, human growth hormone, and ACTH. The hormone produced in excess determines the clinical presentation. The most common and important presentation is the fasting hypoglycemia of the insulin-producing betacytoma. Next in frequency is the Zollinger-Ellison syndrome, followed by pancreatic cholera, glucagon-induced hyperglycemia, and carcinoid syndrome.

Insulinomas can occur at any age but are most often seen in the 30- to 60-year age group and are quite rare before age 20. About 80 percent are solitary and benign, while another 10 percent are multiple and benign. The remaining 10 percent are considered malignant on the basis of distant metastases. About 90 percent of metastases are to the liver and/or periportal lymph nodes. The less common sites for metastases are the peritoneum, adjacent tissues, periaortic lymph nodes, stomach, bone marrow, adrenal, duodenum, spleen, lung, pleura, pericardium, and thyroid. In most instances, beta cell adenomas are hormone producers, whereas only 50 to 75 percent of the carcinomas are functional. Islet cell tumors can arise in any part of the pancreas. Tumor size ranges from millimeters to several centimeters and may extend beyond the surface of the pancreas. Typically they grow concentrically, and commonly outgrow their blood supply, in which case they may be whitish in color. The adenomas are surrounded by a fibrous capsule and almost invariably have wedgelike projections deep into the pancreas. Consequently, at surgery (if possible), a full rim of normal pancreatic tissue around the attached portion of the tumor should be obtained.

The typical clinical presentation is characterized by fasting and/or exercise-induced hypoglycemia. The varied manifestations of hypoglycemia, however, may initially direct investigation away from the pancreas. Early in the course of the illness, the patient may experience only behavioral changes and be advised to have psychiatric evaluation and therapy. Some patients present with seizures, and a neurologic explanation is sought. Further confusion arises from the episodic nature of the attacks, which may be separated by days to months, particularly in the case of adenomas. Weight gain is common, and is usually due to an unrecognized increase in caloric intake to combat chronic or periodic hypoglycemia. Weight gain, though typical, does not invariably occur. The two key clinical features to be looked for when an insulinoma is suspected are (1) signs and symptoms of hypoglycemia occurring in the early morning, late afternoon, or after exercise, and (2) resolution of hypoglycemic manifestations within minutes after the patient ingests glucose.

A definitive diagnosis is often difficult. The following tests have been used to document hyperinsulinemic hypoglycemia: (1) 72-hour fast, (2) tolbutamide tolerance test, (3) leucine tolerance test, (4) glucagon stimulation test, (5) diazoxide inhibition test, and (6) fish or human insulin suppression test. None are ideal or without risk to the patient. Probably the most effective and of least risk to the patient is the human insulin suppression test using the glucose clamp technique. In this procedure the patient's glucose level can be maintained in the euglycemic range and the suppression achieved by insulin infusion as assessed by measuring circulating C peptide as well as insulin and proinsulin by radioimmunoassay. It must be recognized, however, that some insulinoma patients will have equivocal or anomalous results. In most series, adenomas secrete from 3 to 78 percent proinsulin, and functional carcinomas secrete 32 to 89 percent which accounts for 10 percent or less of total insulin secretion. C peptide levels are suppressed in about 90 percent of patients with insulin-secreting islet cell adenomas. The level of C peptide is also useful in evaluating the insulin-dependent diabetic suspected of having an insulinoma, factitious hypoglycemia due to exogenous insulin injection, and in postpancreatectomy follow-up assessments. Fasting is commonly used as a first-line test. About one-third of the patients with an insulinoma develop symptomatic hypoglycemia in the first 12 hours, and an additional one-third in 24 hours. Only occasionally are the patients able to maintain a fast beyond 48 hours. If 12-hour fasting glucose and insulin values are used, about 90 percent of patients have immunoreactive insulin levels that are inappropriately high in comparison to the simultaneous glucose level. When the tolbutamide tolerance test is used, caution must be exercised since profound and prolonged hypoglycemia can occur in insulinoma patients. The leucine tolerance test has the greatest specificity in that excess insulin release is seen only with beta cell tumors; but less than 50 percent of patients respond. Negative fasting and other provocative tests do not completely exclude the diagnosis.

1. Sckein, P. S., DeLellis, R. A., Kahn, C. R., et al. Islet cell tumors: Current concepts and management. *Ann. Intern. Med.* 79:239, 1973.
2. Frerichs, H., and Creutzfeldt, W. Hypoglycemia: I. Insulin secreting tumours. *Clin. Endocrinol. Metab.* 5:747, 1976.
   Two useful reviews (1,2).

3. Scholz, D. Z., ReMine, W. H., and Priestly, J. T. Hyperinsulinism: Review of 95 cases of functional islet cell tumors. *Mayo Clin. Proc.* 35:545, 1970.
   90% were benign insulinomas and 10% were malignant. The varied clinical presentations are discussed.
4. Service, F. J., Dale, A. J. D., Elveback, L. R., et al. Insulinoma. *Mayo Clin. Proc.* 51:417, 1976.
   A useful sequel to article 3. A method for greater accuracy in interpreting intravenous tolbutamide tests is described.
5. Broder, L. E., and Carter, S. K. Pancreatic islet cell carcinoma: I. Clinical features of 52 patients. *Ann. Intern. Med.* 79:101, 1973.
   About 50% of the carcinomas were hormone producers with about 20% producing more than one polypeptide hormone. Almost all patients had metastases to the liver.
6. Dunn, D. C. Diabetes after removal of insulin tumours of pancreas: A long-term follow-up survey of 11 patients. *Br. Med. J.* 1:84, 1971.
   Glucose tolerance was impaired in 3 of the 8 tested. Be aware that with time some patients with benign insulinomas may develop postoperative diabetes.
7. Frawley, T. F., and Pensuwan, S. Hypoglycemia: Tolbutamide and leucine tests in insulinoma. *Med. Clin. North Am.* 52:283, 1968.
   The leucine test can be helpful, but the results are often negative in insulinoma patients.
8. Kumar, D., Mehtalia, S. D., and Miller, L. V. Diagnostic use of glucagon-induced insulin response. *Ann. Intern. Med.* 80:697, 1974.
   Peak serum insulin values were significantly higher in insulinoma patients than in those with hypoglycemia caused by other disorders.
9. Caplan, R. H., Koob, L., Abellera, R. M., et al. Cure of acromegaly by operative removal of an islet cell tumor of the pancreas. *Am. J. Med.* 64:874, 1978.
   Immunoreactive human growth hormone was extracted from the tumor.
10. Heding, L., Turner, R. C., and Harris, E. C-peptide, proinsulin and insulin response to fish insulin induced hypoglycemia in the diagnosis of insulinomas. *Diabetes* 24(Suppl. 2):412, 1975.
11. Rubenstein, A. H., Kuzuya, H., and Horwitz, D. L. Clinical significance of circulating C-peptide in diabetes mellitus and hypoglycemic disorders. *Arch. Intern. Med.* 137:625, 1977.
    These two articles (10,11) demonstrate the usefulness of this peptide, which is secreted in equimolar amounts with insulin.
12. Huggins, G. A. Pancreatic islet cell tumors: Insulinomas, gastrinoma and glucagonoma. *Surg. Clin. North Am.* 59:131, 1979.
    An up-to-date review. Of the 1018 insulinomas collected from the literature about equal numbers were found in the head, middle, and tail of the pancreas.
13. Galbut, D. L., and Markowitz, A. M. Insulinoma: Diagnosis, surgical management and long-term follow up: Review of 41 cases. *Am. J. Surg.* 139:682, 1980.
    In long-term follow-up, significant numbers had neuropsychiatric complaints, diabetes mellitus, and peptic ulcer disease.
14. Tutt, G. O., Jr., Edis, A. J., Service, F. J., et al. Plasma glucose monitoring during operation for insulinoma: A critical reappraisal. *Surgery* 88:351, 1980.
    Rebound hyperglycemia at the operating table does not necessarily indicate the presence of an additional tumor.
15. Nelson, R. L., Rizza, R. A., and Service, F. J. Documented hypoglycemia for 23 years in a patient with insulinoma. *J.A.M.A.* 240:1891, 1978.
    Just a reminder that the diagnosis can be markedly delayed, 25–38% go as long as 3 to 4 years after the onset of symptoms before diagnosis.
16. Kent, R. B., III, Van Heerdan, J. A., and Weiland, L. H. Nonfunctioning islet cell tumors. *Ann. Surg.* 193:185, 1981.
    Patients often presented with abdominal pain and jaundice. The malignancy rate was 92%, but survival was surprisingly long.
17. Berger, M., Bordi, C., Cuppers, H.-J., et al. Functional and morphologic characterization of human insulinomas. *Diabetes* 32:921, 1983.
    A new classification is proposed based on β cell granulation and response to somatostatin and diazoxide.

18. Yasunami, Y., Funakosh, A., Ono, J., et al. In vitro study of cultured human insulinoma cells: Evidence of abnormal sensitivity to glucose. *J. Clin. Endocrinol. Metab.* 65:110, 1987.
    Insensitivity to glucose is documented.
19. Maletti, M., Altman, J.-J., Hoa, D. H. B., et al. Evidence of functional gastric inhibitory polypeptide (GIP) in human insulinoma. *Diabetes* 36:1336, 1987.
    Functional GIP receptors were identified in human insulinomas.
20. Gin, H., Brottier, E., Dupuy, B., et al. Use of the glucose clamp technique for conformation of insulinoma autonomous hyperinsulinism. *Arch. Intern. Med.* 147:985, 1987.
    C peptide levels remained high in insulinoma patients. This technique for human insulin suppression test offers the least risk to patients.
21. Koivisto, V. A., Yki-Jarvinen, H., Hartling, S. G., et al. The effect of exogenous hyperinsulinemia on proinsulin secretion in normal man, obese subjects and patients with insulinomas. *J. Clin. Endocrinol. Metab.* 63:1117, 1986.
    Suppression of proinsulin did not occur in insulinoma patients.
22. Dons, R. F., Hodge, J., Ginsberg, B. H., et al. Anomalous glucose and insulin responses in patients with insulinoma: Caveats for diagnosis. *Arch. Intern. Med.* 145:1861, 1985.
    Fasting did not make the diagnosis in these patients.
23. Benson, E. A., Ho, P., Wang, C., et al. Insulin autoimmunity as a cause of hypoglycemia. *Arch. Intern. Med.* 144:2351, 1984.
    Insulin-binding antibodies can produce clinical and chemical evidence that is a look-alike for insulinoma, a must consideration in fasting hypoglycemia.

64. OBESITY
H. Verdain Barnes

Obesity can be defined as a body weight 20 percent or more over the ideal body weight for height as listed in the 1983 Metropolitan Life Insurance tables or a triceps skin fold thickness equal to or greater than 18 to 19 mm in adult males and 25 to 26 mm or more in adult females. The magnitude of obesity as a potential health problem is evident from the findings of the U.S. Public Health Service's health and nutrition survey. The survey showed the prevalence of obesity to be from about 12 to 30 percent among white men aged 21 to 80 years and 5 to 41 percent among black men. Among females, the prevalence in the same age group ranged from about 9 to 36 percent for whites and 18 to 61 percent for blacks.

Obesity is characterized by an increase in the lipid content of the adipocyte and on occasion an increase in the total number of fat cells. Persons with increased lipid content alone can be categorized as having hypertrophic obesity. This is the most common type, and usually has its onset in adult life. Those with both an increase in lipid content and total fat cell number have hyperplastic-hypertrophic obesity, a type that is most often seen in patients whose obesity begins in early life and/or in patients who are more than 170 percent over ideal body weight. In hyperplastic-hypertrophic obesity, significant nonsurgical weight loss and maintenance is least likely to occur and the complications of obesity are more likely.

The documented direct complications of obesity are increased mortality in relation to age, diabetes mellitus, gallbladder disease, alveolar hypoventilation, cardiovascular and renal disease. The critical cardiovascular component is hypertension. The incidence of hypertension, cardiovascular, and renal disease is highest in normal- or low-weight persons who become obese during adolescence or early adult life. Obesity per se is not a major independent predictor of coronary artery disease. For the overweight patient who is less than 20 percent over ideal body weight, the only known risk is that of becoming progressively heavier and eventually moving into the weight class with known risks.

An impressive array of endocrine-metabolic changes may occur in obesity. They include (1) increase in fasting blood cholesterol, triglyceride, free fatty acid, and amino acid levels; (2) elevated fasting insulin levels, increased insulin release with a glucose load, decreased oral and intravenous glucose tolerance, and an increased resistance of fat and muscle cells to insulin; (3) decreased growth hormone response to glucose and arginine; and (4) increased production rate and metabolism of glucocorticoids while maintaining normal levels of plasma and urinary "free" cortisol and an increased level of the urine metabolites (i.e., 17-hydroxycorticosteroids and 17-ketogenic steroids).

For the vast majority (over 95%) of patients the cause of obesity is a caloric intake in excess of caloric expenditures (exogenous obesity). Nonetheless, the other potential causes of obesity cannot be overlooked in evaluating the overweight individual. Hypothyroidism is a cause of moderate but rarely marked obesity. Patients with hypothyroidism almost invariably have other prominent signs and symptoms of hypometabolism. In children and adolescents linear growth is stunted and the bone age is delayed. Hyperadrenocorticism, Cushing's syndrome, is another rare cause of obesity. These patients have other manifestations of cortisol excess, and in the young linear growth is inhibited. Urinary free cortisol levels are elevated. Hyperinsulinemia due to a benign or malignant insulinoma is often accompanied by obesity. These patients have signs and symptoms of hypoglycemia, along with moderate to marked elevations of serum immunoreactive insulin. Overinsulinization in the treatment of diabetes mellitus occurs relatively frequently. These diabetics often have increased food intake, poor diabetic control, and the Somogyi phenomenon. Acquired hypothalamic obesity results from ventromedial hypothalamic injury. This form of obesity is usually associated with neoplasia (most commonly craniopharyngioma and leukemia), but may occur in association with meningitis, encephalitis, head trauma, or cerebrovascular disease. In these patients satiety is lost, resulting in hyperphagia and with food withdrawal, rage, or extremely aggressive behavior. Reproductive abnormalities are common in the adult, and short stature is usually seen in children. Hypogonadism of hypothalamic, pituitary, or gonadal origin is often associated with obesity. These defects may be congenital or acquired. Polycystic ovary disease probably falls into this category. Obesity is a feature of a variety of syndromes, including (1) Albright's hereditary osteodystrophy, characterized by a round face, short fourth metacarpal, mental retardation, short stature, and pseudohypoparathyroidism; (2) Alström's syndrome, characterized by nerve deafness, retinal degeneration, short stature, hypogonadotropic hypogonadism, and frequently diabetes mellitus and nephropathy; (3) Laurence-Moon-Biedl syndrome, characterized by deafness, retinitis pigmentosa, mental retardation, polydactylism, hypogonadotropic hypogonadism, and short stature; (4) Prader-Labhart-Willi syndrome, associated with mild diabetes mellitus, congenital hypotonia, mental retardation, delayed developmental milestones, short stature, and hypogonadotropic hypogonadism; (5) Morgagni-Stewart-Morel syndrome, which is a disorder primarily of older women who exhibit virilism and hyperostosis of the frontal bone; and (6) Fröhlich's syndrome, usually characterized by a history of central nervous system infection and/or signs and symptoms of an intracranial tumor or degeneration, hypogonadotropic hypogonadism, and short stature. All these syndromes are rare. Finally, all three known types of triglyceride storage disease are associated with obesity.

Therapy for obesity is difficult, and often ends with less than the desired result. The current forms of therapy include diet, exercise, appetite suppressant drugs, and gastric bypass surgery. Therapy of exogenous obesity that results in significant weight loss returns the endocrine and metabolic abnormalities of obesity toward or to normal. In addition, four of the known atherogenic risk factors—blood pressure, cholesterol, blood glucose, and uric acid—are reduced when a 10 percent or better reduction in body weight is achieved. Consequently, although difficult, therapeutic efforts should not be neglected in true obesity.

1. Bray, G. A. *The Obese Patient*. Philadelphia: W. B. Saunders Co., 1976.
   A readable, comprehensive reference.
2. Hirsch, J., and Batchelor, B. Adipose tissue cellularity in human obesity. *Clin. Endocrinol. Metab.* 5:299, 1976.
   A discussion of hypertrophic and hyperplastic obesity.

3. Abraham, S., Collins, G., and Nordsieck, M. Relationship of childhood weight status to morbidity in adults. *HSMHA Health Rep.* 273, 1971.
   The incidence of hypertension and cardiovascular-renal disease was greatest in persons changing from a normal- or low-weight status to obesity during adolescence or young adult life.

4. Bennion, L. J., and Grundy, S. X. Effects of obesity and caloric intake on biliary lipid metabolism in man. *J. Clin. Invest.* 56:996, 1975.
   Obesity is associated with excessive hepatic secretion of cholesterol and hence supersaturated bile, a potential mechanism for the increased incidence of gallstones.

5. Barnes, H. V., and Berger, R. An approach to the obese adolescent. *Med. Clin. North Am.* 59:1507, 1975.
   A useful summary of the differential diagnosis of obesity in teenagers.

6. Bray, G. A., and Gallagher, T. S. Manifestations of hypothalamic obesity in man: A comprehensive investigation of 8 patients and a review of the literature. *Medicine* 54:301, 1975.
   A well-referenced review. The most common cause is central nervous system malignancy.

7. Bell, J. The Laurence-Moon Syndrome. In L. S. Penrose (ed.), *The Treasury of Human Inheritance.* London: Cambridge University Press, 1958. Vol. 5, p. 468.
   The features of this syndrome are detailed.

8. Goldstein, J. L., and Failkow, P. J. The Alström syndrome: Report of three cases with further delineation of the clinical, pathophysiological and genetic aspects of the disorder. *Medicine* 52:53, 1973.
   All of the patients were obese and had retinal degeneration and nerve deafness.

9. Hall, B. D., and Smith, D. W. Prader-Willi syndrome. *J. Pediatr.* 51:286, 1972.
   All the patients had hypotonia, feeding problems, delayed developmental milestones, and (in males) hypogenitalism.

10. Julkunen, H., Heinonen, O. B., Pyorala, K. Hyperostosis of the spine in an adult population: Its relation to hyperglycemia and obesity. *Ann. Rheum. Dis.* 30:605, 1971.
    A discussion of the Morgagni-Stewart-Morel syndrome.

11. Galton, D. J., Gilbert, C., Reekless, J. P., et al. Triglyceride storage disease: A group of inborn errors of trigylceride metabolism. *Q. J. Med.* 43:63, 1974.
    These disorders are associated with varying degrees of obesity.

12. Wiensier, R. L., Fuchs, R. J., Day, T. D., et al. Body fat: Its relationship to coronary heart disease, blood pressure, lipids and other risk factors measured in a large male population. *Am. J. Med.* 61:815, 1976.
    A careful study that confirms obesity as a minor determinant of blood pressure and serum lipid levels.

13. Olefsky, J. M. Insulin resistance and insulin action: An in vitro and in vivo perspective. *Diabetes* 30:149, 1981.
    An excellent review including the insulin resistance of obesity.

14. DeLuise, M., Blackburn, G. L., and Flier, J. S. Reduced activity of the red-cell sodium-potassium pump in human obesity. *N. Engl. J. Med.* 303:1017, 1980.

15. Mir, M. A., Charalambous, R. M., Morgan, K., et al. Erythrocyte sodium-potassium-ATPase and sodium transport in obesity. *N. Engl. J. Med.* 305:1264, 1981.
    Article 14 suggested a possible pathophysiologic component in obesity, but others (15) found just the opposite. Looks like obesity is still a glandular problem for most, if you include the mouth as a gland.

16. Jimenez, J., Zuniga-Guajardo, S., Zinnian, B., et al. Effects of weight loss in massive obesity on insulin and C-peptide dynamics: Sequential changes in insulin production, clearance, and sensitivity. *J. Clin. Endocrinol. Metab.* 64:661, 1987.
    Glucose, C peptide, and insulin moved to normal with sustained weight loss.

17. Hauner, H., Schmid, P., and Pfeiffer, E. F. Glucocorticoids and insulin promote the differentiation of human adipocyte precursor cells into fat cells. *J. Clin. Endocrinol. Metab.* 64:832, 1987.
    Cortisol may play an important role in human hyperplastic obesity.

18. Truglia, J. A., Livingston, J. N., and Lockwood, D. H. Insulin resistance: Receptor

and post-binding defects in human obesity and non–insulin-dependent diabetes mellitus. *Am. J. Med.* 79:13, 1985.
Cellular changes appear to be at the hepatic insulin receptor and peripherally a post-binding defect.

19. Burke, C. M., Kousseff, B. G., Gleeson, M., et al. Familial Prader-Willi syndrome. *Arch. Intern. Med.* 147:673, 1987.
HLA genotype A2 was present in these adult patients.

20. Wittels, E. H. Obesity and hormonal factors in sleep and sleep apnea. *Med. Clin. North Am.* 69:1265, 1985.

21. Messerli, F. H., Nunez, B. D., Ventura, H. O., et al. Overweight and sudden death: Increased ventricular ectopy in cardiopathy of obesity. *Arch. Intern. Med.* 147:1725, 1987.
Two potential complications of obesity (articles 20, 21).

22. Foster, W. R., and Burton, B. T. (eds.). Health implications of obesity: National Institutes of Health consensus development conference. *Ann. Intern. Med.* 103 (Suppl., pt. 2):983, 1985.
The entire supplement provides concise authoritative discussions of multiple aspects of obesity (coronary artery disease, hypertension, cancer, mortality, "ideal body weight," etc.).

23. Elliot, D. L., Goldberg, L., and Girard, D. E. Obesity: Pathophysiology and practical management. *J. Gen. Intern. Med.* 2:188, 1987.
Concise, clinically useful review.

24. Yost, T. J., and Eckel, R. H. Fat calories may be preferentially stored in reduced-obese women: A permissive pathway for resumption of the obese state. *J. Clin. Endocrinol. Metab.* 67;259, 1988.
Gluteal adipose tissue lipoprotein lipase remained elevated and unresponsive to dietary fat after weight loss, perhaps another reason for the failure with dieting.

25. Ravussin, E., Lillioja, S., Knowler, W. C., et al. Reduced rate of energy expenditures as a risk factor for body-weight gain. *N. Engl. J. Med.* 318:467, 1988.
In some families there appears to be a low rate of energy expenditure.

65. OSTEITIS DEFORMANS (PAGET'S DISEASE)
H. Verdain Barnes

Osteitis deformans, or Paget's disease of bone, is a relatively common radiographic finding that is frequently asymptomatic. The disease begins with an increase in osteoclastic bone resorption followed by an increase in osteoblast activity and the formation of new bone. The rapidity of the process of bone resorption and formation is well documented in quantitative microangiographic studies. As the process proceeds, the collagen matrix of the bone loses its normal pattern. Abnormal bone is formed with increased numbers of arterioles and large venous sinuses, resulting in varying degrees of arteriovenous shunting. Bones stressed by weight develop peculiar angulations whereas unstressed bones may become dramatically enlarged; hence the classic clinical deformities. The exact prevalence is unknown, but several studies confirm a 3 percent prevalence in patients over age 40 years, with a maximum occurrence of 5 to 11 percent by the ninth decade. About 80 percent of cases have their clinical presentation in patients between ages 41 and 70 years. Males predominate about 2:1 in most series. The disease is usually slowly progressive with many newly symptomatic patients having had the condition for over 10 years.

The most common complaint among symptomatic patients is bone pain in about 50 percent. The usual areas of pain are the back, lower extremities, pelvis, and hips. Defective hearing, headaches, and urinary tract complaints occur in about 14 percent. Dyspnea and increasing head size may occur. About 45 percent have neuromuscular signs and symptoms. Cardiovascular findings occur in 30 to 40 percent, with peripheral arterial calcification often a striking feature. About 20 to 40 percent have skull or jaw enlargement and/or bowing of the lower extremities. About 5 percent have a palpable mass in involved areas. The skin overlying extensively involved bone is frequently warmer than the surrounding skin. There is no systemic fever, but the increase in skin temperature in involved areas may be as much as 5°F (2.8°C). The oscillometric pulse pressure may be markedly increased in involved as compared to uninvolved extremities.

The diagnosis and extent of involvement (but not of activity) can usually be made radiographically. Involvement is usually symmetric, with the pelvis diseased in 60 percent; skull, vertebral column, and femur in about 40 percent; followed in order by the tibia, humerus, scapula, clavicle, ribs, and mandible. Three types of changes can be seen: osteolytic, sclerotic, or a mixture of the two. There is often a V-shaped lytic edge in long bones. Incomplete or complete pathologic fractures are frequently seen. The usual radiographic findings consist of an irregular woolly-appearing cortical thickening, coarse trabeculae, and deformity. At times these findings must be differentiated from those of osteitis fibrosa cystica and primary or metastatic bone malignancy.

The activity of the disease is difficult to assess. The best current measures are the serum alkaline phosphatase (AP) and urinary hydroxyproline (UHP). The highest levels of AP are recorded in this disease. With increasing disease activity, the AP level rises to a plateau. With sarcomatous change, there is usually no change or a slight decrease in AP values. The level of total UHP correlates well with AP values. These measurements indicate rapid bone turnover and are not specific for Paget's disease. With severe disease, the acid phosphatase may also be elevated. The uptake of radioactive calcium is markedly increased and can be useful in determining the degree of activity. The most promising new techniques for assessing disease activity and bone response to therapy are the bone scintiscan with technetium 99m etidronate (EHDP) and, perhaps, the measurement of osteocalcin by radioimmunoassay. This specific bone protein is elevated in Paget's disease.

The major complications of this abiotrophy of the bone's collagen matrix are sarcomatous degeneration, spinal cord compression, and high output congestive heart failure with or without associated heart block. The incidence of osteosarcomas is about 0.2 percent; when present, 20 percent are multicentric. Vertebral collapse and spinal cord compression are medical emergencies, and rapid surgical decompression may prevent permanent paralysis. Platybasia may also occur, for which surgery may be successful. High output congestive heart failure usually does not occur until 35 percent or more of the skeleton is involved with active disease. Cardiac calcifications are not uncommon and have been reported to involve the aortic or mitral valves or the interventricular septum. Complete heart block with calcification in the bundle of His has been reported. Other complications include malabsorption leading to folic acid deficiency. Hypercalcemia is a rare finding in immobilized patients. Deafness is a relatively common finding; it is usually neural but may be conductive. Finally, there appears to be an increase in the incidence of gout in patients with Paget's disease.

Therapy should be offered to patients with incapacitating bone pain, progressive disease with recurrent fractures or deformity, hypercalciuria with or without hypercalcemia, or congestive heart failure.

1. Paget, J. On a form of chronic inflammation of bones (osteitis deformans). *Med. Chir. Trans.* 60:37, 1877.
   A delightful and thorough clinical discussion.
2. Alvioli, L. V., and Krane, S. M. (eds.). *Metabolic Bone Disease.* New York: Academic Press, 1977. Vol. 1.
   A good general reference.
3. Woodhouse, N. J. Paget's disease of bone. *J. Clin. Endocrinol. Metab.* 1:125, 1972.
   A brief review.
4. Nagant de Deuxchaisnes, C., and Krane, S. M. Paget's disease of bone: Clinical and metabolic observations. *Medicine* 43:233, 1964.
   Alkaline phosphatase and urinary hydroxyproline levels and radioactive calcium turnover rate can be used to determine activity.

5. Poretta, C. A., Dahlin, D. C., and Janes, J. M. Sarcoma in Paget's disease of bone. *J. Bone Joint Surg.* [Am.] 39:1313, 1957.
   20% of the sarcomas are multicentric, and the prognosis is poor.
6. Finneson, B. E., Goluloff, B., and Shenkin, H. A. Sarcomatous degeneration of osteitis deformans causing compression of the cauda equina. *Neurology* 8:82, 1958.
   An uncommon but feared complication.
7. Teng, P., Gross, S. W., and Newman, C. M. Compression of the spinal cord by osteitis deformans (Paget's disease), giant cell tumor and polyostotic fibrous dysplasia (Albright's syndrome) of vertebrae. *J. Neurosurg.* 8:482, 1951.
   A good review of cord compression with and without sarcomatous degeneration.
8. Edholm, O. G., Howarth, S., and McMichael, J. Heart failure and blood flow in osteitis deformans. *Clin. Sci.* 5:249, 1945.
   The cardiac output in the patient described was 13.3 liters per minute.
9. King, M., Huang, J. M., and Glassman, E. Paget's disease with cardiac calcification and complete heart block. *Am. J. Med.* 46:302, 1969.
   The mitral and aortic valves and interventricular septum can be calcified.
10. Sparrow, N. L., and Duvall, A. J. Hearing loss and Paget's disease. *J. Laryngol. Otol.* 81:601, 1967.
    Nerve and/or conduction deafness can be seen.
11. Somayaji, B. N. Malabsorption syndrome in Paget's disease of bone. *Br. Med. J.* 4:278, 1968.
    All had steatorrhea and folate deficiency.
12. Vellegna, C. J. L. R., Pannels, E. K. J., Bijvoet, O. L. M., et al. Evaluation of scintigraphic and roentgenologic studies in Paget's disease under treatment. *Radiol. Clin.* (Basel) 45:292, 1976.
    Technetium 99m EHDP bone scans showed improvement during therapy. A promising new technique.
13. Deftos, L. J., and First, B. P. Calcitonin as a drug. *Ann. Intern. Med.* 95:192, 1981.
    A brief update on therapy with this 32-amino acid peptide hormone.
14. Lluberas-Acosta, G., Hansell, J. R., and Schumacher, R., Jr. Paget's disease of bone in patients with gout. *Arch. Intern. Med.* 146:2389, 1986.
    There appears to be an increased incidence of gout in Paget's patients and an increased incidence of Paget's disease in gout patients.
15. Papapoulos, S. E., Frolich, M., Mudde, A. H., et al. Serum osteocalcin in Paget's disease of bone: Basal concentrations and response to bisphosphonate treatment. *J. Clin. Endocrinol. Metab.* 65:89, 1987.
16. Wilkinson, M. R., Wagstaffe, C., Delbridge, L., et al. Serum osteocalcin concentrations in Paget's disease of bone. *Arch. Intern. Med.* 146:268, 1986.
    Some have found it useful in assessing the activity of Paget's disease (article 16) and some have not (article 15).

66. PHEOCHROMOCYTOMA

H. Verdain Barnes

Pheochromocytoma is a rare tumor of the chromaffin cells, usually of the adrenal medulla. In the vast majority of cases the disease is associated with hypertension, although it is rare among the causes of hypertension, accounting for less than 1 percent of cases in adults. The majority of the tumors produce predominantly norepinephrine, but occasionally epinephrine predominates. Embryologically, chromaffin cells arise from the sympathetic nerve cell precursors of the neural crest and tube. These cells migrate and aggregate along with the cells of the sympathetic nervous system. Aggregations of these cells, therefore, can be found from the neck to the gonads in areas where there are sympathetic nerve plexuses. Pheochromocytomas have been reported in association with the carotid body; the paravertebral sympathetic chains in the cervical, dorsal, and lumbrosacral areas; the periaortic, kidney, bladder, pelvic, prostatic, and gonadal sympathetic plexuses; and the organ of Zuckerkandl.

The classic paroxysmal clinical triad of headache, palpitations, and hyperhydrosis occurs in less than 75 percent of patients. At least 90 percent have hypertension, but in the majority it is sustained rather than paroxysmal. The other major signs and symptoms in decreasing order of frequency are orthostatic hypotension, nausea with or without vomiting, weight loss, visual disturbances, abdominal pain, polyuria and polydipsia, seizures, chest pain, dyspnea, and flushing or warmth. Pheochromocytomas are frequently diagnosed incorrectly as essential hypertension, hyperthyroidism, biliary colic, pancreatitis, carcinoid, diabetes mellitus, myocardial infarction, brain tumor, psychoneurosis, adrenal insufficiency, acute intermittent porphyria, pulmonary embolism, toxemia of pregnancy, and idiopathic seizure disorders. There is a familial tendency. The pattern of inheritance is autosomal dominant with high penetrance. The tumors are commonly seen in association with neurofibromatosis, cerebellar and retinal hemangioblastomatosis, and multiple endocrine neoplasia types II and III.

The diagnosis of a pheochromocytoma can almost invariably be made by the use of the laboratory, drug suppression testing, and medical imaging. The sensitivity and specificity of commonly used tests are plasma norepinephrine (NE) and epinephrine (E) after clonidine suppression—sensitivity 0.97 and specificity 0.99; plasma NE and E—0.94 and 0.97; 24-hour urine metanephrines—0.79 and 0.93; and 24-hour urine vanillymandelic acid (VMA)—0.42 and 1.00. Recently the combined measurement of NE and 3,4-dihydroxyphenylglycol in urine and plasma has been reported to have a sensitivity of 1.00 and 0.82 and a specificity of 0.98 and 0.95, respectively. Computed tomography (CT) of the adrenals with and without accompanying scintigraphy (radioactive iodobenzylguanidine) as well as scintigraphy alone have been reported with high sensitivity and specificity in the diagnosis of pheochomocytoma. Provocative tests (histamine, glucagon, tyramine, and phentolamine) are outmoded and should not be used. It should be noted, however, that other tumors of neural crest origin can produce excess levels of catecholamines and their metabolites. Determination of the urinary homovanillic acid and/or dopamine levels may be of differential help because the levels are frequently elevated by neuroblastomas and ganglioblastomas and almost never with a pheochromocytoma. The procedure used to measure VMA is critical. The colorimetric VMA determination is of no clinical value and should not be used. A chromatographic VMA level, however, can be falsely lowered by monoamine oxidase inhibitors and clofibrate, and it can be spuriously increased by nalidixic acid. Total metanephrine levels can be falsely decreased by monoamine oxidase inhibitors. For initial screening a single voided or overnight urine sample for total metanephrines is probably adequate in most cases. However, if the clinical suspicion is high, full evaluation using several diagnostic methods is needed.

Once the biochemical diagnosis is made, a localization search is imperative since approximately 50 percent of the tumors are bilateral or extraadrenal. The initial evaluation should be noninvasive by CT and scintigraphy. If these are not revealing, an arteriogram can be done after alpha blockade. The arteriographic findings include (1) a fine reticular pattern of the small arteries in the tumor, (2) a homogeneous pattern with distinct borders in the capillary phase, and (3) a venous-phase tumor blush, occasionally with a central radiolucency. These findings are strongly suggestive of pheochromocytoma, but can be seen with other tumors, primarily those of sympathetic origin or a hibernoma. Venous catheterization has also been used to localize tumor areas.

The therapy of choice for pheochromocytoma is surgical removal. Plasma volume is significantly decreased in approximately two-thirds of the patients and should be replaced before surgery. Recent evidence strongly supports the efficacy of several days of alpha-adrenergic blockade prior to surgery to lower operative and postoperative morbidity and mortality. Beta-adrenergic blockade may also be required if there is a significant production and release of epinephrine by the tumor. Today, with these measures the operative and postoperative mortality is less than 15 percent as compared to approximately 50 percent in previous decades.

1. Page, B., and Copeland, R. B. Pheochromocytoma. *D. M.* 1:1, 1968.
   A careful and complete review.
2. Stackpole, R. H., Melicow, M. M., and Uson, A. C. Pheochromocytoma in children:

Report of 9 cases and review of the first 100 published cases with follow-up studies. *J. Pediatr.* 63:315, 1963.
The presentation is essentially the same as in adults, but extraadrenal and multiple tumors are more common.

3. Garcia, R., and Jennings, J. M. Pheochromocytoma masquerading as a cardiomyopathy. *Lancet* 2:126, 1962.
4. Fred, H. L., Allred, D. P., Graber, H. E., et al. Pheochromocytoma masquerading as overwhelming infection. *Am. Heart J.* 73:149, 1967.
Self-explanatory articles (3,4).
5. Page, L. B., Raker, J. W., and Berberich, F. R. Pheochromocytoma with predominant epinephrine secretion. *Am. J. Med.* 47:648, 1969.
Epinephrine can predominate, leading to a clinical picture of excess beta-adrenergic stimulation.
6. Rossi, P., Young, I. S., and Panke, W. F. Techniques, usefulness, and hazards of arteriography of pheochromocytoma: Review of 99 cases. *J.A.M.A.* 205:547, 1968.
Mortality and morbidity can be prevented by prestudy preparation with alpha blockade.
7. Leiphart, C. J., and Nudelman, E. J. Hibernoma masquerading as a pheochromocytoma: A case report. *Radiology* 95:659, 1970.
Arteriography can be misleading.
8. Rashid, M., Khairi, A., Dexter, R. N., et al. Mucosal neuroma, pheochromocytoma and medullary thyroid carcinoma: Multiple endocrine neoplasia, type 3. *Medicine* 54:89, 1975.
The features of multiple endocrine neoplasia.
9. Taubman, I., Pearson, O. H., and Anton, A. H. An asymptomatic catecholamine-secreting pheochromocytoma. *Am. J. Med.* 57:953, 1974.
Almost certainly a rare phenomenon.
10. Cryer, P. E., and Kissane, J. M. (eds.). Metastatic catecholamine-secreting paraganglioma (extra-adrenal pheochromocytoma). *Am. J. Med.* 61:523, 1976.
A good clinicopathologic conference discussion and bibliography.
11. Kaplan, N. M., Kramer, N. J., Holland, O. B., et al. Single-voided urine metanephrine assays in screening for pheochromocytoma. *Arch. Intern. Med.* 137:190, 1977.
Certainly less trouble for the patient.
12. Atuk, N. O., McDonald, T., Wood, T., et al. Familial pheochromocytoma, hypercalcemia, and Von Hippel-Lindau disease. *Medicine* 58:209, 1979.
13. Lips, K. J. M., Van Der Sluys Veer, J. A. A. P., Struynenberg, A., et al. Bilateral occurrence of pheochromocytoma with the multiple endocrine neoplasia syndrome type 2A (Sipple's syndrome). *Am. J. Med.* 70:1051, 1981.
14. Lips, K. J. M., Minder, W. H., Leo, J. R., et al. Evidence of multicentric origin of the multiple Endocrine Neoplasia Syndrome Type 2A (Sipple's syndrome) in a large family in the Netherlands. *Am. J. Med.* 64:569, 1978.
Genetic associations in articles 12–14.
15. Yanase, T., Nawata, H., Kato, K.-I., et al. Studies of adrenorphin in pheochromocytoma. *J. Clin. Endocrinol. Metab.* 64:692, 1987.
Adrenorphin may play an important role in modulating the secretion of catecholamines from pheochromocytomas.
16. Familial extra-adrenal pheochromocytoma: A new syndrome. *Arch. Intern. Med.* 145:257, 1985.
Genetics may determine the site of the pheochromocytoma in some patients.
17. Kullberg, B. J., and Kruseman, A. C. N. Multiple endocrine neoplasia type 2b with a good prognosis. *Arch. Intern. Med.* 147:1125, 1987.
Some type 2b's have as good a prognosis as type 2a's.
18. Chatal, J. F., and Charbonnel, B. Comparison of iodobenzylguanidine imaging with computed tomography in locating pheochromocytoma. *J. Clin. Endocrinol. Metab.* 61:769, 1985.
19. Bravo, E. L., and Gifford, R. W., Jr. Pheochromocytoma: Diagnosis, localization and management. *N. Engl. J. Med.* 311:1298, 1984.
20. Sheps, S. G., Jiang, N.-S., and Klee, G. C. Diagnostic evaluation of pheochromocytoma. *Endocrinol. Metab. Clin. North Am.* 17:397, 1988.

21. Duncan, M. W., Compton, P., Lazarus, L., et al. Measurement of norepinephrine and 3,4-dihydroxyphenylglycol in urine and plasma for the diagnosis of pheochromocytoma. *N. Engl. J. Med.* 319:136, 1988.
   The four articles (18–21) provide an up-to-date discussion of diagnosis.
22. Taylor, H. C., Mayes, D., and Auton, A. H. Clonidine suppression test for pheochromocytoma: Examples of misleading results. *J. Clin. Endocrinol. Metab.* 63:238, 1986.
   No test is perfect, a good reminder for clinicians.
23. Sloand, E. M., and Thompson, T. Propranolol-induced pulmonary edema and shock in a patient with pheochromocytoma. *Arch. Intern. Med.* 144:173, 1984.
24. Goldbaum, T. S., Henochowicz, S., Mustafa, M., et al. Pheochromocytoma presenting with Prinzmetal's angina. *Am. J. Med.* 81:921, 1986.
   Two good reasons (articles 23, 24) to beware of beta blockade in pheochromocytoma patients.
25. Borneman, M., Hill, S. C., and Kidd, G. S., II. Lactic acidosis in pheochromocytoma. *Ann. Intern. Med.* 105:880, 1986.
26. Kunchel, O., Buu, N. T., Larochelle, P., et al. Episodic dopamine discharge in paroxysmal hypertension: Page's syndrome revisited. *Arch. Intern. Med.* 146:1315, 1986.
   Two disorders (articles 25, 26) to add to your differential diagnosis of pheochromocytoma.
27. Ram, C. V. S., Meese, R., and Hill, S. C. Failure of alpha-methyltyrosine to prevent hypertensive crisis in pheochromocytoma. *Arch. Intern. Med.* 145:2114, 1985.
   This inhibitor of tyrosine hydroxylation may be as useful as predicted.
28. Shulkin, B. L., Shapiro, B., and Sisson, J. C. Pheochromocytoma, polycythemia and venous thrombosis. *Am. J. Med.* 83:773, 1987.
29. Hodgson, S. F., Sheps, S. G., Subramanian, R., et al. Catecholamine-secreting paraganglioma of the interstitial septum. *Am. J. Med.* 77:157, 1984.
   Two (articles 28, 29) rare presentations of pheochromocytomas.

67. PRIMARY HYPERPARATHYROIDISM
H. Verdain Barnes

Primary hyperparathyroidism results from an excess production and release of parathyroid hormone by an abnormally functioning parathyroid gland. Pathologically there are four types: (1) parathyroid adenoma, (2) primary chief cell hyperplasia, (3) primary water-clear cell hyperplasia, and (4) parathyroid carcinoma. Histologically a single hyperplastic gland is indistinguishable from an adenoma. A presumptive diagnosis of hyperplasia can be made, however, if three or more parathyroid glands are grossly enlarged. By electron microscopy both the adenoma and primary chief cell hyperplasia have increased numbers of secretory granules, whereas in secondary hyperplasia the number of granules is decreased. Primary water-clear cell hyperplasia is distinctly different by both light and electron microscopy. Parathyroid carcinoma is rare and can usually be identified grossly or microscopically. Excess circulating parathyroid hormone (PTH) almost invariably results in hypercalcemia and hypophosphatemia. PTH increases the urinary excretion of phosphate, decreases the urinary excretion of calcium, accelerates bone demineralization, and increases intestinal tract absorption of calcium. Although PTH decreases the urinary excretion of calcium by increasing the proportion of calcium reabsorbed by the renal tubules, a net calcium loss in the urine occurs when the load of calcium filtered is increased, hence the typical hypercalciuria seen in patients with primary hyperparathyroidism and normal renal function. Severe renal impairment, on the other hand, results in a decreased excretion of calcium regardless of the level of serum calcium.

Regardless of the underlying pathology, the clinical presentation is protean. There may be no early manifestations of hypercalcemia or the patient may have anorexia, thirst, polyuria, perioral and/or peripheral paresthesias, easy fatigue, diminished ability to concentrate, pruritus, and/or the signs and symptoms of urolithiasis or peptic ulcer disease. In most series the incidence of renal calculi is from 50 to 75 percent and peptic ulcer in about 10 percent in symptomatic patients. Later manifestations include nausea, vomiting, constipation, muscle weakness, weight loss, hypertension, drowsiness, stupor, bone pain, anemia, and, on occasion, ectopic calcification in the renal parenchyma, sclerae, conjunctivae, joint capsules, tendons, lungs, and subcutaneous tissue. A rare patient develops cortical blindness, fever of unknown origin, nephrotic syndrome, or seizures. Muscle weakness and pain due to hypotonia may be prominent features and precede other manifestations of the disease. Weakness and/or paresis usually involves the proximal muscles. Electromyographic and muscle biopsy findings are those of a nonspecific myopathy. Bone changes are secondary to bone resorption and are usually seen in patients with a shorter history, larger tumor, and higher calcium level. The initial changes have been described as a moth-eaten appearance most commonly seen in the hands, skull, and acromioclavicular joints. In untreated disease, bone cysts may develop and are typically found in the hands, feet, pelvis, ribs, and occasionally in the jaw. With long-standing disease, vertebral decalcification can lead to compression fractures and marked kyphoscoliosis. A rare patient has osteosclerosis.

A few patients will experience a rapid rise in serum calcium, hyperparathyroid crisis, or storm. In the reported cases the calcium values range from 15 to 26.3 mg/dl with an average of about 17. The majority of patients are in the fifth or sixth decade of life, are occasionally refractory to conventional forms of therapy for hypercalcemia, and have parathyroid adenomas at surgery. Early diagnosis and parathyroid surgery can be critical to survival.

The basic chemical features of primary hyperparathyroidism are discussed in the chapter on hypercalcemia. One point, however, is worth reemphasis—when an elevated calcium level is found or the disease is suspected, repeated serum calcium determinations should be done. A variety of tests are available to help substantiate the diagnosis, but none is ideal. Several studies have assessed the usefulness of a broad spectrum of tests to separate hyperparathyroidism from other causes of hypercalcemia. The tests identified of greatest value in discrimination are the serum calcium, chloride, phosphorus, albumin, cholesterol, alkaline phosphatase, PTH–carboxy-terminal, chloride-phosphate ratio, and hematocrit. Discriminant analysis found albumin, PTH, and chloride to correctly identify 94 percent while in another study serum calcium, chloride, and hematocrit provided a 98 percent degree of accuracy. Nonetheless, incorrect diagnosis by these parameters remains a problem for the clinician. Recent measurements of intact human PTH (1–84), however, appear to hold greater promise for specificity and sensitivity in the diagnosis of parathyroid disease. Enlarged parathyroid gland localization by ultrasound along with thin-needle aspiration biopsy for immunocytochemistry may also prove useful. Both require further evaluation.

A rare patient with primary hyperparathyroidism presents with normocalcemia, has a familial form of the disease, or has multiple endocrine neoplasia type I or II. A wide variety of tumor groupings can be seen in multiple endocrine adenomatosis; the most commonly associated groups are (1) pituitary, pancreatic islet cell, and parathyroid adenoma, and (2) pheochromocytoma, medullary thyroid carcinoma, and parathyroid hyperplasia. The possibility of a pluriglandular syndrome should be considered when primary hyperparathyroidism is the diagnosis.

1. Albright, F. A., Aub, J. C., and Bauer, W. Hyperparathyroidism. *J.A.M.A.* 102:1276, 1934.
   A classic article identifying the protean nature of the disease.
2. Mallette, L. E., Bilezikian, J. P., Heath, D. A., et al. Primary hyperparathyroidism: Clinical and biochemical features. *Medicine* 53:127, 1974.
   An excellent, well-referenced review.
3. Roth, S. I. Recent advances in parathyroid gland pathology. *Am. J. Med.* 50:612, 1971.
   Chief cell secretory granules are increased in primary hyperparathyroidism (HPT).

4. Nathaniels, E. K., Nathaniels, A. M., and Wang, C. Mediastinal parathyroid tumors: A clinical and pathologic study of 84 cases. *Ann. Surg.* 171:165, 1970.
   21% of tumors are ectopic, usually located in the mediastinum.
5. Lloyd, H. M. Primary hyperparathyroidism: An analysis of the role of the parathyroid tumor. *Medicine* 47:53, 1968.
   Patients with bone disease have a shorter history, higher calcium level, and larger tumor than those presenting with urolithiasis.
6. Bischoff, A., and Esslen, E. Myopathy with primary hyperparathyroidism. *Neurology* 15:64, 1965.
   The myopathy may dominate the picture.
7. Purnell, D. C., Smith, L. H., Scholz, D. A., et al. Primary hyperparathyroidism: A prospective clinical study. *Am. J. Med.* 50:670, 1971.
   13.8% of the initially asymptomatic patients required surgery in the first 30 months of the study.
8. Males, J. L., Howard, W. J., Mask, D. R., et al. Primary hyperparathyroidism presenting as a giant cell tumor of the maxilla. *Arch. Intern. Med.* 32:107, 1973.
9. Ehrig, U., and Wilson, D. R. Fibrous dysplasia of bone and primary hyperparathyroidism. *Ann. Intern. Med.* 77:234, 1972.
10. Lomnitz, E., Sepulveda, L., Stevenson, C., et al. Primary hyperparathyroidism simulating rickets. *J. Clin. Endocrinol. Metab.* 26:309, 1966.
11. Genant, H. K., Baron, J. J., Straus, F. H., et al. Osteosclerosis in primary hyperparathyroidism. *Am. J. Med.* 59:104, 1975.
12. Spiegel, A. M., Marx, S. J., Doppman, J. L., et al. Intrathyroidal parathyroid adenoma or hyperplasia: An occasionally overlooked cause of surgical failure in primary hyperparathyroidism. *J.A.M.A.* 234:1029, 1975.
13. Kosinski, K., Roth, S. I., and Chapman, E. H. Primary hyperparathyroidism with 31 years of hypercalcemia. *J.A.M.A.* 236:590, 1976.
   A variety of clinical presentations in this protean disease (articles 8–13).
14. Winnacker, J. L., Becker, K. L., Friedlander, M., et al. Sarcoidosis and hyperparathyroidism. *Am. J. Med.* 46:305, 1969.
   They may occur together.
15. Brown, E. M., Gardner, D. G., Brennan, M. F., et al. Calcium-regulated parathyroid hormone release in primary hyperparathyroidism: Studies in vitro with dispersed parathyroid cells. *Am. J. Med.* 66:923, 1979.
   There appears to be heterogeneous responsiveness to calcium ranging from an elevated set point for response to true autonomous function.
16. Marx, S. J., Stock J. L., Attie, M. F., et al. Familial hypocalciuric hypercalcemia: Recognition among patients referred after unsuccessful parathyroid exploration. *Ann. Intern. Med.* 92:351, 1980.
   Keep this entity in mind before surgery—the family history is key—a calcium creatinine clearance ratio may help in diagnosis.
17. Schnur, M. J., Appel, G. B., and Bilezikian, J. P. Primary hyperparathyroidism and benign monoclonal gammopathy. *Arch. Intern. Med.* 137:1201, 1977.
18. Cohen, A. M., Maxon, H. R., Goldsmith, R. E., et al. Metastatic pulmonary calcification in primary hyperparathyroidism. *Arch. Intern. Med.* 137:520, 1977.
19. Boxer, M., Ellman, L., Geller, R., et al. Anemia in primary hyperparathyroidism. *Arch. Intern. Med.* 137:588, 1977.
   Some (17–19) presentations to remember.
20. Christensson, T., Hellström, K., and Wengle, B. Hypercalcemia and primary hyperparathyroidism: Prevalence in patients receiving thiazides as detected in a health screen. *Arch. Intern. Med.* 137:1138, 1977.
   14 of the 21 patients discovered had parathyroid adenomas.
21. Bayat-Mokhtari, F., Palmieri, G. M. A., Moinuddin, M., et al. Parathyroid storm. *Arch. Intern. Med.* 140:1092, 1980.
   The runaway parathyroid, a life-threatening entity, not to be overlooked, especially in elderly women.
22. Scholz, D. A., and Purnell, D. C. Asymptomatic primary hyperparathyroidism: 10-year prospective study. *Mayo Clin. Proc.* 56:473, 1981.
   A well-done study, but no definitive answer as to who should have early surgery.

23. Roberts, W. C., and Waller, B. F. Effect of hypercalcemia on the heart: An analysis of 18 necropsy patients. *Am. J. Med.* 71:371, 1981.
   Calcification was common, perhaps another reason for not postponing surgery.
24. Lafferty, F. W. Primary hyperparathyroidism. *Arch. Intern. Med.* 141:1761, 1981.
   A concise review and a discriminant analysis of serum chloride, calcium, PTH, and hematocrit levels.
25. Stepan, J. J., Preel, J., Brovlik, P., et al. Serum osteocalcin levels and bone alkaline phosphatase isoenzyme after oophorectomy and in primary hyperparathyroidism. *J. Clin. Endocrinol. Metab.* 64:1079, 1987.
   Osteocalcin and bone alkaline phosphatase isoenzyme were typically elevated in primary hyperparathyroidism.
26. Cantley, L. K., Ontjes, D. A., Cooper, C. W., et al. Parathyroid hormone secretion from dispersed human hyperparathyroid cells: Increased secretion in cells from hyperplastic glands versus adenomas. *J. Clin. Endocrinol. Metab.* 60:1032, 1985.
   Adenomas had an increase in absolute cell number but secreted less PTH in vitro.
27. Diamond, T. W., Botha, J. R., Wing, J., et al. Parathyroid hypertension: A reversible disorder. *Arch. Intern. Med.* 146:1709, 1986.
   Prevalence of hypertension preoperatively was 47%; substantial decreases in mean systolic and diastolic blood pressure occurred in only 54% postoperatively.
28. Martin, P., Bergmann, P., Gillet, C., et al. Partially reversible osteopenia after surgery for primary hyperparathyroidism. *Arch. Intern. Med.* 146:689, 1986.
   Osteopenia was found in both cortical and trabecular bone and neither returned to normal after cure.
29. Fellner, S. K., and Spargo, B. H. Nephrotic syndrome from hypercalcemia in a patient with primary hyperparathyroidism. *Am. J. Med.* 83:355, 1987.
30. Firth, R. G., Grant, C. S., and Riggs, B. L. Development of hypercalcemic hyperparathyroidism after long-term phosphate supplementation in hypophosphatemic osteomalacia. *Am. J. Med.* 78:669, 1985.
31. Sherrard, D. J., Oh, S. M., and Andress, D. L. Pseudohyperparathyroidism: Syndrome associated with aluminum intoxication in patients with renal failure. *Am. J. Med.* 79:127, 1985.
   Some disorders to include in your differential diagnosis (articles 29–31).
32. Boyd, J. C., and Ladenson, J. H. Value of laboratory tests in the differential diagnosis of hypercalcemia. *Am. J. Med.* 77:863, 1984.
   This article differs from article 25 as to which are the most discriminating tests— here albumin, chloride, and PTH.
33. Hackeng, W. H. L., Lips, P., Neterleubos, J. C., et al. Clinical implications of estimation of intact parathyroid hormone (PTH) vs total immunoreactive PTH in normal subjects and hyperparathyroid patients. *J. Clin. Endocrinol. Metab.* 63:447, 1986.
   The two-step human PTH (1–84) assay had more sensitivity and specificity than most regional PTH assays.
34. Mallette, L. E., Malini, S., Rappaport, M. P., et al. Familial cystic parathyroid adenomatosis. *Ann. Intern. Med.* 107:54, 1987.
   A rare form of familial hyperparathyroidism.
35. Winzelberg, G. G. Parathyroid imaging. *Ann. Intern. Med.* 107:64, 1987.
   A good review of computed tomography, high-resolution ultrasound, and thallium 201–technetium 99m subtraction scanning in parathyroid disease diagnosis.
36. Gutekunst, R., Valesky, A. V., Borisch, B., et al. Parathyroid localization. *J. Clin. Endocrinol. Metab.* 63:1390, 1986.
   A potentially promising technique using thin-needle aspiration and immunocytochemistry.
37. Marx, S. J., Vinik, A. I., Sanetn, R. J., et al. Multiple endocrine neoplasia type I: Assessment of laboratory tests to screen for the gene in a large kindred. *Medicine* 65:226, 1986.
   The most common expression of the MEN I gene was primary hyperparathyroidism found in close to 100% by the age of 40 years.
38. Marx, S. J., Fraser, D., and Rapoport, A. Familial hypocalciuric hypercalcemia: Mild

expression of the gene in heterozygotes and severe expression in homozygotes. *Am. J. Med.* 78:15, 1985.
Homozygotes may have severe neonatal primary hyperparathyroidism.
39. Blind, E., Schmidt-Gayk, H., Scharla, S., et al. Two-site assay of intact parathyroid hormone in the investigation of primary hyperparathyroidism and other disorders of calcium metabolism compared with a midregion assay. *J. Clin. Endocrinol. Metab.* 67:353, 1988.
The two-site assay provided the best discrimination for diagnosis.
40. Fitzpatrick, L. A., and Bilezikian, J. P. Acute primary hyperparathyroidism. *Am. J. Med.* 82:275, 1987.
Parathyroid hormone levels were often 20 times normal, 53% had bone and 69% had renal involvement.
41. Palmer, M., Ljunghall, S., Akerstrom, G., et al. Patients with primary hyperparathyroidism operated on over a 24-year period: Temporal trends of clinical and laboratory findings. *J. Chronic Dis.* 40:121, 1987.
Often the signs and symptoms are not classic, especially in older women.

68. RENAL GLYCOSURIA
H. Verdain Barnes

True renal glycosuria (RG) is a rare disorder. The most useful criteria for diagnosis are (1) glycosuria when the blood glucose level is normal (2) glucose in essentially all urine specimens, including the one after an overnight fast, (3) glucose alone inappropriately excreted by the kidney, (4) a normal or slightly flattened oral glucose tolerance curve, and (5) evidence of normal carbohydrate storage and utilization.

Two primary types of RG are known: (1) Type A patients have a low renal threshold and a low level of maximum tubular reabsorption (Tm) for glucose. (2) Type B patients exhibit an exaggerated splay of the renal glucose titration curve, a low renal threshold, and a normal Tm for glucose. The inheritance pattern varies. In some families inheritance appears to be autosomal dominant, and in others autosomal recessive. Both types of RG have been described in the same pedigree, suggesting a degree of genetic heterogeneity. The pathogenetic mechanism for type A appears to be a decreased number of glucose carriers with a normal affinity for glucose. Type B, on the other hand, appears to have a decreased affinity for glucose, but a normal number of carriers. Histologic studies have shown no distinctive structural abnormalities of the kidney, although one study reported nonspecific cellular changes of the proximal convoluted tubules in some patients.

Clinically, RG patients are essentially asymptomatic, although some offer nonspecific complaints, such as easy fatigability and lassitude. Most patients are discovered to have the disease during the second decade of life. Females predominate in most series. Although the course of RG is typically benign, it should be recognized that ketosis and dehydration may develop during starvation or pregnancy. There is no evidence that growth and development are affected even though the excretion of glucose may exceed 100 gm per 24 hours. Using the above criteria, diabetes mellitus during long-term follow-up is no more frequent in RG patients than it is in the general population. However, when less demanding criteria are used, the incidence has been reported to be as high as 63 percent. Consequently, if the less stringent criteria of Lawrence are used for diagnosis, the patient with minimum criteria for diagnosis should be followed closely for the development of true diabetes mellitus. Based on the stricter criteria, the prognosis for a normal life-style and life span in RG is good.

The differential diagnoses of unqualified normoglycemic glycosuria should be kept in mind. These include Fanconi's syndrome, glucoglycinuria, diabetes mellitus, glucose/

galactose malabsorption, and a variety of drug, chemical, or poison exposures or excesses such as those related to phlorhizin, chromium, mercury, uranium, lead, cadmium, lithium, curare, carbon monoxide, caffeine, morphine, strychnine, and chloroform.

1. Krane, S. M. Renal Glycosuria. In J. B. Stanbury, J. B. Wyngaarden, and D. F. Fredrickson (eds.), *The Metabolic Bases of Inherited Disease.* New York: McGraw-Hill, 1982. P. 1536.
   The most comprehensive discussion available.
2. Marble, A. Non-Diabetic Melituria. In A. Marble, P. White, R. A. Bradley, et al. (eds.), *Joslin's Diabetes Mellitus.* Philadelphia: Lea & Febiger, 1971. P. 218.
   If these authors' strict criteria are used, RG is rare.
3. Elsas, L. J., and Rosenberg, L. E. Familial renal glycosuria: A genetic reappraisal of hexose transport by kidney and intestine. *J. Clin. Invest.* 48:1845, 1969.
   This article defines the two primary types of RG.
4. Hjarne, V. A. A study of the orthoglycaemic glycosuria with particular reference to its hereditability. *Acta Med. Scand.* 67:422, 1927.
   In this family, the apparent inheritance pattern was autosomal dominant.
5. Monasterio, B., Oliver, J., Muiesan, G., et al. Renal diabetes as a congenital tubular dysplasia. *Am. J. Med.* 37:44, 1964.
   These authors report the presence of nonspecific histologic changes in the proximal convoluted tubules of two patients with RG.
6. Marble, A., Josli, E. P., Dublin, L. I., et al. Studies in diabetes mellitus VII, non-diabetic glycosuria. *Am. J. Med. Sci.* 197:533, 1939.
   Using strict criteria, the incidence of diabetes mellitus is no greater than in the general population.
7. McPhaul, J. J., and Simonaitis, J. J. Observations on the mechanisms of glycosuria during glucose loads in normal and diabetic subjects. *J. Clin. Invest.* 47:702, 1968.
   The normal renal glucose Tm is 325 ± 36 mg/minute/1.73 sq m body surface.
8. Defronzo, R. A., and Thier, S. O. Inherited tubule disorders. *Hosp. Pract.* 17:111, 1982.
   A concise review of renal tubule disorders.

69. SYNDROME OF INAPPROPRIATE ANTIDIURETIC HORMONE
H. Verdain Barnes

The syndrome of inappropriate antidiuretic hormone (SIADH) is clinically suspected when hyponatremia is encountered. Hyponatremia is seen in patients who are hypervolemic (type I), hypovolemic (type II), and normovolemic (type III). SIADH is a type III disorder which has several subsets: (1) wide erratic fluctuations in arginine vasopressin (ADH) that appear to be unrelated to the normal osmotic control mechanisms; (2) ADH release that appears to correlate with plasma osmolality but with a low osmotic threshold, that is, a resetting of the osmostat; and (3) a nonsuppressible release of ADH which can result from the supraoptic-hypophyseal system, ectopic production, and release of an ADH or ADH-like substance from cells, usually neoplastic, or a pseudo-ADH excess where the action of ADH on the distal renal tubules is enhanced. These subsets do not have a high correlation with the underlying disease process involved except for the last which is associated with drugs such as the oral hypoglycemic agents. Normovolemic hyponatremia accounts for about a third of the cases of inpatient hyponatremia in most larger series.

ADH secretion from the supraoptic-hypophyseal system that is inappropriate for homeostasis may arise as a complication of a variety of central nervous system disorders. These include meningitis, head trauma, brain abscess, central nervous system tumors (primary or metastatic), central nervous system hemorrhage, acute intermittent porphyria, encephalitis, Guillain-Barré syndrome, multiple sclerosis, and a variety of ill-defined central nervous system diseases. This is also the mechanism operative in postoperative patients, head trauma patients, and probably in patients on positive pressure respirators. Finally, inappropriate ADH release can occur after drugs such as the barbiturates haloperidol and narcotics. The most frequently discussed SIADH occurs as a result of ADH or an ADH-like polypeptide produced by malignant tumors. This potential is probably present in many malignancies, of which the following are well documented: oat-cell carcinoma of the lung, histiocytic lymphoma, carcinoma of the pancreas and duodenum, Ewing's sarcoma, olfactory neuroblastoma, and thymoma. A similar mechanism is probably responsible for the syndrome in tuberculosis, other bacterial pneumonias, cavitary aspergillosis, and viral pneumonias. There are occasional patients for whom no cause can be found (idiopathic SIADH). Such patients probably belong to the first group. Finally, the SIADH may occur in patients with hypoadrenolcorticism, but here glucocorticoid and/or thyroid hormone deficiency also has a direct or permissive pathophysiologic role.

The features of classic SIADH are (1) hyponatremia with associated hypoosmolarity of the intravascular and extracellular fluid, (2) urinary osmolarity in excess of serum osmolarity when the serum osmolality is abnormally low, (3) continued urinary excretion of sodium in spite of hyponatremia, (4) suppression of plasma renin and a low aldosterone secretion rate despite a low serum sodium level, and (5) presence of normal skin turgor and blood pressure as well as normal thyroid, renal, and adrenal function. The differential diagnosis of the syndrome can be difficult, especially in combination with liver cirrhosis and/or cardiac failure.

The severity of the hyponatremia is variable, ranging to less than 100 mEq/liter. There is a parallel decline in serum chloride, but no striking changes occur in serum potassium and bicarbonate.

The clinical signs and symptoms are those of water intoxication. It should be noted that obvious pitting edema is rarely a part of the syndrome since there is usually no more than a 4- to 5-liter retention, which is within the interstitium and cells. Individual circumstances may eliminate any one or more of the five classic characteristics described, making the syndrome atypical. These possibilities must be kept in mind when considering the diagnosis. Voluntary fluid restriction may mask the syndrome. Liberal fluid intake early in the syndrome may dilute the urine in relation to the plasma, although maximum dilution does not occur. Salt restriction may result in the urine's being low in sodium, and water loading does not produce the typical rise in urinary sodium. Finally, normal renal function can be compromised by the syndrome itself.

A rare patient will have hypovasopressinemic antidiuresis characterized by low free water clearance despite nonmeasurable ADH levels. The pathophysiologic mechanism is unknown.

1. Schwartz, W. B., Bennett, W., Curelop, S., et al. A syndrome of renal sodium loss and hyponatremia probably resulting from inappropriate secretion of antidiuretic hormone. *Am. J. Med.* 23:529, 1957.
   The initial report of the ectopic ADH syndrome.
2. Bartter, F. C., and Schwartz, W. B. The syndrome of inappropriate secretion of antidiuretic hormone. *Am. J. Med.* 42:790, 1967.
   A good review including pathophysiologic and clinical features.
3. Weissman, P. N., Shenkman, L., and Gregerman, R. I. Chlorpropamide hyponatremia: Drug-induced inappropriate antidiuretic hormone activity. *N. Engl. J. Med.* 284:65, 1971.
   Another cause for the SIADH.
4. Dingman, J. F., Gonzalez-Auvert, C., Ahmed, A. B. J., et al. Plasma antidiuretic hormone in adrenal insufficiency. *J. Clin. Invest.* 44:1041, 1965.
   The syndrome was reversed by glucocorticoid therapy.
5. Vorherr, H., Massry, S. G., Fallet, R., et al. Antidiuretic principle in tuberculous lung tissue of a patient with pulmonary tuberculosis and hyponatremia. *Ann. Intern. Med.* 72:383, 1970.
   An example of nontumor ectopic ADH.

6. Marks, L. J., Berde, B., Klein, L. A., et al. Inappropriate vasopressin secretion and carcinoma of the pancreas. *Am. J. Med.* 45:967, 1968.
   Tumor extracts contained high levels of ADH activity.
7. Mangos, J. A., and Lobeck, C. C. Studies of sustained hyponatremia due to central nervous system infection. *Pediatrics* 34:503, 1964.
   Meningitis can be associated with the syndrome.
8. Conger, J. D., McIntyre, J. A., and Jacoby, W. J., Jr. Central pontine myelinolysis associated with inappropriate antidiuretic hormone secretion. *Am. J. Med.* 47:813, 1969.
9. Cooper, W. C., and Wang, S. Cerebral salt-wasting associated with the Guillain-Barré syndrome. *Arch. Intern. Med.* 116:113, 1965.
   Articles 8–9 report other central nervous system lesions that can produce the syndrome.
10. White, W. A., and Bergland, R. M. Experimental inappropriate ADH secretion by positive-pressure respirators. *J. Neurosurg.* 36:608, 1972.
    Positive pressure respirators can produce the syndrome.
11. Pettinger, W. A., Talner, L., and Ferris, T. F. Inappropriate secretion of antidiuretic hormone due to myxedema. *N. Engl. J. Med.* 272:362, 1965.
    Thyroid hormone alone reversed the syndrome.
12. Robertson, G. L., Bhoopalam, N., and Zelkowitz, L. J. Vincristine neurotoxicity and abnormal secretion of antidiuretic hormone. *Arch. Intern. Med.* 132:717, 1973.
13. Polland, R. B. Inappropriate secretion of antidiuretic hormone associated with adenovirus pneumonia. *Chest* 68:589, 1975.
14. Rosenow, E. C., Segar, W. E., and Zehr, J. E. Inappropriate antidiuretic hormone secretion in pneumonia. *Mayo Clin. Proc.* 47:169, 1972.
    Some more well-documented causes of SIADH (articles 12–14).
15. Cooke, C. R., Turin, M. D., and Walker, W. G. The syndrome of inappropriate antidiuretic hormone secretion (SIADH): Pathophysiologic mechanisms in solute and volume regulation. *Medicine* 58:240, 1979.
    They showed a negative correlation between water intake and cumulative sodium balance and aldosterone secretion.
16. Whitaker, M. D., McArthur, R. G., Corenblum, B., et al. Idiopathic, sustained, inappropriate secretion of ADH with associated hypertension and thirst. *Am. J. Med.* 67:511, 1979.
    A well-studied patient with idiopathic SIADH.
17. Osterman, J., Calhoun, A., Dunham, M., et al. Chronic syndrome of inappropriate antidiuretic hormone secretion and hypertension in a patient with olfactory neuroblastoma: Evidence of ectopic production of arginine vasopressin by the tumor. *Arch. Intern. Med.* 146:1731, 1986.
18. Kern, P. A., Robbins, R. J., Bichet, D., et al. Syndrome of inappropriate antidiuresis in the absence of arginine vasopressin. *J. Clin. Endocrinol. Metab.* 62:148, 1986.
19. Ishikawa, S.-E., Saito, T., Kaneko, K., et al. Hyponatremia responsive to fludrocortisone acetate in elderly patients. *Ann. Intern. Med.* 106:187, 1987.
    Additional settings in which SIADH has been documented (articles 17–19).
20. Zerbe, R., Stropes, L., and Robertson, G. Vasopressin function in the syndrome of inappropriate antidiuresis. *Ann. Rev. Med.* 31:315, 1980.
    Three subsets of SIADH are defined.
21. Vokes, T. J., and Robertson, G. L. Disorders of antidiuretic hormone. *Endocrinol. Metab. Clin. North Am.* 17:281, 1988.
    An up-to-date concise review of SIADH and diabetes insipidus.
22. Anderson, R. J., Chung H.-M., Kluge, R., et al. Hyponatremia: A prospective analysis of its epidemiology and the pathogenetic role of vasopressin. *Ann. Intern. Med.* 102:164, 1985.
    Daily incidence of hyponatremia averaged 0.97% in this hospital of which 34% were normovolemic.
23. Passamonte, P. M. Hypouricemia, inappropriate secretion of antidiuretic hormone, and small cell carcinoma of the lung. *Arch. Intern. Med.* 144:1569, 1984.
    The combination of hypouricemia and hyponatremia was a good predictor of SIADH.

24. Chung, H.-M., Kluge, R., Schrier, R. W., et al. Clinical assessment of extracellular fluid volume in hyponatremia. *Am. J. Med.* 83:905, 1987.
    Clinical assessment identified less than half of those with hypovolemia or normovolemia, but a spot urine sodium was useful in making this separation.
25. Rose, B. D. New approach to disturbances in the plasma sodium concentration. *Am. J. Med.* 81:1033, 1986.
    An excellent review of the physiologic basis for diagnosis and the response to therapy, should be read by all clinicians.
26. Sterns, R. H. Severe symptomatic hyponatremia: Treatment and outcome: A study of 64 cases. *Ann. Intern. Med.* 107:656, 1987.
    A very low serum sodium per se is not an indication for rapid correction.
27. Sterns, R. H., Riggs, J. E., Schochet, S. S., et al. Osmotic demyelination syndrome following correction of hyponatremia. *N. Engl. J. Med.* 314:1535, 1986.
    Do not exceed a correction of more than 12 mmol/liter/day or the patient may pay the price.

70. THYROIDITIS
H. Verdain Barnes

Thyroiditis is the most common thyroid disorder seen in this country. There is a clear female predominance. For clinical purposes, thyroiditis can be grouped as acute, subacute, and chronic. Most appear to have, in total or in part, an autoimmune etiology, while some have an infectious etiology.

Acute thyroiditis is typically suppurative. In acute suppurative thyroiditis, the most common organisms are the β-hemolytic streptococcus, *Staphylococcus aureus,* and pneumococcus. These organisms enter the thyroid as a result of bacteremia or local extension from adjacent areas. Clinically, the patient usually presents with a sudden onset of fever, chills, severe neck pain, and dysphagia. The thyroid and neck are swollen, indurated, and tender and may exhibit overlying erythema, heat, and occasionally fluctuance. Patients are usually euthyroid and remain so, although on occasion a mild degree of clinical and chemical hyperthyroidism is seen. The thyroid scan shows a decreased uptake in areas of acute inflammation which may appear as a cold nodule. In a rare instance, the onset is more insidious, and an erroneous diagnosis of acute nonsuppurative thyroiditis may be made. Rarely the disease is chronic as a result of infection by *Salmonella typhosa, Mycobacterium tuberculosis, Treponema pallidum, Echinococcus,* or a fungus. Major complications include abscess formation and thrombophlebitis of the internal jugular vein.

Subacute thyroiditis (SAT) has a variety of designations in the literature, the most common being acute nonsuppurative, giant cell, granulomatous, and de Quervain's thyroiditis. The precise cause remains uncertain, but viruses such as mumps and Coxsackie appear to be directly linked in some patients. Clinically, the patients usually have pain in the thyroid area, often on both sides of the neck and radiating to the ears. The pain is usually constant and aching. Modest thyroid enlargement is seen in about 30 percent of patients. Sore throat, dysphagia, and hoarseness are not uncommon. Malaise and easy fatigability are almost invariable. Fever occurs in more than 50 percent of patients, but chills are uncommon. About 20 percent have a prior history of an upper respiratory tract infection. Increased nervousness and hyperhydrosis occur in about 50 percent, weight loss in 38 percent, heat intolerance in 30 percent, tachycardia in 18 percent, and tremulousness in 9 percent of patients. On physical examination, the thyroid is usually tender and firm to hard. About 50 percent of patients have clinical manifestations of mild hyperthyroidism in the acute phase of the disease. A modest to marked elevation of the erythrocyte sedimentation rate is common. Thyroglobulin and thyroid microsomal antibody levels are rarely elevated to a significant titer. Serum thyroxine (T_4 and triiodothyronine (T_3) levels may be modestly elevated initially but typically return to normal in 3 to 12 weeks. The serum thyroid-stimulating hormone (TSH) is low, hence the 1- and 24-hour radioiodine uptakes (RAIU) are low. Histologically, the inflammation does not extend beyond the capsule of the thyroid. With light microscopy, microabscesses within the follicles are seen early and are followed by evidence of follicular cell destruction with the appearance of histiocytes and foreign body giant cells. Areas of destruction typically heal by fibrosis.

The process typically lasts from 1 to 3 months, with occasional recurrences. About 20 percent of patients have a transient phase of hypothyroidism following the initial hyperthyroidism, but then typically recover to normal. Hypothyroidism and persistent hyperthyroidism have been reported. Therapy during the acute phase is symptomatic.

Recently, atypical forms of SAT have been described, subacute lymphocytic thyroiditis (SLT) and postpartum SLT. Characteristically, patients with SLT have few if any systemic or constitutional clinical (e.g., pain, fever) manifestations, that is, transient painless thyroiditis, with a lack of giant cells on histologic examination. Otherwise, the course is similar to that of SAT. The postpartum variant is reported to occur in about 10 percent of postpartum women. The etiology of SLT and the postpartum variant is unclear, but may be autoimmune.

Chronic thyroiditis has two primary forms: chronic lymphocytic (Hashimoto's disease) and chronic fibrous (Riedel's disease). Chronic lymphocytic thyroiditis (CLT) accounts for about 87 percent of all cases of thyroiditis in this country. Females predominate by about a 9:1 ratio. A family history of thyroid disease is positive in a substantial majority, but the precise genetic mechanism(s) is not yet known. There is a consensus that CLT is within the spectrum of autoimmune diseases, but the pathophysiologic details remain unclear. Present data suggest that the lymphocytes involved in the process are of polyclonal origin with perhaps a predominance of the cytotoxic/suppressor T8$^+$ phenotype but the potential role of killer cells in the destruction of thyroid cells is not clear.

Clinically, about 90 percent of CLT patients have a goiter. In the majority, the gland is moderately enlarged, but some have marked thyromegaly. Malaise and fatigue are common, while fever, chills, and thyroid tenderness are quite rare. A few patients complain of neck fullness, occasionally associated with a choking sensation or frank dysphagia. At the time of presentation, the patient is usually euthyroid or mildly hypothyroid, with an occasional patient having overt hyperthyroidism. A rare patient has euthyroid exophthalmos. Gland enlargement is typically diffuse and is lobulated and firm on palpation. An occasional patient presents with a solitary nodule that may be homogeneous, cold, or hot on thyroid scan.

The histologic characteristics of CLT include secondary lymphoid follicles, diffuse or localized accumulations of lymphocytes and plasma cells, low cuboidal oxyphilic or tall columnar epithelial cells, fibrosis of varying degrees, and small amounts of colloid. The first two of these features are typical of autoimmune processes. About 90 percent of patients have circulating thyroid antibodies. A variety of antibodies have been reported: thyroglobulin, denatured or denatured and reduced thyroid microsomal antigen, thyroid peroxidase, and several blocking or stimulating immunoglobulins. Of these, antithyroglobulin and antimicrosomal antibodies have the greatest proven value in diagnosing the disease. About 90 percent of CLT patients will have significant titers of thyroglobulin antibodies and about 80 percent microsomal antibodies. On rare occasions, high titers will also be seen in a patient with toxic diffuse goiter, toxic nodular goiter, or thyroid carcinoma.

A variety of diseases have been reported in association with CLT. They include systemic lupus erythematosus, Sjögren's syndrome, diabetes mellitus, rheumatoid arthritis, pernicious anemia, Addison's disease, gonadal dysgenesis, mongolism, Paget's disease of bone, some nephropathies, and cirrhosis of the liver. Of these, only rheumatoid arthritis, diabetes mellitus, gonadal dysgenesis, mongolism, and autoimmune Addison's disease show a clear increase in incidence. All these potential associations, however, must be kept in mind in patients presenting with an atypical picture of CLT and in patients with potential hypothyroidism who also have one of these diseases. The natural history of CLT is difficult to establish from the literature; however, with time hypothyroidism develops in most if not all. Consequently, these patients should be evaluated at least yearly with an immunoassay determination of TSH or perhaps treated for life with replacement doses of thyroid hormone.

Chronic fibrous thyroiditis (CFT) is rare and of unknown etiology. Part or all of the thyroid gland may be replaced by hard fibrous tissue. The fibrosis often spreads beyond the capsule of the thyroid to adjacent structures. Most commonly involved is the trachea which may result in constriction and marked dyspnea. There is frequently an accompanying complaint of intense pressure in the neck that seems disproportionate to the size of the thyroid. The thyroid may be small or large but is typically nontender, fixed, and hard. The thyrometabolic status is usually normal. Patients have been reported to have associated mediastinal fibrosis, retroorbital fibrosis, retroperitoneal fibrosis, and sclerosing cholangitis. These associations should be kept in mind when evaluating and following patients with this disease.

1. Altemeier, W. A. Acute Pyogenic Thyroiditis. In *Transactions of the American Goiter Association.* Springfield, Ill.: Charles C. Thomas, 1952. P. 242.
   The most common organisms are streptococcus, staphylococcus, and pneumococcus.
2. Eylan, E., Zmucky, R., and Sheba, C. Mumps virus and subacute thyroiditis: Evidence for a causal association. *Lancet* 1:1067, 1957.
3. Volpe, R., Row, V. V., and Ezrin, C. Circulating viral and thyroid antibodies in subacute thyroiditis. *J. Clin. Endocrinol. Metab.* 27:1275, 1967.
   In articles 2 and 3, mumps and Coxsackie viruses were documented as the likely pathogens. Other viruses may also be involved.
4. Ogihara, T., Yarnamoto, T., Azukizawa, M., et al. Serum thyrotropin and thyroid hormones in the course of subacute thyroiditis. *J. Clin. Endocrinol. Metab.* 37:602, 1973.
   The serum T_4 and T_3 levels rise and TSH drops in the acute phase, hence the hyperthyroid state. The article depicts the course of the disease in three extensively studied patients.
5. Woolf, P. D. Transient painless thyroiditis with hyperthyroidism: A variant of lymphocytic thyroiditis? *Endocr. Rev.* 1:411, 1980.
   The author favors a variant.
6. Inada, M., Nishikawa, M., Naito, K., et al. Reversible changes of the histological abnormalities of the thyroid in patients with painless thyroiditis. *J. Clin. Endocrinol. Metab.* 52:431, 1981.
7. Willems, J. S., and Lowhagen, T. Fine-needle aspiration cytology in thyroid disease. *Clin. Endrocrinol. Metab.* 10:247, 1981.
   The findings in acute suppurative and nonsuppurative thyroiditis are detailed.
8. Rotenberg, Z., Weinberger, I., Fuchs, J., et al. Euthyroid atypical subacute thyroiditis simulating systemic or malignant disease. *Arch. Intern. Med.* 146:105, 1986.
9. Walfish, P. G., Chan, J. Y. C., Ing, A. D., et al. Esophageal carcinoma masquerading as recurrent acute suppurative thyroiditis. *Arch. Intern. Med.* 145:346, 1985.
   Sometimes you just can't win (articles 8, 9).
10. Madeddu, G., Cosu, A. R., Costanga, C., et al. Serum thyroglobulin levels in the diagnosis and follow-up of subacute "painful" thyroiditis: A sequential study. *Arch. Intern. Med.* 145:243, 1985.
    Serial measurements may be useful.
11. Nikolai, T. F., Turney, S. L., and Roberts, R. C. Postpartum lymphocytic thyroiditis: Prevalence, clinical course and long-term follow-up. *Arch. Intern. Med.* 147:221, 1987.
    Of their patients, 11.3% had thyroid disease, 56% microsomal antibodies, and 48% evidence of continued thyroid disease at 36 months.
12. Hayslip, C. C., Baker, J. R., Jr., Wartofeky, L., et al. Natural killer cell activity and serum autoantibodies in women with postpartum thyroiditis. *J. Clin. Endocrinol. Metab.* 66:1089, 1988.
    No difference in killer cell activity was found, but 33% had antinuclear antibody titers greater than or equal to 1:160, 29% had circulating immune complexes, and 12% TSH receptor antibodies.
13. Smallridge, R. C., DeKeyser, F. M., VanHerle, A. J., et al. Thyroid iodine content and serum thyroglobulin: Cues to the natural history of destruction-induced thyroiditis. *J. Clin. Endocrinol. Metab.* 62:1213, 1986.

Evidence of thyroid gland injury may last for years despite normal hormone levels.

14. Nilsson, L. R., and Doniach, D. Auto-immune thyroiditis in children and adolescents: Clinical studies. *Acta Pediatr.* 53:255, 1964.
    About 91% of patients have demonstrable goiters, usually of medium size.

15. Gluck, F. B., Nusynowitz, M. L., and Plymate, S. Chronic lymphocytic thyroiditis, thyrotoxicosis and low radioactive iodine uptake. *N. Engl. J. Med.* 293:624, 1975.

16. Greenberg, A. H., Czernichow, P., Hung, W., et al. Juvenile chronic lymphocytic thyroiditis: Clinical, laboratory, and histological correlations. *J. Clin. Invest.* 30:293, 1970.
    Some patients with normal serum T_4 levels have elevated thyrotropin and low radioactive iodine uptake levels (articles 15, 16).

17. Winter, J., Eberlin, W. R., and Bongiovanni, A. M. The relationship of juvenile hypothyroidism to chronic lymphocytic thyroiditis. *J. Pediatr.* 69:709, 1966.
    In this study 16 of 18 persons with acquired hypothyroidism were found to have CLT.

18. Bartholomew, L. G., Cain, J. C., Woolner, L. B., et al. Sclerosing cholangitis: Its possible association with Riedel's struma and retroperitoneal fibrosis. *N. Engl. J. Med.* 269:8, 1963.

19. Paphael, H. A., Beahrs, O. H., Woolner, L. B., et al. Riedel's struma associated with fibrous mediastinitis: Report of a case. *Mayo Clin. Proc.* 41:375, 1966.
    Two interesting associations are reported in articles 18, 19.

20. Hay, I. D., Thyroiditis: A clinical update. *Mayo Clin. Proc.* 60:836, 1985.

21. Hamberger, J. I. The various presentations of thyroiditis: Diagnostic considerations. *Ann. Intern. Med.* 104:219, 1986.
    These two articles (20, 21) provide concise well-referenced updates.

22. Wall, T. R. (ed.) Autoimmune thyroid disease. *Endocrinol. Metab. Clin. North Am.* 16:1987.
    This entire volume provides detail about current concepts of pathophysiology.

23. Kaulfersch, W., Baker, J. R., Jr., Burman, K. D., et al. Immunoglobulin and T cell antigen receptor gene arrangements indicate that the immune response in autoimmune thyroid disease is polyclonal. *J. Clin. Endocrinol. Metab.* 66:958, 1988.
    Lymphocyte DNA revealed polyclonal gene rearrangement.

24. Hamada, N., Jaeduck, N. O., Portman, L., et al. Antibodies against denatured and reduced thyroid microsomal antigen in autoimmune thyroid disease. *J. Clin. Endocrinol. Metab.* 64:230, 1987.
    Microsomal antibodies are heterogeneous and may play a role in cell destruction.

25. Kotani, T., Umaki, K., Matsunaga, S., et al. Detection of autoantibodies to thyroid peroxidase in autoimmune thyroid disease by micro-ELISA and immunoblotting. *J. Clin. Endocrinol. Metab.* 62:928, 1986.

26. Sack, J., Baker, J. R., Jr., Weetman, A. P., et al. Killer cell activity and antibody-dependent cell-mediated cytotoxicity are normal in Hashimoto's disease. *J. Clin. Endocrinol. Metab.* 62:1059, 1986.

27. MacKensie, W. A., Schwartz, A. E., Friedman, E. W., et al. Intrathyroidal T cell clones from patients with autoimmune thyroid disease. *J. Clin. Endocrinol. Metab.* 64:818, 1987.

28. DelPrete, G. F., Maggi, E., Mariotti, S., et al. Cytotoxic T lymphocytes with natural killer activity in thyroid infiltrate of patients with Hashimoto's thyroiditis: Analysis at clonal levels. *J. Clin. Endocrinol. Metab.* 62:52, 1986.
    These four articles (25–28) demonstrate the difficulty in assigning a precise etiology for CLT.

29. Rabinoive, S. L., Larsen, P. R., Antman, E. M., et al. Amiodarone therapy and autoimmune thyroid disease: Increase in a new monoclonal antibody–defined T cell subset. *Am. J. Med.* 81:53, 1986.
    This antiarrythmic/antianginal drug may precipitate organ-specific autoimmunity in selected patients.

30. Iwatani, Y., Gerstein, H. C., Iitaka, M., et al. Thyrocyte HLA-DR expression and interferon-gamma production in autoimmune thyroid disease. *J. Clin. Endocrinol. Metab.* 63:695, 1986.
    Does not appear to be induced by nonspecific environmental factors and may normally have a protective function.

71. THYROID NODULES AND CARCINOMA
H. Verdain Barnes

Palpable thyroid nodules are found in about 4 percent of the adult population. Nodules are more frequent in women, particularly those over 40 years of age. In women, the peak incidence is from age 40 to 79 and in men from age 30 to 60. The incidence of nodules in women is about 9:1 greater than in men while the incidence of thyroid carcinoma is about 2:1 greater in men than in women. Nodules may be solitary or multiple. In solitary nodules, the incidence of carcinoma is much higher than in multiple nodules. The primary differential diagnosis of thyroid nodules, solitary or multiple, includes (1) benign adenomas, which may be nonfunctional, functional, or hyperfunctional; (2) colloid cysts; (3) acute thyroiditis; (4) chronic lymphocytic thyroiditis; (5) metastatic carcinoma to the thyroid; (6) thyroid carcinoma; and (7) involvement of the thyroid gland by lymphoma, multiple myeloma, leukemia, or granulomatous processes. There is no noninvasive method for making an unequivocal diagnosis. A thyroid scan with iodine 131 or technetium 99 will usually define nodules of 1 cm or greater and establish whether they are functional or nonfunctional. In most studies, the incidence of primary thyroid carcinoma is much greater in a solitary cold nodule than in a functional solitary nodule or a multinodular gland. Sonography and computed tomography (CT) can usually distinguish between solid and cystic lesions, but only limited usefulness in that some thyroid carcinomas are cystic or may contain sizable hematomas. The use of fine-needle aspiration, an essentially benign invasive technique, for preoperative cytologic examination is frequently useful in selecting patients for surgery. The incidence of false-positive and false-negative aspirations is in the order of 3 to 6 percent and 6 to 10 percent respectively.

There are several clinical points of significance when considering the likelihood of carcinoma. The incidence of thyroid carcinoma appears to be increased if there is (1) a past history of irradiation to the head or neck for acne or for tonsil, adenoid, or thymus enlargement, (2) a painless nodule that is rapidly increasing in size, (3) a hard or fixed thyroid nodule, (4) evidence compatible with lymph node, pulmonary, or bone metastases, (5) vocal cord paralysis, (6) a family history of thyroid carcinoma or multiple endocrine adenomatosis type II or III, and (7) a young age at the time of discovery. The incidence of thyroid nodules is about 30 percent after external irradiation with 500 to 800 rad. In this population, the incidence of thyroid carcinoma in a solitary nodule ranges from 25 to 30 percent; therefore, all patients with a history of low-dose (50–1200 rad) irradiation to the head and neck merit careful evaluation. In postirradiation patients at least 10 percent of nodules are picked up by scan and not by palpation. The general incidence of carcinoma in children and young adults with cold nodules is about 50 percent, as compared to 5 percent in persons in their sixties or older.

Thyroid carcinoma can be classified as differentiated and undifferentiated. The most common differentiated types are papillary and follicular adenocarcinoma. Histologically, about 58 percent of patients show a mixed papillary-follicular, 13 percent a pure follicular, 12 percent a pure papillary picture. About 11 percent show undifferentiated thyroid carcinoma of the giant cell, spindle cell, small cell, or Hürthle cell types. The remaining 5 to 6 percent have medullary thyroid carcinoma arising from the parafollicular cells of the thyroid. Medullary thyroid carcinoma is frequently associated with familial types II and III multiple endocrine adenomatosis. These patients may be diagnosed prior to the presence of observable thyroid abnormalities by documenting an elevated basal serum calcitonin level or by an abnormal calcium or pentagastrin stimulation test. Virtually all patients with medullary thyroid carcinoma have bilateral foci whereas less than two-thirds of patients with other types of thyroid carcinomas have bilateral disease.

The prognosis for thyroid carcinoma depends on tumor histology, the presence or absence of distant metastases, and the age of the patient at onset. Most well-differentiated tumors pursue a relatively benign course. Well-documented studies show that the younger the patient at the onset the higher the 10-year survival. In women under age 40, well-differentiated carcinoma tends to behave as a benign adenoma. About 90 percent of the well-differentiated carcinomas appear to have some dependence on thyroid-stimulating hormone (TSH) for growth; hence they typically respond well to TSH suppression with exogenous thyroid hormone. The prognosis for poorly differentiated carcinoma is much more guarded, with an overall 10-year survival of about 10 percent as compared to about 65 percent in patients with differentiated tumors.

1. Veith, F. J., Brooks, J. R., Grigsby, W. P., et al. The nodular thyroid gland and cancer: A practical approach to the problem. *N. Engl. J. Med.* 270:431, 1964.
   Thyroid carcinoma is more common in men with nodules than in women.
2. Russell, W. O., and Ibanez, M. L. Primary Thyroid Carcinoma: Histiogenesis, Classification and Biologic Behavior Based on Studies of 777 Patients. In *The Endocrine and Nonendocrine Hormone-Producing Tumors.* Chicago: Year Book Medical Publishers, Inc., 1973. P. 363.
   Subserial sections of the thyroid revealed bilateral carcinoma in about two-thirds of the patients.
3. Sanfelippo, P. M., Beahrs, O. H., McConahey, W. M., et al. Indications for thyroidectomy. *Mayo Clin. Proc.* 48:269, 1973.
   15% of patients with multinodular goiters had carcinoma.
4. Mazzaferri, E. L., Young, R. L., Oertel, J. E., et al. Papillary thyroid carcinoma: The impact of therapy in 576 patients. *Medicine* 56:177, 1977.
   An important, up-to-date review.
5. Thijs, L. G., and Wiener, J. D. Ultrasonic examination of the thyroid gland. *Am. J. Med.* 60:96, 1976.
   A careful discussion of the advantages and limitations of this noninvasive technique.
6. McCowen, K. D., Adler, R. A., Ghaed, N., et al. Low dose radioiodine thyroid ablation in postsurgical patients with thyroid cancer. *Am. J. Med.* 61:52, 1976.
   Less than 35 mCi iodine 131 seems to do the job as well as 2 to 3 times that dose.
7. Hamburger, J. I. Solitary autonomously functioning thyroid lesions: Diagnosis, clinical features and pathogenetic considerations. *Am. J. Med.* 58:740, 1975.
   An excellent discussion of a perplexing problem. Large and toxic lesions were found more often in the older population.
8. Mazzaferri, E. L., and Young, R. L. Papillary thyroid carcinoma: A 10-year follow-up report of the impact of therapy in 576 patients. *Am. J. Med.* 70:511, 1981.
   An important continuing follow-up; recurrence was greatest in those with primary tumors greater than 1.5 cm.
9. Selzer, G., Kahn, B. L., and Albertyn, L. Primary malignant tumors of the thyroid gland: A clinicopathologic study of 245 cases. *Cancer* 40:1501, 1977.
   Differentiated tumors may undergo transition to anaplastic—a sobering potential.
10. Schneider, A. B., Pinsky, S., Bekerman, C., et al. Characteristics of 108 thyroid cancers detected by screening in a population with a history of head and neck irradiation. *Cancer* 46:1218, 1980.
    90% were papillary or mixed papillary-follicular, 55% with tissue from both sides were multicentric, and 36% were bilateral.
11. DeGroot, L. J., Reilly, M., Pinnameneni, K., et al. Retrospective and prospective study of radiation-induced thyroid disease. *Am. J. Med.* 74:852, 1983.
12. Samaan, N. A., Schultz, P. N., Ordonez, N. G., et al. A comparison of thyroid carcinoma in those who have and have not had head and neck irradiation in childhood. *J. Clin. Endocrinol. Metab.* 64:219, 1987.
13. Schneider, A. B., Recaut, W., Pinsky, S. M., et al. Radiation-induced thyroid carcinoma: Clinical course and results of therapy in 296 patients. *Ann. Intern. Med.* 105:405, 1986.
14. Schneider, A. B., Shore-Freedman, E., and Weinstein, R. A. Radiation-induced thyroid and other head and neck tumors: Occurrence of multiple tumors and analysis of risk factors. *J. Clin. Endocrinol. Metab.* 63:107, 1986.
    These articles (11–14) discuss the full spectrum of our knowledge about radiation-induced thyroid disease.
15. Werk, E. E., Jr., Vernon, B. M., Gonzales, J. J., et al. Cancer in thyroid nodules: A community hospital survey. *Arch. Intern. Med.* 144:474, 1984.
    Their incidence was 6.5% of those operated on for a solitary nodule.

16. Simpson, W. J., McKinney, S. E., Carruthers, J. S., et al. Papillary and follicular thyroid cancer: Prognostic factors in 1,578 patients. *Am. J. Med.* 83:479, 1987.
    In this Canadian study the most important factors in prognosis in descending order were postoperative status, age at diagnosis, extrathyroid invasion, and presence of distant metastases.
17. Schlumberger, M., Tubiana, M., DeVathaire, F., et al. Long-term results of treatment of 283 patients with lung and bone metastases from differentiated thyroid carcinoma. *J. Clin. Endocrinol. Metab.* 63:960, 1986.
    Early detection and therapy for metastases appear to be important.
18. Schwinberger, M., DeVathaire, F., Travagli, J. P., et al. Differentiated thyroid carcinoma in childhood: Long-term follow-up of 72 patients. *J. Clin. Endocrinol. Metab.* 65:1088, 1987.
    The 20-year survival rate was 90.3%, but the standardized mortality ratio was 8.1.
19. Wells, S. A., Dilley, W. G., Farndon, J. A., et al. Early diagnosis and treatment of medullary thyroid carcinoma. *Arch. Intern. Med.* 145:1248, 1985.
20. Gharib, H., Kao, P. C., and Heath, H., III. Determination of silica-purified plasma calcitonin for the detection and management of medullary thyroid carcinoma: Comparison of two provocative tests. *Mayo Clin. Proc.* 62:373, 1987.
    Early diagnosis and treatment are needed (article 19) and the best methods to accomplish this (article 20) are detailed.
21. Watson, R. G., Brennan, M. D., Goellner, J. R., et al. Invasive Hürthle cell carcinoma of the thyroid: Natural history and management. *Mayo Clin. Proc.* 59:851, 1984.
22. Nel, C. J. C., van Heerden, J. A., Goellner, J. R., et al. Anaplastic carcinoma of the thyroid: A clinicopathologic study of 82 cases. *Mayo Clin. Proc.* 60:51, 1985.
    These two articles (21, 22) review two rare types of thyroid cancer.
23. Ivy, H. K. Cancer metastatic to the thyroid: A diagnostic problem. *Mayo Clin. Proc.* 59:856, 1984.
    The most common were metastases from the kidney, breast, and lung and lymphoma.
24. Smith, S. A., Gharib, H., and Goellner, J. R. Fine-needle aspiration: Usefulness for diagnosis and management of metastatic carcinoma to the thyroid. *Arch. Intern. Med.* 147:311, 1987.
25. Hamberger, J. I. Consistency of sequential needle biopsy findings for thyroid nodules: management implications. *Arch. Intern. Med.* 147:97, 1987.
26. Asp, A. A., Georgitis, W., Waldron, E. J., et al. Fine needle aspiration of the thyroid: Use in an average health care facility. *Am. J. Med.* 83:489, 1987.
    Current uses and usefulness of the thin-needle aspiration biopsy in the diagnosis and management of thyroid nodules are detailed in these articles (24–26).
27. Schneider, A. B., Shore-Freedman, E., Ryo, U. Y., et al. Prospective serum thyroglobulin measurements in assessing the risk of developing thyroid nodules in patients exposed to childhood neck irradiation. *J. Clin. Endocrinol. Metab.* 61:547, 1985.
    Increasing levels of thyroglobulin appear to identify those at risk for developing thyroid nodules and/or cancer.
28. Meyers, F. J., and Goodnight, J. E., Identification of unsuspected thyroid carcinoma using immunoperoxidase for thyroglobulin. *Am. J. Med.* 81:177, 1986.
    Two patients with a cancer of unknown primary were shown to have metastatic thyroid cancer.
29. Filetti, S., Belfiore, A., Amir, S. M., et al. The role of thyroid-stimulating antibodies of Graves' disease in differentiated thyroid cancer. *N. Engl. J. Med.* 318:753, 1988.
    Human thyroid-stimulating antibodies may be pathogenic in selected patients with Graves' disease, a sobering potential.
30. Gharib, H., and Goellner, J. R. Evaluation of nodular thyroid disease. *Endocrinol. Metab. Clin. Am.* 17:511, 1988.
    A concise review touting thin-needle aspiration biopsy as the first step in diagnosis.

V. DISEASES OF THE GASTROINTESTINAL TRACT

72. ACUTE PANCREATITIS

Jerry L. Spivak

Acute pancreatitis can be caused by biliary tract disease, chronic alcohol abuse, hyperlipemia (types I, IV, and V), hyperparathyroidism, viral hepatitis, mumps, arteritis, trauma, hypothermia, uremia, iatrogenic factors (surgery, endoscopy), and drugs (e.g., furosemide, tetracycline, L-asparaginase, estrogens, azathioprine, thiazides, sulfonamides). In a small group of patients, the disease occurs on a hereditary basis, often with aminoaciduria. In over 10 percent of cases, the cause of the acute pancreatitis is not apparent. Alcoholic pancreatitis differs from the other varieties because chronic destructive changes are present in the gland at the time of the initial clinical manifestations; acute alcohol abuse itself probably does not result in the clinical syndrome of acute pancreatitis unless it precipitates type V hyperlipemia.

Since the signs and symptoms of acute pancreatitis mimic those of surgically correctable intraabdominal disorders, the diagnosis of acute pancreatitis is one of exclusion. Other diseases to be considered are perforated peptic ulcer, mesenteric thrombosis, intestinal obstruction, dissecting aneurysm, peritonitis, acute cholecystitis, and appendicitis. The diagnostic process is complicated by the fact that hyperamylasemia can occur in disorders other than pancreatic inflammation. These include all the diseases mentioned, as well as ectopic pregnancy, parotitis, carcinoma of the lung, posterior penetrating ulcer, ruptured aortic aneurysm, and opiate administration. Although amylase values greater than 1000 units have been said to occur principally in conditions requiring surgery (e.g., biliary tract disease), this distinction is not absolute. In addition, a normal serum amylase value does not exclude the presence of acute pancreatitis; here urinary amylase determinations may be of help since in acute pancreatitis renal clearance of amylase is increased. In such cases the serum should also be examined for lactescence since hyperlipemia can interfere with the serum amylase determination. The type of lipemia can be simply confirmed by refrigerating a sample of blood. With refrigeration the plasma lipids separate, with chylomicrons layering on top. In type V hyperlipoproteinemia, the plasma beneath the chylomicron layer will be lactescent; in type I, the plasma will be clear. Diabetic ketoacidosis, hyperosmolar nonketotic coma, or jaundice may accompany pancreatitis and occasionally obscure the diagnosis. Jaundice is usually the result of a common duct stone, edema of the head of the pancreas (in which case pain precedes the jaundice), or diffuse parenchymal liver disease (alcoholic, viral). X-ray studies may reveal a "sentinel loop" or a "colonic cutoff" sign with the colonic gas pattern stopping abruptly at the splenic flexure. Computed tomography is also a useful diagnostic technique in detecting acute pancreatitis and is particularly helpful in the evaluation of its complications. Ultrasonography is, however, superior for the detection of gallstones. Atelectasis, pneumonitis, or pleural effusion (which can be bilateral) can also be seen. It should be remembered, however, that an elevated pleural fluid amylase can occur with carcinoma or esophageal rupture.

The mechanisms by which different stimuli cause pancreatic inflammation are unknown. Current hypotheses include cell membrane damage by the inciting stimulus leading to calcium influx, cell death, and release of degradative enzymes, or injury-mediated intrapancreatic activation of trypsin with the subsequent activation of elastase, phospholipase A, and the kallikrein system. Kallikrein system activity causes edema and vasodilation; elastase and phospholipase A produce vascular damage and tissue necrosis, in part due to the conversion of bile lecithin to the toxic compound lysolecithin.

Therapy in acute pancreatitis is initially directed at correcting fluid, electrolyte, acid-base, and metabolic abnormalities. While it is commonly held that putting the pancreas at rest by removal of intestinal secretions is an important component of the immediate therapy of acute pancreatitis, gastric suction alone may be inadequate since considerable fluid pools in the upper small intestine. In confirmation of this, it has been demonstrated that nasogastric suction was not beneficial in mild to moderately severe pancreatitis (*Br. Med. J.* 2:659, 1978 and *Surgery* 100:500, 1986). Another study (*Surg. Gynecol. Obstet.* 148:206, 1979) has indicated that anticholinergic therapy is without effect on the course of the acute pancreatitis, and cimetidine was not found to be better than a placebo in this disorder (*Gastroenterology* 77:687, 1979). The enzyme inhibitors aprotinin and glucagon, which suppress both gastric acid secretion and pancreatic exocrine function, appeared to influence neither the mortality nor the clinical course of acute pancreatitis (*Lancet* 2:632, 1977; *Gastroenterology* 74:489, 1978; *Gut* 21:334, 1978). Early use of total parenteral nutrition also does not appear to influence the clinical outcome of acute pancreatitis (*Am. J. Surg.* 153:117, 1987). In the absence of documented infection, antibiotics should not be employed. Fluid losses due to vomiting, pooling of fluid in the bowel, fever, and retroperitoneal and peritoneal burns can be massive. In patients who are hypotensive, the deficit can be 6 to 8 liters. Acidosis usually responds to the correction of the fluid deficit. Peritoneal lavage has been used successfully to remove toxic and necrotic products of the inflammatory process, but its role in the treatment of acute pancreatitis has not been established. Indeed, it can be concluded that the optimal method for managing acute pancreatitis has not been established, but with newer diagnostic techniques and means of intervention it should be possible in the future to define optimal therapy for this disorder.

Abnormalities of the bowel may complicate acute pancreatitis. They include ileus, duodenal obstruction, and colonic necrosis or stricture formation. Pulmonary insufficiency is a common complication of acute pancreatitis and may be occult or manifest as the adult respiratory distress syndrome. Activation of the complement system may be involved in the pathogenesis of this complication. Pseudocysts and abscess formation are two other complications of acute pancreatic necrosis, both of which may have a fatal outcome. If other causes of acute abdominal pain can be excluded, surgery should be deferred in patients with acute pancreatitis until the inflammatory process has subsided. Since some pseudocysts will resolve spontaneously within 4 to 6 weeks and approximately 6 weeks is required for cyst wall maturation, surgical intervention for the treatment of pseudocysts is best delayed for at least 6 weeks.

1. Geokas, M. C., Baltaxe, H. A., Banks, P. A., et al. Acute pancreatitis. *Ann. Intern. Med.* 103:86, 1985.
   Comprehensive review of all aspects of acute pancreatitis. (See also Am. J. Gastroenterol. 83:597, 1988.)
2. Mossa, A. R. Diagnostic tests and procedures in acute pancreatitis. *N. Engl. J. Med.* 311:639, 1984.
   Critical evaluation of the tests employed in the diagnosis of acute pancreatitis. (See also Arch. Pathol. Lab. Med. 109:316, 1985 and Ann. Intern. Med. 102:576, 1985.)
3. Renner, I. G., Rinderknecht, H., and Douglas, A. P. Profiles of pure pancreatic secretions in patients with acute pancreatitis: The possible role of proteolytic enzymes in pathogenesis. *Gastroenterology* 75:1090, 1978.
   Duct obstruction and intraductal zymogen activation implicated in the etiology of acute pancreatitis.
4. Acosta, J. M., and Ledesma, C. L. Gallstone migration as a cause of acute pancreatitis. *N. Engl. J. Med.* 290:484, 1974.
   Pancreatitis due to transient obstruction of the ampulla by gallstones. (See also Arch. Surg. 118:901, 1983.)
5. McMahon, M. J., and Pickford, I. R. Biochemical prediction of gallstones early in an attack of acute pancreatitis. *Lancet* 2:541, 1979.
   An elevated AST (SGOT) in the absence of alcohol consumption suggests gallstones as the cause of pancreatitis.
6. Corfield, A. P., Cooper, M. J., Williamson, R. C., et al. Prediction of severity in acute pancreatitis: prospective comparison of three prognostic indices. *Lancet* 2:403, 1985.
   Combined use of clinical assessment, laboratory tests, and peritoneal lavage in the evaluation of pancreatitis (For the laboratory criteria, see Surg. Gynecol. Obstet. 139:69, 1974.)
7. Williamson, R. C. N. Early assessment of severity in acute pancreatitis. *Gut* 25:1331, 1984.
   Concise review with useful guidelines.
8. Mallory, A., and Kern, F., Jr. Drug-induced pancreatitis: A critical review. *Gastroenterology* 78:813, 1980.

Azathioprine, thiazides, sulfonamides, furosemide, estrogens, and tetracycline sub-stantiated as causing pancreatitis. The evidence implicating other drugs such as cor-ticosteroids is less convincing. (See also Lancet *1:706, 1979 and* N. Engl. J. Med. *282:380, 1970).*

9. Steinberg, W. M., and Lewis, J. H. Steroid-induced pancreatitis: Does it really exist? *Gastroenterology* 81:799, 1981.
   Steroids might prove to be beneficial in acute pancreatitis.

10. Mixter, C. G., Keynes, W. M., and Cope, O. Further experience with pancreatitis as a diagnostic clue to hyperparathyroidism. *N. Engl. J. Med.* 266:265, 1962.
    Normal serum calcium in acute pancreatitis or pancreatic calculi should suggest parathyroid disease.

11. Achard, J. L. Acute pancreatitis with infectious hepatitis. *J.A.M.A.* 205:837, 1968.
    An easily overlooked complication of infectious hepatitis. (See also Johns Hopkins Med. J. *133:156, 1973.)*

12. Cameron J. L., Capuzzi, D. M., Zuidema, G. D., et al. Acute pancreatitis with hyper-lipemia. *Am. J. Med.* 56:482, 1974.
    High incidence of fasting hypertriglyceridemia and abnormal serum lipoproteins found in patients with a history of pancreatitis.

13. Davidoff, F., Tishler, S., and Rosoff, C. Hyperlipidemia and pancreatitis associated with oral contraceptive therapy. *N. Engl. J. Med.* 289:552, 1973.
    A complication in patients with type IV hyperlipoproteinemia.

14. Potts, D. E., Mass, M. F., and Iseman, M. D. Syndrome of pancreatic disease, sub-cutaneous fat necrosis and polyserositis. *Am. J. Med.* 58:417, 1975.
    Comprehensive review.

15. McKenna, J. M., Chandrasekhar, A. J., Skorton, D., et al. The pleuropulmonary com-plications of pancreatitis. *Chest* 71:197, 1977.
    Review of the clinical features (see also Chest *73:360, 1978.)*

16. Rovner, A. J., and Westcott, J. L. Pulmonary edema and respiratory insufficiency in acute pancreatitis. *Radiology* 118:513, 1976.
    A serious complication of acute pancreatitis. (For a discussion of abdominal x-ray findings, see Radiology *118:535, 1976.)*

17. Jacob, H. S., Goldstein, I. M., Shapiro, I., et al. Sudden blindness in acute pancrea-titis. *Arch. Intern. Med.* 141:134, 1981.
    Leukoembolization due to complement activation. (See also Am. J. Med. Sci. *275:257, 1978.)*

18. Salt, W. B., II, and Schenker, S. Amylase: Its clinical significance: A review of the literature. *Medicine* 55:269, 1976.
    All the important information about amylase in one article.

19. Levitt, M. D., Ellis, C. J., and Meiar, P. B. Extrapancreatic origin of chronic unex-plained hyperamylasemia. *N. Engl. J. Med.* 302:670, 1980.
    Persistent hyperamylasemia is usually due to nonpancreatic causes such as salivary gland disorders or metastatic tumor.

20. Berk, J. E., Shimamura, J., and Fridhandler, L. Amylase changes in disorders of the lung. *Gastroenterology* 74:1313, 1978.
    Hyperamylasemia can be produced by a variety of pulmonary disorders. The amylase is of the salivary type.

21. Levitt, M. D., and Johnson, S. G. Is the $C_{am}/C\%_r$ ratio of value for the diagnosis of pancreatitis? *Gastroenterology* 75:118, 1978.
    This is not a specific test for acute pancreatitis.

22. Hansen, H. R., Van Kley, H., and Knight, W. A. Macroamylasemia due to binding by protein. *Am. J. Med.* 52:712, 1972.
    Binding of amylase by immunoglobulin.

23. Adams, J. T., Libertino, J. A., and Schwartz, S. I. Significance of an elevated serum amylase. *Surgery* 63:877, 1968.
    A serum amylase greater than 1000 units suggests the presence of a surgically cor-rectable lesion. (See also Surg. Obstet. Gynecol. Obstet. *161:139, 1985.)*

24. Warshaw, A. L., Feller, E. R., and Lee, K.-H. On the cause of raised serum-amylase in diabetic ketoacidosis. *Lancet* 1:929, 1977.
    The amylase is salivary, not pancreatic.

25. Robertson, G. M., Jr., Moore, E. W., Switz, D. M., et al. Inadequate parathyroid response in acute pancreatitis. *N. Engl. J. Med.* 294:512, 1976.
Relative parathyroid insufficiency thought to account for hypocalcemia.
26. Russell, J. C., Welch, J. P., and Clark D. G. Colonic complications of acute pancreatitis and pancreatic abscess. *Am. J. Surg.* 146:558, 1983.
Colonic involvement is an uncommon but serious complication.
27. Beger, H. G., Bittner, R., Block S., et al. Bacterial contamination of pancreatic necrosis. A prospective clinical study. *Gastroenterology* 91:433, 1986.
This occurs early and frequently in the presence of pancreatic necrosis; abscess formation occurs much later. (See also Dig. Dis. Sci. *32:1082, 1987.)*
28. Clavien, P. A., Hauser, H., Meyer, P., et al. Value of contrast-enhanced computerized tomography in the early diagnosis and prognosis of acute pancreatitis. A prospective study of 202 patients. *Am. J. Surg.* 155:457, 1988.
A useful test. (See also Radiology *156:767, 1985.)*
29. van Sonnenberg, E., Wittich, G. R., Casola, G., et al. Complicated pancreatic inflammatory disease: Diagnostic and therapeutic role of interventional radiology. *Radiology* 155:335, 1985.
An effective alternative to surgery. (See also Radiology *167:435, 1988.)*
30. Winship, D. Pancreatitis: Pancreatic pseudocysts and their complications. *Gastroenterology* 73:593, 1977.
Comprehensive review. (See also Am. J. Surg. *156:159, 1988.)*
31. Czaja, A., Fisher, M., and Marin, G. A. Spontaneous resolution of pancreatic masses (pseudocysts?). *Arch. Intern. Med.* 135:558, 1975.
A mass associated with pancreatitis that resolves rapidly is usually a phlegmon, not a pseudocyst.
32. Frey, C. F. Pancreatic pseudocyst-operative strategy. *Ann. Surg.* 188:652, 1978.
Angiography recommended to identify patients with pseudoaneurysms who are at risk of hemorrhage.
33. Donahue, P. E., Nyhus, L. M., and Baker, R. T. Pancreatic abscess after alcoholic pancreatitis. *Arch. Surg.* 115:905, 1980.
A fatal disorder if undiagnosed. Surgery may be a contributing factor to the development of pancreatic infection. (See Surgery *82:99, 1977.)*
34. Kodesch, R., and Dupont, H. K. Infectious complications of acute pancreatitis. *Surg. Gynecol. Obstet.* 136:763, 1973.
Prophylactic antibiotics do not prevent infection.
35. Warshaw, A. L. Pancreatic abscesses. *N. Engl. J. Med.* 287:1234, 1972.
Late complication of pancreatitis requiring surgical drainage. (See also Ann Surg. *194:545, 1981.)*
36. Steinberg, W. M., and Schlesselman, S. E. Treatment of acute pancreatitis. Comparison of animal and human studies. *Gastroenterology* 93:1420, 1987.
Critical review; most studies are statistically unsatisfactory and even negative results may be in error.
37. Neoptolemos, J. P., Carr-Locke, D. L., London, N. J., et al. Controlled trial of urgent endoscopic retrograde cholangiopancreatography [ERCP] and endoscopic spincterotomy versus conservative treatment for acute pancreatitis due to gallstones. *Lancet* 2:979, 1988.
ERCP found to be useful in gallstone pancreatitis.
38. Mayer, A. D., McMahon, M. J., Corfield, A. P., et al. Controlled clinical trial of peritoneal lavage for the treatment of severe acute pancreatitis. *N. Engl. J. Med.* 312:399, 1985.
In this trial, peritoneal lavage did not influence the clinical course.
39. Reynolds, J. C., Inman, R. D., Kimberly, R. P., et al. Acute pancreatitis in systemic lupus erythematosus: report of twenty cases and a review of the literature. *Medicine* 61:25, 1982.
A not uncommon complication.
40. Ranson, J. H. C. Surgical treatment of acute pancreatitis. *Dig. Dis. Sci.* 25:453, 1980.
Surgery for cholelithiasis is best performed after pancreatic inflammation has subsided.

73. ANTIBIOTIC-ASSOCIATED DIARRHEA
John G. Bartlett

Antibiotic-associated diarrhea represents one of the penalties paid for the use and abuse of antimicrobial agents. *Clostridium difficile* is the most important identifiable agent involved and the organism most frequently responsible for serious complications.

Nearly any antimicrobial agent that alters the intestinal flora has been implicated as a cause of antibiotic-associated diarrhea. The frequency of this complication is highly variable depending on the agent, the host, and on the definition of diarrhea. The best information is available for clindamycin and ampicillin where prospective studies show rates of 10 to 30 percent and 5 to 10 percent, respectively. The other major category of drugs in antibiotic-associated diarrhea is the cephalosporins for which the rate of diarrhea ranges from 2 to 10 percent. Higher rates are noted when the definition of diarrhea is two or more loose stools for 2 or more consecutive days versus three or more loose stools for 3 or more days. There is also the expected increased frequency with oral versus parenteral administration. Nevertheless, many drugs that are given parenterally reach substantial concentrations in the gastrointestinal tract as a result of biliary excretion.

There is considerable variation in the frequency, volume, and duration of diarrhea. At one end of the spectrum is a benign, self-limited bout of "nuisance diarrhea" characterized by a few loose bowel movements that promptly subside when antibiotics are discontinued. At the other end of the spectrum are patients with up to 20 or 30 stools a day and a course that may be protracted for several months. The onset of changes in bowel habits usually occurs during the course of antibiotic administration, but as many as one-third of patients with antibiotic-associated colitis never note substantial changes until the implicated drug has been discontinued.

Clinical features of antibiotic-associated diarrhea usually consist of loose or water stools that may contain mucus and rarely contain blood. Grossly bloody stools (hemorrhagic colitis) are most common with ampicillin. The greatest concern is for patients who have inflammation of the colon characterized by fecal leukocytes and verified by the demonstration of an inflammatory reaction by colonic biopsy. A relatively infrequent but severe form of antibiotic-associated colitis is pseudomembranous colitis (PMC) which is almost invariably due to *C. difficile*. Common associated findings in patients with antibiotic-associated colitis include systemic findings of fever and leukocytosis. The fever is often low grade in the 100°F to 102°F (37.7–38.8°C) range, but it may be as high as 105°F (40.5°C). The peripheral leukocyte count is often 10,000 to 15,000 per microliter, but there may be a leukemoid reaction with counts of 50,000 or higher. Late and serious complications include ileus, toxic megacolon, intestinal perforation, electrolyte imbalance due to fluid losses, and hypoalbuminemia sometimes associated with anasarca. The most common agent associated with these severe complications is *C. difficile*, which is important to recognize due to the potential severity of the syndrome associated with it as well as the fact that it is readily treatable.

Antibiotic-associated diarrhea and colitis were described as complications of antibiotic administration soon after these agents were introduced in the late 1940s. The implication of *Staphylococcus aureus* at that time is not surprising since it was a major nosocomial pathogen, and its recovery in stool with the antibiotics used was not surprising. In fact, stool cultures yield *S. aureus* in 20 to 30 percent of healthy persons and in up to 90 percent of patients taking commonly used antibiotics, even in the absence of a change in bowel habits. A retrospective review of the information published at that time casts doubts on the etiologic role of *S. aureus*.

C. difficile is now recognized as the most common identifiable agent of antibiotic-associated diarrhea and colitis. The frequency of this organism is dependent directly on the severity of the disease process. Among patients who have uncomplicated antibiotic-associated diarrhea, it is implicated in 15 to 25 percent, meaning that the majority are due to some other mechanism. For those who have evidence of colitis by endoscopy the frequency is 50 to 70 percent, and in those with pseudomembranous colitis, it is 90 to 100 percent. Causes of antibiotic-associated diarrhea and colitis in which *C. difficile* is not implicated are often enigmatic.

It is possible that *S. aureus* may actually be occasionally involved, although this is a matter of considerable debate and extremely difficult to prove given the frequency with which *S. aureus* is found in the stools of healthy persons. There are occasional cases of what appears to be antibiotic-associated diarrhea in which salmonella can be recovered in stool. In large outbreaks of salmonella infections, it has been frequently noted that the majority of patients who have the disease are those who were taking antibiotics for diverse indications. The only other microbial agent that has been occasionally found is *Clostridium perfringens,* which is also frequently associated with food poisoning.

For the majority of patients who have antibiotic-associated diarrhea with no evidence of *C. difficile,* the mechanism of the diarrhea is not known. The popular notion is that it represents a poorly understood alteration in the intestinal bacterial flora that presumably maintains homeostasis and is sometimes referred to as "dysbiosis." Most of these patients have diarrhea without colitis, the diarrhea starts during antibiotic therapy, it is usually not devastating, and it is dose-related with prompt resolution when the implicated agent is either reduced in dose or discontinued.

The best understood form of antibiotic-associated diarrhea and colitis is *C. difficile*–induced disease. There are four interrelated factors that participate in the pathogenesis of this complication:

1. Altered intestinal flora: The common denominator here is exposure to antibiotics. The major culprits are ampicillin, amoxicillin, clindamycin, and cephalosporins, although almost any antibiotic that alters the normal flora has been implicated including tetracycline, chloramphenicol, erythromycin, and trimethoprim-sulfamethoxazole. Antibiotics active only against parasites, fungi, viruses, or mycobacteria are not responsible. Aminoglycosides given parenterally do not appear to cause this complication, presumably because they are not excreted into the gut. The pivotal role of drugs is the effect they have on the intestinal flora.

2. A source of *C. difficile* is obviously required. Approximately 3 percent of healthy adults harbor *C. difficile* in their normal flora, and these individuals are presumably susceptible when antibiotics are given. It has also been noted that there may be epidemics of *C. difficile*–induced diarrhea and colitis in hospitals and chronic care facilities. Here the organism appears to be acquired from environmental sources, and the outbreaks occur as a reflection of the clustering of large numbers of patients rendered susceptible by the frequent use of antibiotics.

3. There must be toxin produced by *C. difficile.* This is a toxin-mediated complication in which there is no microbial invasion of the gut. *C. difficile* actually produces two distinct protein toxins referred to as toxin A and toxin B. Toxin B is a powerful cytotoxin which is responsible for the changes in the standard toxin assay for detecting *C. difficile.* However, toxin A appears to be responsible for the pathologic effects since only this toxin reproduces the changes noted in the colon in experimental infection. Both toxins are reproduced during log-phase growth. Translating these observations to the clinical setting, the assumption is that the antibiotic distorts the normal flora to produce an environmental setting in which *C. difficile* has an opportunity to replicate and produce toxin. Most strains of *C. difficile* produce both toxin A and toxin B, although there appear to be strain variations in the amount of toxin produced which may account for differences in the disease severity.

4. Age-related susceptibility is also an important consideration. Most enteric pathogens are far more common in the young, reflecting frequent exposure and immunologic naiveté, but observations with infants and *C. difficile* are a bit of a paradox. Repeated studies show that children less than 3 months of age often harbor *C. difficile* and its toxins with no associated antibiotic usage and no clinical consequences. Following the development of the usual flora at 6 to 12 months of age, the carrier rate of *C. difficile* is low and the toxins are virtually never encountered except with antibiotic exposure. The frequency of clinical expression with diarrhea and colitis subsequently shows a direct correlation with age, so that older adults are especially vulnerable.

These four factors account for the composite clinical picture of *C. difficile*–induced diarrhea and colitis. The usual patient is an adult, and the most serious disease is encountered in the elderly. The patient is either previously colonized with *C. difficile* or acquires the organism from an exogenous source such as a hospital or nursing home. This by itself is of little importance except in the presence of antibiotic exposure. Assuming the organism has toxigenic potential and the antibiotic given has a sufficient impact on the normal flora, *C. difficile* has the opportunity to replicate, produce toxin, and ultimately cause clinical disease. Variations in the clinical disease may be due to the amount of toxin produced, other virulence factors of the organism, and the susceptibility of the host.

Many cases of *C. difficile*–induced enteric disease are isolated events and represent sporadic disease. However, as noted, this organism may also produce epidemics or outbreaks within hospitals and nursing homes, or it may be endemic within an institution, meaning there is an increased rate of this complication that persists over a sustained period of time. The epidemic or endemic strain may be highly virulent and cause severe disease or it may be of relatively low virulence so that large numbers of cases are apparent only when this diagnosis is carefully sought.

Two different methods are used to evaluate antibiotic-associated diarrhea, one directed at identifying the etiologic agent and the second at defining anatomic changes.

The decision to perform a diagnostic evaluation depends on the severity of the symptoms and the epidemiology. Antibiotic-associated diarrhea is often trivial and subsides promptly when the implicated drug is discontinued. There is little reason to perform any further tests in such individuals unless multiple patients are affected. The major justifications for a diagnostic evaluation in the patient with antibiotic-associated diarrhea are (1) severe diarrhea with large volumes of stool; (2) diarrhea that occurs in association with systemic changes such as fever and leukocytosis; (3) chronic diarrhea that persists despite discontinuation of the implicated antibiotics; and (4) outbreaks in which the reason to pursue less severe cases is for infection control purposes.

The first therapeutic maneuver is discontinuation of the implicated agent. Patients who do not respond and satisfy the criteria noted above warrant a diagnostic evaluation. Fecal leukocyte examinations are easily performed, but are not particularly rewarding in this setting. Approximately half of the patients with *C. difficile*–induced disease have fecal leukocytes, but this is viewed as a nonspecific finding compatible with many other forms of infectious diarrhea, and the absence of this finding certainly does not exclude the diagnosis. Stool cultures in most hospital laboratories include studies to detect salmonella, *Shigella,* and *Campylobacter jejuni.* None of these are common agents of antibiotic-associated diarrhea. Stool cultures for *C. difficile* are sometimes done, but most hospital laboratories do not offer this type of culturing, and the best clinical correlations are with detection of the toxin. The preferred test is a tissue culture assay to detect a cytopathic toxin that is neutralized with *C. difficile* or *Clostridium sordellii* antitoxin. (The neutralization of this toxin by *C. sordellii* antitoxin represents an antigenic cross-reaction.) There are other methods to assess for *C. difficile* toxins, but none are as sensitive or specific as the tissue culture assay, which is regarded as the gold standard.

The second type of test that is often performed is endoscopy to define the nature of pathologic changes in the colon. This is often accomplished with sigmoidoscopy, but pseudomembranes are beyond the reach of the sigmoidoscope in up to one-third of cases, and colonoscopy is regarded as the most definitive procedure. Typical findings in the patient with antibiotic-associated colitis are erythema, edema, and often friability of the colonic mucosa. The most characteristic feature of *C. difficile* colitis is the detection of pseudomembranes characterized by white or grayish plaques which stud the intestinal mucosa, often with skip areas. Pseudomembranes colitis (PMC) was actually described in the preantibiotic era and not all cases are antibiotic-associated, but the great majority are and most authorities consider the observation of PMC sufficiently compelling to assume *C. difficile* is responsible. The toxin assay is regarded as the most definitive method to implicate this organism and is certainly preferred on the basis of cost, patient convenience, and sensitivity since many patients have a rather serious illness with nonspecific findings on endoscopy.

The indications for specific forms of treatment directed against *C. difficile* are similar to those suggested for the diagnostic evaluation based primarily on the severity and chronicity of the symptoms. Patients who have modest illnesses often respond well when the implicated antibiotic is simply discontinued. With more severe disease or persistent disease, the favored drugs are vancomycin given orally in a dose of 125 mg 4 times daily, or metronidazole given orally in a dose of 500 mg 3 times daily. The usual duration of treatment is 10 to 15 days. Vancomycin is generally preferred for patients who are seriously ill. The main reason for interest in metronidazole is the high cost of vancomycin which runs $200 to $600 per course compared to $10 to $20 for metronidazole.

The anticipated response to either agent is dramatic. Patients with fever, including those with high fevers, usually become afebrile within 24 to 48 hours. Diarrhea generally resolves with the return to normal bowel habits in an average of 5 to 7 days. There are occasional failures with metronidazole, but this is rarely a problem with vancomycin unless the patient has an ileus or toxic megacolon which prevents the drugs from reaching the site of infection. Vancomycin is not absorbed when given orally, but this is appropriate since *C. difficile* does not invade the intestinal mucosa. For patients who cannot take oral medication, there is no specific treatment with well-established merit. Anecdotal case reports suggest intravenous metronidazole may be helpful, but oral treatment should be instituted as soon as feasible.

The major problems associated with either vancomycin or metronidazole treatment are relapses following discontinuation of treatment. Typically, the patient responds well, but then has recurrence of similar symptoms at several days or up to 1 month after the drug was discontinued. The agent selected and the dose and duration of treatment have essentially no influence on the frequency of relapse. Relapses have been reported in 5 to 55 percent of patents, but the usual rate is around 25 percent. Patients who relapse usually respond when either of the drugs is given again, but there may be subsequent relapses, and occasionally patients have a "multiple relapse pattern" characterized by five or more relapses with each successive course of antibiotics. The best method to manage relapses is to give the usual antibiotic course for 10 to 14 days; once the patient is stabilized, a second course of treatment is given consisting of oral administration of lactobacilli, low-dose vancomycin (125 mg every other day), or cholestyramine. This second course of treatment should follow the initial course and should not be given concurrently. The intent here is to stabilize the patient with the initial course of treatment and to continue stabilization while the normal flora become reestablished. Lactobacilli are given to assist in restoring the normal flora, cholestyramine works by binding the toxin produced by *C. difficile,* and the low dose of vancomycin permits control of *C. difficile* with minimal impact on the normal flora. All three have enthusiastic advocates and they seem to work most of the time, but none are universally successful.

For the patient with antibiotic-associated diarrhea or colitis without *C. difficile* toxin, there is no specific form of therapy that can be advocated except for supportive care. Nevertheless, occasional patients appear to respond to oral vancomycin as described above. Suggested explanations for response in this setting are the possibility that the disease would have resolved with no treatment, the toxin assay may have been falsely negative, or there may be another organism such as another clostridial species or even *S. aureus* that may be responsible.

1. Bartlett, J. G., Chang, T. W., Gurwith M., et al. Antibiotic-associated pseudomembranous colitis due to toxin producing clostridia. *N. Engl. J. Med.* 298:531, 1978.
   The original report implicating C. difficile *in antibiotic-associated colitis.*
2. Mogg, G. M., Keighley, M., Burdon, D., et al. Antibiotic-associated colitis: A review of 66 cases. *Br. J. Surg.* 66:738, 1979.
   A review of clinical features of antibiotic-associated colitis from a surgical group in England.
3. Tedesco F. J. Clindamycin-associated colitis: Review of the clinical spectrum of 47 cases. *Dig. Dis.* 21:26, 1976.
   A review of clinical features of antibiotic-associated colitis from a surgical group in England.
4. Prohaska, J. V., Jacobson, M. J., Drake, C. T., et al. Staphylococcal enterotoxin enteritis. *Surg. Gynecol. Obstet.* 108:73, 1959.
5. Tedesco, F. J., Barton R. W., Alpers, H. D. Clindamycin-associated colitis. *Ann. Intern. Med.* 81:429, 1974.
   The original Barnes Hospital report of clindamycin-associated colitis in what was subsequently viewed as an epidemic.

6. Bartlett, J. G., Taylor, N. W., Chang, T. W., et al. Clinical and laboratory observations in *Clostridium difficile* colitis. *Am. J. Clin. Nutr.* 33:2521, 1981.
   A large series reviewing the clinical, microbiologic, and toxin assays for C. difficile *in patients with diarrhea.*
7. Bartlett, J. G. Antimicrobial agents implicated in *Clostridium difficile* toxin associated diarrhea or colitis. *Johns Hopkins Med. J.* 149:6, 1981.
   A review of antibiotics implicated in over 300 patients with antibiotic-associated diarrhea or colitis due to C. difficile.
8. Bartlett, J. G., Onderdonk, A. B., Cisneros, A. B., et al. Clindamycin-associated colitis due to toxin producing species of *Clostridium* in hamsters. *J. Infect. Dis.* 136:701, 1977.
   The original report of C. difficile *as the agent of antibiotic-associated hemorrhagic cecitis in hamsters.*
9. George. W. L., Sutter, V. L., Citron, D., et al. Selective and differential medium for isolation of *Clostridium difficile*. *J. Clin. Microbiol.* 9:214, 1979.
   A review of methods to culture C. difficile.
10. Fekety, R., Kim, K.-H., Brown, D., et al. Epidemiology of antibiotic-associated colitis. *Am. J. Med.* 70:906, 1981.
    A large-scale epidemiologic survey of hospitals for C. difficile.
11. Taylor, N. S., Thorne, G. M., and Bartlett, J. G. Comparison of two toxins produced by *Clostridium difficile*. *Infect. Immun.* 34:1036, 1981.
    This is the original report of a second toxin produced by C. difficile.
12. Viscidi, R., Willey, S., and Bartlett, J. G. Isolation rates and toxigenic potential of *Clostridium difficile* isolates from various patient populations. *Gastroenterology* 81:5, 1981.
    A review of clinical and microbiologic data dealing with C. difficile.
13. Mulligan, M. E., George, W. L., Rolfe, R. D., et al. Epidemiological aspects of *Clostridium difficile*–induced diarrhea and colitis. *Am. J. Clin. Nutr.* 33:2533, 1981.
    An epidemiologic study showing high isolation rates of C. difficile *in case-associated areas.*
14. Chang, T. W., Lauermann, M., and Bartlett, J. G. Cytotoxicity assay in antibiotic-associated colitis. *J. Infect. Dis.* 140:765, 1979.
    The standard tissue culture assay to detect C. difficile *toxin is reviewed.*
15. Tedesco, F. J. Antibiotic-associated pseudomembranous colitis with negative proctosigmoidoscopy examination. *Gastroenterology* 7:295, 1980.
    The author notes the importance of colonoscopy in place of sigmoidoscopy for detecting PMC in some cases.
16. Bartlett, J. G. Treatment of *Clostridium difficile* colitis. *Gastroenterology* 89:1192, 1985.
    A review of the treatments for C. difficile–*induced colitis.*
17. Teasley, D. G., Gerding, D. N., Olson, M. M., et al. Prospective randomized trial of metronidazole versus vancomycin for *Clostridium difficile*–induced diarrhoea and colitis. *Lancet* 1:1843, 1983.
    A comparison of metronidazole and vancomycin shows them to be equally effective in treating C. difficile–*induced colitis.*

74. ASCITES
Jerry L. Spivak

Ascites is a complication of many diseases, but recognition of ascites by physical examination is often difficult. Shifting dullness and fluid waves are not specific and may be elicited in the presence of a distended viscus, pelvic cyst, neoplasm, or hydramnios. Abdominal shape is not helpful since massive ascites may be present without bulging flanks. Needle aspiration may be negative because of failure to appreciate the thickness of the panniculus or because of loculation or mucinous consistency of the ascitic fluid. Ultrasound can be helpful, but peritoneoscopy may be necessary to confirm the clinical impression.

Evaluation of the cause of ascites begins with examination of the ascitic fluid, with attention to color; specific gravity; cell count and differential; protein, glucose, and amylase determinations; cytology; Gram's and acid-fast stains; and cultures.

The best test for distinguishing exudative from transudative ascites is not the total ascitic fluid protein concentration but rather the serum-ascites albumin concentration gradient (serum albumin–ascites albumin). A concentration gradient greater than 1.1 suggests a transudate. The gradient is not helpful, however, in distinguishing the cause of exudative ascites or defining situations in which the ascites has both exudative and transudative components.

The mechanism for transudative ascites is still under debate. One school of thought holds that excessive hepatic lymph formation results in intraperitoneal fluid accumulation, a diminution in plasma volume, and an attendant retention of salt and water leading to ascites (underfill theory). Another school holds that salt and water retention are primary (overflow theory). Of course, the necessary underlying abnormality in splanchnic and hepatic hemodynamics must be present in either case, and it is likely that elements of both "underfill" and "overflow" are involved in transudative ascites. It is also thought that systemic arteriovenous fistulas which occur in cirrhosis are involved in this process.

The most common cause of ascites is obstruction to hepatic venous outflow, usually due to diffuse hepatic disease and less commonly to hepatic vein or inferior vena cava obstruction by web, thrombosis, or tumor (Budd-Chiari syndrome). The absence of jaundice is no guarantee that the ascites is not due to an intrahepatic process since regenerating nodules can provide adequate liver function while causing postsinusoidal obstruction to blood flow. A low ascitic fluid protein level is also no assurance that infection is not present. Ascitic fluid protein is usually less than 3 gm/dl in the spontaneous bacterial peritonitis of cirrhosis, but the cloudy appearance and elevated leukocyte count of the fluid should leave no doubt about the presence of infection. Ascites may occasionally result in hydrothorax, which is more frequently observed on the right side but may occur bilaterally. The origin of the hydrothorax is not completely understood. The condition may be due to diaphragmatic defects, lymphatic communications, or abnormalities of pleural venous or lymphatic drainage. Meigs' syndrome is the association of ovarian tumors with ascites and hydrothorax in the absence of metastases. Hydrothorax, however, is not always present. Exudative ascites is usually the result of an infectious, inflammatory, or neoplastic process within the peritoneal cavity. An exception to this is the ascites associated with myxedema, in which the protein content may be more than 4 gm/dl; the fluid is ascitic and not myxedematous. When an exudative fluid is found, the possibility of tuberculous peritonitis must always be considered.

Amylase determination will avoid missing a pancreatic cause for ascites, particularly since a history of acute pancreatitis is often lacking. Bloody ascites may be due to a traumatic tap, tuberculosis, sarcoidosis, metastatic carcinoma, or hepatoma. The difficulty of distinguishing tumor cells from mesothelial cells with Wright's stain necessitates the use of special cytologic techniques. In this regard, the initial fluid withdrawn may not be as helpful as a second specimen into which fresh cells have been shed. A careful rectal examination is also important; it may reveal induration of the rectal shelf. Chylous ascites may have a high or low protein content without regard to cause and may occur with cirrhosis, lymphoma, intraabdominal and metastatic carcinoma, and the nephrotic syndrome.

Therapy of ascites is directed toward the underlying disease. Paracentesis is useful for both diagnostic and therapeutic purposes. Removal of fluid therapeutically may be employed when ascites compromises respiration, to assist in initiating a diuresis, or to lower portal pressure when there is bleeding from varices. As in the case of pericardial tamponade, removal of only a small amount of fluid can produce a significant increase in cardiac output by increasing venous return. Although it was formerly held that large-volume paracentesis could result in significant hypovolemia, this appears not to be the case, particularly in edematous patients in whom paracentesis with the intravenous infusion of albumin can be an effective means of initiating diuresis. In the nonedematous patient, removal of more than 750 ml of ascites may cause a fall in plasma volume. The physician should also be aware that the paracentesis needle track can provide a path for continued fluid drainage, which may proceed externally or dissect internally along tissue planes, resulting in subcutaneous or scrotal edema. A small needle should be used and inserted through the linea alba. Bleeding is a hazard if other locations are used, and massive retroperitoneal hemorrhage can occur with a lateral approach. Repeated paracentesis can result in hypoproteinemia and dilutional hyponatremia due to stimulation of antidiuretic hormone (ADH) secretion. When ascites is the result of sodium retention, reduction of sodium chloride intake to 500 mg/day prevents continued formation. Diuretic therapy, if administered judiciously and with adequate potassium chloride supplementation, can result in a reduction of ascites. Hypovolemia and electrolyte imbalance are complications of diuretic therapy and, in the patient with liver failure, encephalopathy can be precipitated. Ascites due to portal hypertension is not predictably alleviated following portacaval shunt, particularly with an end-to-side anastomosis.

The peritoneovenous shunt is an alternate method for the treatment of ascites that avoids the dangers of electrolyte imbalance and renal insufficiency. The shunt consists of a perforated tube, embedded subcutaneously, which links the peritoneal cavity with the superior vena cava. By virtue of a one-way pressure-sensitive valve, ascites fluid moves from the abdomen to the bloodstream during inspiration. Complications include fever, shunt blockage, disseminated intravascular coagulation (DIC), infection, leakage of peritoneal fluid, circulatory overload, variceal hemorrhage, and superior vena cava thrombosis. DIC or a reduction in fibrinogen survival is virtually an inevitable consequence of the peritoneovenous shunt. Clinically, significant hemorrhage is not uncommon and has proved fatal, but its occurrence is unpredictable. Peritoneovenous shunting may have a role in the management of malignant ascites but should be used with caution in patients with cirrhosis and hepatic decompensation. In these patients, the liver is least able to either clear activated clotting factors or compensate for their increased consumption.

1. Rocco, V. K., and Ware, A. J. Cirrhotic ascites. *Ann. Intern. Med.* 105:573, 1986.
   Comprehensive review of pathophysiology, differential diagnosis, and treatment.
2. Rector, W. G., Jr., and Reynolds, T. B. Superiority of the serum-ascites albumin difference over ascites total protein concentration in separation of "transudative" and "exudative" ascites. *Am. J. Med.* 77:83, 1984.
   The total ascitic fluid protein concentration is not as informative in distinguishing between transudates and exudates as the difference between the serum albumin and ascitic fluid albumin concentrations (see also Gastroenterology 85:240, 1983 *and* Hepatology 8:1104, 1988).
3. Frakes, J. T. Physiologic considerations in the medical management of ascites. *Arch. Intern. Med.* 140:620, 1980.
   Salt and water restriction with the judicious use of diuretics is usually effective.
4. Hyman, S., Villa, F., and Steigman, F. Mimetic aspects of ascites. *J.A.M.A.* 183:651, 1963.
   Similar clinical presentations of cirrhosis, metastatic tumor, tuberculous peritonitis, and hepatoma.
5. Baker, A., Kaplan, M., and Wolfe, H. Central congestive fibrosis of the liver in myxedema ascites. *Ann. Intern. Med.* 77:927, 1972.
   Myxedema must always be considered in the differential diagnosis of exudative ascites.
6. Takeuchi, J., Takada, A., Hasumura, Y., et al. Budd-Chiari syndrome associated with obstruction of the inferior vena cava. *Am. J. Med.* 51:11, 1971.
   Painless ascites and edema without jaundice.
7. Cameron, J. Chronic pancreatic ascites and pancreatic pleural effusions. *Gastroenterology* 74:134, 1978.
   Ascites is usually due to the formation of a pancreatic fistula; medical therapy should be employed first.
8. Gluck, Z., and Nolph, K. D. Ascites associated with end-stage renal disease. *Am. J. Kidney Dis.* 10:9, 1987.

A difficult diagnostic and therapeutic problem. (See also Arch. Intern. Med. *148:1577, 1988 and* Surgery *101:161, 1987.)*

9. Clinicopathologic Conference. Massive ascites due to Meigs' syndrome. *Am. J. Med.* 47:125, 1969.
   Pathogenesis of Meigs' syndrome.

10. Lindenbaum, J., and Scheidt, S. S. Chylous ascites and the nephrotic syndrome. *Am. J. Med.* 44:830, 1968.
    An interesting association.

11. Pockros, P. J., and Reynolds, T. B. Rapid diuresis in patients with ascites from chronic liver disease: the importance of peripheral edema. *Gastroenterology* 90:1827, 1986.
    Rapid diuresis is most safe in patients with edema. (See also Gastroenterology *90:2022, 1986 and* Lancet *1:775, 1988.)*

12. Reynolds, T. B. Therapeutic paracentesis. Have we come full circle? *Gastroenterology* 93:386, 1987.
    Large-volume paracentesis can be performed safely. (See also Gastroenterology *93:234, 1987.)*

13. Pinto, P. C., American, J., and Reynolds, T. B. Large-volume paracentesis in non-edematous patients with tense ascites: its effect on intravascular volume. *Hepatology* 8:207, 1988.
    A 5-liter paracentesis did not reduce the plasma volume. (See also Hepatology *8:1167, 1988.)*

14. Gauthier, A., Levy, V. G., Quinton, A., et al. Salt or no salt in the treatment of cirrhotic ascites: a randomized study. *Gut* 27:705, 1986.
    Salt restriction is important.

15. Rector, W. G., Jr. "Diuretic-resistant" ascites. Observations on pathogenesis. *Arch. Intern. Med.* 146:1597, 1986.
    Renal function is a major determinant of diuretic responsiveness. (See also Canad. Med. Assoc. J. *135:481, 1986.)*

16. Black, M., and Friedman, A. C. Ultrasound examination in the patient with ascites. *Ann. Intern. Med.* 110:253, 1989.
    Ultrasound is useful not only to identify ascites but to determine the presence of hepatic or portal venous obstruction. (See also Gastroenterology *104:377, 1986.)*

17. Lawson, J. D., and Weissbein, A. S. The puddle sign: An aid in the diagnosis of minimal ascites. *N. Engl. J. Med.* 260:652, 1959.
    A simple test for a difficult diagnostic problem.

18. Jolles, H., and Coulam, C. M. CT of ascites: Differential diagnosis. *AJR* 135:315, 1980.
    Computed tomography scanning can detect ascites with a high degree of accuracy.

19. Gregory, P. B., Broekelschen, P. H., Hill, M. D., et al. Complications of diuresis in the alcoholic patient with ascites: A controlled trial. *Gastroenterology* 73:534, 1977.
    Diuresis was accomplished without serious side effects due to the diuretics.

20. Llach, J., Gines, P., Arroyo, V., et al. Prognostic value of arterial pressure, endogenous vasoactive systems, and renal function in cirrhotic patients admitted to the hospital for the treatment of ascites. *Gastroenterology* 94:482, 1988.
    Blood pressure and renal function are the most important variables.

21. Mallory, A., and Schaefer, J. W. Complications of diagnostic paracentesis in patients with liver disease. *J.A.M.A.* 239:628, 1978.
    Hemorrhage, bowel perforation, and infection.

22. Fischer, D. S. Abdominal paracentesis for malignant ascites. *Arch. Intern. Med.* 139:235, 1979.
    Catheter drainage for malignant ascites. (See also J.A.M.A. *225:1361, 1973.)*

23. Conn, H. O. Unilateral edema and jaundice after portacaval anastomosis. *Ann. Intern. Med.* 76:459, 1972.
    Dissection of ascitic fluid through the surgical wound to dependent areas.

24. Wilcox, C. M., and Dismukes, W. E. Spontaneous bacterial peritonitis. *Medicine* 66:447, 1987.
    Ascites from any cause is a risk factor and an ascitic fluid neutrophil count of >500 per microliter is suggestive.

25. Rimland, D., and Hand, W. L. Spontaneous peritonitis: a reappraisal. *Am. J. Med. Sci.* 30:285, 1987.
    Invasive procedures appear to predispose to this complication. (See also Am. J. Gastroenterol. *81:1156, 1986.)*
26. Gerding, D. N., Hall, W. H., and Schierl, E. A. Antibiotic concentrations in ascitic fluid of patients with ascites and bacterial peritonitis. *Ann. Intern. Med.* 86:708, 1977.
    Direct instillation is not usually necessary but there is a lag time for achieving therapeutic levels after systemic administration.
27. Haight, J. B., and Ockner, S. A. *Chlamydia trachomatis* perihepatitis with ascites. *Am. J. Gastroenterol.* 83:323, 1988.
    An interesting version of the Fitz-Hugh–Curtis syndrome. (See also Br. J. Med. *293:5, 1986.)*
28. Wapnich, S., Grosberg, S., Kenney, M., et al. LaVeen continuous peritoneal-jugular shunt. *J.A.M.A.* 237:131, 1977.
    Description of the LeVeen shunt.
29. Epstein, M. Peritoneovenous shunt in the management of ascites and the hepatorenal syndrome. *Gastroenterology* 82:790, 1982.
    Peritoneovenous shunting found to be effective in relieving intractable ascites but should only be employed after medical therapy fails.
30. Tempero, M. A., Davis, R. B., Reed, E., et al. Thrombocytopenia and laboratory evidence of disseminated intravascular coagulation after shunts for ascites in malignant disease. *Cancer* 55:2718, 1985.
    A common problem with peritoneovenous shunts. (See also Cancer *55:1973, 1985 and* Ann. Intern. Med. *90:774, 1979.)*
31. Stein, S. F., Fulenwider, T., Ansley, J. D., et al. Accelerated fibrinogen and platelet destruction after peritoneovenous shunting. *Arch. Intern. Med.* 141:1149, 1981.
    Evaluation of the mechanism of the coagulopathy associated with peritoneovenous shunts.
32. Straus, A. K., Roseman, D. L., and Shapiro, T. M. Peritoneovenous shunting in the management of malignant ascites. *Arch. Surg.* 114:489, 1979.
    Effective palliation achieved. (See also J. Surg. Oncol. *33:31, 1986.)*
33. Epstein, M. Treatment of refractory ascites. *N. Engl. J. Med.* 321:1675, 1989.
    *Medical therapy including large volume paracentesis is preferable to a mechanical shunt. Shunts do not prolong survival (*N. Engl. J. Med. *321:1632, 1989).*

75. CHRONIC PANCREATITIS
Jerry L. Spivak

Chronic pancreatic insufficiency is most commonly caused by chronic alcohol abuse. Other etiologic factors include malnutrition, hypercalcemia, vascular disease, hemochromatosis, cystic fibrosis, stenosis of the sphincter of Oddi, and hereditary pancreatitis. In some cases no predisposing condition can be identified. There is good evidence that recurrent bouts of acute pancreatitis, such as that associated with gallstones, rarely result in irreversible destructive changes in the pancreas. The clinical presentation of chronic pancreatitis may be one of weight loss, steatorrhea, glucose intolerance, and pancreatic calcification or recurrent attacks of abdominal pain indistinguishable from acute pancreatitis and with the attendant complications, such as pseudocyst formation.

The mechanism by which ethanol abuse results in chronic destructive changes in the pancreas is unknown. Suggested possibilities include protein malnutrition, abnormal bile formation with an increase in free bile acids that cause pancreatic cell damage, a direct toxic effect, increased pancreatic secretion in combination with duct obstruction, and sphincter atony with reflux of duodenal contents. Morphologically there is obstruction and dilatation of the smaller pancreatic ducts and atrophy, fibrosis, and calcification of glandular tissue. The importance of protein malnutrition is indicated by the fact that dietary protein repletion can correct an abnormal pancreatic response to secretin in the presence of continued ethanol ingestion. Loss of pancreatic exocrine function results in malabsorption of fat, protein, and carbohydrate. Weight loss is usually marked despite a good appetite, and a characteristic of the steatorrhea is the presence of gross oil in the stool. In contrast to nontropical sprue, anorexia, weakness, edema, tetany, vitamin K deficiency, and osteomalacia are uncommon. This may be a reflection of the shorter duration of illness in patients with chronic pancreatitis, the presence of a normal intestinal mucosa, or the ability of bile salts alone to facilitate the absorption of fat-soluble vitamins. The reserve capacity of the pancreas is such that over 90 percent of the gland must be destroyed before steatorrhea or nitrogen loss becomes significant.

Chronic pancreatitis, particularly the painless variety, must be distinguished from other causes of malabsorption, such as tropical and nontropical sprue, Whipple's disease, intestinal diverticuli, abdominal lymphoma, diabetic steatorrhea, and pancreatic carcinoma. Pancreatic function tests require specialized facilities, but x-ray studies, small bowel biopsy, and glucose tolerance and D-xylose absorption tests usually distinguish pancreatic disease from the other possibilities. It should be noted, however, that D-xylose absorption can be abnormal in the presence of pancreatic disease. Differentiation of pancreatic carcinoma from pancreatic inflammation can be more difficult. Occult intestinal blood loss, anorexia, jaundice with a palpable gallbladder, and migratory phlebitis are helpful signs. Angiography is the most rewarding x-ray study, but in the final analysis nothing can replace a tissue diagnosis.

Therapy of chronic pancreatitis begins with determination of the cause and removal of the noxious stimulus. Cessation of alcohol ingestion usually results in alleviating pain; destruction of the gland continues but at a lesser rate. Therapy with insulin, pancreatic extracts, sodium bicarbonate, antibiotics, antimotility agents, medium-chain triglycerides, and vitamins (including B_{12}) must be tailored to the individual patient. The optimal surgical management for patients with intractable pain and debility is unsettled. Decompression of the pancreatic duct provides relief of pain but does not prevent continued destruction of the gland. Near-total (80–95%) pancreatectomy relieves pain but produces insulin dependence. Lesser degrees of pancreatic extirpation are not as effective. Islet autotransplantation is a promising new adjunct to near-total pancreatectomy but is still at the experimental stage.

1. Niederau C., and Grendell, J. H. Diagnosis of chronic pancreatitis. *Gastroenterology* 88:1973, 1985.
   Comprehensive review with an approach differentiating between pancreatitis and pancreatic carcinoma. (See also Am. J. Gastroenterol. 81:153, 1986.).
2. Strum, W. B., and Spiro, H. M. Chronic pancreatitis. *Ann. Intern. Med.* 74:264, 1971.
   Alcohol causes chronic changes before the first painful episode occurs.
3. Nagata, A., Homma, T., Tamai, K., et al. A study of chronic pancreatitis by serial endoscopic pancreatography. *Gastroenterology* 81:884, 1981.
   Pancreatic ductal lesions were progressive in alcoholic pancreatitis even with abstinence. (See also Gastroenterology 95:1063, 1985.)
4. Jones, S. N., Lees, W. R., and Frost, R. A. Diagnosis and grading of chronic pancreatitis by morphological criteria derived by ultrasound and pancreatography. *Clin. Radiol.* 39:43, 1988.
   Ultrasound is more useful than computed tomography scanning.
5. Warshaw, A. L., Heizer, W. D., and Laster, L. Pancreatic insufficiency as the presenting feature of hyperparathyroidism. *Ann. Intern. Med.* 68:161, 1969.
   Unusual correctable cause of pancreatic insufficiency.
6. Coates, E. O. Characteristics of cystic fibrosis in adults: A report of seven patients. *Dis. Chest* 49:195, 1966.
   Pulmonary symptoms usually mask pancreatic insufficiency.
7. Banks, P. A., and Janowitz, H. D. Some metabolic aspects of exocrine pancreatic disease. *Gastroenterology* 56:601, 1969.
   Antecedents and consequences of pancreatic insufficiency.
8. Mezey, E., Jow, E., Slavin, R. E., et al. Pancreatic function and intestinal absorption in chronic alcoholism. *Gastroenterology* 59:657, 1970.

Protein malnutrition is in part responsible for malabsorption in chronic alcoholism.

9. Clinicopathologic Conference. Chronic relapsing pancreatitis with cardiac and renal disease. *Am. J. Med.* 53:335, 1972.
   Atheroembolic pancreatitis.

10. McElroy, R., and Christiansen, P. A. Hereditary pancreatitis in a kinship associated with portal vein thrombosis. *Am. J. Med.* 52:228, 1972.
    Familial pancreatitis, portal hypertension, and sudden death.

11. DiMagno, E. P., Go, V. L. W., and Summerskill, W. H. J. Pancreatic enzyme outputs and malabsorption in pancreatic insufficiency. *N. Engl. J. Med.* 288:813, 1973.
    Steatorrhea and creatorrhea occur only when pancreatic function is reduced to 10% of normal.

12. Evans, W. B., and Wollaeger, E. E. Incidence and severity of nutritional deficiency states in chronic exocrine pancreatic insufficiency: Comparison with nontropical sprue. *Am. J. Dig. Dis.* 11:594, 1966.
    Gross oil in the stool suggested as a sign of pancreatic insufficiency.

13. Bank, S., Marks, I. N., Farman, J., et al. Further observations on calcified medullary bone lesions in chronic pancreatitis. *Gastroenterology* 51:224, 1966.
    Osteolytic and calcified lesions in calcific pancreatitis.

14. Longstreth, G. F., Newcomer, A. D., and Green, P. A. Extrahepatic portal hypertension caused by chronic pancreatitis. *Ann. Intern. Med.* 75:903, 1971.
    Portal hypertension without liver disease in chronic alcoholics. (See also Arch. Surg. *122:410, 1987.)*

15. Cameron, J. L. Chronic pancreatic ascites and pancreatic pleural effusions. *Gastroenterology* 74:134, 1978.
    Pancreatic ascites occurs as a consequence of pancreatic duct disruption with fistula formation. (See also Medicine *53:183, 1974.)*

16. Snope, W. J., Long, W. B., Trotman, B. W., et al. Marked alkaline phosphatase elevation with partial common bile duct obstruction due to calcific pancreatitis. *Gastroenterology* 70:70, 1976.
    Elevated alkaline phosphatase, with a normal bilirubin and BSP (sulfobromophthalein). (See also Surgery *82:303, 1977.)*

17. Toskes, P. P., Dawson, W., Curington, C., et al. Non-diabetic retinal abnormalities in chronic pancreatitis. *N. Engl. J. Med.* 300:942, 1979.
    Impaired dark adaptation and night vision in the absence of steatorrhea.

18. Marcoullis, G., Parmentier, Y., Nicolas, J.-P., et al. Cobalamin malabsorption due to nondegradation of R proteins in the human intestine. *J. Clin. Invest.* 66:430, 1980.
    Explanation of the mechanism of vitamin B_{12} malabsorption in pancreatic insufficiency.

19. Ammann, R. W., Muench, R., Otto, R., et al. Evolution and regression of pancreatic calcification in chronic pancreatitis. A prospective long-term study of 107 patients. *Gastroenterology* 95:1018, 1988.
    Spontaneous dissolution of stones occurs. (See also Gastroenterology *95:1144, 1988).*

20. Meyer, J. H. The ins and outs of oral pancreatic enzymes. *N. Engl. J. Med.* 296:1347, 1977.
    A brief review of pancreatic enzyme replacement therapy.

21. DiMagno, E. P. Medical treatment of pancreatic insufficiency. *Mayo Clin. Proc.* 54:435, 1979.
    Part of a symposium on the pancreas and its diseases.

22. DiMagno, E. P. Controversies in the treatment of exocrine pancreatic insufficiency. *Dig. Dis. Sci.* 27:481, 1982.
    Useful advice.

23. Angelini, G., Merigo, F., Degani, G., et al. Association of chronic alcoholic liver and pancreatic disease: a prospective study. *Am. J. Gastroenterol.* 80:998, 1985.
    Different factors appear to be involved in each disorder. (See also Am. J. Clin. Nutr. *48:148, 1988.)*

24. Sarles, H., Bernard, J. P., Johnson, C., et al. Pathogenesis and epidemiology of chronic pancreatitis. *Annu. Rev. Med.* 40:453, 1989.
    Comprehensive review.

25. Frey, C. F., Child, C. G., III, and Fry, W. Pancreatectomy for chronic pancreatitis. *Ann. Surg.* 184:403, 1976.
   Resection of less than 80% of the gland results in lower morbidity and mortality but probably less relief of pain. (See also Ann. Surg. 189:217, 1979.)
26. Warshaw, A. L., Popp, J. W., Jr., and Schapiro, R. H. Long-term patency, pancreatic function and pain relief after lateral pancreaticojejunostomy for chronic pancreatitis. *Gastroenterology* 79:289, 1980.
   Pancreatic duct decompression relieves pain but does not prevent continued tissue destruction.
27. Aldrete, J. S., Jimenez, H., and Halpern, N. B. Evaluation and treatment of acute and chronic pancreatitis. *Ann. Surg.* 191:664, 1980.
   The surgical management of patients with chronic pancreatitis is still a controversial subject. (See also Mayo Clin. Proc. 54:443, 1979.)
28. Balart, L. A., and Ferrante, W. A. Pathophysiology of acute and chronic pancreatitis. *Arch. Intern. Med.* 142:113, 1982.
   Concise review.

76. DIVERTICULOSIS
Jerry L. Spivak

Diverticulosis is a common asymptomatic condition which is usually discovered incidentally when a barium enema is done for other reasons. A few scattered diverticula may be seen, or the colon may be shortened and narrowed, with loss of haustral markings. The shortening is not due to inflammation but only to the excessive loss of mucosal surface by diverticular herniation. Herniation usually occurs at sites where vessels interrupt muscular continuity. The majority of diverticula occur in the sigmoid colon, where high pressures are generated prior to release of feces into the rectum. The increased incidence of diverticular disease in Western countries has led to the suggestion that the low-residue Western diet results in a less viscous stool, requiring greater sigmoid pressure to maintain continence. Other factors must also be involved since diverticula are not a constant feature of the irritable colon syndrome, in which very high intracolonic pressure is generated.

In 20 percent of individuals with diverticulosis (with females predominating) symptomatic diverticulitis may occur. It is always due to perforation of a diverticulum with resultant pericolic inflammation. Usually the leak seals quickly, but occasionally fecal soilage of the peritoneum occurs. The symptoms of diverticulitis—fever, abdominal pain, and a change in bowel functions—are not specific and can occur with other diseases affecting the colon or pelvic organs. The abdominal pain is usually localized to the left lower quadrant, but may be generalized if peritonitis has occurred. In addition, right lower quadrant pain, simulating appendiceal inflammation, may occur in women when drainage from a ruptured diverticulum is diverted to the right pelvis by the uterus. Sigmoidoscopy findings are usually normal in diverticulitis but can be normal in granulomatous colitis as well. On barium enema, it may be difficult to differentiate diverticulitis, colonic carcinoma, and granulomatous colitis. In general, granulomatous colitis tends to involve a greater segment of the bowel. Fever and abdominal pain in patients under age 40, in men, or when there is a history or presence of anal or perianal lesions also suggest granulomatous colitis as the likely diagnosis. In some instances, surgery is required to differentiate diverticulitis from other diseases. In this regard, it should be noted that a distended bladder pressing on the lower colon may mimic the signs of bowel disease, both clinically and radiologically.

The complications of diverticulitis are pericolic inflammation, fecal peritonitis, pelvic abscess, obstruction, fistula formation, and bleeding. Most patients with acute diverticulitis respond well to antibiotics and conservative therapy; surgery is not indicated unless appendicitis is suspected or peritonitis or a pelvic abscess is present. Indications for surgery after the acute episode has subsided are less clearly defined. Recurrent episodes of diverticulitis are not common. Surgical intervention is indicated for fistula, obstruction, persistence of a mass, particularly with continued fever, and when carcinoma or colitis cannot be excluded. The exact surgical approach for correction of diverticulitis is also controversial. It is, however, clear that a diverting colostomy with drainage is inadequate. Primary resection with the primary anastomosis appears to be the optimal approach, but in many instances the infectious and inflammatory complications prevent a primary anastomosis and a staged procedure must be employed.

Bleeding is an uncommon complication of diverticulosis, occurring in only 3 percent of the cases. However, diverticular bleeding is one of the causes of massive rectal hemorrhage. Angiodysplasia of the colon is another recognized cause of massive hemorrhage. Frequently, angiodysplasia coexists with diverticulosis. Other causes of bleeding include polyps, cancer, ischemic colitis, anticoagulation therapy, and thrombocytopenia. It should also be remembered that massive hemorrhage from the small bowel may present as rectal bleeding. In addition, massive hemorrhoidal hemorrhage may reflux in a retrograde fashion into the colon before any blood is expelled from the anus, thus obscuring the true site of hemorrhage. Due to the capacity of the colon, colonic hemorrhage is usually manifested as sudden evacuation of a large quantity of blood. The reservoir effect of the colon also makes it difficult to assess accurately the rate of bleeding. Initial management of the patient with brisk rectal hemorrhage should include gastric aspiration to rule out upper gastrointestinal hemorrhage, and sigmoidoscopy to rule out anal or rectal lesions. In most patients, bleeding will stop spontaneously. In patients who continue to bleed briskly, angiography should be employed to localize the site of bleeding. The intravascular catheter can also serve as a conduit for infusion of vasopressin. Colonoscopy is probably best reserved for patients who have stopped bleeding or are bleeding at a very slow rate. If either angiography or colonoscopy fails to reveal the site of bleeding, a barium enema should be performed. Bleeding frequently stops following a barium enema. However, colonic hemorrhage frequently stops spontaneously, so the significance of this observation is unclear. If a bleeding site is not demonstrable and particularly when angiodysplasia coexists with diverticulosis, subtotal colectomy is the recommended surgical procedure.

1. Almy, T. P., and Howell, D. A. Diverticular disease of the colon *N. Engl. J. Med.* 302:324, 1980.
   State-of-the-art review.
2. Slack, W. W. Diverticula of the colon and their relation to the muscle layers and blood vessels. *Gastroenterology* 39:708, 1960.
   Herniation occurs along vascular pathways.
3. Muir, E. Diverticulitis. *Lancet* 1:195, 1966.
   Diverticulitis often occurs without a history of symptoms.
4. Fleischner, F. G. Diverticular disease of the colon. *Gastroenterology* 60:316, 1971.
   X-ray findings in diverticulosis.
5. Chappuis, C. W., and Cohn, I., Jr. Acute colonic diverticulitis. *Surg. Clin. North Am.* 68:301, 1988.
   Useful review. (See also Dis. Colon Rectum *28:317, 1985.)*
6. Larson, D. M., Masters, S. S., and Spiro, H. M. Medical and surgical therapy in diverticular disease. *Gastroenterology* 71:734, 1976.
   In most patients diverticulitis is a single, nonrecurring event. Surgery is reserved for complications.
7. Feczko, P. J., Nish, A. D., Craig, B. M., et al. Acute diverticulitis in patients under 40 years of age: Radiologic diagnosis. *Am. J. Roentgenol.* 150:1311, 1988.
   Men predominate. (See also Dis. Colon Rectum *29:639, 1986.)*
8. Chodak, G. W., Rangel, D. M., and Passaro, E., Jr. Colonic diverticulitis in patients under age 40: Need for earlier diagnosis. *Am. J. Surg.* 141:699, 1981.
   Early barium enema advocated to distinguish between diverticulitis and appendicitis. (See also Am. J. Surg. *125:308, 1973.)*
9. Walker, J. D., Gray, L. A., and Polk, H. C., Jr. Diverticulitis in women. *Ann. Surg.* 185:402, 1977.
   Diverticulitis is frequently overlooked as a cause of a pelvic mass in women.

10. Arrington, P., and Judd, C. S., Jr. Cecal diverticulitis. *Am. J. Surg.* 142:56, 1981.
    The incidence of this type of diverticulitis is higher in younger individuals and Orientals.

11. Graham, S. M., and Ballantyne, G. H. Cecal diverticulitis. A review of the American experience. *Dis. Colon Rectum* 30:821, 1987.
    A difficult diagnostic problem. (See also Radiology *162:79, 1987;* Surg. Gynerol. Obstet. *166:99, 1988; and* Am. J. Gastroenterol. *81:1104, 1986).*

12. Johnson, C. D., Baker, M. E., Rice, R. P., et al. Diagnosis of acute colonic diverticulitis: Comparison of barium enema and CT. *Am. J. Roentgenol.* 148:541, 1987.
    These techniques are complementary.

13. Green, G. J., Schuman, B. M., and Barron, J. Ehlers-Danlos syndrome complicated by acute hemorrhagic sigmoid diverticulitis with an unusual mitral valve abnormality. *Am. J. Med.* 41:622, 1966.
    An unusual cause of diverticulosis.

14. Scheff, R. T., Zuckerman, G., Harter, H., et al. Diverticular disease in patients with chronic renal failure due to polycystic kidney disease. *Ann. Intern. Med.* 92:202, 1980.
    Patients with polycystic renal disease and renal failure have a high incidence of diverticulosis and diverticulitis.

15. Staniland, J. R., Ditchburn, J., and DeDombal, F. T. Clinical presentation of diseases of the large bowel. *Gastroenterology* 70:22, 1976.
    Detailed study of diverticulitis, ulcerative colitis, Crohn's colitis, and carcinoma.

16. Meyers, M. A., Alonso, D. R., Morson, B. C., et al. Pathogenesis of diverticulitis complicating granulomatous colitis. *Gastroenterology* 74:24, 1978.
    Diverticulitis can be produced by granulomatous colitis.

17. Marshak, R. H., Janowitz, H. D., and Present, D. H. Granulomatous colitis in association with diverticula. *N. Engl. J. Med.* 283:1080, 1970.
    Longitudinal fistulous tracts are not pathognomonic for granulomatous bowel disease.

18. Parks, T. G., and Connell, A. M. The outcome in 455 patients admitted for treatment of diverticular disease of the colon. *Br. J. Surg.* 57:775, 1970.
    Surgery does not guarantee freedom from recurrence. (See also Br. Med. J. *1:1205, 1966.)*

19. Klein, S., Mayer, L., Present, D. H., et al. Extraintestinal manifestations in patients with diverticulitis. *Ann. Intern. Med.* 108:700, 1988.
    Diverticulitis can mimic inflammatory bowel disease. (For other extraabdominal manifestations, see Am. J. Gastroenterol. *80:346, 1985.)*

20. Neff, C. C., van Sonnenberg, E., Casola, G., et al. Diverticular abscesses: percutaneous drainage. *Radiology* 163:15, 1987.
    A useful adjunct to surgery. (See also Radiology *164:321, 1987 and* Arch. Surg. *121:475, 1986.)*

21. Meyers, M. A., Volberg, F., Katzen, B., et al. The angioarchitecture of colonic diverticula. *Radiology* 108:249, 1973.
    Mechanism of diverticular hemorrhage examined.

22. Meyers, M. A., Alonso, D. R., and Baer, J. W. Pathogenesis of massively bleeding colonic diverticulosis: New observations. *AJR* 127:901, 1976.
    Asymmetric rupture of the vas rectum in the absence of inflammation.

23. Baum, S., Athanasoulis, C. A., Waltman, A. C., et al. Angiodysplasia of the right colon: A cause of gastrointestinal bleeding. *AJR* 129:789, 1977.
    Vascular ectasia can only be identified by angiography.

24. Boley, S. J., Sammartano, R., Adams, A., et al. On the nature and etiology of vascular ectasias of the colon: Degenerative lesions of aging. *Gastroenterology* 72:650, 1977.
    An important review.

25. Wright, H. K. Massive colonic hemorrhage. *Surg. Clin. North Am.* 60:1297, 1980.
    Good advice. (See also Am. J. Surg. *141:478, 1981.)*

26. Giacchino, J. L., Geis, W. P., Pickelman, J. R., et al. Changing perspectives in massive lower intestinal hemorrhage. *Surgery* 86:368, 1979.
    In 77% of patients, hemorrhage was not due to diverticulosis or angiodysplasia.

27. Tedesco, F. J., Waye, J. D., Raskin, J. B., et al. Colonoscopic evaluation of rectal bleeding. *Ann. Intern. Med.* 89:907, 1978.
Colonoscopy revealed a significant number of lesions in patients in whom barium enema and sigmoidoscopy were normal.

28. Maxfield, R. C., and Maxfield, C. M. Colonoscopy as a primary diagnostic procedure in chronic gastrointestinal tract bleeding. *Arch. Surg.* 121:401, 1986.
Colonoscopy was more informative than barium enema. (See also Dis. Colon Rectum *31:107, 1988.)*

29. Koval, G., Benner, K. G., Rosch, J., et al. Aggressive angiographic diagnosis in acute lower gastrointestinal hemorrhage. *Dig. Dis. Sci.* 32:248, 1987.
Use of pharmacologic agents to increase the incidence of extravasation. (See also Ann. Surg. *204:530, 1986 and* Radiology *168:375, 1988.)*

30. Cello, J. P., and Grendell, J. H. Endoscopic laser treatment for gastrointestinal vascular ectasias. *Ann. Intern. Med.* 104:352, 1986.
A useful technique, particularly for colonic lesions. (See also Br. J. Surg. *75:256, 1988.)*

31. Baum, S., Rosch, J., Dotter, C. T., et al. Selective mesenteric arterial infusions in the management of massive diverticular hemorrhage. *N. Engl. J. Med.* 288:1269, 1973.
Successful pharmacologic control of lower intestinal tract hemorrhage.

32. Brodribb, A. J. M. Treatment of symptomatic diverticular disease with a high-fibre diet. *Lancet* 1:664, 1977.
A high-fiber diet was effective in relieving symptomatic diverticular disease.

33. Drossman, D. A., Powell, D. W., and Sessions, J. T., Jr. The irritable bowel syndrome. *Gastroenterology* 73:811, 1977.
Comprehensive review. (See also Lancet *2:557, 1978;* Ann. Intern. Med. *90:431, 1979; and* Dig. Dis. Sci. *25:401, 1980.)*

34. Imperiale, T. F., and Ransohoff, D. F. Aortic stenosis, idiopathic gastrointestinal bleeding, and angiodysplasia: Is there an association? *Gastroenterology* 95:1607, 1988.
A definitive association has not been demonstrated.

77. GASTRIC ULCER DISEASE

H. Verdain Barnes

Gastric ulcers account for 15 to 20 percent of all peptic ulcers. They may occur anywhere in the stomach, but the majority are in the antrum, near its junction with the acid- and pepsin-secreting oxyntic mucosa. The other sites are, in order of frequency, the prepylorus, pylorus, and fundus. The exact pathophysiology is not known. Multiple factors have been suggested as etiologic by themselves or in combination; these include abnormal pyloroduodenal motility with or without bile acid and lysolecithin reflux from the duodenum; abnormal gastric mucosa, as in gastritis with or without associated infection as with *Campylobacter pyloris*; abnormal gastric mucosal barrier; genetic predisposition (i.e., association with blood group A, first-degree relatives, etc.); response to ulcerogenic drugs such as the nonsteroidal anti-inflammatory agents; and delayed gastric emptying with or without chronic outlet obstruction. Gastric ulcer patients may present with typical signs and symptoms of duodenal ulcer disease, but often exhibit atypical features; for example, the pain is frequently constant, radiates to the back, and is likely to be aggravated by the ingestion of food. In addition, gastric ulcer patients tend to be older, with the peak incidence between ages 45 and 55 years. These patients often come from the lower socioeconomic groups, have associated chronic diseases (such as chronic pulmonary or cardiovascular disease), and abuse alcohol and analgesics. Men predominate over women about 3.5:1. About 20 percent have an accompanying duodenal ulcer and these patients may have associated acid hypersecretion. A significant number are asymptomatic until a complication occurs. About 10 to 25 percent present with a major complication.

An important concern in gastric ulcer disease is whether the ulcer is benign or malignant. When an ulcer is demonstrated radiographically carcinoma can often be correctly identified if (1) the ulcer crater fails to project beyond the lumen of the stomach, (2) there is an irregular mound around an eccentrically placed ulcer, (3) the ulcer margin is irregular, rounded, and rolled, and (4) the ulcer bed is nodular. It is a myth that the size and location are reliable distinguishing criteria.

At least 15 percent of gastric ulcers are missed by a routine upper gastrointestinal series. Diagnostic accuracy and the differentiation of benign and malignant ulcers can be improved to over 98 percent with the addition of fiberoptic gastroscopy, and cytologic and histologic examination. Endoscopy alone is capable of making an accurate distinction in up to 95 percent and can often detect ulcers missed radiographically. On endoscopy the malignant ulcer has an irregular margin, a nodular base, a steplike depression at its margin, and an associated tumor mass or distinctly abnormal adjacent mucosa with clubbed rigid rugae. The benign ulcer's features are essentially the opposite. A biopsy taken at the time of gastroscopy can be diagnostic if positive for tumor, but malignancy is not ruled out if only chronic inflammation is seen since the biopsy may not have been deep enough to penetrate the inflammatory process to the tumor. Cells for cytology should be obtained at the time of endoscopy by lavage or brushing. The accuracy of cytologic differentiation depends on the handling of the specimen, the technique, and the experience of the cytologist. If any one of the three factors is inadequate, accuracy is no greater than about 40 percent, whereas it is about 85 percent when all are present.

It is true that the majority of benign ulcers—unless they are fairly large—show 50 percent or more healing after 2 weeks of intensive medical management. About 75 percent show complete radiographic healing in 12 weeks. Neither response, however, can be considered diagnostic since malignant ulcers may follow an identical pattern.

The major complications of gastric ulcer are, in descending order of frequency, hemorrhage, which may be massive; perforation; penetration, with or without gastrocolic fistula formation; and obstruction. The clinical aspects of hemorrhage are covered in Chapter 12. Perforation and penetration require further comment. About 27 percent of all gastric ulcers perforate, and 7 percent have simultaneous bleeding. Severe pain is almost invariably present with perforation, but it may not be classically sudden in onset. Vomiting is common and syncope occurs in up to 16 percent. Physical signs include a silent, rigid, tender abdomen in the majority. Evidence for free air may be found on physical examination by the absence of liver dullness or Lui's popping sign. About 75 percent have free air demonstrable on upright abdominal x ray. The best prognosis is seen with perforations into the lesser peritoneal sac, which occur in only about 13 percent. The most common site of perforation is into the greater peritoneal sac. Rare perforations into the pericardium, ventricles, aorta, colon, common bile duct, gallbladder, renal pelvis, and external abdominal wall have been reported. Overall mortality is between 10 and 15 percent, with much higher rates seen in the elderly. A medical and surgical team approach is a necessity in managing these patients. The development of a gastrocolic fistula occurs in about 4 percent of patients with a mortality rate of close to 15 percent. These patients usually present with watery diarrhea and weight loss. Complete obstruction is an uncommon complication of gastric ulcer, occurring in 1 percent or less.

A variety of stress situations and drugs are known to be associated with gastric ulcer formation. In general, stress ulcers are most likely to arise with major surgery, trauma, severe burns, and central nervous system disorders. These ulcers are typically multiple with a gastric ulcer in about 62 percent and a single gastric ulcer in about 19 percent. Mortality is in the range of 60 percent. The drugs that have been documented to produce gastric ulceration include salicylates, phenylbutazone, cinchophen, acetophenetidin, colchicine, reserpine, and the multiple nonsteroidal anti-inflammatory agents. These ulcers are often asymptomatic until a major complication occurs, usually hemorrhage.

1. Bynum, T. E., Hartsuck, J., and Jacobson, E. D. Gastric ulcer. *Gastroenterology* 62:1052, 1972.

A concise overview of the gastric ulcer problem.

2. Grossman, M. I., Guth, P. H., Isenberg, J. I., et al. A new look at peptic ulcer. *Ann. Intern. Med.* 84:57, 1976.
   Diffuse gastritis is commonly seen. A well-referenced review that also discusses diagnosis and therapy.
3. Wenger, J., Brandborg, L. L., and Spellman, F. A. Cancer: Clinical aspects. *Gastroenterology* 61:598, 1971.
   3.9% of the ulcers were malignant. The history and symptoms were of shorter duration in malignant cases.
4. Prolla, J. C., Xavier, R. G., and Kirsner, J. B. Exfoliative cytology in gastric ulcer. *Gastroenterology* 63:33, 1972.
   In this series, all gastric carcinomas were diagnosed by the combination of cytology and gastroscopy.
5. Roth, H. P. Healing of initial ulcers in relation to age and race. *Gastroenterology* 61:570, 1971.
   46.1% healed in 3 weeks, an additional 24.3% by 6 weeks, and 5.5% more by 12 weeks.
6. Sakita, T., Aguro, Y., Takasu, S., et al. Observations of the healing of ulcerations in early gastric cancer. *Gastroenterology* 60:835, 1971.
   70.8% of malignant ulcers heal to some degree and on rare occasions initially heal completely.
7. Hanscom, D. H., and Buchman, E. The follow-up period. *Gastroenterology* 61:585, 1971.
   41.9% of those with benign ulcers have a recurrence after successful medical therapy, 50% of these within 6 months.
8. Littman, A., and Hanscom, D. H. The course of recurrent ulcer. *Gastroenterology* 61:592, 1971.
   42.5% had a second recurrence.
9. Palmer, E. D. Perforation of gastroduodenal ulcer. *Arch. Intern. Med.* 130:957, 1972.
   27% of ulcers perforate. 7% have a simultaneous hemorrhage.
10. Lui, A. H. F. An unusual sign in perforated peptic ulcer. *Am. J. Surg.* 93:876, 1957.
    A pop is heard when testing for rebound tenderness.
11. Akwari, O., Edis, A. J., and Wollaeger, E. E. Gastrocolic fistula complicating benign unoperated gastric ulcer. *Mayo Clin. Proc.* 51:233, 1976.
    75% had watery diarrhea. Mortality was 16%.
12. Crawford, F. A., Hammon, J. W., and Shingleton, W. W. The stress ulcer syndrome: A clinical and pathologic review. *Am. J. Surg.* 121:644, 1971.
    62% of ulcers are gastric and multiple. In autopsy series, incidence was 3.6%, with more than 50% undiagnosed at time of death.
13. Boyle, J. D. Multiple gastric ulcers. *Gastroenterology* 61:628, 1971.
    2.3% incidence in garden variety gastric ulcer.
14. Wald, A., and Burbige, E. J. Benign gastric ulcers occurring with persistent histamine-fast achlorhydria. *Johns Hopkins Med. J.* 135:436, 1974.
    Not all gastric ulcers with achlorhydria are malignant.
15. Stabile, B. E., and Passaro, E. Recurrent peptic ulcer. *Gastroenterology* 70:124, 1976.
    An excellent, well-referenced discussion of the problem.
16. Conn, H. O., and Blitzer, B. L. Nonassociation of adrenocorticosteroid therapy and peptic ulcer. *N. Engl. J. Med.* 294:473, 1976.
    Corticosteroids do not cause peptic ulcers.
17. Storey, D. W., Bown, S. G., Swain, C. P., et al. Endoscopic prediction of recurrent bleeding in peptic ulcers. *N. Engl. J. Med.* 305:915, 1981.
    Rebleeding occurs primarily in those patients with visible bleeding vessels at endoscopy.
18. Elashoff, J. D., and Grossman, M. I. Trends in hospital admissions and death rates for peptic ulcer in the United States from 1970 to 1978. *Gastroenterology* 78:280, 1980.
    Gastric ulcer has changed little while duodenal ulcer has substantially decreased.
19. Grossman, M. I., Kurata, J. H., Rotter, J. I., et al. Peptic ulcer: New therapies, new diseases. *Ann. Intern. Med.* 95:609, 1981.
    An up-to-date discussion of the heterogeneity of peptic ulcer disease.

20. Brooks, F. P., Cohen, S., and Soloway, R. D. (eds.) *Peptic Ulcer Disease. Contemporary Issues in Gastroenterology.* New York: Churchill Livingstone, Inc., 1985. Vol. 3.
21. Robert A. Cytoprotection of the gastrointestinal mucosa. *Adv. Intern. Med.* 28:325, 1983.
22. Drumm, B., Sherman, P., Cutz, E., et al. Association of *Campylobacter pyloris* on the gastric mucosa with antral gastritis in children. *N. Engl. J. Med.* 316:1557, 1987.
    Articles 20–22 discuss current concepts in the pathophysiology of gastric ulcer.
23. Gabrielsson, N. Benign and malignant gastric ulcers: Evaluation of the differential diagnostics in roentgen examination and endoscopy. *Endoscopy* 4:73, 1972.
    Good comparative data; endoscopy alone is better than upper gastrointestinal series alone.
24. Jorde, R., Bostad, L., and Burhol, P. G. Asymptomatic gastric ulcer: A follow-up study in patients with previous gastric ulcer. *Lancet* 1:119, 1986.
    Asymptomatic gastric ulcer was found in about a quarter of these patients.
25. Selling, J. A., Hogan, D. L., Aly, A., et al. Indomethacin inhibits duodenal mucosal bicarbonate secretion and endogenous prostaglandin E_2 output in human subjects. *Ann. Intern. Med.* 106:368, 1987.
    This article demonstrates the loss of an important duodenal defense system.
26. Spindel, E., Harty R. F., Leibach, J. R., et al. Decision analysis in evaluation of hypergastrinemia. *Am. J. Med.* 80:11, 1986.
    An important article to keep in mind when evaluating peptic ulcer patients for a gastrinoma.
27. Jensen, R. T., Gardner, J. D., Raufman, J.-P., et al. Zollinger-Ellison syndrome: Current concepts and management. *Ann. Intern. Med.* 98:59, 1983.
    A comprehensive, well-referenced review of this rare disease.
28. Battaglia, G., DiMario, F., Piccoli, A., et al. Clinical markers of slow healing and relapsing gastric ulcer. *Gut* 28:210, 1987.
    Cigarette smoking was the most important risk factor for nonhealing.
29. Hazell, S. L., and Lee A. *Campylobacter pyloris*, urease, hydrogen ion back diffusion, and gastric ulcers. *Lancet* 2:15, 1986.
    This bacterium may be implicated as an etiologic agent for gastric ulcer.

78. GRANULOMATOUS BOWEL DISEASE (CROHN'S DISEASE)
Edward J. Levine
Theodore M. Bayless

Granulomatous bowel disease is an idiopathic inflammatory bowel disease that was clinically recognized in 1932 by Dr. Burrill B. Crohn. The disease occurs most frequently between ages 20 to 40, with a second peak beginning at about age 50. Crohn's disease occurs more frequently in Jews. Roughly 20% of patients have a positive family history of inflammatory bowel disease. Recent epidemiologic data suggest that the incidence of Crohn's disease is between 1 and 7 per 100,000, and is probably increasing. Crohn's disease may involve any portion of the gastrointestinal tract; however, involvement of the upper digestive tract is uncommon (less than 5% of patients). A wide range of extraintestinal manifestations can occur. These include peripheral arthritis (20%), ankylosing spondylitis (10–20%), erythema nodosum (15%), pyoderma gangrenosum (1%), uveitis (2%), and liver abnormalities (up to 90%), including fatty infiltration, pericholangitis, granulomatous hepatitis, and sclerosing cholangitis. Patients with terminal ileal disease have an increased incidence of gallstones because of bile salt malabsorption as well as hyperoxaluria and urinary oxalate stones. Other less common systemic manifestations include fever, aphthous stomatitis, amyloidosis, and myositis.

Clinically, Crohn's disease has a number of different patterns. Ileocolitis is the most common form (55% of patients), while isolated colonic involvement occurs in 10–30% of patients. Isolated small intestinal involvement occurs in 30%. Intestinal obstruction, fistulae, abscesses, perforation, and bleeding occur in all forms of the disease. Crohn's disease recurs in the majority of patients after intestinal resection, and tends to recur proximally to the intestinal anastomosis.

The most common presenting manifestations of Crohn's disease are abdominal pain and diarrhea, or both. The more occult types of presentation include fever of unknown origin and acute arthritis. Included in the differential diagnosis of Crohn's disease are appendicitis, diverticulitis, pelvic inflammatory disease, ischemic bowel disease, adenocarcinoma, lymphoma, ulcerative colitis, bacillary dysentery, intestinal amebiasis, and irritable bowel syndrome. Clinical features distinguishing Crohn's colitis from ulcerative colitis include rectal sparing, extensive small bowel involvement, predominantly right-sided colitis, segmental disease, and perianal fistulae. Twenty percent of idiopathic inflammatory colitis patients cannot be differentiated into Crohn's colitis or ulcerative colitis, and are classified having "indeterminant colitis." Toxic megacolon occurs with both disorders, although much more commonly with ulcerative colitis.

In contrast to ulcerative colitis, which is primarily a mucosal disease, Crohn's disease involves the entire bowel wall. The diagnosis of Crohn's disease occasionally is made at laparotomy for presumed acute appendicitis; however, the diagnosis is more commonly made after months to years of vague abdominal symptoms. An important clue for the physician is the occurrence of anal lesions, such as fistulae, abscesses, or fissures. Such lesions occur in up to 90% of patients, and may precede the onset of symptomatic bowel involvement by several years.

Sulfasalazine, corticosteroids, metronidazole, and azathioprine are the mainstays of medical therapy. Sulfasalazine is most beneficial in mild disease and those patients with colonic involvement. Prednisone is used for moderate and severe disease and is most useful with small intestinal disease, although it is also used for colonic disease. Often, combination therapy with corticosteroids and sulfalazine seems to allow some steroid sparing. Metronidazole is often used for patients with fistulae and colonic involvement. A reversible peripheral neuropathy is a troublesome side effect that occurs after 8–10 weeks with doses over 1 gm/day. The role of azathioprine and its metabolite 6-mercaptopurine (6-MP) is controversial but appears to be gaining wider acceptance. These agents are used for diffuse, small intestinal disease, severe colonic and perianal involvement, and patients requiring large doses of corticosteroids in order to achieve a steroid sparing effect. These agents are directly toxic to the bone marrow and have also been rarely associated with the development of leukemia and lymphoma in patients with renal transplants.

Surgery is indicated in patients with intestinal obstruction, perforation, toxic megacolon, dysplasia, and failure of medical therapy. Nutritional support is also very important in patient management. Enteral feeding using an elemental diet and nutritional supplements have a role in both the acute and chronic settings. Parenteral nutrition can be used preoperatively in the malnourished patient and in providing bowel rest for patients with an acute exacerbation of their disease. Rarely, patients with diffuse disease and previous massive resections who are not operative candidates can be maintained on long-term home hyperalimentation.

1. Summers, R. W., Switz, D. M., Sessions, J. T., Jr., et al. National Cooperative Crohn's Disease Study: Results of drug treatment. *Gastroenterology* 77:847, 1979.
   Part of a massive 5-year study. Other articles in this issue discuss drug toxicity, natural history, radiology, and extraintestinal manifestations.
2. Mekhjian, H. S., Switz, D. M., Melnyk, C. S., et al. Clinical features and natural history of Crohn's disease. *Gastroenterology* 77:898, 1979.
3. Lashner, B. A., Evans, A. A., Kirsner, J. B., et al. Prevalence and incidence of inflammatory bowel disease in family members. *Gastroenterology* 91:1396, 1986.
   Twenty-two percent of family members from 40 proband families had confirmed inflammatory bowel disease. Risk for first-, second-, or third-degree family members is low (5%).
4. Sommers, S. C. Ulcerative and granulomatous colitis. *A.J.R.* 130:817, 1978.
   Excellent review of the pathology of these diseases.

5. Bull, D. M., Peppercorn, M. A., Glotzer, D. J., et al. Crohn's disease of the colon. *Gastroenterology* 76:607, 1979.
   Comprehensive clinical review.
6. Kirsner, J. B., and Shorter, R. G. Recent developments in "nonspecific" inflammatory bowel disease. *N. Engl. J. Med.* 306:775, 837, 1982.
   Comprehensive review.
7. Farmer, R. G., Whelan, G., Fazio, V. W. Long term follow-up of patients with Crohn's disease. Relationship between the clinical pattern and prognosis. *Gastroenterology* 88:1818, 1985.
   Reviews the Cleveland Clinic experience regarding the initial anatomic involvement of Crohn's disease and how it relates to prognosis.
8. Cooke, W. T., and Swan, C. H. J. Diffuse jejuno-ileitis of Crohn's disease. *Q. J. Med.* 43:583, 1974.
   Edema due to protein-losing enteropathy may be the presenting feature.
9. Greenstein, A. J., Janowitz, H. D., and Sachar, D. B. The extra-intestinal complications of Crohn's disease and ulcerative colitis: A study of 700 patients. *Medicine* 55:401, 1976.
   Joint, skin, eye, and mouth lesions are more common with colonic disease.
10. Marshak, R. H. Granulomatous disease of the intestinal tract (Crohn's disease). *Radiology* 114:3, 1975.
    Roentgenographic and clinical features reviewed.
11. Eade, M. N., Cooke, W. T., Brooke, B. N., et al. Liver disease in Crohn's colitis. *Ann. Intern. Med.* 74:518, 1971.
    Fatty infiltration, granulomas, inflammatory infiltrates, amyloidosis, and cirrhosis.
12. Haslock, I., and Wright, V. The musculoskeletal complications of Crohn's disease. *Medicine* 52:217, 1973.
    Synovitis, ankylosing spondylitis, sacroiliitis, and clubbing.
13. Frayha, R., Stevens, M. B., and Bayless, T. M. Destructive monoarthritis and granulomatous synovitis as the presenting manifestations of Crohn's disease. *Johns Hopkins Med. J.* 137:151, 1975.
    Granulomatous joint involvement. (For bone and muscle involvement, see N. Engl. J. Med. *294:262, 1976 and 295:818, 1976.)*
14. Morris, R. I., Metzger, A. L., Bluestone, R., et al. HL-A-W27: A useful discriminator in the arthropathies of inflammatory bowel disease. *N. Engl. J. Med.* 290:1117, 1974.
    Spondylitis occurs mainly in W27-positive patients; peripheral arthritis occurs alone in W27-negative patients.
15. Present, D. H., Rabinowitz, J. G., Banks, P. A., et al. Obstructive hydronephrosis in granulomatous disease of the bowel. *N. Engl. J. Med.* 280:523, 1969.
    Symptoms referable to the urinary tract are absent and routine IVP is recommended in patients with granulomatous bowel disease.
16. Javett, S. L., and Brooke, B. N. Acute dilation of colon in Crohn's disease. *Lancet* 2:126, 1970.
    Toxic megacolon in granulomatous colitis. (See also Lancet *1:480, 1979.)*
17. Dyer, N. H., Child, J. A., Mollin, D. L., et al. Anemia in Crohn's disease. *Q. J. Med.* 41:419, 1972.
    Megaloblastic anemia due to folate deficiency is not uncommon.
18. Pounder, R. E., Craven, E. R., Henthorn, J. S., et al. Red cell abnormalities associated with sulphasalazine maintenance therapy for ulcerative colitis. *Gut* 16:181, 1975.
    Red cell abnormalities are dose related.
19. Mir-Madjlessi, S. H., Brown, C. H., and Hawk, W. A. Amyloidosis associated with Crohn's disease. *Am. J. Gastroenterol.* 58:563, 1972.
    Amyloid nephropathy.
20. Earnest, D. L., Johnson, G., Williams, H. E., et al. Hyperoxaluria in patients with ileal resection: An abnormality in dietary oxalate absorption. *Gastroenterology* 66:1114, 1974.
    Oxalate absorption and the risk of nephrolithiasis increases with the length of bowel removed and the degree of steatorrhea.

21. Lock, M. R., Farmer, R. G., Fazio, V. W., et al. Recurrence and reoperation for Crohn's disease. *N. Engl. J. Med.* 304:1586, 1981.
The risk of recurrence declines after 8 years; recurrences requiring surgery are highest with ileocolic disease. (See also the accompanying editorial on p. 1602).

22. Meyers, S., Wolfish, J. S., Sachar, D. B., et al. Quality of life after surgery for Crohn's disease: A psychosocial survey. *Gastroenterology* 78:1, 1980.
Surgery is perceived by patients as improving their quality of life.

23. Bernstein, L. H., Frank, M. S., Brandt, L. S., et al. Healing of perineal Crohn's disease with metronidazole. *Gastroenterology* 79:357, 1980.
An interesting and possibly important observation. (See also the accompanying editorial on p. 393.)

24. Present, D. H., Korelitz, B. I., Wisch, N., et al. Treatment of Crohn's disease with 6-mercaptopurine. *N. Engl. J. Med.* 302:981, 1980.
6-MP was effective when administered for more than 3 months. (See also the accompanying editorial on p. 1024.)

25. Donoghue, D. P., Dawson, A. M., Powell-Tuck, J., et al. Double-blind withdrawal trial of azathioprine as maintenance treatment for Crohn's disease. *Lancet* 2:955, 1978.
Reduction in relapse rate observed with azathioprine therapy.

26. Das, K. M., Eastwood, M. A., McManus, J. P. A., et al. Adverse reactions during salicylazosulfapyridine therapy and the relations with drug metabolism and acetylator phenotype. *N. Engl. J. Med.* 289:491, 1973.
Toxicity is due to absorption of sulfapyridine in slow acetylators.

27. LaMont, J. T., and Trnka, Y. M. Therapeutic implications of clostridium difficile toxin during relapse of chronic inflammatory bowel disease. *Lancet* 1:381, 1980.
Vancomycin eradicated the toxin. (See also the editorial on p. 402.)

28. Halsted, C. H., Gandhi, G., and Tamura, T. Sulfasalazine inhibits the absorption of folates in ulcerative colitis. *N. Eng. J. Med.* 305:1513, 1981.
Sulfasalazine inhibits both polyglutamate hydrolysis and folate absorption.

29. Donaldson, R. M. Management of medical problems in pregnancy-inflammatory bowel disease. *N. Engl. J. Med.* 312:1616, 1985.
Review of the patient with inflammatory bowel disease during pregnancy.

30. Matuchansky, C. Parenteral nutrition in inflammatory bowel disease. *Gut* 27:51, 81, 1986.
Reviews the literature and emphasizes that the precise role of total parenteral nutrition has yet to be defined.

31. McIntyre, P. B., Powell-Tuck, J., Wood, S. R., et al. Controlled trial of bowel rest in the treatment of severe acute colitis. *Gut* 27:481, 1986.
No difference in operative or mortality rate between total parenteral nutrition group or oral diet group. Ulcerative colitis and Crohn's disease behaved differently in the acute attack.

79. HEPATOLENTICULAR DEGENERATION (WILSON'S DISEASE)
H. Verdain Barnes

Wilson's disease (WD) is a rare autosomal recessive disorder of copper metabolism. In this disease, serum copper, copper-binding protein (ceruloplasmin), and biliary excretion of copper are decreased and urinary copper excretion is increased. The net effect is an increased body copper load with primary deposition in the brain and liver, resulting in central nervous system degeneration and cirrhosis, respectively.

The onset of symptoms is usually during the second and third decades of life. Presentation of the disease tends to occur earlier in women than in men. In most series cirrhosis is the predominant manifestation in younger patients and neurologic abnormalities the predominant manifestation in older patients, although both the central nervous system and liver are usually dysfunctional to some degree in a majority of patients. Renal tubular or glomerular dysfunction is common. The most frequent signs and symptoms and their approximate incidence are the Kayser-Fleischer ring (97% of patients), neuropsychiatric dysfunction (74%), skeletal demineralization (66%), thrombocytopenia (52%), hyperpigmentation of the legs (50%), splenomegaly (44%), easy bruising (40%), hepatomegaly (36%), edema, arthralgias, and leukopenia (30%), osteoarthritis (25%), small liver (20%), jaundice (19%), ascites (18%), sunflower cataracts (17%), nephrolithiasis (16%), fever, hematemesis, or melena (10%), and Coombs-negative hemolytic anemia (2%). The greenish-yellow to golden-brown pigmentation in Descemet's membrane at the corneal limbus junction—the Kayser-Fleischer ring—has in the past been considered pathognomonic of WD, but it is now recognized that such rings may occur in some patients with primary biliary cirrhosis, neonatal hepatitis, and other causes of chronic active hepatitis. The most frequent neurologic manifestations are a lack of coordination, psychologic problems, tremor, dysarthria, dysphagia, masked facies, ridigity, and gait disturbances. Dementia, dystonia, hypertonia, drooling, choreoathetosis, coma, blurred vision, headaches, and convulsions are less common. Minimal to marked renal dysfunction is seen in more than 50% of the patients. These abnormalities range from hematuria to proteinuria to mild azotemia to decreased concentrating ability to aminoaciduria to a complete Fanconi's syndrome. Bone and joint abnormalities are, in order of frequency, osteoporosis, subarticular cysts, bone fragmentation, and osteoarthritis.

The diagnosis of WD can usually be confirmed by one or more of the following: a serum copper of less than 80 μg/dl, a ceruloplasmin level of less than 20 mg/dl, a liver copper concentration of over 250 μg/gm of dry liver weight, or a 24-hour urinary excretion of over 100 μg of copper. On occasion the diagnosis may be obscured during active liver necrosis when blood copper and ceruloplasmin levels may be normal or increased; however, urine and liver copper levels usually remain increased. During hemolysis, serum copper levels may be normal, but the other diagnostic parameters remain abnormal. In an occasional patient with nondiagnostic blood, urine, and liver copper levels, radioactive copper turnover studies may substantiate the diagnosis. Finally, it must be remembered that (1) a low serum copper and ceruloplasmin concentration can be seen in some patients with nephrotic syndrome, celiac disease, sprue, and kwashiorkor; (2) an increased renal copper excretion can occur in nephrotic syndrome, Laennec's cirrhosis, and biliary cirrhosis; and (3) liver copper levels can be high in biliary cirrhosis. Other common laboratory abnormalities in WD include a prolonged prothrombin time (80% of patients), bromosulfophthalein (BSP) retention (66%), decreased total protein and albumin (about 25%), elevated bilirubin (34%), thrombocytopenia, leukopenia, and anemia. Hemolytic anemia, often episodic, may be the presenting manifestation. Hyperchloremia, hypokalemia, hypouricemia, hypophosphatemia, and decreased serum carbon dioxide content are not uncommon. An occasional patient has mild hypocalcemia.

The clinical presentation and course are extremely variable. Previously asymptomatic patients may present with hepatic coma, sudden onset of hepatic necrosis, hematemesis and melena, transient hemolytic anemia, or insidious new or chronic progressive neurologic or psychiatric dysfunction. Any child, adolescent, or young adult with unexplained chronic active hepatitis, incoordination, psychiatric dysfunction, osteoporosis, or nonspherocytic Coombs-negative hemolytic anemia should be screened for WD, as should all siblings of patients with WD. The importance of early diagnosis cannot be overemphasized since in the vast majority penicillamine therapy prevents the progression of the disease and reverses much and on occasion all existing pathologic changes. The most frequent causes of death are hepatic coma, massive hematemesis, and intracranial hemorrhage.

1. Cartwright, E. E., and Lee, G. R. The pathogenesis and evolution of Wilson's disease. *Epatologia* 20:51, 1974.
2. Strickland, G. T., and Leu, M. L. Wilson's disease: Clinical and laboratory manifestations of 40 patients. *Medicine* 54:113, 1975.
   Articles 1 and 2 offer comprehensive coverage of the subject.
3. Wilson, S. A. K. Progressive lenticular degeneration: A familial nervous disease associated with cirrhosis of the liver. *Brain* 34:295, 1912.
   A medical classic.

4. Sternlieb, I., Van Den Hamer, C. J. A., Morell, A. J., et al. Lysosomal defect of hepatic copper excretion in Wilson's disease (hepatolenticular degeneration). *Gastroenterology* 64:99, 1973.
   The excretion of copper in bile is markedly diminished and a hepatic lysosomal enzyme defect is postulated.
5. Strickland, G. T., Forommer, D., Leu, M. L., et al. Wilson's disease in the United Kingdom and Taiwan: I. General characteristics of 142 cases and prognosis. II. A genetic analysis of 88 cases. *Q. J. Med.* 42:619, 1973.
   The disorder is inherited as an autosomal recessive.
6. Cox, D. W., Fraser, F. C., and Sass-Kortsak, A. A genetic study of Wilson's disease: Evidence for heterogeneity. *Am. J. Hum. Genet.* 24:646, 1972.
   Heterogeneity is demonstrated. Young patients are found to have a higher incidence of liver dysfunction, and older patients a higher incidence of neurologic dysfunction.
7. Fleming, C. R., Dsekson, R., Wahner, H. W., et al. Pigmented corneal rings in non-Wilsonian liver disease. *Ann. Intern. Med.* 86:285, 1977.
   The Kayser-Fleischer ring is not pathognomonic of WD. It can be seen in some patients with primary biliary cirrhosis and other causes of chronic aggressive hepatitis with cirrhosis.
8. Leu, M. L., Strickland, G. T., and Gutman, R. A. Renal function in Wilson's disease: Response to penicillamine therapy. *Am. J. Med. Sci.* 260:381, 1970.
   Improvement in most abnormalities is seen with therapy.
9. Morgan, H. G., Stewart, W. K., Lowe, K. G., et al. Wilson's disease and the Fanconi syndrome. *Q. J. Med.* 31:361, 1962.
   A significant number of the patients have Fanconi's renal tubular acidosis.
10. Mindelzun, R., Elkin, M., Scheinberg, I. H., et al. Skeletal changes in Wilson's disease. A radiographical study. *Radiology* 94:127, 1970.
    A variety of bony changes may be seen, the most common one being osteoporosis.
11. Deiss, A., Lee, G. R., and Cartwright, E. E. Hemolytic anemia and Wilson's disease. *Ann. Intern. Med.* 73:413, 1970.
    Transient hemolytic anemia generally antedates other manifestations of the disease. In the patient described the process was due to increased oxidative stress resulting from the accumulation of copper in the erythrocytes.
12. Sternlieb, I., and Feldmann, G. Effects of anti-copper therapy on hepatocellular mitochondria in patients with Wilson's disease. *Gastroenterology* 71:457, 1976.
    There was improvement in the characteristic mitochondrial abnormalities of the hepatocyte after therapy.
13. Sternlieb, I., and Scheinberg, I. H. Chronic hepatitis as a first manifestation of Wilson's disease. *Ann. Intern. Med.* 76:59, 1972.
    An important observation. All children, adolescents, and young adults with chronic hepatitis should be screened for WD.
14. LaRusso, N. F., Summerskill, W. H. J., and McCall, J. T. Abnormalities of chemical tests for copper metabolism in chronic active hepatitis: Differentiation from Wilson's disease. *Gastroenterology* 70:653, 1976.
    The only differential feature was the low plasma ceruloplasmin level in WD.
15. Owen, C. A., Goldstein, N. P., and Bowie, J. W. Platelet function and coagulation in patients with Wilson's disease. *Arch. Intern. Med.* 136:148, 1976.
    Over 90% of the patients had abnormal platelet aggregation studies.
16. Dobyns, W. B., Goldstein, N. P., and Gordon, H. Clinical spectrum of Wilson's disease (hepatolenticular degeneration). *Mayo Clin. Proc.* 54:35, 1979.
    17% presented with liver disease alone and 33% with brain disease alone.
17. Hoagland, H. C., and Goldstein, N. P. Hematologic (cytopenic) manifestations of Wilson's disease (hepatolenticular degeneration). *Mayo Clin. Proc.* 53:498, 1978.
    The cytopenic manifestations rarely improved with therapy.
18. Golding, D. N., and Walshe, J. M. Arthropathy of Wilson's disease. *Ann. Rheum. Dis.* 36:99, 1977.
    Acute polyarthritis in their patients followed penicillamine therapy.
19. Wiebers, D. O., Hollenhorst, R. W., and Goldstein, N. P. The ophthalmologic manifestations of Wilson's disease. *Mayo Clin. Proc.* 52:409, 1972.
    Sunflower cataracts were seen in 17%.

20. Wiebers, D. O., Wilson, D. M., McLeod, R. A., et al. Renal stones in Wilson's disease. *Am. J. Med.* 67:249, 1979.
   16% had nephrolithiasis.
21. Spechler, S. J., and Koff, R. S. Wilson's disease: Diagnostic difficulties in the patient with chronic hepatitis and hypoceruloplasminemia. *Gastroenterology* 78:803, 1980.
   The differential can be extraordinarily difficult.
22. Cartwright, G. E. Diagnosis of treatable Wilson's disease. *N. Engl. J. Med.* 298:1347, 1978.
   A concise statement. Progressive Wilson's disease and phenothiazine effects can look alike.
23. Winge, D. R. Normal physiology of copper metabolism. *Semin. Liver Dis.* 4:239, 1984.
24. Walshe, J. M. Copper: Its role in the pathogenesis of liver disease. *Semin. Liver. Dis.* 4:252, 1984.
   These articles (23, 24) discuss current concepts of copper metabolism and disease.
25. Deiss, A. Treatment of Wilson's disease. *Ann. Intern. Med.* 99:398, 1983.
26. Scheinberg, I. H., Jaffe, M. E., and Sternlieb, I. The use of trientine in preventing the effects of interrupting penicillamine therapy in Wilson's disease. *N. Engl. J. Med.* 317:209, 1987.
   Two important articles (25, 26) on the current therapy of Wilson's disease.

80. HEPATIC ENCEPHALOPATHY
H. Franklin Herlong

Hepatic encephalopathy is a complex neuropsychiatric syndrome that can complicate both acute and chronic liver disease. Although the exact pathogenesis of hepatic encephalopathy remains obscure, it represents either direct or indirect exposure of the central nervous system to toxic substances normally cleared by the liver. Many potentially comagenic toxins are produced in the gut, largely from bacterial action on luminal contents. With cirrhosis and portal hypertension these toxins bypass extraction by the liver and are diverted via the systemic circulation to the brain where they cause coma. While hepatic encephalopathy occurs most commonly in cirrhosis, it may complicate acute liver failure. Factors which cause encephalopathy in fulminant hepatic failure are likely different from those in chronic liver disease, but the clinical manifestations are similar.

The components of the syndrome of hepatic encephalopathy include impairment in the level of consciousness (delirium), decreased intellectual function, alterations in personality and behavior, and neuromuscular abnormalities (hyperreflexia, asterixis, tremor). Semiquantitative stages of hepatic encephalopathy (Parsons-Smith scale) are based on the severity of the alteration in level of consciousness. The presence of asterixis is commonly associated with hepatic encephalopathy. This flapping tremor of the outstretched hand is caused by impaired descending reticular system function. It is not specific for hepatic encephalopathy and may be seen with pulmonary disease, uremia, or malnutrition. The electroencephalogram is characteristically abnormal in hepatic encephalopathy. A normal electroencephalogram makes the diagnosis of hepatic encephalopathy suspect. While triphasic waves are seen with hepatic encephalopathy, they may also occur with other disorders such as uremia, cerebral anoxia, and electrolyte abnormalities. Most commonly, the electroencephalogram is characterized by diffuse slow waves of increased amplitude. The degree of slowing correlates with the severity of the grade of encephalopathy.

Since an elevated concentration of ammonia is found in the blood of most patients with hepatic encephalopathy, it has been incriminated as the major toxin. Supporting ammonia's comagenic potential is the observation that children with urea cycle abnormalities, but otherwise normal livers, develop marked hyperammonemia and a syndrome with the clinical features of hepatic encephalopathy. Importantly, improvement in mental status generally follows therapy directed at lowering ammonia concentration. While ammonia is undoubtedly important, the pathogenesis of hepatic encephalopathy is likely multifactorial. Synergism between ammonia and endogenous or exogenous comagenic substances such as short chain fatty acids and mercaptans contributes to ammonia's capacity to induce coma.

Other as yet unproven theories on the pathogenesis of hepatic encephalopathy include altered neurotransmitter synthesis secondary to abnormalities in plasma amino acid concentrations. With portal systemic shunting as in cirrhosis, the plasma amino acid profile is characterized by reduction in branched chain amino acids (leucine, isoleucine, and valine) and elevation in aromatic amino acid levels (phenylalanine and tryptophan). Excessive transport of aromatic amino acids into the brain favors synthesis of false neurotransmitters causing altered CNS function.

Other investigators feel that abnormal inhibitory neurotransmission in the brain caused by various neuroinhibitory substances such as gamma-aminobutyric acid (GABA) may be important. Receptors for benzodiazepine and phenobarbital have been identified in close proximity to the GABA receptor complex. These observations suggest that endogenous or exogenous benzodiazepine-like substances may contribute to the development of hepatic encephalopathy. Supporting this hypothesis are the observations that benzodiazepine antagonists have been reported to improve the alteration in mental status in animals and patients with coma due to severe liver disease.

While the exact etiology for hepatic encephalopathy remains to be established, its therapy is based on the premise that substances in the gastrointestinal tract are acted on by intestinal bacteria and converted to toxins that are absorbed into the blood. These toxins bypass the liver via collateral circulation, enter the brain, and presumably induce encephalopathy. Based on these principles, therapy is directed at (1) decreasing the colonic substrate for comagenic toxins, (2) reducing the bacteria capable of producing these toxins, (3) managing the influx of these compounds into the CNS, and (4) decreasing the effect of these compounds on neurotransmitter activity and metabolism.

Hepatic encephalopathy is often precipitated by complicating conditions frequently seen in cirrhotic patients. Gastrointestinal bleeding is the most common. Blood in the gastrointestinal tract not only decreases hepatic and renal perfusion, but provides many potential comagenic substrates. Rapid catharsis of the gut is essential in patients who develop encephalopathy after a gastrointestinal bleed.

Restricting dietary protein can reduce the nitrogenous load and substrate for toxin production. Supplying adequate carbohydrate calories is necessary to minimize protein catabolism. The administration of antibiotics such as neomycin or metronidazole inhibits bacterial production of comagenic substances.

The metabolic alkalosis caused by potassium depletion, often seen in cirrhotic patients receiving diuretic therapy, may induce encephalopathy. This acid-base disturbance is associated with a pH gradient which favors intracellular transport of ammonia, and hence worsening of hepatic encephalopathy. Potassium supplementation may be all that is required to reverse the encephalopathy in such patients.

The mainstay of therapy for hepatic encephalopathy is lactulose. This nonabsorbable disaccharide works by several mechanisms. Its cathartic action increases toxin elimination. Bacterial metabolism of lactulose acidifies the colonic contents, favoring the conversion of ammonia to its ionized and less absorbable form. Lactulose may be administered orally or as a retention enema in obtunded patients. For patients with chronic recurrent encephalopathy a combination of protein restriction and lactulose is used as maintenance therapy to reduce the number of symptomatic episodes. Some studies suggest that vegetable protein may be less comagenic than animal protein. The lesser toxicity of vegetable compared with meat protein may be related to a lower ammonia content of vegetable protein or perhaps due to the cathartic action of indigestible polysaccharides in vegetables which have an effect like lactulose.

Several specific therapies for hepatic encephalopathy have been proposed. Nutritional supplementation (Hepatic Aid, Hepatamine) designed to correct plasma amino acid abnormalities in patients with hepatic encephalopathy are available. However, controlled trials have failed to demonstrate conclusively that these supplements are of benefit in patients with hepatic encephalopathy. Recent reports showing reversal of the mental status changes in patients with encephalopathy by benzodiazepine receptor antagonists are promising, but require further research.

1. Atterbury, C. E., Maddrey, W. C., Conn, H. O., et al. Neomycin-sorbitol and lactulose in the treatment of acute portal systemic encephalopathy: A controlled double blind clinical trial. *Am. J. Dig. Dis.* 23:398, 1978.
   This study confirms the efficacy of lactulose in the treatment of portal systemic encephalopathy. Its beneficial effect was equal to that of a combination of sorbitol and neomycin.
2. Bansky, G., Meier, P. H., Zeigler, W. H., et al. Reversal of hepatic coma by benzodiazepine antagonist (RO 15-1788). *Lancet* 1:1324, 1985.
   This article describes improvement in the symptoms of hepatic encephalopathy with therapy using an antagonist to the benzodiazepine receptor. This report suggests the hypothesis that endogenous benzodiazepine-like substances may play a role in the pathogenesis of hepatic encephalopathy.
3. Batshaw, M. L. Inherited hyperammonemia: An algorithm for diagnosis. *Hepatology* 7:1381, 1987.
   A comprehensive review of disorders of ammonia metabolism and their clinical manifestations.
4. Bassett, M. L., Mullen, K. D., Skolnick, P., et al. Amelioration of hepatic encephalopathy by pharmacologic antagonism of the GABA-benzodiazepine receptor complex in a rabbit model of fulminant hepatic failure. *Gastroenterology* 93:1069, 1987.
   In this experimental model of fulminant hepatic failure, amelioration of hepatic encephalopathy was produced using an agent which blocked the benzodiazepine receptor.
5. Bernthal, P., Hays, A., and Tarter, R. E. Cerebral CT scan abnormalities in cholestatic and hepatocellular disease and their relationship to neuropsychological test performance. *Hepatology* 7:107, 1987.
   This study showed no difference in computed tomography (CT) abnormalities in patients with hepatocellular and cholestatic diseases. Both groups of patients had evidence of cerebral atrophy. The changes seen on CT scan correlated with impairment in psychomotor testing.
6. Cerra, F. B., Cheung, N. K., Fischer, J. E., et al. Disease specific amino acid infusion (FO80) in hepatic encephalopathy: A prospective randomized double blind controlled trial. *J. P. E. N.* 9:288, 1985.
   This randomized controlled trial suggests that branched chain amino acid supplementation in hepatic encephalopathy is beneficial. The control groups received lactulose.
7. Conn, H. O. The Hepatic Encephalopathies. In H. O. Conn and J. Bircher (eds.), *Hepatic Encephalopathy: Management with Lactulose and Related Carbohydrates.* East Lansing, Mich: Medi-Ed Press, 1988. P. 3.
   An excellent review of the clinical symptoms and classification of encephalopathy.
8. Conn, H. O. The Theoretic Therapy of Hepatic Encephalopathy. In H. O. Conn and J. Bircher (eds.), *Hepatic Encephalopathy: Management with Lactulose and Related Carbohydrates.* East Lansing, Mich.: Medi-Ed Press, 1988. P. 83.
   A comprehensive review of the rationale of various therapies used to treat hepatic encephalopathy.
9. Conn, H. O. Complications of Portal Hypertension. In G. Gitnick (ed.), *Current Hepatology,* 9th ed. Chicago: Year Book Medical Publishers, Inc., 1989. P. 254.
10. Conn, H. O., Leevy, C. M., Vlahcevic, Z. R., et al. Comparison of lactulose and neomycin in the treatment of chronic portosystemic encephalopathy: A double blind control trial. *Gastroenterology* 72:573, 1977.
    This study compares the results of treatment of hepatic encephalopathy with lactulose and neomycin. It confirms the efficacy of both of these agents in ameliorating the symptoms of hepatic encephalopathy.
11. Eriksson, L. S. Branched-Chain Amino Acids in the Treatment of Hepatic Encephalopathy. In H. O. Conn and J. Bircher (eds.) *Hepatic Encephalopathy: Management*

with Lactulose and Related Carbohydrates. East Lansing, Mich.: Medi-Ed Press, 1988. P. 129.
Altered plasma concentrations of amino acids have been proposed to play a role in the pathogenesis of hepatic encephalopathy. This article reviews the various reports of therapies using branched chain amino acid preparations to treat hepatic encephalopathy.

12. Ferenci, P., Grimm, G., Meryn, S., et al. Successful long-term treatment of chronic hepatic encephalopathy with a benzodiazepine antagonist. *Hepatology* 7:1064, 1987.
This report describes long-term therapy with an agent that blocks the benzodiazepine receptor.

13. Fraser, C. L., and Arieff, A. I. *Hepatic encephalopathy. N. Engl. J. Med.* 313:865, 1985.
Comprehensive review of pathogenesis and therapy of hepatic encephalopathy.

14. Herlong, H. F. Hepatic Encephalopathy. In R. T. Johnson (ed.), *Current Therapy in Neurologic Disease* Toronto: B. C. Decker Inc., 1987. Vol. 2, p. 303.
A general article on the practical therapy of hepatic encephalopathy.

15. Hsia, Y. E. Inherited hyperammonemic syndromes. *Gastroenterology* 67:347, 1974.
This article describes disorders of the urea cycle resulting in hyperammonemia and the symptomatology resulting from these disorders.

16. Jones, E. A., and Schafer, D. F. Hepatic encephalopathy: a neurochemical disorder. *Prog. Liver Dis.* 8:525, 1986.

17. Jones, E. A., and Gammal, S. H. In I. M. Arias, W. B. Jakoby, H. Popper, et al. (eds.), *The Liver: Biology and Pathobiology,* 2nd ed. New York: Raven Press, 1988. P. 985.
These two articles (16, 17) review the neurochemical abnormalities proposed by some to be important in the pathogenesis of hepatic encephalopathy. The GABA receptor model, as well as the benzodiazepine receptor model, is discussed.

18. Pappas, S. C., and Jones, E. A. Methods for assessing hepatic encephalopathy. *Semin. Liver Dis.* 3:298, 1983.
A practical review article summarizing the assessment of the severity of hepatic encephalopathy based on routinely available diagnostic techniques.

19. Schenker, S., and Bradley, C. E. Pathogenesis of Hepatic Encephalopathy. In H. O. Conn and J. Bircher (eds.), *Hepatic Encephalopathy: Management with Lactulose and Related Carbohydrates.* East Lansing, Mich.: Medi-Ed Press, 1988. P. 15.
This review article summarizes many current theories of the pathogenesis of hepatic encephalopathy with an extensive well-supported bibliography.

20. Warren, K. S., Iber, F. L., Dolle, W., et al. Effective alterations in blood pH on distribution of ammonia from blood to cerebral spinal fluid in patients with hepatic coma. *J. Lab. Clin. Med.* 56:687, 1960.
This study shows the effect of pH on ammonia metabolism. These results help explain why a metabolic alkalosis induced by hypokalemia can worsen hepatic encephalopathy.

21. Uribe, M., Marquez, M. A., Garcia Ramos, G., et al. Treatment of chronic portal systemic encephalopathy with vegetable and animal protein diet: A control crossover study. *Dig. Dis. Sci.* 27:119, 1982.
This article compares animal and vegetable protein diets in the treatment of hepatic encephalopathy. Patients receiving protein primarily from vegetable sources have an improvement in symptoms of hepatic encephalopathy, suggesting a beneficial effect from this dietary manipulation.

22. Zieve, L., Doizaki, W. M., and Zieve, F. Synergism between mercaptans and ammonia or fatty acids in the production of coma: A possible role of mercaptans in the pathogenesis of hepatic coma. *J. Lab. Clin. Med.* 83:16, 1974.
This study suggests that hepatic encephalopathy is multifactorial. It demonstrates synergism between several proposed toxins in the development of the clinical syndrome of hepatic encephalopathy.

81. MALABSORPTION
H. Verdain Barnes

Malabsorption can occur in a variety of diseases, result from surgery, or from the ingestion of certain drugs. For normal homeostasis, man requires the absorption of proteins, carbohydrates, fat, vitamins, and minerals. Protein and carbohydrate absorption occur primarily in the proximal small bowel. Ingested proteins require the action of gastric, small intestine, and pancreatic enzymes for proper hydrolysis to amino acids and small peptides. These hydrolyzed molecules are actively transported into the mucosal cells of the jejunum and ileum where they pass directly into the portal blood system. A similar process occurs with carbohydrates, which initially are partially hydrolyzed by the pancreatic amylases. After absorption, carbohydrates also move directly into the portal circulation.

Fat absorption is more complex, requiring at least two additional steps. Ingested fat is primarily in the form of triglyceride, which generally remains intact until hydrolyzed by pancreatic lipase in the proximal small bowel. Two amphopaths are formed, namely, fatty acids and β-monoglycerides. They are made water-soluble by being dissolved in the macromolecular clusters of bile constituents called micelles. From these complexes, the fatty acids and β-monoglycerides passively diffuse into the cell, where the triglyceride is reformed and associated with protein, cholesterol, cholesterol ester, and phospholipid to form a chylomicron. The chylomicron moves into the central lacteal of the intestinal villus and ultimately through the lymphatic system into the bloodstream, where it is delivered to the liver, muscle, and adipose tissue. Any process that alters the availability of the pancreatic enzymes or bile constituents, small bowel cellular structure and function, lymphatic integrity, and/or increases the rate of passage through the small bowel can produce varying degrees of fat malabsorption. Fat malabsorption (steatorrhea) is more common than protein malabsorption, which in turn is more frequent than carbohydrate.

Pancreatic enzyme deficiency is seen most often in chronic pancreatitis, usually of alcoholic origin, but it may also occur with pancreatic carcinoma, cystic fibrosis, and following pancreatic resection. Deficiencies in the availability of bile constituents are seen in intrahepatic and extrahepatic biliary obstruction, hepatocellular diseases with or without jaundice, cholecystocolonic fistulas, and the blind loop syndrome with excessive bacterial overgrowth. A number of diseases can specifically result in small bowel destruction or in defective intracellular enzyme activity. These diseases include celiac disease, tropical sprue, Whipple's disease, amyloidosis, lymphoma, abetalipoproteinemia, intestinal lymphangiectasia, jejunitis, eosinophilic gastroenteritis, food allergy, dermatitis herpetiformis, exfoliative dermatitis, eczema, erythrodermic psoriasis, small intestinal ischemia due to atherosclerosis, vasculitides, Köhlmeier-Degos syndrome, and hyperviscosity, as in polycythemia vera and the dysproteinemias. A mixture of defects or poorly understood processes have been reported to produce malabsorption in the following conditions: scleroderma; irradiation enteritis; Zollinger-Ellison syndrome; extensive ileal resection; regional enteritis; hypogammaglobulinemia; parasitic infestation with *Giardia, Strongyloides,* hookworm, *Capillaria,* and schistosomes; mast cell disease; tuberculosis; coccidioidomycosis; and a variety of endocrinopathies, such as diabetes mellitus, carcinoid, hyperthyroidism, hypoadrenocortisolism, hypoparathyroidism, and pseudohypoparathyroidism.

Malabsorption can be documented with appropriate tests. The determination of fecal nitrogen excretion provides a reliable but indirect measure of protein absorption. A 72-hour stool collection is analyzed for nitrogen while the patient is on a diet providing 80 to 100 gm of protein per day. The primary pitfall is the falsely elevated nitrogen levels seen in the severe protein-losing enteropathies. To document fat malabsorption, the standard is still the 72-hour fecal fat determination, but the triolein breath test and oxalate loading test appear to be sensitive screening tests with excellent specificity. To perform a diagnostic fecal fat determination, the patient must (1) be on a 60- to 100-gm fat diet for 3 to 5 days prior to and during the 72-hour collection period, (2) have bowel movements at least daily, (3) collect a complete stool collection, (4) not ingest castor and nut oils, and (5) have a chemical determination of the stool fat.

A biopsy of the small bowel is probably the single most valuable tool in diagnosing malabsorption in celiac disease, Whipple's disease, amyloidosis, mast cell disease, primary intestinal lymphoma, eosinophilic gastroenteritis, intestinal immunodeficiency diseases, giardiasis, coccidiosis, strongyloidiasis, lymphangiectasis, and abetalipoproteinemia since each of these processes has a distinctive histologic picture. The biopsy can provide supportive evidence in cases due to tropical sprue, scleroderma, hypogammaglobulinemia, dermatitis herpetiformis, irradiation enteritis, and other parasitic infestations. Evidence for the functional cellular integrity of the jejunum and the ileum can be obtained by the D-xylose and Schilling tests, respectively. Lactose malabsorption can be demonstrated by the lactose tolerance test or a radioactive lactose breath test.

The possibility of excessive bacterial overgrowth requires consideration, since it can be the sole or a contributing cause of malabsorption and is readily treatable. The D-xylose and Schilling tests are abnormally low in the presence of severe overgrowth. Probably the most sensitive test for overgrowth is the radioisotope breath test, which gives abnormal results in the presence of an increased deconjugation of bile salts in the small bowel or the degradation of xylose. This increase can result from bacterial overgrowth or ileal resection. Radioactive glycine-1-cholate or xylose is given by mouth and the expired air is examined for the presence of radioactive carbon dioxide metabolite.

Evidence of significant malabsorption of the fat-soluble vitamins should be sought. Hyperkeratosis follicularis is almost invariably present in vitamin A deficiency. Hypocalcemia is seen in vitamin D deficiency and a prolonged prothrombin time with vitamin K deficiency. A number of other tests are available but offer less specific or less reliable data. A specific etiologic diagnosis of malabsorption is usually possible by aggressive appropriate testing.

1. Brandenborg, L. L. Histologic diagnosis of diseases of malabsorption. *Am. J. Med.* 67:999, 1979.
   An update on histologic diagnosis from peroral small bowel biopsy.
2. Corcino, J. J., Waxman, S., and Herbert, V. Absorption and malabsorption of vitamin B_{12}. *Am. J. Med.* 48:562, 1970.
   A detailed discussion of the setting for vitamin B_{12} malabsorption.
3. Benson, G. D., Kowlessar, O. D., and Sleisenger, M. H. Adult celiac disease with emphasis upon response to the gluten-free diet. *Medicine* 43:1, 1964.
4. Mann, J. G., Brown, W. R., and Kern, F. The subtle and variable clinical expressions of gluten-induced enteropathy. *Am. J. Med.* 48:357, 1970.
5. Mawhinney, H., and Tomkin, G. H. Gluten enteropathy associated with selective IgA deficiency. *Lancet* 1:121, 1971.
6. Johnson, R. L., Van Arsdel, P. P., Tobe, A. D., et al. Adult hypogammaglobulinemia with malabsorption and iron deficiency anemia. *Am. J. Med.* 43:935, 1967.
7. Knarer, C. M., and Svoboda, A. C. Malabsorption and jejunal diverticulosis. *Am. J. Med.* 44:606, 1968.
8. Lake, B., and Andrews, G. Rheumatoid arthritis with secondary amyloidosis and malabsorption syndrome. *Am. J. Med.* 44:105, 1968.
9. Brow, J. R., Parker, F., Weinstein, W. M., et al. The small intestinal mucosa in dermatitis herpetiformis. *Gastroenterology* 60:355, 1971.
10. Trier, J. S., Phelps, P. C., Eidelman, S., et al. Whipple's disease: Light and electron microscope correlation of jejunal mucosal histology with antibiotic treatment and clinical status. *Gastroenterology* 48:684, 1965.
11. Gilat, T., Revach, M., and Sohar, E. Deposition of amyloid in the gastrointestinal tract. *Gut* 10:98, 1969.
12. Klein, N. C., Hargrove, R. L., Sleisenger, M. H., et al. Eosinophilic gastroenteritis. *Medicine* 49:299, 1970.
13. Carron, D. B., and Douglas, A. P. Steatorrhea in vascular insufficiency of the small intestine. *Q. J. Med.* 34:331, 1965.
14. Ways, P. O., Parmentier, C. M., Kayden, H. J., et al. Studies on the absorptive defect for triglyceride in abetalipoproteinemia. *J. Clin. Invest.* 46:35, 1967.

15. Eidelman, S., Parkin, R. A., and Rubin, C. E. Abdominal lymphoma presenting as malabsorption: A clinicopathologic study of nine cases in Israel and a review of the literature. *Medicine* 45:111, 1966.

16. Shimoda, S. S., Saunders, D. R., and Rubin, C. E. The Zollinger-Ellison syndrome with steatorrhea. *Gastroenterology* 55:705, 1968.

17. McBrien, D. J., and Mummery, H. E. L. Steatorrhea in progressive systemic sclerosis (scleroderma). *Br. Med. J.* 2:1653, 1962.

18. Broilman, S. A., McGray, R. S., May, J. C., et al. Mastocytosis and intestinal malabsorption. *Am. J. Med.* 48:383, 1970.

19. Dobbins, W. O., III. Drug-induced steatorrhea. *Gastroenterology* 54:1193, 1968.

20. Levin, D. M., Lipsky, P. E., and Kirkpatrick, C. H. Selective hypogammaglobulinemia with persistence of IgE, malabsorption and a nutritionally dependent, reversible defect in cell-mediated immunity. *Am. J. Med.* 58:129, 1975.
    Articles 3–20 present a spectrum of the known causes of malabsorption.

21. Bossart, R., Henry, K., Booth, C. C., et al. Subepithelial collagen in intestinal malabsorption. *Gut* 16:18, 1975.
    Increased subepithelial collagen is not uncommon in adult celiac sprue, hence "collagenous sprue" is probably not a separate entity.

22. Bayless, T. M., Rothfeld, B., Massa, C., et al. Lactose and milk intolerance: Clinical implications. *N. Engl. J. Med.* 292:1156, 1975.
    Abnormal lactose tolerance was found in 81% of the blacks tested and was not uncommon in whites.

23. Newcomer, A. D., Hofmann, A. F., DiMagno, E. P., et al. Triolein breath test: A sensitive and specific test for fat malabsorption. *Gastroenterology* 76:6, 1979.

24. Rampton, D. S., Kasidas, G. P., Rose, G. A., et al. Oxalate loading test: A screening test for steatorrhea. *Gut* 20:1089, 1979.
    Two impressive screening tests for fat malabsorption (articles 23, 24), a breath of fresh air for gastrointestinal laboratories.

25. Haeney, M. R., Culank, L. S., Montgomery, R. D., et al. Evaluation of xylose absorption as measured in blood and urine: A one-hour blood xylose screening test in malabsorption. *Gastroenterology* 75:393, 1978.
    Another improvement in screening tests for malabsorption.

26. Baer, A. N., Bayless, T. M., and Yardley, J. H. Intestinal ulceration and malabsorption syndromes. *Gastroenterology* 79:754, 1980.
    A potentially fatal complication of celiac disease to keep in mind.

27. Anderson, C. M. Malabsorption in children. *Clin. Gastroenterol.* 6:355, 1977.
    A useful review for those who see children and adolescents.

28. Orchard, J. L., Luparello, F., and Brunskill, D. Malabsorption syndrome occurring in the course of disseminated histoplasmosis: Case report and review of gastrointestinal histoplasmosis. *Am. J. Med.* 66:331, 1979.

29. Dawson, J., Hodgson, H. J. F., Papys, M. B., et al. Immunodeficiency, malabsorption and secretory diarrhea: A new syndrome. *Am. J. Med.* 67:540, 1979.
    Both rare and one new etiology for malabsorption (articles 28, 29).

30. Sleisenger, M. H., and Glickman, R. M. Symposium on malabsorption. *Am. J. Med.* 67:979, 1979.
    An excellent symposium update on pathophysiology, diagnosis, and selected specific diseases of malabsorption (includes fat, vitamin D and calcium, nutrition in the short bowel syndrome, protein, vitamin B_{12}, folate, bacterial overgrowth, parasites, drugs, alcohol, intestinal immunity, gluten-sensitive enteropathy, and eosinophilic gastroenteropathy).

31. King, C. E., Toskes, P. P., Spivey, J. C., et al. Detection of small intestinal bacterial overgrowth by means of a ^{14}C-D-xylose breath test. *Gastroenterology* 77:75, 1979.
    Discusses the tests for the overgrowth of bacteria in the small bowel.

32. Ryan, M. E., and Olsen, W. A. A diagnostic approach to malabsorption syndromes: A pathophysiologic approach. *Clin. Gastroenterol.* 12:533, 1983.

33. Russell, R. I., and Lee, F. D. Tests of small-intestinal function—digestion, absorption, secretion. *Clin. Gastroenterol.* 7:277, 1978.
    Two (articles 32, 33) well-done, comprehensive, well-referenced reviews for the clinician.

34. Bo-Linn, G. W., and Fordtran, J. S. Fecal fat concentration in patients with steatorrhea. *Gastroenterology* 87:319, 1984.
    A fecal fat concentration of greater than 9.5% in a patient who loses 21 gm of fat per day or more points to pancreatic insufficiency as the cause.
35. Borgstrom, B. Relative colipase deficiency as a cause of fat malabsorption in humans and the importance of the law of mass action for clinical medicine. *Gastroenterology* 86:194, 1984.
    Yet another cause of steatorrhea.

82. TOXIC MEGACOLON

H. Verdain Barnes

Toxic megacolon (TM) occurs as a complication in up to 6 percent of patients with minimal to moderate ulcerative colitis and in 10 to 20 percent of those patients with severe ulcerative colitis. Mortality ranges from 10 to 50 percent, depending on the patient's age and the aggressiveness of the treatment. Toxic megacolon is seen only in the presence of active disease. Five to twenty-five percent develop TM with their initial attack of ulcerative colitis, whereas 16 to 31 percent develop the complication during its chronic course. Women show a slight predominance. Patient age is variable, although about 20 percent are over 60 years of age.

Toxic megacolon is not consistently defined in the literature, but the patients all have one or more of the following features of toxicity: pyrexia greater than 39.7°C (103.5°F), tachycardia over 120 beats per minute, leukocyte count greater than 10,500 cells per microliter with a shift to the left, anemia with a hematocrit of less than 28 percent, hypotension, mental changes, electrolyte disturbances, and/or dehydration. The primary electrolyte problem is potassium deficiency, with most patients having values of less than 3.5 mEq/liter. About 50 percent require over 150 mEq of potassium replacement per day for maintenance. Dehydration may be severe and hypoproteinemia profound in the presence of persistent moderate or severe diarrhea. The mental state may be one of confusion, incoherence, agitation, or apathy.

The diarrhea is usually severe but on occasion is mild. Proctoscopic examination usually reveals severe bowel changes, but on occasion is misleading, showing only minimal changes. In addition to toxicity, the sine qua non is dilatation of the colon. This can be documented by a plain x ray of the abdomen. An air-filled segment of bowel with a transverse diameter of over 6 cm is abnormal. Radiographically there is also a loss of haustral markings and most patients show broad-based nodular interluminal projections—pseudopolyps. The clinical evidence of dilatation is abdominal distention and/or rebound tenderness. These features are by no means invariably present, occurring in less than 50 percent in some series. The vast majority of patients have a pancolitis. The transverse colon is the most commonly dilated segment, with occasional dilatation of the ascending colon and (rarely) the sigmoid. Associated small bowel and gastric distention is not uncommon.

Several precipitating or contributing factors have been reported. Hypokalemia has been implicated since it produces a decrease in colonic muscle tone. In many cases there is a definite temporal relationship between the development of TM and the starting of anticholinergic or opiate therapy, or preparation for a barium enema. Consequently in a severe attack of ulcerative colitis, serum potassium levels should be maintained, anticholinergics and opiates used with extreme caution or not at all, and in general barium enemas avoided.

The most frequent complication of TM is colon perforation, occurring in about one-third of patients. Perforation can be insidious and difficult to assess since these patients are severely ill and are frequently receiving high-dose steroids and antibiotics. Free peritoneal air is radiographically demonstrable in only 20 to 50 percent, and there may be no significant change found on physical examination. Perforation should be suspected in any intensively treated patient who shows no response or continues to clinically deteriorate. The mortality is clearly higher in this group. The second most frequent complication is gram-negative septicemia, which occurs in about one-third of patients. Finally, massive colonic hemorrhage occurs in about 10 percent.

Most patients who die do so within 10 days of diagnosis. With maximum medical therapy, if deterioration continues after 24 to 48 hours or if colonic dilatation persists for longer than 48 to 72 hours, surgery should be undertaken without delay. Some authors advocate early surgery regardless of the clinical course; this, however, seems to overstate the case for surgery.

In TM the primary histologic lesion is the formation of deep ulcers with inflammation and destruction of the muscularis propria of the colon. The factors that cause this transmural extension in a primarily mucosal disease are not understood.

The other diseases reported to produce toxic megacolon are Crohn's disease, amebic colitis, typhoid fever, Chagas' disease, cholera, pseudomembranous enterocolitis, lymphoma, bacillary dysentery, *Yersinia* enterocolitis, connective tissue disease, and ischemic colitis. Ischemic colitis should routinely be considered as the potential etiology of TM in elderly patients without a history of ulcerative colitis.

1. Norland, C. C., and Kirsner, J. B. Toxic dilatation of colon (toxic megacolon): Etiology, treatment and prognosis in 42 patients. *Medicine* 48:229, 1969.
2. Jalan, K. N., Sircus, W., Card, W. I., et al. An experience of ulcerative colitis: I. Toxic dilation in 55 cases. *Gastroenterology* 57:68, 1969.
   Articles 1 and 2 provide good general reviews of the entity, with an emphasis on clinical presentation and management.
3. Colin, E. M., Copit, D., and Tumen, H. J. Ulcerative colitis with hypopotassemia. *Gastroenterology* 30:950, 1956.
   Hypokalemia may be a key factor in toxic megacolon.
4. Smith, F. W., Law, D. H., Nickel, W. F., et al. Fulminant ulcerative colitis with toxic dilation of the colon. *Gastroenterology* 42:233, 1962.
   TM can be precipitated by anticholinergics and opiates.
5. Odyniec, N. A., Judd, E. S., and Sauer, W. G. Toxic megacolon. *Arch. Surg.* 94:638, 1967.
   Barium enema can be a precipitating factor. Perforation was diagnosed preoperatively in only one-third of cases.
6. Tumen, H. J. Toxic megacolon in fulminating disease. *J.A.M.A.* 191:838, 1965.
   Silent perforation is not uncommon, and it can occur in the patient with or without steroid therapy.
7. Margolis, I. B., Faro, R. S., Howells, E. M., et al. Megacolon in the elderly: Ischemic or inflammatory? *Ann. Surg.* 190:40, 1979.
   Ischemia should regularly be in the differential diagnosis of TM in the elderly.
8. Mogan, G. R., Sachar, D. B., Bauer, J., et al. Toxic megacolon in ulcerative colitis complicated by pneumomediastinum: Report of two cases. *Gastroenterology* 79:559, 1980.
   Unusual and rare to say the least.
9. Brown, J. W. Toxic megacolon associated with loperamide therapy. *J.A.M.A.* 241:501, 1979.
   Yet another drug that can precipitate TM in ulcerative colitis.
10. Truelove, S. C., Willoughby, C. P., Lee, E. G., et al. Further experience in treatment of severe attacks of ulcerative colitis. *Lancet* 2:1086, 1978.
    A medical approach to therapy.
11. Gonzales, A., Vargas, V., Guarner, L., et al. Toxic megacolon in typhoid fever. *Arch. Intern. Med.* 145:2120, 1985.
    A well-documented case of this rare disorder.
12. Ferreiro, J. E., Busse, J. C., and Saldana, M. J. Megacolon in a collagen vascular overlap syndrome. *Am. J. Med.* 80:307, 1986.
    The connective tissue diseases can be an etiology.

83. ULCERATIVE COLITIS
H. Verdain Barnes

Ulcerative colitis (UC) is a chronic inflammatory disease of the colonic mucosa. The cause(s) remains unknown. The general incidence ranges from about 3.9 to 7.3 new cases per year per 100,000 population. Women show a variable predominance, and an increased incidence has been confirmed in the white and Jewish populations. Ten to twenty percent have a positive family history of inflammatory bowel disease. The typical histologic picture is abscess formation in the crypts of Lieberkühn, with accompanying polymorphonuclear leukocytic and round cell infiltration. As the disease progresses, scarring occurs, resulting in a loss of mucosa and a shortened narrow colon.

The onset of UC may be acute or insidious. The most common presenting complaint is rectal bleeding, usually with diarrhea. In an acute presentation, the bleeding is usually associated with varying degrees of toxicity, fever, abdominal pain and distention, anorexia, weight loss, and tenesmus. Rarely a more fulminant picture is seen with massive colonic hemorrhage or sepsis as hallmarks. Toxic megacolon may accompany these symptoms. Clinically the disease can be categorized as ulcerative proctitis, acute ulcerative colitis, acute intermittent ulcerative colitis, fulminant ulcerative colitis, or chronic unremitting ulcerative colitis. Acute ulcerative proctitis, the mildest form of the disease, commonly presents with recurrent blood and pus in an otherwise normal stool. Sigmoidoscopic examination shows normal bowel above 10 to 15 cm. When the rectum is involved, fecal urgency is common. Complications other than rectal fistulas are rare and the prognosis is good. In acute ulcerative colitis, involvement extends above 15 cm by sigmoidoscopic examination, and is frequently pancolonic. Local and systemic complications are more common and the prognosis is guarded. The fulminant form occurs in 1 to 5 percent of the patients with UC. In most reports, death from the disease is most common in the first 8 weeks of medical therapy, especially if toxic megacolon is present. Chronic unremitting ulcerative colitis is usually insidious in onset. The initial bout is most often characterized by malaise, anorexia, weight loss, fever, abdominal cramping after eating, fecal urgency, and tenesmus.

The differential diagnoses include amebic colitis, ischemic colitis, bacillary dysentery, lymphogranuloma venereum, uremic colitis, diverticulitis, *Campylobacter fetus* colitis, pseudomembranous enterocolitis, carcinoma of the colon, metastatic carcinoma, tuberculosis of the bowel, laxative colon, collagenous colitis, and Crohn's disease of the colon.

There are a wide variety of complications of UC. Local complications include hemorrhoids, perianal abscesses, strictures, rectovaginal fistulas, pseudopolyps, perforation with abscess formation, localized peritonitis, generalized peritonitis, and carcinoma. The incidence of colon carcinoma in UC is probably near 10 percent. Recent studies find the primary risk factors to be the extent and duration of the disease. The cumulative probability of cancer developing is 30 to 40 percent at 25 years. The majority who develop cancer have pancolitis and an average disease duration of about 21 years. Rectal and multiple colon biopsies during colonoscopy may identify patients with precancerous mucosal dysplasia.

Complications arising outside the bowel involve the eyes, skin, liver, kidneys, joints, blood, and blood vessels. The most common complications involve the hepatobiliary system. The histologic lesions of the liver are, in decreasing order of frequency, fatty infiltration, chronic active hepatitis, postnecrotic cirrhosis, focal necrosis, amyloidosis, primary sclerosing cholangitis syndrome, hemosiderosis, and hyaline degeneration. These lesions are most often seen in combination, with the dominant lesion being small-duct or large-duct pericholangitis. Microscopic features differentiate pericholangitis into acute, subacute, and chronic forms. The more extensive the disease, the greater the incidence of these changes, which may be seen with the initial attack or during the course of UC. Some cases progress to cirrhosis. The exact cause is unknown, but recurrent portal bacteremia and/or autoimmunity have been postulated.

Rheumatic complaints occur in as high as 45 percent, with frank arthritis occurring in 10 to 20 percent. The specific arthritis of UC consists of recurrent acute synovitis, which is usually an asymmetric monoarticular involvement of the knee or ankle. Subcutaneous nodules and tendon sheath effusions are not seen. Arthritis is more often seen in patients with extensive long-standing bowel involvement. Exacerbations tend to parallel the activity of the bowel disease. Sacroiliitis occurs in 18 percent and bears no relationship to the extent, duration, activity, or other complications of UC. Ankylosing spondylitis is seen in about 5 percent, possibly on a genetic basis.

Skin manifestations include generalized pustular dermatitis, erythema nodosum, erythema multiforme, pyoderma gangrenosum, and severe aphthous ulcers in the mouth. Ocular complications are iritis, episcleritis, marginal corneal ulcers, uveitis, and conjunctivitis.

Anemia and hypercoagulability are common. The anemia is predominantly due to iron deficiency. When the sigmoidoscopic examination reveals a hemorrhagic mucosa, blood loss typically exceeds 200 ml/week. Even in the presence of nonhemorrhagic mucosa, blood loss may exceed 50 to 100 ml/week. Anemia, therefore, may be more severe than expected on purely clinical grounds since often no blood is observed by the patient when losses range from 50 to 150 ml/week. The hypercoagulable state is due to increased factor VIII activity, thromboplastin generation, and fibrinogen. This is at least in part the cause of the migratory thrombophlebitis occasionally seen in UC. A qualitative platelet defect has been suggested, but not proved, and thrombocytosis has been reported.

Finally, there is an increased incidence of nephrolithiasis in these patients. Renal stones occur primarily in patients who have had an ileostomy within the preceding 16 months. The causative mechanism may be the increased absorption of dietary oxylate.

1. Shorter, R. G., and Shepard, D. A. E. (eds.). Frontiers in inflammatory bowel disease. *Am. J. Dig. Dis.* 20:540, 639, 1975.
   A comprehensive, well-referenced article.
2. Perrett, A. D., Higgins, G., Johnston, H. H., et al. The liver in ulcerative colitis. *Q. J. Med.* 40:211, 1971.
   A thorough study of the liver changes in 300 patients, along with hematologic, biochemical, bacteriologic, and immunologic profiles.
3. Eade, M. N., and Brooke, B. N. Portal bacteremia in cases of ulcerative colitis submitted to colectomy. *Lancet* 1:1008, 1969.
   24% of patients have portal bacteremia. The most common bacterium is Escherichia coli.
4. Wright, V., and Watkinson, G. The arthritis of ulcerative colitis. *Br. Med. J.* 2:670, 1965.
   45% have rheumatic complaints and 11.5% in this series had the specific arthritis of UC.
5. Wright, V., and Watkinson, G. Sacro-iliitis and ulcerative colitis. *Br. Med. J.* 2:676, 1965.
   Sacroiliitis is a common finding and seemingly has no relation to the extent, duration, or activity of UC.
6. Ellis, P. P., and Gentry, J. H. Ocular complications of ulcerative colitis. *Am. J. Ophthalmol.* 58:779, 1964.
   A good discussion of the eye manifestations of UC.
7. Beal, R. W., Skyring, A. P., McRae, J., et al. The anemia of ulcerative colitis. *Gastroenterology* 45:589, 1963.
   A good general discussion.
8. Stack, H. R., Smith, T., Jones, J. H., et al. Measurement of blood and iron loss in colitis with a whole body counter. *Gut* 10:769, 1969.
   In nonhemorrhagic-appearing bowel, blood loss can range from 0–200 ml/week.
9. Lee, J. C. L., Spittell, J. A., Sauer, W. G., et al. Hypercoagulability associated with chronic colitis: Changes in blood coagulation factors. *Gastroenterology* 54:76, 1968.
   Factor VIII, thromboplastin generation, and fibrinogen are commonly increased, whereas in active disease, factors VII and X are often decreased.
10. Fawaz, K. A., Glotzer, D. J., Goldman, H., et al. Ulcerative colitis and Crohn's disease of the colon: A comparison of the long term postoperative courses. *Gastroenterology* 71:372, 1976.

Colectomy and ileostomy work well in UC but not so well in Crohn's disease of the colon.

11. Tucker, P. C., Webster, P. D., and Kilpatrick, Z. M. Amebic colitis mistaken for inflammatory bowel disease. *Arch. Intern. Med.* 135:681, 1975.
    Entamoeba histolytica should be searched for routinely.
12. Meyers, M. A., Oliphant, M., Teixidor, H., et al. Metastatic carcinoma simulating inflammatory bowel disease. *Am. J. Roentgenol. Radium Ther. Nucl. Med.* 123:74, 1975.
    A potential look-alike.
13. Kraft, S. C., Earle, R. H., Roesler, M., et al. Unexplained bronchopulmonary disease with inflammatory bowel disease. *Arch. Intern. Med.* 136:454, 1976.
    Another potential complication of this systemic disease.
14. Greenstein, A. J., Sachar, D. B., Smith, H., et al. Cancer in universal and left-sided ulcerative colitis: Factors determining risk. *Gastroenterology* 77:290, 1979.
    The risks were the extent and duration of the disease.
15. Sharon, P., Ligumsky, M., Rachmilewitz, D., et al. Role of prostaglandins in ulcerative colitis: Enhanced production during active disease and inhibition by sulfasalazine. *Gastroenterology* 75:638, 1978.
16. Rampton, D. S., Sladen, G. E., and Youlten, L. J. F. Rectal mucosal prostaglandin E_2 release and its relation to disease activity, electrical potential difference and treatment and ulcerative colitis. *Gut* 2:591, 1980.
    Prostaglandin E_2 may play an important role in this disease (articles 15, 16).
17. Mee, A. S., and Jewell, D. P. Factors inducing relapse in inflammatory bowel disease. *Br. Med. J.* 3:801, 1978.
    60% of UC relapse had had a recent upper respiratory tract infection.
18. Basler, R. S. W. Ulcerative colitis and the skin. *Med. Clin. North Am.* 64:941, 1980.
    An up-to-date comprehensive review.
19. Loss, R. W., Jr., Mangla, J. C., and Pereira, M. *Campylobacter* colitis presenting as inflammatory bowel disease with segmental colonic ulcerations. *Gastroenterology* 79:138, 1980.
    Another look-alike to keep in mind.
20. Rosekrans, P. C. M., Meijer, C. J. L. M., Van Der Wal, A. M., et al. Allergic proctitis: A clinical and immunopathological entity. *Gut* 21:1017, 1980.
    An apparent subgroup among patients with isolated proctitis.
21. Barot, L. R., Rombeau, J. L., Steinberg, J. J., et al. Energy expenditure in patients with inflammatory bowel disease. *Arch. Surg.* 116:460, 1981.
    An objective method of estimating the daily caloric needs of these patients using the simple Harris-Benedict equation.
22. Mogadam, M., Dobbins, W. O., III, Korelitz, B. I., et al. Pregnancy in inflammatory bowel disease: Effect of sulfasalazine and corticosteroids on fetal outcome. *Gastroenterology* 80:72, 1981.
    There was no adverse effect; it appears that pregnant women can be treated just like nonpregnant women.
23. Goldman, H. N., and Antonioli, D. A. Mucosal biopsy of the rectum, colon and distal ileum. *Hum. Pathol.* 70:981, 1982.
    Reviews biopsy as a method of diagnosis.
24. Rickert, R. R. The important "imposters" in the differential diagnosis of inflammatory bowel disease. *J. Clin. Gastroenterol.* 6:153, 1984.
    Beware of these.
25. Wee, A., and Ludwig, J. Pericholangitis in chronic ulcerative colitis: Primary sclerosing cholangitis of the small bile ducts. *Ann. Intern. Med.* 102:581, 1985.
    Pericholangitis and primary sclerosing cholangitis may represent a spectrum of the same disease process. About 7% of these patients developed bile duct cancer.
26. Greenstein, A. J., Janowitz, H. D., and Sachar, D. B. The extraintestinal complications of Crohn's disease and ulcerative colitis: A study of 700 patients. *Medicine* 55:401, 1976.
    A comprehensive review of these complications and an assessment of their correlation with disease activity.

27. Rams, H., Rogers, A. I., and Ghandur-Mnaymneh, L. Collagenous colitis. *Ann. Intern. Med.* 106:108, 1987.
   Review of a disease that falls into the differential diagnosis of UC.
28. Lashner, B. A., Hanauer, S. B., and Silverstein, M. D. Optimal timing of colonoscopy to screen for cancer in ulcerative colitis. *Ann. Intern. Med.* 108:274, 1988.
   These authors propose the use of patient-specific hazard rates to assess the need for screen colonoscopy.
29. Chapman, R. W., Cottone, M., Selby, W. S., et al. Serum autoantibodies, ulcerative colitis and primary sclerosing cholangitis. *Gut* 27:86, 1986.
   Anticolon antibodies were found in 62.5% of patients with ulcerative colitis and primary sclerosing cholangitis.
30. Zimmerman, J., Gavish, D., and Rachmilewitz, D. Early and late onset ulcerative colitis: Distinct clinical features. *J. Clin. Gastroenterol.* 7:492, 1985.
   Late-onset disease (>50 years old) patients more often presented with proctocolitis and more liver disease than early-onset patients (<31 years old).
31. Stonnington, C. M., Phillips, S. F., Melton, L. J., III, et al. Chronic ulcerative colitis: Incidence and prevalence in a community. *Gut* 28:402, 1987.
   In this population the rate was 15/100,000 person-years with a male-female ratio of 15:1.

84. VIRAL HEPATITIS
H. Verdain Barnes

Viral hepatitis is a major health problem, occurring at a rate of about 25 cases per 100,000 population in the United States. The estimated economic cost is close to $650 million annually. A variety of viruses are known to produce hepatitis, but the majority of cases appear to be caused by the hepatitis A (HAV), B (HBV), or non-A, non-B (NA/NBH) viruses. HAV and HBV can be differentiated to a degree on an epidemiologic and definitely on an immunologic basis. NA/NBH is a diagnosis of exclusion, that is, no evidence of HAV, HBV, cytomegalovirus, and Epstein-Barr viral infection. Hepatitis A (infectious hepatitis, or Willowbrook MS-1) typically has an average incubation time of 25 to 30 days, a peak incidence in the winter and spring, and an increased frequency in persons under age 15 years. The clinical onset is usually abrupt, the course is short, the disease is mild, complications are uncommon, and the mortality is about 0.1 percent. The virus can be cultured from the stool until approximately 1 week after the onset of jaundice.

Hepatitis B (serum hepatitis or Willowbrook MS-2) typically has an average incubation period of 60 to 90 days, no seasonal variation, and no age predilection. The clinical onset is usually insidious, the course is long, the severity is variable, complications are common, and the mortality is 1 to 10 percent. The virus has not been cultured from the stool. It should be noted that the long-held epidemiologic distinction based on the route of infection is no longer tenable. Infection can occur for either type by the oral or parenteral route although the former is rare for hepatitis B.

NA/NBH has been shown to account for 60 to 90 percent of posttransfusion hepatitis, while the incidence of nontransfusion-related disease remains unknown. The posttransfusion incubation period ranges from 5 to 20 weeks with an average of about 8 weeks. It appears that the majority have anicteric disease (approximately 60–70%). The clinical presentation is variable. It may be acute with symptoms similar to HBV or insidious with few if any symptoms. The ALT (SGPT) is routinely elevated and often remains so for a year or more. Those anicteric patients with a peak ALT of more than 300 IU/liter appear to be at greatest risk to develop chronic active or chronic persistent hepatitis. By actuarial analysis, no more than 54 percent of those predicted have a spontaneous biochemical remission within 3 years. Patients with icteric or anicteric disease have about an equal chance of developing chronic hepatitis.

In many respects the clinical courses of HAV and HBV disease are similar. Both typ-ically have a flulike prodrome consisting of malaise, fatigue, headache, and minimal to severe nausea. Some well-documented but poorly recognized features that can occur in the prodromal phase are (1) symmetric nonmigratory polyarthritis with or without ef-fusion (occurring in up to 15%), (2) mild to severe degree of hyposmia, dysosmia, hypo-geusia, or dysgeusia, (3) urticaria with or without an associated maculopapular skin rash, (4) polyarteritis, or (5) thrombophlebitis. Hepatitis B surface antigen (HB$_s$Ag) is positive in patients with polyarteritis alone and in most cases of polyarthritis and urti-caria. The basic underlying process appears to be circulating immune complexes. The synovial fluid of the arthritic joints characteristically has a positive HB$_s$Ag titer and low complement, as does the serum.

The signs and symptoms of the prodromal phase begin to abate with the onset of jaun-dice and for the most part totally subside during the icteric phase. Jaundice usually increases rapidly to a peak over a period of 7 to 14 days and then slowly declines over a period of from 1 to 8 weeks. During the icteric phase, occasional intravascular coagula-tion or hemolytic anemia develops. The anemia usually subsides along with the other manifestations of the disease but on occasion is protracted. In the reported cases of he-molytic anemia there is frequently an underlying glucose-6-phosphate dehydrogenase deficiency. A rare patient has fulminant hepatic necrosis or acute yellow atrophy in this phase of the disease. If the bilirubin level is still rising or the clinical signs and symp-toms have not begun to abate in 14 days, the development of subacute or fulminant hepatitis should be suspected. In fulminant hepatitis the mortality exceeds 90 percent, regardless of the mode of therapy used.

After a typical icteric phase, there is a variable recovery time for all clinical and chem-ical abnormalities. In HAV, all but 10 percent of patients are completely well at the end of 3 months, whereas in HBV the recovery period is longer and complete recovery less likely. During the recovery phase, about 15 percent of patients have clinical or chemical relapses that rarely last longer than 1 month.

In summary, the outcome of acute HAV and HBV disease may be (1) complete recovery, (2) carrier state, (3) nonspecific reactive hepatitis, (4) chronic persistent hepatitis, (5) chronic active hepatitis, (6) bridging necrotic hepatitis, (7) fulminant hepatic necrosis, (8) cirrhosis, and (9) hepatoma. The precise course the disease may take in a patient is not initially predictable.

Sophisticated serologic testing is now available for HAV and HBV disease, but not for NA/NBH. The current immunologic characteristics and their interpretations are:

Hepatitis A (HA)	
HA antigen (anti-HA)	Presence in feces equals acute infection in prog-ress. Absence in feces does not rule out acute infec-tion.
HA antibody (IgM anti-HA)	Presence in serum equals acute infection or infec-tion within the past year.
Hepatitis B (HB)	
HB surface antigen (HB$_s$Ag)	Presence in serum equals acute or recent infection. High titer in acute phase persisting for longer than 6 weeks appears to increase the risk of developing chronic hepatitis.
HB core antigen (HB$_c$Ag)	Presence in serum equals recent or very old infec-tion.
DNA polymerase (DNA poly)	Presence in serum reflects active viral replication and high infectivity.
HB surface antibody (HB$_s$Ab)	Presence in serum equals prior infection and prob-ably immunity.
HB core antibody (HB$_c$Ab)	Presence in serum suggests recent or ongoing in-fection. HB$_s$Ag carriers have high titers.

Some evidence for predicting the long-term outcome can be obtained from a histologic examination of the liver and determination of the status of the HB$_s$Ag titers over time. Typically, in viral hepatitis the areas of hepatocellular necrosis are small and widely distributed, which is indicative of a good prognosis. On the other hand, if the foci of necrosis are larger and bridge portal triads, central veins, and/or extend into adjacent lobules (i.e., if subacute hepatic necrosis exists), the prognosis is guarded. Approximately 25 percent of these patients die, and an additional one-third develop cirrhosis. Only rarely do patients show a transition from the typical to the subacute form. The subacute picture is seen most often in hepatitis B but fortunately is uncommon. Typically the HB_sAg appears from 2 to 8 weeks before the icteric phase. In about 4 percent the titer persists beyond 13 weeks. In a majority of these patients chronic aggressive hepatitis or, less commonly, chronic persistent hepatitis ensues.

An anicteric form of HAV and HBV disease is well documented. In some screening series, up to 7.4 percent have had serologic and/or histologic evidence of viral hepatitis without clinical jaundice. The most commonly associated clinical features are a poorly defined right upper quadrant discomfort or epigastric fullness made worse by activity, liver enlargement and/or tenderness, anorexia, weight loss, malaise, and nausea with or without vomiting. The prognosis is in general good; however, some patients develop chronic liver disease.

In recent years an increasing incidence of delta agent viral hepatitis (HDV) has been recognized, particularly in the high-risk groups for HBV infection. HDV is a partial RNA viral particle which requires HB_sAg for transmission and survival. HDV can produce nonfulminant hepatitis in association with acute or chronic hepatitis B, fulminant hepatitis in association with acute or chronic hepatitis B, or can result in chronic hepatitis D in association with chronic hepatitis B. In some studies, the incidence of fulminant hepatitis has been as high as 23 percent accounting for 59 percent of the deaths. The development of chronic active hepatitis is common. Diagnosis is by a positive serology for anti-HD.

1. Krugman, S., Giles, J. P., and Hammond, J. Infectious hepatitis: Evidence for two distinctive clinical, epidemiological, and immunological types of infection. *J.A.M.A.* 200:365, 1967.
   A classic study.
2. Koff, R. S., and Isselbacher, K. J. Changing concepts in the epidemiology of viral hepatitis. *N. Engl. J. Med.* 278:1371, 1968.
   Hepatitis A and B can be transmitted parenterally and by fecal-oral contamination.
3. Heukin, R. I., and Smith, F. R. Hyposmia in acute viral hepatitis. *Lancet* 1:823, 1971.
   Abnormalities of smell and taste may be prominent factors in the anorexia of hepatitis patients.
4. Alpert, E., Isselbacher, K. J., and Schur, P. H. Pathogenesis of arthritis associated with viral hepatitis: Complement component studies. *N. Engl. J. Med.* 285:185, 1971.
   Patients with arthritis most often have high HB – Ag titers and low C3 levels.
5. Fernandez, R., and McCarty, D. J. The arthritis of viral hepatitis. *Ann. Intern. Med.* 74:207, 1971.
   Arthritis as a prodrome can be seen also in HB – Ag-negative patients.
6. Salen, G., Goldstein, F., Haurani, F., et al. Acute hemolytic anemia complicating viral hepatitis in patients with glucose-6-phosphate dehydrogenase deficiency. *Ann. Intern. Med.* 65:1210, 1966.
   Hyperbilirubinemia is out of proportion to the degree of hepatic function abnormalities. Hemolysis is probably due to oxidative destruction of the red cell.
7. Green, A. J., and Novak, L. J. Thrombophlebitic prodrome in hepatitis. *N. Engl. J. Med.* 285:1322, 1971.
   Thrombophlebitis is a rare feature of the prodromal phase.
8. Tolsma, D. D., and Bryan, J. A. The economic impact of viral hepatitis in the United States. *Public Health Rep.* 91:349, 1976.
   The estimate is about $650 million yearly.
9. Villarejos, V. M., Visona, K. A., Gutierrez, A., et al. Role of saliva, urine and feces in transmission of type B hepatitis. *N. Engl. J. Med.* 291:1375, 1974.
   About 60% carried the antigen in their saliva, probably the main route of nonparenteral infection.

10. Ray, M. B., Desmet, V. J., Bradburne, A. F., et al. Differential distribution of hepatitis B surface antigen and hepatitis B core antigen in the liver of hepatitis B patients. *Gastroenterology* 71:462, 1976.
    Different degrees of HB$_s$Ag and HB$_c$Ag accumulation in the liver correlate with the histologic picture.
11. Hagler, L., Pastore, R. A., and Bergin, J. A. Aplastic anemia following viral hepatitis. *Medicine* 54:139, 1975.
    An important complication that occurs predominantly in males. A well-referenced, provocative review.
12. Dienstag, J. L., Alaama, A., Mosley, J. W., et al. Etiology of sporadic hepatitis B surface antigen: Negative hepatitis. *Ann. Intern. Med.* 87:1, 1977.
    About half were non-A, non-B viral hepatitis.
13. Deinhardt, F. Predictive value of markers of hepatitis virus infection. *J. Infect. Dis.* 141:299, 1980.
    A concise update regarding the significance of most of the markers.
14. Nisman, R. M., Ganderson, A. P., Valahceric, R., et al. Acute viral hepatitis with bridging hepatic necrosis: An overview. *Arch. Intern. Med.* 139:1289, 1979.
    This finding may have a more benign prognosis than previously thought.
15. Maynard, J. E. Nosocomial viral hepatitis. *Am. J. Med.* 70:439, 1981.
    A concise review of this problem with a focus on those at risk and modes of transmission.
16. Blumberg, B. S., and London, W. T. Hepatitis B virus and the prevention of primary hepatocellular carcinoma. *N. Engl. J. Med.* 304:782, 1981.
17. Shafritz, D. A., Shouval, D., Sherman, H. I., et al. Integration of hepatitis B virus DNA into the genome of liver cells in chronic liver disease and hepatocellular carcinoma. *N. Engl. J. Med.* 305:1067, 1981.
    These two articles (16, 17) provide provocative updates and new data regarding the causal relationship between HBV and primary hepatocellular carcinoma. There is at least a 22-fold increase in this cancer in HBV carriers.
18. Szmuness, W., Stevens, C. E., Harley, E. J., et al. Hepatitis B vaccine: Demonstration in a controlled clinical trial in a high-risk population in the United States. *N. Engl. J. Med.* 303:833, 1980.
    A major advance in preventive medicine.
19. Hollinger, F. B., Mosley, J. W., Szmuness, R. D., et al. Transfusion-transmitted viruses study: Experimental evidence for two non-A, non-B hepatitis agents. *J. Infect. Dis.* 142:400, 1980.
    A well-done study that leaves little doubt that there are at least two NA/NBH agents.
20. Berman, M., Alter, H. J., Ishak, K. G., et al. The chronic sequelae of non-A, non-B hepatitis. *Ann. Intern. Med.* 91:1, 1979.
    The anicteric patients with peak ALT (SGPT) levels over 300 IU/liter had the greatest risk of developing chronic hepatitis.
21. Omata, M., Afroudakis, A., Liew, C.-T., et al. Comparison of serum hepatitis B surface antigen (HB$_s$Ag) and serum anticore with tissue HB$_s$Ag and hepatitis B core antigen (HB$_c$Ag). *Gastroenterology* 75:1003, 1978.
    HBV appears to be the cause of at least one-third of the cases of cryptogenic cirrhosis.
22. Klugman, S., Overby, L. R., Mushahwar, I. K., et al. Viral hepatitis, type B: Studies on natural history and prevention reexamined. *N. Engl. J. Med.* 300:101, 1979.
    Viremia can occur within 6 days of exposure; therefore, prophylaxis is needed immediately after exposure.
23. DeFranchis, R., D'Arminio, A., Vecchi, M., et al. Chronic asymptomatic HB$_s$Ag carriers: Histologic abnormalities and diagnostic and prognostic value of serologic markers of the HBV. *Gastroenterology* 79:521, 1980.
    HB$_e$Ag did not correlate well with histology or course.
24. Chadwick, R. G., Galizzi, J., Jr., Heathcote, J., et al. Chronic persistent hepatitis: Hepatitis B virus markers and histologic follow-up. *Gut* 20:372, 1979.
    Chronic persistent hepatitis continues to be a benign process.
25. Tiollais, P., Pourcel, C., and Dejean, A. The hepatitis B virus. *Nature* 317:489, 1985.
    Details our current knowledge of this virus.

26. Dienstag, J. L. Non-A, non-B hepatitis. *Gastroenterology* 85:439, 743, 1983.
   A comprehensive review.
27. Rizzetto, M., Verme, G., Gerin, J. L., et al. Hepatitis delta virus disease. *Prog. Liver Dis.* 8:417, 1986.
   A concise review by the discoverer of HDV.
28. Kunches, L. M., Croven, D. E., and Werner, B. G. Seroprevalence of hepatitis B virus and delta agent in parenteral drug abusers: Immunogenecity of hepatitis B vaccine. *Am. J. Med.* 81:591, 1986.
   A high-risk population: 87.5% were HBV-positive of which 10.6% were HDV-positive.
29. Cade, R., Wagemaker, H., Vogel, S., et al. Hepatorenal syndrome: Studies of the effect of vascular volume and intraperitoneal pressure on renal and hepatic function. *Am. J. Med.* 82:427, 1987.
   Improvement in intraperitoneal pressure produced an improvement in renal function.
30. Seeff, L. B., and Hoofnagle, J. H. Passive and active immunoprophylaxis of hepatitis B. *Gastroenterology* 86:958, 1984.
   A comprehensive, well-referenced review.
31. Lai, K. N., Lai, F.M.-M., Lo, S. T. H., et al. IgA and membranous nephropathy associated with hepatitis B surface antigenemia. *Hum. Pathol.* 18:411, 1987.
   Another complication of HBV.
32. Rakela, J., Lange, S. M., Ludwig, J., et al. Fulminant hepatitis: Mayo Clinic experience with 34 cases. *Mayo Clin. Proc.* 60:289, 1985.
   The survival rate was 6%.
33. Osmon, D. R., Melton, J., III, Keys, T. F., et al. Viral hepatitis: A population-based study in Rochester, Minn, 1971–1980. *Arch. Intern. Med.* 147:1235, 1987.
   The incidence was 28.6 per 100,000 person-years.
34. Colombo, M., Cambieri, R., Rumi, M. G., et al. Long term delta superinfection in hepatitis B surface antigen carriers and its relation to the course of chronic hepatitis. *Gastroenterology* 85:235, 1983.
   Prognosis is guarded.
35. DeCock, K. M., Govindarajan, S., Chin, K. P., et al. Delta hepatitis in the Los Angeles area: A report of 126 cases. *Ann. Intern. Med.* 105:108, 1986.
   The overall fatality rate was 23%.
36. Jensen, D. M., Dickerson, D. D., Linderman, M. A., et al. Serum alanine aminotransferase levels and prevalance of hepatitis A, B, and delta in outpatients. *Arch. Intern. Med.* 147:1734, 1987.
   51% were previously undiagnosed.
37. Denniston, K. J., Hoyer, B. H., Smedile, A., et al. Cloned fragment of the hepatitis delta virus RNA genome: Sequence and diagnostic application. *Science* 232:873, 1986.
   A sensitive radioactive probe for diagnosis.
38. Kao, H. W., Ashcovai, M., Redeker, A. G., et al. The persistence of hepatitis A IgM antibody after clinical hepatitis A. *Hepatology* 4:933, 1984.
   The IgM antibody lingered for 7 months in 13%.
39. Sjogren, M. H., Tanno, H., Fay, O., et al. Hepatitis A virus in stool during clinical relapse. *Ann. Intern. Med.* 106:221, 1986.
   Hepatitis A virus appears to be the culprit in relapse.

VI. DISEASES OF HEMATOPOIESIS AND HEMOSTASIS

85. ACUTE LEUKEMIA
Judith E. Karp

In acute leukemia unregulated accumulation of immature leukocytes results in a compromise of organ function most marked in the bone marrow but also occurring in other tissues that become infiltrated with the immature cells. The pathophysiology and clinical presentation of acute leukemia relate to two factors: bone marrow failure due to tumor-related suppression of normal hematopoiesis and the clinical expression of the malignant hematopoietic clone. The growth of blood cell precursors arrested at an immature stage of differentiation suppresses production of normal bone marrow elements, resulting in anemia, infection, and bleeding, and the metabolic effects of increased cell turnover. Increased growth of leukemic cells and infiltration of virtually all organ systems completes the pathophysiologic complex. The signs and symptoms of bone marrow failure and infiltration of the central nervous system, liver, spleen, testes, ovaries, lymph nodes, skin, and gastrointestinal tract, with varied degrees of failure of each organ, may contribute to the overall symptom complex at presentation.

The cause of de novo acute leukemia is unknown, but both genetic and environmental factors are important. The acute phase may be preceded by antecedent prodromes of variable duration such as paroxysmal nocturnal hemoglobinuria, chronic myelogenous leukemia, or the myelodysplastic syndromes; alternatively, acute leukemia can also arise following exposure to specific mutagens, usually alkylating agent chemotherapy and/or radiotherapy for a previous malignancy such as Hodgkin's or non-Hodgkin's lymphoma, ovarian or breast cancer, multiple myeloma, or myeloproliferative disorders such as polycythemia vera and idiopathic myelofibrosis. Other potential leukemogenic insults include exposure to benzene or marrow aplasia-inducing agents such as chloramphenicol, arsenic, or phenylbutazone.

The diagnosis of acute leukemia is usually easily established by demonstration of marrow replacement by immature cells. This finding effectively eliminates a leukemoid reaction, but problems may arise occasionally in distinguishing a leukemic marrow from that of megaloblastic anemia or a marrow recovering from aplasia caused by a drug, hepatitis, or infection, particularly viral. The major diagnostic dilemma, however, revolves around classification of the specific cell of origin and lineage of the leukemic process. This morphologic identification is important in terms of selecting specific drug therapy and predicting the response to therapy and the overall prognosis. Although acute lymphocytic leukemia is more common in childhood and acute myelogenous leukemia predominates in adults, these relationships are of no help in the individual patient. Distinction between the myeloblast and lymphoblast by light microscopy is often not possible unless Auer rods are present or there has been differentiation to the level of the promyelocyte. Lymphoblasts, in common with monoblasts, stain with the nonspecific esterase, acid phosphatase, and PAS although the staining pattern is different. Myeloblasts stain with peroxidase, Sudan black, and the specific (chloroacetate) esterase. Monoblasts stain with the nonspecific (naphthyl) esterase, acid phosphatase, and PAS. The monocyte-nonspecific esterase is inhibited by fluoride in contrast to the myelocyte-specific esterase. Monoblasts stain weakly or not at all with peroxidase and Sudan black while cells with characteristics of both myeloblasts and monoblasts stain with peroxidase, Sudan black, specific and nonspecific esterases, acid phosphatase, and PAS. There is a poor correlation between classification by Wright's stain and histochemical stains, and when electron microscopy is employed it appears that the bulk of acute nonlymphocytic leukemia in the adult is either monocytic or mixed myelomonocytic leukemia while pure myelocytic variants represent only a minority of cases.

The differentiation between myeloid and lymphoid leukemias has recently been facilitated with the ability to determine the immunophenotype of individual leukemic populations by detecting the presence of specific surface antigenic markers. These markers, detected by monoclonal antibodies directed against cell surface proteins, can identify both the lineage and the level of differentiation vs. aberrant maturation of the leukemic population. Specific patterns of aberrant differentiation states, mixed lineage clones, or primitive stem cell involvement can be associated with disease that is refractory to antileukemic therapy.

The ability to determine the genotype as well as the morphologic and surface antigenic phenotype of a leukemic clone can have major prognostic significance in terms of initial response to therapy and overall duration of that response. For example, as prophase banding techniques have improved, it is clear that the majority of adults with acute myelogenous leukemias have at least one karyotypic abnormality with either a balanced translocation, deletion, or addition. Some of these specific genotypic derangements can be closely associated with specific morphologic variants and clinical syndromes or with certain hematologic prodromes or mutagen-induced leukemias. The most common abnormalities involve chromosomes 5, 7, or 8, either individually or in combination, or involve other chromosomes by reciprocal translocation. Detection of the Philadelphia chromosome (t[9;22]) in either acute myelogenous or acute lymphocytic leukemia portends a poor prognosis; in contrast, specific translocations in acute myelogenous leukemias, such as (8;21), (15;17), and inversions within the long arm of chromosome 16, are associated with sensitivity to antileukemic therapy, while partial or total deletions of chromosomes 5 or 7 are often associated with antecedent myelodysplasia or mutagen-induced leukemias that reflect damage to a primitive stem cell and drug resistance.

By combining morphology, histochemistry, immunophenotyping by monoclonal antibodies to cell surface differentiation antigens, and cytogenetic analysis, the leukemic process can be categorized and the appropriate therapy selected. While the combination of marrow failure and organ barrier breakdown from tumor invasion determines the clinical presenting features of acute leukemia, the aspects of clonal expression based on tumor mass, specific leukemia cell characteristics, and the rate of cell turnover determine both the need for prompt intervention and the initial therapy-related complications. Paradoxically, rapid cell kill with intensive drug treatment results in the appearance or exacerbation of severe metabolic imbalances that are sometimes difficult to correct. Survival also depends on the recognition of both disease- and treatment-related complications and the rational use of supportive measures that permit both disease eradication and treatment survival.

Patients presenting with massive hyperleukocytosis (WBC counts >200,000/µl) are at high risk for cerebral vascular occlusions with intracranial hemorrhage and pulmonary leukostasis. Patients with acute lymphocytic leukemia have a very high incidence of meningeal leukemia, and frequently abnormal cells may be identified in the spinal fluid before the onset of symptoms. The incidence of CNS involvement in acute nonlymphocytic leukemia is 20 percent. While in acute lymphocytic leukemia bone pain and infarction or marrow necrosis may be prominent and hypercalcemia may develop, hyperuricemia and hyperphosphatemia are more common and if not treated can result in obstructive uropathy. Additional renal problems may be present in myelogenous or myelomonocytic leukemia. Many patients have hypergammaglobulinemia and proteinuria. Some have azotemia, lysozymuria, hypokalemia without renal tubular acidosis, and a defect in both glomerular filtration and proximal tubular function related to lysozyme-induced damage. The leukemic patient is at risk from hemorrhage due to thrombocytopenia, and this risk is increased when infection is present. In addition, patients with acute myelogenous leukemia, particularly progranulocytic or monoblastic, may develop a consumptive coagulopathy that has the clinical and laboratory hallmarks of disseminated intravascular coagulation.

The most common problem in the patient with acute leukemia is infection. Leukemic patients infect themselves with their own flora but usually do so with nosocomially acquired organisms, particularly *Escherichia coli*, *Klebsiella*, and *Pseudomonas*. When steroids, immunosuppressive agents, or antibiotics have been employed, fungal invasion by *Candida* or *Aspergillus* is not uncommon. The signs of infection in acute leukemia may be muted by lack of the usual inflammatory response. The rectal area is a frequent site of infection and should be carefully examined when fever occurs. The rapid recognition and treatment of infection is essential to successful outcome of intensive antileukemic chemotherapy. Prophylaxis against gastrointestinal-based infection with oral antibiotics that act against aerobic bacteria, such as norfloxacin, will control endogenous host gram-negative organisms once the patient is rendered aplastic by disease or by cytotoxic drugs. Surveillance cultures of the stool give advanced warning of impending overgrowth and systemic invasion. The febrile granulocytopenic patient should be treated with combination antibiotics (i.e., ticarcillin and an aminoglycoside) and the antibiotics should be continued during the period of granulocytopenia. If the patient does not improve or if improvement is followed by relapse and recurrent fever without an evident cause, amphotericin B should be administered.

Recent clinical trials in adults with acute myelogenous leukemia indicate that remissions can be achieved in more than 70 percent of those receiving intensive induction chemotherapy with cytosine arabinoside plus an anthracycline. New agents that hold promising activity include amsacrine and etoposide, both of which interact with topoisomerases to inhibit DNA synthesis and exert eventual cytotoxicity. Further intensive therapy administered early in complete remission, at the time of minimal residual disease which has not been allowed time to acquire multidrug resistance by random mutation, has resulted in prolonged (>5-year) disease-free survival rates in more than 40 percent of patients treated in this manner. This curative approach can employ either high-dose chemotherapy or bone marrow transplantation. Less aggressive therapies that use maintenance approaches have not yielded such prolongations of remission.

Unfortunately, chemotherapy of any kind is difficult to deliver to patients older than 60 years. In this population, which is more likely to experience myelodysplastic prodromes with leukemic progression or monocytic leukemia with a poor prognosis, alternate therapy must be sought. With evidence that clonal maturation can be achieved after intensive therapy, noncytotoxic drugs may be found that will cause maturation. To date, retinoic acid, low-dose cytosine arabinoside, and vitamin D have had little success. However, with products of genetic engineering now available to the clinician, humoral regulators such as the colony-stimulating activities hold the hope of the reestablishment of normal stimulation of proliferation and maturation. These noncytotoxic agents may biomodulate patients in remission to terminally mature their minimal residual tumor and allow recovery of normal polyclonal stem cells.

1. Bennett, J. M., Catovsky, D., and Daniel, M. T. Proposed revised criteria for the classification of acute myeloid leukemia. *Ann. Intern. Med.* 103:626, 1985.
   Morphologic classification of acute leukemia. (See also Ann. Intern. Med. *87:740, 1977.)*
2. Mertelsmann, R., Thaler, H. T., To, L., et al. Morphological classification, response to therapy, and survival in 263 adult patients with acute nonlymphoblastic leukemia. *Blood* 56:773, 1980.
3. Champlin, R., and Gale, R. P. Acute lymphoblastic leukemia: Recent advances in biology and therapy. *Blood* 73:2051, 1989.
4. Chan, L. C., Pegram, S. M., and Greaves, M. F. Contribution of immunophenotype to the classification and differentiation diagnosis of acute leukemia. *Lancet* 1:475, 1985.
   Immunologic classification of acute leukemia.
5. Foon, K. A., and Todd, R. F., III. Immunologic classification of leukemia and lymphoma. *Blood* 68:1, 1986.
   See also N. Engl. J. Med. *316:111, 1987.*
6. Bloomfield, C. D., and de la Chapelle, A. Chromosome abnormalities in acute nonlymphocytic leukemia: clinical and biological significance. *Semin. Oncol.* 14:372, 1987.
   Genotypic classification of acute leukemia. (See also Blood *73:263, 1989,* Leukemia *2:403, 1988, and* Br. J. Haematol. *68:189, 1988.)*
7. Fearon, E. R., Burke, P. J., Schiffer, C. A. et al. Differentiation of leukemic cells to polymorphonuclear leukocytes in patients with acute nonlymphocytic leukemia. *N. Engl. J. Med.* 315:15, 1986.
   See also Blood *57:1068, 1981.*
8. Keating, M. J., Cork, A., Broach, Y., et al. Toward a clinically relevant cytogenetic classification of acute myelogenous leukemia. *Leuk. Res.* 11:119, 1987.
9. Look, A. T. The emerging genetics of acute lymphoblastic leukemia: Clinical and biologic implications. *Semin. Oncol.* 12:92, 1985.

10. Cunningham, I., Gee, T. S., Reich, L. M., et al. Acute promvelocytic leukemia: Treatment results during a decade at Memorial Hospital. *Blood* 73:1116, 1989.
    Clinical manifestations of acute leukemia: Specific subtypes. (See also Am. J. Med. *80:789, 1986,* Blood *71:690, 1988, and* Cancer *55:18, 1985.)*
11. Kantarjian, H. M., and Keating, M. J. Therapy-related leukemia and myelodysplastic syndrome. *Semin. Oncol.* 14:435, 1987.
12. Peterson, B. A., and Levine, E. G. Uncommon subtypes of acute nonlymphocytes leukemia: Clinical feature and management of FAB M5, M6 and M7. *Semin Oncol.* 14:425, 1987.
    For megakaryocytocytic leukemia, see also Blood *72:402, 1988.*
13. Ribeiro, R. C., and Pui, C. H. The clinical and biological correlates of coagulopathy in children with acute leukemia. *J. Clin. Oncol.* 4:1212, 1986.
14. Straus, D. J., Mertelsmann, R., Koziner, B., et al. The acute monocytic leukemias: Multidisciplinary studies in 45 patients. *Medicine* 59:409, 1980.
    See also J. Clin. Invest. *49:1694, 1970.*
15. Bunin, N. J., and Pui, C. H. Differing complications of hyperleukocytosis in children with acute lymphoblastic or acute nonlymphoblastic leukemia. *J. Clin. Oncol.* 3:1590, 1985.
    Clinical manifestations of acute leukemia: Hyperleukocytosis.
16. Dutcher, J. P., Schiffer, C. A., and Wiernik, P. H. Hyperleukocytosis in adult acute nonlymphocytic leukemia: Impact on remission rate and duration, and survival. *J. Clin. Oncol.* 5:1364, 1987.
    See also Cancer *52:773, 1983.*
17. Lester, T. J., Johnson, J. W., and Cuttner, J. Pulmonary leukostasis as the single worst prognostic factor in patients with acute myelocytic leukemia and hyperleukocytosis. *Am. J. Med.* 79:43, 1985.
18. Lichtman, M. A. The Relationship of Excessive White Cell Count to Vascular Insufficiency in Patients with Leukemia. In H. J., Meiselman, M. A. Lichtman, and P. L. LaCelle, (eds.), *White Cell Mechanics: Basic Science and Clinical Aspects.* New York: Alan R. Liss, 1984. P. 295.
19. McKee, L. C., and Collins, R. D. Intravascular leukocyte thrombi and aggregates as a cause of morbidity in leukemia. *Medicine* 53:463, 1974.
20. Meyer, R. J., Ferreira, P. P. C., Cuttner, J., et al. Central nervous system involvement at presentation in acute granulocytic leukemia. *Am. J. Med.* 68:691, 1980.
    Clinical manifestations of acute leukemia: Central nervous system complications.
21. Rivera, G. R., and Mauer, A. M. Controversies in the management of childhood acute lymphoblastic leukemia: Treatment intensification, CNS leukemia, and prognostic factors. *Semin. Hematol.* 24:1, 1987.
22. Stewart, D. T., Keating, M. J., McCredie, K. B., et al. Natural history of central nervous system acute leukemia in adults. *Cancer* 47:184, 1981.
    See also Blood *55:199, 1980.*
23. Cadman, E. C., Lundberg, W. B., and Bertino, J. R. Hyperphosphatemia and hypocalcemia accompanying rapid cell lysis in a patient with Burkitt's lymphoma and Burkitt cell leukemia. *Am. J. Med.* 62:283, 1987.
    Clinical manifestations of acute leukemia: Tumor lysis syndrome.
24. Dauber, L. G., and Scharschmidt, L. A. Hyperphosphatemic renal failure following treatment of acute nonlymphatic leukemia. *Cancer Treat. Rep.* 69:563, 1985.
    See also Am. J. Hematol. *16:185, 1984.*
25. Donehower, R. C., Karp, J. W., and Burke, P. J. Pharmacology and toxicity of high-dose cytosine arabinoside by 72 hour continuous infusion. *Cancer Treat. Rep.* 70:1056, 1986.
    Antileukemic drug toxicity.
26. Haupt, H. M., Hutchins, G. M., and Moore, G. W. Ara C–lung: Noncardiogenic pulmonary edema complicating cytosine arabinoside therapy of leukemia. *Am. J. Med.* 70:256, 1981.
27. Young, R. C., Ozols, R. F., and Myers, C. E. The anthracycline antineoplastic drugs. *N. Engl. J. Med.* 305:139, 1981.

28. Burch, P. A., Karp, J. E., and Merz, W. G. Favorable outcome of invasive aspergillosis in patients with acute leukemia. *J. Clin. Oncol.* 5:1985, 1987.
    Management of infectious complications.
29. Karp, J. E., Merz, W. G., Hendrickson, C., et al. Multivariate analysis of factors associated with invasive fungal disease during remission induction therapy for acute myelogenous leukemia and granulocytopenia. *Ann. Intern. Med.* 106:1, 1987.
30. Pizzo, P. A., Robichaud, K. J., Gill, F. A., et al. Antibiotic and antifungal therapy for cancer patients with prolonged fever and granulocytopenia. *Am. J. Med.* 72:101, 1982.
31. Schwartz, R. S., Mackintosh, F. R., Schrier, S. L., et al. Multivariate analysis of factors associated with invasive fungal disease during remission induction therapy for acute myelogenous leukemia. *Cancer* 53:411, 1984.
32. Hoelzer, D., and Gale, R. P. Acute lymphoblastic leukemia in adults: Recent progress, future directions. *Semin. Hematol.* 24:27, 1987.
    Chemotherapy reviewed.
33. Keating, M. J., Smith, T. L., Gehan, E. A., et al. Factors related to length of complete remission in adult acute leukemia. *Cancer* 45:2017, 1980.
34. Mayer, R. J. Current chemotherapeutic treatment approaches to the management of previously untreated adults with de novo acute myelogenous leukemia. *Semin. Oncol.* 14:384, 1987.
35. Rai, K. A., Holland, J. F., Glidewell, O. J., et al. Treatment of acute myelocytic leukemia: A study by Cancer and Leukemia Group B. *Blood* 58:1203, 1981.
36. Rohatiner, A. Z. S., Gregory, W. M., Bassan, R., et al. Short-term therapy for acute myelogenous leukemia. *J. Clin. Oncol.* 6:218, 1988.
    See also Cancer Treat. Rep. *71:2, 1987.*
37. Vaughan, W. P., Karp, J. E., and Burke, P. J. Two cycle timed-sequential chemotherapy for adult acute non-lymphocytic leukemia. *Blood* 64:975, 1984.
38. Cliff, R. A., Buckner, C. S., Thomas, E. D., et al. The treatment of acute non-lymphocytic leukemia by allogeneic marrow transplantation. *Bone Marrow Transplantation* 2:243, 1987.
    Bone marrow transplantion in acute leukemia. (See also Semin. Hematol. *24:55, 1987.)*
39. Proctor, S. J., Hamilton, P. J., Taylor, P., et al. A comparative study of combination chemotherapy versus marrow transplant in first remission in adult acute lymphoblastic leukemia. *Br. J. Haematol.* 69:35, 1988.
40. Yeager, A. M., Kaizer, H., Santos, G. W., et al. Autologous bone marrow transplantation in patients with acute nonlymphocytic leukemia, using ex vivo marrow treatment with 4-hydroperoxycyclophosphamide. *N. Engl. J. Med.* 315:141, 1986.

---

86. ACUTE NONLYMPHOCYTIC LEUKEMIA

Michael A. Baumann

Acute nonlymphocytic leukemia (ANLL) is an acquired disease of hematopoietic stem cells characterized by accumulation in the bone marrow and peripheral blood of clonal primitive myeloid cells with commensurate reduction of normally formed elements. The disease occurs in all age groups, but the median age at diagnosis is 63 years. As many as 25 percent of patients may have an antecedent history of myelodysplasia (preleukemia) lasting months or years.

The level of stem cell involvement in ANLL may vary, but it has been demonstrated by cytogenetic analysis or by study of isoenzyme composition of cells in glucose 6-phosphate dehydrogenase (G-6-PD) heterozygotes that transformation often occurs in a cell pluripotent for erythroid, myeloid, and megakaryocytic cell lines. It has been established that the malignant cells do not divide more rapidly than normal, but that they accumulate as the result of the large growth fraction (percentage of cells having the capacity for self-renewal) of the malignant clone compared to the normal hematopoietic population. Although the hallmark of the disease is the accumulation of morphologically immature cells, the malignant clone may retain some capacity for differentiation. Remission hematopoiesis has been shown to remain clonal in some instances, and sensitive cDNA probes have been used to demonstrate aneuploidy in mature neutrophils of some patients analogous to that found in their leukemic blasts.

Clinical symptoms of ANLL most commonly relate to reduction of normal marrow myeloid, erythroid, and megakaryocytic elements with resultant peripheral neutropenia, anemia, and thrombocytopenia. Presenting complaints include fatigue, poor exercise tolerance, dyspnea, palpitations, bleeding into the skin or mucous membranes, and fever and chills with or without evidence of localized infection. Less often, symptoms are related to the mechanical effects of tumor cell burden and include lymphadenopathy, hepatosplenomegaly, and skin or gingival lesions. Patients with very high circulating blast counts (>100,000/μl) may develop leukostasis in small blood vessels with resultant central nervous system dysfunction, pulmonary infiltrates, or cardiac decompensation.

The French-American-British Cooperative Group (FAB) recognizes seven variants of ANLL, based primarily on morphologic criteria. Certain clinical features are associated with FAB subclass. Patients with the promyelocytic variant (M3) often present with disseminated intravascular coagulation (DIC) and systemic fibrinolysis that may be aggravated by cytotoxic treatment with resultant increased release of intracellular procoagulants or plasminogen activators. Patients with monocytic morphology (M4, M5) are more likely to evidence tissue invasion by leukemic blasts, manifested as gingival hyperplasia or cutaneous lesions. In spite of these clinical differences, it has not been convincingly shown that FAB subclassification bears upon ultimate outcome. However, karyotype is an independent prognostic indicator, and certain karotypes are closely associated with FAB morphologic subgroups. A t(8;21) chromosomal translocation is associated with myeloblastic (M2) morphology, while t(15;17) is associated with the promyelocytic (M3) variant and risk of coagulopathy. Abnormalities of chromosome 16 are associated with myelomonocytic (M4) morphology and dysplastic marrow eosinophilia. These karyotypes are associated with a relatively good prognosis, while t(9;22) and abnormalities of chromosomes 5 or 7 are associated with a lesser chance of obtaining remission and a shorter remission duration.

Great progress has been achieved in the treatment of ANLL over the past 20 years, and a significant proportion of patients may now be expected to enjoy prolonged disease-free survival. Vigorous supportive care is essential for a favorable outcome and includes transfusion of red cells and platelets, treatment of documented or suspected infection with synergistic broad-spectrum antibiotics, attention to adequate hydration, and correction of hyperuricemia with allopurinol. Patients having laboratory evidence of DIC or M3 morphology are treated with heparin and replacement of coagulation factors as needed. The addition of epsilon-aminocaproic acid may be warranted in patients with significant evidence of fibrinolysis. Intensive combination chemotherapy, usually with a combination of daunorubicin and cytosine arabinoside, results in complete remission in more than 75 percent of patients. Remission rates are lower in elderly patients and in those who have antecedent myelodysplastic disorders or secondary leukemias. The optimal postremission therapy remains unclear, but some amount of additional chemotherapy is necessary for best results. The median survival from diagnosis is about 18 months, but 5-year disease-free survivals of over 30 percent have been reported in numerous studies. Many of these patients may be cured. Early results of several trials employing much higher doses of cytosine arabinoside suggest the possibility of 45 to 55 percent disease-free survival at 2 years in selected patients.

The role of allogenic bone marrow transplantation following marrow ablative therapy for the treatment of ANLL remains controversial. The procedure is generally limited to those patients under 45 years of age who have an HLA-matched sibling (about 10% of patients), although roughly equivalent overall results are being obtained using single-antigen mismatched grafts. About 50 percent of patients who undergo marrow transplantation while in first remission will be alive and free of leukemia 5 years later, but they are at higher risk of dying during the first 6 months after treatment because of transplant-related problems of infection, interstitial pneumonitis, and graft-versus-host disease (GVH). Recent prospective studies have not shown a convincing superiority of transplantation in first remission over treatment with chemotherapy alone. There is currently consensus that eligible patients who relapse after chemotherapy should receive transplants, because up to 20 percent may be salvaged. Graft-versus-host disease appears to be the major impediment to progress in allogeneic transplantation. Ironically, GVH may have an antileukemic effect. Depletion of T-lymphocytes from donor marrow appears to reduce the incidence and severity of GVH but also results in an increased number of graft rejections and leukemic relapses. Recent trials of transplantation using HLA-identical non-related donors have shown promising early results suggesting that the procedure may become an option for a greater proportion of patients.

1. Rowley, J. D., and de la Chapelle, A. Chromosome abnormalities in acute non-lymphocytic leukemia: Clinical and biologic significance. *Semin. Oncol.* 14:372, 1987.

2. Koeffler, H. P. Syndromes of acute nonlymphocytic leukemia. *Ann. Intern. Med.* 107:748, 1987.

3. Misawa, S., Lee, E., Schiffer, C. A., et al. Association of the translocation (15;17) with malignant proliferation of promyelocytes in acute leukemia and chronic myelogenous leukemia at blastic crisis. *Blood* 67:270, 1986.

4. Hogge, D. E., Misawa, S., Parsa, N. Z., et al. Abnormalities of chromosome 16 in association with acute myelomonocytic leukemia and dysplastic bone marrow eosinophils. *J. Clin. Oncol.* 2:550, 1984.
   Karyotype is an independent prognostic indicator. Certain karyotypes are closely associated with FAB morphologic subgroups (articles 1–4).

5. Fialkow, P. J., Singer, J. W., Adamson, J. W., et al. Acute nonlymphocytic leukemia. Expression in cells restricted to granulocytic and monocytic differentiation. *N. Engl. J. Med.* 301:1, 1979.

6. Fialkow, P. J., Singer, J. W., Adamson, J. W., et al. Acute nonlymphocytic leukemia: Heterogeneity of stem cell origin. *Blood* 57:1068, 1981.
   The level of stem cells affected in ANLL may vary (articles 5,6).

7. Jacobson, R. J., Temple, M. J., Singer, J. W., et al. A clonal complete remission in a patient with acute nonlymphocytic leukemia originating in a multipotent stem cell. *N. Engl. J. Med.* 310:1513, 1984.

8. Kere, J., Ruttu, T., and de la Chapelle, A. Monosomy 7 in granulocytes and monocytes in myelodysplastic syndrome. *N. Engl. J. Med.* 316:499, 1987.

9. Fearon, E. R., Burke, P. J., Schiffer, C. A., et al. Differentiation of leukemia cells to polymorphonuclear leukocytes in patients with acute nonlymphocytic leukemia. *N. Engl. J. Med.* 315:15, 1986.
   The leukemic clone may retain some capacity for differentiation (articles 7,8,9).

10. Bennett, J., Catovsky, D., and Daniel, M. T. Proposed revised criteria for the classification of acute myeloid leukemia. *Ann. Intern. Med.* 103:626, 1985.

11. Bennett, J., Catovsky, D., Daniel, M. T., et al. Criteria for the diagnosis of acute leukemia of megakaryocytic lineage (M7). A report of the French-American-British Cooperative Group. *Ann. Intern. Med.* 103:460, 1985.
   Subclassification (articles 10,11) of ANLL proposed by the FAB group.

12. Van Slyck, E. J., Rebuck, J. W., Waddell, C. C., et al. Smoldering acute granulocytic leukemia. Observations on its natural history and morphologic characteristics. *Arch. Intern. Med.* 143:37, 1983.

13. Greenberg, P. L. The smouldering myeloid leukemic states: Clinical and biologic features. *Blood* 61:1035, 1983.
    It may occasionally be difficult (articles 12, 13) to distinguish ANLL from a more indolent myelodysplastic disorder.

14. Cordonnier, C., Vernant, J. P., Brun, B., et al. Acute promyelocytic leukemia in 57 previously untreated patients. *Cancer* 55:18, 1985.
15. Kantarjian, H. M., Keating, M. J., and Walters, R. S. Acute promyelocytic leukemia: MD Anderson Hospital experience. *Am. J. Med.* 80:789, 1986.
16. Cunningham, I., Gee, T. S., Reich, L. M., et al. Acute promyelocytic leukemia: Treatment results during a decade at Memorial Hospital. *Blood* 73:1116, 1989.
17. Schwartz, B. S., Williams, E. C., Conlan, M. G., et al. Epsilon-aminocaproic acid in the treatment of patients with acute promyelocytic leukemia and acquired alpha-2-plasmin inhibitor deficiency. *Ann. Intern. Med.* 105:873, 1986.
    The propensity of patients with this variant of ANLL to develop DIC and systemic fibrinolysis requires careful clinical and laboratory monitoring (articles 14, 15, 16, 17). Heparin should be considered prophylactically, possibly in combination with epsilon-aminocaproic acid.
18. Champlin, R., and Gale, R. P. Acute myelogenous leukemia: Recent advances in therapy. *Blood* 69:1551, 1987.
19. Mayer, R. J. Current chemotherapeutic treatment approaches to the management of previously untreated adults with de novo acute myelogenous leukemia. *Semin. Oncol.* 14:384, 1987.
20. Kahn, S. B., Bogg, C. B., Mazza, J. J., et al. Full-dose versus attenuated-dose daunorubicin, cytosine arabinoside and 6-thioguanine in the treatment of acute nonlymphocytic leukemia in the elderly. *J. Clin. Oncol.* 2:865, 1984.
21. Gajewski, J. L., Ho, W. G., Nimer, S. D., et al. Efficacy of intensive chemotherapy for acute myelogenous leukemia associated with a preleukemic syndrome. *J. Clin. Oncol.* 7:1637, 1989.
22. Rohatiner, A. Z. S., Gregory, W. M., Bassan, R., et al. Short-term therapy for acute myelogenous leukemia. *J. Clin. Oncol.* 8:218, 1988.
23. Wolff, S. N., Herzig, R. H., Fay, J. W., et al. High-dose cytarabine and daunorubicin as consolidation therapy for acute myeloid leukemia in first remission: Long-term follow-up and results. *J. Clin. Oncol.* 7:1260, 1989.
24. Appelbaum, F. R., Fisher, I. D., and Thomas, E. D. Chemotherapy vs. marrow transplantation for acute nonlymphocytic leukemia. A 5-year followup. *Blood* 72:179, 1988.
25. International Bone Marrow Transplant Registry. Transplant or chemotherapy in acute myelogenous leukaemia. *Lancet* 1:1119, 1989.
26. Butturini, A., and Gale, R. P. Chemotherapy versus transplantation in acute leukemia. *Brit. J. Haematol.* 72:1, 1989.
27. Mayer, R. J. Allogeneic transplantation versus intensive chemotherapy in first-remission acute leukemia: is there a "best choice?" *J. Clin. Oncol.* 6:1532, 1988.
28. Appelbaum, F. R., Clift, R. A., Buckner, C. D., et al. Allogeneic bone marrow transplantation for non-lymphoblastic leukemia after first relapse. *Blood* 61:949, 1983.
    Results of chemotherapy of ANLL continue to improve. The role of allogeneic bone marrow transplantation (articles 24, 25, 26, 27) in first remission remains unsettled. Transplantation is indicated (article 28) for eligible patients in first relapse.
29. Butturini, A., Bortin, M. M., and Gale, R. P. Graft-versus-leukemia following bone marrow transplantation. *Bone Marrow Transplantation* 2:233, 1987.
30. Sullivan, K. M., Weiden, P. L., Storb, R., et al. Influence of acute and chronic graft-versus-host disease on relapse and survival after bone marrow transplantation from HLA-identical siblings as treatment of acute and chronic leukemia. *Blood* 73:1720, 1989.
    Graft-versus-host disease following transplantation apparently has a graft-versus-leukemia effect (articles 29, 30). Depletion of T-cells from donor marrow reduces chronic GVH but may result in increased leukemic relapse.
31. Beatty, P. G., Hansen, J. A., and Thomas, E. D. Marrow grafting for HLA matched unrelated donors. *Blood* 74:[Suppl. 1]:122a, 1989.
32. Ash, R. C., Casper, J. T., Chitambar, C. R., et al. Successful allogeneic transplantation of T-cell depleted bone marrow from closely HLA-matched unrelated donors. *N. Engl. J. Med.* 322:485, 1990.
    Encouraging early results are being obtained in trials of transplantation using HLA-matched unrelated donors.

87. ANEMIA AND CHRONIC DISEASE
Jerry L. Spivak

Anemia occurs with many systemic diseases. In some instances, the anemia results from blood loss, hemolysis, vitamin deficiencies, impaired renal function, or as a consequence of therapy. With hypopituitarism or primary hypothyroidism, tissue oxygen demands are reduced and the stimulus for red cell production declines. Anemia in these situations, as in the case of a hemoglobin with a low oxygen affinity (such as hemoglobin Seattle), is not inappropriate since oxygen transport is probably adequate to meet tissue demands. With chronic infections, inflammatory disorders, or malignancies, an anemia often develops that cannot be accounted for by any of the obvious mechanisms mentioned. Despite the diverse nature of the underlying diseases, this anemia, which has been designated the anemia of chronic disease, has certain constant features. They include a low plasma iron and total iron-binding capacity, decreased transferrin saturation, elevated serum ferritin, normal or increased reticuloendothelial iron stores, increased red cell free–protoporphyrin, and a low reticulocyte index. Red cell life span is usually reduced while the plasma iron turnover is rapid and erythrocyte iron utilization is increased. The increased erythropoiesis, however, is inadequate to compensate for the shortened red cell survival, although such compensation would normally be well within the capacity of the bone marrow.

Failure of marrow compensation may be due to changes in hemoglobin-oxygen affinity, and a reduction in erythropoietin production can also be uniformly implicated. Another important factor limiting erythropoiesis is a relative iron deficiency, since iron extracted from senescent red cells by the reticuloendothelial system is not available for reutilization by the marrow. The cause of the reticuloendothelial iron blockade is unknown but may be due to the increased synthesis of lactoferrin and its binding to macrophages. Lactoferrin binds iron more avidly than transferrin but does not release bound iron for utilization, and this cannot be overcome by administration of iron orally or parenterally. In addition to adequate stores of reticuloendothelial iron, the anemia of chronic disease also differs from true iron deficiency with regard to both the serum ferritin level, which is high, and the serum transferrin level, which is usually low. The low serum transferrin level implies a defect in protein synthesis, but whether the defect is involved in the cause of the anemia or is merely another manifestation of chronic illness is unknown. A normal serum ferritin level in a patient with the anemia of chronic disease suggests that true iron deficiency is also present. The role of monokines and lymphokines such as interleukin-1 (IL-1), tumor necrosis factor, and interferon-gamma in the anemia of chronic disease is undefined, but all of these can inhibit erythropoiesis under experimental conditions.

The anemia of chronic disease is generally mild but can be severe. Correction of the underlying disease alleviates the anemia. It is important to remember, however, that patients with the anemia of chronic disease, in whom erythropoiesis is limited, are prone to superimposed iatrogenic anemia in the form of repeated bleeding for diagnostic studies.

Recently, clinical trials with recombinant human erythropoietin have demonstrated that this hormone can correct anemia and ameliorate transfusion requirements in patients with anemia due to inflammation or infection, suggesting that not only does erythropoietin lack an important component of the anemia of chronic disease but also that the anemia is amenable to correction even if the disease process cannot be corrected.

1. Douglas, S. W., and Adamson, J. W. The anemia of chronic disorders: Studies of marrow regulation and iron metabolism. *Blood* 45:55, 1975.
   An inadequate supply of iron is a cause of impaired erythropoiesis in the anemia of chronic disease.
2. Cartwright, G. E., and Lee, G. R. The anemia of chronic disorders. *Br. J. Haematol.* 49:147, 1971.
   A brief review.

3. Finch, C. A., Deubelbeiss, K., Cook, J. D., et al. Ferrokinetics in man. *Medicine* 49:17, 1970.
   Increased red cell production is coupled with a limited iron supply and shortened red cell survival in the anemia of chronic disease.
4. Barrett-Connor, E. Anemia and infection. *Am. J. Med.* 52:242, 1972.
   A comprehensive review.
5. Haurani, F. I., Burke, W., and Martiez, E. J. Defective reutilization of iron in the anemia of inflammation. *J. Lab. Clin. Med.* 65:560, 1965.
   Iron is retained by the reticuloendothelial system and is unavailable for reutilization.
6. Rodriguez, J. M., and Shahidi, N. T. Erythrocyte 2,3 diphosphoglycerate in adaptive red-cell volume deficiency. *N. Engl. J. Med.* 285:479, 1971.
   Red cell 2,3-diphosphoglycerate levels are reduced in panhypopituitarism.
7. Stamatoyannopoulos, G., Parer, J. T., and Finch, C. A. Physiologic implications of a hemoglobin with decreased oxygen affinity (hemoglobin Seattle). *N. Engl. J. Med.* 285:915, 1969.
   Decreased hemoglobin-oxygen affinity was associated with anemia but not elevated erythropoietin titers.
8. Das, K. C., Mukherjee, M., Sarkar, T. K., et al. Erythropoiesis and erythropoietin in hypo- and hyperthyroidism. *J. Clin. Endocrinol. Metab.* 40:211, 1975.
   Anemia may not be evident in hypothyroidism since the plasma volume as well as the red cell mass may be reduced.
9. Kurnick, J. E., Ward, H. P., and Pickett, J. C. Mechanism of the anemia of chronic disorders. *Arch. Intern. Med.* 130:323, 1972.
   Impaired protein synthesis postulated to be causally related to the anemia, although it could be just a concomitant of chronic illness.
10. Paine, C. J., Polk, A., and Eichner, E. R. Analysis of anemia in medical inpatients. *Am. J. Med. Sci.* 268:37, 1974.
    Anemia associated with chronic disorders was the most common form of anemia seen on a large medical service.
11. Ferrari, E., Ascari, E., Bossolo, P. A., et al. Sheehan's syndrome with complete bone marrow aplasia: Long-term results of substitution therapy with hormones. *Br. J. Haematol.* 33:575, 1976.
    The severity of the hematologic disturbance in this patient is unusual; the long delay in diagnosis is not.
12. Horton, L., Coburn, R. J., England, J. M., et al. The haematology of hypothyroidism. *Q. J. Med.* 45:101, 1976.
    Anemia, macrocytosis, acanthocytosis, and a low-serum iron without an increase in total iron-binding capacity.
13. Rivlin, R. S., and Wagner, H. N., Jr. Anemia in hyperthyroidism. *Ann. Intern. Med.* 70:507, 1969.
    Impaired iron utilization demonstrated in some anemic patients with hyperthyroidism.
14. Utiger, R. D. Decreased extrathyroidal triiodothyronine production in nonthyroidal illness: Benefit or harm. *Am. J. Med.* 69:807, 1980.
    Decreased extrathyroidal triiodothyronine production is an adaptive phenomenon that might explain in part the anemia of chronic disease. (See also J. Lab. Clin. Med. 98:860, 1981.)
15. Boxer, M., Ellman, L., Geller, R., et al. Anemia in primary hyperparathyroidism. *Arch. Intern. Med.* 137:588, 1977.
    Anemia is usually seen with advanced disease and myelofibrosis.
16. Lund, C. J., and Donovan, J. C. Blood volume during pregnancy: Significance of plasma and red cell volumes. *Am. J. Obstet. Gynecol.* 98:393, 1967.
    In the absence of complications, the hematocrit in pregnancy reflects changes occurring in the plasma volume.
17. Schuman, J. E., Tanser, C. L., Peloquin, R., et al. The erythropoietic response to pregnancy in β-thalassaemia minor. *Br. J. Haematol.* 25:249, 1973.
    A frequently unsuspected cause of refractory anemia in pregnant females.
18. Freedman, M. L., and Marcus, D. L. Anemia and the elderly: Is it physiology or pathology? *Am. J. Med. Sci.* 280:81, 1980.
    Anemia in the elderly cannot be dismissed as a consequence of aging.

19. Crosby, W. H. Reticulocyte counts. *Arch. Intern. Med.* 141:1747, 1981.
    Good advice.

20. Owen, J. S., Brown, D. J. C., Harry, D. S., et al. Erythrocyte echinocytosis in liver disease. Role of abnormal plasma high density lipoproteins. *J. Clin. Invest.* 76:2275, 1985.
    Spur formation in liver disease appears to be due to the incorporation of an abnormal high-density lipoprotein. (See also J. Lipid Res. 24:1612, 1983 and Nature 298:290, 1982.)

21. Kimber, C., Deller, D. J., Ibbotson, R. N., et al. The mechanism of anaemia in chronic liver disease. *Q. J. Med.* 34:33, 1965.
    Bleeding, hemolysis, decreased red cell production, and nutritional deficiency alone or in combination contribute to the anemia of chronic liver disease. (See also J. Clin. Invest. 34:3901, 1955.)

22. Salen, G., Goldstein, F., Haurani, F., et al. Acute hemolytic anemia complicating viral hepatitis in patients with glucose 6-phosphate dehydrogenase deficiency. *Ann. Intern. Med.* 65:1210, 1966.
    Hyperbilirubinemia out of proportion to other hepatic function tests in viral hepatitis should suggest hemolysis of glucose 6-phosphate dehydrogenase–deficient red cells.

23. Caldwell, P. R. B., Fritts, H. W., and Cournand, A. Oxyhemoglobin dissociation curve in liver disease. *J. Appl. Physiol.* 20:316, 1965.
    Oxyhemoglobin dissociation curve is shifted to the right, and there is a decrease in oxygen affinity of hemoglobin.

24. Dainiak, N., Kulkarni, V., Howard, D., et al. Mechanisms of abnormal erythropoiesis in malignancy. *Cancer* 51:1101, 1983.
    Erythroid progenitor cells are normal but erythropoietin levels are low.

25. Roodman, G. D., Horadam, V. W., and Wright, T. L. Inhibition of erythroid colony formation by autologous bone marrow adherent cells from patients with the anemia of chronic disease. *Blood* 62:406, 1983.
    Macrophages in chronic inflammatory states inhibit erythropoiesis.

26. Mamus, S. W., Beck-Schroeder, S., and Zanjani, E. D. Suppression of normal human erythropoiesis by gamma interferon in vitro: role of macrophages. *J. Clin. Invest.* 75:1496, 1985.
    Interferon inhibits erythropoiesis and will synergize with tumor necrosis factor in this regard.

27. Kluger, M. J., and Rothenburg, B. A. Fever and reduced iron: their interaction as a host defense response to bacterial infection. *Science* 203:374, 1979.
    Mechanism for the low serum iron in the anemia of chronic disease.

28. The pathogenesis of the anaemia associated with rheumatoid disease. *Ann. Rheum. Dis.* 47:972, 1988.
    Implication of IL-1 in the anemia associated with inflammation.

29. Hochberg, M. C., Arnold, C. M., Hogans, B. B., et al. Serum immunoreactive erythropoietin in rheumatoid arthritis: impaired response to anemia. *Arthritis Rheum.* 31:1318, 1988.
    An important component of the anemia of chronic disease is depression of erythropoietin production. (See also Br. J. Haematol. 66:559, 1987.)

30. Fahey, J. L., Rahbar, S., Farbstein, M. J., et al. Microcytosis in Hodgkin disease associated with unbalanced globin chain synthesis. *Am. J. Hematol.* 23:123, 1986.
    An interesting mechanism for anemia associated with malignancy.

88. ANEMIA AND RENAL DISEASE

Jerry L. Spivak

Normally, erythropoiesis is regulated by erythropoietin, a glycoprotein hormone produced in the kidneys and to a small extent in the liver. Renal disease usually results in a reduction in erythropoietin production and a variable degree of anemia (exceptions include some cases of renal artery stenosis, focal glomerulonephritis, and polycystic kidney disease), while the anephric state is associated with severe anemia. Even in the latter condition, however, erythropoiesis persists although transfusions are required to maintain the hematocrit at an acceptable level. The persistence of erythropoiesis in the anephric state is probably due to erythropoietin production by the liver. The correlation between renal excretory function and renal erythropoietin production is not precise. In general, anemia is usually present when the creatinine clearance is reduced below 40 ml/minute, but following renal transplantation erythropoietin production can be increased at a time when renal excretory function is still profoundly impaired.

With acute renal failure, anemia is usually the result of the disease causing the renal disorder. Such diseases include glucose 6-phosphate dehydrogenase (G-6-PD) deficiency, malaria, clostridial sepsis, vasculitis, and thrombotic thrombocytic purpura (TTP). With a prolonged state of renal failure, marrow hypoproliferation due to lack of erythropoietin production develops. In addition, red cell survival is shortened, apparently due in part to the uremic environment since the life span of normal red cells is reduced in uremic recipients while the survival of uremic red cells is improved in normal recipients. In some patients, a defect in the hexose monophosphate shunt has been identified. The severity of this defect correlates well with the degree of anemia and is not corrected with dialysis. Other factors associated with depression of red cell formation include inanition, infection, toxins in dialysis fluids, iron deficiency due to blood loss from diagnostic phlebotomy and from dialysis, and folic acid loss during dialysis. In some patients, overtransfusion has been demonstrated to depress endogenous erythropoiesis, suggesting that a feedback mechanism is still maintained. Attempts to demonstrate uremic toxins that might be responsible for a reduction in erythropoiesis have led to the recognition that in some patients, marrow fibrosis resulting from secondary hyperparathyroidism contributes to the anemia. In such patients, parathyroidectomy has led to an improvement in hematocrit and a reduction in the degree of marrow fibrosis. However, elevation of the serum parathyroid hormone level does not provide assurance that erythropoiesis will improve following parathyroidectomy. Neither parathyroid hormone nor uremic toxins can be considered to have a central role in the anemia of uremia, since erythropoiesis in uremic animals can be restored entirely to normal by adequate replacement of erythropoietin. Furthermore, in a unique patient with polycythemia vera who developed chronic renal failure, erythropoiesis was not inhibited to a significant degree even after bilateral nephrectomy.

Maintenance dialysis in conjunction with supportive care (replacement of iron and folic acid, treatment of infection, attention to nutrition, and the composition of the dialysis bath) eventually results in an improvement in red cell production rate and survival. These changes are not, however, generally sufficient to elevate the red cell mass to tolerable levels in most patients. In addition, the P_{50} and 2,3-DPG levels of uremic red cells are lower than would be expected for the same degree of anemia in a normal individual, and this defect is not corrected by dialysis. Until recently, transfusions were the mainstay of therapy for symptomatic anemia in chronic renal disease, but were obviously unsatisfactory, considering the risk of allergic reactions, sensitization to blood group and HLA antigens, immunosuppression, transfer of hepatitis viruses and other infectious agents (Epstein-Barr virus, cytomegalovirus, toxoplasmosis, human immunodeficiency virus, and malaria), and the expense. Acquisition of the hepatitis antigen by renal dialysis patients results in an asymptomatic carrier rate of approximately 15 percent and thus a reservoir for infection of the dialysis staff and family members, among whom clinical hepatitis is common.

Through recombinant DNA technology, the erythropoietin gene has been now cloned and recombinant human erythropoietin has been produced in adequate quantities for clinical trials. Recombinant human erythropoietin is biochemically, immunologically, and biologically identical to native human erythropoietin. In over 3 years of clinical trials, it has not proved to be antigenic in man and has been uniformly successful in correcting anemia and alleviating transfusion requirements in patients with end-stage renal disease in a dose-dependent fashion whether administered intravenously or subcutaneously. The hormone also has been employed successfully in predialysis renal failure, and correction of anemia in this situation has not been associated with an acceleration of renal insufficiency. The major adverse effects of recombinant human erythropoietin in patients with end-stage renal disease have been exacerbation of preexisting hypertension, de novo hypertension, and seizures. The exact incidence of these complications awaits the completion of double-blind trials. Erythropoietin per se has no intrinsic pressor activity but is an extremely potent hormone, and its toxicity may be related to overly rapid expansion of the red cell mass with or without a comcomitant reduction of the plasma volume. With expansion of the red cell mass, iron deficiency may also be unmasked, and most patients receiving recombinant erythropoietin will require supplemental iron therapy. Erythropoietin does not cause an increase in white cells or platelets, and its effect may be blunted in the presence of infection, inflammation, aluminum overload, renal osteodystrophy, and hypersplenism. It is now the therapy of choice for the correction of anemia in patients with renal failure.

1. Eschbach, J. W., and Adamson, J. W. Recombinant human erythropoietin: implications for nephrology. *Am. J. Kidney Dis.* 11:203, 1988.
   Concise review.
2. Watson, A. J., and Spivak, J. L. Recombinant human erythropoietin therapy in end stage renal failure. *J. Clin. Pharmacol.* 28:1086, 1988.
   Brief review.
3. Winearls, C. G., Pippard, M. J., Downing, M. R., et al. Effect of human erythropoietin derived from recombinant DNA on the anaemia of patients maintained by chronic haemodialysis. *Lancet* 2:1175, 1986.
   Correction of the anemia of end-stage renal disease by recombinant erythropoietin.
4. Eschbach, J. W., Egrie, J. C., Downing, M. R., et al. Correction of the anemia of end-stage renal disease with recombinant human erythropoietin: results of a combined phase I and II clinical trial. *N. Engl. J. Med.* 316:73, 1987.
   The rate and extent of correction of anemia depends on the supply of iron.
5. Raine, A. E. G. Hypertension, blood viscosity, and cardiovascular morbidity in renal failure: implications of erythropoietin therapy. *Lancet* 1:97, 1988.
   Potential hazards of erythropoietin therapy in renal disease.
6. Lichtman, M. A., Murphy, M. S., Byer, B. J., et al. Hemoglobin affinity for oxygen in chronic renal disease: The effect of hemodialysis. *Blood* 43:417, 1974.
   Hemoglobin-oxygen affinity is higher in patients with uremia than would be expected for the degree of anemia; dialysis produces only a small increase in oxygen binding by hemoglobin.
7. Hocken, A. G., and Marwak, P. K. Iatrogenic contribution to anaemia of chronic renal failure. *Lancet* 1:164, 1971.
   Insidious iron loss by "diagnostic" phlebotomy and dialysis.
8. Walle, A. J., Wong, G. Y., Clemons, G. K., et al. Erythropoietin-hematocrit feedback circuit in the anemia of end-stage renal disease. *Kidney Int.* 31:1205, 1987.
   The feedback circuit is intact.
9. Nathan, D. G., Schupak, E., Stohlman, F., Jr., et al. Erythropoiesis in anephric man. *J. Clin. Invest.* 43:2158, 1964.
   Erythropoiesis is maintained but at a markedly reduced rate in the anephric state.
10. Denny, W. F., Flanigan, W. J., and Zukoski, C. F. Serial erythropoietin studies in patients undergoing renal homotransplantation. *J. Lab. Clin. Med.* 67:386, 1966.
    There is no correlation between renal excretory function and erythropoietin production.
11. Swales, J. D., and Evans, D. B. Erythraemia in renal transplantation. *Br. Med. J.* 1:80, 1969.
    A complication, often requiring phlebotomy, that is not necessarily associated with rejection.
12. Meyrier, A., Simon, P., Boffa, G., et al. Uremia and the liver. *Nephron* 29:3, 1981.
    Hepatitis, either infectious or toxic, can be associated with an increase in serum erythropoietin.
13. Bondurant, M. C., and Koury, M. J. Anemia induces accumulation of erythropoietin mRNA in the kidney and liver. *Mol. Cell. Biol.* 6:2731, 1986.
    Erythropoietin production is regulated at the level of gene expression.
14. Lacombe, C., Da Silva, J.-L., Bruneval, P., et al. Peritubular cells are the site of

erythropoietin synthesis in the murine hypoxic kidney. *J. Clin. Invest.* 81:620, 1988.
See also Blood *71:524, 1988. For studies of the correlation of recruitment of erythropoietin-producing cells and the hematocrit, see* Blood *74:645, 1989.*

15. Whitehead, V. M., Comty, C. H., Posen, G. A., et al. Homeostasis of folic acid in patients undergoing maintenance hemodialysis. *N. Engl. J. Med.* 279:970, 1968.
An adequate diet compensates for loss of folic acid during dialysis. (See also Clin. Pharmacol. Ther. *18:200, 1975.)*

16. Jakal, R., Millard, P. R., Weatherall, D. J., et al. Iron metabolism in haemodialysis patients. *Q. J. Med.* 48:369, 1979.
Iron absorption is normal in patients with chronic renal failure.

17. Stenzel, K. H., Cheigh, J. S., Sullivan, J. F., et al. Clinical effects of bilateral nephrectomy. *Am. J. Med.* 58:69, 1975.
Nephrectomy results in severe anemia, impaired blood pressure regulation, and occasionally hypocalcemia.

18. Zappacosta, A. R., Caro, J., and Erslev, A. Normalization of hematocrit in patients with end-stage renal disease on continuous ambulatory peritoneal dialysis [CAPD]. *Am. J. Med.* 72:53, 1982.
CAPD can restore erythropoiesis to normal if erythropoietin production is adequate. (See also Nephron *46:312, 1987.)*

19. Caro, J., Brown, S., Miller, O., et al. Erythropoietin levels in uremic nephric and anephric patients. *J. Lab. Clin. Med.* 93:449, 1979.
Erythropoietin levels can be normal or elevated in uremic patients.

20. Segal, G. M., Eschbach, J. W., Egrie, J. C., et al. The anemia of end-stage renal disease: hematopoietic progenitor cell response. *Kidney Int.* 33:983, 1988.
Erythroid progenitor cells are normally responsive to erythropoietin, and uremic inhibitors do not appear to be a significant factor in the anemia of renal disease.

21. Lim, V. S., DeGowin, R. L., Zavala, D., et al. Recombinant human erythropoietin in pre-dialysis patients. *Ann. Intern. Med.* 110:108, 1989.
Erythropoietin corrects anemia in predialysis patients.

22. Moia, M., Vizzotto, L., Cattaneo, M., et al. Improvement in the haemostatic defect of uraemia after tretment with recombinant human erythropoietin. *Lancet* 2:1227, 1987.
Improvement but not correction.

23. Weinberg, S. G., Lubin, A., Wiener, S. N., et al. Myelofibrosis and renal osteodystrophy. *Am. J. Med.* 63:755, 1977.
A cause of anemia in some patients with chronic renal failure.

24. Barbour, G. L. Effect of parathyroidectomy on anemia in chronic renal failure. *Arch. Intern. Med.* 139:889, 1979.
Parathyroidectomy does not always improve erythropoiesis in uremic patients. (See also Arch. Intern. Med. *138:1650, 1978.)*

25. Mansell, M., and Grimes, A. J. Red and white cell abnormalities in chronic renal failure. *Br. J. Haematol.* 42:169, 1979.
Review of the biochemical abnormalities.

26. Swartz, R., Dombrouski, J., Burnatowska-Hledin, M., et al. Microcytic anemia in dialysis patients: reversible marker of aluminum toxicity. *Am. J. Kidney Dis.* 9:217, 1987.
Use of deferoxamine to correct anemia.

27. Eschbach, J. W., Abdulhadi, M. H., Browne, J. K., et al. Recombinant human erythropoietin in anemic patients with end-stage renal disease. *Ann. Intern. Med.* 111:992, 1989.
Results of a phase III clinical trial involving 333 patients.

28. Spivak, J. L. Erythropoietin: A brief review. *Nephron* 52:289, 1989.

89. APLASTIC ANEMIA
Jerry L. Spivak

Pancytopenia can be produced by a variety of disorders. They include leukemia, lymphoma, carcinoma metastatic to the marrow, myelofibrosis, vitamin B_{12} or folic acid deficiency, paroxysmal nocturnal hemoglobinuria, thymoma, and hypersplenism associated with parenchymal liver disease, granulomatous diseases, lipidoses, and infections. The diagnosis of aplastic anemia is made only after exclusion of these other possible causes of pancytopenia. A bone marrow aspirate, whether dry or productive of cellular particles, is inadequate for assessment of marrow cellularity, and a bone marrow biopsy should always be done. In aplastic anemia, the biopsy may reveal varying degrees of cellularity, ranging from complete aplasia with only lymphocytes present to scattered islands of hematopoietic activity, with megakaryocytes absent or markedly reduced in number. The bone marrow aspirate frequently does not correlate with the biopsy, and it may reveal cellular particles when the biopsy is hypocellular. This is probably due to sampling error, with the aspirate picking up a small island of hematopoietic tissue. If there is any doubt, other areas can be biopsied. A marrow scan may also be of help. Pancytopenia associated with a hypercellular marrow on biopsy should not be considered as part of the aplastic anemia spectrum. Some of these cases are myelodysplastic in etiology while others may be due to hypersplenism. Occasionally benzene toxicity can result in a phase of marrow hypercellularity with pancytopenia, but in most cases of benzene toxicity the marrow is hypoplastic. The presence of splenomegaly should also raise doubt about the diagnosis of aplastic anemia. Splenomegaly occurs in true aplastic anemia as a result of transfusion hemosiderosis but is not an early feature of the disease.

Tuberculosis is often cited as causing a syndrome difficult to distinguish from aplastic anemia. Review of such cases reveals a lack of critical evaluation. Pancytopenia may occur with tuberculosis as a result of hypersplenism, but if marrow aplasia is present, it is usually the result of some other process complicated by a tuberculous infection. The only exception to this is disseminated infection with certain atypical mycobacteria.

The cause of aplastic anemia is often difficult to ascertain, and in most series no cause is established in up to 50 percent of cases. In the rest, although an absolute cause and effect is difficult to prove, drugs appear to be the most common offending agents. Often the issue is clouded because the patient is the victim of polypharmacy. Statistical evidence implicates chiefly quinacrine, phenylbutazone, mephenytoin, gold, trimethadione, organic arsenicals, and chloramphenicol. Many other compounds have also been implicated (a reference citing these has been provided). The development of aplastic anemia during drug therapy seems to be an idiosyncratic reaction, and there is also evidence of a genetic predisposition to this.

Aplastic anemia can also be produced by insecticides, such as DDT and lindane, and by organic solvents, with benzene the leading offender. Usually exposure is chronic. Glue sniffing has been associated with aplastic anemia, presumably because the glue contains toluene. An association of aplastic anemia with viral hepatitis is well recognized. The patients have usually been young, and the hepatitis was resolving when marrow aplasia developed.

Paroxysmal nocturnal hemoglobinuria (PNH) must always be considered when aplastic anemia is discovered; it may develop during the course of aplastic anemia, or marrow aplasia may complicate PNH. Recurrent abdominal pain or thrombotic episodes are clues to the diagnosis.

When the diagnosis of aplastic anemia is established, the patient's environment, including the medicine cabinet, must be thoroughly evaluated for all possible offending agents. This may provide information about the cause of the marrow aplasia and prevent continuing toxic exposure.

The course of untreated aplastic anemia is usually grim. Mortality is highest in the elderly and in those with profound leukopenia and thrombocytopenia. Fifty percent of deaths occur within the first 2 years from hemorrhage or infection. Recovery, when it occurs, is often incomplete, with persisting thrombocytopenia, and some patients, particularly those with marrow aplasia due to chloramphenicol, develop acute leukemia.

Many modes of therapy for aplastic anemia have been tried, including corticosteroids, splenectomy, and androgens. In mild forms of the disorder, androgens may be effective, but several months of therapy are required before a response is evident. Severely affected patients will not survive long enough for a beneficial effect, if any, to be observed. No androgen preparation is superior to any other in terms of its therapeutic-toxic ratio, but oral agents are more likely to cause liver damage. Corticosteroids and splenectomy appear to have little effect on the course of the disease. Most often aplastic anemia is due to a quantitative or qualitative defect of hematopoietic stem cells and when possible marrow transplantation (HLA-identical sibling or identical twin) is the treatment of choice. For patients who have not been transfused, a survival rate of 80 percent has been achieved. Antithymocyte or lymphocyte globulin has proved to be an effective form of therapy in patients who lack a suitable donor or who are by age ineligible for bone marrow transplantation. The mechanism by which these agents work is undefined but effects other than immunosuppression are probably involved. The role of other forms of therapy for aplastic anemia such as cyclosporin and hematopoietic growth factors is still under investigation.

1. Rozman, C., Nomdedeu, B., Marin, P., et al. Criteria for severe aplastic anemia. *Lancet* 2:955, 1987.
   Brief review.
2. Camitta, B. M., Storb, R., and Thomas, E. D. Aplastic anemia: Pathogenesis, diagnosis, treatment, and prognosis. *N. Engl. J. Med.* 306:645, 712, 1982.
   A comprehensive review.
3. Hoffman, R., Zanjani, E. D., Lutton, J. D., et al. Suppression in aplastic anemia by erythroid-colony formation by lymphocytes. *N. Engl. J. Med.* 296:10, 1977.
   Suppressor lymphocytes implicated in the pathogenesis of this disease.
4. Hoffman, R., Dainiak, N., Sibrock, L., et al. Antibody-mediated aplastic anemia and diffuse fasciitis. *N. Engl. J. Med.* 300:718, 1979.
   An unusual constellation of events occurring in the setting of a lymphoproliferative disorder.
5. Kelton, J. G., Huang, A. T., Mold, N., et al. The use of in vitro technics to study drug-induced pancytopenia. *N. Engl. J. Med.* 301:621, 1979.
   Quinidine-induced aplasia.
6. Roodman, G. D., Ascensao, J. L., Banisadre, M., et al. Autoimmune pancytopenia: Lymphocyte inhibition of autologous but not allogenic bone marrow growth in vitro. *Am. J. Med.* 69:325, 1980.
   Lymphocyte-mediated aplasia.
7. Ajlouni, K., and Doeblin, T. D. The syndrome of hepatitis and aplastic anemia. *Br. J. Haematol.* 27:345, 1974.
   Young age, 4- to 10-week latency after onset of hepatitis, and poor prognosis. (See also Medicine 54:139, 1975.)
8. Lewis, S. M., and Dacie, J. V. The aplastic anemia–paroxysmal nocturnal hemoglobinuria syndrome. *Br. J. Haematol.* 13:236, 1967.
   Acid hemolysis can be weak and transient.
9. Rosse, W. F. Paroxysmal nocturnal haemoglobinuria in aplastic anaemia. *Clin. Haematol.* 7:541, 1978.
   Summary of the clinical experience.
10. Williams, D. M., Lynch, R. E., and Cartwright, G. E. Drug-induced aplastic anemia. *Semin. Haematol.* 10:195, 1973.
    Review of offending agents and their toxicity.
11. Nagao, T., and Mauer, A. M. Concordance for drug-induced aplastic anemia in identical twins. *N. Engl. J. Med.* 281:7, 1969.
    Evidence that chloramphenicol-induced aplastic anemia is genetically conditioned.
12. Scott, J. L., Fitzgerald, S. M., Belkin, G. A., et al. A controlled double blind study of the hematologic toxicity of chloramphenicol. *N. Engl. J. Med.* 272:1137, 1965.
    Reversible dose-related toxicity of chloramphenicol.
13. Roodman, G. D., Reese, E. P., Jr., and Cardamone, J. M. Aplastic anemia associated with rubber cement used by a marathon runner. *Arch. Intern. Med.* 140:703, 1980.
    Benzene-induced aplasia.

14. Bacon, B. R., Treuhaft, W. H., and Goodman, A. M. Azathioprine-induced pancyto-penia: Occurrence in two patients with connective-tissue diseases. *Arch. Intern. Med.* 141:223, 1981.
    Reversible pancytopenia due to azathioprine. (See also Ann. Intern. Med. *93:560, 1980.)*

15. Inman, W. H. W. Study of fatal bone marrow depression with special reference to phenylbutazone and oxyphenbutazone. *Br. Med. J.* 1:1500, 1977.
    Phenylbutazone and oxyphenbutazone are important causes of aplastic anemia in the aged.

16. Needleman, S. W., Burns, P., Dick, F. R., et al. Hypoplastic acute leukemia. *Cancer* 48:1410, 1981.
    Something to consider in the patient with pancytopenia.

17. Horn, N. L., Bennett, L. R., and Marciano, D. Evaluation of aplastic anemia with indium chloride in 111 scannings. *Arch. Intern. Med.* 140:1299, 1980.
    Bone marrow scanning correlates well with biopsy evidence of hypoplasia.

18. Camitta, B. M., Thomas, E. D., Nathan, D. G., et al. A prospective study of androgens and bone marrow transplantation for treatment of severe aplastic anemia. *Blood* 53:504, 1979.
    Androgens are not effective in the treatment of severe aplastic anemia.

19. Bagheri, S. A., and Boyer, J. L. Peliosis hepatis associated with androgenic-anabolic steroid therapy. *Ann. Intern. Med.* 81:610, 1974.
    Many of the patients with this complication should not have been receiving andro-gens. (See also Lancet *1:430, 1972.)*

20. Appelbaum, F. R, Fefer, A., Cheever, M. A., et al. Treatment of aplastic anemia by bone marrow transplantation in identical twins. *Blood* 55:1033, 1980.
    In some twin transplants, immunosuppression is required to achieve a successful graft.

21. Anasetti, C., Doney, K. C., Storb, R., et al. Marrow transplantation for severe aplas-tic anemia: long term outcome in fifty "untransfused" patients. *Ann. Intern. Med.* 104:461, 1986.
    Untransfused patients have an 80% probability of surviving 10 years.

22. McGlave, P. B., Haake, R., Miller, W., et al. Therapy of severe aplastic anemia in young adults and children with allogeneic bone marrow transplantation. *Blood* 70:1325, 1987.
    In this series, prior transfusions did not have an adverse impact.

23. Klingemann, H.-G., Storb, R., Fefer, A., et al. Bone marrow transplantation in pa-tients aged 45 years and older. *Blood* 67:770, 1986.
    The complication rate, particularly interstitial pneumonia, is higher in older pa-tients.

24. Hows, J. M., Yin, J. L., Marsh, J., et al. Histocompatible unrelated volunteer donors compared with HLA nonidentical family donors in marrow transplantation for aplas-tic anemia and leukemia. *Blood* 68:1322, 1986.
    These donors proved to be effective. (See also N. Engl. J. Med. *313:765, 1985.)*

25. Baldwin, J. L., Storb, R., and Thomas, E. D. Bone marrow transplantation in pa-tients with gold-induced marrow aplasia. *Arthritis Rheum.* 20:1043, 1977.

26. Young, N., Griffith, P., Brittain, E., et al. A multicenter trial of antithymocyte glob-ulin in aplastic anemia and related diseases. *Blood* 72:1861, 1988.
    Antithymocyte globulin (ATG) is an effective form of therapy in aplastic anemia.

27. Hunter, R. F., Roth, P. A., and Huang, A. T. Predictive factors for response to anti-thymocyte globulin in acquired aplastic anemia. *Am. J. Med.* 79:73, 1985.
    Early administration was the most effective.

28. Champlin, R. E., Ho, W. G., Feig, S. A., et al. Do androgens enhance the response to antithymocyte globulin in patients with aplastic anemia? A prospective randomized trial. *Blood* 66:184, 1985.
    Androgens were not beneficial.

29. Means, R. T., Jr., Krantz, S. B., Dessypris, E. N., et al. Re-treatment of aplastic anemia with antithymocyte globulin or antilymphocyte serum. *Am. J. Med.* 84:678, 1988.
    Retreatment increased the number of responders.

30. Tichelli, A., Gratwohl, A., Wursch, A., et al. Late haematological complications in severe aplastic anaemia. *Br. J. Haematol.* 69:413, 1988.
    Development of myelodysplasia following therapy with antilymphocyte globulin. (See also Br. J. Haematol *70:55, 1988 and* Lancet *1:1425, 1989.)*
31. Bielory, L., Gascon, P., Lawley, T. J., et al. Human serum sickness: a prospective analysis of 35 patients treated with equine anti-thymocyte globulin for bone marrow failure. *Medicine* 67:40, 1988.
    Serum sickness is not necessary for the therapeutic response to ATG. (See Br. J. Haematol. *63:729, 1986.)*
32. Vadhan-Raj, S., Buescher, S., Broxmeyer, H. E., et al. Stimulation of myelopoiesis in patients with aplastic anemia by recombinant human granulocyte-macrophage colony-stimulating factor. *N. Engl. J. Med.* 319:1628, 1988.
    Not everyone responds. (See Blood *72:2045, 1988.)*
33. Bridges, R., Pineo, G., and Blahey, W. Cyclosporin A for the treatment of aplastic anemia refractory to antithymocyte globulin. *Am. J. Hematol.* 26:83, 1987.
    Another treatment alternative, as yet of unproved value. (See also Br. J. Haematol. *61:267, 1985.)*
34. Graft-versus-host disease after marrow transplantation. *Lancet* 1:491, 1984.
    A major debilitating complication. (See also Am. J. Med. *66:611, 1979.)*
35. Vogelsang, G. B., Hess, A. D., and Santos, G. W. Acute graft-versus-host disease: clinical characteristics in the cyclosporine era. *Medicine* 67:163, 1988.
    Comprehensive review.
36. Wingard, J. R., Mellits, E. D., Sostrin, M. B., et al. Interstitial pneumonitis after allogeneic bone marrow transplantation. Nine-year experience at a single institution. *Medicine* 67:175, 1988.
    An important posttransplantation complication.
37. Winston, D. J., Gale, R. P., Meyer, D. V., et al. Infectious complications of human bone marrow transplantation. *Medicine* 58:1, 1979.
    Comprehensive review.
38. Fohlmeister, I., Fischer, R., Modder, B., et al. Aplastic anaemia and the hypocellular myelodysplastic syndrome: histomorphological, diagnostic, and prognostic features. *J. Clin. Pathol.* 38:1218, 1985.
    For operational purposes, pancytopenia with a hypocellular marrow is aplastic anemia.
39. Champlin, R. Bone marrow aplasia due to radiation accidents: pathophysiology, assessment and treatment. *Clin. Haematol.* 2:69, 1989.
    Radiation accidents are occurring with increasing frequency making this a timely review.

90. CHRONIC LYMPHOCYTIC LEUKEMIA
Jerry L. Spivak

In chronic lymphocytic leukemia (CLL), a gradual and progressive accumulation of mature-appearing lymphocytes results in an increase in the number of circulating lymphocytes, enlargement of lymph nodes and spleen, and infiltration of the bone marrow and occasionally other organs such as the skin and respiratory tract. CLL is the most common form of chronic leukemia. It occurs most often in individuals over age 50 with a higher incidence in men than women, in whites than blacks, in Jews than non-Jews, and is rare in Orientals. A familial tendency is more evident with CLL than with other leukemias, and autoimmune disorders occur with greater frequency in relatives of patients with CLL than they do in the general population. The onset of the disease is insidious, and symptoms arise from the mechanical effects of the accumulated lymphocyte mass, a loss of normal immune function, the development of autoantibodies to red cells or platelets, or as a consequence of products produced by the leukemic lymphocytes.

A mild lymphocytosis is usually the earliest sign of the disorder and, at this stage, only with studies of surface markers can CLL be distinguished from benign disorders causing lymphocytosis. Advanced disease may be discovered fortuitously in an asymptomatic patient and occasionally the presenting manifestations of the disorder may be adenopathy or splenomegaly without any increase in the number of circulating lymphocytes. In the usual situation, however, there is a correlation between the height of the lymphocyte count and the presence of adenopathy, splenomegaly, and constitutional symptoms. When the lymphocyte count is greater than 50,000 per microliter, extensive involvement of the marrow is usually found. CLL is a clonal disorder most often due to the uncontrolled proliferation of a committed B lymphocyte progenitor. Rarely, the disorder may arise as a consequence of the neoplastic transformation of a T lymphocyte. In contrast to B cell CLL, T cell CLL appears to occur with equal frequency in men and women and with a high incidence in Orientals. In general, T cell CLL is a more aggressive disease than B cell CLL and is characterized by a high circulating lymphocyte count, marked splenomegaly, frequent involvement of the skin, and less frequent tumor infiltration of the bone marrow.

The circulating lymphocytes in CLL usually consist of a homogeneous population of normal-appearing small lymphocytes with a minor component of larger, less mature cells. Peripheral blood smears usually contain a large number of smudge cells that are thought to arise because of the absence from the surface of the neoplastic lymphocyte of a large, cold-insoluble globulin. In a small fraction of patients, the predominant circulating lymphocyte is larger with more abundant cytoplasm, and an irregular or clefted nucleus often containing a distinct nucleolus. This cell has been designated the prolymphocyte and is characteristically seen in the setting of a marked lymphocytosis and massive splenomegaly. Prolymphocytes may arise from either B cells or T cells. Prolymphocytic conversion may occur at any time during the course of CLL and independently of therapy. It is usually an aggressive disorder and difficult to control.

As in the case of other forms of leukemia, the rate of cell proliferation in CLL is less than normal, and the disorder is due to an accumulation of functionally impaired lymphocytes. In contrast to the normal situation, in CLL there are more lymphocytes circulating in the peripheral blood than in the thoracic duct lymph indicating an impaired ability of the leukemic cells to gain access to the normal routes for lymphocyte recirculation. The rate of increase in the concentration of circulating lymphocytes in untreated CLL is variable and may be a reflection of the functional properties of the particular transformed clone.

The diagnosis of CLL is usually easily made on the basis of examination of the patient and the peripheral blood smear but occasionally difficulties may arise in distinguishing CLL from leukemic reticuloendotheliosis ("hairy-cell" leukemia), Waldenström's macroglobulinemia, or mu heavy chain disease. There is no merit in employing lymph node biopsy to distinguish between CLL and lymphocytic lymphoma. The lymph node biopsy may reveal pathology characteristic of either well-differentiated lymphoma or poorly differentiated lymphoma but the response to therapy in either case appears to be the same. In earlier literature, a distinction was made between CLL and lymphosarcoma cell leukemia (LSCL). In the latter disorder, the circulating lymphocytes appear less mature than those found in typical CLL and their surface immunofluorescence is more intense. It is likely that many cases of LSCL are in reality examples of prolymphocytic leukemia.

The clinical course of CLL may be indolent or progressive depending on the stage of the disease in which the diagnosis is made. Based on the clinical findings, it is possible to separate the disorder into distinct stages that correlate well with length of survival. In general, patients with lymphocytosis and adenopathy survive longer than patients with lymphocytosis and splenomegaly, hepatomegaly, anemia, or thrombocytopenia. CLL in which the lymphocytes bear κ rather than λ chains may have a more benign course.

Abnormalities of the immune system are an important feature of CLL. In general, there is loss of ability to mount either a cellular or humoral response to most antigenic stimuli. Previously acquired cellular immunity is intact, however. Hypogammaglobulinemia is common but may not be present early in the course of the disease. Isohemagglutinins may be absent. In approximately 6 percent of patients, a monoclonal macroglobulinemia involving excess IgM production may be found, and paradoxically, Coombs-positive hemolytic anemia develops in approximately 35 percent of patients. With the development of tests for platelet antibodies, it is now apparent that autoimmune thrombocytopenia is not infrequent in patients with CLL. Indeed, both autoimmune hemolytic anemia and autoimmune thrombocytopenia may exist together in the same patient. Both of these disorders respond to prednisone therapy. Although anemia and thrombocytopenia are considered poor prognostic signs in staging patients with CLL, autoimmune hemolytic anemia and autoimmune thrombocytopenia do not confer a poor prognosis.

Recurrent pyogenic infection is a common complication in CLL and is not always related to the degree of hypogammaglobulinemia. Leukemic pulmonary disease, although uncommon, is more frequent in CLL than in other leukemias. It may appear as a unilateral pleural effusion or an alveolar capillary block syndrome. It should be emphasized, however, that respiratory infections are the most common causes of pulmonary infiltration in CLL. In contrast to chronic myelogenous leukemia, transition to an acute leukemic phase is not a usual feature of CLL; coexistent acute leukemia has been described with CLL as has development of multiple myeloma and, more commonly, the development of diffuse histiocytic lymphoma (Richter's syndrome). The development of diffuse histiocytic lymphoma in patients with CLL appears to be independent of treatment or disease duration and is manifested by the development of fever, increasing adenopathy, weight loss, and abdominal pain. Diffuse histiocytic lymphoma occurring in the setting of CLL usually responds poorly to chemotherapy. It should also be noted that patients with CLL have a higher incidence of other malignancies than the general population.

Therapy in patients with CLL is usually directed at controlling the disorder and not at producing a remission. Survival is sufficiently long in patients with early stages of the disease that it is difficult to determine whether aggressive chemotherapy prolongs life. There is no evidence that chemotherapy can provoke autoimmune phenomena. In general, patients are treated initially with a single alkylating agent, usually chlorambucil. Corticosteroids, while enhancing the response of the alkylating agent when used in combination, have not been shown to prolong survival. However, they are a valuable adjunct when there is autoimmune hemolytic anemia or thrombocytopenia. The physician should be aware, however, that the introduction of steroids may produce a marked increase in the circulating lymphocyte count that will decline with time. Since lymphocytes are smaller than granulocytes, steroid-induced lymphocytosis does not result in a significant increase in blood viscosity or in leukostatic phenomena, in spite of marked elevation of the white count. Biweekly chlorambucil given as a single pulse produces less hematologic toxicity than daily oral chlorambucil and provides the same degree of tumor control. In patients refractory to a single alkylating agent, the combination of cyclophosphamide (Cytoxan), vincristine, and prednisone has proved very effective. Cyclophosphamide, vincristine, Adriamycin, and prednisone (CHOP) is another regimen which can be employed effectively in treating late-stage CLL or prolymphocytic leukemia. Recently, evidence has been presented that monthly administration of intravenous gamma globulin reduces the incidence of infection in patients with CLL. Other new promising drugs which are currently under investigation include fludarabine, chlorodeoxyadenosine, and deoxycoformycin (pentostatin).

1. Gale, R. P., and Foon, K. A. Chronic lymphocytic leukemia. *Ann. Intern. Med.* 103:101, 1985.
   Comprehensive review.
2. Rai, K. R., Sawitsky, A., Cronkite, E. P., et al. Clinical staging of chronic lymphocytic leukemia. *Blood* 46:219, 1975.
   A simple staging procedure with important prognostic implications. (See also Cancer *48:1302, 1981.)*
3. Binet, J.-L., Catovsky, D., Chandra, P., et al. Chronic lymphocytic leukaemia: proposals for a revised prognostic staging system. *Br. J. Haematol.* 48:365, 1981.
   An alternative to the Rai classification.
4. Pangalis, G. A., Roussou, P. A., Kittas, C., et al. B-chronic lymphocytic leukemia. *Cancer* 59:767, 1987.
   Prognosis according to bone marrow histology.

5. Montserrat, E., Sanchez-Bisono, J., Vinolas, N., et al. Lymphocyte doubling time in chronic lymphocytic leukaemia: analysis of its prognostic significance. *Br. J. Haematol.* 62:567, 1986.
   A doubling time of less than 12 months signifies a poor prognosis.
6. Han, T., Ozer, H., Gavigan, M., et al. Benign monoclonal B cell lymphocytosis. A benign variant of CLL: clinical, immunologic, phenotypic, and cytogenetic studies in 20 patients. *Blood* 64:244, 1984.
   An interesting observation.
7. Gordon, D. S., Jones, B. M., Browning, S. W., et al. Persistent polyclonal lymphocytosis of B lymphocytes. *N. Engl. J. Med.* 307:232, 1982.
   This emphasizes the importance of clonality in diagnosing CLL.
8. Han, T., Barcos, M., Emrich, L., et al. Bone marrow infiltration patterns and their prognostic significance in chronic lymphocytic leukemia: Correlations with clinical, immunologic, phenotypic, and cytogenetic data. *J. Clin. Oncol.* 2:562, 1984.
   Marrow histology was useful in predicting disease progression.
9. Rozman, C., Montserrat, E., Feliu, E., et al. Prognosis of chronic lymphocytic leukemia: A multivariate survival analysis of 150 cases. *Blood* 59:1001, 1982.
   A leukocyte count of greater than 50,000 confers a poor prognosis (see also Blood *59:1191, 1982).*
10. Baldini, L., Mozzana, R., Cortelezzi, A., et al. Prognostic significance of immunoglobulin phenotype in B cell chronic lymphocytic leukemia. *Blood* 65:340, 1985.
    A μ phenotype confers a poor prognosis (see also Blood *62:256, 1983).*
11. Han, T., Ozer, H., Sadamori, N., et al. Prognostic importance of cytogenetic abnormalities in patients with chronic lymphocytic leukemia. *N. Engl. J. Med.* 310:288, 1984.
    Trisomy 12 is the commonest abnormality.
12. Mintzer, D. M., and Hauptman, S. P. Lymphosarcoma cell leukemia and other non-Hodgkin's lymphomas in leukemic phase. *Am. J. Med.* 75:110, 1983.
    Blood involvement is not infrequent but may not affect prognosis (see also Cancer *52:1220, 1983.)*
13. Fialkow, P. J., Najfeld, V., Lakshma Reddy, A., et al. Chronic lymphocytic leukemia: Clonal origin in a committed B-lymphocyte progenitor. *Lancet* 2:444, 1978.
    Clonal origin of B cell CLL established using glucose 6-phosphate dehydrogenase isoenzymes.
14. Conley, C. L., Misiti, J., and Laster, A. J. Genetic factors predisposing to chronic lymphocytic leukemia and to autoimmune disease. *Medicine* 59:323, 1980.
    CLL and autoimmune diseases occur more frequently in relatives of patients with CLL than in the general population.
15. Pangales, G. A., Nathwani, B. N., and Rappaport, H. Malignant lymphoma, well differentiated lymphocytic. *Cancer* 39:999, 1977.
    Well-differentiated lymphocytic lymphoma (WDLL), WDLL with monoclonal gammopathy, and CLL are all part of the spectrum of B cell neoplasia and cannot always be clearly separated.
16. Kubo, R. T., Grey, H. M., and Pirosky, B. IgD: A major surface immunoglobulin on the surface of lymphocytes from patients with chronic lymphatic leukemia. *J. Immunol.* 112:1952, 1974.
    CLL lymphocytes can have IgD and/or IgM on their surface.
17. Bearman, R. M., Pangalis, G. A., and Rappaport, H. Prolymphocytic leukemia. *Cancer* 42:2360, 1978.
    Marked lymphocytosis, massive splenomegaly, minimal adenopathy, large lymphocytes, and a poor prognosis.
18. Dighiero, G., Charron, D., Debre, P., et al. Identification of a pure splenic form of chronic lymphocytic leukemia. *Br. J. Haematol.* 41:169, 1979.
    CLL with massive splenomegaly in the absence of anemia, thrombocytopenia, and superficial adenopathy carries a good prognosis. (See also Arch. Intern. Med. *127:259, 1971.)*
19. Safai, B., and Good, R. A. Lymphoproliferative disorders of the T cell series. *Medicine* 59:335, 1980.
    A comprehensive review.

20. Griesser, H., Tkachuk, D., Reis, M. D., et al. Gene rearrangements and translocations in lymphoproliferative diseases. *Blood* 73:1402, 1989.
   These are useful in establishing clonality in lymphoproliferative disorders. (See also Arch. Pathol. Lab. Med. *112:117, 1988.)*

21. Loughran, T. P., Jr., and Starkebaum, G. Large granular lymphocyte leukemia. *Medicine* 66:397, 1987.
   This is an important but poorly understood syndrome. (See also Leukemia *2:617, 1988 and* Cancer *60:2971, 1987.)*

22. Jaffe, E. S., Bookman, M. A., and Longo, D. L. Lymphocytic lymphoma of intermediate differentiation—mantle zone lymphoma: a distinct subtype of B-cell lymphoma. *Hum. Pathol.* 18:877, 1987.
   Prognosis is reasonably good with this disorder.

23. Toben, H. R., and Smith, R. G. T lymphocytes bearing complement receptors in a patient with chronic lymphocytic leukemia. *Clin. Exp. Immunol.* 27:292, 1977.
   T cell CLL is rare and may mimic B cell CLL; but it generally is more aggressive, with higher white cell counts, greater tumor mass, skin lesions, and less marrow infiltration. (See also Blood *53:1066, 1979.)*

24. Hoffman, R., Kopel, S., Hsu, S. D., et al. T cell chronic lymphocytic leukemia: Presence in bone marrow and peripheral blood of cells that suppress erythropoiesis in vitro. *Blood* 52:255, 1978.
   Anemia due to suppression of erythropoiesis by malignant T lymphocytes.

25. Cone, L., and Uhr, J. W. Immunological deficiency disorders associated with chronic lymphocytic leukemia and multiple myeloma. *J. Clin. Invest.* 43:2241, 1964.
   Hypogammaglobulinemia and absence of primary or secondary immune response with retention of previously acquired delayed hypersensitivity occurs in CLL.

26. Weed, R. I. Exaggerated delayed hypersensitivity to mosquito bites in chronic lymphocytic leukemia. *Blood* 26:257, 1965.
   Cellular immune response in CLL can be inappropriately reactive.

27. Green, R. A., and Nichols, N. J. Pulmonary involvement in leukemia. *Am. Rev. Respir. Dis.* 80:833, 1959.
   Pleural involvement with effusions is not uncommon.

28. Kaden, B. R., Rosse, W. F., and Hauch, T. W. Immune thrombocytopenia in lymphoproliferative diseases. *Blood* 53:545, 1979.
   Immune thrombocytopenia is not uncommon in CLL, does not have a poor prognosis, and may be associated with immune hemolysis. (See also Am. J. Med. *71:729, 1981.)*

29. Chikkappa, G., Zarrabi, M. H., and Tsan, M.-F. Pure red-cell aplasia in patients with chronic lymphocytic leukemia. *Medicine* 65:339, 1986.
   This complication can occur early in the disease.

30. Chandra, P., Sawitsky, A., Chanana, A. D., et al. Correlation of total body potassium and leukemic cell mass in patients with chronic lymphocytic leukemia. *Blood* 43:594, 1979.
   Use of total body potassium to assess tumor cell mass in unemaciated patients with CLL. Lymphocytes in CLL have an increased potassium content. (See Br. J. Cancer *28:354, 1973 and* Cancer *36:926, 1975.)*

31. Shaw, R. K., Boggs, D. R., Silberman, H. R., et al. A study of prednisone therapy in chronic lymphocytic leukemia. *Blood* 17:182, 1960.
   A transient reduction in adenopathy and splenomegaly and a marked increase in circulating lymphocytes produced by steroids.

32. Liepman, M., and Votaw, M. L. The treatment of chronic lymphocytic leukemia with COP chemotherapy. *Cancer* 41:1664, 1978.
   The combination of cyclophosphamide, vincristine, and prednisone is an effective form of therapy in patients refractory to daily chlorambucil.

33. Knospe, W. H., Loeb, V., Jr., and Huguley, C. M., Jr. Biweekly chlormabucil treatment of chronic lymphocytic leukemia. *Cancer* 33:555, 1974.
   Hematologic toxicity is less when chlorambucil is given orally as a single pulse every 2 weeks, and the response rate is similar to daily treatment.

34. Trump, D. L., Mann, R. B., Phelps, R., et al. Richter's syndrome: Diffuse histiocytic

lymphoma in patients with chronic lymphocytic leukemia. *Am. J. Med.* 68:539, 1980.
Fever, increasing adenopathy, weight loss, and abdominal pain in a patient with CLL should suggest the presence of Richter's syndrome. (See also Cancer *48:1302, 1981.)*

35. McDonnell, J. M., Beschorner, W. E., Staal, P., et al. Richter's syndrome with two different B cell clones. *Cancer* 58:2031, 1986.
In Richter's syndrome, the aggressive lymphoma does not always arise from the existing one.

36. Zarrabi, M. H., Grunwald, H. W., and Rosner, F. Chronic lymphocytic leukemia terminating in acute leukemia. *Arch. Intern. Med.* 137:1059, 1977.
*In untreated patients both disorders have been seen simultaneously (*Br. J. Haematol. *43:369, 1979).*

37. Amamoo, D. G., Moayeri, H., Takita, H., et al. Bronchogenic carcinoma in chronic lymphocytic leukemia. *Chest* 75:174, 1979.
Pulmonary neoplasms are common in patients with CLL.

38. Alexanian, R. Monoclonal gammopathy in lymphoma. *Arch. Intern. Med.* 135:62, 1975.
6% of patients with CLL had a monoclonal gammopathy in this series. (See also Blood *52:532, 1978.)*

39. Brouet, J.-C., Seligmann, M., Danon, F., et al. M-chain disease. *Arch. Intern. Med.* 139:672, 1979.
This disease may mimic CLL but vacuolated plasma cells in the marrow and Bence Jones proteinuria should suggest the diagnosis.

40. Turner, A., and Kjeldsberg, C. R. Hairy cell leukemia: A review. *Medicine* 57:477, 1978.
Splenomegaly, pancytopenia, and a "dry marrow aspirate" without lymphadenopathy should suggest the diagnosis. (See also Ann. Intern. Med. *89:677, 1978.)*

41. Glaspy, J. A., Jacobs, A. D., and Golde, D. W. Evolving therapy of hairy cell leukemia. *Cancer* 59:652, 1987.
Splenectomy, interferon-alpha and deoxycoformycin. (See also Cancer *57:644, 1986.)*

42. Delpero, J. R., Gastaut, J. A., Letreut, Y. P., et al. The value of splenectomy in chronic lymphocytic leukemia. *Cancer* 59:340, 1987.
Splenectomy may be required for autoimmune cytopenias.

43. Roncadin, M., Arcicasa, M., Trovo, M. G., et al. Splenic irradiation in chronic lymphocytic leukemia. *Cancer* 60:2624, 1987.
This is a palliative procedure which does not prolong survival. (See also Am. J. Hematol. *19:177, 1985.)*

44. Cash, J., Fehir, K. M., and Pollack, M. S. Meningeal involvement in early stage chronic lymphocytic leukemia. *Cancer* 59:798, 1987.
This is unusual.

45. Blayney, D. W., Jaffe, E. S., Fisher, R. I., et al. The human T-cell leukemia/lymphoma virus (HTLV), lymphoma, lytic bone lesions, and hypercalcemia. *Ann. Intern. Med.* 98:144, 1983.
A very aggressive T cell neoplasm due to HTLV-I.

46. Ratner, L., and Poiesz, B. J. Leukemias associated with human T-cell lymphotropic virus type I in a non-endemic region. *Medicine* 67:401, 1988.
These leukemias can be acute or chronic. (See also Lancet *2:633, 1985.)*

47. Lukes, R. J., and Tindle, B. H. Immunoblastic lymphadenopathy. *N. Engl. J. Med.* 292:1, 1975.
An unusual disorder which may progress to lymphoma. (See also Cancer *52:318, 1983.)*

48. Bunch, C., et al. Intravenous gammaglobulin for the prevention of infection in chronic lymphocytic leukemia. *N. Engl. J. Med.* 319:902, 1988.
Intravenous IgG given every 3 weeks reduces the incidence of bacterial infection, particularly pneumonia.

49. Keating, M. J., Kantarjian, H., Talpaz, M., et al. Fludarabine: A new agent with major activity against chronic lymphocytic leukemia. *Blood* 74:19, 1989.

One of several new drugs for treating CLL. For deoxycoformycin, see Ann. Int. Med. *108:733, 1988. For chlorodeoxyadenosine, see* Blood 72:1069, 1988.

91. CHRONIC MYELOGENOUS LEUKEMIA
Judith E. Karp

Chronic myelogenous leukemia (CML) is an acquired clonal disorder of a pluripotent hematopoietic stem cell which is characterized by a marked increase in the production of granulocytes and platelets and occasionally red blood cells. The disorder is most common in individuals between 40 and 60 years of age and analysis of the natural history of CML suggests that by the time it is clinically manifest, it has been present for approximately 8 years. CML must be distinguished from other disorders that cause leukocytosis. They include idiopathic myelofibrosis, polycythemia vera, neoplasms such as hypernephroma and hepatoma, and the recovery phase of agranulocytosis or megaloblastic anemia.

Two laboratory tests can be employed to distinguish CML from other disorders associated with leukocytosis. Leukocyte alkaline phosphatase (LAP) is decreased or absent in CML neutrophils as compared to normal neutrophils. However, with infection, inflammation, corticosteroid therapy, following remission induction, or with the development of myelofibrosis or blast crisis, the LAP of CML cells may rise to normal or high levels. A more useful diagnostic test because of its specificity is cytogenetic analysis of blood or marrow cells. The cytogenetic hallmark of CML is the presence of a shortened chromosome 22 (the Philadelphia, or Ph[1], chromosome) which results from translocation of a portion of the long arm of chromosome 9 containing the c-abl protooncogene to the bcr gene region of chromosome 22, and the reciprocal translocation of a portion of the long arm of chromosome 22 containing the c-sis protooncogene 22 to chromosome 9 (t [9;22] [q34;q11]). While transcription of c-sis and its gene product, platelet-derived growth factor, does not appear to be consistently affected by its translocation to chromosome 9, the heat-to-tail juxtaposition of the 5'-end of c-abl with the truncated 3'-end of the bcr gene on chromosome 22 results in a new transcriptional unit producing a novel bcr-abl fusion mRNA transcript. The translocational product of this hybrid 8.5 mRNA is a 210-kilodalton protein with tyrosine kinase activity. By analogy with murine disease model systems, where v-abl functions as a transforming gene, it is likely that the bcr-abl p210 product plays an important role in CML disease progression.

This clonal rearrangement and DNA fusion with its unique gene product is present in all hematopoietic cells, including those of the lymphoid series, and can be detected in most patients during the stable phase of the disease, even despite apparent clinical remission, and in the blastic phase of the illness. However, in approximately 10 percent of patients with the clinical features of CML, the hematopoietic cells do not contain the Ph[1] chromosome. Ph[1]-negative CML is also a clonal disorder of a pluripotent hematopoietic stem cell but its clinical course differs from that of Ph[1]-positive CML. Patients with Ph[1]-negative CML are usually older, have lower white cell and platelet counts, a less satisfactory response to therapy, and a shorter survival time. It is of interest, nonetheless, that some Ph[1]-negative patients have a clonal rearrangement of the bcr gene with an associated p210 tyrosine kinase–like protein, despite the absence of the full Ph[1] translocation; these patients tend to have a more favorable overall clinical course, behaving like those with Ph[1]-positive CML.

While most patients with CML present with a marked leukocytosis representing granulocytes in all stages of maturation but with a preponderance of mature, normally functioning cells, some patients may present with myelofibrosis, or acute leukemia with either myeloid, lymphoid, or biphenotypic characteristics. The latter presentation, which may account for 25 percent of all newly diagnosed acute lymphoblastic leukemia (particularly in adults), is a much more drug-resistant variant than its de novo non–Ph[1]-positive myeloid or lymphoid counterparts, with refractory disease and exceedingly short survival. In some cases of Ph[1]-positive acute lymphoblastic leukemia, a novel clonal bcr rearrangement has been detected, with an unusual tyrosine kinase–like protein of lesser molecular weight (p185); how this relates to pathogenesis, perpetuation, and/or disease aggressiveness is at present intriguing but unknown.

During the early phase of CML, the patient may be asymptomatic or suffer from the consequences of the large turnover of marrow cells with hypermetabolism, hyperuricemia, and problems related to rapid enlargement of the spleen. During this phase of the disease, oscillations of the white cell and platelet counts may be observed with a cycle of approximately 60 days. During its chronic phase, CML can be controlled with an alkylating agent such as busulfan or with hydroxyurea, both of which can be taken orally. Hydroxyurea is less toxic than busulfan and produces a more rapid reduction in white cell and platelet counts but the duration of its effects are transient and daily therapy is usually required. The effect of busulfan on the white cell count takes several weeks to become evident and continues for several weeks after the drug is discontinued. Busulfan's toxicities include not only marrow aplasia, which can persist for a prolonged period, but also amenorrhea, alopecia, hyperpigmentation, Addisonian-like symptoms, and porphyrinuria. Busulfan also produces a siccalike syndrome that can be distressing to the patient and persists long after the drug has been discontinued. Next to marrow aplasia, however, the most important toxicity of busulfan is pulmonary injury. This may develop insidiously with a clinical picture of pulmonary fibrosis, or acutely and resemble a pneumonic process. The chest x ray may not indicate the extent of pulmonary involvement and lung biopsy may be necessary to establish the basis for the pneumonitis. The role of corticosteroid therapy in this situation is uncertain but should be considered in busulfan-treated patients with acute noninfectious interstitial pneumonitis since progression of the process can be rapid.

Recently it has been demonstrated that a normal hematopoietic clone can be detected in many patients with stable-phase CML and that this clone can transiently and at least partially repopulate the bone marrow after intensive chemotherapy. Along these lines, the in vitro demonstration that the interferons (IFN) could suppress the growth and differentiation of CML marrow precursors has led to promising clinical trials of IFN. In particular, IFN-alpha can clinically suppress the Ph[1]-positive clone and decrease the proportion of Ph[1]-positive marrow metaphases for up to 3 years with continuous therapy. To date, however, while significant complete remissions can be achieved with long-term INF-alpha therapy, the effect on overall survival has yet to be determined.

Eventually, the chronic (stable) phase of CML transforms to an aggressive, therapy-resistant phase characterized by progressive marrow failure, hypermetabolism, myelofibrosis, basophilia, aneuploidy on karyotypic analysis, and frequently the development of lymphadenopathy and skin lesions. Bone pain associated with hypercalcemia and osteolytic lesions may be observed. In some but not all patients, a blast crisis occurs with increasing anemia, thrombocytopenia, and a leukocytosis due to an increase in circulating blast cells. Blast crisis in CML can be due to proliferation of myeloblasts or lymphoblasts. A characteristic feature of the blast crisis of CML is the poor response obtained with chemotherapeutic agents, which are uniformly effective in acute myelogenous leukemia (AML) not associated with CML. An exception to this occurs when the blast cells have the features of lymphoblasts, particularly with respect to the presence of terminal deoxynucleotidyl transferase and the common acute lymphocytic leukemia (ALL) antigen. Patients whose blast cells have these features may transiently respond to anti-ALL therapy, but eventually relapse, often with a drug-resistant population of cells that has changed its phenotypic characteristics. Even for those patients who respond to chemotherapy, the duration of survival with blast crisis is extremely short.

The refractoriness of blastic crisis to all therapeutic modalities (including bone marrow transplantation) has led to the evaluation of the role of allogeneic and/or autologous bone marrow transplant as potential curative therapy while the disease is still in the early chronic phase. Allogeneic bone marrow transplantation in young patients in stable phase with HLA-identical sibling donors has produced continuing long-term disease-free survival in 50 percent of patients treated. Innovative approaches to autologous bone marrow transplantation for CML include infusion of bone marrow cells harvested after conversion to the Ph[1]-negative state by in vivo interferon therapy, infusion of bone marrow cells grown in long-term liquid culture, and infusion of marrow treated ex vivo with chemotherapeutic agents or cytokines. There is evidence in CML for persistence of normal Ph[1]-negative hematopoietic precursors which are suppressed by clonal expansion of abnormal cells with a proliferative advantage. The aim of therapy is to reduce the number of abnormal cells to allow functional recovery of the more differentiated committed precursor cells. Whether the Ph[1]-negative cells that emerge after the annihilation of the leukemic cells are normal or merely neoplastic cells in a preleukemic phase is unknown. That malignant cells themselves can proliferate and differentiate in both CML and AML has been demonstrated by isoenzyme studies, cytogenetics, and restriction fragment–length polymorphisms. The prevalence of maturation of leukemia cells following chemotherapy is as yet unknown but it does indicate that drugs which force maturation rather than incur cytotoxicity should be of value in the treatment of this malignancy.

1. Kardinal, G. C., Bateman, J. R., and Weiner, J. Chronic granulocytic leukemia. *Arch. Intern. Med.* 136:305, 1976.
   Diagnosis, staging and prognosis: clinical parameters.
2. Monfardini, S., Gee, T., Fried, J., et al. Survival in chronic myelogenous leukemia: Influence of treatment and extent of disease at diagnosis. *Cancer* 31:492, 1973.
3. Sokal, J. E., Cox, E., Baccarani, M., et al. Prognostic discrimination in "good-risk" chronic granulocytic leukemia. *Blood* 63:789, 1984.
4. Tura, S., Baccarni, M., Corbelli, G., et al. Staging of chronic myeloid leukemia. *Br. J. Haemat.* 47:105, 1981.
5. Brodsky, I., Fuscaldo, K. E., Kahn, S. B., et al. Myeloproliferative disorders: II. CML: Clonal evolution and its role in management. *Leuk. Res.* 3:379, 1979.
   CML as a clonal hematologic malignancy.
6. Fialkow, P. J., Martin, P. J., Najfield, V., et al. Evidence for a multistep pathogenesis of chronic myelogenous leukemia. *Blood* 58:158, 1981.
7. Singer, J. W., Adamson, J. W., Zalmen, A. A., et al. Chronic myelogenous leukemia. *J. Clin. Invest.* 67:1593, 1981.
8. Singer, J. W., Arlin, Z. A., Najfield, V., et al. Restoration of nonclonal hematopoiesis in chronic myelogenous leukemia (CML) following a chemotherapy-induced loss of the Ph[1] chromosome. *Blood* 56:356, 1980.
9. Sokal, J. E., and Gomez, G. A. The Philadelphia chromosome and Philadelphia chromosome mosaicism in chronic granulocytic leukemia. *J. Clin. Oncol.* 4:104, 1986.
10. Collins, S. J., and Groudine, M. T. Chronic myelogenous leukemia: Amplification of a rearranged c-abl oncogene in both chronic phase and blast crisis. *Blood* 69:893, 1987.
    Molecular genetics of the Philadelphia chromosome.
11. Kurzrock, R., Gutterman, J. U., and Talpaz, M. The molecular genetics of Philadelphia chromosome–positive leukemias. *N. Engl. J. Med.* 319:990, 1988.
12. Stam, K., Heisterkamp, N., Grosveld, G., et al. Evidence of a new chimeric bcr/c-abl mRNA in patients with chronic myelocytic leukemia and the Philadelphia chromosome. *N. Engl. J. Med.* 313:1429, 1985.
13. Ezdinli, E. Z., Sokal, J. E., Crosswhite, L., et al. Philadelphia-chromosome–positive and –negative chronic myelocytic leukemia. *Ann. Intern. Med.* 72:175, 1970.
    Philadelphia chromosome–negative CML.
14. Fialkow, P. J., Jacobson, R. J., Singer, J. W., et al. Philadelphia chromosome (Ph[1])–negative chronic myelogenous leukemia (CML): A clonal disease with origin in a multipotent stem cell. *Blood* 56:70, 1980.
15. Ganesan, T. S., Raddool, F., Guo, K. H., et al. Rearrangement of the bcr gene in Philadelphia chromosome–negative chronic myeloid leukemia. *Blood* 68:957, 1986.
16. Kantarjian, H. M., Shtalrid, M., Kurzrock, R., et al. Significance and correlations of molecular analysis results in patients with Philadelphia chromosome–negative chronic myelogenous leukemia and chronic myelomonocytic leukemia. *Am. J. Med.* 85:639, 1988.
17. Kurzrock, R., Blick, M. B., Talpaz, M., et al. Rearrangement in the breakpoint cluster

region and the clinical course in Philadelphia–negative chronic myelogenous leukemia. *Ann. Intern. Med.* 105:673, 1986.

18. Wiedmann, L. M., Karhi, K. K., Shivji, M. K. K., et al. The correlation of breakpoint cluster region rearrangement and p210 phl/abl expression with morphological analysis of Ph-negative chronic myeloid leukemia and other myeloproliferative diseases. *Blood* 71:349, 1988.

19. Chabner, B. A., Haskell, C. M., and Canellos, G. P. Destructive bone lesions in chronic granulocytic leukemia. *Medicine* 48:401, 1969.

Blastic crisis of CML: Clinical features and staging.

20. Kantarjian, H. M., Keating, M. J., Talpaz, M., et al. Chronic myelogenous leukemia in blast crisis. *Am. J. Med.* 83:445, 1987.

21. Peterson, L. C., Bloomfield, C. D., and Brunning, R. D. Blast crisis as an initial or terminal manifestation of chronic myeloid leukemia. *Am. J. Med.* 60:209, 1976.

22. Rosenthal, S., Canellos, G. P., Whang-Peng, J., et al. Blast crisis of chronic granulocytic leukemia. *Am. J. Med.* 63:542, 1977.

23. Sadamori, N., Gomez, G. A., and Sandberg, A. A. Therapeutic and prognostic value of initial chromosomal findings at the blastic phase of Ph[1]-positive chronic myeloid leukemia. *Blood* 61:935, 1983.

24. Klein, A. D., Hagemeijer, A., Bartram, C. R., et al. bcr rearrangement and translocation of the c-abl oncogene in Philadelphia positive acute lymphoblastic leukemia. *Blood* 68:1369, 1986.

Lymphoid blast crisis.

25. Duval, C. P., Carbone, P. P., Bell, W. R., et al. Chronic myelocytic leukemia with two Philadelphia chromosomes and prominent peripheral lymphadenopathy. *Blood* 29:652, 1967.

26. Marks, S. M., Baltimore, D., and McCaffrey, R. Terminal transferase as a predictor of initial responsiveness to vincristine and prednisone in blastic chronic myelogenous leukemia. *N. Engl. J. Med.* 298:812, 1978.

27. Miller, W. J., Gonzalez-Sarmiento, R., and Kersey, J. H. Immunoglobulin and T-cell receptor gene rearrangement in blast crisis of chronic myelocytic leukemia. *Exp. Hematol.* 16:884, 1988.

28. Bolin, R. W., Robinson, W. A., Sutherland, J., et al. Busulfan versus hydroxyurea in long-term therapy of chronic myelogenous leukemia. *Am. Cancer Soc.* 50:1683, 1982.

Therapy of CML: Chemotherapy. (See also Arch. Intern. Med. *136:1181, 1976, and* J.A.M.A. *246:1449, 1981.)*

29. Champlin, R. E., and Golde, D. W. Chronic myelogenous leukemia: Recent advances. *Blood* 65:1039, 1985.

30. Griffin, J. D. Management of chronic myelogenous leukemia. *Semin. Hematol.* 23:20, 1986.

31. Kantarjian, H. M., Smith, T. L., McCredie, K. B., et al. Chronic myelogenous leukemia: A multivariate analysis of the associations of patient characteristics and therapy with survival. *Blood* 66:1326, 1985.

Interferon therapy.

32. Talpaz, M., Kantarjian, H. M., McCredie, K. B., et al. Chronic myelogenous leukemia: Hematologic remissions and cytogenetic improvements induced by recombinant alpha A interferon. *N. Engl. J. Med.* 314:1065, 1986.

33. Goldman, J. M., Gale, R. P., Horowitz, M. M., et al. Bone marrow transplantation for chronic myelogenous leukemia in chronic phase. *Ann. Intern. Med.* 108:806, 1988.

Bone marrow transplantation.

34. Lemonnier, M. P., Gorin, N. C., Laporte, J. P., et al. Autologous marrow transplantation for patients with chronic myeloid leukemia in accelerated or blastic phase: Report of 14 cases. *Exp. Hematol.* 14:658, 1986.

35. McGlave, P., Arthur, D., Hoake, R., et al. Therapy of chronic myelogenous leukemia with allogeneic bone marrow transplantation. *J. Clin. Oncol.* 5:1033, 1987.

36. Thomas, E. D., and Clift, R. A. Indications for marrow transplantation in chronic myelogenous leukemia. *Blood* 73:861, 1989.

37. Vogler, W. R., Winton, E. F., James, S., et al. Autologous marrow transplantation after karyotypic conversion to normal in blastic phase of chronic myelocytic leukemia. *Am. J. Med.* 75:1080, 1983.

92. DISSEMINATED INTRAVASCULAR COAGULATION
Jerry L. Spivak

Acquired deficiency of coagulation factors is usually the result of impaired production (liver disease, vitamin K lack, anticoagulant therapy) or increased extravascular loss (massive blood loss and replacement, amyloidosis, nephrotic syndrome). Inappropriate intravascular utilization of coagulation factors is normally prevented by continuous rapid blood flow, circulating inhibitors of procoagulants, and removal of activated clotting factors and thromboplastic substances by the liver. When these homeostatic mechanisms are impaired or overwhelmed following activation of the clotting cascade, intravascular consumption of coagulation factors occurs, with variable degrees of reduction in their blood concentration. This sequence of events has been termed *disseminated intravascular coagulation (DIC)*, consumption coagulopathy, or the defibrinogenation syndrome. Factors responsible for triggering or potentiating intravascular coagulation include release of thromboplastic material into the circulation, endothelial cell damage, endotoxemia, antigen-antibody reactions, hypotension, hypoxia, acidosis, and reticuloendothelial blockage.

Diseases or therapeutic maneuvers in which DIC has been documented include infections with bacteria (gram-positive and gram-negative), viruses, rickettsiae, *Mycobacterium tuberculosis*, fungi, and *Plasmodium falciparum;* splenectomy; septic abortion; hypertonic saline abortion; amnionitis; abruptio placentae; amniotic fluid embolism; retained dead fetus; toxemia; carcinomatosis; acute nonlymphocytic leukemia; hemolytic transfusion reactions; anaphylaxis; chemotherapy; cardiac arrest; heat stroke; snake bite; hemangioendotheliomas (Kasabach-Merritt syndrome); massive pulmonary embolism; aortic aneurysm; acute hepatic necrosis; brain damage; and thrombotic thrombocytopenic purpura.

In the classic situation, fibrinogen, factors V and VIII, and platelets are reduced, and fibrinogen-fibrin degradation products are elevated due to secondary activation of the fibrinolytic system. All of the "classic" findings may not always be present, however, if marked elevation of the level of fibrinogen (an acute-phase reactant) and other coagulation factors are present before the onset of DIC, or if production of clotting factors is able to compensate for consumption. In one such instance, thrombotic thrombocytopenic purpura, fibrinogen, and coagulation factor levels are usually normal, and the only evidence of DIC is thrombocytopenia and elevated levels of fibrinogen-fibrin degradation products. It must also be emphasized that none of the coagulation abnormalities produced by DIC are specific for that disorder and can be observed in other situations in which no intravascular consumption of coagulation factors is occurring. They include liver disease and extravascular accumulations of blood.

The complications of DIC depend on the rapidity and extent to which the coagulation changes occur. Chronic DIC may be manifest as recurrent ecchymoses or phlebitis. Acute DIC results in superficial hemorrhage and bleeding from the mucous membranes and venipuncture sites. Intravascular deposition of fibrin thrombin may cause traumatic hemolysis (microangiopathy) and, in the presence of hypotension, renal cortical necrosis. In postinfectious DIC, purpura fulminans may occur. Hemorrhage may be the result of marked reduction in levels of coagulation factors or platelets, but more often these are not markedly depressed and the bleeding diathesis results from the anticoagulant effect of the fibrinogen-fibrin degradation products.

Therapy in the patients with DIC should be directed toward the underlying disease that triggered the process—evacuation of the uterus in septic abortion or retained dead fetus, correction of hypotension, acidosis, and hypoxia, administration of antibiotics in infections, and administration of estrogen in patients with prostatic carcinoma. These maneuvers usually result in prompt elevation of the clotting factor levels within 10 hours and reduction in split products (half-life 9 hours), although platelets take longer to respond. If bleeding is brisk, fresh blood should be used for replacement. The role of fibrinogen, platelets, and specific clotting factor replacement is less clear, particularly in view of the risk of volume overload, hepatitis, and continued presence of fibrin degradation products. The use of prothrombin complex concentrates that contain activated clotting factors should be avoided.

Much interest has been given to the use of heparin in the therapy of DIC. Considerable clinical evidence has been accumulated, suggesting that heparin can stop consumption, with a resultant elevation of coagulation factor levels. On the other hand, it cannot be emphasized too strongly that DIC is a fluctuating process with spontaneous remissions and that no controlled study of the efficacy of heparin has ever been performed. In addition, heparin can cause DIC, thrombocytopenia, and serious, occasionally fatal, hemorrhage. Heparin is also not always able to reverse the coagulopathy. This may be due to the fact that the level of antithrombin III, a cofactor for heparin, is reduced in DIC. Clinical experience suggests that in patients with DIC, correction of the underlying disease is prognostically the most important therapeutic maneuver. Heparin is most likely to benefit those individuals with Trousseau's syndrome in whom the tumor can either not be located or is unresponsive to therapy. In such cases, coumarin derivatives are usually not effective in controlling thrombotic events and heparin must be employed, usually by continuous infusion. There is little evidence that ε-aminocaproic acid (EACA) has any role in the management of DIC with the possible exception of the Kasabach-Merritt syndrome.

1. Schafer, A. I. The hypercoagulable states. *Ann. Intern. Med.* 102:814, 1985.
   Excellent review of a complex subject.
2. Mant, M. J., and King, E. G. Severe, acute disseminated intravascular coagulation: A reappraisal of its pathophysiology, clinical significance and therapy based on 47 patients. *Am. J. Med.* 67:557, 1979.
   Heparin is rarely beneficial in acute DIC and may exacerbate hemorrhage.
3. Harker, L. A., and Slichter, S. J. Platelet and fibrinogen consumption in man. *N. Engl. J. Med.* 2871269, 1972.
   The circulating levels of platelets and fibrinogen do not always reflect their turnover rates.
4. Yoshikawa, T, Tanaka, K. R., and Guze, L. B. Infection and disseminated intravascular coagulation. *Medicine* 50:237, 1971.
   DIC can occur as a complication of infections with gram-positive and gram-negative bacteria, viruses, rickettsiae, tuberculosis, aspergillosis, malaria, and kala azar. (See also Arch. Intern. Med. 137:844, 1977.)
5. Satterwhite, T. K., Hawiger, J., Burklow, S. L., et al. Degradation products of fibrinogen and fibrin in bacteremia due to gram-negative rods. *J. Infect. Dis.* 127:437, 1973.
   Transient subclinical DIC is common with gram-negative rod bacteremia.
6. Bauer, K. A., and Rosenberg, R. D. The pathophysiology of the prethrombotic state in humans: insights gained from studies using markers of hemostatic system activation. *Blood* 70:343, 1987.
   Biochemical basis for hypercoagulability.
7. Rickles, F. R., and Edwards, R. L. Activation of blood coagulation in cancer: Trousseau's syndrome revisited. *Blood* 62:14, 1983.
   Mechanisms for thrombosis reviewed. (See also Human Pathol. 18:275, 1989.)
8. Lopex, J. A., Ross, R. S., Fishbein, M. C., et al. Nonbacterial thrombotic endocarditis: a review. *Am. Heart J.* 113:773, 1987.
   Comprehensive review.
9. Clouse, L. H., and Comp, P. C. The regulation of hemostasis: the protein C system. *N. Engl. J. Med.* 314:1298, 1986.
   Comprehensive review. (See also N. Engl. J. Med. 319:1265, 1988 and Lancet 1:435, 1988.)
10. Comp, P. C., and Esmon, C. T. Recurrent venous thromboembolism in patients with a partial deficiency of protein S. *N. Engl. J. Med.* 311:1525, 1984.
    An inherited hypercoagulable state, but protein S levels can be reduced nonspecifically by a variety of disorders. (See J. Clin. Invest 81:1445, 1988.)
11. McGehee, W. G., Klotz, T. A., Epstein, D. J., et al. Coumarin necrosis associated with hereditary protein C deficiency. *Ann. Intern. Med.* 101:59, 1984.
    Protein C deficiency should be considered in patients with coumarin necrosis.

12. Cosgriff, T. M., Bishop, D. T., Hershgold, E. J., et al. Familial antithrombin III deficiency: its natural history, genetics, diagnosis and treatment. *Medicine* 62:209, 1983.
    This deficiency state is not rare.
13. Nielsen, L. E., Bell, W. R., Borkon, A. M., et al. Extensive thrombus formation with heparin resistance during extracorporeal circulation: a new presentation of familial antithrombin III deficiency. *Arch. Intern. Med.* 147:149, 1987.
    An unusual presentation of an inherited predisposition to thrombosis.
14. Elias, M., and Eldor, A. Thromboembolism in patients with the "lupus"-type circulating anticoagulant. *Arch. Intern. Med.* 144:510, 1984.
    Successful use of anticoagulants.
15. Bisno, A. L., and Freeman, J. C. The syndrome of asplenia, pneumococcal sepsis and disseminated intravascular coagulation. *Ann. Intern. Med.* 72:389, 1970.
    Pneumococcal infection in asplenic persons is frequently associated with overwhelming sepsis and DIC.
16. Ten Cate, J. W., Timmers, H., and Becker, H. E. Coagulopathy in ruptured or dissecting aortic aneurysms. *Am. J. Med.* 59:171, 1975.
    DIC complicating aneurysmal disease. (See also Arch. Surg. *118:1252, 1983.)*
17. Goodnight, S. H., Kenoyer, G., Rapaport, S. I., et al. Defibrination after brain-tissue destruction. *N. Engl. J. Med.* 290:1043, 1974.
    Transient DIC associated with brain damage.
18. Spicer, T. E., and Rau, J. M. Purpura fulminans. *Am. J. Med.* 61:566, 1976.
    Postinfectious DIC, which can occur in adults. (See also Arch. Intern. Med. *146:497, 1986.)*
19. Sack, G. H., Jr., Levin, J., and Bell, W. R. Trousseau's syndrome and other manifestations of chronic disseminated coagulopathy in patients with neoplasms: Clinical, pathophysiologic and therapeutic features. *Medicine* 56:1, 1977.
    A comprehensive review.
20. Bell, W. R., Starksen, N. F., Tong, S., et al. Trousseau's syndrome: devastating coagulopathy in the absence of heparin. *Am. J. Med.* 79:423, 1985.
    Emphasizes the need to use heparin and not a coumarin derivative in this situation.
21. Lerner, R. G., Nelson, J. C., Corines, P., et al. Disseminated intravascular coagulation: Complication of LeVeen peritoneovenous shunts. *J.A.M.A.* 240:2064, 1978.
    The usefulness of this shunting procedure is diminished by a high incidence of DIC.
22. Robboy, S. J., Colman, R. W., and Minna, J. D. Pathology of disseminated intravascular coagulation (DIC). *Hum. Pathol.* 3:327, 1972.
    Deposition of fibrin is most frequent in kidney, skin, lungs, and testes, but it is easily overlooked.
23. Putnam, C. E., Minagi, H., and Blaisdell, F. W. The roentgen appearance of disseminated intravascular coagulation (DIC). *Radiology* 109:13, 1973.
    The x-ray picture mimics that of simple pulmonary edema.
24. Schwartzman, R. J., and Hill, J. B. Neurologic complications of disseminated intravascular coagulation. *Neurology* 32:791, 1982.
    Large-vessel thrombosis and subarachnoid or intracerebral hemorrhage.
25. Bull, B. S., and Kuhn, I. N. The production of schistocytes by fibrin strands (a scanning electron microscope study). *Blood* 35:104, 1970.
    Pathogenesis of microangiopathic hemolytic anemia.
26. Jacobson, R. J., and Jackson, D. P. Erythrocyte fragmentation in defibrination syndromes. *Ann. Intern. Med.* 81:207, 1974.
    Red cell fragmentation is associated with significant organ damage.
27. Merksey, C. Defibrination syndrome or . . .? *Blood* 41:599, 1973.
    An important reminder that defibrinogenation may not always be due to intravascular coagulation.
28. Bloom, A. L. Intravascular coagulation and the liver. *Br. J. Haematol.* 30:1, 1975.
    A well-balanced review. The evidence for DIC occurring in liver disease is controversial. (See also Semin. Thromb. Hemost. *4:29, 1977.)*
29. Mant, M. J., Hirsh, J., Pineo, G. F., et al. Prolonged prothrombin time and partial

thromboplastin time in disseminated intravascular coagulation not due to deficiency of factors V and VIII. *Br. J. Haematol.* 24:725, 1973.
Vitamin K deficiency or liver disease complicating DIC.

30. Feinstein, D. I. Diagnosis and management of disseminated intravascular coagulation: the role of heparin therapy. *Blood* 60:284, 1982.
Excellent advice. Heparin is rarely indicated. (See also Med. Clin. North. Am. *56:193, 1972 and* Semin. Thromb. Hemost. *14:351, 1988.)*

31. Goldberg, M. A., Ginsburg, D., Mayer, R. J., et al. Is heparin administration necessary during induction chemotherapy for patients with acute promyelocytic leukemia? *Blood* 69:187, 1987.
Heparin is not recommended.

32. Bell, W. R., Tomasulo, P. A., Alving, B. M., et al. Thrombocytopenia occurring during the administration of heparin. *Ann. Intern. Med.* 85:155, 1976.
Heparin-induced DIC and thrombocytopenia.

33. Corrigan, J. J., and Jordan, C. M. Heparin therapy in septicemia with disseminated intravascular coagulation. *N. Engl. J. Med.* 283:778, 1970.
Correction of hypotension is more important than heparin therapy in improving survival.

34. Green, D., Seeler, R. A., Allen, N., et al. The role of heparin in the management of consumption coagulopathies. *Med. Clin. North Am.* 56:193, 1972.
An important warning about the dangers of heparin therapy.

35. Straub, P. W. A case against heparin therapy of intravascular coagulation. *Thromb. Diath. Hemorrh.* 33:107, 1974.
Many other disease processes can mimic DIC.

36. Bell, W. R. Heparin-associated thrombocytopenia and thrombosis. *J. Lab. Clin. Med.* 111:600, 1988.
Comments by an expert.

37. Litt, M. R., Bell, W. R., and Lepor, H. A. Disseminated intravascular coagulation in prostatic carcinoma reversed by ketoconazole. *J.A.M.A.* 258:1361, 1987.
An interesting new therapeutic approach.

38. Neidhart, J. A., and Roach, R. W. Successful treatment of skeletal hemangioma and Kasabach-Merritt syndrome with aminocaproic acid. *Am. J. Med.* 73:434, 1982.
A situation in which EACA may be useful. (See also N. Engl. J. Med. *313:309, 1985.)*

39. Cole, M. S., Minifee, P. K., and Wolma, F. J. Coumarin necrosis—a review of the literature. *Surgery* 103:271, 1988.
A useful review.

93. ERYTHROCYTOSIS AND POLYCYTHEMIA
Jerry L. Spivak

Under normal circumstances, the production of red blood cells is regulated to maintain the circulating red cell mass within narrow limits that differ for men and women. Red blood cell production is regulated by the hormone erythropoietin. When tissue oxygen demands exceed oxygen supply and the deficit cannot be corrected by adjustments of blood flow, respiration, or hemoglobin-oxygen affinity, there is an increase in erythropoietin production, which leads to an increase in erythropoiesis and eventually an elevation of the red cell mass, if tissue hypoxia is not corrected. Although the erythrocytosis serves to increase blood oxygen-carrying capacity, if the red cell mass exceeds a certain limit, systemic oxygen transport declines due to the increase in blood viscosity. An elevated hematocrit is usually the first clue to the presence of erythrocytosis. However, the hematocrit merely reflects the ratio of the red cell mass to the plasma volume and thus is not itself sufficient to establish the diagnosis of an absolute erythrocytosis. For this purpose, an independent determination of the red cell mass must be performed. Red cell mass is usually determined by isotope dilution, a technique that can give falsely low results in a patient with erythrocytosis, particularly when there is substantial splenomegaly associated with it, unless at least 90 minutes is allowed for equilibration of the radiolabeled red cells within the expanded blood pool. Determination of the red cell mass by extrapolation based on a direct determination of the plasma volume is unsatisfactory for establishing the presence of erythrocytosis. Relative erythrocytosis due to profound dehydration can occur from a variety of causes (diarrhea, diuretics, diaphoresis, deprivation of water, emesis, ethanol ingestion, and polyuria). A red cell mass determination is most valuable in distinguishing true erythrocytosis from pseudo or spurious erythrocytosis (Geisböck's syndrome). The latter, which is due to the combination of a low plasma volume and a normal red cell mass, is most often seen in individuals who have chronically elevated levels of carbon monoxide levels in the blood as a consequence of cigarette smoking.

True erythrocytosis is due to either an increase in erythropoietin production or an autonomous increase in erythropoiesis. Erythropoietin production is normally stimulated by tissue hypoxia. Disorders that impair tissue oxygen delivery and cause polycythemia include intrinsic pulmonary disease, intrapulmonic or intracardiac right-to-left shunts, impaired ventilation due to neuromuscular disease or obesity, abnormal hemoglobin with altered oxygen affinity or impaired binding of 2,3-diphosphoglycerate (2,3-DPG), reduced 2,3-DPG production, and renal ischemia. The most common cause of hypoxic erythrocytosis encountered in clinical practice is an elevation in the concentration of carboxyhemoglobin. Chronic elevation of the carboxyhemoglobin level may be due to environmental or occupational exposure, but cigarette smoking alone (one to two packs/day) can result in carboxyhemoglobin elevations of 10 to 20 times normal. These levels are high enough to significantly alter tissue oxygen delivery and promote erythrocytosis. The pathophysiology of this disorder is discussed in Chapter 11. Androgen therapy, particularly in women, is another correctable cause of erythrocytosis.

Inappropriate secretion of erythropoietin by certain tumors can result in erythrocytosis. Tumors associated with erythrocytosis include hypernephroma, hepatoma, uterine leiomyomata, cerebellar hemangioblastoma, adrenal adenoma, and pheochromocytoma. It is of interest that hypernephroma, cerebellar hemangioblastoma, and pheochromocytoma can all be seen as part of the von Hippel-Lindau syndrome.

In polycythemia vera, the increase in red cell mass is due to an autonomous proliferation of red cells that are responsive to erythropoietin but appear not to require it for proliferation. Using patients heterozygous for the isoenzymes of glucose-6-phosphate dehydrogenase (G-6-PD) it has been established that polycythemia vera is a clonal disorder of a pluripotent hematopoietic stem cell. An increase in the number of circulating red cells, white cells, and platelets is usual in this disorder but it is the increase in red cell mass that is responsible for the bulk of the clinical manifestations. Polycythemia vera is a disease of individuals over the age of 60. In most patients, the disorder presents as a panmyelopathy, but in some, erythrocytosis may be the only manifestation. Differentiation of erythropoietin-mediated erythrocytosis and the inappropriate erythrocytosis of polycythemia vera can usually be made by plasma erythropoietin assay. Unless there is a complicating feature, such as congestive failure, pulmonary embolization, pulmonary parenchymal disease, or central nervous system lesions, the arterial oxygen saturation in polycythemia vera is always above 90 percent. Other helpful features are the presence of leukocytosis, thrombocytosis, basophilia, hyperuricemia, elevation of both leukocyte alkaline phosphatase and unsaturated vitamin B_{12}–binding capacity, and splenomegaly. Patients with polycythemia vera have an increased incidence of peptic ulcer disease, and the diagnosis may initially be obscured by the presence of iron-deficiency anemia.

The development of an increased red cell mass in polycythemia vera is usually accompanied by an increase in the plasma volume, a compensatory increase in cardiac output and a decrease in peripheral vascular resistance. As a result the increase in blood viscosity is offset and tissue oxygen delivery is maintained. The cardiovascular response to polycythemia is conditioned by the state of the cardiovascular system. With cardiac disease or atherosclerosis, compensation for the increased blood viscosity is incomplete. As the hematocrit rises above 65 percent, tissue oxygen delivery is also reduced, even under normal circumstances. In addition, in cyanotic congenital heart disease or smoker's erythrocytosis, the increase in red cell mass is usually associated with a reduction in plasma volume, leading to further impairment of tissue oxygen delivery.

Once the presence of an elevated red cell mass has been established, attention should be directed toward defining the cause of the erythrocytosis and at the same time reducing the red cell mass. Even when the erythrocytosis is secondary to cardiopulmonary disease, a reduction in the red cell mass leads to symptomatic improvement. While in patients with cardiopulmonary disorders it is usually sufficient to reduce the hematocrit to below 55, in patients with polycythemia vera sufficient blood should be removed to bring the hematocrit below 45 in men and 42 in women. With continuous phlebotomy, a state of iron deficiency can be induced so that only periodic phlebotomy is necessary to maintain a hematocrit at the desired limit. The reduction in red cell mass reduces the risk of thrombosis and hemorrhage in these patients, and no patient with polycythemia vera should undergo any surgical procedure until the red cell mass has been lowered. In older persons with cardiac failure or atherosclerosis, it may be necessary to remove less than 500 ml at one time and replace the blood removed with a volume expander. This will avert an abrupt lowering of the blood volume without changing the hematocrit and the attendant possibility of a stroke.

As part of the natural history of polycythemia vera, there is gradual expansion of the abnormal clone with suppression of hematopoiesis by normal precursors. Eventually, the proliferative capacity of the abnormal clone declines. Ineffective erythropoiesis increases and myelofibrosis with extramedullary hematopoiesis ensues. Acute leukemia appears to be a terminal event in some patients. The frequency with which this occurs appears to depend on whether the patient has been treated with either phosphorus 32 or an alkylating agent. A large cooperative study has indicated that the use of either phosphorus 32 or alkylating agents such as chlorambucil does not lead to improved survival when compared to treatment by vigorous phlebotomy alone. These agents, however, do lead to an increased incidence of acute leukemia. The cornerstone of therapy for polycythemia vera is phlebotomy but sufficient blood must be removed to lower the hematocrit below 45 and maintain it there. If this is done, the incidence of thromboembolic events in patients with polycythemia vera is not increased over the general population even when thrombocytosis is present. Hydroxyurea may have a role in patients who are too incapacitated to undergo repeated phlebotomy. On the other hand, there appears to be no role for alkylating agents in this disorder and there is sufficient clinical evidence to support the contention that it is the elevated red cell mass and not the thrombocytosis that is responsible for the vascular complications in patients with polycythemia vera. These patients do, of course, suffer from excessive histamine production and hyperuricemia. They will benefit from the use of antihistamines and, when necessary, allopurinol. Salicylates may be dangerous and should be avoided. Finally, it should be remembered that in the patient with erythrocytosis, the amount of anticoagulant necessary for blood collection is less than for individuals with a normal red cell mass. Failure to appreciate this fact will result in abnormal values for coagulation tests such as the prothrombin time.

1. Adamson, J. W., Fialkow, P. J., Murphy, S., et al. Polycythemia vera: Stem cell and probable clonal origin of the disease. *N. Engl. J. Med.* 295:913, 1976.
   Isoenzymes of G-6-PD used to establish the clonal nature of polycythemia vera.
2. Golde, D. W., Hocking, W. G., Koeffler, H. P., et al. Polycythemia mechanisms and management. *Ann. Intern. Med.* 95:71, 1981.
   Comprehensive review with important information on cell kinetics in polycythemia vera.
3. Smith, J. R., and Landau, S. A. Smokers' polycythemia. *N. Engl. J. Med.* 298:6, 1978.
   Carboxyhemoglobin levels are sufficiently elevated to produce hypoxemia, erythrocytosis and a reduced plasma volume.
4. Conley, C. L. Polycythemia vera. Diagnosis and treatment. *Hosp. Pract.* 22(March):181, 1987.
   Comments by an expert.

5. Adamson, J. W. The erythropoietin/hematocrit relationship in normal and polycy-themic man: Implications of narrow regulation. *Blood* 32:597, 1968.
   In polycythemia vera, erythropoietin is undetectable until the hematocrit is reduced to normal.
6. Cotes, P. M., Doré, C. J., Liu Yin, J. T., et al. Determination of serum immunoreactive erythropoietin in the investigation of erythrocytosis. *N. Engl. J. Med.* 315:283, 1986.
   Use of an accurate erythropoietin assay to identify patients with secondary erythro-cytosis. (For cyanotic congenital heart disease, see Blood *70:822, 1987.)*
7. Spivak, J. L., and Cooke, C. R. Polycythemia vera in an anephric man. *Am. J. Med. Sci.* 272:339, 1976.
   Erythropoietin is not required for erythropoiesis in polycythemia vera.
8. Silverstein, M. N. Post-polycythemia myeloid metaplasia. *Arch. Intern. Med.* 134:113, 1974.
   Occasionally myeloid metaplasia precedes the onset of erythrocytosis.
9. Balcerzak, S. P., and Bromberg, P. A. Secondary polycythemia. *Semin. Hematol.* 12:353, 1975.
   Part of a symposium on polycythemia.
10. Prchal, J. T., Crist, W. M., Goldwasser, E., et al. Autosomal dominant polycythemia. *Blood* 66:1208, 1985.
    Interesting but unexplained cases of familial erythrocytosis. (See also Blood *56:233, 1980 and 58:1155, 1981.)*
11. Moore-Gillon, J. C., Treacher, D. F., Gaminara, E. J., et al. Intermittent hypoxia in patients with unexplained polycythaemia. *Br. J. Haematol.* 293:588, 1986.
    Something to remember.
12. Hutchison, D. C. S., Sapru, R. P., and Seimerling, M. D. Cirrhosis, cyanosis, and polycythemia: Multiple pulmonary arteriovenous anastomoses. *Am. J. Med.* 45:139, 1968.
    Venous admixture effect resulting in hypoxia and secondary polycythemia.
13. Thorling, E. B. Paraneoplastic erythrocytosis and inappropriate erythropoietin pro-duction. *Scand. J. Haematol. (Suppl.)* 17:13, 1972.
    The best reference on the topic.
14. Wu, K. K., Gibson, T. P., Freeman, R. M., et al. Erythrocytosis after renal transplan-tation. *Arch. Intern. Med.* 132:898, 1973.
    Erythrocytosis appears to be more common with cadaver kidneys.
15. Sonneborn, R., Perez, G. O., Epstein, M., et al. Erythrocytosis associated with the nephrotic syndrome. *Arch. Intern. Med.* 137:1068, 1977.
    Focal sclerosing glomerulonephritis appears to be associated with erythrocytosis.
16. Kaplan, J. P., Sprayregan, S., Ossias, A. L., et al. Erythropoietin-producing renal cyst and polycythemia vera: Clarification of their relationship. *Am. J. Med.* 54:819, 1973.
    Polycythemia vera is usually the cause of erythrocytosis in patients with renal cysts.
17. Stephens, A. D. Polycythaemia and high affinity haemoglobins. *Br. J. Haematol.* 36:153, 1977.
    Brief review.
18. Weil, J. V., Jamieson, G., Brown, D. W., et al. The red cell mass–arterial oxygen relationship in normal man. *J. Clin. Invest.* 47:1627, 1968.
    Oxygen saturation, not oxygen tension, is the important determinant of the erythro-poietic response to hypoxia.
19. Murray, J. F. Arterial studies in primary and secondary polycythemic disorders. *Am. Rev. Respir. Dis.* 92:435, 1965.
    Oxygen saturation in uncomplicated polycythemia vera is always greater than 90%.
20. Wasserman, L. R., and Gilbert, H. S. Surgery in polycythemia vera. *N. Engl. J. Med.* 269:1226, 1963.
    High incidence of hemorrhage or thrombosis unless the red cell volume is reduced to normal.
21. Clain, D., Freston, J., Kreel, L., et al. Clinical diagnosis of the Budd-Chiari syn-drome. *Am. J. Med.* 43:544, 1967.
    Polycythemia vera is a common cause of hepatic vein thrombosis.

22. Pearson, T. C., and Wetherley-Mein, G. Vascular occlusive episodes and venous hae-matocrit in primary proliferative polycythaemia. *Lancet* 2:1219, 1978.
    Thromboembolism correlated with the hematocrit and not the platelet count.
23. Thomas, D. J., Marshall, J., Russell, R. W. R., et al. Cerebral blood-flow in polycy-thaemia. *Lancet* 2:161, 1977.
    Cerebal blood flow improved when the hematocrit was reduced below 46%.
24. Oldershaw, P. J., and Sutton, M. G. Haemodynamic effects of hematocrit reduction in patients with polycythemia secondary to cyanotic congenital heart disease. *Br. Heart J.* 44:584, 1980.
    Phlebotomy improves circulatory dynamics.
25. York, E. L., Jones, R. L., Sproule, B. J., et al. Management of secondary polycythemia with hypoxic lung disease. *Am. Heart J.* 100:267, 1980.
    Symptomatic improvement with phlebotomy was attributed to improved cerebral blood flow. (See also Chest 68:785, 1975.)
26. Sivolin, B., Weinfeld, A., and Westin, M. A prospective, long-term cytogenetic study in polycythemia vera in relation to treatment and clinical course. *Blood* 72:386, 1988.
    An abnormal karyotype is common in this disorder but was not predictive of myelo-fibrosis or acute leukemia. (See Cancer Genet. Cytogenet. 25:233, 1987.)
27. Modan, B., and Lilienfeld, A. M. Polycythemia vera and leukemia: The role of radia-tion treatment. *Medicine* 44:305, 1965.
    X-ray or phosphorus 32 therapy associated with an increased incidence of acute leu-kemia. (See also Blood 52:350, 1978.
28. Berk, P. D., Goldberg, J. D., Silverstein, M. N., et al. Increased incidence of acute leukemia in polycythemia vera associated with chlorambucil therapy. *N. Engl. J. Med.* 304:441, 1981.
    Phlebotomy is the therapy of choice in polycythemia vera. Alkylating agents are con-traindicated. (See also Cancer 61:89, 1988.
29. Meytes, D., Katz, D., and Ramot, B. Preleukemia and leukemia in polycythemia vera. *Blood* 47:237, 1976.
    A sideroblastic preleukemic phase preceded the onset of acute leukemia.
30. Kaplan, M. E., Mack, K., Goldberg, J. D., et al. Long-term management of polycy-themia vera with hydroxyurea. *Semin. Hematol.* 23:167, 1986.
    Hydroxyurea is not without risks.
31. Najean, Y., Deschamps, A., Dresch, C., et al. Acute leukemia and myelodysplasia in polycythemia vera. *Cancer* 61:89, 1988.
    The clinical features are similar to other secondary leukemias.
32. Tartaglia, A. P., Goldberg, J. D., Berk, P. D., et al. Adverse effects of antiaggregating platelet therapy in the treatment of polycythemia vera. *Semin. Hematol.* 23:172, 1986.
    Salicylates and dipyridamole should be avoided in patients with polycythemia vera. Phlebotomy is the key.

94. FOLIC ACID DEFICIENCY
Jerry L. Spivak

Folic acid, like vitamin B_{12}, is an essential vitamin. However, in contrast to vitamin B_{12}, conservation of folic acid in man is not efficient, and interruption of supply results in a deficiency state within 4 months. The deficiency state is accelerated if body stores of folic acid are low, if there is concurrent ethanol ingestion, or if demands for the vitamin are substantially increased. Folic acid deficiency can develop with (1) ingestion of a diet lacking in liver, leafy vegetables, and fresh fruits, (2) excessive boiling of food, (3) intestinal malabsorption, (4) hemodialysis, (5) drug antagonism, and when (6) there is an imbalance between supply and demand (e.g., in pregnancy, thyrotoxicosis, hemolytic anemia, and exfoliative dermatitis). The deficiency state results in changes in epithelial and hematopoietic cells that are indistinguishable from those occurring with vitamin B_{12} lack. Folic acid deficiency does not itself result in damage to nervous tissue, but neurologic abnormalities may be present when the deficiency state is due to conditions such as malnutrition or ethanol abuse. In addition, since both folate deficiency and ethanol abuse impair vitamin B_{12} absorption, a combined deficiency state may occur. Serum vitamin B_{12} and red cell folate levels may not always be helpful in determining the cause of megaloblastic hematopoiesis. The serum vitamin B_{12} level is falsely low in approximately 50 percent of patients with folic acid deficiency while red cell folate may be falsely low in patients with vitamin B_{12} deficiency. When iron deficiency coexists with folic acid deficiency, red cell folate levels can be normal and megaloblastic changes in erythroid cells are suppressed. In this instance, neutrophil hypersegmentation may be the only clue to the presence of folic acid deficiency. Since the level of folic acid in the serum is influenced by dietary intake, it cannot be used as a measure of tissue folate stores. The serum folate level may also be falsely high when there is coexisting folate and vitamin B_{12} deficiency. When the serum vitamin B_{12} level is falsely low in a patient with folic acid deficiency, it will increase with folic acid replacement. Since serum vitamin B_{12} and red cell folate levels will not be available at the time of treatment, it is advisable in the acutely ill patient to administer both vitamins initially. The possibility of vitamin B_{12} malabsorption can be evaluated after the patient is stable.

Absorption and utilization of folic acid are antagonized by a number of drugs in common use. Many chemotherapeutic agents exert their effects by inhibiting folate metabolism. They include methotrexate, pyrimethamine, trimethoprim, and pentamidine. The diuretic triamterene is structurally similar to these agents and has occasionally been associated with megaloblastic anemia. Folic acid is not effective in reducing toxicity due to the chemotherapeutic agents, but folinic acid (citrovorum factor), which bypasses the metabolic block, may alleviate toxicity without interfering with the therapeutic effect of the antimetabolite. Anticonvulsants appear to increase the catabolism of folic acid while oral contraceptives may increase its excretion. Folic acid deficiency does not occur in either instance, unless the diet is markedly deficient in folic acid. Therapy with folic acid does not impair seizure control. Ethanol does not impair absorption of unconjugated folic acid, but its effect on food folate is unknown. Folate deficiency occurring with ethanol abuse is due to a combination of dietary inadequacy and interference with folate metabolism by ethanol. In addition to folate deficiency, such patients are usually deficient in other vitamins, such as thiamine, niacin, pyridoxine, and ascorbic acid. Multivitamin therapy is thus indicated.

1. Herbert, V. Experimental nutritional folate deficiency in man. *Trans. Assoc. Am. Physicians* 75:307, 1962.
   A classic study.
2. Sullivan, L. W., and Herbert, V. Suppression of hematopoiesis by ethanol. *J. Clin. Invest.* 43:2048, 1964.
   An important study of the interaction of ethanol and folic acid.
3. Eichner, E. R., and Hillman, R. S. The evolution of anemia in alcoholic patients. *Am. J. Med.* 50:218, 1971.
   Explanation of the spectrum of hematologic abnormalities seen with alcohol abuse.
4. Eichner, E. R., and Hillman, R. S. Effect of alcohol on serum folate level. *J. Clin. Invest.* 52:584, 1973.
   Inhibition of folic acid metabolism by alcohol.
5. Halsted, C. H., Robles, E. A., and Mezey, E. Decreased jejunal uptake of labeled folic acid (^{3}H-PGA) in alcoholic patients: Roles of alcohol and nutrition. *N. Engl. J. Med.* 285:701, 1971.
   Alcohol does not impair absorption of unconjugated folic acid.
6. Lindenbaum, J., and Klipstein, F. A. Folic acid deficiency in sickle-cell anemia. *N. Engl. J. Med.* 269:875, 1963.
   The requirement for folic acid is increased with hemolytic anemia.

7. Hershko, C., Grossowicz, N., Rachmilewitz, M., et al. Serum and erythrocyte folates in combined iron and folate deficiency. *Am. J. Clin. Nutr.* 28:1217, 1975.
   Red cell but not serum folate levels are a reliable index of tissue folate stores.
8. Van Der Weyden, M. B., Rother, M., and Firken, B. G. The metabolic significance of reduced serum B_{12} in folate deficiency. *Blood* 40:23, 1972.
   Vitamin B_{12} does not correct an anemia due to folic acid deficiency.
9. Hermos, J. A., Adams, W. H., Liu, Y. K., et al. Mucosa of the small intestine in folate-deficient alcoholics. *Ann. Intern. Med.* 76:957, 1972.
   Severity of intestinal lesion correlates with severity of marrow megaloblastosis.
10. Rose, M., and Johnson, I. Reinterpretation of the haematological effects of anticonvulsant treatment. *Lancet* 1:1349, 1978.
    Macrocytic anemia in patients taking anticonvulsants is due to poor nutrition.
11. Corcino, J., Waxman, S., and Herbert, V. Mechanism of triamterene-induced megaloblastosis. *Ann. Intern. Med.* 73:419, 1970.
    Inhibition of folate reduction by a structurally similar drug.
12. Waxman, S., and Herbert, V. Mechanism of pyrimethamine-induced megaloblastosis in human bone marrow. *N. Engl. J. Med.* 380:1316, 1969.
    Drug effect is corrected by folinic acid.
13. Kabinsky, N. L., and Ramsay, N. K. C. Acute megaloblastic anemia induced by high-dose trimethroprim-sulfamethoxazole. *Ann. Intern. Med.* 94:789, 1981.
    Pancytopenia and megaloblastic maturation occurred in a setting of impaired food intake and increased demand for folic acid.
14. Skoutakis, V. A., Acchiardo, S. R., Meyer, M. C., et al. Folic acid dosage for chronic hemodialysis patients. *Clin. Pharmacol. Ther.* 18:200, 1975.
    Administration of 1 mg of folic acid after each dialysis prevents deficiency.
15. Hild, D. H. Folate losses from the skin in exfoliative dermatitis. *Arch. Intern. Med.* 123:51, 1969.
    Significant amounts of folic acid can be lost with exfoliation.
16. Carmel, R. The laboratory diagnosis of megaloblastic anemias. *West. J. Med.* 128:294, 1978.
    An important review of the pitfalls and problems in the diagnosis of folic acid and vitamin B_{12} deficiency.
17. Lindenbaum, J. Status of laboratory testing in the diagnosis of megaloblastic anemia. *Blood* 61:624, 1983.
    Concise review.
18. Herbert, V. Making sense of laboratory tests of folate status: Folate requirements to sustain normality. *Am. J. Hematol.* 26:199, 1987.
19. Carmel, R. Artifactual radioassay results due to serum contamination by intravenous radioisotope administration: Falsely low serum vitamin B_{12} and folic acid results. *Am. J. Clin. Pathol.* 70:364, 1977.
    Technetium 99m and gallium 67 can interfere with the serum assays for vitamin B_{12} and folic acid.
20. Breedveld, F. C., Bieger, R., and van Wermeskerken, R. K. A. The clinical significance of macrocytosis. *Acta Med. Scand.* 209:319, 1981.
    Macrocytosis can occur in a variety of disorders.
21. Wu, A., Chanarin, I., and Levi, A. J. Macrocytosis of chronic alcoholism. *Lancet* 1:829, 1974.
    Macrocytosis unrelated to folate deficiency is a common finding with chronic ethanol abuse.
22. Bessman, J. D., and Banks, D. Spurious macrocytosis: A common clue to erythrocyte cold agglutinins. *Am. J. Clin. Pathol.* 74:797, 1980.
    Another situation in which the electronic particle counter provides a spurious result.
23. Spivak, J. L. Masked megaloblastic anemia. *Arch. Intern. Med.* 142:2111, 1982.
    Masked megaloblastic anemia is not uncommon; neutrophil hypersegmentation is an important clue. (See also Br. J. Haematol. 44:511, 1980.)
24. Nath, B. J., and Lindenbaum, J. Persistence of neutrophil hypersegmentation during recovery from megaloblastic granulopoiesis. *Ann. Intern. Med.* 90:757, 1979.
    The persistence of neutrophil hypersegmentation is a valuable clue to previous megaloblastic hematopoiesis in a patient treated with folic acid or vitamin B_{12}.

25. Lindenbaum, J. Folate and vitamin B_{12} deficiencies in alcoholism. *Semin. Hematol.* 17:119, 1980.
    Brief review.
26. Halsted, C. H., Gandhi, G., and Tamura, T. Sulfasalazine inhibits the absorption of folates in ulcerative colitis. *N. Engl. J. Med.* 305:1513, 1981.
    Supplemental folic acid should be given to patients taking sulfasalazine.
27. Feussner, J. R., Shelburne, J. D., Bredehoeft, S., et al. Arsenic-induced bone marrow toxicity. *Blood* 53:820, 1979.
    An unusual cause of megaloblastic erythropoiesis.

95. GRANULOCYTOPENIA
Jerry L. Spivak

Evaluation of the granulocytopenic patient is facilitated by an understanding of granulocyte physiology. In the bone marrow, granulocytes can be divided into two pools, mitotic and storage. The mitotic pool consists of all cells up to the myelocyte stage. These cells are capable of DNA synthesis and cell division. The storage pool, which normally contains enough cells to maintain the blood neutrophil level for 4 days in the absence of production by the mitotic pool, consists of metamyelocytes and juvenile and polymorphonuclear granulocytes. The orderly release of granulocytes from the marrow appears to be governed in part by a decrease in cell size and surface charge and an increase in cell deformability, adhesiveness, and motility—changes that normally occur during cell maturation. Other factors, such as marrow architecture, blood flow, and humoral agents (corticosteroids, endotoxin, and lithium), also affect granulocyte release. The relationship of granulocyte production and release to the size of the blood neutrophil pool is still undefined.

Blood granulocytes can also be divided into two pools. The blood neutrophil count reflects only the circulating granulocyte pool, which is in equilibrium with a marginating granulocyte pool. The latter consists of granulocytes that do not participate in axial blood flow and are presumably marginated along vessel walls. The proportion of cells in each pool is approximately equal under normal circumstances but may be altered in disease. The mature neutrophil spends a very short time in the bloodstream; its circulating half-life is approximately 7 hours. Neutrophils leave the bloodstream randomly and not from senescence.

Granulocytopenia may occur on a genetic basis or may be produced by drugs, toxins, vitamin deficiencies, hypersplenism, hematologic disorders, or systemic diseases that secondarily affect the marrow. Prior granulocyte counts are helpful in establishing the duration of the problem. Inquiry directed to the onset of infectious complications is also helpful in determining the duration of granulocytopenia and its severity. Granulocytopenia is usually associated with infections in "dirty" areas, such as the mouth, rectum, and sites of superficial trauma. The family history should be examined carefully for evidence of a genetic basis. The investigation may require granulocyte counts in relatives. Familial neutropenia may be cyclic or noncyclic and variable in expression with respect to age of onset, severity of the neutropenia, and incidence and severity of infections. In general, the severity of infections declines with increasing age. It is important to recognize that blacks, particularly males, may have neutrophil counts less than 1500 per microliter. The history should also place emphasis on arthritic symptoms, particularly in women, since granulocytopenia may occur in early rheumatoid arthritis without the other features of Felty's syndrome.

Physical examination of the granulocytopenic patient may reveal arthritic deformities, splenomegaly, or the adipose lesions of Weber-Christian disease. Bony tenderness should suggest leukemia or marrow necrosis.

Examination of a bone marrow aspirate may reveal normal granulopoiesis, a paucity of granulocyte precursors, absence of mature granulocytes (the storage pool), megaloblastic maturation, or leukemic cells. Rarely, necrotic marrow may be obtained. The presence of normal granulopoietic activity provides no assurance that either marrow production or granulocyte reserves are adequate. A paucity or absence of mature neutrophils (storage pool) with the persistence of immature forms (mitotic pool) is the pattern incorrectly described as "maturation arrest." This pattern may be seen when the storage pool is exhausted or when the marrow is recovering from granulocyte hypoplasia. True maturation arrest occurs only in leukemia or with deficiency of vitamin B_{12} or folic acid. If marrow cannot be aspirated, the physician should suspect the existence of reticulin fibrosis. This may be the presenting sign of acute leukemia in the adult. Although a high serum muramidase level may be found in myelofibrosis and in untreated megaloblastic anemia in which ineffective granulopoiesis is occurring, measurement of this enzyme is usually of little aid in the differential diagnosis of granulocytopenia. With granulocytopenia, measurement of leukocyte alkaline phosphatase is difficult, but the possibility of paroxysmal nocturnal hemoglobinuria can be pursued with a sucrose hemolysis test.

The single most important cause of neutropenia is drug ingestion. In addition to chemotherapeutic agents, the following can produce profound granulocytopenia: sulfonamides, oral hypoglycemic agents, methicillin, nafcillin, carbenicillin, gentamicin, thiazides, phenylbutazone, dapsone, phenothiazines, propylthiouracil, methimazole, phenindione, phenytoin, procainamide and other antiarrhythmic agents, cimetidine, and chloramphenicol. Granulocytopenia due to chloramphenicol as a dose-related effect is much less common than anemia or thrombocytopenia. Although phenothiazines have been shown to inhibit DNA synthesis, with most other drugs the granulocytopenia appears to be idiosyncratic and due to the development of antineutrophil antibodies. Many patients taking phenothiazines or antithyroid agents develop a slightly low neutrophil count but this is not an indication for stopping therapy. There is no correlation between this mild neutropenia and the development of agranulocytosis. Often the neutrophil count returns to normal with or without a reduction in drug dose. A review of the literature indicates that some patients with mild granulocytopenia while taking these drugs had low neutrophil counts before starting therapy. In addition to drugs, exposure to toxins such as benzene and arsenic should be investigated.

Regardless of the cause of the granulocytopenia, the physician should treat the patient, not the neutrophil count. Patients have been described with long-standing granulocytopenia but without recurrent infections. A normal or low circulating blood granulocyte count may even be associated with an enlarged marginating granulocyte pool. The important point is that neutrophils be mobilized to the area of microbial invasion early, in adequate numbers, and with phagocytic capability. Examination of an inflammatory exudate should provide an indication of a patient's ability to mobilize neutrophils.

Recent studies employing in vitro clonal assays for hematopoietic progenitor cells and sensitive techniques for neutrophil antibodies have not only established that immune-associated neutropenia may involve committed granulocyte progenitor cells alone or in addition to circulating neutrophils but also have provided a means for identifying the mechanism of neutropenia in situations where this was not formerly possible. Furthermore, these assays can provide a sound basis for therapeutic decisions such as administering corticosteroids to a neutropenic patient and for monitoring such therapy.

Neutropenic patients are most at risk of infection when the absolute granulocyte count is below 500 per microliter in the presence of an underlying disorder such as acute leukemia, which compromises host defenses. Isolation under the appropriate conditions and administration of antibiotics that reduce pathogenic aerobic gut flora appear to reduce the incidence of infection. Simple protective isolation as practiced on general medical wards does not. Antibiotics should not be administered unless there are clinical signs of infection. Most granulocytopenic patients respond to infection with fever, but the inflammatory response is otherwise muted. Induration is found when swelling or fluctuation might be expected. Careful examination of "dirty" areas (mouth, anus) is mandatory.

Much attention has been directed at the management of severe neutropenia, particularly in patients receiving cancer chemotherapy, with a view to maximizing antibiotic effectiveness and minimizing the toxicity of these drugs and avoiding superinfection with bacterial or fungal organisms. At present, in the severely granulocytopenic patient, administration of combination therapy (an anti-*pseudomonas* penicillin and an aminoglycoside) appears prudent. Granulocyte transfusions can be beneficial but not prophylactically.

The role of recombinant granulocyte–colony stimulating factor (G-CSF) and granulocyte macrophage–colony stimulating factor (GM–CSF) in the treatment of various forms of neutropenia is currently under intensive investigation. Studies in neutropenic patients with acquired immunodeficiency syndrome (AIDS) or aplastic anemia or in patients receiving chemotherapy have been promising.

1. Dancey, J. T., Deubelbeiss, K. A., Harker, L. A., et al. Neutrophil kinetics in man. *J. Clin. Invest.* 58:705, 1976.
   A detailed study of granulocyte production and life span.
2. Dale, D. C., Guerry, D., IV, Wewerka, J. R., et al. Chronic neutropenia. *Medicine* 58:128, 1979.
   A comprehensive evaluation of 29 patients. (See also Blood *55:915, 1980.)*
3. Kyle, R. A., and Linman, J. W. Chronic idiopathic neutropenia. *N. Engl. J. Med.* 279:1015, 1968.
   A benign syndrome usually seen in women. (For a follow-up of these patients see N. Engl. J. Med. *302:908, 1980.)*
4. Wright, D. G., Dale, D. C., Fauci, A. S., et al. Human cyclic neutropenia: Clinical review and long term follow-up of patients. *Medicine* 60:1, 1981.
   The most complete review of this disorder.
5. Mason, B. A., Lessin, L., and Schechter, G. P. Marrow granulocyte reserves in black Americans. *Am. J. Med.* 67:201, 1979.
   Neutropenia in some black individuals appears to be due to a reduction in granulocyte release from the marrow.
6. Joyce, R. A., and Boggs, D. R. Visualizing the marrow granulocyte reserve. *J. Lab. Clin. Med.* 93:101, 1979.
   If mature neutrophils (bands and segmented forms) constitute less than 25% of the nucleated cells, the neutrophil reserve pool is inadequate.
7. Dunlop, W. M., Watson-James, G., III, and Hume, D. M. Anemia and neutropenia caused by copper deficiency. *Ann. Intern. Med.* 80:470, 1974.
   Vacuolization of marrow precursors, sideroblasts, and granulocytopenia. (See also Am. J. Hematol. *3:177, 1977.)*
8. Arneborn, P., and Palmblad, J. Drug-induced neutropenias in the Stockholm region 1976–1977. *Acta Med. Scand.* 206:241, 1979.
   Sulfonamides, antithyroid drugs, and phenothiazines were the most common offenders.
9. Weitzman, S. A., Stossel, T. P., and Desmond, M. Drug-induced immunological neutropenia. *Lancet* 1:1068, 1978.
   Identification of antibodies as a cause of drug-induced neutropenia. (See also Am. J. Med. Sci. *291:51, 1986 and* Am. J. Med. *85:264, 1988.)*
10. Wiberg, J. J., and Nuttal, F. Q. Methimazole toxicity from high doses. *Ann. Intern. Med.* 77:414, 1972.
    Granulocytopenia may precede the use of the drug. (See also Am. Intern. Med. *86:60, 1977.)*
11. Wing, S. S., and Fantus, I. G. Adverse immunologic effects of antithyroid drugs. *Can. Med. Assoc. J.* 136:121, 1987.
    Immunologic abnormalities are not limited to granulocytopenia.
12. Fibbe, W. E., Claas, F. H., Van der Star-Dijkstra, W., et al. Agranulocytosis induced by propylthiouracil: evidence of a drug dependent antibody reacting with granulocytes, monocytes, and haematopoietic progenitor cells. *Br. J. Haematol.* 64:363, 1986.
    See also Am. J. Med. *85:725, 1988.*

13. Levitt, L. J. Chlorpropamide-induced pure white cell aplasia. *Blood* 69:394, 1987.
    An antibody-mediated phenomenon. For an additional case involving ibuprofen, see
    N. Engl. J. Med. *314:624, 1986.*
14. Homayouni, H., Gross, P. A., Setia, N., et al. Leukopenia due to penicillin and ceph-
    alosporin homologues. *Arch. Intern. Med.* 139:827, 1979.
    With high-dose therapy, the risk of leukopenia increases. (See also Br. Heart J.
    36:216, 1974.)
15. Reyes, M. P., Palutke, M., and Lerner, A. M. Granulocytopenia associated with car-
    benicillin. *Am. J. Med.* 54:413, 1973.
    A direct cytotoxic effect on the marrow is postulated.
16. Markowitz, S. M., Rothkopf, M., Holden, F. D., et al. Nafcillin-induced agranulocy-
    tosis. *J.A.M.A.* 232:1150, 1975.
    *Nafcillin now joins a growing list of drugs capable of producing neutropenia. Gen-
    tamicin can also be added (*J.A.M.A. *232:1155, 1975).*
17. Mordenti, J., Ries, C., Brooks, G. F., et al. Vancomycin-induced neutropenia compli-
    cating bone marrow recovery in a patient with leukemia. Case report and review of
    the literature. *Am. J. Med.* 80:333, 1986.
    An interesting observation. (See also Am. J. Med. *81:1059, 1986 and* Am. J. Med. Sci.
    294:110, 1987.)
18. Logue, G. L., and Shimm, D. S. Autoimmune granulocytopenia. *Annu. Rev. Med.*
    31:191, 1980.
    Comprehensive review. (See also Br. J. Haematol. *43:595, 1979.)*
19. Blaschle, J., Goehen, N. E., Thompson, J. S., et al. Acquired agranulocytosis with
    granulocyte specific cytotoxic autoantibody. *Am. J. Med.* 66:717, 1979.
    Splenectomy was effective in correcting the neutropenia; steroids were not.
20. Loughran, T. P., Jr., Clark, E. A., Price, T. H., et al. Adult-onset cyclic neutropenia
    is associated with increased large granular lymphocytes. *Blood* 68:1082, 1986.
    *The expansion of the large granular lymphocyte population is usually clonal. (See
    also* J. Exp. Med. *164:2089, 1986.)*
21. Winton, E. F., Chan, W. C., Check, I., et al. Spontaneous regression of a monoclonal
    proliferation of large granular lymphocytes associated with reversal of anemia and
    neutropenia. *Blood* 67:1427, 1986.
    An interesting observation. (See also Blood *69:1204, 1987.)*
22. Kundel, D. W., Brecher, G., Borley, G. P., et al. Reticulin fibrosis and bone infarction
    in acute leukemia: Implications for prognosis. *Blood* 23:526, 1964.
    A cause of leukopenia and "dry" marrow aspiration.
23. Brown, C. H. Bone marrow necrosis: A study of seventy cases. *Johns Hopkins Med.
    J.* 131:189, 1972.
    An unusual cause of leukopenia.
24. Nauseef, W. M., and Maki, D. G. A study of the value of simple protective isolation
    in patients with granulocytopenia. *N. Engl. J. Med.* 304:448, 1981.
    Protective isolation alone is without benefit.
25. Bodey, G. R., Buckley, M., Sathe, Y. S., et al. Quantitative relationships between
    circulating leukocytes and infection in patients with acute leukemia. *Ann. Intern.
    Med.* 64:328, 1966.
    Risk of infection increases with granulocyte levels less than 1000/µl.
26. Sickles, E. A., Greene, W. H., and Wiernik, P. H. Clinical presentation of infection in
    granulocytopenic patients. *Arch. Intern. Med.* 135:715, 1975.
    Fever, erythema, and pain without swelling or pus.
27. Gill, F. A., Robinson, R., Maclowry, J. D., et al. The relationship of fever, granulocy-
    topenia, and antimicrobial therapy to bacteremia in cancer patients. *Cancer*
    39:1704, 1977.
    Bacteremia did not occur in the absence of fever.
28. Rubin, R. H. Empiric antibacterial therapy in granulocytopenia induced by cancer
    chemotherapy. *Ann. Intern. Med.* 108:134, 1988.
    *A β-lactam and an aminoglycoside should be employed initially if granulocytopenia
    is severe. Vancomycin should only be used when specifically indicated. (See also* Br.
    Med. J. *293:406, 1986.)*

29. Young, L. S. Empirical antimicrobial therapy in the neutropenic host. *N. Engl. J. Med.* 315:580, 1986.
   A balanced view in an area of controversy.
30. Rubin, M., Halthorn, J. W., Marshall, D., et al. Gram-positive infections and the use of vancomycin in 550 episodes of fever and neutropenia. *Ann. Intern. Med.* 108:30, 1988.
   Staphylococcal infections are common (Acta Med. Scand. 222:465, 1987) but vancomycin should not be employed empirically. Others advocate empiric vancomycin (Am. J. Med. 81:237, 1986).
31. DiNubile, M. J. Stopping antibiotic therapy in neutropenic patients. *Ann. Intern. Med.* 108:289, 1988.
   This is a difficult issue for which there is no "correct" answer. (See also Am. J. Med. 76:450, 1984.)
32. Talbot, G. H., Provencher, M., and Cassileth, P. A. Persistent fever after recovery from granulocytopenia in acute leukemia. *Arch. Intern. Med.* 148:129, 1988.
   Visceral fungal infections were the leading cause of fever.
33. Starnes, H. F., Jr., Moore, F. D., Jr., Mentzer, S., et al. Abdominal pain in neutropenic cancer patients. *Cancer* 57:616, 1986.
   Conservative management advocated (see also Am. J. Surg. 151:563, 1986) with radiologic follow-up (see Am. J. Roentgenol. 149:731, 1987) but others advocate a more aggressive approach (Arch Surg. 121:571, 1986).
34. Ognibene, F. P., Martin, S. E., Parker, M. M., et al. Adult respiratory distress syndrome in patients with severe neutropenia. *N. Engl. J. Med.* 315:547, 1986.
   Neutropenia does not protect against adult respiratory distress syndrome. (See also Am. Rev. Respir. Dis. 133:313, 1986 and Am. J. Med. Sci. 80:1022, 1986.)
35. Dana, B. W., Durie, B. G. M., White, R. F., et al. Concomitant administration of granulocyte transfusions and amphotericin B in neutropenic patients: Absence of significant pulmonary toxicity. *Blood* 57:90, 1981.
   For an opposing view see N. Engl. J. Med. 304:1185, 1981.
36. Herzig, R. H., Poplack, D. G., and Yankee, R. A. Prolonged granulocytopenia from incompatible platelet transfusion. *N. Engl. J. Med.* 290:1220, 1974.
   A hazard of unmatched platelets in patients with marrow suppression.
37. Three antibiotic regimens in the treatment of infection in febrile granulocytopenic patients with cancer. *J. Infect. Dis.* 137:14, 1978.
   Carbenicillin or ticarcillin plus an aminoglycoside provided the best therapeutic-toxic ratio.
38. Forlenza, S. W. *Capnocytophaga* sepsis: A newly recognised clinical entity in granulocytopenic patients. *Lancet* 1:567, 1980.
   Clindamycin or carbenicillin appeared to be effective against this organism.
39. Wright, D. G., Fauci, A. S., Dale, D. C., et al. Correction of human cyclic neutropenia with prednisolone. *N. Engl. J. Med.* 298:295, 1978.
   Alternate-day prednisolone restored myelopoiesis to normal.
40. Hammond, W. P., IV, Price, T. H., Souza, L. M., et al. Treatment of cyclic neutropenia with granulocyte colony-stimulating factor. *N. Engl. J. Med.* 320:1306, 1989.
   This may become the treatment of choice.
41. Jakubowski, A. A., Souza, L., Kelly, F., et al. Effects of human granulocyte colony-stimulating factor in a patient with idiopathic neutropenia. *N. Engl. J. Med.* 320:38, 1989.
   Correction of neutropenia with recombinant G-CSF. For correction of congenital agranulocytosis, see N. Engl. J. Med. 320:1574, 1989.
42. Gabrilove, J. L., Jakubowski, A., Scher, H., et al. Effect of granulocyte colony-stimulating factor on neutropenia and associated morbidity due to chemotherapy for transitional-cell carcinoma of the urothelium. *N. Engl. J. Med.* 318:1414, 1988.
   Use of a recombinant growth factor to offset the toxicity of chemotherapy. (See also Lancet 1:667, and 2:471, 1988.)
43. Bagby, G. C., Jr., Lawrence, H. J., and Neerhout, R. C. T-lymphocyte–mediated granulopoietic failure. *N. Engl. J. Med.* 309:1073, 1983.
   A correctable cause of neutropenia.

44. Talcott, J. A., Finberg, R., Mayer, R. J., et al. The medical course of cancer patients with fever and neutropenia. *Arch. Intern. Med.* 148:2561, 1988. *Identification of a low-risk subgroup.*

96. HEMOLYTIC ANEMIA
Jerry L. Spivak

Disorders resulting in increased red blood cell destruction can be classified as intracorpuscular or extracorpuscular and congenital or acquired. In the adult most intracorpuscular defects resulting in hemolysis are congenital. These include disorders of the red cell membrane (hereditary spherocytosis and elliptocytosis), hemoglobinopathies (thalassemia, sickle hemoglobin, hemoglobin C, and unstable hemoglobins such as Zurich, Köln, and Seattle), and enzyme defects (most commonly glucose-6-phosphate dehydrogenase [G-6-PD] deficiency and pyruvate kinase deficiency). Acquired intracorpuscular disorders include deficiency states (iron, vitamin B_{12}, and folic acid), the hemoglobinopathy occurring with myeloproliferative disorders (hemoglobin H), and paroxysmal nocturnal hemoglobinuria (PNH).

Extracorpuscular disorders resulting in red blood cell destruction include hypersplenic states, toxins (naphthalene and heavy metals), infection (clostridia, hemophilus, and malaria), liver disease, trauma (march or exercise, hemoglobinuria, disseminated intravascular coagulation [DIC], vasculitis, vascular tumors, carcinomatosis, thrombotic thrombocytopenic purpura [TTP], prosthetic valves, acquired valvular disease, eclampsia, and malignant hypertension), and immune hemolysis. Immune hemolysis can be produced by a variety of drugs (penicillin, α-methyldopa, cephalothin, phenacetin, ρ-aminosalicylic acid, quinidine, quinine, isoniazid, sulfonamides, chlorpropamide, stibophen, antithymocyte globulin, and chlorpromazine). A positive Coombs' test, however, does not always signify the presence of hemolysis, particularly when associated with hypergammaglobulinemia as in acquired immunodeficiency syndrome (AIDS) or with the use of cephalothin, levodopa, or α-methyldopa, while drugs such as the sulfonamides can hemolyze normal cells via nonimmune mechanisms. Other disorders in which red blood cell antibodies are produced include lymphomas, ovarian tumors, systemic lupus erythematosus (SLE), infections (atypical pneumonia, infectious mononucleosis, and syphilis), bone marrow transplantation, and transfusion reactions. As in the case of drug-induced immune hemolysis, a positive Coombs' test does not always indicate active hemolysis, nor does a negative Coombs' test assure the absence of a hemolytic process. The erythrocyte coating substance may be either IgG or complement or a combination of these two. When autoimmune hemolytic anemia complicates SLE, complement is usually present on the red cell surface while in certain drug-induced hemolytic anemias complement is not fixed to the red cell by the offending antibody. In many cases of autoimmune hemolytic anemia, the IgG coating antibody has been found to have a specificity for the Rh system, a finding that is true of the red cell antibody associated with α-methyldopa as well. IgM cold agglutinins, however, react specifically with the erythrocyte I antigen, except in infectious mononucleosis, in which the antibody is directed against the i antigen.

Evaluation of the patient suspected of having a hemolytic process begins with a careful family history, which should include inquiry about gallbladder disease as well as jaundice, anemia, and splenectomy. A detailed drug history is extremely important, as is the occupational and travel history. Data from prior hematologic studies help to date the onset of the patient's illness.

The most important initial laboratory test is examination of a well-made blood smear. Characteristic abnormalities suggesting a hemolytic process include spherocytes, fractured cells, spur cells, agglutinated cells, or blister cells. Blister cells owe their unique appearance to denaturation of only a portion of the cell's hemoglobin, and they are usually seen when there is oxidant injury to the red cell, as in G-6-PD deficiency. Hypochromic microcytic red cells will not lead one away from the diagnosis of a hemolytic process if it is remembered that disorders such as PNH and microangiopathic hemolytic anemia produce iron deficiency through intravascular hemolysis. Polychromatophilia and basophilic stippling representing the reticulocyte response are absent early in the course of an acute hemolytic process or when folic acid deficiency, iron deficiency, or an aplastic crisis supervenes during a chronic hemolytic disorder. Leukocytosis and thrombocytosis often accompany brisk hemolysis, but changes in both processes are influenced by the presence of underlying disease (splenomegaly, infection, hematologic malignancy, collagen-vascular disease, and vitamin B_{12} or folic acid deficiency) or by the hemolytic disorder (PNH, TTP, drugs, or autoimmune disease).

Although the indirect bilirubin level is usually elevated, the abnormality is obviously not specific for hemolytic anemia. Haptoglobin determination is helpful if it is found to be reduced or absent, but a normal level does not exclude the presence of a hemolytic process since haptoglobin is an acute-phase reactant. Hemopexin is not usually reduced in the presence of a normal haptoglobin level. Coagulation studies should be performed to exclude the presence of DIC. In patients with a compensated hemolytic anemia, a red cell survival study may be necessary to establish the presence of hemolysis. In a similar fashion, a normal G-6-PD level in the presence of an elevated reticulocyte count does not exclude a deficiency of this enzyme. Physical examination may also be misleading since in many patients with hemolytic anemia splenomegaly is absent.

Therapy in patients with hemolytic anemia is directed toward the underlying disorder or is supportive if there is no correctable problem. With autoimmune hemolytic anemia, corticosteroids are the initial therapy of choice. Splenectomy is reserved for treatment failures. In hereditary spherocytosis, the indications for splenectomy are more apparent in children than in adults, in whom decisions concerning splenectomy must be individualized. In other situations red blood cell sequestration studies may be of benefit, but negative findings do not preclude a successful result from splenectomy. A quick and simple test for possible splenic sequestration is measurement of the body-venous hematocrit ratio. If this is greater than unity, sequestration is strongly suggested. Crossmatching for transfusion in immune hemolytic states can present problems; often cautious infusion of the most compatible blood is the only solution. Therapy of immune hemolysis with steroids is not without hazard, particularly from infection, which is often due to opportunistic organisms. The role of high-dose intravenous gamma globulin in the treatment of autoimmune hemolysis is not yet clear.

1. Frank, M. M., Schreiber, A. D., Atkinson, J. P., et al. Pathophysiology of immune hemolytic anemia. *Ann. Intern. Med.* 87:210, 1977.
   An important review of the mechanisms by which red cell antibodies cause hemolysis. (For a review of cold agglutinins, see also N. Engl. J. Med. 297:538 and 583, 1977.)
2. Chaplin, H., Jr. Clinical usefulness of specific antiglobulin reagents in autoimmune hemolytic anemias. *Prog. Hematol.* 8:25, 1973.
   Critical evaluation of the Coombs' test.
3. Bohnen, R. F., Ultmann, J. E., Gorman, J. G., et al. The direct Coombs' test: Its clinical significance. *Ann. Intern. Med.* 68:19, 1968.
   Highest incidence of Coombs' test positivity was found in collagen-vascular disease, in lymphomas, and after blood transfusion.
4. Eyster, M. E., and Jenkins, D. E. Erythrocyte coating substances in patients with positive direct antiglobulin reactions. *Am. J. Med.* 46:360, 1969.
   Most patients with a positive Coombs' test in this series had an underlying disease.
5. Gilliland, B. C., Baxter, E., and Evans, R. S. Red-cell antibodies in Coombs' negative hemolytic anemia. *N. Engl. J. Med.* 285:252, 1971.
   Immune hemolysis not detected by Coombs' test.
6. Liesveld, J. L., Rowe, J. M., and Lichtman, M. A. Variability of the erythropoietic response in autoimmune hemolytic anemia: Analysis of 109 cases. *Blood* 69:820, 1987.
   Reticulocytopenia is not uncommon in autoimmune hemolytic anemia.

7. Berlin, N. I., and Beck, P. D. Quantitative aspects of bilirubin metabolism for hematologists. *Blood* 57:983, 1981.
   Comprehensive review. (See also Gastroenterology *78:821, 1980.)*
8. Jones, S. E. Autoimmune disorders and malignant lymphoma. *Cancer* 31:1092, 1973.
   Autoimmune hemolytic anemia complicates only 2% of lymphomas.
9. Conley, C. L., Lippman, S. M., and Ness, P. Autoimmune hemolytic anemia with reticulocytopenia: A medical emergency. *J.A.M.A.* 244:1688, 1980.
   This is a medical emergency in which transfusion can be lifesaving. (For a study of the mechanism see N. Engl. J. Med. 306:281, 1982.)
10. Goldfinger, D. Acute hemolytic transfusion reactions: A fresh look at pathogenesis and considerations regarding therapy. *Transfusion* 17:85, 1977.
    Advocates the use of furosemide, not mannitol. (See also J.A.M.A. 244:1333, 1980.)
11. Pineda, A. A., Taswell, H. F., and Brzica, S. M., Jr. Delayed hemolytic transfusion reaction: An immunologic hazard of blood transfusion. *Transfusion* 18:1, 1978.
    An important complication of blood transfusion that is frequently unrecognized. (See also J.A.M.A. 239:729, 1978.)
12. Schmidt, P. J., and Holland, P. V. Pathogenesis of the acute renal failure associated with incompatible transfusion. *Lancet* 2:1169, 1967.
    Transfusion of incompatible stroma results in acute renal failure.
13. Garratty, G., and Petz, L. D. Drug-induced immune hemolytic anemia. *Am. J. Med.* 58:398, 1975.
    The mechanism for hemolysis varies with the offending drug.
14. Kerr, R. O., Cardamone, J., Dalmasso, A. P., et al. Mechanisms of erythrocyte destruction in penicillin-induced hemolysis. *N. Engl. J. Med.* 287:1322, 1972.
    Complement-mediated injury of red cells not coated with penicillin.
15. Snyder, E. L., and Spivack, M. Clinical and serologic management of patients with methyldopa-induced positive antiglobulin tests. *Transfusion* 19:313, 1979.
    This is generally a laboratory curiosity.
16. Woodruff, A. W., Ansdell, V. E., and Petitt, L. E. Cause of anaemia in malaria. *Lancet* 1:1055, 1979.
    Immune complex–mediated hemolysis.
17. Jacobsen, L. B., Longstreth, G. F., and Edgington, T. S. Clinical and immunological features of transient cold agglutinin hemolytic anemia. *Am. J. Med.* 54:514, 1973.
    Cold agglutinins associated with infection are polyclonal; anti-i for mononucleosis and anti-I for atypical pneumonia.
18. Silberstein, L. E., Berkman, E. M., and Schreiber, A. D. Cold hemagglutinin disease associated with IgG cold-reactive antibody. *Ann. Intern. Med.* 106:238, 1987.
    In contrast to IgM-mediated cold agglutination, IgG-induced disease is steroid-responsive but probably very rare. (See also N. Engl. J. Med. 296:1490, 1977.)
19. Shirey, R. S., Kickler, T. S., Bell, W., et al. Fatal immune hemolytic anemia and hepatic failure associated with a warm-reacting IgM autoantibody. *Vox Sang* 52:219, 1987.
    Erythrocyte agglutination occurred at 37°C (98.6°F).
20. Abdulgabar, S., and Mueller-Eckhardt, C. The role of metabolite-specific antibodies in nomifensine-dependent immune hemolytic anemia. *N. Engl. J. Med.* 313:469, 1985.
    Antibodies to metabolites can cause hemolysis.
21. Eyster, E., Mayer, K., and McKenzie, S. Traumatic hemolysis with iron deficiency anemia in patients with aortic valve lesions. *Ann. Intern. Med.* 68:995, 1968.
    Hemolysis increases as the hematocrit falls, creating a vicious cycle. Thus both transfusions and iron replacement are required as therapy.
22. Fabry, M. E., Kaul, D. K., Raventos, C., et al. Some aspects of the pathophysiology of homozygous Hb CC erythrocytes. *J. Clin. Invest.* 67:1284, 1981.
    CC hemoglobin aggregates with deoxygenation.
23. Forman, S. J., Kumar, K. S., Redeker, A. G., et al. Hemolytic anemia in Wilson's disease: Clinical findings and biochemical mechanisms. *Am. J. Hematol.* 9:269, 1980.
    An adverse effect of a high serum copper level.
24. Bird, G. W. G. Paroxysmal cold haemoglobinuria. *Br. J. Haematol.* 37:167, 1977.
    The hemolysin is an IgG, usually an anti-P.

25. Hirono, A., Forman, L., and Beutler, E. Enzymatic diagnosis in nonspherocytic hemolytic anemia. *Medicine* 67:110, 1988.
   A diagnosis is not established in the majority of patients. (See also Blood *54:1, 549, 1979).*
26. Burka, E. R., Weaver Z., and Marks, P. A. Clinical spectrum of hemolytic anemia associated with glucose-6-phosphate dehydrogenase deficiency. *Ann. Intern. Med.* 64:817, 1966.
   Heterozygotes are also at risk from hemolysis.
27. Gordon-Smith, E. C., and White, J. M. Oxidative hemolysis and Heinz body hemolytic anaemia. *Br. J. Haematol.* 26:513, 1974.
   A concise review.
28. Agre, P., Asimos, A., Casella, J. F., et al. Inheritance pattern and clinical response to splenectomy as a reflection of erythrocyte spectrin deficiency in hereditary spherocytosis. *N. Engl. J. Med.* 315:1579, 1986.
   Spectrin deficiency is a cause of one type of hereditary spherocytosis.
29. McGuire, M., and Agre, P. Clinical disorders of the erythrocyte membrane skeleton. *Hematol. Pathol.* 2:1, 1988.
   Review of the molecular basis of hereditary disorders of the red cell skeleton.
30. Schmidt, P. J. Hereditary hemolytic anemias and the null blood types. *Arch. Intern. Med.* 139:570, 1979.
   "Null" blood types are associated with morphologic abnormalities and hemolytic anemia. (See also Am. J. Hematol. *24:267, 1987.)*
31. Spira, M. A., and Lynch E. C. Autoimmune hemolytic anemia and carcinoma: An unusual association. *Am. J. Med.* 67:753, 1979.
   An association between carcinoma and idiopathic thrombocytopenic purpura has also been observed.
32. Antman, K. H., Skarin, A. T., Mayer, R. J., et al. Microangiopathic hemolytic anemia and cancer: A review. *Medicine* 58:377, 1979.
   Mechanisms other than DIC may be responsible for microangiopathic red cell changes in patients with cancer.
33. Fairbanks, V. F., Opfell, R. W., and Burgert, E. O. Three families with unstable hemoglobinopathies (Köln, Olmsted and Santa Ana) causing hemolytic anemia with inclusion bodies and pigmenturia. *Am. J. Med.* 46:344, 1969.
   Pigmenturia due to pyrrole excretion.
34. Macpherson, A. I. S., Richmond, J., Donaldson, G. W. K., et al. The role of the spleen in congenital spherocytosis. *Am. J. Med.* 50:35, 1971.
   Splenic "conditioning" of red cells results in an increased susceptibility to hemolysis.
35. Lefrere, J.-J., Courouce, A.-M., Bertrand, Y., et al. Human pavovirus and aplastic crisis and chronic hemolytic anemias: A study of 24 observations. *Am. J. Hematol.* 23:271, 1986.
   An important reminder.
36. Selby, G. B., and Eichner, E. R. Endurance swimming, intravascular hemolysis, anemia, and iron depletion: New perspective on athlete's anemia. *Am. J. Med.* 81:791, 1986.
   Running is not the only exercise associated with hemolysis.
37. Eichner, E. R. Spider bite hemolytic anemia: Positive Coombs' test, erythrophagocytosis, and leukoerythroblastic smear. *Am. J. Clin. Pathol.* 81:683, 1984.
   An unusual cause of hemolysis.
38. Jacob, H. S. Hypersplenism: Mechanisms and management. *Br. J. Haematol.* 27:1, 1974.
   Guidelines for splenectomy in hemolytic disorders. (See also Q. J. Med. *41:261, 1972.)*
39. Besa, E. C. Rapid transient reversal of anemia and long-term effects of maintenance intravenous immunoglobin for autoimmune hemolytic anemia in patients with lymphoproliferative disorders. *Am. J. Med.* 84:691, 1988.
   The role of intravenous IgG in treating immune hemolysis has not been established. (See also Scand. J. Haematol. *34:394, 1985.)*
40. Levine, R. A., and Klatskin, G. Unconjugated hyperbilirubinemia in the absence of overt hemolysis. *Am. J. Med.* 36:541, 1964.

Unconjugated hyperbilirubinemia occurs in a wide variety of nonhematologic illnesses.

41. Marchand, A., Galen, R. S., and Van Lente, F. The predictive value of serum haptoglobin in hemolytic disease. *J.A.M.A.* 243:1909, 1980.
   Haptoglobin measurements can be useful in the diagnosis of hemolysis.
42. Muller-Eberhard, U. Hemopexin. *N. Engl. J. Med.* 283:1090, 1970.
   Use of plasma hemopexin levels in the evaluation of hemolytic anemia.
43. Bartholomew, J. R., Bell, W. R., and Shirey, R. S. Cold agglutinin hemolytic anemia: Management with an environmental suit. *Ann. Intern. Med.* 106:243, 1987.
   An interesting therapeutic maneuver.
44. Beutler, E. Glucose-6-phosphate dehydrogenease: New Perspectives. *Blood* 73:1397, 1989.
   State-of-the-art review.
45. Hirono, A., Forman, L., and Beutler, E. Enzymatic diagnosis in nonspherocytic hemolytic anemia. *Medicine* 67:110, 1988.
   The diagnosis was established in only 28% of these patients and pyruvate kinase and G-6-PD deficiency were the most common causes.

97. HEMOPHILIA AND ALLIED DISORDERS
Jerry L. Spivak

The hemostatic mechanisms of the body are delicately balanced to maintain the integrity of the blood volume by preventing bleeding while at the same time maintaining the integrity of blood flow by preventing thrombosis. Abnormalities of either the vessel wall, the blood platelets, or the proteins involved in the coagulation pathway can upset this balance and lead to hemorrhage or thrombosis. Hereditary disorders of the coagulation proteins that lead to thrombosis are uncommon but include the dysfibrinogenemias and antithrombin 3 deficiency as well as deficiency of protein C and protein S. Most often disorders leading to thromboembolic disease do not involve the coagulation system directly. They include homocystinuria, paroxysmal nocturnal hemoglobinuria, sickle cell disease, Behçet's syndrome, erythrocytosis from any cause, diabetes mellitus, mucinous adenocarcinoma, ingestion of oral contraceptives, and pregnancy.

Hereditary disorders of the coagulation proteins leading to hemorrhage usually involve a single protein although there are exceptions to this rule. They include deficiency of the plasma inhibitor of protein C that leads to simultaneous factor V and VIII deficiencies, simultaneous deficiencies of factors VIII and IX, and combined deficiencies of the vitamin K–dependent clotting factors. Deficiency of a coagulation protein does not always produce a hemorrhagic disorder as is the case with factor XII (Hageman factor) deficiency, and the severity of the hemorrhagic disorder can be variable. For example, factor XI deficiency, which occurs predominately in Jewish individuals, is frequently discovered for the first time at surgery or with major trauma. Factor VII deficiency may also have a mild clinical course.

In evaluating patients for a bleeding tendency the best single test is a careful history, particularly with respect to bleeding in other members of the family and the patient's response to previous surgical procedures such as tooth extractions or tonsillectomy, both of which involve disruption of arterial vessels. Two coagulation tests, the prothrombin time (PT) and the partial thromboplastin time (PTT), are commonly used to evaluate the function of coagulation proteins. The PT is influenced by the level and function of fibrinogen; prothrombin; and factors V, VII, and X. Prothrombin and factors VII and X are vitamin K–dependent coagulation factors. The other vitamin K–dependent coagulation factor, factor IX, is not measured by the PT. The PTT measures the function of all coagulation proteins except factor VII. A normal PT and a prolonged PTT indicate that the coagulation abnormally involves factors VIII, IX, XI, XII, or proteins of the kallikrein and kininogen pathways. A normal PTT and a prolonged PT indicates factor VII deficiency. It is important to remember that when the fibrinogen concentration falls below 100 mg/dl, neither the PT nor the PTT provides a reliable measure of the activity of the other coagulation factors. Neither the PTT nor the PT measures the activity of factor XIII. This factor is assayed by testing the solubility of the fibrin clot in 5M urea.

Prolongations of the PT and PTT can be caused by circulating anticoagulants as well as by deficiencies of the various clotting factors. Circulating anticoagulants may take the form of fibrin split products in disseminated intravascular coagulation (DIC), or the monoclonal protein produced during the course of multiple myeloma or macroglobulinemia. They may also occur post partum; in association with collagen-vascular disorders, inflammatory bowel disease, drug reactions, or skin disorders such as pemphigus; or spontaneously in older individuals without any underlying disease being present. Circulating anticoagulants are most often directed against factor VIII but may be directed against other clotting factors, particularly V, IX, XI, and XIII. The so-called lupus anticoagulant, which can occur in association with lymphomas, following exposure to certain drugs, or for no apparent reason, as well as in patients with lupus or other collagen vascular diseases, appears to be directed against phospholipid epitopes rather than a specific clotting factor. Paradoxically, while it causes a prolongation of the PT and PTT, it is not associated with hemorrhagic phenomena but rather an increased tendency to thrombosis. Circulating inhibitors to specific coagulation factors are also seen in approximately 10 percent of patients with classic hemophilia (factor VIII deficiency) or Christmas disease (factor IX deficiency).

It should be emphasized with respect to the PT and PTT that these tests are not sensitive to a reduction in procoagulant activity until the level falls below 20 percent of normal. The whole blood clotting time will be normal with a factor VIII level of 5 percent. Therefore, these tests are not reliable for screening purposes.

The most common hereditary disorder of blood coagulation is classic hemophilia (factor VIII deficiency). The next most common disorders are Christmas disease (factor IX deficiency) and von Willebrand's disease, both of which occur at approximately one-fourth the frequency of classic hemophilia. Both classic hemophilia and Christmas disease are X-linked recessive disorders in which only males are clinically affected while females are obligate carriers. While most of the remaining congenital abnormalities of blood coagulation are inherited as autosomal recessive traits, von Willebrand's disease and factor XI deficiency can be inherited in either an autosomal dominant or autosomal recessive manner. In most hereditary coagulopathies the severity of the disorder is proportional to the extent of the deficiency of the clotting factor or factors involved. In a mild deficiency state, up to 25 percent of the activity of the particular clotting factor may be preserved. In severe deficiency states, the activity of the involved procoagulant is usually reduced to less than 1 percent of normal.

Patients with hereditary deficiencies of coagulation factors are usually subject to spontaneous hemorrhages, usually in the joints and soft tissues. Knees, elbows, and ankles are most frequently affected and recurrent hemarthrosis can result in joint destruction and immobility. Bleeding into the soft tissues may result in nerve entrapment while retroperitoneal hemorrhage and central nervous system bleeding have a substantial mortality. In patients with factor VIII deficiency, upper gastrointestinal bleeding is commonly due to peptic ulcer disease. Paradoxically, hereditary deficiency of a coagulation factor does not protect against atherosclerosis, coronary artery disease, or thromboembolic phenomena.

In contrast to the factor VIII deficiency occurring in classic hemophilia, factor VIII deficiency associated with von Willebrand's disease is characterized not by spontaneous hemarthroses but rather by mucous membrane bleeding from the nose and gastrointestinal tract. Although telangiectasia has been observed in patients with von Willebrand's disease, more commonly mucous membrane bleeding is attributable to coagulation factor abnormalities. In contrast to classic hemophilia, the bleeding time in patients with von Willebrand's disease is usually prolonged. The differences between these two deficiency states of factor VIII can be explained by the complex nature of the factor VIII molecule. This molecule is actually a complex of two proteins, the factor VIII procoagulant protein or antihemophiliac factor and the factor VIII–related protein or von Willebrand's factor. Each is under separate genetic control. The factor VIII procoagulant protein (factor VIII-C) is controlled by the X chromosome, while the von Willebrand's factor (factor VIII-R) is controlled by an autosomal gene. VIII-C is involved in the coagulation cascade in the enzymatic activation of factor X by activated factor IX. VIII-R is involved in platelet function, and its behavior can be measured in vitro using the antibiotic ristocetin. VIII-R contains ristocetin cofactor activity and appears to be synthesized in endothelial cells as well as in megakaryocytes. The site of synthesis of VIII-C is unknown. The mechanism by which VIII-C and VIII-R interact is unsettled. VIII-R has a molecular weight of greater than 10^6 and is composed of multimers of smaller subunits while VIII-C has a molecular weight in the unactivated state of approximately 285,000. It is currently thought that the interaction of VIII-R and VIII-C serves to protect the VIII-C from proteolytic degradation in the plasma. Using both immunologic and procoagulant assays it can be demonstrated that patients with classic hemophilia have normal levels of von Willebrand's factor (VIII-R) but extremely low levels of factor VIII procoagulant activity (VIII-C), while most patients with von Willebrand's disease have low levels of both VIII-R and VIII-C. Some patients with classic hemophilia have detectable VIII-C antigen in their plasma (cross-reacting material) while others do not. In both instances the procoagulant activity of factor VIII-C is abnormal. Thus, in classic hemophilia, some patients synthesize dysfunctional factor VIII-C molecules while others make no factor VIII-C or make a factor that lacks both procoagulant activity and normal antigenic determinants.

Von Willebrand's disease can occur in a variety of patterns. The classic form is inherited as an autosomal dominant trait and has been divided into two types. In type I, factors VIII-C and VIII-R and ristocetin cofactor activity are reduced, but the VIII-R molecule appears to be normal. In type II disease there is a qualitative abnormality of VIII-R with a loss of the larger multimers from both plasma and platelets. The absolute levels of VIII-C and VIII-R may be reduced or normal. A subtype of type II von Willebrand's disease, type IIB, has recently been identified. In type IIB disease, also an autosomal dominant, ristocetin cofactor activity is increased. However, the bleeding time remains prolonged and there are both qualitative and quantitative abnormalities of VIII-R with a loss of larger-molecular-weight multimers, but only from the plasma. In contrast to type IIA, in type IIB disease there is a heightened interaction between VIII-R and platelets as measured by ristocetin-induced platelet aggregation, and desmopressin (DDAVP) can cause thrombocytopenia. Since bleeding occurs in both IIA and IIB, it is apparent that ristocetin cofactor activity in vitro does not always reflect the clinical situation. The most severe form of von Willebrand's disease (type III) is not inherited as an autosomal dominant as is the case of types I and IIA and IIB but rather as a recessive trait with factor VIII-R levels of less than 1 percent of normal. In addition to abnormalities of the quantitative production of VII-R, abnormalities of carbohydrate composition have also been identified in some patients with von Willebrand's disease. Additional subclasses of type II von Willebrand's disease include IID and IIE, which have different multimer patterns, and IIC, which is inherited as an autosomal recessive like type III and has a unique multimer pattern on electrophoresis. In pseudo-von Willebrand's disease, the defect is on the platelet membrane, and changes in circulating multimers occur as a consequence of this. Acquired forms of von Willebrand's disease have been observed with lymphoproliferative disorders, autoimmune disorders, and solid tumors.

The ability to administer concentrates of various coagulation factors has greatly simplified the treatment of patients with coagulation factor deficiencies. The type and quantity of procoagulant administered depends on the location of the hemorrhage and its severity. Hemarthroses, which occur in a closed space providing some measure of tamponade, only require elevation of the deficient coagulation factor to at least 10 percent of normal. Soft tissue hemorrhage and dental extractions require 20 to 50 percent levels while major surgery or central nervous system hemorrhage requires levels of greater than 50 percent for a period of 10 to 14 days. For dental extraction, ε-aminocaproic acid (EACA) has been used effectively in conjunction with factor replacement. Desmopressin, an analogue of arginine vasopressin, has been used successfully to raise factor VIII levels in patients with mild factor VIII deficiency. As a general rule, replacement of one unit of a clotting factor per kilogram raises the plasma concentration by approximately 2 percent. In administering coagulation factors, the volume of distribution of these factors with respect to the plasma volume must be taken into consideration. For example, the volume of distribution of factor VIII is 1.5 while that of factor IX is approximately 2.5. The half-life of a particular coagulation factor is also an important consideration in maintaining the factor at a therapeutic level. Recent studies suggest that continuous infusion, once an adequate procoagulant level has been obtained by bolus injection, may prove to be the most satisfactory way of maintaining hemostatic levels of factor VIII. It should be noted with respect to von Willebrand's disease that factor VIII concentrate, which lacks high-molecular-weight multimers, does not correct the hemorrhage tendency but cryoprecipitate does. The recognition in recent years that patients with hemophilia were subject to human immunodeficiency virus (HIV) infection via factor VIII replacement therapy has led to the development of factor VIII concentrates that are free from this virus.

A circulating anticoagulant is one of the most difficult complications to deal with in the management of patients with hereditary deficiencies of procoagulant proteins. Circulating anticoagulants develop most commonly in patients with the most severe deficiency state. Most occur in childhood or adolescence but some arise in adults. Some patients produce only low titers of the inhibitor whereas others produce high titers. Most inhibitors are of the IgG class, particularly IgG4, which does not fix complement. Treatment of patients with circulating anticoagulants should be symptomatic. In patients with surface hemorrhage, local measures and, if necessary, transfusion with washed red cells, may be sufficient. In patients with a low titer of inhibitor, a large quantity of the particular factor can be administered in the hope of exceeding the titer of the antibody. This is done with the knowledge that an anamnestic response can be expected in which inhibitor titers may increase markedly. In patients with high-titer inhibitors to factor VIII, factor IX concentrates, both activated and unactivated, have been employed. In several control studies these seem to be effective though their mechanism of action is still a matter of controversy. Immunosuppressive agents have been employed but the tendency of some circulating anticoagulants to disappear spontaneously has made results of such therapy difficult to interpret. Plasmapheresis has also been successfully employed as has high-dose continuous infusion of factor VIII and high-dose intravenous gamma globulin. Danazol should be avoided.

1. Furie, B., and Furie, B. C. The molecular basis of blood coagulation. *Cell* 53:505, 1988.
   State-of-the-art review. (See also Trends Genet. *4:233, 1988.)*
2. Hoyer, L. W. Molecular pathology and immunology of factor VIII (hemophilia A and factor VIII inhibitors). *Hum Pathol.* 18:153, 1987.
   A critical review.
3. Zimmerman, T. S., and Ruggeri, Z. M. von Willebrand disease. *Blood* 70:895, 1987.
   State-of-the-art review. (See also Hum. Pathol. *18:140, 1987.)*
4. Mannucci, P. M., Lombardi, R., Bader, R., et al. Studies of the pathophysiology of acquired von Willebrand's disease in seven patients with lymphoproliferative disorders or benign monoclonal gammopathies. *Blood* 64:614, 1984.
   Desmopressin may be useful in treating these patients.
5. Rapaport, S. I. Preoperative hemostatic evaluation: Which tests, if any? *Blood* 61:229, 1983.
   Excellent advice. (See also Ann. Surg. *208:554, 1988.)*
6. Bennett, B., and Ratnoff, O. D. Studies on the response of patients with classic hemophilia to transfusion with concentrates of antihemophilia factor. *J. Clin. Invest.* 151:2593, 1971.
   Transfused factor VIII–like antigen disappears more slowly than clot-promoting activity.
7. Bennett, B., Ratnoff, O. D., and Levin, J. Immunologic studies in von Willebrand's disease. *J. Clin. Invest.* 51:2597, 1972.
   Transfused factor VIII–like antigen disappears more rapidly than clot-promoting activity.
8. Lusher, J. M., and McMillan, C. W. Severe factor VIII and factor IX deficiencies in females. *Am. J. Med.* 65:637, 1978.

Clinical review of the causes for factor VIII or IX deficiency in females. (See also Am. J. Med. *60:138, 1976.)*

9. Hay, C. R. M., Triger, D. R., Preston, F. E., et al. Progressive liver disease in hae-mophilia: An understood problem? *Lancet* 1:1495, 1985.
This can be a significant problem even when cryoprecipitate is the major treatment product. (See also Lancet *2:146, 1982 and* Blood *66:1317, 1985.)*

10. Mittal, R., Spero, J. A., Lewis, J. H., et al. Patterns of gastrointestinal hemorrhage in hemophilia. *Gastroenterology* 88:515, 1985.
Duodenal ulcer is the most common, but other anatomic lesions are also found.

11. Eyster, M. E., Gill, F. M., Blatt, P. M., et al. Central nervous bleeding in hemophil-iacs. *Blood* 51:1179, 1978.
After trauma there can be a symptom-free interval of several days before bleeding occurs; recurrent hemorrhage occurred in 26%.

12. Hasegawa, D. K., Bennett, A. J., Coccia, P. F., et al. Factor V deficiency in Philadelphia-positive chronic myelogenous leukemia. *Blood* 56:585, 1980.
Factor V deficiency appears to be associated with a large hematopoietic cell mass.

13. Yorke, A. J., and Mant, M. J. Factor VII deficiency and surgery. *J.A.M.A.* 238:424, 1977.
Surgical bleeding is uncommon in factor VII deficiency.

14. Seligsohn, U. High gene frequency of factor XI (PTA) deficiency in Ashkenazi Jews. *Blood* 51:1223, 1978.
This disorder may be asymptomatic until trauma or surgery.

15. Marlar, R. A., and Griffin, J. H. Deficiency of protein C inhibitor in combined factor V/VIII deficiency disease. *J. Clin. Invest.* 66:1186, 1980.
The biologic basis for combined deficiency of factors V and VIII is lack of the inhibitor of protein C.

16. Griffin, J. H., and Cochrane, C. G. Recent advances in the understanding of contact activation reactions. *Semin. Thromb. Hemost.* 5:254, 1979.
Review of the contact phase of coagulation.

17. Hougie, C., McPherson, R. A., and Brown, J. E., et al. The Passavoy defect. *N. Engl. J. Med.* 298:1045, 1978.
A defect of the contact phase of coagulation associated with a bleeding diathesis.

18. Brown, C. H., Kvols, L. K., Hsu, T. H., et al. Factor IX deficiency and bleeding in a patient with Sheehan's syndrome. *Blood* 39:650, 1972.
Corticosteroid-dependent factor IX deficiency. (See also N. Engl. J. Med. *273:1057, 1965.)*

19. Furie, B., Voo, L., McAdam, K. P. W. J., et al. Mechanism of factor X deficiency in systemic amyloidosis. *N. Engl. J. Med.* 304:827, 1981.
Amyloid fibrils bind factor X and also factors II and IX. Splenectomy can correct the deficiency state (N. Engl. J. Med. *301:1050, 1979).*

20. Natelson, E. A., Lynch, E. C., Hettig, R. A., et al. Acquired factor IX deficiency in the nephrotic syndrome. *Ann. Intern. Med.* 73:373, 1970.
Loss of factor IX in the urine.

21. Pickering, N. J., Brody, J. I., and Barrett, M. J. Von Willebrand syndrome and mitral valve prolapse: Linked mesenchymal dysplasias. *N. Engl. J. Med.* 305:131, 1981.
An interesting association.

22. Ratnoff, O. D., and Forman, W. B. Criteria for the differentiation of dysfibrinoge-nemic states. *Semin. Hematol.* 13:141, 1976.
A thorough review of a complex topic.

23. Weiss, H. J., Meyer, D., Rabinowitz, R., et al. Pseudo-von Willebrand's disease. *N. Engl. J. Med.* 306:326, 1982.
The accompanying editorial on page 360 provides prospective on this addition to the coagulopathies.

24. Palascak, J. E., and Martinez, J. Dysfibrinogenemia associated with liver disease. *J. Clin. Invest.* 60:89, 1977.
Defective fibrin monomer polymerization in liver disease.

25. Kitchens, C. S., and Newcomb, T. F. Factor XIII. *Medicine* 58:413, 1979.
Comprehensive review.

26. Agle, D. P., Ratnoff, O. D., and Spring, G. K. The anticoagulant malingerer. *Ann. Intern. Med.* 73:67, 1970.
   A not uncommon problem among paramedical personnel.
27. McMillan, C. W., Shapiro, S. S., Whitehurst, D., et al. The natural history of factor VIII:C inhibitors in patients with hemophilia A: A national cooperative study. II. Observations on the initial development of factor VIII:C inhibitors. *Blood* 71:344, 1988.
   A genetic predisposition appears to be involved. (For VIII:Ag inhibitors, see Blood *72:116, 1988.)*
28. Lottenberg, R., Kentro, T. B., and Kitchens, C. S. Acquired hemophilia. *Arch. Intern. Med.* 147:1077, 1987.
   Expectant treatment worked well in these patients.
29. Reece, E. A., Clyne, L. P., Romero, R., et al. Spontaneous factor XI inhibitors. Seven additional cases and a review of the literature. *Arch. Intern. Med.* 144:525, 1984.
   An unusual occurrence. For a drug-induced example, see Arch. Intern. Med. *137:1471, 1977.*
30. Nilsson, I. M., Berntorp, E., and Zettervall, O. Introduction of immune tolerance in patients with hemophilia and antibodies to factor VIII by combined treatment with intravenous IgG, cyclophosphamide, and factor VIII. *N. Engl. J. Med.* 318:947, 1988.
   Successful treatment for alloantibody to factor VIII. For a balanced review of therapy for inhibitors, see Prog. Hemost. Thromb. *9:57, 1989. For immunosuppressive therapy for spontaneous inhibitors, see* Ann. Intern. Med. *110:744, 1989.*
31. Sultan, Y., Maisonneuve, P., Kazatchkine, M. D., et al. Anti-idiotypic suppression of autoantibodies to factor VIII (antihaemophilic factor) by high-dose intravenous gammaglobulin. *Lancet* 2:765, 1984.
   See also Arch. Pathol. Lab. Med. *112:143, 1988 and* Proc. Natl. Acad. Sci. U.S.A. *84:828, 1987.*
32. Thiagarajan, P., Shapiro, S. S., and DeMarco, L. Monoclonal immunoglobulin Mλ coagulation inhibitor with phospholipid specificity. *J. Clin. Invest.* 66:397, 1980.
   Explanation of the mechanism of action of the "lupus" anticoagulant.
33. Mueh, J. R., Herbst, K. D., and Rapaport, S. I. Thrombosis in patients with the lupus anticoagulant. *Ann. Intern. Med.* 92:156, 1980.
   Thrombosis, not hemorrhage, is observed with the "lupus" anticoagulant.
34. Allain, J.-P. Dose requirement for replacement therapy in hemophilia A. *Thromb. Haemost.* 42:825, 1979.
   A minimum dose of 0.26 U/kg of factor VIII is suggested.
35. Zauber, N. P., and Levin, J. Factor IX levels in patients with hemophilia B (Christmas disease) following transfusion with concentrates of factor IX or fresh frozen plasma (FFP). *Medicine* 56:213, 1977.
   Initially, transfusion therapy should be based on a $t^{1/2}$ for factor IX of 6–8 hours.
36. Orringer, E. P., Koury, M. J., Blatt, P. M., et al. Hemolysis caused by factor VIII concentrates. *Arch. Intern. Med.* 136:1018, 1976.
   A complication associated with intensive therapy. (See also Am. J. Med. *69:953, 1980.)*
37. Mannucci, P. M. Desmopressin: a nontransfusional form of treatment for congenital and acquired bleeding disorders. *Blood* 72:1449, 1988.
   A useful review. Tachyphylaxis is a significant problem. (See also Lancet *1:1145, 1984.)*
38. Sjamsoedin, L. J. M., Heijnen, L., Mauser-Bunschoten, E. P., et al. The effect of activated prothrombin-complex concentrate (FEIBA) on joint and muscle bleeding in patients with hemophilia A and antibodies to factor VIII. *N. Engl. J. Med.* 305:717, 1981.
   Activated prothrombin complex is effective in controlling hemorrhage as is a nonactivated complex. (See also N. Engl. J. Med. *303:421, 1980.) For a logical approach to therapy see the editorial on page 757. For an adverse effect see* Am. J. Med. *85:245, 1988.*
39. Cederbaum, A. I., Blatt, P. M., and Roberts, H. R. Intravascular coagulation with use of human prothrombin complex concentrates. *Ann. Intern. Med.* 84:683, 1976.

Liver disease is a contraindication to the use of concentrates containing activated factors. (See also N. Engl. J. Med. 304:670, 1981.)

40. Kitchens, C. S. Surgery in hemophilia and related disorders. A prospective study of 100 consecutive procedures. *Medicine* 65:34, 1986.
    Factor VIII inhibitors are the major contraindication to surgery. (See also J.A.M.A. 253:1279, 1985.)

41. Ratnoff, O. D. Some complications of the therapy of classic hemophilia. *J. Lab. Clin. Med.* 103:653, 1984.
    Allergic reactions, factor VIII antibodies, hepatitis, and acquired immunodeficiency syndrome (AIDS).

42. Goodnough, L. T., Saito, H., and Ratnoff, O. D. Thrombosis or myocardial infarction in congenital clotting factor abnormalities and chronic thrombocytopenias: A report of 21 patients and a review of 50 previously reported cases. *Medicine* 62:248, 1983.
    An interesting clinical paradox.

43. Soff, G. A., and Levin, J. Familial multiple coagulation factor deficiencies. *Semin. Thromb. Hemost.* 7:112, 1981.
    State-of-the-art review. (See also the accompanying review on page 149.)

44. White, G. C., II, and Shoemaker, C. B. Factor VIII gene and hemophilia A. *Blood* 73:1, 1989.
    The molecular genetics of factor VIII deficiency.

45. Allain, J.-P., Laurian, Y., Paul, D. A., et al. Long-term evaluation of HIV antigen and antibodies to p24 and gp41 in patients with hemophilia. *N. Engl. J. Med.* 317:1114, 1987.
    HIV antigenemia implies a poor prognosis. See also Ann. Intern. Med. 110:963, 1989.)

46. Giles, A. R., Hoogendoorn, H., and Benford, K. Type IIB von Willebrand's disease presenting as thrombocytopenia during pregnancy. *Br. J. Haematol.* 67:349, 1987.
    An interesting and reversible complication.

98. IRON DEFICIENCY
Jerry L. Spivak

Iron deficiency is one of the most common causes of anemia encountered in clinical practice. Since the body has the ability to facilitate iron absorption but lacks a physiologic mechanism for iron excretion, iron deficiency in the adult is usually due to blood loss or is a complication of pregnancy and lactation. Dietary inadequacy is not a consideration, particularly in view of the fortification of many foods with iron. Iron deficiency may, however, occur with intestinal malabsorption or clay ingestion. In the latter instance, iron and other substances such as potassium are chelated and made unavailable for absorption. Hemoglobinuria and pulmonary hemosiderosis are more unusual causes of iron deficiency. In the latter, diagnosis may be delayed unless it is realized that hemoptysis is often not a prominent feature and that pulmonary infiltrates can be evanescent. The sputum should be searched for hemosiderin-laden macrophages. Chronic intravascular hemolysis leading to iron loss in the urine occurs in paroxysmal nocturnal hemoglobinuria (PNH) and with anatomic cardiac abnormalities, such as aortic valve disease, atrial myxoma, and unseated prosthetic valves.

The diagnosis of iron deficiency requires demonstration of absent iron stores in the marrow. Iron losses are replaced from this storage pool and a reduction in reticuloendothelial iron is the earliest manifestation of iron deficiency. Absence of stainable marrow iron is, however, not seen solely with iron deficiency but also occurs in polycythemia vera due to expansion of the red blood cell mass. Except for mild anisocytosis and poikilocytosis, little change occurs in red cell morphology or indices in early iron-deficiency anemia. Overt hypochromia and microcytosis do not occur for several months after the development of iron deficiency due to the long life span of the normal red cell, and microcytosis occurs before hypochromia. Usually a reduction in tissue iron stores is followed by a decrease in serum iron and percent saturation of transferrin, an increase in serum transferrin levels, and an increase in free erythrocyte protoporphyrin. However, in catabolic states or with protein loss, serum transferrin may not increase. Decreased serum iron and percent saturation and elevated free erythrocyte protoporphyrin also occur with chronic inflammation, a state in which tissue iron stores are usually normal or increased.

The serum ferritin level is a valuable alternative to the serum iron and iron-binding capacity for the diagnosis of iron deficiency. Serum ferritin measurements also serve as a convenient method for monitoring tissue iron repletion during iron replacement therapy. In the absence of inflammation, malignancy, or liver disease, serum ferritin correlates directly with tissue iron stores ($1\mu g$/liter is the equivalent of 8 mg of storage iron). With reduction in tissue iron, the serum ferritin level declines before changes occur in serum iron, iron-binding capacity, or erythrocyte protoporphyrin. When the serum ferritin is less than 12 μg/liter, tissue iron stores are depleted. When the serum ferritin is between 15 and 50 μg/liter in the presence of inflammation, tissue iron deficiency is likely. In most patients with inflammation, malignancy, or liver disease, however, marrow iron stores must be examined directly to establish the presence of iron deficiency. A marrow iron stain is also necessary to demonstrate ringed sideroblasts in patients with microcytic, hypochromic red cells on this basis.

Microcytosis with or without hypochromia is a feature of α- and β-thalassemia minor. Many of these patients also have an elevated red cell count. In β-thalassemia minor, the level of hemoglobin A_2 is also elevated. Elevation of the hemoglobin F level in β-thalassemia minor is sufficiently infrequent to lack usefulness as a diagnostic test; basophilic stippling is also not a constant finding. Serum ferritin and erythrocyte-free protoporphyrin are normal in α- and β-thalassemia minor in the absence of iron deficiency or systemic disease. In some patients with β-thalassemia minor, however, iron deficiency produces a reduction in the level of hemoglobin A_2. Therefore, when the serum ferritin is low, the presence of β-thalassemia minor cannot be excluded on the basis of a normal level of hemoglobin A_2.

Iron deficiency is often accompanied by thrombocytosis, but since this may occur with infection, inflammation from any cause, collagen-vascular disease, and carcinoma, its diagnostic significance is diminished.

When the diagnosis of iron deficiency is established, it is the responsibility of the physician to determine its exact cause. A carefully taken drug history, particularly with reference to aspirin, phenylbutazone, indomethacin, steroids, and alcohol, may be rewarding. The skin lesions of pseudoxanthoma elasticum and hereditary telangiectasia must be looked for. Iron deficiency may be an early sign of neoplasia. The classic example is carcinoma of the ascending colon, in which the liquid consistency of the stool prevents obstruction, and occult bleeding may be the only manifestation. A vigorous diagnostic evaluation of the gut is recommended if it is the suspected site of blood loss. This may require flexible fiberoptic endoscopy and mesenteric arteriography, as well as conventional contrast x-ray studies. If hemoglobinuria is suspected, the urine should be examined for hemosiderin-laden cells. If the process is chronic, renal shadows may be dense on plain x rays due to deposition of iron. If no source of iron loss is established, therapy may be initiated with iron but only to the point at which the hematocrit returns to normal. If therapy is then stopped, tissue iron stores will not be repleted, and if bleeding recurs, the hematocrit will fall and diagnostic studies to determine the bleeding site can be reinitiated.

Ferrous sulfate is the most effective form of iron for oral therapy. If gastric upset occurs, the dose can be decreased or given with meals. In this instance the meal should always contain animal protein, which facilitates inorganic iron absorption; vegetable products may impair it. In patients who have undergone gastric surgery, liquid iron (taken through a straw to avoid dental staining) is more effective than the tablet form. In the unreliable patient and the patient with malabsorption or inflammatory bowel disease, parenteral iron is indicated, but fever or allergic reactions should be anticipated. Enteric-coated iron is of no value. Iron absorption is blocked by some antacids and iron binds to tetracycline and prevents absorption of the antibiotic.

1. Cook, J. D. Clinical evaluation of iron deficiency. *Semin. Hematol.* 19:6, 1982.
   Advice from an expert.
2. Finch, C. A., and Huebers, H. Perspectives in iron metabolism. *N. Engl. J. Med.* 306:1520, 1982.
   Comprehensive review.
3. Conrad, M. E., and Crosby, W. H. The natural history of iron deficiency induced by phlebotomy. *Blood* 20:173, 1962.
   Description of the red cell changes induced by iron deficiency and the events following iron repletion. (See also Blood 56:786, 1980.)
4. Hillman, R. S., and Henderson, P. A. Control of marrow production by the level of iron supply. *J. Clin. Invest.* 48:454, 1969.
   Marrow red cell production is proportional to the amount of iron available.
5. Engel, J. P., Schein, O. D., and Conley, C. L. Bone marrow hemosiderin does not always reflect body iron stores. *Arch. Intern. Med.* 142:287, 1982.
   Splenic accumulation with absent marrow iron during a hemolytic anemia.
6. Bjorn-Rasmussen, E. Iron absorption: Present knowledge and controversies. *Lancet* 1:914, 1983.
   Brief review.
7. Cook, J. D., and Lynch, S. R. The liabilities of iron deficiency. *Blood* 68:803, 1986.
   Review of the potentially deleterious effects of iron deficiency.
8. Rector, W. G., Jr., Fortuin, N. J., and Conley, C. L. Non-hematologic effects of chronic iron deficiency. *Medicine* 61:382, 1982.
   In adults, iron deficiency without anemia has no clinically deleterious effects.
9. Lipschitz, D. A., Cook, J. D., and Finch, C. A. A clinical evaluation of serum ferritin as an index of iron stores. *N. Engl. J. Med.* 290:1213, 1974.
   A useful test for the diagnosis of iron deficiency.
10. Bessman, J. D. Microcytic polycythemia: Frequency of nonthalassemic causes. *J.A.M.A.* 238:2391, 1977.
    An elevated red cell count with microcytosis is a feature of thalassemia minor or polycythemia vera.
11. Cunningham, L. O., and Rising, J. A. Erythrocytic microcytosis: Clinical implications in 100 patients. *Am. J. Med. Sci.* 273:149, 1977.
    Iron deficiency was the most common cause of microcytosis in this series.
12. England, J. M., and Fraser, P. Discrimination between iron-deficiency and hetero-zygous-thalassemia syndromes in differential diagnosis of microcytosis. *Lancet* 1:145, 1979.
    An approach for distinguishing between thalassemia minor and iron deficiency.
13. Hancock, D. E., Onstad, J. W., and Wolf, P. C. Transferrin loss into the urine with hypochromic, microcytic anemia. *Am. J. Clin. Pathol.* 65:73, 1976.
    An unusual cause of iron-deficient erythropoiesis.
14. DeGowin, R. L., Sorensen, L. B., Charleston, D. B., et al. Retention of radioiron in the lungs of a woman with idiopathic pulmonary hemosiderosis. *Ann. Intern. Med.* 69:1213, 1968.
    Interesting cause of iron-deficiency anemia.
15. Hamilton, R. W., Schwartz, E., Atwater, J., et al. Acquired hemoglobin H disease. *N. Engl. J. Med.* 285:1217, 1971.
    Unusual cause of hypochromic anemia associated with a myeloproliferative disorder.
16. Layrisse, M., Martinez-Torres, C., Cook, J. D., et al. Iron fortification of food: Its measurement by the extrinsic tag method. *Blood* 41:333, 1973.
    Ingestion of animal protein facilitates iron absorption, but ingestion of vegetables impairs it.
17. Schade, S. G., Cohen, R. J., and Conrad, M. E. Effect of hydrochloric acid on iron absorption. *N. Engl. J. Med.* 279:672, 1968.
    Gastric acid facilitates absorption of ferric food iron.
18. Cook, I. J., Pavli, P., Riley, J. W., et al. Gastrointestinal investigation of iron deficiency anaemia. *Br. Med. J.* 292:1380, 1986.
    Benign lesions in the upper gastrointestinal tract may be associated with malignant ones in the colon.

19. Reynolds, R. D., Binder, H. J., Miller, M. B., et al. Pagophagia and iron-deficiency anemia. *Ann. Intern. Med.* 69:435, 1968.
    Craving for ice associated with iron-deficiency anemia.
20. Crosby, W. H. Food pica and iron deficiency. *Arch. Intern. Med.* 127:960, 1971.
    Curious dietary habits should suggest iron deficiency.
21. Roselle, H. A. Association of laundry starch and clay ingestion with anemia in New York City. *Arch. Intern. Med.* 125:57, 1970.
    Possible role for starch ingestion in the production of iron deficiency.
22. Elwood, P. C., Jacobs, A., and Pitman, R. G. Epidemiology of the Paterson-Kelly syndrome. *Lancet* 2:716, 1964.
    Lack of correlation between postcricoid dysphagia and iron deficiency.
23. Kann, H. E., Jr., Mengel, C. E., and Wall, R. C. Paroxysmal nocturnal hemoglobinuria obscured by the presence of iron deficiency. *Ann. Intern. Med.* 67:593, 1967.
    Negative Ham's test in the presence of iron deficiency. Iron deficiency also masks folic acid deficiency in PNH.
24. Wheby, M. S. Effect of iron therapy on serum ferritin levels in iron-deficiency anemia. *Blood* 56:138, 1980.
    Serum ferritin can be employed to assess repletion of iron stores during iron replacement therapy.
25. Hamstra, R. D., Block, M. H., and Schocket, A. L. Intravenous iron dextran in clinical medicine. *J.A.M.A.* 243:1726, 1980.
    Allergic reactions, immediate or delayed, are uncommon and unpredictable.
26. Kernoff, L. M., Dommisse, J., and du Toit, E. D. Utilization of iron dextran in recurrent iron deficiency anaemia. *Br. J. Haematol.* 30:419, 1975.
    Ultimately, all the iron dextran is utilized.
27. Dudrick, S. J., O'Donnell, J. J., Raleigh, D. P., et al. Rapid restoration of red blood cell mass in severely anemic surgical patients who refuse transfusion. *Arch. Surg.* 120:721, 1985.
    Use of parenteral iron therapy.
28. Payne, S. M., and Finkelstein, R. A. The critical role of iron in host-bacterial interactions. *J. Clin. Invest.* 61:1428, 1978.
    Bacterial virulence correlates with ability to acquire iron. (See also Science 203:374, 1979.)
29. Klausner, R. D. From receptors to genes—insights from molecular iron metabolism. *Clin. Res.* 36:494, 1988.
    Review of the regulation of iron metabolism at the level of gene expression.
30. Huebers, H. A., and Finch, C. A. Transferrin: Physiologic behavior and clinical implications. *Blood* 64:763, 1984.
    Brief review.
31. Auerbach, M., Witt, D., Toler, W., et al. Clinical use of the total dose intravenous infusion of iron dextran. *J. Lab. Clin. Med.* 111:566, 1988.
    Excellent advice.
32. Huebers, H. A., Beguin, Y., Pootrakul, P., et al. Intact transferrin receptors in human plasma and their relation to erythropoiesis. *Blood* 75:102, 1990.
    Use of circulating transferrin receptors as a measure of erythropoiesis.

99. IRON OVERLOAD
Jerry L. Spivak

Iron absorbed from the gastrointestinal tract is normally transported by transferrin to developing marrow erythroblasts; excess iron is stored in the reticuloendothelial system (RES). When the plasma iron level increases and transferrin saturation exceeds 60 percent, iron is deposited in parenchymal cells. RES iron deposition is not harmful; parenchymal iron deposition, however, eventually results in tissue dysfunction. Parenchymal iron overload occurs in the following conditions: hereditary hemochromatosis, alcoholic cirrhosis with or without portacaval shunting, ineffective erythropoiesis (thalassemia, sideroblastic and refractory anemias), porphyria cutanea tarda (PCT), chronic transfusion therapy, chronic iron ingestion, and congenital atransferrinemia.

Hereditary hemochromatosis is an autosomal recessive disorder in which the responsible gene is located on chromosome 6. The gene is tightly linked to the HLA-A locus, and by HLA typing individuals within a given pedigree who are at risk of developing hemochromatosis and those who are heterozygous for the disorder can be identified. The frequency of the gene in the general population is about 10 percent and the frequency of hereditary hemochromatosis is 0.5 percent. In hereditary hemochromatosis, there is both an increase in iron absorption and defective handling of the iron by the RES. Consequently, parenchymal iron overload develops without an initial increase in RES iron. In PCT, which is also a hereditary disorder, iron overload also involves parenchymal cells predominantly, while in the other disorders associated with iron overload, both the RES and parenchymal cells are involved.

Parenchymal deposition of iron is most marked in the liver and pancreas, but it also occurs in the heart, the pituitary, adrenal, parathyroid, and thyroid glands, the joints, and the eye. Clinically, therefore, iron overload can be manifested in a number of ways. These include cirrhosis (with little evidence of functional impairment by laboratory tests), diabetes mellitus, skin pigmentation (more often due to melanin and thinning of the epidermis than to iron), cardiac arrhythmias, testicular atrophy and loss of libido (due to pituitary insufficiency), chondrocalcinosis, hypothyroidism, and, rarely, hypoparathyroidism or hypoaldosteronism. In hereditary hemochromatosis, the disease generally does not present until the fourth or fifth decade since accumulation of approximately 30 to 50 gm of iron is required for the clinical manifestations. Men are more commonly clinically affected than women, in part due to the protective effect of menstruation while ethanol abuse accelerates iron accumulation. With transfusion-induced iron overload, parenchymal iron accumulation and tissue damage are detectable after approximately 100 units of blood has been transfused.

The presence of iron overload due to hemochromatosis is suggested in men by a transferrin saturation of 62 percent or more in the fasting state; the comparable transferrin saturation for premenopausal women is less certain but is probably lower. Concomitant elevation of the serum ferritin is an indication for liver biopsy. Serum ferritin, alone, is not a useful test since it may be normal in some patients with tissue iron overload or elevated nonspecifically by inflammatory disorders or hepatocellular injury. Direct evaluation of liver iron is important since there appears to be a critical iron concentration at which cirrhosis or fibrosis develops. Deferoxamine iron excretion is an insensitive test and is not recommended. The extent of tissue damage can also be assessed by a glucose tolerance test, echocardiography, and skeletal x rays which may show chondrocalcinosis and osteoporosis. When a diagnosis of hemochromatosis is established in the absence of a clinical illness predisposing to iron overload, it is incumbent on the physician to examine the patient's family to determine if other members suffer from excessive but clinically inapparent iron overload.

Phlebotomy is the therapy of choice in tissue iron overload from any cause. In patients with iron overload secondary to ineffective erythropoiesis, anemia may prevent the use of phlebotomy. In this instance, continuous subcutaneous infusion of deferoxamine can be beneficial. Removal of iron improves survival, reverses hepatic damage, decreases skin pigmentation, and improves cardiac failure, glucose tolerance and testicular function, but has little effect on the arthropathy. The degree of saturation of transferrin is a convenient guide to the effectiveness of phlebotomy. In PCT, phlebotomy often results in clinical improvement, even after iron stores are normalized. Patients with hereditary hemochromatosis who develop cirrhosis are at risk from hepatocellular carcinoma. This is not affected by phlebotomy. A clue to the presence of this complication is a fall in the serum iron and transferrin saturation. Anemia or erythrocytosis may also develop although the latter can be obscured by an increased plasma volume.

1. Edwards, C. Q., Griffen, L. M., Goldgar, D., et al. Prevalence of hemochromatosis among 11,065 presumably healthy blood donors. *N. Engl. J. Med.* 318:1355, 1988. *Screening of men in the third decade using transferrin saturation is advocated.*

2. Dadone, M. M., Kushner, J. P., Edwards, C. Q., et al. Hereditary hemochromatosis: Analysis of laboratory expression of the disease by genotype in 18 pedigrees. *Am. J. Clin. Pathol.* 78:196, 1982.
A transferrin saturation of 62% or greater identifies individuals homozygous for hemochromatosis. (See also Ann. Intern. Med. *101:707, 1984.)*

3. Simon, M., Le-Mignon, L., Fauchet, R., et al. A study of 609 HLA haplotypes marking for the hemochromatosis gene: (1) mapping of the gene near the HLA-A locus and characters required to define a heterozygous population and (2) hypothesis concerning the underlying cause of hemochromatosis-HLA association. *Am. J. Hum. Genet.* 41:89, 1987.
Only HLA-A3 is an independent marker for hemochromatosis. (See also Am. J. Hum. Genet. *38:805, 1986.)*

4. Cartwright, G. E., Edwards, C. Q., Kravitz, K., et al. Hereditary hemochromatosis: Phenotypic expression of the disease. *N. Engl. J. Med.* 301:175, 1979.
HLA-A3, -B14, and -B7 are observed with increased frequency in patients with hemochromatosis.

5. Edwards C. Q., Cartwright, G. E., Skolnick, M. H., et al. Homozygosity for hemochromatosis: Clinical manifestations. *Ann. Intern. Med.* 93:519, 1980.
Very few patients have the classic triad of hepatomegaly, diabetes mellitus, and hyperpigmentation. Arthralgia but not arthritis is an important early manifestation.

6. Beaumont, C., Simon, M., Smith, P. M., et al. Hepatic and serum ferritin concentrations in patients with idiopathic hemochromatosis. *Gastroenterology* 79:877, 1980.
Serum ferritin levels can be normal early in the disease.

7. Bassett, M. M., Halliday, J. W., Ferris R. A., et al. Diagnosis of hemochromatosis in young subjects: Predictive accuracy of biochemical screening tests. *Gastroenterology,* 87:628, 1984.
The combination of serum ferritin and transferrin saturation is reliable for screening purposes.

8. Edwards, E. Q., Carroll, M., Bray, P., et al. Hereditary hemochromatosis. *N. Engl. J. Med.* 297:7, 1977.
Estimation of liver iron is the most sensitive method for detecting early disease.

9. Bassett, M. L., Halliday, J. W., and Powell, L. W. Value of hepatic iron measurements in early hemochromatosis and determination of the critical iron level associated with fibrosis. *Hepatology* 6:24, 1986.
Accumulation of more than 20 mg iron per gram of liver is associated with hepatic fibrosis.

10. Brink, B., Disler, P., Lynch, S., et al. Patterns of iron storage in dietary iron overload and idiopathic hemochromatosis. *J. Lab. Clin. Med.* 88:725, 1976.
In hemochromatosis, liver iron increases without a comparable rise in marrow iron. (See also Gastroenterology 75:886, 1978.)

11. Prieto, J., Barry M., and Sherlock, S. Serum ferritin in patients with iron overload and with acute and chronic liver diseases. *Gastroenterology* 68:525, 1975.
In the presence of liver disease, the serum ferritin level does not correlate well with body iron stores.

12. Cook, J. D., Skikne, B. S., Lynch, S. R., et al. Estimates of iron sufficiency in the US population. *Blood* 68:726, 1986.
In adult men, iron overload may be more common than iron deficiency.

13. Jacobs, A. Metabolic consequences of iron overload. *Br. J. Haematol.* 34:1, 1976.
Lipid peroxidation, lysosomal damage, and ascorbic acid depletion, which can lead to osteoporosis.

14. Howard, J. M., Ghent, L. N., Carey, L. S., et al. Diagnostic efficacy of hepatic computed tomography in the detection of body iron overload. *Gastroenterology* 84:209, 1983.
Computed tomography is not a sensitive method for evaluating hepatic iron stores.

15. Jensen, P. S. Hemochromatosis: A disease often silent but not invisible. *Am. J. Roentgenol. Radium Ther. Nucl. Med.* 126:343, 1976.
Arthritic changes involving the hand and wrist, as well as generalized chondrocalcinosis, are characteristic findings.

16. Cawley, E. P., Hsu, Y. T., Wood B. T., et al. Hemochromatosis and the skin. *Arch. Dermatol.* 100:1, 1969.
    Pigmentation is usually due to melanin.
17. Dymock, I. W., Cassar, J., Pyke, D. A., et al. Observations on the pathogenesis, complications and treatment of diabetes in 115 cases of hemochromatosis. *Am. J. Med.* 52:203, 1972.
    All the complications of diabetes, including insulin resistance, occur in hemochromatosis.
18. Iyer, R., Duckworth, W. C., and Solomon, S. S. Hypogonadism in idiopathic hemochromatosis: endocrine studies. *Arch. Intern. Med.* 141:517, 1981.
    Hypothalamic-pituitary dysfunction is the cause of gonadal failure and can be reversed with iron depletion. (See also Ann. Intern. Med. *101:629, 1984 and* J. Clin. Endocrinol. Metab. *65:585, 1987.)*
19. Edwards, C. Q., Kelly, T. M., Ellweis, G., et al. Thyroid disease in hemochromatosis. Increased incidence in homozygous men. *Arch. Intern. Med.* 143:1890, 1983.
    Iron-induced hypothyroidism is seen primarily in men.
20. Sherman, L. A., Pfefferbaum, A., and Brown, E. B. Hypoparathyroidism in a patient with longstanding iron storage disease. *Ann. Intern. Med.* 73:259, 1970.
    An unusual complication of iron overload. (See also Am. J. Med. Sci. *276:363, 1978.)*
21. Cutler, D. J., Isner, J. M., Bracey, A. W., et al. Hemochromatosis heart disease: An unemphasized cause of potentially reversible restrictive cardiomyopathy. *Am. J. Med.* 69:923, 1980.
    Hemochromatosis is an important cause of reversible, restrictive cardiomyopathy. (See also Am. J. Med. *70:1275, 1981 and* Gastroenterology 76:178, 1979.)
22. Olson, L. J., Edwards, W. D., McCall, J. T., et al. Cardiac iron deposition in idiopathic hemochromatosis: Histologic and analytic assessment of 14 hearts from autopsy. *J. Am. Coll. Cardiol.* 10:1239, 1987.
    Parenchymal deposition of iron documented.
23. Olson, L. J., Baldus, W. P., Tajik, A. J. Echocardiographic features of idiopathic hemochromatosis. *Am. J. Cardiol.* 60:885, 1987.
    Use of two-dimensional-echocardiography to evaluate cardiac function.
24. Dabestani, A., Child, J. S., Henze, E., et al. Primary hemochromatosis: anatomic and physiologic characteristics of the cardiac ventricles and their response to phlebotomy. *Am. J. Cardiol.* 54:153, 1984.
    Phlebotomy improves cardiac function.
25. Grisaru, D., Golfarb, A. W., Gotsman, M. S., et al. Deferoxamine improves left ventricular function in β-thalassemia. *Arch. Intern. Med.* 146:2344, 1986.
    Use of chelation therapy in transfusion hemosiderosis.
26. Askari, A. D., Muir, W. A., Rosner, I. A., et al. Arthritis of hemochromatosis. *Am. J. Med.* 75:957, 1983.
    Arthritis classically involves the first three metacarpophalangeal joints but may not be an early manifestation of the disease. (See also Arthritis Rheum. *30:1137, 1987.)*
27. Johnson, B. F. Hemochromatosis resulting from prolonged oral iron therapy. *N. Engl. J. Med.* 278:1100, 1968.
    A rare occurrence. (See also Am. J. Pathol. *96:611, 1979.)*
28. Sauer, G. F., and Funk, D. D. Iron overload in cutaneous porphyria. *Arch. Intern. Med.* 124:190, 1969.
    Hepatic localization of iron is similar to that of hemochromatosis.
29. Beaumont, C., Fauchet, R., Phung, L. N., et al. Porphyria cutanea tarda and HLA-linked hemochromatosis. *Gastroenterology* 92:1833, 1987.
    There is no association between HLA-A3 and PCT.
30. Felsher, B. F., and Kushner, J. P. Hepatic siderosis and porphyria cutanea tarda: Relation of iron excess to the metabolic defect. *Semin. Hematol.* 14:243, 1977.
    PCT is a hereditary disorder in which ethanol need not have a role.
31. Rumsay, C. A., Magnus, I. A., Turnbull, A., et al. The treatment of porjhyria cutanea tarda by venesection. *Q. J. Med.* 43:1, 1974.
    Phlebotomy is an effective form of therapy.
32. Schafer, A. I., Cheron, R. G., Dluhy, R., et al. Clinical consequences of acquired transfusional iron overload in adults. *N. Engl. J. Med.* 304:319, 1981.

Transfusion-induced iron overload can cause widespread tissue damage in a manner similar to hereditary hemochromatosis.

33. Pippard, M. J., Callender, S. T., Warner, G. T., et al. Iron absorption and loading in β-thalassaemia intermedia. *Lancet* 2:819, 1979.
    The risk of iron overload from increased absorption is significant in thalassemia intermedia.

34. Hakim, R. M., Stivelman, J. C., Schulman, G., et al. Iron overload and mobilization in long-term hemodialysis patients. *Am. J. Kidney Dis.* 10:293, 1987.
    This is not an HLA-linked problem.

35. Wallack, M. K., and Winkelstein, A. Acute iron intoxication in an adult. *J.A.M.A.* 229:1333, 1974.
    An uncommon occurrence in adults.

36. Niederau, C., Fischer, R., Sonnenberg, A., et al. Survival and causes of death in cirrhotic and in noncirrhotic patients with primary hemochromatosis. *N. Engl. J. Med.* 313:1256, 1985.
    If treatment is begun in the precirrhotic phase, life expectancy is normal.

37. Hoffbrand, A. V., Gorman, A., Laulicht, M., et al. Improvement in iron status and liver function in patients with transfusional iron overload with long-term subcutaneous desferrioxamine. *Lancet* 1:947, 1979.
    Subcutaneous administration of deferoxamine is effective in reducing tissue iron content. (See also N. Engl. J. Med. 297:418, 1977.)

38. Pippard, M. J., Callender, S. T., Letsky, E. A., et al. Prevention of iron loading in transfusion-dependent thalassaemia. *Lancet* 1:1178, 1978.
    Use of subcutaneous deferoxamine in thalassemia major. (For the use of intravenous deferoxamine see J.A.M.A. 239:2149, 1978 and Annu. Rev. Med. 33:509, 1982.)

39. Olivieri, N. F., Buncic, J. R., Chew, E., et al. Visual and auditory neurotoxicity in patients receiving subcutaneous deferoxamine infusions. *N. Engl. J. Med.* 314:869, 1986.
    An avoidable complication.

40. Nienhuis, A. W. Vitamin C and iron. *N. Engl. J. Med.* 304:170, 1981.
    Vitamin C augments iron chelation by deferoxamine but can also mobilize iron from the reticuloendothelial system making it available for deposition in other organs. (See also N. Engl. J. Med. 304:158, 1981.)

41. Weintraub, L. R., Edwards, C. Q., and Krikker, M. Hemochromatosis. *Ann. N. Y. Acad. Sci.* 526:1, 1988.
    A major symposium on hemochromatosis.

42. Finch, C. A., and Huebers, H. Perspectives in iron metabolism. *N. Engl. J. Med.* 306:1520, 1982.
    Excellent review of this subject.

---

100. MYELOFIBROSIS
Jerry L. Spivak

Under normal circumstances, the bone marrow contains a network of reticulin fibers that serves as part of its supporting stroma. Viewed with special stains, this reticulin network is incomplete and most prominent around blood vessels. Under certain conditions, the content of marrow reticulin increases, often to the point of forming large collagenous bands and new bone within the marrow cavity with displacement of normal hematopoietic elements. The development of significant marrow fibrosis occurs in widely disparate conditions. They include acute leukemia, both lymphocytic and non-lymphocytic, leukemic reticuloendotheliosis ("hairy-cell" leukemia), non-Hodgkin's lymphoma, Hodgkin's disease, chronic myelogenous leukemia (CML), idiopathic myelofibrosis (IMF), polycythemia vera (PV), multiple myeloma, carcinoma metastatic to the bone marrow, chronic renal failure, infection, irradiation or chemotherapy, thorium dioxide (Thorotrast) intoxication, and certain autoimmune disorders such as pure red cell aplasia, scleroderma, and systemic lupus erythematosus. The presence of myelofibrosis is usually recognized when bone marrow aspiration fails to yield any marrow particles. When bone marrow aspiration is performed in a technically satsifactory manner, failure to obtain marrow particles is usually a consequence of either marrow aplasia, myelofibrosis, osteosclerosis, or replacement of normal marrow elements by metastatic tumor. The concept that a marrow tightly packed with hematopoietic cells is resistant to aspiration is incorrect since the most crowded marrows are usually observed with megaloblastic anemia, a situation in which difficulty in aspirating an adequate sample is almost never encountered. The presence of myelofibrosis is established by examination of a bone marrow biopsy using special stains for reticulin and collagen fibers. A slight increase in reticulin content is usually encountered when the degree of marrow cellularity is increased, but a marked increase in reticulin content, particularly away from blood vessels, is of pathologic significance.

Myelofibrosis should always be considered as a reactive process secondary to a disorder involving the bone marrow. Clear-cut examples of this include carcinoma metastatic to the marrow, thorium dioxide intoxication in which intense radiation of the marrow by alpha rays occurs as a consequence of aggregation of thorium deposited in marrow macrophages, and the fibrosis occurring within the marrow as part of the metabolic bone disease associated with the hyperparathyroidism of renal failure. Myelofibrosis most commonly occurs in the setting of myeloproliferative disorders. It is seen in a high percentage of patients with acute leukemia (both lymphocytic and nonlymphocytic) where it may be asymptomatic or associated with bone pain and bone infarcts. Patients with CML often develop myelofibrosis during the course of that disease and in some patients myelofibrosis may be present at the onset of CML. Patients with PV not uncommonly develop myelofibrosis, myeloid metaplasia, and ineffective erythropoiesis as their disease runs its course. Some patients develop a syndrome in which myelofibrosis and myeloid metaplasia are associated without evidence of erythrocytosis or CML, and this syndrome has been termed *idiopathic myelofibrosis (IMF)*. CML, PV, and IMF all share one feature in common other than myelofibrosis. Namely, they are clonal disorders of hematopoietic stem cells. In CML, the disease appears to arise in the stem cell pluripotent for lymphocyte progenitors as well as erythroid, myeloid, and megakaryocytic progenitors. In PV and IMF, the progeny of the neoplastic stem cell are limited to erythroid, myeloid, and megakaryocytic precursors. In each of these conditions, it has been amply demonstrated that bone marrow fibroblasts do not arise from the neoplastic clone but appear to represent part of the bone marrow reaction to the clonal proliferation. In spite of certain similarities, CML appears to be an entirely separate disorder from IMF. It is noteworthy, however, that transitions do occur between PV and IMF, often to the extent that it is difficult to distinguish the two disorders. For example, patients with IMF have developed erythrocytosis following splenectomy, and as mentioned above many patients with PV eventually develop myelofibrosis, myeloid metaplasia, and anemia, a clinical picture indistinguishable from IMF.

The generally indolent and chronic course of IMF with myeloid metaplasia must be distinguished from certain disorders with myelofibrosis that have a much more fulminant course. The term *acute* ("malignant") *myelosclerosis* has been used to describe a group of patients with pancytopenia, minimal or absent anisocytosis and poikilocytosis, a dry bone marrow aspirate, a marked increase in marrow reticulin content, hyperplasia and immaturity of erythroid, myeloid and megakaryocytic cell lines (i.e., a panmyelopathy), minimal to absent splenomegaly, and a rapidly progressive course. Acute myelosclerosis is thought to be distinguishable from acute leukemia with myelofibrosis. Such a distinction, however, seems artificial. For example, acute leukemia of the nonlymphocytic variety can arise in either the common hematopoietic stem cell or in the granulocyte-macrophage progenitor cell. In either case, the end result is the same, acute leukemia, and it is not possible from the phenotypic expression of the disorder to determine the site of the malignant transformation any more than it is possible without cytogenetic studies to distinguish CML presenting as blast crisis from acute leukemia. Furthermore, progression from a panmyelopathy with hyperplasia of all marrow elements to a marrow that is totally replaced by blast cells has been observed. It, therefore, seems more rational to consider acute myelosclerosis as acute leukemia presenting with myelofibrosis. The absence of splenomegaly cannot be used to differentiate between the acute and chronic forms of myelofibrosis since a number of patients with chronic myelofibrosis, for unknown reasons, do not develop splenomegaly, at least early in the course of their disease. A much more important differential point in acute myelofibrosis associated with acute leukemia is the absence of teardrop-shaped red cells in the peripheral blood. These are a hallmark of chronic myelofibrosis. Teardrop forms are usually not seen in carcinoma metastatic to the marrow, however; metastatic carcinoma may be associated with a microangiopathic hemolytic anemia.

IMF is a chronic disorder with a symptom complex that includes weakness, progressive weight loss, and gastrointestinal discomfort due to the mechanical effects of massive splenomegaly and splenic infarction. Complications of IMF include anemia due to ineffective erythropoiesis, hypersplenism leading to the thrombocytopenia, hyperuricemia with gout or renal stones as a consequence of the high turnover of hematopoietic cells, folic acid deficiency due to the increased demand for this vitamin by hematopoietic tissue, and portal hypertension and ascites as a consequence of sinusoidal obstruction by extramedullary hematopoiesis, venous thrombosis, or increased splenic blood flow. Patients with IMF have an increased incidence of bacterial infections and, in the early literature, tuberculosis, particularly of the disseminated variety, was not uncommon. In some patients, extramedullary hematopoiesis causes serious organ dysfunction. Proliferating hematopoietic cells can occlude hepatic sinusoids and cause spinal cord compression, increased intracranial pressure, small bowel or ureteral obstruction, and recurrent pulmonary thrombosis. In less than 10 percent of patients, acute leukemia occurs as a terminal event. In some of these patients, IMF was preceded by PV and a majority of the patients had been treated with either alkylating agents, irradiation, or both. The diagnosis of acute leukemia cannot be established on the basis of a high white count or the presence of circulating blast cells since both of these are features characteristic of IMF in the absence of leukemic transformation.

The etiology of myelofibrosis is unknown. The persistence of megakaryocytes in contrast to other hematopoietic cells within the myelofibrotic area of the marrow and the association of myelofibrosis with myeloproliferative disorders has led to the interesting postulate that the fibrosis may be secondary to the leakage of platelet-derived growth factor from dysfunctional megakaryocytes of the myeloproliferative clone. Since platelet-derived growth factor is known to stimulate fibroblast proliferation and fibroblasts are not derived from the transformed clone, this is an attractive hypothesis. It does not, however, explain the lack of fibrosis associated with other disorders in which there is an expanded bone marrow pool of megakaryocytes, nor does it explain the observation that some patients with IMF do not have significant fibrosis within the bone marrow. Other unexplained features of myelofibrosis are its occurrence in patients with collagen-vascular disease and an appreciable incidence of autoimmune phenomena occurring in patients with IMF and myelofibrosis in the absence of overt collagen-vascular disease. The possibility that myelofibrosis in some instances is due to autoimmune phenomena or immune complexes is worthy of consideration.

The treatment of myelofibrosis should be directed at the condition causing the disorder. In patients with acute leukemia, myelofibrosis can be eradicated by chemotherapy. It has also been reversed with bone marrow transplantation. In patients with uremia and secondary hyperparathyroidism, parathyroidectomy often ameliorates the condition. In patients with chronic myelofibrosis associated with myeloid metaplasia, treatment is generally symptomatic since these patients are sensitive to the effects of alkylating agents or irradiation. The role of agents such as the interferons in the treatment of IMF is currently under evaluation. Splenectomy is occasionally necessary because of mechanical problems or hypersplenism. Death in IMF is usually a consequence of infection, heart failure, hemorrhage, or acute leukemia.

---

1. Varki, A., Lottenberg, R., Griffith, R., et al. The syndrome of idiopathic myelofibrosis. A clinicopathologic review with emphasis on the prognostic variables predicting survival. *Medicine* 62:353, 1983.

Anemia, thrombocytopenia, and constitutional symptoms are prognostic signs. (See also Medicine 50:357, 1971.)

2. Jacobson, R. J., Solo, A., and Fialkow, P. J. Agnogenic myeloid metaplasia: A clonal proliferation of hematopoietic stem cells with secondary myelofibrosis. Blood 51:189, 1978.
   IMF is a clonal disorder of the hematopoietic stem cell and marrow fibroblasts are not involved.

3. Manoharan, A. Myelofibrosis: Prognostic factors and treatment. Br. J. Haematol. 69:295, 1988.
   A brief review.

4. Demory, J. L., Dupriez, B., Fenaux, P., et al. Cytogenetic studies and their prognostic significance in agnogenic myeloid metaplasia: A report on 47 cases. Blood 72:855, 1988.
   Chromosome abnormalities are associated with a poor prognosis.

5. Burston, J., and Pinniger, J. L. The reticulin content of bone marrow in haematological disorders. Br. J. Haematol. 7:172, 1963.
   A survey of the reticulin content of the marrow in various blood diseases. (See also Am. J. Clin. Pathol. 56:24, 1971.)

6. Bentley, S. A., and Herman, C. J. Bone marrow fibre production in myelofibrosis: A quantitative study. Br. J. Haematol. 42:51, 1979.
   Marrow fiber content does not correlate with spleen weight or duration of clinical illness. (See also Br. J. Haematol. 59:1, 1985.)

7. Glew, R. H., Haese, W. H., and McIntyre, P. A. Myeloid metaplasia with myelofibrosis: The clinical spectrum of extramedullary hematopoiesis and tumor formation. Johns Hopkins Med. J. 132:253, 1973.
   Complications produced by aggressive extramedullary hematopoiesis.

8. Ligumski, M., Polliack, A., and Benbasset, J. Nature and incidence of liver involvement in agnogenic myeloid metaplasia. Scand. J. Haematol. 21:83, 1978.
   Portal hypertension, ascites, and abnormal liver function tests as a consequence of myeloid metaplasia and increased portal blood flow. (See also Eur. J. Haematol. 40:355, 1988.)

9. Kuo, T.-T., Uhlemann, J., and Reinhard, E. H. Cutaneous extramedullary hematopoiesis. Arch. Dermatol. 112:1302, 1976.
   An unusual site of hematopoiesis in myeloid metaplasia.

10. Kosmidis, P. A., Palacas, C. G., and Axelrod, A. R. Diffuse purely osteolytic lesions in myelofibrosis. Cancer 46:2263, 1980.
    Usually osteosclerosis is observed.

11. Ligumski, M., Polliack, A., Benbassat, J. Myeloid metaplasia of the central nervous system in patients with myelofibrosis and agnogenic myeloid metaplasia. Am. J. Med. Sci. 275:99, 1978.
    CNS complications of extramedullary hematopoiesis reviewed.

12. Price, R., and Bell, H. Spinal cord compression due to extramedullary hematopoiesis. Successful treatment in a patient with long-standing myelofibrosis. J.A.M.A. 253:2876, 1985.
    A review.

13. Murphy, S., Davis, J. L., Walsh, P. N., et al. Template bleeding time and clinical hemorrhage in myeloproliferative disease. Arch. Intern. Med. 138:1251, 1978.
    A prolonged bleeding time is not uncommon in IMF.

14. Manaharan, A., Horsley, R., and Pitney, W. R. The reticulin content of bone marrow in acute leukemia in adults. Br. J. Haematol. 43:185, 1979.
    Myelofibrosis occurs in both lymphocytic and nonlymphocytic leukemia.

15. Bearman, R. M., Pangalis, G. A., and Rappaport, H. Acute ("malignant") myelosclerosis. Cancer 43:279, 1979.
    Absence of teardrop-shaped red cells and splenomegaly used to distinguish acute leukemia with myelofibrosis from IMF.

16. Truong, L. D., Saleem, A., and Schwartz, M. R. Acute myelofibrosis. Medicine 63:182, 1984.
    A form of acute leukemia. (See also Br. J. Haematol. 42:9, 1979.)

17. Spector, J. I., and Levine, P. H. Carcinomatous bone marrow invasion simulating acute myelofibrosis. *Am. J. Med. Sci.* 266:145, 1973.
    A problem in differential diagnosis.
18. Wolf, B. C., and Neiman, R. S. Myelofibrosis with myeloid metaplasia: Pathophysiologic implications of the correlation between bone marrow changes and progression of splenomegaly. *Blood* 65:803, 1985.
    Progression of fibrosis and disease duration are not related.
19. Rosenthal, D. S., and Moloney, W. C. Occurrence of acute leukemia in myeloproliferative disorders. *Br. J. Haematol.* 36:373, 1977.
    Acute leukemia in IMF is usually associated with alkylating agents or irradiation.
20. Gordon, B. R., Coleman, M., Kohen, P., et al. Immunologic abnormalities in myelofibrosis with activation of the complement system. *Blood* 58:904, 1981.
    Complement activation occurs in patients with IMF and myelofibrosis.
21. Cooper, B., Fishler, P. V., Atkins, L., et al. Loss of Rh antigen associated with acquired Rh antibodies and a chromosome translocation in a patient with myeloid metaplasia. *Blood* 54:642, 1979.
    Acquired Rh mosaicism is not uncommon in myeloproliferative disorders.
22. Kaelin, W. G., Jr., and Spivak, J. L. Systemic lupus erythematosus and myelofibrosis. *Am. J. Med.* 81:935, 1986.
    For another example of autoimmune myelofibrosis, see Am. J. Hematol. *25:225, 1987.*
23. Vandermolen, L., Rice, L., and Lynch, E. G. Plasma cell dyscrasia with marrow fibrosis. Clinicopathologic syndrome. *Am. J. Med.* 79:297, 1985.
    An uncommon presentation. (See also Am. J. Clin. Pathol. *89:63, 1989.)*
24. Broe, P. J., Conley, C. L., and Cameron, J. L. Thrombosis of the portal vein following splenectomy for myeloid metaplasia. *Surg. Gynecol. Obstet.* 152:488, 1981.
    Portal vein thrombosis may occur several years after splenectomy but is unrelated to the height of the platelet count.
25. Mason, B. A., Kressel, B. R., Cashdollar, M. R., et al. Periostitis associated with myelofibrosis. *Cancer* 43:1568, 1979.
    An unusual complication palliated by irradiation.
26. Wagner, H., Jr., McKeough, P. G., Desforges, J., et al. Splenic irradiation in the treatment of patients with chronic myelogenous leukemia or myelofibrosis with myeloid metaplasia. Results of daily and intermittent fractionation with and without concomitant hydroxyurea. *Cancer* 58:1204, 1986.
    The toxicity of this approach is not small.

101. NONTHROMBOCYTOPENIC PURPURA
Jerry L. Spivak

Purpura in the absence of thrombocytopenia is the result of either defective platelet plug formation or an abnormality of vascular or connective tissue. Abnormalities of platelet function resulting in defective plug formation can be either congenital or acquired. Congenital abnormalities include impaired platelet adhesiveness (Bernard-Soulier syndrome, von Willebrand's disease), impaired platelet aggregation (Ehlers-Danlos syndrome, thrombasthenia), and impairment of secretion (storage pool disease, albinism, Wiskott-Aldrich syndrome, Chédiak-Higashi syndrome, and a heterogeneous group of disorders in which prostaglandin synthesis is impaired). Acquired platelet dysfunction is seen in the myeloproliferative disorders (idiopathic myelofibrosis, preleukemia, polycythemia vera, and idiopathic thrombocythemia), uremia, alcoholism, postcardiopulmonary bypass, dysproteinemias, vitamin C and vitamin B_{12} deficiency, and with administration of certain drugs. Dextran and dipyridamole impair platelet adhesiveness.

Penicillin and its derivatives may interfere with platelet membrane receptors. Aspirin, phenylbutazone, sulfinpyrazone, and indomethacin impair platelet aggregation and endogenous adenosine diphosphate (ADP) release. The effect of aspirin is irreversible and lasts the life span of the platelet. In uremia a prolonged bleeding time is associated with impaired platelet adhesion, aggregation, and factor III release. The defect is not completely corrected by dialysis. The substance(s) responsible for abnormal platelet function is unknown but urea, guanidinosuccinic acid, and phenolic acids have been implicated. Dysproteinemias are commonly associated with a hemorrhagic diathesis, which may be due to temperature-induced protein precipitation (cryoglobulinemia), increased blood viscosity (macroglobulinemia), reduction in clotting factor levels, or a circulating anticoagulant, but which has been best correlated with abnormal platelet adhesiveness and a prolonged bleeding time. Bleeding occurs most often in Waldenström's macroglobulinemia and IgA myeloma.

Connective tissue disorders associated with nonthrombocytopenic purpura include Marfan's syndrome, Ehlers-Danlos syndrome, and osteogenesis imperfecta. Abnormal-appearing platelets can be seen in patients with these conditions and platelet aggregation may be impaired. Structural abnormalities of vascular and connective tissue are probably important in the hemorrhagic diathesis, and a recent study suggests that in some patients defective fibronectin is responsible for both the platelet dysfunction and joint hypermobility. Acquired disorders of connective tissue producing purpura include Cushing's syndrome, exogenous steroid administration, amyloidosis, and scurvy. Steroids appear to have an adverse effect on vascular fragility, presumably due to their catabolic action. Scorbutic bleeding is the result of both a platelet and a connective tissue defect. Characteristically, hemorrhage is perifollicular but, in contrast to most purpuric syndromes, deep tissue bleeding is not uncommon and perineural hematomas causing nerve entrapment have been described. Amyloidosis is an uncommon but interesting cause of vascular purpura. It is due to amyloid infiltration of small superficial vessels. In contrast to many forms of purpura that show a dependent distribution, amyloid purpura is most common on the upper part of the body. The bleeding tendency in amyloidosis may also be enhanced by acquired factor IX or X deficiency due to binding of these factors by amyloid fibrils.

Vasculitis is a common cause of nonthrombocytopenic purpura, and when the origin of the purpura is unclear, a skin biopsy is often helpful. Drug hypersensitivity is a frequent cause of vasculitic purpura, and it is important to be aware of the unusual reactions caused by coumarin congeners. In contrast to purpura associated with dysproteinemias, purpura occurring in the benign hyperglobulinemia of Waldenström appears to be due to a vasculitis. In this syndrome the presence of circulating IgG or IgM–anti-IgG complexes is probably more important than the actual concentration of gamma globulin in the serum. Purpura is a component of the Henoch-Schönlein syndrome, in which vasculitis also involves the joints, lungs, gastrointestinal tract, and kidneys. It is unclear whether the syndrome should be considered a separate entity or a part of the spectrum of necrotizing vasculitis due to drugs, toxins, and infectious agents.

A peculiar syndrome that cannot be classified with any of the conditions mentioned is psychogenic purpura. Patients with this interesting disorder develop painful ecchymoses that can often be reproduced by intracutaneous injection of their own blood. The most striking component of the illness is the underlying personality disorder. It is important to remember, however, when evaluating a patient for psychogenic purpura, that Cushing's syndrome and systemic lupus erythematosus can also present with purpura and a psychiatric disturbance.

Finally, certain infections may also cause nonthrombocytopenia purpura. They include smallpox, typhoid, rickettsial infections, meningococcemia, and bacterial endocarditis.

1. Kitchens, C. S. The purpuric disorders. *Semin. Thromb. Hemost.* 10:173, 1984.
   Brief review.
2. Katz, P. Vasculitic purpura: Differential diagnosis and therapy. *Semin. Thromb. Hemost.* 10:202, 1984.
   For a review of the pathology of immune-mediated vasculitis, see Semin. Thromb. Hemost. *10:196, 1984.*

3. Weiss, H. J. Congenital disorders of platelet function. *Semin. Hematol.* 17:228, 1980.
   Comprehensive review.
4. Malpass, T. W., and Harker, L. A. Acquired disorders of platelet function. *Semin. Hematol.* 17:242, 1980.
   Comprehensive review.
5. Harker, L. A., and Slichter, S. J. The bleeding time as a screening test for evaluation of platelet function. *N. Engl. J. Med.* 287:155, 1972.
   Correlation of bleeding time with platelet function rather than with number.
6. Ratnoff, O. D., and Agle, D. P. Psychogenic purpura: A re-evaluation of the syndrome of autoerythrocyte sensitization. *Medicine* 47:475, 1968.
   Painful ecchymoses associated with multiple somatic complaints and a characteristic personality disorder.
7. O'Reilly, R. A., and Aggeler, P. M. Covert anticoagulant ingestion: Study of 25 patients and review of world literature. *Medicine* 55:389, 1976.
   These patients are mostly women, often are paramedical personnel, and are self-destructive or malingering.
8. Estes, J. W. Platelet size and function in the hereditable disorders of connective tissue. *Ann. Intern. Med.* 68:1237, 1968.
   Abnormal platelet morphology found but not correlated with hemostatic abnormalities.
9. Arneson, M. A., Hammerschmidt, D. E., Furcht, L. T., et al. A new form of Ehlers-Danlos syndrome. *J.A.M.A.* 244:144, 1980.
   Defective fibronectin postulated to be the cause of platelet and connective tissue abnormalities.
10. Czapek, E. E., Deykin, D., Salzman, E., et al. Intermediate syndrome of platelet dysfunction. *Blood* 52:103, 1978.
    A thrombocytopathic defect unmasked by aspirin and similar drugs.
11. Kyle, R. A., Gleich, G. J., Bayrd, E. D., et al. Benign hypergammaglobulinemic purpura of Waldenström. *Medicine* 50:113, 1971.
    Polyclonal gammopathy with IgG–anti-IgG complexes, purpura, and a tendency to develop collagen-vascular disease.
12. Fauci, A. S., Haynes, B. F., and Katz, P. The spectrum of vasculitis. *Ann. Intern. Med.* 89:660, 1978.
    Clinical review.
13. Barth, W. F., Willerson, J. J., Waldmann, T. A., et al. Primary amyloidosis: Clinical immunochemical and immunoglobulin metabolism studies in fifteen patients. *Am. J. Med.* 47:259, 1969.
    Purpura is most common on the upper part of the body.
14. Furie, B., Voo, L., McAdam, K. P., et al. Mechanism of factor X deficiency in systemic amyloidosis. *N. Engl. J. Med.* 304:827, 1981.
    Amyloid fibrils bind factor X and occasionally IX and II. (See also Am. J. Hematol. 11:443, 1981.)
15. Perkins, H. A., Mackenzie, M. R., and Fudenberg, H. H. Hemostatic defects in dysproteinemias. *Blood* 35:695, 1970.
    Hemorrhagic diathesis is best correlated with abnormal bleeding time or abnormal platelet adhesiveness.
16. Brouet, J.-C., Clavel, J.-P., Danon, F., et al. Biologic and clinical significance of cryoglobulins. *Am. J. Med.* 57:775, 1974.
    Nonthrombocytopenic purpura is the most common manifestation.
17. Ferreiro, J. E., Pasarin, G., Quesada, R., et al. Benign hypergammaglobulinemic purpura of Waldenström associated with Sjögren's syndrome. *Am. J. Med.* 81:734, 1986.
    See also Am. J. Kidney Dis. 9:172, 1987.
18. Roth, D. A., Wilz, D. R., and Theil, G. B. Schönlein-Henoch syndrome in adults. *Q. J. Med.* 55:145, 1985.
    An IgA-mediated immune complex disorder.
19. Ballard, H. S., Eisinger, R. P., and Gallo, G. Renal manifestations of the Henoch-Schönlein syndrome in adults. *Am. J. Med.* 49:328, 1970.
    Crescent formation is indicative of a poor prognosis. (See also Q. J. Med. 41:241, 1972.)

20. Waldo, F. B. Is Henoch-Schönlein purpura the systemic form of IgA nephropathy? *Am. J. Kidney Dis.* 12:373, 1988.
    An interesting hypothesis. (See also N. Zl. Med. J. 99:534, 1986.)
21. Hene, R. J., Velthuis, P., van de Wiel, A., et al. The relevance of IgA deposits in vessel walls of clinically normal skin. *Arch. Intern. Med.* 146:745, 1986.
    A useful diagnostic maneuver.
22. Cwazka, W. F., Sprenger, J. D., Nagawa, S. N., et al. Cryofibrinogenemia in Henoch-Schönlein purpura. *Arch. Intern. Med.* 139:592, 1979.
    Cryofibrinogenemia observed to parallel disease activity.
23. Greer, J. M., Longley, S., Edwards, L., et al. Vasculitis associated with malignancy. *Medicine* 67:220, 1988.
    An unusual but not rare association.
24. Janson, P. A., Jubelirer, S. T., Weinstein, M. J., et al. Treatment of the bleeding tendency in uremia with cryoprecipitate. *N. Engl. J. Med.* 303:1318, 1980.
    Reduction in bleeding time and control of hemorrhage achieved with cryoprecipitate. (See also N. Engl. J. Med. 308:8, 1983.)
25. Remuzzi, G. Bleeding in renal failure. *Lancet* 1:1205, 1988.
    Comprehensive review.
26. Slagel, G. A., and Lupton, G. P. Postproctoscopic periorbital purpura. Primary systemic amyloidosis. *Arch. Dermatol.* 122:464, 1986.
    Something to remember.
27. Wallerstein, R. O., and Wallerstein, R. O., Jr. Scurvy. *Semin. Hematol.* 13:211, 1976.
    Hemorrhage can be deep as well as superficial. (See also Lancet 1:975, 1967.)
28. Shattil, S. J., Bennett, J. S., McDonough, M., et al. Carbenicillin and penicillin G inhibit platelet function in vitro by impairing the interaction of agonists with the platelet surface. *J. Clin. Invest.* 65:329, 1980.
    A mechanism by which penicillin and its derivatives can produce platelet dysfunction (See also N. Engl. J. Med. 291:265, 1974 and Lancet 2:1039, 1976.)
29. Hammerschmidt, D. E. Szechwan purpura. *N. Engl. J. Med.* 302:1191, 1980.
    A hemorrhagic diathesis is part of the "Chinese restaurant syndrome."
30. Greene, M. H., Macher, A. M., Hernandez, A. D., et al. Disseminated cryptococcosis presenting as palpable purpura. *Arch. Intern. Med.* 138:1412, 1978.
    Intravascular aggregation of cryptococci in a thrombocytopenic patient. (See also Am. J. Med. 80:679, 1986 for purpura associated with Candida sepsis.)
31. Hautekeete, M. L., Berneman, Z. N., Bieger, R., et al. Purpura fulminans in pneumococcal sepsis. *Arch. Intern. Med.* 146:497, 1986.
    Immune complexes implicated in the pathogenesis.
32. Harker, L. A., Malpass, T. W., Branson, H. E., et al. Mechanism of abnormal bleeding in patients undergoing cardiopulmonary bypass: Acquired transient platelet dysfunction associated with selective α-granule release. *Blood* 56:824, 1980.
    Bleeding in these patients responds to platelet transfusions.
33. Weiss, H. J., Rosove, M. H., Lages, B. A., et al. Acquired storage pool deficiency with increased platelet-associated IgG: Report of five cases. *Am. J. Med.* 69:711, 1980.
    Immune-induced bleeding tendency with a normal platelet count.
34. Feder, W., and Auerbach, R. "Purple toes": An uncommon sequela of oral coumarin drug therapy. *Ann. Intern. Med.* 55:91, 1961.
    This lesion should not be confused with ischemic necrosis.

102. PAROXYSMAL NOCTURNAL HEMOGLOBINURIA
Jerry L. Spivak

Paroxysmal nocturnal hemoglobinuria (PNH) is an acquired disorder of a pluripotent hematopoietic stem cell. Its cause is uncertain, its manifestations are protean, and it is characterized by an episodic impairment of proliferation of one or more of the formed elements of the blood, as well as by a surface membrane defect resulting in red cell hemolysis. The sine qua non of PNH is an abnormal sensitivity of the red blood cells to the lytic effects of complement. Platelets and white cells are also sensitive to damage by complement, but the damage does not result in a shortened life span of either. PNH spares no age, sex, or racial group, but it is most common in young adults. Because it is a panmyelopathy with impairment of cellular proliferation and increased cell destruction, PNH can present in a variety of ways. Classic attacks of PNH occur in fewer than 25 percent of patients initially, but hemoglobinuria (not always nocturnal or paroxysmal) occurs at some point in most patients. A more constant finding resulting from chronic intravascular hemolysis is hemosiderinuria. PNH may masquerade as iron-deficiency anemia, especially since lack of iron can prevent expression of the red cell defect. It can also present as aplastic anemia. In some patients, the disease is manifested by multiple thrombotic episodes. In others, the development of leukopenia and/or thrombocytopenia is the initial sign of the disorder. A chronic, Coombs-negative, hemolytic anemia without gross hemoglobinuria is a common form of presentation. Obviously, if one relies on the classic description of the disorder, the diagnosis will be frequently overlooked.

The red cells in PNH vary in their sensitivity to the lytic effects of complement. Some are highly sensitive, others only moderately sensitive, while some cannot be distinguished from normal with respect to complement lysis. Most patients have at least two subpopulations of red cells that differ in complement sensitivity. Some have three subpopulations but only rarely is a single population of red cells, uniform in complement sensitivity, observed. The severity of hemolysis depends on the number of abnormal red cells and their degree of complement sensitivity. This varies from patient to patient and even in the same patient during the course of the illness. In some patients, the abnormal cell populations may eventually vanish altogether. In spite of the documented mosaicism of the red cells with respect to complement sensitivity, the disease appears to be clonal in origin. In vitro studies of hematopoietic colony-forming cells in PNH have demonstrated that these cells fail to express decay-accelerating factor (DAF) and have the same sensitivity to the lytic effects of complement as their mature end-stage progeny. Based on the expression of DAF, the level of hematopoietic progenitor cell involvement varies in different patients.

Lysis of the complement-sensitive red cell population occurs via the alternative (properdin) pathway of complement activation. In contrast to the classic pathway of complement activation, the alternative pathway does not require the presence of an antibody, fixation of the first, second, and fourth components of complement, or calcium. It can be activated in the fluid phase by a number of substances, including complex polysaccharides and endotoxin. The activity of the alternative pathway is sensitive to pH, temperature, and the concentration of magnesium. Activation of the alternative pathway by lowering the pH is the basis of the classic test for PNH, Ham's acidified serum test. PNH cells characteristically lack a group of proteins such as DAF, C8 binding protein, and Fc receptor type III, which are anchored within the cell membrane by phosphatidylinositol glycans, the so-called PIG tails. DAF deficiency permits the accumulation of C3b on the cell membrane, and lack of the C8 binding protein enhances the binding and lytic activity of the C5–9 membrane attach complex, particularly the polymerization of C9. For red cells, this leads to intravascular hemolysis and possibly destruction of erythroid progenitor cells in the marrow. Platelets, rather than being lysed, may be activated leading to thrombotic complications. Defective granulocyte function may also involve complement activation or insufficient Fc receptor activity.

Other laboratory abnormalities in this disease include low red cell acetylcholinesterase activity (proportional to the number of complement-sensitive cells), heat instability of the red cells as 37°C (98.6°F), and low leukocyte alkaline phosphatase (LAP) levels. Based on complement sensitivity, two subpopulations of granulocytes can be identified. PNH granulocytes when sensitized by complement demonstrate impaired chemotaxis.

The diagnosis of PNH in an untransfused patient can be established with either Ham's acidified serum test or the sucrose hemolysis test. The sucrose hemolysis test, which relies on low ionic strength conditions to activate complement, is easier to perform and more sensitive than Ham's test but less specific. However, a falsely positive Ham's test can be obtained in patients with type II congenital dyserythropoietic anemia

(HEMPAS). In this disorder, however, the sucrose hemolysis test is negative and in contrast to PNH, patients' serum cannot be used to lyse their own red cells.

Heat-induced (37°C[98.6°F]) hemolysis is not specific for PNH, but its absence should rule out the diagnosis. The inulin test is another simple diagnostic test that relies on activation of the alternative pathway of complement. The presence of hemosiderinuria is a valuable clue to the source of iron loss and the presence of intravascular hemolysis; if absent, the diagnosis of PNH is unlikely.

The clinical course of PNH is quite variable, depending on the proliferative potential of the abnormal clone and the proportion of highly complement-sensitive red cells. Marrow aplasia can be recurrent, as can isolated defects in the production of any of the formed elements. Folic acid deficiency can occur because of the increased demand for red cell production. Cholelithiasis and peptic ulceration are two other disorders with an increased incidence in patients with PNH. Thrombosis and thromboembolic events are among the serious complications of the disease. The thrombi or emboli may involve any organ, but the most devastating ones occur in the brain and liver. Diffuse hepatic vein thrombosis is a common cause of death, but patients have survived after development of the Budd-Chiari syndrome. Patients with PNH have an increased susceptibility to infection, and since infections can activate the alternative pathway of complement, these patients are doubly at risk. Fever and acidosis obviously accelerate hemolysis. A small number of patients have developed acute leukemia. Recurrent headaches and back and abdominal pain have been attributed to thrombotic episodes, and occasionally the symptoms may simulate the presence of a "surgical abdomen." Only rarely, however, is a surgically correctable lesion present.

Therapy for PNH is dictated by the clinical manifestations of the disorder. Acidosis (as may occur with the use of acetazolamide and salicylates), cold, and overexertion should be avoided. Oral contraceptives may also be dangerous. Iron therapy, either oral or parenteral, can precipitate hemolysis and should not be given unless the patient has been given transfusions to suppress endogenous erythropoiesis. Since whole blood transfusions can precipitate hemolysis, saline-washed or frozen red cells should be used. The role of dextran in limiting hemolysis is unclear. A beneficial effect of androgens on hemolysis has been observed that appears to be independent of its effect on erythropoiesis. In some patients, corticosteroid therapy has been effective in reducing hemolysis. Heparin is more effective than warfarin (Coumadin) in treating thrombotic events but must be given in therapeutic amounts because at low concentrations it enhances complement activation. Streptokinase has also been used to treat thrombosis in PNH patients without exacerbating hemolysis. Since PNH is uncommon and its clinical progression quite variable, it has been difficult to document the actual benefits of any form of therapy. Both pregnancy and surgery can be dangerous in these patients.

1. Oni, S. B., Osunkoya, B. O., and Luzzatto, L. Paroxysmal nocturnal hemoglobinuria: Evidence for monoclonal origin of abnormal red cells. *Blood* 36:145, 1970.
   Evidence using glucose 6-phosphate dehydrogenase enzymes for the clonal nature of this disorder. (See also Annu. Rev. Med. *28:187, 1977.)*
2. Rosse, W. F. The control of complement activation by the blood cells in paroxysmal nocturnal hemoglobinuria. *Blood* 67:268, 1986.
   Brief review.
3. Dessypus, E. N., Clark, D. A., McKee, L. C., Jr., et al. Increased sensitivity to complement of erythroid and myeloid progenitors in paroxysmal nocturnal hemoglobinuria. *N. Engl. J. Med.* 309:690, 1983.
   Expression of the PNH defect at the progenitor cell level.
4. Kanamaru, A., Okuda, K., Ueda, E., et al. Different distribution of decay-accelerating factor on hematopoietic progenitors from normal individuals and patients with paroxysmal nocturnal hemoglobinuria. *Blood* 72:507, 1988.
   DAF is not expressed by PNH hematopoietic progenitor cells.
5. Nicholson-Weller, A., Spicer, D. B., and Austen, K. F. Deficiency of the complement regulatory protein, "decay-accelerating factor," on membranes of granulocytes, monocytes, and platelets in paroxysmal nocturnal hemoglobinuria. *N. Engl. J. Med.* 25:312, 1985.
   One of the important membrane defects leading to complement sensitivity in PNH.

6. Dockter, M. E., and Morrison, M. Paroxysmal nocturnal hemoglobinuria erythrocytes are of two distinct types: Positive or negative for acetylcholinesterase. *Blood* 67:540, 1986.
   Use of flow cytometry to detect defective red cells in PNH. Acetylcholinesterase-negative cells also lack DAF. (DAF and LAP behave in the same fashion in granulocytes. See Blood *71:1086, 1988.)*

7. Packman, C. H., Rosenfeld, S. I., Jenkins, D. E., et al. Complement lysis of human erythrocytes: Differing susceptibility of two types of paroxysmal nocturnal hemoglobinuria cells to C5b–9. *J. Clin. Invest.* 64:428, 1979.
   The most complement-sensitive cell population exhibits a greater sensitivity to C5b–9 as well as to C3.

8. Hansch, G. M., Schonermark, S., and Roelcke, D. Paroxysmal nocturnal hemoglobinuria type III. Lack of an erythrocyte membrane protein restricting the lysis by C5b–9. *J. Clin. Invest.* 80:7, 1987.
   A second membrane defect in PNH. (See also J. Exp. Med. *165:572, 1987 and* Proc. Natl. Acad. Sci. U.S.A. *82:5520, 1985.)*

9. Devine, D. V., Siegel, R. S., and Rosse, W. F. Interactions of the platelets in paroxysmal nocturnal hemoglobinuria with complement. Relationship to defects in the regulation of complement and to platelet survival in vivo. *J. Clin. Invest.* 79:131, 1987.
   Mechanism for "platelet sparing" in PNH. See also J. Immunol. *140:3045, 1988 for possible role of platelets in PNH thrombosis.*

10. Verwilghen, R. L., Lewis, S. M., Dacie, J. V., et al. HEMPAS: Congenital dyserythropoietic anaemia (type II). *Q. J. Med.* 42:257, 1973.
    An unusual disorder that may not be recognized until adulthood and in which Ham's test is positive. (See also J. Clin. Invest. *53:31, 1974.)*

11. Conrad, M. E., and Barton, J. C. The aplastic-anemia–paroxysmal nocturnal hemoglobinuria syndrome. *Am. J. Hematol.* 7:61, 1979.
    Patients with this syndrome may have a better survival than patients with aplastic anemia alone. (See also Br. J. Haematol. *13:236, 1967.)*

12. Hertz, I. H., and Keller, R. Paroxysmal nocturnal hemoglobinuria: Small bowel findings. *AJR* 136:204, 1981.
    Description of radiographic findings during an acute attack.

13. Valla, D., Dhumeaux, D., Babany, G., et al. Hepatic vein thrombosis in paroxysmal nocturnal hemoglobinuria. A spectrum from asymptomatic occlusion of hepatic venules to fatal Budd-Chiari syndrome. *Gastroenterology* 93:569, 1987.
    A not uncommon problem which can be recognized at an early stage. (See also Br. J. Haematol. *64:737, 1986.)*

14. Zimmerman, D., and Bell, W. R. Venous thrombosis and splenic rupture in paroxysmal nocturnal hemoglobinuria. *Am. J. Med.* 68:275, 1980.
    An unusual occurrence.

15. Sholar, P. W., and Bell, W. R. Thrombolytic therapy for inferior vena cava thrombosis in paroxysmal nocturnal hemoglobinuria. *Ann. Intern. Med.* 103:539, 1985.
    Successful use of thrombolytic therapy.

16. Hirsch, V. J., Neubach, P. A., Parker, D. M., et al. Paroxysmal nocturnal hemoglobinuria: Termination in acute myelomonocytic leukemia and reappearance after leukemic remission. *Arch. Intern. Med.* 141:525, 1981.
    Recurrence of the PNH clone following remission induction of acute leukemia.

17. Clark, D. A., Butler, S. A., Braren, V., et al. The kidneys in paroxysmal nocturnal hemoglobinuria. *Blood* 57:83, 1981.
    Renal involvement due to thrombosis can be substantial.

18. Brubaker, L. H., Essig, L. J., and Mengel, C. E. Neutrophil life span in paroxysmal nocturnal hemoglobinuria. *Blood* 50:657, 1977.
    In spite of increased sensitivity to complement, neutrophil life span was normal.

19. Craddock, P. R., Fehr, J., and Jacob, H. S. Complement-mediated granulocyte dysfunction in paroxysmal nocturnal hemoglobinuria. *Blood* 47:931, 1976.
    Impairment of granulocyte chemotaxis in PNH by complement.

20. Hartmann, R. C., Jenkins, D. E., Jr., and Arnold, A. B. Diagnostic specificity of su-

crose hemolysis test for paroxysmal nocturnal hemoglobinuria. *Blood* 35:462, 1970.
Evaluation of the sucrose hemolysis test.

21. Kann, H. E., Jr., Mengel, C. E., and Wall, R. C. Paroxysmal nocturnal hemoglobinuria obscured by the presence of iron deficiency. *Ann. Intern. Med.* 67:593, 1967.
Iron deficiency obscuring Ham's test.

22. Solal-Celigny, P., Tertian, G., Fernandex, H., et al. Pregnancy and paroxysmal nocturnal hemoglobinuria. *Arch. Intern. Med.* 148:593, 1988.
A nice review of this problem.

23. Baumann, M. A., Pacheco, J., Paul, C. C., et al. Paroxysmal nocturnal hemoglobinuria associated with the acquired immunodeficiency syndrome. *Arch. Intern. Med.* 148:212, 1988.
An interesting association.

24. Antin, J. H., Ginsburg, D., Smith, B. R., et al. Bone marrow transplantation for paroxysmal nocturnal hemoglobinuria: Eradication of the PNH clone and documentation of complete lymphohematopoietic engraftment. *Blood* 66:1247, 1985.
Cure by marrow transplantation.

25. Logue, G. L. Effect of heparin on complement activation and lysis of paroxysmal nocturnal hemoglobinuria (PNH) red cells. *Blood* 50:239, 1977.
Low concentrations of heparin enhance complement activation; high concentrations inhibit it.

26. Hartmann, R. C., Jenkins, D. E., Jr., McKee, L. C., et al. Paroxysmal nocturnal hemoglobinuria: Clinical and laboratory studies relating to iron metabolism and therapy with androgen and iron. *Medicine* 45:331, 1966.
Comprehensive treatise on iron metabolism and the use of androgens in PNH.

27. Issaragrisil, S., Piankijagum, A., and Tang-naitrisorana, Y. Corticosteroid therapy in paroxysmal nocturnal hemoglobinuria. *Am. J. Hematol.* 25:77, 1987.
The response is not uniform.

103. PLASMA CELL DYSCRASIAS
Jerry L. Spivak

Human immunoglobulins can be divided into five classes on the basis of their physicochemical properties. Listed according to their serum concentration, the classes are IgG, IgA, IgM, IgD, and IgE. The IgG class constitutes the bulk of the serum immunoglobulins. IgA immunoglobulins are present in both the blood and external secretions. IgM is a macroglobulin and constitutes the usual class of antibodies produced in response to a primary antigenic challenge. The exact physiologic function of IgD globulins has not been established, although they are present along with IgM on lymphocyte (B cell) surface membranes. IgE is the reaginic antibody.

Immunoglobulins, like hemoglobin, are composed of two pairs of polypeptide chains. One pair consists of the heavy chains, which are unique for each immunoglobulin class; the other pair, the light chains, are common to all immunoglobulin classes. There are two different types of light chains, kappa (κ) and lambda (λ). Each immunoglobulin, therefore, has class-specific heavy chains and either κ or λ light chains. Within some immunoglobulin classes, subclasses exist (four for IgG, and two for IgA) that may be functionally different (e.g., in their ability to fix complement). IgG, IgD, and IgE exist as monomers, while IgM and some IgA globulins exist as polymers in conjunction with a protein called the J chain. Secretory IgA also contains a protein designated the secretory component.

Marked increases in serum immunoglobulin levels can occur in a variety of disorders. These include bacterial, viral, fungal, and parasitic infections, cirrhosis, sarcoidosis, collagen-vascular disorders, and arteritis. In these situations the increase in serum immunoglobulin concentration is polyclonal, involving a number of immunoglobulin classes. Under certain circumstances, there is a selective increase in only one immunoglobulin class, and the proteins produced are identical, indicating a monoclonal origin. In certain cases the monoclonal protein is associated with another disorder, such as Gaucher's disease, acute leukemia, polycythemia vera, and rectosigmoid, gastric, or breast carcinoma. In others, no underlying disease is present, and the concentration of the monoclonal protein is generally less than 3 gm/dl, does not change with time, and is not associated with proteinuria, bone lesions, anemia, reduction in the other serum immunoglobulins, or plasmacytosis in the marrow. These patients may be said to have a benign monoclonal gammopathy, but that diagnosis can be made only in retrospect. In some patients, the antibody activity of the monoclonal protein is such that it produces a particular syndrome, such as the benign hyperglobulinemic purpura of Waldenström's disease (IgG–anti-IgG activity), Meltzer's syndrome (IgM–anti-IgG activity), or cold agglutinin disease. The most common monoclonal gammopathies, however, are those resulting from neoplasia of the lymphoid system, and with such tumors a monoclonal gammopathy involving any of the immunoglobulin classes, or even heavy or light chains alone, can occur.

Myeloma is characterized by plasma cell proliferation with overproduction of either IgG, IgA, IgD, or IgE with or without free light chain production (Bence Jones protein). The monoclonal gammopathy is associated with underproduction of other immunoglobulins, a factor predisposing the patients to recurrent infections, often pneumococcal or gram-negative. In some patients only light chains are produced, and no serum monoclonal protein is observed. Rarely, no protein is secreted by the tumor. Myeloma is, of course, not always multiple; it can be solitary (usually in the spine or pelvis), although dissemination eventually occurs. Occasionally, plasma cell leukemia may develop.

In Waldenström's macroglobulinemia, the monoclonal protein is an IgM, and the tumor cell type may be lymphocytic, plasmacytic, or intermediate in morphology. Contrary to published dogma, bone lesions are not uncommon in this disorder. In addition, some patients with chronic lymphocytic leukemia or lymphoma have also been observed to have a monoclonal macroglobulinemia.

Monoclonal gammopathies involving three of the five heavy chain classes have also been described. Gamma heavy chain disease is characterized by cervical and axillary adenopathy and palatal edema caused by involvement of Waldeyer's ring. Alpha heavy chain disease, also known as Mediterranean lymphoma, generally presents with malabsorption and abdominal pain. Mu heavy chain disease generally occurs in the setting of chronic lymphocytic leukemia. Vacuolated plasma cells in the marrow are a characteristic feature of this disorder.

Amyloidosis, a disease characterized by deposition of light chains or β_2-microglobulin in various tissues, occurs in approximately 15 percent of patients with myeloma. Amyloidosis may, of course, occur in the absence of myeloma either secondary to a chronic infectious or inflammatory disorder, as a familial disorder, or as a primary disorder with a monoclonal gammopathy but without significant plasmacytosis. Recent studies have failed to confirm an earlier belief that the various types of amyloidosis can be segregated on the pattern of tissue involvement by the amyloid.

Signs and symptoms in the plasma cell dyscrasias are a consequence of the tumor mass, its secretory products, and the presence of amyloid deposits. The complications attributed to these include anemia, leukopenia, thrombocytopenia, hypercalcemia, hyperuricemia, renal failure, neuropathy, skeletal fractures, the hyperviscosity syndrome, infection, organ dysfunction due to infiltration by tumor or amyloid, and renal tubular acidosis. The monoclonal proteins may exhibit antibody behavior resulting in cold agglutinin hemolysis, anti-factor VIII activity, hyperlipidemia, and vascular purpura. They may also exhibit thermal instability as cryoglobulins or pyroglobulins. Substances such as tumor necrosis factor are also produced that stimulate bone resorption and hypercalcemia, or inhibit antibody formation by normal lymphocytes.

The hyperviscosity syndrome is usually due to an IgM globulin but if IgA or IgG levels are high enough, or if aggregation of IgG3 or light chains occurs, the syndrome can also develop. Clinically there are epistaxis and other hemorrhagic manifestations, congestive heart failure, and neurologic signs (such as dizziness, tinnitus, deafness, and vertigo), visual disturbances (hemorrhagic glaucoma), encephalopathy, and neuropathy (Bing-Neel syndrome). Bedside measurements of serum viscosity can be made with a red cell pipet. Plasmapheresis can be employed to control hyperviscosity until chemotherapy takes effect.

The diagnosis of a plasma cell dyscrasia is usually not difficult. Patients with unexplained renal failure, recurrent or atypical infections, proteinuria, or hypogammaglobulinemia should always be evaluated for this possibility. In patients with Bence Jones proteinuria alone, the diagnosis may be missed if only the standard tests for urine protein and the heat test are relied on. Immunochemical analysis of concentrated urine is generally required to document the presence of these proteins. Sia's water test is a simple way to confirm the presence of a macroglobulin since these serum proteins often (but not always) form a precipitate in water that can be redissolved in saline.

The prognosis in plasma cell dyscrasias varies with the clinical syndrome. Plasma cell leukemia, light chain disease, amyloidosis, and IgD myeloma all have a poor prognosis. In general, severe anemia, hypercalcemia, azotemia, and high serum myeloma protein level are associated with a shortened life span. Age does not appear to influence the response to therapy.

1. Barlogie, B., Epstein, J., Selvanayagam, P., et al. Plasma cell myeloma—new biological insights and advances in therapy. *Blood* 73:865, 1989.
   Comprehensive review. (See also J.A.M.A. *27:258, 1987.)*
2. Rubio-Felix, D., Giralt, M., Giraldo, M. P., et al. Nonsecretory multiple myeloma. *Cancer* 59:1847, 1987.
   This disorder responds to therapy in the same fashion as secretory myeloma.
3. Kyle, R. A. "Benign" monoclonal gammopathy. *J.A.M.A.* 251:1849, 1984.
   A proportion develop myeloma, macroglobinemia or amyloidosis. (See also Acta Med. Scand. *219:519, 1986.)*
4. Durie, B. G. M., Salmon, S. E., and Moon, T. E. Pretreatment tumor mass, cell kinetics, and prognosis in multiple myeloma. *Blood* 55:364, 1980.
   A high pretreatment labeling index indicates a poor prognosis.
5. Endo, T., Okumura, H., and Kikuchi, K., et al. Immunoglobulin E (IgE) multiple myeloma. *Am. J. Med.* 70:1127, 1981.
   IgE myeloma is characterized by a younger age of onset, male predominance, osteosclerosis, and a short survival.
6. Noel, P., and Kyle, R. A. Plasma cell leukemia: An evaluation of response to therapy. *Am. J. Med.* 83:1062, 1987.
   An uncommon and not very responsive disorder.
7. Duston, M. A., Skinner, M., Shirahama, J., et al. Diagnosis of amyloidosis by abdominal fat aspiration. *Am. J. Med.* 82:412, 1987.
   A high degree of positive results in patients with clinical findings suggestive of amyloidosis.
8. Rossi, J. F., Bataille, R., Chappard, D., et al. B cell malignancies presenting with unusual bone involvement and mimicking multiple myeloma. *Am. J. Med.* 83:10, 1987.
   An interesting observation.
9. Alexanian, R., Barlogie, B., and Dixon, D. Prognosis of asymptomatic multiple myeloma. *Arch. Intern. Med.* 148:1963, 1988.
   In the absence of lytic lesions or a high concentration of monoclonal protein, therapy can be withheld.
10. Kyle, R. A., and Greipp, P. R. Smouldering multiple myeloma. *N. Engl. J. Med.* 302:1347, 1980.
    Patients with greater than 3 dl of monoclonal protein in whom there was no disease progression and no need for chemotherapy. (See also Blood *56:521, 1980.)*
11. Suchman, A. L., Coleman, M., Mouradian, J., et al. Aggressive plasma cell myeloma: A terminal phase. *Arch. Intern. Med.* 141:1315, 1981.
    Myeloma can exhibit an aggressive terminal phase.
12. Riddell, S., Traczyk, Z., Paraskevas, F., et al. The double gammopathies. *Medicine* 65:135, 1986.
    Myeloma with 2 M proteins.

13. Blattner, F. R., and Tucker, P. W. The molecular biology of immunoglobulin D. *Nature* 307:417, 1984.
    Its function remains a mystery.

14. Greipp, P. R., Katzmann, J. A., O'Fallon, W. M., et al. Value of β_2-microglobulin level and plasma cell labeling indices as prognostic factors in patients with newly diagnosed myeloma. *Blood* 72:219, 1988.
    The β_2-microglobulin level is an important prognostic indicator. (See also Br. J. Haematol. 69:47, 1988 and 61:611, 1985.)

15. Frangione, B., and Franklin, E. C. Heavy chain diseases: Clinical features and molecular significance of the disordered immunoglobulin structure. *Semin. Hematol.* 10:53, 1973.
    Part of a symposium on dysproteinemias. (See also Arch. Intern. Med. 139:672, 1979.)

16. Seligman, M. Immunochemical, clinical, and pathological features of α-chain disease. *Arch. Intern. Med.* 135:78, 1975.
    Malabsorption, pain, and enteric lymphadenopathy. (See also Cancer 41:1161, 1978.)

17. Solomon, A. Clinical implications of monoclonal light chains. *Semin. Oncol.* 13:341, 1986.
    Tubular and glomerular disease and amyloidosis. (See also Am. J. Med. 80:98, 1986.

18. Pascali, E., and Pezzoli, A. The clinical spectrum of pure Bence Jones proteinuria. *Cancer* 62:2408, 1988.
    This can be seen in a variety of lymphomas in addition to myeloma and amyloidosis. For Bence Jones proteins in the serum, see Br. J. Haematol. 62:689, 1986.

19. Corwin, J., and Lindberg, R. D. Solitary plasmacytoma of bone vs. extramedullary plasmacytoma and their relationship to multiple myeloma. *Cancer* 43:1007, 1979.
    Extramedullary plasmacytoma has a better prognosis than solitary plasmacytoma of bone.

20. De Troyer, A., Stolarczyk, A., Zegers de Beyl, D., et al. Value of anion-gap determination in multiple myeloma. *N. Engl. J. Med.* 296:859, 1977.
    A low anion gap is a specific feature of IgG myeloma.

21. Busse, J. C., Gelbard, M. A., Byrnes, J. J., et al. Pseudohyperphosphatemia and dysproteinemia. *Arch. Intern. Med.* 147:2045, 1987.
    A test tube artifact. (See also Am. J. Kidney Dis. 11:260, 1988.)

22. Broder, S., Humphrey, R., Durm, M., et al. Impaired synthesis of polyclonal immunoglobulins in myeloma. *N. Engl. J. Med.* 293:887, 1975.
    Cell-mediated suppression of normal immunoglobulin synthesis in myeloma.

23. Carter, A., Hocherman, I., Linn, S., et al. Prognostic significance of plasma cell morphology in multiple myeloma. *Cancer* 60:1060, 1987.
    Morphology could be correlated with survival duration. (See also Medicine 54:225, 1975.)

24. Vandermolen, L., Rice, L., and Lynch, E. C. Plasma cell dyscrasia with marrow fibrosis. *Am. J. Med.* 79:297, 1985.
    Not a rare complication. (See also Am. J. Clin. Pathol. 89:63, 1988.)

25. Perez-Soler, R., Esteban, R., Allende, E., et al. Liver involvement in multiple myeloma. *Am. J. Hematol.* 20:25, 1985.
    Liver involvement is usually not significant but the alkaline phosphatase can be elevated in 40%. (See Arch. Intern. Med. 132:195, 1973.)

26. Silverstein, A., and Doniger, D. E. Neurologic complications of myelomatosis. *Arch. Neurol.* 9:534, 1963.
    Compression, infiltration, infection, amyloid, and metabolic changes are responsible for neurologic deficits. (See Arch. Intern. Med. 140:256, 1980 for meningeal myeloma.)

27. Kyle, R. A., Pierre, R. V., and Bayrd, E. D. Multiple myeloma and acute leukemia associated with alkylating agents. *Arch. Intern. Med.* 135:185, 1975.
    An association being recognized with increasing frequency and possibly more with melphalan than cyclophosphamide (Cytoxan) (Ann. Intern. Med. 105:360, 1986. (See also N. Engl. J. Med. 301:743, 1979.)

28. Farhangi, M., and Osserman, E. F. Myeloma and xanthoderma due to an IgG monoclonal anti-flavin antibody. *N. Engl. J. Med.* 294:177, 1976.

Interesting effect of a monoclonal antibody. For another, see J. Lab. Clin. Med. *88:375, 1976.*

29. Holt, P. J. A., Davies, M. G., Saunders, K. C., et al. Pyoderma gangrenosum: Clinical and laboratory findings in 15 patients with special reference to polyarthritis. *Medicine* 59:114, 1980.
    Pyoderma gangrenosum can be associated with IgA myeloma.

30. Bardwick, P. A., Zvaifler, N. J., Gill, G. N., et al. Plasma cell dyscrasia with polyneuropathy, organomegaly, endocrinopathy, M protein, and skin changes: The POEMS syndrome. *Medicine* 59:311, 1980.
    A usual symptom complex associated with osteosclerosis. (See also Arch. Intern. Med. *146:993, 1986.)*

31. DeFronzo, R. A., Cooke, R., Wright, J. R., et al. Renal function in patients with multiple myeloma. *Medicine* 57:151, 1978.
    Bence Jones proteins exert a direct toxic effect on the renal tubules.

32. Rota, S., Mougenot, B., Baudouin, B., et al. Multiple myeloma and severe renal failure: A clinicopathologic study of outcome and prognosis in 34 patients. *Medicine* 66:126, 1987.
    Nonsteroidal anti-inflammatory agents and infection may play a role; renal biopsy and an aggressive therapeutic approach is advocated, but see Lancet *1:1202, 1988.*

33. Rao, D. S., Parfitt, A. M., Villanueva, A. R., et al. Hypophosphatemic osteomalacia and adult Fanconi syndrome due to light-chain nephropathy. *Am. J. Med.* 82:333, 1987.
    Fanconi's syndrome can precede the development of myeloma or amyloidosis. (See also Am. J. Med. *58:354, 1975.)*

34. Solomon, A. Homogeneous (monoclonal) immunoglobulins in cancer. *Am. J. Med.* 63:169, 1977.
    A monoclonal gammopathy is most commonly associated with adenocarcinoma of the rectosigmoid, prostate, lung, or gallbladder.

35. Mackenzie, M. R., and Fudenberg, H. H. Macroglobulinemia: An analysis for forty patients. *Blood* 39:874, 1972.
    The bone marrow may contain a mixture of plasma cells, lymphocytes, and lymphocytoid plasma cells—or any one of these may predominate. Mast cells are often increased. (See also Blood *35:695, 1970 and* Lancet *2:311, 1985.)*

36. Vermess, M., Pearson, D. D., Einstein, A. B., et al. Osseous manifestations of Waldenström's macroglobulinemia. *Radiology* 102:497, 1972.
    Osteoporosis and destructive bone lesions are not uncommon.

37. Winterbauer, R. H., Riggins, R. C. K., Greisman, F. A., et al. Pleuropulmonary manifestations of Waldenström's macroglobulinemia. *Chest* 66:368, 1974.
    Effusions and nodular and diffuse infiltrates.

38. Bedine, M. S., Yardley, J. H., Elliott, H. L., et al. Intestinal involvement in Waldenström's macroglobulinemia. *Gastroenterology* 65:308, 1973.
    Malabsorption due to deposition of macroglobin in the intestinal villi.

39. Brody, J. I., Haidar, M. E., and Rossman, R. E. A hemorrhagic syndrome in Waldenström's macroglobulinemia secondary to immunoadsorption of factor VIII. *N. Engl. J. Med.* 300:408, 1979.
    Immunoadsorption of factor VIII to malignant lymphocytes.

40. Wright, D. J., and Jenkins, D. E., Jr. Simplified method for estimation of serum and plasma viscosity in multiple myeloma and related disorders. *Blood* 36:516, 1970.
    Use of a red cell pipet to measure viscosity at the bedside.

41. Bloch, K. J., and Maki, D. G. Hyperviscosity syndromes associated with immunoglobulin abnormalities. *Semin. Hematol.* 10:113, 1973.
    Most often hyperviscosity occurs with IgM or IgA, but it may occur with IgG if the protein level is high enough or aggregation occurs (IgG3).

42. Glenner, G. G. Amyloid deposits and amyloidosis. *N. Engl. J. Med.* 302:1283, 1333, 1980.
    Comprehensive review. (See also Lab. Invest. *58:122, 1988.)*

43. Kyle, R. A., and Bayrd, E. D. Amyloidosis: Review of 236 cases. *Med.* 54:271, 1975.
    Amyloidosis classified as (1) primary (no coexisting disease), (2) associated with my-

eloma, (3) associated with chronic inflammation or infection, (4) localized, and (5) familial.

44. Yood, R. A., Skinner, M., Rubinow, A., et al. Bleeding manifestations in 100 patients with amyloidosis. *J.A.M.A.* 249:1322, 1983.
    Bleeding was most often due to vessel infiltration.

45. Gertz, M. A., Kyle, R. A., Griffing, W. L., et al. Jaw claudication in primary systemic amyloidosis. *Medicine* 65:173, 1986.
    For another type of muscle involvement, see Am. J. Med. *83:175, 1987.*

46. Fielder, K., and Durie, B. G. M. Primary amyloidosis associated with multiple myeloma. *Am. J. Med.* 80:413, 1986.
    Chemotherapy is worthwhile in primary amyloidosis. (See also Arch. Intern. Med. *142:1445, 1982.)*

47. Kelly, J. J., Jr., Kyle, R. A., O'Brien, P. C., et al. The natural history of peripheral neuropathy in primary systemic amyloidosis. *Ann. Neurol.* 6:1, 1979.
    A progressive distal sensorimotor and autonomic neuropathy.

48. Benson, M. D., and Cohen, A. S. Serum amyloid A protein in amyloidosis, rheumatic, and neoplastic diseases. *Arthritis Rheum.* 22:36, 1979.
    Amyloid A protein is elevated in a variety of disorders.

49. Piette, W. W. Myeloma, paraproteinemias, and the skin. *Med. Clin. North. Am.* 70:155, 1986.
    Review of the various skin lesions associated with dysproteinemias.

50. Ludwig, H., Fruhwald, F., Tscholakoff, D., et al. Magnetic resonance imaging of the spine in multiple myeloma. *Lancet* 2:364, 1987.
    A sensitive method for detecting osseous involvement. (See also Am. J. Roentgenol. *146:353, 1986; for computed tomography, see* Arch. Intern. Med. *145:1451, 1985.)*

51. Gould, J., Alexanian, R., Goodacre, A., et al. Plasma cell karotype in multiple myeloma. *Blood* 71:453, 1988.
    Hypodiploidy was associated with resistance to therapy. (See also Blood *66:380, 1985.)* *Common acute lymphoblastic leukemia antigen positivity also has a poor prognosis* (Blood *66:229, 1985).*

52. Kyle, R. A., and Jowsey, J. Effect of sodium fluoride, calcium carbonate, and vitamin D on the skeleton in multiple myeloma. *Cancer* 45:1669, 1980.
    Bone mass increases.

53. Durie, B. G. M., Russell, D., and Solmon, S. E. Reappraisal of plateau phase in myeloma. *Lancet* 2:65, 1980.
    Recognition of the stable state following treatment can avoid unnecessary chemotherapy. (See also Blood *51:1005, 1978.)*

54. Kyle, R. A., and Greipp, P. R. "Idiopathic" Bence Jones proteinuria. *N. Engl. J. Med.* 306:564, 1982.
    "Idiopathic" Bence Jones proteinuria may evolve into multiple myeloma.

55. Barlogie, B., Alexanian, R., Dicke, K. A., et al. High-dose chemoradiotherapy and autologous bone marrow transplantation for resistant multiple myeloma. *Blood* 70:869, 1987.
    An aggressive approach which is effective in some patients.

56. Coupland, R. W., Pontifex, A. H., and Salinas, F. A. Angioimmunoblastic lymphadenopathy with dysproteinemia. *Cancer* 55:1902, 1985.
    An unusual disorder with polyclonal hyperglobulinemia which can progress to lymphoma.

104. THE PORPHYRIAS
Jerry L. Spivak

The porphyrias are a clinically diverse group of hereditary and acquired disorders of heme biosynthesis which have as their basis the overproduction of one or more of the metabolic precursors of heme, the essential prosthetic group of proteins involved in oxygen transport and biologic oxidation reactions.

The porphyrias can be classified anatomically on the basis of the tissues in which their overproduction predominates, that is, hepatic, erythroid, or both, or clinically into acute and nonacute forms. With the exception of the rare erythropoietic porphyria, which is an autosomal recessive trait, and hepatoerythropoietic porphyria, a homozygous disorder, both of which are expressed in childhood, all other porphyrias are inherited as autosomal dominant traits which are not usually expressed until puberty and characteristically can be latent for many years after that.

Central to understanding the porphyrias is knowledge of the heme biosynthetic pathway which is illustrated in Figure 104-1.

The heme biosynthetic pathway is intramitochrondrial with respect to the synthesis of ALA and for all the intermediates after coproporphyrinogen; the rest are synthesized

Fig. 104-1. Heme synthetic pathway. *Spontaneously cyclizes to form uroporphyrinogen I.

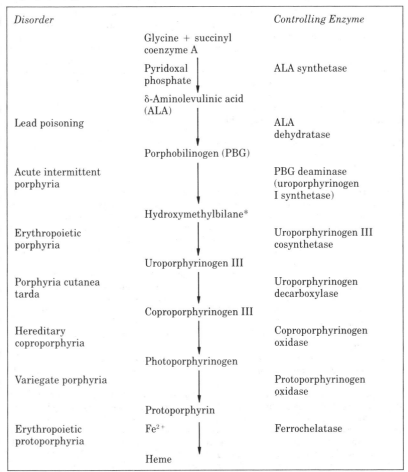

Disorder		Controlling Enzyme
	Glycine + succinyl coenzyme A	
	Pyridoxal phosphate ↓	ALA synthetase
	δ-Aminolevulinic acid (ALA)	
Lead poisoning	↓	ALA dehydratase
	Porphobilinogen (PBG)	
Acute intermittent porphyria	↓	PBG deaminase (uroporphyrinogen I synthetase)
	Hydroxymethylbilane*	
Erythropoietic porphyria	↓	Uroporphyrinogen III cosynthetase
	Uroporphyrinogen III	
Porphyria cutanea tarda	↓	Uroporphyrinogen decarboxylase
	Coproporphyrinogen III	
Hereditary coproporphyria	↓	Coproporphyrinogen oxidase
	Photoporphyrinogen	
Variegate porphyria	↓	Protoporphyrinogen oxidase
	Protoporphyrin	
Erythropoietic protoporphyria	Fe^{2+} ↓	Ferrochelatase
	Heme	

in the cell cytoplasm. The overriding feature of the heme biosynthetic pathway is feedback inhibition of heme synthesis by heme itself which controls the activity of the rate-limiting enzyme in the pathway, δ-aminolevolinic acid (ALA) synthetase. All porphyrias can be understood as due to an elevation of ALA synthetase activity, as a consequence of the absence of sufficient heme for its repression; the difference between the acute and nonacute forms of porphyria appears to be related to the activity of the next enzyme in the pathway, porphobilinogen (PBG) deaminase, which is elevated in the nonacute porphyrias but normal or low in the acute forms. The presence of cutaneous manifestations depends on the overproduction of porphyrins which absorb light in the Soret band (400 nm).

All of the acute porphyrias—acute intermittent porphyria (AIP), variegate porphyria (VP), and hereditary coproporphyria (HC)—are due to overproduction of porphyrin precursors in the liver, the most important of these being ALA and PBG. Because the biochemical lesions of VP and HC occur more distally than that of AIP, photosensitizing porphyrins accumulate and skin lesions are a feature of VP and HC. Otherwise, clinically these three disorders are identical, and AIP, which is the most common, can serve as a paradigm for them. The acute porphyrias are more common, occur at an earlier age in women, and like other disorders with multiple organ system involvement such as paroxysmal nocturnal hemoglobinuria (PNH), their diagnosis may not be entertained at the time of the initial presentation or even for many years thereafter. Indeed, for this reason, AIP has been designated the "little imitator." The frequency and duration of attacks vary greatly as does their age of onset. In 40 percent of attacks, no inciting cause is identified. For the rest, as might be expected for disorders of hepatic heme metabolism, drugs, including ethanol, are an important cause as are infections, starvation, and the hormonal changes associated with menses and pregnancy. The list of drugs which are hazardous to the patient with acute porphyria is long and as yet incomplete. They include barbiturates, estrogens, oral contraceptives, sulfonamides, and their derivatives such as chlorpropamide, hydantoin, phenylbutazone, griseofulvin, methyldopa, chlordiazepoxide, glutethimide, meprobamate, imipramine, carbamazepine, and chloroquine. It is likely that many of these drugs induce an acute attack by stimulating hepatic heme metabolism. "Safe" drugs include salicylates, chlorpromazine, atropine, chloral hydrate, digoxin, diazepam, iodine, morphine, meperidine, propranolol, diphenhydramine, dicumarol, and corticosteroids.

The acute porphyric attack may be manifested by abdominal, back, or chest pain, nausea, vomiting, constipation, paresthesias, weakness, mental confusion, hallucinations, seizures, cranial and bulbar nerve palsies, and coma. Typically, pain and neuromuscular symptoms are initially most common in the shoulder and pelvic girdle regions. The autonomic nervous system may be prominently involved producing hypertension, postural hypotension, tachycardia, ileus, bladder dysfunction, and dyshidrosis. Restless legs are another manifestation of these disorders. Although dark urine is frequently cited as a useful sign in the acute porphyrias, the urine is colorless until PBG is oxidized to a porphyrin derivative. While this may occur in the bladder, it is more usual after the urine has been exposed to light. Important laboratory abnormalities include hyponatremia which may be due to inappropriate release of antidiuretic hormone (ADH), EEG abnormalities, a reduced blood volume, hypercholesterolemia, or elevated thyroid-binding globulin. The excretion of ALA and PBG in the urine is always increased during an acute attack in AIP, VP, and HC, but normal levels may be found between acute attacks in VP and HC. In contrast to lead poisoning, PBG excretion exceeds that of ALA in the acute porphyrias.

During an acute attack, the presence of ALA and PBG in increased amounts in the urine establishes the presence of a hepatic porphyria. To distinguish between AIP, VP, and HC in the absence of skin lesions, measurements of fecal protoporphyrin (for VP) and coproporphyrin (for HC) are necessary. It is important to remember that PBG is unstable in acid conditions and in light. Therefore, freshly voided urine is the best substrate. PBG reacts with Ehrlich's reagent to form a red compound which, unlike urobilinogen, is water-soluble. This is the basis of the Watson-Schwartz test for PBG in the urine in which the reaction mixture is extracted with chloroform, and optimally with butanol as well, to remove urobilinogen and avoid a false-positive result.

During the latent phase of AIP, PBG and usually ALA will be elevated in the urine but may be missed when only qualitative screening tests are employed. As an alternative in screening for AIP, in addition to a careful family history, measurement of red cell PBG deaminase is a convenient test. A positive test should be confirmed with quantitative determinations of urinary PBG and ALA. It is important to remember, however, that the molecular basis of AIP is heterogeneous, and in some kindreds red cell PBG deaminase levels are normal even when urinary PBG and ALA levels are increased. Therefore, a normal red cell PBG deaminase level does not exclude the diagnosis of AIP. For VP and HC, as mentioned above, measurements of fecal porphyrin levels are necessary for diagnostic purposes during the latent phases of these disorders as urine PBG and ALA levels may not be elevated.

The nonacute porphyrias include those disorders in which skin lesions and liver disease are the major abnormalities. The most common nonacute porphyria is porphyria cutanea tarda (PCT), a disorder which may be hereditary or acquired and rarely manifest in a homozygous fashion as hepatoerythropoietic porphyria. PCT is due to a deficiency of uroporphyrinogen decarboxylase and occurs in two forms: familial, in which the enzyme activity is reduced in both hepatocytes and erythrocytes, and sporadic, in which the erythrocyte enzyme activity is normal. Usually manifest in middle-aged individuals, PCT is characterized by a light-sensitive dermatitis, bullous skin lesions, hypertrichosis, increased mechanical fragility of the skin, dermal sclerosis, hyperpigmentation, and alopecia. Environmental factors are important in the expression of latent PCT. They include ethanol abuse, estrogens, iron overload, and exposure to certain chemicals. In sporadic PCT, heterozygosity for the hemochromatosis gene has been suggested as the basis for the disorder, but iron loading is not the only inciting factor for PCT as its incidence is not increased in idiopathic hemochromatosis nor does phlebotomy affect the activity of the mutant enzyme.

The distinction between PCT and the other porphyrias which produce skin lesions, erythropoietic protoporphyria (EPP), VP, and HC, is made by chemical analysis. This is particularly germane with respect to VP where skin lesions can occur in the absence of an acute attack. Erythrocyte protoporphyrin levels are elevated in EPP but erythrocyte porphyrins are normal in PCT, VP, and HC. Urine PBG is normal in PCT as well as in quiescent VP, while in HC skin lesions usually do not occur in the absence of an acute attack. In PCT, urine uroporphyrin is increased in excess of coproporphyrin in contrast to VP, and fecal isocoproporphyrin is also increased. In familial PCT, measurement of red cell uroporphyrinogen decarboxylase activity may be employed for diagnostic purposes.

The best therapy for the porphyrias is prevention. In the case of the acute porphyrias, this involves avoiding ethanol, any drugs not known to be safe, as well as maintaining an adequate caloric intake. For the nonacute forms, avoidance of ethanol, estrogens, iron overload, and exposure to sunlight are important. Once an acute porphyria attack has begun, adequate hydration, electrolyte balance, adequate sedation, and analgesia should be maintained. Carbohydrates repress ALA synthetase activity and ingestion of at least 300 gm/day is recommended. If there is vomiting, the carbohydrate can be given intravenously with care taken to avoid sudden lowering of the carbohydrate load since this can be associated with rebound effects. Propranolol may be useful to control autonomic activity, but tachycardia is a good indicator of disease activity. Since a prolonged attack may lead to severe neurologic deficits with a prolonged convalescence, if carbohydrate loading does not alleviate symptoms or neurologic manifestations appear, therapy with hematin should be instituted. Hematin is thought to act by inhibiting ALA synthetase and is an effective agent, although not without side effects, particularly with respect to anticoagulant activity when given in high concentrations.

For the cutaneous, nonacute porphyrias, phlebotomy and chloroquine therapy are effective remedies. In EPP, where liver failure due to accumulation of protoporphyrin may occur, iron therapy may be effective.

1. Hindmarsh, J. T. The porphyrias: Recent advances. *Clin. Chem.* 32:1255, 1986.
   A useful review.
2. Brodie, M. J., Moore, M. R., and Goldberg, A. Enzyme abnormalities in the porphyrias. *Lancet* 2:699, 1977.
   A brief review.

3. Gibson, S. L. M., MacKenzie, J. C., and Goldberg, A. The diagnosis of industrial lead poisoning. *Br. J. Ind. Med.* 25:40, 1968.
   A review of the biochemical changes associated with inorganic lead poisoning. (See also Ann. Clin. Biochem. *21:453, 1984, and for organic lead poisoning,* Lancet *2:12, 1972.)*

4. Stein, J. A., and Tschudy, D. P. Acute intermittent porphyria: A clinical and biochemical study of 46 patients. *Medicine* 49:1, 1970.
   A comprehensive review of the clinical features of AIP.

5. Tishler, P. V., Woodward, B., O'Connor, J., et al. High prevalence of intermittent acute porphyria in a psychiatric patient population. *Am. J. Psychiatry* 142:1430, 1985.
   An interesting observation.

6. Desnick, R. J., Ostasiewicz, L. T., Tishler, P. A., et al. Acute intermittent porphyria: Characterization of a novel mutation in the structural gene for porphobilinogen deaminase. *J. Clin. Invest.* 76:865, 1985.
   An important study describing the varied molecular basis for AIP and providing an explanation for normal red cell PBG deaminase in some patients.

7. Pierach, C. A., Weimer, M. K., Cardinal, R. A., et al. Red blood cell porphobilinogen deaminase in the evaluation of acute intermittent porphyria. *J.A.M.A.* 257:60, 1987.
   Red cell PBG deaminase levels are not always reduced in patients with AIP.

8. Lamon, J., With, T. K., and Redeker, A. G. The Hoesch test: Bedside screening for urinary porphobilinogen in patients with suspected porphyria. *Clin. Chem.* 20:1438, 1974.
   A simple bedside test for the acute porphyrias.

9. Becker, D. M., and Kramer, S. The neurological manifestations of porphyria. *Medicine* 56:411, 1977.
   Review of possible mechanisms by which overproduction of PBG and ALA or impaired heme synthesis could cause neurologic abnormalities.

10. Brodie, M. J., Moore, M. R., Thompson, G. G., et al. Pregnancy and the acute porphyrias. *Br. J. Obstet. Gynaecol.* 84:726, 1977.
    Pregnancy can exacerbate acute porphyria, but the interaction of the two conditions is not necessarily deleterious.

11. Lamon, J. M., Frykholm, B. C., Hess, R. A., et al. Hematin therapy for acute porphyria. *Medicine* 58:252, 1979.
    A comprehensive study of hematin therapy.

12. Lamon, J. M., Frykholm, B. C., Bennett, M., et al. Prevention of acute porphyric attacks by intravenous haematin. *Lancet* 2:492, 1978.
    Use of hematin prophylactically to prevent AIP associated with the menstrual cycle.

13. Goetsch, C. A., and Bissell. Instability of hematin used in the treatment of acute hepatic porphyria. *N. Engl. J. Med.* 315:235, 1986.
    *Important observations on hematin toxicity, particularly with respect to its anticoagulant effects. (Heme arginate [*Br. Med. J. *293:538, 1986] is a more stable derivative for therapeutic purposes.)*

14. Douer, D., Weinberger, A., Pinkhas, J., et al. Treatment of acute intermittent porphyria with large doses of propranolol. *J.A.M.A.* 240:766, 1978.
    Propranolol may be useful in controlling the autonomic side effects of AIP.

15. Anderson, K. E., Spitz, I. M., Sassa, S., et al. Prevention of cyclical attacks of acute intermittent porphyria with a long-acting agonist of luteinizing hormone–releasing hormone. *N. Engl. J. Med.* 311:643, 1984.
    Further proof that suppression of ovarian hormone production can prevent exacerbations of AIP in susceptible individuals.

16. Grossman, M. E., Bickers, D. R., Poh-Fitzpatrick, M. B., et al. Porphyria cutanea tarda. *Am. J. Med.* 67:277, 1979.
    Comprehensive review.

17. Kushner, J. P., Barbuto, A. J., and Lee, G. R. An inherited enzymatic defect in porphyria cutanea tarda. Decreased uroporphyrinogen decarboxylase activity. *J. Clin. Invest.* 58:1089, 1976.
    Description of the enzyme defect in PCT: decreased uroporphyrinogen decarboxylase activity.

18. Elder, G. H., Sheppard, D. M., Tovey, J. A., et al. Immunoreactive uroporphyrinogen decarboxylase in porphyria cutanea tarda. *Lancet* 1:1301, 1983.
    Red cell uroporphyrinogen decarboxylase activity is decreased in some patients with PCT but not others. (See also N. Engl. J. Med. 306:766, 1982.)
19. Kushner, J. P., Edwards, C. O., Dadone, M. M., et al. Heterozygosity for HLA-linked hemochromatosis as a likely cause of the hepatic siderosis associated with sporadic porphyria cutanea tarda. *Gastroenterology* 88:1232, 1985.
    A possible mechanism for the hepatic siderosis in patients with sporadic PCT.
20. Lynch, R. E., Lee, G. R., and Kushner, J. P. Porphyria cutanea tarda associated with disinfectant misuse. *Arch. Intern. Med.* 135:549, 1975.
    An interesting toxic cause for PCT.
21. Epstein, J. H., Tuffanelli, D. L., Epstein, W. L., et al. Cutaneous changes in the porphyrias. A microscopic study. *Arch. Dermatol.* 107:689, 1973.
    Anatomic basis for the skin lesions in the porphyrias.
22. Rocchi, E., Gibertini, P., Cassanelli, M., et al. Serum ferritin in the assessment of liver iron overload and iron removal therapy in porphyria cutanea tarda. *J. Lab. Clin. Med.* 107:36, 1986.
    The serum ferritin can be used to monitor liver iron stores in patients with PCT.
23. Toback, A. C., Sassa, S., Poh-Fitzpatrick, M. B., et al. Hepatoerythropoietic porphyria: clinical, biochemical, and enzymatic studies in a three-generation family lineage. *N. Engl. J. Med.* 316:645, 1987.
    A rare disorder resulting from homozygous inheritance of a defective uroporphyrinogen decarboxylase gene, the same gene responsible for PCT. (See also Lancet 1:916, 1981.)
24. de Verneuil, H., Grandchamp, B., Romeo, P. H., et al. Molecular analysis of uroporphyrinogen decarboxylase deficiency in a family with two cases of hepatoerythropoietic porphyria. *J. Clin. Invest.* 77:431, 1986.
    The molecular basis of the disease in these patients was rapid degradation of the mutant enzyme.
25. Gordeuk, V. R., Brittenham, G. M., Hawkins, C. W., et al. Iron therapy for hepatic dysfunction in erythropoietic protoporphyria. *Ann. Intern. Med.* 105:27, 1986.
    While beta carotene, transfusions, and cholestyramine (Yale, J. Biol. Med. 52:39, 1979) are useful in this disease, iron therapy may have an important role in preventing fatal liver failure.
26. Pimstone, N. R., Gandhi, S. H., and Mukerji, S. K. Therapeutic efficacy of oral charcoal in congenital erythropoietic porphyria. *N. Engl. J. Med.* 316:390, 1987.
    Oral activated charcoal appeared to be more effective than transfusions or cholestyramine in reducing plasma porphyrin levels.
27. Harber, L. C., and Bickers, D. R. Porphyria and pseudoporphyria. *J. Invest. Dermatol.* 82:207, 1984.
    Brief review of PCT and disorders which mimic it.
28. Day, R. S., and Eales, L. Porphyrins in chronic renal failure. *Nephron* 26:90, 1980.
    Description of the abnormalities of porphyrin metabolism associated with renal failure which may explain the bullous dermatitis seen in this condition. These patients may also have true PCT (N. Engl. J. Med. 299:292, 1978).
29. Pierach, C. A., Bossenmaier, I. C., Cardinal, R. A., et al. Pseudo-porphyria in a patient with hepatocellular carcinoma. *Am. J. Med.* 76:545, 1984.
    No clinical symptoms were associated with the overproduction of PBG in this patient with a hepatoma.
30. Mustajoki, P., Tenhunen, R., Pierach, C., et al. Heme in the treatment of porphyrias and hematological disorders. *Semin. Hematol.* 26:1, 1989.
    Part of a symposium on porphyria.

105. PRELEUKEMIA (MYELODYSPLASTIC SYNDROME)
Jerry L. Spivak

Preleukemia is the term used to designate the panmyelopathy involving red cells, white cells, and platelets, which usually terminates in acute leukemia if the patient does not die first from hemorrhage or infection. The term is a poor one since it implies that there exists a prodromal syndrome that eventually transforms into acute leukemia when in fact the disorder is a form of acute leukemia in which the cells have a differentiation advantage. The term preleukemia would be better employed to describe those disorders that predispose to acute leukemia but are not themselves leukemic. They include Down's syndrome, Bloom's syndrome, Fanconi's anemia, ataxia telangiectasia, drug-induced aplastic anemia, idiopathic refractory sideroblastic anemia, paroxysmal nocturnal hemoglobinuria, polycythemia vera, multiple myeloma, and exposure to chemotherapeutic agents or irradiation. Chronic myelogenous leukemia is also a preleukemic disorder since it terminates as acute leukemia in most patients. The term preleukemia as currently used is of course preferable to other names employed to describe the panmyelopathy. They include erythroleukemia, chronic erythremic myelosis, Di Guglielmo's syndrome, refractory anemia with excessive blasts, and chronic monocytic leukemia. None of these represents a distinct disease entity but only describes the various morphologic abnormalities that occur in the preleukemic syndrome, any of which can be seen at various times in a single patient. The fallacy of using morphologic abnormalities as evidence of leukemic transformation becomes evident when it is recognized that many of the same morphologic abnormalities are observed in a variety of benign, congenital, or acquired dyserthropoietic states. They include the congenital dyserythropoietic anemias with multinuclearity, vitamin B_{12} or folic acid deficiency, and idiopathic refractory sideroblastic anemia. By definition acute leukemia is a clonal disorder and designation of cells as leukemic requires proof that they are part of the malignant clone. With the use of chromosomal markers and the isoenzymes of glucose-6-phosphate dehydrogenase, it has become apparent that acute leukemia may involve the common hematopoietic stem cell or the granulocyte-monocyte progenitor cell. When the neoplastic transformation takes place at the level of the common hematopoietic stem cell, red cells and megakaryocytes will be involved as well as white cells. This appears to be the usual situation in adults. On the other hand, when the leukemic transformation occurs at the level of the granulocyte-monocyte progenitor cell, as is the case in children with acute nonlymphocytic leukemia, erythroid precursors and megakaryocytes are not a part of the leukemic process. Light microscopy alone cannot distinguish between these possibilities. Since cell-cell interactions play a role in the mechanisms by which a leukemic cell population establishes its growth advantage, morphologically abnormal erythroid precursors in the marrow of a patient with acute leukemia could just as well be derived from a normal clone as from the leukemic clone but the difference could not be detected on the basis of morphologic abnormalities. Therefore, it seems better to abandon uncritical terms such as erythroleukemia, chronic erythremic myelosis, or chronic monocytic leukemia since they are based on subjective criteria.

The preleukemia syndrome can occur at any age but is seen most often in patients over the age of 60. Most patients are anemic and neutropenic and many are thrombocytopenic as well. In over 50 percent of patients circulating erythroblasts are observed. Macrocytosis and poikilocytosis are common and hypochromia may also be present. The latter may be seen when there is an abnormality of iron metabolism resulting in ringed sideroblasts or when there is a disturbance in globin production resulting in the synthesis of hemoglobin H. There may be abnormalities in the activity of red cell enzymes and in the expression of red cell surface antigens. Circulating granulocytes may be hyposegmented resembling the granulocytes of the Pelger-Huët anomaly. Granulocyte alkaline phosphatase and myeloperoxidase levels may be reduced. Monocytosis is not uncommon and giant platelets are frequently observed. The bone marrow of patients with preleukemia is usually normocellular or hypercellular. There may be marked abnormalities of erythroid maturation with megaloblastoid or frankly megaloblastic changes and giant multinucleated erythroblasts. There is usually a shift to the left in the myeloid series with an increase in monocytes. Megakaryocytes may exhibit morphologic abnormalities, particularly with respect to hypolobulation and a reduction in size. Iron stain may reveal ringed sideroblasts. Chromosome abnormalities are observed in over 50 percent of patients. The common ones are 5q-, 7-, and trisomy 8. The development of additional chromosome abnormalities usually heralds the terminal phase of the disorder with loss of the capacity to differentiate and development of the typical features of acute leukemia.

Studies of hematopoietic progenitor cell growth in vitro have indicated that patients with the preleukemic syndrome, in common with patients with acute leukemia, have defective colony formation by granulocyte-macrophage progenitor cells. The growth of erythroid progenitor cells in vitro, however, is usually normal.

The most difficult problem in evaluating patients with the preleukemic syndrome is distinguishing that syndrome from other disorders that cause similar morphologic abnormalities. Chromosome studies are helpful but will be normal in approximately 50 percent of cases. Less than 10 percent of patients with idiopathic refractory sideroblastic anemia develop acute leukemia. Hemoglobin H has been suggested as a marker for those patients who will. Other markers include a low reticulocyte count, a high transfusion requirement, and thrombocytopenia. In patients with another malignancy who have been treated with chemotherapy and/or radiotherapy, development of sideroblastic anemia or dyserythropoiesis can usually be considered as evidence of a preleukemic syndrome.

The mean duration of the preleukemic syndrome is approximately 2 years. Some patients, however, have a much shorter survival and a few have been described who have lived as long as 10 years from the time of diagnosis. One may reasonably question, however, whether those patients did indeed have a preleukemic syndrome and not another dyserythropoietic syndrome. Although the preleukemic syndrome should be considered as a form of acute leukemia, it does not respond to therapy as well as the more classic form of disease. A particularly difficult problem in the management of these patients is deciding when to initiate treatment. Many of the patients are in reasonably good health when first seen and given the poor response to chemotherapy, it is difficult to initiate it at that stage in the disorder. However, once the terminal phase occurs, the disease progresses rapidly and is often refractory to therapy. In addition, many patients develop severe infections that further complicate treatment with cytotoxic agents. In the absence of established guidelines for therapy, each patient must be managed on an individual basis. Numerous attempts to predict prognosis based on a variety of scoring systems using multiple clinical and laboratory markers have been published. It is generally accepted that those patients without excessive blasts have the most favorable prognosis. Chromosome abnormalities do not necessarily predict the likelihood of transformation but are extremely useful in establishing the presence of a clonal disorder of hematopoiesis and avoiding the pitfalls of "phenotypic prognostication" in assisting patients to understand their disease.

1. Bennett, J. M., Catovsky, D., Daniel, M. T., et al. Proposals for the classification of the myelodysplastic syndromes. *Br. J. Haematol.* 51:189, 1982.
   The French-American-British (FAB) classification for myelodysplastic syndromes.
2. Greenberg, P. L. The smoldering myeloid leukemic states: Clinical and biologic features. *Blood* 61:1035, 1983.
   A comparison of the various myelodysplastic syndromes.
3. Koeffler, H. P., and Golde, D. W. Human preleukemia. *Ann. Intern. Med.* 93:347, 1980.
   Comprehensive review.
4. Linman, J. W., and Bagby, G. C. The preleukemic syndrome (hemopoietic dysplasia). *Cancer* 42:854, 1978.
   The preleukemic syndrome is a panmyelopathy.
5. Weber, R. F. A., Geraedts, J. P. M., Kerkhofs, H., et al. The preleukemic syndrome. *Acta Med. Scand.* 207:391, 1980.
   Two-thirds of the patients in this series died from infection, hemorrhage, or other causes without developing overt leukemia.

6. Fisher, W. B., Armentrout, S. A., Weisman, R., Jr., et al. "Preleukemia." *Arch. Intern. Med.* 132:226, 1973.
   In this series splenic enlargement was associated with the appearance of the leukemic phase.
7. Anderson, R. L., Bagby, G. C., Jr., Richert-Boe, K., et al. Therapy-related preleukemic syndrome. *Cancer* 47:1867, 1981.
   This form of preleukemia is being seen with increasing frequency.
8. Solal-Celigny, P., Desaint, B., Herrera, A., et al. Chronic myelomonocytic leukemia according to FAB classification: Analysis of 35 cases. *Blood* 63:634, 1984.
   This is probably the most distinct of the myelodysplastic syndromes and actually may have a long survival.
9. Cazzola, M., Barosi, G., Gobbi, P. G., et al. Natural history of idiopathic refractory sideroblastic anemia. *Blood* 71:305, 1988.
   Multilineage defects portend a poor prognosis but most patients have a reasonable survival. (See also Cancer *44:724, 1979.)*
10. Clark, R., Peters, S., Hoy, T., et al. Prognostic importance of hypodiploid hemopoietic precursors in myelodysplastic syndromes. *N. Engl. J. Med.* 314:1472, 1986.
    Hypodiploidy by flow cytometry suggests a poor prognosis.
11. Foucar, K., Langdon, II, R. M., Armitage, J. O., et al. Myelodysplastic syndromes. A clinical and pathologic analysis of 109 cases. *Cancer* 56:553, 1985.
    Use of FAB classification for prognosis; refractory anemia (RA) and refractory anemia with ringed sideroblasts (RARS) had the longest survival.
12. Garcia, S., Sanz, M. A., Amigo, V., et al. Prognostic factors in chronic myelodysplastic syndromes. *Am. J. Hematol.* 27:163, 1988.
    Hemoglobin, platelet count, age, nucleated erythroblasts, and dyserythropoiesis are important prognostic factors. (For chromosome analysis, see Br. J. Haematol. *68:189, 1988.)*
13. Nowell, P., and Finan, J. Chromosome studies in preleukemic states. *Cancer* 42:2254, 1978.
    Cytogenic abnormalities, particularly if multiple, are associated with the development of overt leukemia.
14. Wisniewski, L. P., and Hirschhorn, K. Acquired partial deletions of the long arm of chromosome 5 in hematologic disorders. *Am. J. Hematol.* 15:295, 1983.
    This can be associated with indolent or progressive marrow abnormalities. (See also Cancer Genet. Cytogenet. *17:189, 1985.) It is of great interest that the long arm of chromosome 5 contains genes for several hematopoietic growth factors and certain growth factor receptors.*
15. Boehme, W. M., Piira, T. A., Kurnick, J. E., et al. Acquired hemoglobin H in refractory sideroblastic anemia. *Arch. Intern. Med.* 138:603, 1978.
    Hemoglobin H may be a marker for leukemia in patients with sideroblastic anemia.
16. Valentine, W. N., Konrad, P. N., and Paglia, D. E. Dyserythropoiesis, refractory anemia, and "preleukemia": Metabolic features of the erythrocytes. *Blood* 41:857, 1973.
    Red cell enzyme abnormalities occur in preleukemia.
17. Hartz, J. W., Buss, D. H., White, D. R., et al. Marked elliptocytosis and schistocytosis in hematopoietic dysplasia. *Am. J. Clin. Pathol.* 82:354, 1984.
    This can occasionally be a striking finding.
18. Adamson, J. W., and Finch, C. A. Erythropoietin and the regulation of erythropoiesis in di Guglielmo's syndrome. *Blood* 36:590, 1970.
    Erythropoiesis is not autonomous in "erythroleukemia." (See also Arch. Intern. Med. *123:60, 1969.)*
19. Fialkow, P. J., Singer, J. W., Adamson, J. W., et al. Acute nonlymphocytic leukemia: Heterogeneity of stem cell origin. *Blood* 57:1068, 1981.
    In children, acute nonlymphocytic leukemia arises at the level of the granulocyte-monocyte progenitor cell. In adults, it appears to arise at the level of the hematopoietic stem cell.
20. Blackstock, A. M., and Garson, O. M. Direct evidence for involvement of erythroid cells in acute myeloblastic leukaemia. *Lancet* 2:1178, 1974.
    A method for identifying leukemic erythroblasts.

21. Greenberg, P. L., and Mara, B. The preleukemic syndrome: Correlation of in vitro parameters of granulopoiesis with clinical features. *Am. J. Med.* 66:951, 1979.
   Impairment of in vitro granulocyte-macrophage colony formation was predictive of a short survival.
22. Koeffler, H. P., Cline, M. J., and Golde, D. W. Erythropoieseis in preleukemia. *Blood* 51:1013, 1978.
   In contrast to erythropoiesis in vivo, erythropoiesis in vitro was normal in this series.
23. Davies, A. R., and Schmitt, R. G. Auer bodies in mature neutrophils. *J.A.M.A.* 203:895, 1968.
   Leukemic cells are capable of differentiation.
24. Bainton, D. F. Abnormal neutrophils in acute myelogenous leukemia: Identification of subpopulations based on analysis of azurophil and specific granules. *Blood Cells* 1:191, 1975.
   Normal-appearing neutrophils can be functionally abnormal.
25. Cohen, J. R., Creger, W. P., Greenberg, P. L., et al. Subacute myeloid leukemia: A clinical review. *Am. J. Med.* 66:959, 1979.
   Anemia, hepatosplenomegaly, and leukocytosis or thrombocytopenia were poor prognostic signs. Chemotherapy did not improve survival.
26. Buzaid, A. C., Garewal, H. S., and Greenberg, B. R. Management of myelodysplastic syndromes. *Am. J. Med.* 80:1149, 1986.
   There are few treatment options. (See also Lancet *2:717, 1987.)*
27. Bolwell, B. J., Cassileth, P. A., and Gale, R. P. Low dose cytosine arabinoside in myelodysplasia and acute myelogenous leukemia: A review. *Leukemia* 1:575, 1987.
   It is important to remember that hematologic toxicity can be severe. This is not an outpatient regimen.
28. Kufe, D. W., Griffin, J. D., and Spriggs, D. R. Cellular and clinical pharmacology of low-dose ara-C. *Semin. Oncol.* 12:200, 1985.
   Comprehensive review.
29. Clark, R. E., Lush, C. J., Jacobs, A., et al. Effect of 13-cis-retinoic acid on survival of patients with myelodysplastic syndrome. *Lancet* 1:763, 1987.
   This was not effective when blasts were prominent.
30. Appelbaum, F. R., Storb, R., Ramberg, R. E., et al. Treatment of preleukemic syndromes with marrow transplantation. *Blood* 69:92, 1987.
   This is the treatment of choice for de novo myelodysplasia without myelofibrosis.
31. Ganser, A., Volkers, B., Greher, J., et al. Recombinant human granulocyte-macrophage colony-stimulating factor [GM-CSF] in patients with myelodysplastic syndromes—A phase I/II trial. *Blood* 73:31, 1989.
   In this study, GM-CSF stimulated the leukemic clone to expand.
32. Negrin, R. S., Haeuber, D. H., Nagler, A., et al. Treatment of myelodysplastic syndromes with recombinant human granulocyte colony-stimulating factor [G-CSF]. *Ann. Intern. Med.* 110:976, 1989.
   G-CSF appears more promising than GM-CSF.

106. PURE RED CELL APLASIA
Jerry L. Spivak

The syndrome of pure red cell aplasia (PRCA) is characterized by a normochromic, normocytic anemia with absent or a markedly reduced number of reticulocytes, normal leukocyte and platelet counts, a virtual absence of erythroid precursors in the marrow, or less commonly an arrest of erythropoiesis at the pronormoblast level, and normal marrow myelopoiesis and megakaryocytopoiesis. Occasionally, an increase in marrow lymphocytes and eosinophils is observed. PRCA may be congenital (the Diamond-Blackfan syndrome) or acquired. PRCA has occurred with renal insufficiency; infections and in particular parvovirus infection; malnutrition; riboflavin deficiency; with a variety of neoplasms including oat-cell carcinoma, Hodgkin's and non-Hodgkin's lymphomas, and chronic lymphocytic leukemia (CLL); with systemic lupus erythematosus (SLE) and rheumatoid arthritis; autoimmune hemolytic anemia; and thymoma. A variety of drugs have also been implicated in the production of PRCA. They include phenytoin, isoniazid, chlorpropamide, tolbutamide, phenylbutazone, azathioprine, halothane, sulfonamides, penicillin, phenobarbital, cephalothin, and probenecid. In a small proportion of patients, PRCA occurs in the absence of any disease or drug ingestion. In approximately 50 percent of these cases, an immunoglobulin cytotoxic to nucleated erythroid precursors has been identified. Another interesting feature of patients with this form of acquired PRCA is the coexistence of a wide variety of immunologic abnormalities. They include hypogammaglobulinemia, monoclonal gammopathy, and autoantibodies against red cells or platelets.

A striking feature of acquired PRCA is the high frequency with which this disorder is associated with a thymoma. Fifty percent of patients with PRCA will be found to have a thymoma, while approximately 5 percent of patients with thymoma develop PRCA. Isolated red cell aplasia is the most common hematologic disorder occurring with thymoma. In a small proportion of patients, thrombocytopenia, leukopenia, or pancytopenia may occur. Most patients with the syndrome of thymoma and PRCA are women, generally over the age of 50. The PRCA never precedes the thymoma but the tumor may be present many years before the onset of anemia, and PRCA has been observed after removal of such tumors. The histology of the thymoma does not appear to correlate with the development of PRCA or other clinical syndromes known to be associated with thymomas. These include myasthenia gravis, SLE, aplastic anemia, hypogammaglobulinemia, rheumatoid arthritis, polymyositis, Cushing's syndrome, autoimmune hemolytic anemia, and monoclonal gammopathy. These paraneoplastic syndromes appear to be interrelated since a number of patients have been described in whom thymoma and PRCA have been complicated by myasthenia and SLE. In other patients, in the absence of a documented thymoma, PRCA has been associated with either autoimmune hemolytic anemia or autoimmune thrombocytopenia and SLE, suggesting an autoimmune basis for the disorder even in the absence of a lymphoid neoplasm.

The diagnosis of PRCA is established by examination of a bone marrow aspirate. While this might appear routine, because marrow cellularity in PRCA is usually normal, the absence of erythroblasts has not infrequently been overlooked, and in patients in whom there is an associated disorder such as myelofibrosis, CLL, or chronic myelogenous leukemia (CML), a marked reduction or even the absence of erythroid precursors may not be noticed.

Once the presence of PRCA has been established, it is necessary to determine its etiology. In view of the high frequency with which thymomas cause red cell aplasia, it is important to evaluate all patients for the presence of this tumor with appropriate radiographic procedures. A careful history of drug exposure is also important since removal of the offending agent will result in correction of the PRCA. In patients with underlying malignancies such as lymphoma, CLL, CML, or Hodgkin's disease, treatment of the malignancy usually results in remission of the PRCA. Patients with thymoma have a remission rate of approximately 30 percent following thymectomy, although it must be remembered that in some patients PRCA develops after the tumor has been removed. Only rarely has irradiation of a thymic tumor resulted in remission of PRCA. Even though thymectomy does not always result in remission, it is generally necessary if the patients are to respond to treatment with other agents such as prednisone and cyclophosphamide. Without thymectomy, steroids appear to be ineffective and indeed the disorder has occurred in patients on steroid therapy. After thymectomy, however, steroids appear to be an effective form of therapy. The role of splenectomy in patients with thymoma is unclear. Splenectomy alone appears to offer little benefit but may be useful as an adjunct to immunosuppressive agents. The prognosis of patients with thymoma appears to depend more on the size of the tumor and its invasiveness than its histology. PRCA in association with small tumors appears to respond less well than with larger tumors; invasive tumors have a poorer prognosis than encapsulated tumors but prolonged survival has been observed with an invasive thymoma.

Since PRCA can be caused by viral infections as well as by many drugs, patients with his disorder unassociated with thymoma or another illness should be observed for several months before considering the use of immunosuppressive agents. Although antibodies cytotoxic for erythroid progenitor cells have been identified in approximately 50 percent of patients with PRCA unassociated with other diseases, it is noteworthy that even when erythroblast antibodies cannot be demonstrated, responses can be obtained with immunosuppressive therapy. Recently, in patients with PRCA, a correlation has been observed between the ability of their marrow cells to form erythroid colonies in vitro and responsiveness to therapy. This is an important advance in predicting which patients might benefit from immunosuppressive therapy since such therapy is not without risks. Prednisone is the initial drug of choice for acquired PRCA. If no response is seen, then cyclophosphamide should be employed in conjunction with prednisone. Other drugs, such as azathioprine and 6-mercaptopurine, have also been used successfully as has antithymocyte globulin (ATG). It should be remembered that spontaneous remissions have been observed in patients with PRCA, while chemotherapy-induced remissions are not always sustained. In a few patients, particularly those in whom there have been an appreciable number of proerythroblasts in the marrow, splenectomy has been beneficial when immunosuppressive agents have not been effective. In some patients, maintenance therapy may be required to sustain a remission. In a few patients repeated plasmapheresis produced a prolonged remission. Other therapeutic agents which have been employed include danazol, cyclosporin, and intravenous gamma globulin, but experience with these is still anecdotal.

1. Saarinen, U. M., Chorba, T. L., Tattersall, P., et al. Human parvovirus B19–induced epidemic acute red cell aplasia in patients with hereditary hemolytic anemia. *Blood* 67:1411, 1986.
   Human parvovirus is the cause of transient red cell aplasia in patients with hemolytic anemia. (See also Science *233:883, 1986 and* J. Clin. Invest. *79:1486, 1987.)*
2. Ammus, S. S., and Yunis, A. A. Acquired pure red cell aplasia. *Am. J. Hematol.* 24:311, 1987.
   Comprehensive review. (See also Med. Clin. North Am. *60:945, 1976.)*
3. Krantz, S. B. Pure red cell aplasia. *N. Engl. J. Med.* 291:345, 1974.
   Cytotoxicity of pretreatment IgG for erythroblasts demonstrated in some patients with PRCA.
4. Beard, M. E. J., Krantz, S. B., Johnson, S. A. N., et al. Pure red cell aplasia. *Q. J. Med.* 47:339, 1978.
   Prednisone and cyclophosphamide alone or in combination produced a remission in PRCA in the absence of detectable erythroblast antibodies.
5. Hirst, E., and Robertson, T. I. The syndrome of thymoma and erythroblastopenia anemia. *Medicine* 46:225, 1967.
   50% of patients with PRCA have a thymoma.
6. Verley, J. M., and Hollmann, K. H. Thymoma. *Cancer* 55:1074, 1985.
   A review of 200 patients.
7. MacKechnie, H. L. N., Squires, A. H., Plotts, M., et al. Thymoma, myasthenia gravis, erythroblastopenic anemia and systemic lupus erythematosus in one patient. *Can. Med. Assoc. J.* 109:733, 1973.
   Unusual constellation of disorders of autoimmunity.
8. Zaentz, S. D., Krantz, S. B., and Sears, D. A. Studies on pure red cell aplasia: VII. Presence of erythroblasts and response to splenectomy: A case report. *Blood* 46:261, 1975.
   Splenectomy-induced remission following failure of immunosuppressive therapy.
9. Zaentz, S. D., Krantz, S. B., and Brown, E. B. Studies on pure red cell aplasia: VIII. Maintenance therapy with immunosuppressive drugs. *Br. J. Haematol.* 32:47, 1976.
   Maintenance therapy may be required in some patients with PRCA.
10. Cavalcant, J., Shadduck, R. K., Winkelstein, A., et al. Red-cell hypoplasia and increased bone marrow reticulin in systemic lupus erythematosus: Reversal with corticosteroid therapy. *Am. J. Hematol.* 5:253, 1978.
    Coexistent myelofibrosis and red cell aplasia.

11. Meyer, R. J., Hoffman, R., and Zanjani, E. D. Autoimmune hemolytic anemia and periodic pure red cell aplasia. *Am. J. Med.* 65:342, 1978.
    Red cell eluates contained a factor that impaired erythroid colony formation in vitro.
12. Fox, R. M., and Firkin, F. C. Sequential pure red cell and megakaryocyte aplasia associated with chronic liver disease and ulcerative colitis. *Am. J. Hematol.* 4:79, 1978.
    An interesting association since red cells and megakaryocytes are thought to share a common stem cell.
13. Dessypris, E. N., McKee, C. L., Jr., Metzantonakis, C., et al. Red cell aplasia and chronic granulocytic leukemia. *Br. J. Haematol.* 48:217, 1981.
    PRCA can precede, occur at the onset, or during the course of CML.
14. Chikkappa, G., Zarrabi, M. H., and Tsan, M.-F. Pure red cell aplasia in patients with chronic lymphocytic leukemia. *Medicine* 65:339, 1986.
    PRCA can occur early or late in the illness and can be drug-induced (chlorambucil).
15. Nagasawa, T., Abe, T., and Nakagawa, T. Pure red cell aplasia and hypogamma-globulinemia associated with T-cell chronic lymphocytic leukemia. *Blood* 57:1025, 1981.
    Suppression of erythroid colony formation and gamma globulin production by malignant T cells. (See also Nature 266:57, 1977 and J. Clin. Invest. 70:1148, 1982.)
16. Morgan, E., Pang, K. M., and Goldwasser, E. Hodgkin's disease and red cell aplasia. *Am. J. Hematol.* 5:71, 1978.
    PRCA of immune origin that resolved with chemotherapy.
17. Sears, D. A., George, J. N., and Gold, M. S. Transient red blood cell aplasia in association with viral hepatitis: Occurrence four years apart in siblings. *Arch. Intern. Med.* 135:1585, 1975.
    Unusual occurrence suggesting a genetic predisposition. (See also Ann. Intern. Med. 92:196, 1980.)
18. Dessypris, E. N., Redline, S., Harris, J. W., et al. Diphenylhydantoin-induced pure red cell aplasia. *Blood* 65:789, 1985.
    Immunologic mediation by a drug-dependent antibody.
19. Planas, A. T., Kranwinkel, R. N., and Soletsky, H. B. Chlorpropamide-induced pure RBC aplasia. *Arch. Intern. Med.* 140:707, 1980.
    Direct toxic effect suggested since the dose of chloropropamide was excessive.
20. McGrath, B. P., Ibels, L. S., Raik, E., et al. Erythroid toxicity of azathioprine. *Q. J. Med.* 44:57, 1975.
    PRCA is a dose-related toxic effect of azathioprine.
21. Old, C. W., Flannery, E. P., Grogan, T. M., et al. Azathioprine-induced pure red cell aplasia. *J.A.M.A.* 240:552, 1978.
    Substitution of cyclophosphamide permitted recovery of erythropoiesis.
22. Lacombe, C., Casadevall, N., Muller, O., et al. Erythroid progenitors in adult chronic pure red cell aplasia: Relationship of in vitro erythroid colonies to therapeutic response. *Blood* 64:71, 1984.
    Use of in vitro clonal assays to predict response in PRCA.
23. Dessypris, E. N., Fogo, A., Russell, M., et al. Studies on pure red cell aplasia: X. Association with acute leukemia and significance of bone marrow karyotype abnormalities. *Blood* 56:421, 1980.
    Abnormal karyotypes in PRCA are uncommon and may presage the development of acute leukemia.
24. Clark, D. A., Dessypris, E. N., and Krantz, S. B. Studies on pure red cell aplasia. XI. Results of immunosuppressive treatment of 37 patients. *Blood* 63:277, 1984.
    66% remission rate but the relapse rate was high as was the incidence of infection.
25. Abkowitz, J. L., Powell, J. S., Nakamura, J. M., et al. Pure red cell aplasia: Response to therapy with anti-thymocyte globulin. *Am. J. Hematol.* 23:363, 1986.
    Erythroid colony formation in vitro may be predictive of who will respond to ATG.
26. Messner, H. A., Fauser, A. A., Curtis, J. E., et al. Control of antibody-mediated pure red cell aplasia by plasmapheresis. *N. Engl. J. Med.* 304:1334, 1981.
    Plasmapheresis produced a prolonged remission after failure of immunosuppressive therapy. (See also Scand. J. Haematol. 34:13, 1985.)
27. Kurtzman G., Frickhofen N., Kimball S., et al. Pure red cell aplasia of 10 years'

duration due to persistent parvovirus B19 infection and its cure with immunoglobulin therapy. *N. Engl. J. Med.* 321:519, 1989.
See also N. Engl. J. Med. *317:1004, 1987.*
28. Lenarksy, C., Weinberg, K., Guinan, E., et al. Bone marrow transplantation for constitutional pure red cell aplasia. *Blood* 71:226, 1988.
An extreme measure for young patients with refractory PRCA.

107. SICKLE CELL ANEMIA
Jerry L. Spivak

Substitution of valine for glutamic acid in the sixth position on the β chain of hemoglobin results in a molecule (hemoglobin S) whose solubility is reduced on deoxygenation.
The loss of solubility is due to the formation of linear aggregates of hemoglobin, which
align to form twisted rodlike structures or tactoids (liquid crystals). This sol-to-gel
transformation of the deoxygenated hemoglobin S results in the characteristic sickle
deformity of the red cell membrane. Repeated episodes of sickling result in loss of cell
surface area, increased rigidity, sequestration, and hemolysis. In addition to low oxygen
tension, other factors promoting sickling are low pH, elevated temperature, increased
osmolarity, and a high concentration of hemoglobin S within the red cell. In homozygous
sickle cell disease, in which 80 percent or more of the hemoglobin is S, sickling occurs
in vivo at physiologic tissue oxygen tensions. In sickle trait, in which less than 50 percent of the red cell hemoglobin is S, sickling does not occur unless oxygen tension falls
below physiologic levels.

The sickling phenomenon is also moderated by the presence of other hemoglobins.
Cells containing both hemoglobin S and C sickle at higher oxygen tensions than S-A
cells, even though the concentration of S is the same in both. Cells containing S and D
may sickle as readily as S-S cells, despite the fact that the concentration of S is less than
50 percent. On the other hand, hemoglobin F does not interact with S, and cells containing S and F do not sickle readily, even though the concentration of S is 70 percent. Since
the clinical severity in sickling disorders is related to the rate of sickling, these facts
explain the variability of the disease in patients carrying the sickle gene. Patients with
both sickle cell anemia and hereditary persistence of fetal hemoglobin have a very mild
illness, as do some patients with sickle cell–β-thalassemia. Patients with S-D hemoglobin, however, can have a disease as severe as the S-S homozygote.

Although the molecular defect in sickle cell disease is limited to the red cell, its effect
is seen in every organ and tissue in the body. The patient with sickle cell anemia exists
in a precarious balance. As a result of intrapulmonic shunts, the oxygen saturation of
arterial blood is often reduced. In addition, hemoglobin S has a lower affinity for oxygen
than can be accounted for by the concentration of red cell 2,3-diphosphoglycerate. Increased cardiac output, increased plasma volume, and anemia tend to offset both the
tendency to sickle and the increased viscosity of the sickled cells. This equilibrium is
threatened by ischemic damage to the renal medulla, which results in hyposthenuria
and impaired ability to excrete an acid load. The spleen is a particular target organ due
to its unique anatomy, and with repeated infarction it becomes atrophic. Splenomegaly
in an adult with sickle cell disease should suggest the presence of a mixed hemoglobinopathy (S-C, S-F, or S-thalassemia) or another illness, such as sarcoidosis. As a result
of splenic atrophy and defective complement activation, there is an increased incidence
of infection in patients with sickle cell anemia. In younger patients, fulminant meningitis and bacteremia are common. In older patients, pneumonia, urinary tract infections,
and osteomyelitis, particularly with salmonella, occur.

The diagnosis of infection is often difficult since pain, fever, and leukocytosis occur
with vasoocclusive crises, and marrow infarction and aseptic necrosis of bone are not
uncommon. Pulmonary infiltrates and pleuritis are often due to embolization of fat,

marrow, and sickle thrombi. Jaundice also provides diagnostic difficulties and can be due to stasis of hepatic sinusoidal blood flow with hypoxic damage, congestive heart failure, hemolysis, hepatic vein thrombosis, hemochromatosis, viral hepatitis, or cholelithiasis. Liver biopsy may not be helpful because intrahepatic cholestasis can occur without ductal obstruction. Emergency surgery is rarely warranted since common duct obstruction by stones is extremely uncommon. Complications of the chronic hemolysis also include leg ulcers, skeletal deformities, megaloblastic anemia due to increased utilization of folic acid, and aplastic crises. The aplastic crises appear to be due to parvovirus infection, often occur in clusters in a particular family, and can result in a rapid fall in hematocrit if not appreciated. Hyperhemolytic crises are due to superimposed glucose-6-phosphate dehydrogenase (G-6-PD) deficiency, which occurs with increased frequency in S-S disease. This condition may be missed with the usual screening tests because of the elevated reticulocyte count. Sequestration crises rarely occur in adults. Hyperuricemia is a consequence of the increased turnover of red cells in the presence of impaired urate excretion.

In managing the symptomatic patient it is important to avoid hypoxia, acidosis, and dehydration. Sickling begins in vivo at a PO_2 of 60 mm Hg. Arterial blood gas measurements are a valuable tool in assessing the adequacy of oxygenation. Patients with pneumonia or pulmonary embolism who have impaired oxygenation may require exchange transfusion. This will not abort a painful crisis, but it will prevent exacerbation of the sickling process until the patient has recovered. It must be remembered, however, that transfusion carries the risk of febrile reactions which may increase the patient's symptoms. Clinical judgment cannot always be relied on to determine the presence of infection, and serial blood cultures may be useful in this regard. The therapy for vasoocclusive crises otherwise remains unsatisfactory, numerous remedies having been tried without success. Adequate analgesia (without impairing respiration) is important.

In recent years much attention has been paid to identifying individuals with sickle trait. Ordinarily, they are asymptomatic and not anemic. Rarely, they may develop thrombotic complications (aseptic bone necrosis, pulmonary and splenic infarcts). Their major problem is hematuria due to renal medullary necrosis. Many remedies have been tried, but without success—usually the bleeding stops spontaneously. Unless some other lesion is suspected, surgery should be avoided. Finally, the diagnosis of sickle trait by electrophoretic techniques should always be confirmed by a sickle preparation since other hemoglobins migrate in the same fashion.

1. Dean, J., and Schechter, A. N. Sickle cell anemia: Molecular and celluar bases of therapeutic approaches. *N. Engl. J. Med.* 299:752, 804, 863, 1978.
   Comprehensive review of all aspects of sickle cell anemia. (See also Blood *58:1057, 1981.*
2. Steinberg, M. H., and Hebbel, R. P. Clinical diversity of sickle cell anemia. *Am. J. Hematol.* 14:405, 1983.
   Genetic factors are important. (See also N. Engl. J. Med. *312:880, 1985 and* Am. J. Hematol. *20:195, 1985.)*
3. Charache, S. Treatment of sickle cell anemia. *Annu. Rev. Med.* 32:195, 1981.
   Excellent advice by an expert.
4. Huisman, T. H. J. Sickle cell anemia as a syndrome: A review of diagnostic features. *Am. J. Hematol.* 6:173, 1979.
   Use of the laboratory in the diagnosis of sickling disorders.
5. Charache, S., and Conley, C. L. Rate of sickling of red cells during deoxygenation of blood from persons with various sickling disorders. *Blood* 24:25, 1964.
   The viscosity of sickled blood is proportional to the square of the hematocrit.
6. Karayalcin, G., Rosner, F., Kim, K. Y., et al. Sickle cell anemia: Clinical manifestations in 100 patients and review of the literature. *Am. J. Med. Sci.* 269:51, 1975.
   A source of useful information. For x-ray findings, see Am. J. Med. Sci. *271:132, 1976.*
7. Ballas, S. K., Lewis, C. N., Noone, A. M., et al. Clinical, hematological, and biochemical features of Hb SC disease. *Am. J. Hematol.* 13:37, 1982.
   Comprehensive review. (See also Am. J. Hematol. *18:261, 1985.)*
8. Comer, P. B., and Fred, H. L. Diagnosis of sickle-cell disease by ophthalmoscopic inspection of the conjunctiva. *N. Engl. J. Med.* 271:544, 1964.

Conjunctival vascular lesions are diagnostic for sickle-cell disease.

9. Barrett-Connor, E. Bacterial infection and sickle cell anemia. *Medicine* 50:97, 1971.
   Increased incidence of infection in sickle cell anemia.

10. Charache, S., Scott, J. C., and Charache, P. Acute chest syndrome in adults with sickle cell anemia: Microbiology, treatment, and prevention. *Arch. Intern. Med.* 139:67, 1979.
    Pulmonary infarction is more likely than infection in adults with sickle cell anemia and an acute pulmonary disorder. (See also Am. Rev. Respir. Dis. 103:858, 1971.)

11. Statius Van Eps, L. W., Pinedo-Veels, C., de Vries, G. H., et al. Nature of concentrating defect in sickle cell nephropathy. *Lancet* 1:450, 1970.
    Loss of vasa recta resulting in impaired concentrating capacity.

12. Strauss, J., Zilleruelo, G., and Abitbol, C. The kidney and hemoglobin S. *Nephron* 43:241, 1986.
    A variety of renal lesions occur.

13. Diamond, H. S., Meisel, A. D., and Holden, D. The natural history of urate overproduction in sickle cell anemia. *Ann. Intern. Med.* 90:752, 1979.
    Hyperuricemia results from overproduction of uric acid in the presence of diminished renal function.

14. Friedman, E. A., Sreepada Rao, T. K., Sprung, C. L., et al. Uremia in sickle-cell anemia treated by maintenance hemodialysis. *N. Engl. J. Med.* 291:431, 1974.
    Dialysis is tolerated well by sickle-cell patients.

15. Johnson, C. S., Omata, M., Tong, M. J., et al. Liver involvement in sickle cell disease. *Medicine* 64:349, 1985.
    A variety of causes other than sickling are responsible for liver disease in these patients. (See also Am. J. Med. 69:833, 1980 and Br. Med. J. 290:744, 1985.)

16. Cameron, J. L., Maddrey, W. C., and Zuidema, G. D. Biliary tract disease in sickle cell anemia. *Ann. Surg.* 174:702, 1971.
    Advocates biliary tract surgery only if cholelithiasis is symptomatic. (See also Br. Med. J. 295:234, 1987.)

17. Falk, R. H., and Hood, W. B., Jr. The heart in sickle cell anemia. *Arch. Intern. Med.* 142:1680, 1982.
    Left ventricular failure due to sickle cell disease is uncommon.

18. Powars, D., Weidman, J. A., Odom-Maryon, I., et al. Sickle cell chronic lung disease: prior morbidity and the risk of pulmonary failure. *Medicine* 67:66, 1988.
    Progressive pulmonary hypertension whose progression is inexorable.

19. Espinoza, L. R., Spilberg, I., and Osterland, C. K. Joint manifestations of sickle cell disease. *Medicine* 53:295, 1974.
    Acute polyarthritis of short duration involving large joints is most common.

20. Hutchinson, R. M., Merrick, M. V., and White, J. M. Fat embolism in sickle cell disease. *J. Clin. Pathol.* 26:620, 1973.
    An unusual cause of respiratory distress.

21. Charache, S., and Page, D. L. Infarction of bone marrow in the sickle cell disorders. *Ann. Intern. Med.* 67:1195, 1967.
    Marrow necrosis associated with aseptic necrosis of femoral head and bone infarcts.

22. Portnoy, B. A., and Herion, J. C. Neurological manifestations in sickle-cell disease. *Ann. Intern. Med.* 76:643, 1972.
    High incidence of hemiplegia. For S-C disease see Arch. Neurol. 41:289, 1984.

23. Stockman, J. A., Negro, M. D., Mishkin, M. M., et al. Occlusion of large cerebral vessels in sickle cell anemia. *N. Engl. J. Med.* 287:846, 1972.
    Neurologic damage due to carotid artery occlusion.

24. Powars, D., Wilson, B., Imbus, C., et al. The natural history of stroke in sickle cell disease. *Am. J. Med.* 65:461, 1978.
    Strokes tend to reoccur within a limited time span and then cease. In adults, hemorrhage is more common than thrombus.

25. Russell, M. O., Goldberg, H. I., Hodson, A., et al. Effect of transfusion therapy on arteriographic abnormalities and on recurrence of stroke in sickle cell disease. *Blood* 63:162, 1984.
    Transfusion therapy is effective in reducing recurrent strokes and vascular abnormalities.

26. Welch, R. B., and Goldberg, M. F. Sickle-cell hemoglobin and its relation to fundus abnormality. *Arch. Ophthalmol.* 75:353, 1966.
   Retinal lesions of S-S, S-C, S-A, and A-C reviewed. (See also Arch. Intern. Med. *137:325, 1977.)*
27. Green, R. L., Huntsman, R. G., and Serjeant, G. R. The sickle-cell and altitude. *Br. Med. J.* 4:593, 1971.
   Patients with S-C disease are at the greatest risk from crisis with air travel.
28. Watson, R. J., Lichtman, H. C., and Shapiro, H. D. Splenomegaly in sickle cell anemia. *Am. J. Med.* 20:196, 1956.
   Splenomegaly is usually found in association with S-C, S-thalassemia, or S-F disease.
29. Emond, A. M., Holmam, R., Hayes, R. J., et al. Priapism and impotence in homozygous sickle cell disease. *Arch. Intern. Med.* 140:1434, 1980.
   (See also J. Urol. 119:610, 1978.)
   Priapism is common and varies in severity.
30. Sears, D. A. The morbidity of sickle cell trait. *Am. J. Med.* 64:1021, 1978.
   Hyposthenuria and hematuria are the common complications of sickle cell trait. (See also N. Engl. J. Med. 268:969, 1963.)
31. Kark, J. A., Posey, D. M., Schumacher, H. R., et al. Sickle-cell trait as a risk factor for sudden death in physical training. *N. Engl. J. Med.* 317:781, 1987.
   Evidence to support sickle trait as a risk factor for exercise-associated sudden death.
32. Lane, P. A., and Githens, J. H. Splenic syndrome at mountain altitudes in sickle cell trait: Its occurrence in nonblack persons. *J.A.M.A.* 253:2251, 1985.
   Phenotypic expression of sickle trait in whites.
33. Heller, P., Best, W. R., Nelson, R. B., et al. Clinical implications of sickle-cell trait and glucose-6-phosphate dehydrogenase deficiency in hospitalized black male patients. *N. Engl. J. Med.* 300:1001, 1979.
   G-6-PD deficiency does not have an adverse effect on patients with sickle trait. (See also N. Engl. J. Med. 290:826, 1974.)
34. Sherwood, J. B., Goldwasser, E., Chilcote, R., et al. Sickle cell anemia patients have low erythropoietin levels for their degree of anemia. *Blood* 67:46, 1986.
   This appears to be related to increasing age and could reflect ongoing renal damage.
35. Ahonkhai, V. I., Landesman, S. H., Fikrig, S. M., et al. Failure of pneumococcal vaccine in children with sickle-cell disease. *N. Engl. J. Med.* 301:26, 1979.
   Because of a suboptimal antibody response, penicillin prophylaxis is also recommended in susceptible individuals.
36. Koshy, M., Burd, L., Wallace, D., et al. Prophylactic red-cell transfusions in pregnant patients with sickle cell disease. *N. Engl. J. Med.* 319:1447, 1988.
   In this randomized study, prophylactic red cell transfusions were not beneficial to either the mother or the fetus.
37. Cox, J. V., Steane, E., Cunningham, G., et al. Risk of alloimmunization and delayed hemolytic transfusion reactions in patients with sickle cell disease. *Arch. Intern. Med.* 148:2485, 1988.
   Delayed transfusion reactions are not uncommon but easy to miss.
38. Charache, S., Dover, G. J., Moyer, M. A., et al. Hydroxyurea-induced augmentation of fetal hemoglobin production in patients with sickle cell anemia. *Blood* 69:109, 1987.
   A potentially promising therapy for sickle cell anemia.

108. SIDEROBLASTIC ANEMIA
Jerry L. Spivak

Iron not used in the synthesis of hemoglobin appears in the red cell cytoplasm as ferritin. Normally aggregates of this nonheme iron can be seen with Prussian blue staining in

30 to 50 percent of developing red cells in the marrow. Such cells, designated as sidero-cytes or, if nucleated, as sideroblasts, are markedly reduced during iron deficiency and increased when iron supply exceeds utilization, as in the arrested maturation of mega-loblastic anemia or in thalassemia where hemoglobin synthesis is defective. Such intra-cellular aggregates cause rigidity of the red cell membrane and are usually removed when the cell passes through the spleen. Consequently siderocytes are rarely seen in the blood of adults, except when the spleen is absent or atrophic or when there is he-molysis with an increased delivery of reticulocytes containing siderotic granules to the peripheral blood. Although siderocytes may be tentatively identified in Wright-stained preparations, absolute identification requires the use of the Prussian blue stain for fer-ric iron. This stain permits distinction between siderocytes and stippled red cells. The latter are reticulocytes whose ribosomal RNA has been precipitated by the staining pro-cess. The degree of stippling, coarse or fine, appears to depend in part on the technique used in drying and staining the blood smear. Stippling may also be conditioned by dis-ordered hemoglobin synthesis since an increase in stippled cells is characteristic of lead poisoning and thalassemia.

Occasionally iron accumulation in the red cell occurs not in the cytoplasm but in the mitochondria, which in erythroblasts are normally arranged in a perinuclear distribu-tion. With Prussian blue staining such cells appear to have a ring of iron granules around the nucleus and thus are called ringed sideroblasts. Recognition of ringed sid-eroblasts and their clinical implications is relatively recent, and understanding of their pathophysiology is still incomplete. These cells may be seen in a variety of disease states, including myeloproliferative disorders, megaloblastic anemia, thalassemia, leu-kemia, and multiple myeloma. In addition, exposure to certain drugs and toxins may produce ringed sideroblasts and anemia; these include isoniazid (INH), cycloserine, pyr-azinamide, chloramphenicol, and alcohol. Anemia associated with ringed sideroblasts can also occur in the absence of drugs, toxins, or underlying disease. Such cases may be classified as hereditary or acquired and as pyridoxine-responsive or -unresponsive.

In addition to ringed sideroblasts, sideroblastic anemia is characterized by an in-crease in body iron stores, hyperferremia, increased transferrin saturation, and marrow erythroid hyperplasia, usually normoblastic but occasionally megaloblastic. Red blood cells may be macrocytic, normocytic, or microcytic, and poikilocytosis can be marked. Hypochromia is either generalized or limited to a subpopulation of red cells, producing a dimorphic pattern. Stippling is common and is characteristically prominent in the hypochromic cells; iron stain reveals circulating siderocytes. Occasionally in acquired idiopathic sideroblastic anemia, neutropenia, monocytosis, or thrombocytopenia occurs; leukocyte alkaline phosphatase is often low and splenomegaly of a mild degree may be encountered.

The mechanism for production of ringed sideroblasts is unknown but multiple factors appear to be involved. A number of enzymatic defects have been identified in patients with sideroblastic anemia of both the hereditary and acquired variety. They include im-pairment of δ-aminolevolinic acid (ALA) synthetase, heme synthetase, and mitochon-drial serine protease activity. In addition, in a study employing the isoenzymes of glu-cose 6-phosphate dehydrogenase (G-6-PD) idiopathic refractory sideroblastic anemia was identified as a clonal disorder of the pluripotent hematopoietic stem cell. In patients with hereditary sideroblastic anemia, the response to pyridoxine may be incomplete when iron overload is present; in such patients phlebotomy may produce a further in-crease in the hematocrit. Sideroblastic anemia has been associated with erythropoietic porphyria as well, further implicating abnormal porphyrin metabolism as a cause of sideroblastic abnormalities. Although pyridoxine metabolism is disturbed by isoniazid, cycloserine, and ethanol, pyridoxine deficiency appears to have no role in the majority of patients with acquired sideroblastic anemia. Sideroblastic anemia can be a feature of the pre-leukemic syndrome and not uncommonly precedes the development of leukemia in patients treated with chemotherapy for another malignancy. However, 90 percent of patients with an acquired idiopathic refractory sideroblastic anemia do not develop leu-kemia. The small fraction who do can be identified by a more severe anemia, a lower reticulocyte count, a high transfusion requirement, and thrombocytopenia.

The course of sideroblastic anemia is related to its cause. Reversible causes should always be sought and the offending drug or toxin removed. However, pyridoxine replacement has been successful during the continued administration of isoniazid. Patients with increased iron stores should be phlebotomized if the hematocrit permits, to prevent hemochromatosis. In most patients, pyridoxine therapy produces little response or a suboptimal one, regardless of dose or route of administration. Folic acid is also usually without effect, even when megaloblastoid changes are present.

1. Jacobs, A. Primary acquired sideroblastic anaemia. *Br. J. Haematol.* 64:415, 1986.
   Brief review.
2. Cartwright, G. E., and Deiss, A. Sideroblasts, siderocytes, and sideroblastic anemia. *N. Engl. J. Med.* 292:185, 1975.
   Pathogenesis of sideroblasts reviewed.
3. Cazzola, M., Barosi, G., Gobbi, P. G., et al. Natural history of idiopathic refractory sideroblastic anemia. *Blood* 71:305, 1988.
   Transfusion dependence leads to iron overload; leukemia or marrow failure occurred in 27%.
4. Kushner, J. P., Lee, G. R., Wintrobe, M. M., et al. Idiopathic refractory sideroblastic anemia: Clinical and laboratory investigation of 17 patients and review of the literature. *Medicine* 50:139, 1971.
   Excellent study demonstrating a median survival of 10 years, with a 7% incidence of acute leukemia.
5. Pierce, H. I., McGuffin, R. G., and Hillman, R. S. Clinical studies in alcoholic sideroblastosis. *Arch. Intern. Med.* 136:283, 1976.
   Diet, alcohol, and folate all play a role in the development of sideroblasts.
6. Eichner, E. R., and Hillman, R. S. The evolution of anemia in alcoholic patients. *Am. J. Med.* 50:218, 1971.
   Sideroblastic changes follow closely the development of megaloblastic erythropoiesis.
7. Cullen, M. R., Robins, J. M., and Eskenazi, B. Adult inorganic lead intoxication: Presenation of 31 new cases and a review of recent advances in the literature. *Medicine* 62:221, 1983.
   Significant anemia is not encountered in adults.
8. Beritic, T. Siderotic granules and the granules of punctate basophilia. *Br. J. Haematol.* 9:185, 1963. *Siderotic granules differ from basophilic stippling in staining, morphology, and intracellular position.*
9. Weintraub, L. R., Conrad, M. E., and Crosby, W. H. Iron-loading anemia. *N. Engl. J. Med.* 275:169, 1966.
   Use of vitamin B_6 and phlebotomy to prevent excessive accumulation of iron.
10. Simon, M., Beaumont, C., Briere, J., et al. Is the HLA-linked haemochromatosis allele implicated in idiopathic refractory sideroblastic anaemia? *Br. J. Haematol.* 64:415, 1986.
    The hemochromatosis allele was not implicated.
11. Peto, T. E. A., Pippard, M. J., and Weatherall, D. J. Iron overload in mild sideroblastic anaemias. *Lancet* 1:375, 1983.
    Iron overload in the absence of transfusions.
12. Prchal, J. T., Throckmorton, D. W., Carroll, A. J., III, et al. A common progenitor for human myeloid and lymphoid cells. *Nature* 274:590, 1978.
    Idiopathic refractory sideroblastic anemia is a clonal disorder of the pluripotent hematopoietic stem cell.
13. Aoki, Y. Multiple enzymatic defects in mitochondria in hematological cells of patients with primary sideroblastic anemia. *J. Clin. Invest.* 66:43, 1980.
    Demonstration of mitochondrial enzyme defects in patients with various types of sideroblastic anemia.
14. McCurdy, P. R., and Donohoe, R. F. Pyridoxine responsive anemia conditioned by isonicotinic acid hydrazide. *Blood* 27:352, 1966.
    Isoniazid-induced sideroblastic anemia.
15. Khaleek, M., Keane, W. M., and Lee, G. R. Sideroblastic anemia in multiple myeloma. *Blood* 41:17, 1973.
    Appearance of anemia with ringed sideroblasts before development of acute leukemia.
16. Brown, G. O. Chronic erythromonocytic leukemia. *Am. J. Med.* 47:785, 1969.
    Sideroblastic anemia is not uncommon in the preleukemic syndrome.

17. Kitahara, M., Cosgriff, T. M., and Eyre, H. J. Sideroblastic anemia as a preleukemic event in patients treated for Hodgkin's disease. *Ann. Intern. Med.* 92:625, 1980.
    Another example of sideroblastic anemia as a leukemic marker.
18. Yoo, D., Schechter, G. P., Amigable, A. N., et al. Myeloproliferative syndrome with sideroblastic anemia and acquired hemoglobin H disease. *Cancer* 45:78, 1980.
    Sideroblastic anemia associated with an acquired hemoglobinopathy. Hemoglobin H may be a preleukemic marker. (See Arch. Intern. Med. 138:603, 1978.)
19. Cheng, D. S., Kushner, J. P., and Wintrobe, M. M. Idiopathic refractory sideroblastic anemia: Incidence and risk factors for leukemic transformation. *Cancer* 44:724, 1979.
    The overall incidence of leukemia was 10%; a low reticulocyte count, thrombocytopenia, and a high transfusion requirement are poor prognostic signs.
20. Lumeng, L., and Li, T. K. Vitamin B_6 metabolism in chronic alcohol abuse: Pyridoxal phosphate levels in plasma and the effects of acetaldehyde on pyridoxal phosphate synthesis and degradation in human erythrocytes. *J. Clin. Invest.* 53:693, 1974.
    Acetaldehyde-induced degradation of erythrocyte pyridoxine.
21. Chillar, R. K., Johnson, C. S., and Beutler, E. Erythrocyte pyridoxine kinase levels in patients with sideroblastic anemia. *N. Engl. J. Med.* 295:881, 1976.
    Pyridoxal phosphate formation is not defective in alcoholic and nonalcoholic sideroblastic anemia.
22. Barton, J. L., Conrad, M. E., and Parmley, R. T. Acute lymphoblastic leukemia in idiopathic refractory sideroblastic anemia. *Am. J. Hematol.* 9:109, 1980.
    Further evidence for the clonal origin of idiopathic refractory sideroblastic anemia. (See also Blood 70:1003, 1982.)
23. Hall, R., and Losowsky, M. S. The distribution of erythroblast iron in sideroblastic anaemias. *Br. J. Haematol.* 12:334, 1966.
    In acquired sideroblastic anemia, ringed sideroblasts occur at all stages of erythroblast maturation. This distribution is unusual in hereditary sideroblastic anemia.

109. SPLENOMEGALY
Jerry L. Spivak

The spleen is the major in-line filter of the circulation, processing approximately 5 percent of the blood volume per minute or over 300 liters of blood each day. Once an organ of mystery, the functions of the spleen are now well understood. In the embryo and under certain circumstances in the adult, the spleen serves as a site of hematopoiesis. It remodels reticulocytes, reducing their surface area and culling from them nuclear remnants (Howell-Jolly bodies), iron granules, and other debris. The ability of the spleen to perform this culling function is due to its unique anatomy and circulation, which causes the red cells to pass through narrow pores before reentering the circulation. Spherocytes or other types of rigid red cells are unable to pass easily through these pores and eventually are destroyed in the spleen. The spleen is the site of synthesis of immunoglobulins, proteins involved in the complement system, and tuftsin, a tetrapeptide involved in neutrophil phagocytosis. The spleen participates in the removal of immune complexes, microorganisms, and particulate antigens from the bloodstream. In the nonimmune state and in the absence of opsonins, the spleen is the principal organ responsible for removing encapsulated organisms from the bloodstream. Consequently, in the asplenic state, there is an increased risk of infection, particularly with pneumococci, *Haemophilus*, and meningococci. Furthermore, when bacterial infection does occur, it is frequently fulminant and associated with disseminated intravascular coagulation and a high mortality. In addition to loss of filtering capacity, removal of the spleen results in a reduction in plasma IgM levels for up to 4 years, a poor immune response to certain bacterial capsular antigens, impairment of the alternative pathway of complement, and a reduction in tuftsin.

The postsplenectomy state can be mimicked by a variety of conditions that cause hyposplenism. They include sickle cell anemia, inflammatory bowel disease, celiac disease, dermatitis herpetiformis, amyloidosis, disorders associated with the formation of immune complexes such as systemic lupus erythematosus (SLE), administration of corticosteroids, thorium dioxide (Thorotrast), and therapeutic irradiation. Depending on the degree of splenic hypofunction, patients with these disorders may be at risk of overwhelming sepsis.

Splenomegaly is an important sign of disease and can occur through a variety of mechanisms. Splenomegaly is a feature of acute infections such as infectious mononucleosis and of chronic infections such as subacute bacterial endocarditis. It occurs in patients with immune complex disorders such as SLE or Felty's syndrome; in infiltrative or granulomatous disorders such as sarcoidosis, Gaucher's disease, and amyloidosis; and when there is chronic destruction of red cells as in hereditary spherocytosis or autoimmune hemolytic anemia. Splenic enlargement also occurs as a consequence of extramedullary hematopoiesis in thalassemia major and in the myeloproliferative disorders, polycythemia vera, and idiopathic myelofibrosis. The spleen is usually involved in acute and chronic leukemias as well as Hodgkin's and non-Hodgkin's lymphomas. Hepatic cirrhosis with portal hypertension also produces splenomegaly.

Hypersplenism is a frequent complication of splenomegaly. In patients with portal hypertension or massive splenomegaly, there is increased pooling of circulating formed elements in the organ, although there may not be increased destruction of these cells. In patients with hairy-cell leukemia, the retention of the rigid neoplastic cells within the spleen results in trapping of normal formed elements. In disorders in which there is an increased destruction of cells, such as autoimmune hemolytic anemia or congenital hemolytic anemia, splenomegaly results from work hypertrophy and in the presence of another stimulus such as an acute infection, the degree of splenic sequestration and cell destruction may increase markedly.

Mild splenomegaly occurs in a variety of disorders while marked splenomegaly is a feature of relatively few illnesses. They include splenic lymphoma, idiopathic myelofibrosis, chronic myelogenous leukemia, Felty's syndrome, hairy-cell leukemia, sarcoidosis, Gaucher's disease, and parasitic infections.

The decision to perform a splenectomy is not one to be taken lightly. The spleen is a difficult organ to approach surgically, and hemorrhage, infection, and portal vein thrombosis are not infrequent complications. Massive spleens are particularly difficult to remove due to their size and the presence of adhesions. The indications for splenectomy include (1) hereditary spherocytosis in children; (2) autoimmune thrombocytopenia or autoimmune hemolytic anemia that cannot be controlled with corticosteroids; (3) to obtain tissue for diagnosis or staging; (4) to correct hypersplenism in disorders such as thalassemia, Gaucher's disease, Felty's syndrome, hairy-cell leukemia, splenic vein thrombosis, and hemodialysis splenomegaly; and (5) because of symptoms due to organomegaly. Postsplenectomy, there is usually a leukocytosis consisting of an increase in lymphocytes, monocytes, and granulocytes, which generally subsides with time. Thrombocytosis is also a feature of the postsplenectomy state but has not been demonstrated to cause any morbidity. The peripheral blood smear postsplenectomy is also striking for the presence of Howell-Jolly bodies in all patients as well as siderocytes and spur cells in approximately 25 percent of the patients.

In view of the increased incidence of infection postsplenectomy, and in particular the risk of overwhelming pneumococcal sepsis in which death can occur within 24 hours, patients undergoing splenectomy should receive pneumococcal vaccine. The vaccine alone cannot be considered a panacea since it only contains the antigens of 23 capsular types and is at best probably 80 percent effective. Therefore, in individuals who are at high risk of pneumococcal infection, namely school-age children or those associated with them, prophylactic penicillin therapy should also be employed. It is, of course, well to remember that these patients are at risk of infection with other bacteria as well. Since viral infections often predispose to bacterial infections, influenza vaccine should also be administered. There is no incompatibility or a reduction in antibody response when the vaccines are given simultaneously. It is also worth noting that patients with Hodgkin's disease who have been treated with chemotherapy or irradiation have an impaired antibody response to pneumococcal vaccine for approximately 3 years after treatment, while patients with sickle cell anemia have a variable response to the vaccine. The vaccine is also not without side effects, particularly acute febrile reactions. It is thought that a single vaccination usually produces protection for at least 3 years and in some instances longer.

1. Eichner, E. R. Splenic function: Normal, too much and too little. *Am. J. Med.* 66:311, 1979.
   An excellent review.
2. Eichner, E. R., and Whitfield, C. L. Splenomegaly: An algorithmic approach to diagnosis. *J.A.M.A.* 246:2858, 1981.
   A step-by-step, diagnostic approach.
3. Crosby, W. H. Splenic remodeling of red cell surfaces. *Blood* 50:643, 1977.
   Brief review.
4. McIntyre, O. R., and Ebaugh, F. G., Jr. Palpable spleens in college freshmen. *Ann. Intern. Med.* 66:301, 1967.
   A palpable spleen in a normal individual is unusual; substantial splenic enlargement can occur without palpable splenomegaly.
5. Chen, L. T. Microcirculation of the spleen: An open or closed circulation? *Science* 201:157, 1978.
   Both open and closed circulation exists in the spleen but the majority of blood flow occurs by the open circulation.
6. Pearson, H. A., Spencer, R. P., and Cornelius, E. A. Functional asplenia in sickle-cell anemia. *N. Engl. J. Med.* 281:923, 1969.
   Absence of splenic function in the presence of splenomegaly in S-S disease but not in S-C or S-β-thalassemia.
7. Neilan, B. A., and Perry, J. F., Jr. Persistence of vacuolated RBCs after splenectomy in adults. *J.A.M.A.* 243:1741, 1980.
   Adult spleens are not born again.
8. Dailey, M. O., Coleman, C. N., and Kaplan, H. S. Radiation-induced splenic atrophy in patients with Hodgkin's disease and non-Hodgkin's lymphomas. *N. Engl. J. Med.* 302:215, 1980.
   Splenic irradiation can predispose to overwhelming pneumococcal sepsis and disseminated intravascular coagulation.
9. Ryan, F. P., Smart, R. C., Holdsworth, C. D., et al. Hyposplenism in inflammatory bowel disease. *Gut* 19:50, 1978.
   Hyposplenism is common in ulcerative colitis but not in Crohn's disease.
10. Marsh, G. W., and Stewart, J. S. Splenic function in adult coeliac disease. *Br. J. Haematol.* 19:445, 1970.
    The degree of hypofunction varies but can be severe.
11. Hurd, W. W., and Katholi, R. E. Acquired functional asplenia: Association with spontaneous rupture of the spleen and fatal spontaneous rupture of the liver in amyloidosis. *Arch. Intern. Med.* 140:844, 1980.
    Amyloidosis causes hyposplenia.
12. Lockwood, C. M., Worlledge, S., Nicholas, A., et al. Reversal of impaired splenic function in patients with nephritis or vasculitis (or both) by plasma exchange. *N. Engl. J. Med.* 300:524, 1979.
    Splenic hypofunction can be produced by immune complexes but this is not always the case. (See Am. J. Med. 69:80, 1980.)
13. Jandl, J. H., Jacob, H. S., and Daland, G. A. Hypersplenism due to infection: A study of five cases manifesting hemolytic anemia. *N. Engl. J. Med.* 264:1063, 1961.
    Prolonged antigenic stimulation associated with infection led to hypersplenism.
14. Hess, C. E., Ayers, C. R., Sandusky, W. R., et al. Mechanism of dilutional anemia in massive splenomegaly. *Blood* 47:231, 1976.
    Portal hypertension with expansion of the portal vascular bed provokes salt and water retention and hemodilution.
15. Foghill, P. J., and Green, S. Splenic influences on the blood in chronic liver disease. *Q. J. Med.* 48:613, 1979.
    There was no consistent relationship between splenomegaly and hematologic abnormalities.

16. Dacie, J. V., Galton, D. A. G., Gordon-Smith, E. C., et al. Non-tropical idiopathic splenomegaly. *Br. J. Haematol.* 38:185, 1978.
    Most of these patients eventually develop a lymphoma.
17. Narang, S., Wolf, B. C., and Neiman, R. S. Malignant lymphoma presenting with prominent splenomegaly. *Cancer* 55:1948, 1985.
    A common presentation for intermediate cell lymphoma. (See also Arch. Pathol. Lab. Med. *109:1076, 1985.)*
18. Chun, C. H., Raff, M. J., Contreras, L., et al. Splenic abscess. *Medicine* 59:50, 1980.
    Infective endocarditis was the most common cause.
19. Schilling, R. F. Hereditary spherocytosis: A study of splenectomized persons. *Semin. Hematol.* 13:169, 1976.
    Serum IgM levels are reduced and spherocytosis persists.
20. Beahrs, J. R., and Stephens, D. H. Enlarged accessory spleens: CT appearance in postsplenectomy patients. *AJR* 135:483, 1980.
    Computed tomography scanning is useful in identifying accessory spleens.
21. Davis, H. H., II, Varki, A., Heaton, W. A., et al. Detection of accessory spleens with indium 111-labeled autologous platelets. *Am. J. Hematol.* 8:81, 1980.
    In this report, removal of accessory spleens did not alter the immune thrombocytopenia.
22. Appel, M. F., and Bart, J. B. The surgical and hematologic significance of accessory spleens. *Surg. Gynecol. Obstet.* 143:191, 1976.
    When the spleen is removed in childhood, a missed accessory spleen may subsequently become important.
23. Giuliano, A. E., and Lim, R. C., Jr. Is splenic salvage safe in the traumatized patient? *Arch. Surg.* 116:651, 1981.
    The spleen should be salvaged whenever possible.
24. Rice, H. M., and James, P. D. Ectopic splenic tissue failed to prevent fatal pneumococcal septicaemia after splenectomy for trauma. *Lancet* 1:565, 1980.
    Splenosis is not protective against sepsis.
25. Hosea, S. W., Brown, E. J., Hamburger, M. I., et al. Opsonic requirements for intravascular clearance after splenectomy. *N. Engl. J. Med.* 304:245, 1981.
    Clearance requires increased quantities of antibody following splenectomy.
26. Hosea, S. W., Burch, C. G., Brown, E. J., et al. Impaired immune response of splenectomised patients to polyvalent pneumococcal vaccine. *Lancet* 1:804, 1981.
    If possible, the vaccine should be administered before splenectomy.
27. Francke, E. L., and Neu, H. C. Postsplenectomy infection. *Surg. Clin. North Am.* 61:135, 1981.
    Comprehensive review.
28. Gopal, V., and Bisno, A. Z. Fulminant pneumococcal infections in normal asplenic hosts. *Arch. Intern. Med.* 137:1526, 1977.
    Comprehensive review. (See also Am. J. Hematol. *2:193, 1977.)*
29. Reed, W. P., Chick, T. W., Jutila, K., et al. Pulmonary leukostasis in fatal human pneumococcal bacteremia without pneumonia. *Am. Rev. Respir. Dis.* 130:1184, 1984.
    The ultimate consequence of the asplenic state.
30. Chaikof, E. L., and McCabe, C. J. Fatal overwhelming postsplenectomy infection. *Am. J. Surg.* 149:534, 1985.
    The incidence was 10 times higher in children than adults. (See also Q. J. Med. *63:523, 1987.)*
31. Minor, D. R., Schiffman, G., and McIntosh, L. S. Response of patients with Hodgkin's disease to pneumococcal vaccine. *Ann. Intern. Med.* 90:887, 1979.
    Complete protection with vaccination is not obtained if administered within 3 years of antitumor therapy. (See also N. Engl. J. Med. *299:442, 1978.)*
32. Gabor, E. P., and Seeman, M. Acute febrile systemic reaction to polyvalent pneumococcal vaccine. *J.A.M.A.* 242:2208, 1979.
    A probable Arthus reaction.
33. Linnemann, C. C., Jr., First, M. R., and Schiffman, G. Revaccination of renal transplant and hemodialysis recipients with pneumococcal vaccine. *Arch. Intern. Med.* 146:1554, 1986.
    Revaccination was achieved without significant side effects in these patients.

34. Kehoe, J. E., Daly, J. M., Straus, D. J., et al. Value of splenectomy in non-Hodgkin's lymphoma. *Cancer* 55:1256, 1985.
   A palliative procedure.
35. McBride, J. A., Dacie, J. V., and Shapley, R. The effect of splenectomy on the leukocyte count. *Br. J. Haematol.* 14:225, 1968.
   Lymphocytes, monocytes, and granulocytes are elevated.
36. Coon, W. W., Penner, J. Clagett, G. P., et al. Deep venous thrombosis and postsplenectomy thrombocytosis. *Arch. Surg.* 113:429, 1978.
   Thrombocytosis postsplenectomy does not lead to venous thrombosis. (See also Arch. Surg. *113:808, 1978.)*

110. THROMBOCYTOPENIA
Jerry L. Spivak

Thrombocytopenia can be due to decreased marrow platelet production, increased platelet utilization or destruction on either an immune or a nonimmune basis, or a combination of these. Decreased production may be due to marrow aplasia, infiltration with tumor or fibrosis, deficiency of vitamin B_{12} or folic acid, paroxysmal nocturnal hemoglobinuria, infection, drugs, or toxins (cytotoxic agents, irradiation, ethanol, thiazides, benzene). Increased platelet utilization or nonimmune destruction occurs in disseminated intravascular coagulation (DIC), thrombotic thrombocytopenic purpura, hypersplenic states, infection, and occasionally with heparin therapy.

Immune thrombocytopenia is most commonly due to drugs, particularly sulfonamides, oral hypoglycemic agents, gold, quinidine, quinine, digitoxin, and sedatives. In drug-induced immune thrombocytopenia the drug acts as a haptene, binding to a plasma protein and eliciting an antibody response. Antigen-antibody complexes form and attach to platelets, resulting in premature removal of the platelets from the circulation. IgG, IgA, and IgM globulins have all been implicated in such immunologic reactions. Drug antibodies have not been demonstrated, however, in all cases of drug-induced thrombocytopenia. Recent evidence suggests that in some instances this is because antibody is produced only against a metabolite of the drug and not against the drug itself. Immune thrombocytopenia also occurs during the course of many diseases, including systemic lupus erythematosus, rheumatoid arthritis, human immunodeficiency virus (HIV) infection, and lymphomas. Rarely, immune thrombocytopenia can occur from blood transfusion; and when more than 10 units of bank blood have been transfused, dilutional thrombocytopenia is often seen.

When no cause of the thrombocytopenia is evident, the condition has been called *idiopathic*. By definition, patients with idiopathic thrombocytopenic purpura (ITP) have no discernible underlying disease, no other disturbance of coagulation, no history of drug ingestion, abundant megakarocytes in the marrow, and no splenic enlargement. In general, most patients with ITP have been found to have an antibody directed against their platelets, sometimes against major membrane glycoproteins such as Ib and IIb/IIIa. Antibody-coated platelets are removed from the circulation by the spleen, which also participates in the process by producing the antiplatelet antibody. When antibody titers are high, platelets are also sequestered in the liver. Bleeding cannot, however, be attributed solely to thrombocytopenia since qualitative defects in platelet function (impaired aggregation) have also been demonstrated. The course of ITP may be acute, chronic, or recurrent. Acute ITP occurs most often in children, is frequently preceded by a viral illness, and usually remits spontaneously or with therapy within 6 months. Chronic ITP is usually seen in adults, rarely remits spontaneously, and may be refractory to both steroid therapy and splenectomy.

Evaluation of the patient with thrombocytopenia should include careful examination of red cell morphology on a peripheral blood smear, a prothrombin time, partial thromboplastin time and fibrin split products determination, bone marrow examination,

Coombs' test, and an antinuclear antibody assay. The patient must be carefully questioned concerning drug or toxin exposure, and the sites and extent of bleeding and the presence or absence of adenopathy or organomegaly determined on physical examination. Large friable oral submucosal hematomas are characteristic of thrombocytopenic bleeding although they are frequently misinterpreted as tumors or fungal infestations. An acute fall in the platelet count is usually accompanied by diffuse petechial hemorrhage; this is less common with thrombocytopenia of more gradual onset. Intracranial hemorrhage is the most feared event in the thrombocytopenic patient; it is usually heralded by the onset of mucous membrane bleeding.

Corticosteroids at a dose of 60 mg/day are the initial treatment of choice in patients with immune thrombocytopenia. Even if the platelet count does not initially respond, there is usually a reduction in bleeding or bruising. Platelet transfusions perhaps preceded by intravenous IgG (*Ann. Int. Med.* 104:808, 1986) should be reserved for serious and otherwise intractable hemorrhage. Splenectomy may be necessary on an emergency basis if steroid therapy is not effective in controlling hemorrhage. Otherwise, splenectomy is reserved on an elective basis for patients who are either unresponsive or require continuous corticosteroid therapy to maintain the platelet count at a hemostatic level. A response to corticosteroids should be evident within the first 2 weeks of therapy. Once a satisfactory platelet count is obtained, the corticosteroids can be tapered. It is important to emphasize the failure to achieve a complete remission is not an indication for splenectomy. A platelet count of 30,000 per microliter is hemostatic, and splenectomy has sufficient disadvantages that it should be avoided if possible. Splenectomy removes both a site of antibody formation and platelet sequestration. In some patients in whom neither steroids nor splenectomy has produced a satisfactory remission, immunosuppressive therapy has been tried with either cyclophosphamide, azathioprine, or vincristine. The response rate has not been very high. A short course of high-dose corticosteroids (dexamethasone 10 mg PO qid) has been effective in some patients as has high-dose intravenous gamma globulin, although the effect of the latter is usually transient. Other recently introduced therapies for this troublesome disorder include danazol, ascorbic acid, α interferon, colchicine, and cyclosporin. The broad array of disparate therapeutic agents employed reflects the difficulty encountered in treating immune thrombocytopenia. HIV-infected patients now represent an increasing component of the ITP population. These patients appear to respond to conventional therapy like HIV-negative patients. The role of zidovudine in the treatment of HIV-associated ITP is under investigation.

1. Thompson, C. B., and Jakubowski, J. A. The pathophysiology and clinical relevance of platelet heterogeneity. *Blood* 72:1, 1988.
   Heterogeneity of platelet size is not age-related, but younger platelets are more functionally active.
2. Berchtold, P., and McMillan, R. Therapy of chronic idiopathic thrombocytopenic purpura in adults. *Blood* 74:2309, 1989.
   State of the art review of all forms of therapy.
3. Moss, R. A. Drug-induced immune thrombocytopenia. *Am. J. Hematol.* 9:439, 1980.
   Brief review.
4. Court, W. S., Bozeman, J. M., Soong, S.-J., et al. Platelet surface-bound IgG in patients with immune and nonimmune thrombocytopenia. *Blood* 69:278, 1987.
   Use of platelet-associated IgG to differentiate immune from nonimmune thrombocytopenia. (See also Blood *60:1050, 1982.)*
5. Kaden, B. R., Rosse, W. F., and Houch, T. W. Immune thrombocytopenia in lymphoproliferative diseases. *Blood* 53:545, 1979.
   Immune thrombocytopenia is not uncommon in lymphoproliferative disorders, does not carry a poor prognosis, and should be treated like ITP.
6. Shashaty, G. G., and Rath, C. E. Idiopathic thrombocytopenic purpura in the elderly. *Am. J. Med. Sci.* 276:263, 1978.
   ITP is not uncommon in elderly individuals.
7. Kim, H. D., and Boggs, D. R. A syndrome resembling idiopathic thrombocytopenic purpura in 10 patients with diverse forms of cancer. *Am. J. Med.* 67:371, 1979.

ITP was thought to be related to the development of carcinoma in these patients. (See also Am. J. Med. Sci. *278:153, 1979.)*

8. Adrouny, A., Sandler, R. M., and Carmel, R. Variable presentation of thrombocytopenia in Graves' disease. *Arch. Intern. Med.* 142:1460, 1982.
   The mechanism for the thrombocytopenia varies. (See also Ann. Intern. Med. *94:27, 1981.)*

9. McMillan, R., Longmire, R. C., Tavassoli, M., et al. In vitro platelet phagocytosis by splenic leukocytes in idiopathic thrombocytopenic purpura. *N. Engl. J. Med.* 290:249, 1974.
   The spleen is a site of antiplatelet antibody production, platelet sequestration, and platelet phagocytosis.

10. Clancy, R., Jenkins, E., and Firkin, B. Qualitative platelet abnormalities in idiopathic thrombocytopenic purpura. *N. Engl. J. Med.* 286:622, 1972.
    Impaired aggregation with immunologically damaged platelets.

11. Onder, O., Weinstein, A., and Hoyer, L. W. Pseudothrombocytopenia caused by platelet agglutinins that are reactive in blood anticoagulated with chelating agents. *Blood* 56:177, 1980.
    EDTA-induced pseudothrombocytopenia can be caused by a variety of different antibodies.

12. Bell, W. R., and Royall, R. M. Heparin-associated thrombocytopenia: A comparison of three heparin preparations. *N. Engl. J. Med.* 303:902, 1980.
    The incidence of thrombocytopenia was highest with beef lung–derived heparin.

13. Sullivan, L. W., Adams, W. H., and Liu, Y. K. Induction of thrombocytopenia by thrombopheresis in man. *Blood* 49:197, 1977.
    Ethanol-induced thrombocytopenia is due to suppression of platelet production.

14. Neame, P. B., Kelton, J. G., Walker, I. R., et al. Thrombocytopenia in septicemia: The role of disseminated intravascular coagulation. *Blood* 56:88, 1980.
    DIC cannot always be implicated. (See also N. Engl. J. Med. *300:760, 1979.)*

15. Young, R. C., Nachman, R. L., and Horowitz, H. I. Thrombocytopenia due to digitoxin. *Am. J. Med.* 41:605, 1966.
    A well-studied case.

16. Belkin, G. A. Cocktail purpura. *Ann. Intern. Med.* 66:583, 1967.
    An unusual case of quinine-induced purpura. (See also Br. Med. J. *2:1551, 1979.)*

17. Eisner, E. V., and Shahidi, N. T. Immune thrombocytopenia due to a drug metabolite. *N. Engl. J. Med.* 287:376, 1972.
    Drug metabolite was implicated when drug was found to be immunogically inert.

18. Levin, H. A., McMillan, R., Tavassoli, M., et al. Thrombocytopenia associated with gold therapy. *Am. J. Med.* 59:274, 1975.
    Immune mechanism for thrombocytopenia demonstrated; only splenectomy was effective.

19. Deren, B., Masi, R., Weksler, M., et al. Gold-associated therombocytopenia. *Arch. Intern. Med.* 134:1012, 1974.
    Advocates the use of steroid therapy only. (For the use of dimercaprol (BAL) therapy see J.A.M.A. *195:782, 1966.)*

20. Kelton, J. G., Meltzer, D., Moore, J., et al. Drug-induced thrombocytopenia is associated with increased binding of IgG to platelets both in vivo and in vitro. *Blood* 58:524, 1981.
    Platelet-associated IgG is usually elevated in drug-induced thrombocytopenia. (See also Blood *72:1155, 1988.)*

21. Morse, E. E., Zinkham, W. H., and Jackson, D. P. Thrombocytopenic purpura following rubella infection in children and adults. *Arch. Intern. Med.* 117:573, 1966.
    Steroids did not shorten the clinical course.

22. Kelton, J. G. Vaccination-associated relapse of immune thrombocytopenia. *J.A.M.A.* 245:369, 1981.
    Relapses of ITP observed with administration of pneumococcal or influenza vaccine.

23. Kickler, T. S., Ness, P. M., Heaman, J. H., et al. Studies on the pathophysiology of posttransfusion purpura. *Blood* 68:347, 1986.
    Soluble transfused PL^{A1} antigen binds to PL^{A1}-negative platelets leading to antibody

recognition and destruction. For a brief review of this syndrome see Br. J. Haematol. 64:419, 1986, and for other involved antigens, see Blood 71:894, 1988 and Am. J. Hematol. 29:38, 1988.

24. Lau, P., Sholtis, C. M., and Aster, R. H. Post-transfusion purpura: An enigma of alloimmunization. *Am. J. Hematol.* 9:331, 1980.
    Plasma exchange was effective in this patient but has not been in others. (See Arch. Intern. Med. *138:998, 1978.)*

25. Stoll, D., Cines, D. B., Aster, R. H., et al. Platelet kinetics in patients with idiopathic thrombocytopenic purpura and moderate thrombocytopenia. *Blood* 65:584, 1985.
    Platelet production may not be increased in ITP. (See also Blood *67:86, 1986.)*

26. Kelton, J. G., Blanchette, V., Wilson, W. E., et al. Neonatal thrombocytopenia due to passive immunization. *N. Engl. J. Med.* 302:1401, 1980.
    Simultaneous measurement of platelet-associated IgG and serum anti-platelet IgG employed to distinguish between alloimmune and passive autoimmune neonatal thrombocytopenia.

27. Aster, R. H. Pooling of platelets in the spleen: Role in the pathogenesis of "hypersplenic" thrombocytopenia. *J. Clin. Invest.* 45:645, 1966.
    Normally up to 30% of the blood platelets are pooled in the spleen.

28. Pizzuto, J., and Ambriz, R. Therapeutic experience on 934 adults with idiopathic thrombocytopenic purpura: Multicentric trial of the cooperative Latin American group on hemostasis and thrombosis. *Blood* 64:1179, 1984.
    See also Q. J. Med. *58:153, 1986.*

29. Thompson, R. L., Moore, R. A., Hess, L. E., et al. Idiopathic thrombocytopenic purpura. *Arch. Intern. Med.* 130:730, 1972.
    A good response to steroids usually indicates a good response to splenectomy.

30. Bellucci, S., Charpak, Y., Chastang, C., et al. Low doses vs conventional doses of corticoids in immune thrombocytopenic purpura (ITP): Results of a randomized clinical trial in 160 children, 223 adults. *Blood* 71:1165, 1988.
    In this study, 0.25 mg/kg of prednisone was as effective as 1.0 mg/kg in adults.

31. Bussell, J. B., Pham, L. C., Aledort, L., et al. Maintenance treatment of adults with chronic refractory immune thrombocytopenic purpura using repeated intravenous infusion of gamma globulin. *Blood* 72:121, 1988.
    Therapy to complete or partial remission in some adult patients with ITP. This form of therapy is also effective in HIV-infected patients (see Am. J. Hematol. *28:79, 1988 and* Br. J. Haematol. *68:303, 1988).*

32. Branda, R. F., Tate, D. Y., McCullough, J. J., et al. Plasma exchange in the treatment of fulminant idiopathic (autoimmune) thrombocytopenic purpura. *Lancet* 1:688, 1978.
    Success is not always the rule with plasma exchange in ITP. (See Arch. Intern. Med. *140:1101, 1980.) When successful, it is possible that immune complexes are responsible for the thrombocytopenia. (*Br. J. Haematol. *44:645, 1980).*

33. Fehr, J., Hofmann, V., and Kappeler, U. Transient reversal of thrombocytopenia in idiopathic thrombocytopenic purpura by high-dose intravenous gamma globulin. *N. Engl. J. Med.* 306:1254, 1982.
    Rapid but transient reversal of thrombocytopenia was achieved.

34. Ratner, L. Human immunodeficiency virus–associated autoimmune thrombocytopenic purpura: a review. *Am. J. Med.* 86:194, 1989.
    Immune thrombocytopenia is a common complication of HIV infection. (See also Ann. Intern. Med. *109:190, 1988.)*

35. Hoffman, R., Bruno, E., Elwell, J., et al. Acquired amegakaryocytic thrombocytopenic purpura: A syndrome of diverse etiologies. *Blood* 60:1173, 1982.
    A rare etiology for thrombocytopenia. (See also Q. J. Med. *263:243, 1989.)*

36. Oksenbendler, E., Bierling, P., Ferchal, F., et al. Zidovudine for thrombocytopenic purpura related to human immunodeficiency virus (HIV) infection. *Ann. Intern. Med.* 110:365, 1989.
    Zidovudine caused an increase in the platelet count. (See also J.A.M.A. *260:3045, 1988 and* Ann. Intern. Med. *109:718, 1988.)*

37. West, S. G., and Johnson, S. C. Danazol for the treatment of refractory autoimmune thrombocytopenia in systemic lupus erythematosus. *Ann. Intern. Med.* 108:703, 1988.

Danazol has also been used in ITP not due to systemic lupus erythematosus (SLE) (N. Engl. J. Med. *308:1396, 1983) but the results are less impressive (see also* Arch. Intern. Med. *145:2251, 1985).*

38. Coon, W. W. Splenectomy for cytopenias associated with systemic lupus erythematosus. Am. J. Surg. 155:391, 1988.
    Splenectomy for ITP is not always successful in SLE.
39. Burrows, R. F., and Kelton, J. G. Incidentally detected thrombocytopenia in healthy mothers and their infants. N. Engl. J. Med. 319:142, 1988.
    Mild thrombocytopenia is common but clinically not harmful. (See also Am. J. Hematol. *21:397, 1986 and* Am. J. Obstet. Gynecol. *157:109, 1987.)*
40. Averbuch, M., Koifman, B., and Levo, Y. Lupus anticoagulant, thrombosis and thrombocytopenia in systemic lupus erythematosus. Am. J. Med. Sci. 293:2, 1987.
    Association of the lupus anticoagulant and thrombocytopenia. (See also Arch. Intern. Med. *146:2153, 1986.)*
41. Manoharan, A. Slow infusion of vincristine in the treatment of idiopathic thrombocytopenic purpura. Am. J. Hematol. 21:135, 1986.
    An alternate approach to vinicristine administration.
42. Morris, L., Distenfeld, A., Amorosi, E., et al. Autoimmune thrombocytopenic purpura in homosexual men. Ann. Intern. Med. 96:714, 1982.
    Another disturbance of immunity in homosexual individuals.
43. Kelton, J. G., McDonald, J. W. D., Barr, R. M., et al. The reversible binding of vinblastine to platelets: Implications for therapy. Blood 57:431, 1981.
    Vinblastine elutes rapidly from platelets and thus vinblastine-loaded platelets may not achieve the effect desired.
44. Carr, J. M., Kruskall, M. S., Kaye, J. A., et al. Efficacy of platelet transfusions in immune thrombocytopenia. Am. J. Med. 80:1051, 1986.
    Effectiveness of platelet transfusions in ITP confirmed.
45. Salama, A., Kiefel, V., and Mueller-Eckhardt, C. Effect of IgG anti-Rho(D) in adult patients with chronic autoimmune thrombocytopenia. Am. J. Hematol. 22:241, 1986.
    Another therapeutic approach to ITP.
46. Picozzi, V. J., Roeshe, W. R., and Creger, W. P. Fate of therapy failures in adult idiopathic thrombocytopenia purpura. Am. J. Med. 69:690, 1980.
    Spontaneous recovery observed in patients with ITP who had failed all forms of therapy.
47. Howard, J. E., and Perkins, H. A. The natural history of alloimmunization to platelets. Transfusion 18:496, 1978.
    Cytotoxic antibodies form in approximately 70% of patients receiving random-donor platelet transfusions.
48. Daly, P. A., Schiffer, C. A., Aisner, J., et al. Platelet transfusion therapy: One-hour posttransfusion increments are valuable in predicting the need for HLA-matched preparations. J.A.M.A. 243:435, 1980.
    The 1-hour posttransfusion platelet increment correlates well with the presence of alloimmunization.
49. Edelson, R. N., Chernik, N. L., and Posner, J. B. Spinal subdural hematomas complicating lumbar puncture. Arch. Neurol. 31:134, 1974.
    In the thrombocytopenic patient, lumbar puncture should be done with a small needle and if the platelet count is less than 20,000, platelets should be administered.
50. Bartholomew, J. R., Salgia, R., and Bell, W. R. Control of bleeding in patients with immune and nonimmune thrombocytopenia with aminocaproic acid. Arch. Intern. Med. 149:1959, 1989.
    See also J.A.M.A. *243:35, 1980.*
51. Gernsheimer, T, Stratton, J., Ballem, P. J., et al. Mechanisms of response to treatment in autoimmune thrombocytopenic purpura. N. Engl. J. Med. 320:974, 1989.
    Prednisone increases platelet production: splenectomy when effective prolongs platelet survival.
52. Proctor, S. J., Jackson, G., Carey, P., et al. Improvement of platelet counts in steroid-unresponsive idiopathic immune thrombocytopenic purpura after short-course therapy with recombinant α2b interferon. Blood 74:1894, 1989.
    Another form of therapy for the refractory patient.

111. THROMBOCYTOSIS
Jerry L. Spivak

The platelet count may be elevated in a variety of conditions. Transient elevations occur following exercise, acute blood loss, or administration of epinephrine. The rise is due in part to release of platelets from the spleen, but other platelet pools are also involved since exercise-induced thrombocytosis can occur in asplenic persons. Splenectomy results in an elevation in platelet count beginning within 2 weeks of surgery and lasting approximately 3 months. Persistent elevation of the platelet count following splenectomy for hemolytic anemia is usually associated with the persistence of the anemia, but the mechanism for the thrombocytosis is undefined. Thrombocytosis occurring with iron-deficiency anemia can be reversed with iron replacement.

A sustained increase in platelet number may occur with acute or chronic infections or inflammatory processes. The latter include rheumatoid arthritis, celiac disease, ulcerative colitis, regional enteritis, and sarcoidosis. Fluctuations in the platelet count correlate with the activity of the underlying disease. Thrombocytosis is commonly seen with malignancies. Occasionally the elevation in platelet count precedes the discovery of the neoplastic process. Transient thrombocytosis occurs during the recovery from thrombocytopenia. It may occur following replacement of vitamin B_{12} or folic acid, withdrawal from alcohol or other toxins, and correction of immune thrombocytopenia by splenectomy.

Thrombocytosis is also a feature of the myeloproliferative disorders polycythemia vera (PV), idiopathic myelofibrosis (IMF), chronic myelogenous leukemia (CML), and essential thrombocytosis (ET). All of these are clonal disorders of pluripotent hematopoietic stem cells which differ in their clinical course. PV, IMF, and ET have considerable overlap and may be interrelated illnesses, while CML is a distinctly different disorder with a unique chromosomal abnormality. Since there is no clinically available clonal marker for PV, IMF, and ET, the diagnosis of ET is usually assumed upon exclusion of the former disorders on clinical grounds and exclusion of CML by cytogenetic analysis of the marrow. This test is extremely important and should be performed on all patients with ET since a small proportion of these patients express the Ph[1] chromosome abnormality characteristic of CML and the other clinical features of CML will eventually evolve, including blast crisis. In patients with ET who lack the Ph[1] chromosome, a chronic indolent course can be expected. The leukocyte alkaline phosphatase is not a useful discriminant between ET and CML presenting with thrombocytosis alone.

In the myeloproliferative disorders, large and bizarre platelet forms and circulating megakaryocyte fragments are frequently seen, but electron microscopic studies have not revealed striking ultrastructural abnormalities. Coagulation studies, including determination of bleeding time and clot retraction, are usually normal. Platelet aggregation in response to epinephrine and adenosine diphosphate (ADP) is impaired, but aggregation on exposure to collagen is not. Hemorrhagic phenomena appear to correlate best with platelet size, which can be evaluated simply by observing the thickness of the buffy coat if the white count is not elevated. Spurious hyperkalemia is an interesting benign complication of thrombocytosis. It occurs in vitro as a result of release of potassium from platelets during clotting. The phenomenon becomes evident only when there is an increase in total platelet mass; it is not a result of an increased platelet potassium concentration. No clinical evidence of hyperkalemia is found.

In most instances, thrombocytosis is a benign phenomenon but thrombotic episodes have been reported, particularly when the platelet count exceeds 1 million per microliter. Our experience is that both bleeding and thrombosis are uncommon; bleeding is usually associated with the use of anti-inflammatory drugs and thrombosis occurs most often in the presence of an elevated red cell mass or in elderly individuals, particularly those with a history of vascular disease. A number of articles have stressed the association of thrombocytosis with abnormalities within the arterial circulation, leading to either neurologic symptoms or digital ischemia. In some reports, thrombotic events were associated with platelet hyperaggregability. In others, no abnormality in platelet function could be detected nor was there a clear correlation between the height of the platelet count and thrombotic events. Given the age of most of the patients, the possibility of other causes for peripheral vascular or cerebrovascular disease is highly likely in some, while others may have had erythromelalgia, a disorder of unknown etiology characterized by increased temperature, erythema, and burning pain of the extremities without an apparent deficit in the arterial circulation. In view of the lack of any controlled studies of the relationship of the platelet count to peripheral or cerebrovascular disease and, indeed, a lack of any direct correlation between the height of the platelet count and the presence of thrombotic events, it is difficult to give credence to reports of treatment based on the platelet count alone, particularly since such treatment may be more hazardous than the thrombocytosis itself. This is not to claim that thrombocytosis is not in certain circumstances associated with vasoocclusive events or migrainelike syndromes but rather that reflex therapy based on a platelet count alone is totally inappropriate. In patients with PV and thrombocytosis, it has been clearly demonstrated that it is the red cell mass, not the platelet count, which is the major determinant of thrombotic events and that antiplatelet agents can be very harmful in these patients. Patients with ET are sensitive to salicylates which can provoke bleeding and their routine use cannot be condoned. Acute leukemia has complicated ET treated with alkylating agents, and when it is deemed necessary to reduce the platelet count hydroxyurea is the agent of choice, although even it is not without risk in this regard.

1. Levin, J., and Conley, C. L. Thrombocytosis associated with malignant disease. *Arch. Intern. Med.* 114:497, 1964.
   A common association.
2. Davis, W. M., and Mendez Ross, A. O. Thrombocytosis and thrombocytopenia. *Am. J. Clin. Pathol.* 59:243, 1973.
   Malignancy, myeloproliferative disorders, splenectomy, iron deficiency, and inflammatory disease account for most cases of thrombocytosis.
3. Stoll, D. B., Peterson, P., Exten, R., et al. Clinical presentation and natural history of patients with essential thrombocytopenia and the Philadelphia chromosome. *Am. J. Hematol.* 27:77, 1988.
   Cytogenetic analysis should be performed in all patients with ET.
4. Iland, H. J., Laszlo, J., Case, Jr., D. C., et al. Differentiation between essential thrombocythemia and polycythemia vera with marked thrombocytosis. *Am. J. Hematol.* 25:191, 1987.
   Clinical features of ET reviewed. (See also Cancer *61:1207, 2487, 1988.)*
5. Ginsburg, A. D. Platelet function in patients with high platelet counts. *Ann. Intern. Med.* 82:506, 1975.
   Defective platelet aggregation is common in the myeloproliferative disorders.
6. Kaywin, P., McDonough, M., Insel, P. A., et al. Platelet function in essential thrombocythemia. *N. Engl. J. Med.* 299:505, 1978.
   A deficiency of alpha-adrenergic receptors was demonstrated but no clinical abnormality of blood coagulation was present.
7. Buss, D. H., Stuart, J. J., and Lipscomb, G. E. The incidence of thrombotic and hemorrhagic disorders in association with extreme thrombocytosis: An analysis of 129 cases. *Am. J. Hematol.* 20:365, 1985.
   Bleeding was more common with ET than in reactive thrombocytosis but the incidence of thrombosis was the same and infrequent.
8. Schloesser, L. C., Kipp, M. A., and Wenzel, F. J. Thrombocytosis in iron deficiency anemia. *J. Lab. Clin. Med.* 66:107, 1965.
   Thrombocytosis reduced with iron therapy.
9. Knizley, H., and Noyes, W. D. Iron deficiency, anemia, papilledema, thrombocytosis and transient hemiparesis. *Arch. Intern. Med.* 129:483, 1972.
   An interesting case report.
10. Morowitz, A. D., Allen, L. W., and Kirsner, J. B. Thrombocytosis in chronic inflammatory bowel disease. *Ann. Intern. Med.* 68:1013, 1968.
    Elevation of platelet count with disease activity.
11. Hirsh, J., and Dave, J. V. Persistent postsplenectomy thrombocytosis and throm-

boembolism: A consequence of continuing anaemia. *Br. J. Haematol.* 12:44, 1966.
The height of the platelet count after splenectomy is related to the level of the hematocrit.

12. Hartman, R. C., Auditore, J. V., and Jackson, D. P. Studies on thrombocytosis: 1. Hyperkalemia due to release of potassium from platelets during coagulation. *J. Clin. Invest.* 37:699, 1958.
Spurious hyperkalemia resulting from an increase in platelet mass. (See also Am. J. Kidney Dis. *12:116, 1988.*

13. Kessler, C. M., and Klein, H. G. Untreated thrombocythemia in chronic myeloproliferative disorders. *Br. J. Haematol.* 50:157, 1982.
Bleeding was usually associated with the use of aspirin; thrombosis was rare.

14. Pearson, T. C., and Wetherly-Mein, G. Vascular occlusive episodes and venous haematocrit in primary proliferative polycythaemia. *Lancet* 2:1219, 1978.
There was a high correlation of thrombosis with elevations in the hematocrit but no correlation between the platelet count and thrombotic episodes.

15. Hoagland, H. C., and Silverstein, M. N. Primary thrombocythemia in the young patient. *Mayo Clin. Proc.* 53:578, 1978.
Thrombocytosis was unassociated with bleeding or thrombosis in this group of patients.

16. Kurzrock, R., and Cohen, P. R. Erythromelalgia and myeloproliferative disorders. *Arch. Intern. Med.* 149:105, 1989.
An uncommon syndrome which responds to low-dose acetylsalicylic acid or hydroxyurea.

17. Welford, C., Spies, S. M., and Green, D. Priapism in primary thrombocythemia. *Arch. Intern. Med.* 141:807, 1981.
An unusual complication that responded to thrombectomy.

18. Preston, F. E., Martin, J. F., Steward, R. M., et al. Thrombocytosis, circulating platelet aggregates, and neurological dysfunction. *Br. Med. J.* 2:1561, 1979.
A cause-and-effect relationship has not been established.

19. Barbui, T., Buelli, M., Cortelazzo, S., et al. Aspirin and risk of bleeding in patients with thrombocythemia. *Am. J. Med.* 83:265, 1987.
Salicylates increase the bleeding time more in patients with ET.

20. Coon, W. W., Penner, J., Clagett, G. P., et al. Deep venous thrombosis and postsplenectomy thrombocytosis. *Arch. Surg.* 113:429, 1978.
Thrombocytosis is not associated with venous thrombosis.

21. Boxer, M. A., Braun, J., Ellman, L. Thromboembolic risk of post-splenectomy thrombocytosis. *Arch. Surg.* 113:808, 1978.
There was no correlation in this study between the platelet count and venous thrombosis.

22. Taft, E. G., Babcock, R. B., Scharfman, W. B., et al. Plateletpheresis in the management of thrombocytosis. *Blood* 50:927, 1977.
Use of thrombocytopheresis for acute relief of vascular obstruction due to thrombocytosis.

23. Goldfinger, D., Thompson, R., Lowe, C., et al. Long-term plateletpheresis in the management of primary thrombocytosis. *Transfusion* 19:336, 1979.
Chronic thrombocytopheresis is an inefficient method for reducing the platelet count.

24. Kaplan, K. L., and Owen, J. Plasma levels of β-thromboglobulin and platelet factor 4 as indices of platelet activation in vivo. *Blood* 57:199, 1981.
Beta thromboglobulin can be used as a measure of in vivo platelet activation.

25. Kempczinski, R. F. Lower-extremely arterial emboli from ulcerating atherosclerotic plaques. *J.A.M.A.* 241:807, 1979.
An important cause of distal vascular insufficiency.

26. Fialkow, P. J., Faquet, G. B., Jacobson, R. J., et al. Evidence that essential thrombocythemia is a clonal disorder with origin in a multipotent stem cell. *Blood* 58:916, 1981.
Clonal origin of essential thrombocythemia established.

27. Murphy, S., Davis, J. L., Walsh, P. N., et al. Template bleeding time and clinical hemorrhage in myeloproliferative disease. *Arch. Intern. Med.* 138:1251, 1978.

There was no correlation between bleeding time, platelet aggregation, or clinical hemorrhage.
28. Sedlacek, S. M., Curtis, J. L., Weintraub, J., et al. Essential thrombocythemia and leukemic transformation. *Medicine* 65:353, 1986.
Evidence that phosphorus 32 or alkylating agents can increase the risk of leukemia in ET patients. Treatment of asymptomatic ET is unjustified until well-controlled studies prove otherwise.
29. Hehlmann, R., Jahn, M., Baumann, B., et al. Essential thrombocythemia. *Cancer* 61:2487, 1988.
Life expectancy was not compromised in this series.
30. Schafer, A. I. Bleeding and thrombosis in the myeloproliferative disorders. *Blood* 64:1, 1984.
Excellence advice concerning the therapy for thrombocytosis.

112. THROMBOTIC THROMBOCYTOPENIC PURPURA
Jerry L. Spivak

Thrombotic thrombocytopenic purpura (TTP) is a syndrome characterized by thrombocytopenia, purpura, hemolytic anemia, neurologic signs, fever, renal dysfunction, and widespread hyaline occlusions of terminal arterioles and capillaries. TTP is uncommon but not rare. Both sexes are affected, but the syndrome occurs predominantly in women in the reproductive age. Initial symptoms are usually nonspecific and include headache, weakness, vomiting, and fever; purpura, seizures, an acute organic brain syndrome, hemorrhage, or jaundice are more likely to bring the patient to the doctor. Due to the diffuse distribution of the vascular lesions and the population involved, the internist is often not the first physician consulted. The disease may occur during pregnancy, and vaginal bleeding as an initial manifestation is not uncommon. Abdominal pain is a frequent complaint and some patients undergo surgery before the diagnosis is made. Occasionally retrospective evaluation of tissue obtained at the time of laparotomy has revealed arteriolar and capillary lesions that were initially overlooked. Although TTP is usually a progressive illness, the disease process can fluctuate; coma may remit and carefully elicited neurologic abnormalities may be undemonstrable a few minutes later. High fever, coma, or generalized seizures are ominous features and usually indicate the terminal phase of the illness.

The diagnosis of TTP will never be overlooked if a peripheral blood smear is always examined as part of the physical examination. Marked red cell fragmentation and distortion are present, as is a reduction in platelet number. If the hemolytic process is severe, the indirect bilirubin level is elevated, but the Coombs' test is negative. Leukocytosis is often present, but it is rarely due to infection. Unless there is bleeding into the subarachnoid space, the cerebrospinal fluid is normal. Although thrombocytopenia is present, fibrinogen and the other coagulation factors are usually normal, which has been taken as evidence against disseminated intravascular coagulation (DIC). However, elevated levels of fibrin split products have been found in patients with TTP, indicating that DIC does occur and contributes to the bleeding diathesis. Normal levels of the various coagulation factors are only a reflection of the fact that consumption of these factors has not exceeded synthetic capacity. The hyaline arteriolar occlusions found in TTP appear to result from the process of DIC and are not specific for the syndrome. They may be found in other situations in which DIC occurs. Thus, the clinical and laboratory findings of TTP are nonspecific, and the diagnosis is made by exclusion of other diseases that may damage vessel walls or produce DIC or thrombocytopenia. These include idiopathic thrombocytopenic purpura (ITP), Evans's syndrome, systemic lupus erythematosus, infectious mononucleosis, periarteritis nodosa, eclampsia, posttransfusion purpura, disseminated carcinomatosis, nonbacterial thrombotic endocarditis, sepsis with

DIC, and reactions to drugs and toxins. Since the vascular lesion of TTP is nonspecific, there is no justification for invoking a special relationship between TTP and other diseases in which a similar lesion is seen, as has been done with systemic lupus erythematosus and TTP.

The cause of TTP is unknown. Occurrences of the disorder in siblings suggest a genetic predisposition while a report of TTP developing in a husband and a wife suggests an infectious etiology. The contention that a rickettsial agent might be involved has not been substantiated. Drugs, particularly penicillin and its derivatives, have been implicated in the pathogenesis of TTP. Elevated platelet-associated IgG, vascular deposition of complement, and circulating immune complexes have also been described, suggesting that in some instances the disease may have an immunologic basis. Since the vascular lesion associated with TTP is not specific for the disorder, it is not unlikely that a variety of factors—toxic, immune, infectious, and genetic—may be involved.

Until recently, the prognosis of patients with TTP was grim with a mortality of greater than 90 percent. With the application of plasma exchange and plasma infusion, in addition to corticosteroid therapy and splenectomy, survival rates of greater than 50 percent have been reported. Due to the tendency of the disorder to fluctuate in severity and the occurrence of spontaneous remissions, as well as the uncontrolled retrospective nature of most reports and the simultaneous use of multiple therapeutic approaches, it is unclear at present what constitutes the most effective form of therapy for TTP. Analysis of the problem is, of course, complicated by the possibility that the disorder may have multiple etiologies, each of which responds differently to a particular type of therapy. In some patients with TTP, a factor that aggregates platelets and is inhibited by normal plasma has been observed. These observations fit in well with the beneficial effect of exchange transfusion. The possibility that plasma prostacyclin (PGI_2) deficiency might be responsible for the manifestations of TTP has been evaluated. Low PGI_2 levels and accelerated degradation of plasma PGI_2 have been observed but infusion of PGI_2 has not reversed the clinical manifestations of the disorder. Furthermore, in some patients exchange transfusion is beneficial while plasma infusion alone is not. In others, plasmapheresis alone without plasma replacement has been effective suggesting the possibility that immune complexes are involved in these instances. In other patients, including some of our own, plasmapheresis without plasma replacement has not been an effective form of therapy. Splenectomy appears to be effective in some patients but it is noteworthy that the disease has been observed in splenectomized individuals. Most recently, vincristine has been observed to have a beneficial effect with a high response rate but the number of patients reported is too small for any definitive conclusions to be made.

At the present time, it appears reasonable to treat patients with TTP with a layered approach. In the patient without severe neurologic manifestations, corticosteroid therapy, at doses greater than 100 mg/day, seems reasonable. In the presence of significant neurologic abnormalities, such as coma or seizures, or if steroid therapy alone has not been effective, plasma exchange and replacement with fresh-frozen plasma should be initiated. Serum LDH should be monitored to determine the adequacy of the plasma exchange procedure while the reticulocyte count, platelet count, and clinical status as well as the degree of red cell fragmentation will provide evidence of disease response. If a beneficial effect is not obtained, antiplatelet agents should be employed with splenectomy reserved for those patients who fail to respond to the previous measures. Treatment of TTP in pregnancy is no different from that in the nonpregnant individual. The fetus is not generally affected and there is no evidence that removal of the products of conception will ameliorate the illness. Until the pathophysiology of TTP is understood, controversies over the most effective method of treatment are likely to continue.

1. Ridolfi, R. L., and Bell, W. R. Thrombotic thrombocytopenic purpura. Report of 25 cases and review of the literature. *Medicine* 60:413, 1981.
   A comprehensive review.
2. Weiner, C. P. Thrombotic microangiopathy in pregnancy and the postpartum period. *Semin. Hematol.* 24:119, 1987.

The distinction between TTP and preeclampsia can be difficult. For the hemolysis, elevated liver enzymes, and low platelet count (HELLP) syndrome, see Am. J. Obstet. Gynecol. *142:159, 1982.*

3. Umlas, J., and Kaiser, J. Thrombohemolytic thrombocytopenic purpura: A disease or syndrome? *Am. J. Med.* 49:723, 1970.
   Lesions of TTP are not specific and can be seen with DIC due to other causes.
4. Berkowitz, L. R., Dalldorf, F. G., and Blatt, P. M. Thrombotic thrombocytopenic purpura. *J.A.M.A.* 241:1709, 1979.
   The pancreas was the most severely affected organ in this series.
5. Goodman, A., Ramos, R., Petrelli, M., et al. Gingival biopsy in thrombotic thrombocytopenic purpura. *Ann. Intern. Med.* 89:501, 1978.
   Only 39% of biopsies in this series were positive. The skin appears to be a better site. (See also Semin. Thromb. Hemost. *5:184, 1979.)*
6. Ridolfi, R. L., Hutchins, G. M., and Bell, W. R. The heart and cardiac conduction system in thrombotic thrombocytopenic purpura. *Ann. Intern. Med.* 91:357, 1979.
   The heart is a target organ in this disease with only the pancreas and adrenal showing more involvement.
7. Mitch, W. E., Spivak, J. L., Spangler, D. B., and Bell, W. R. Thrombotic thrombocytopenic purpura presenting with gynecologic manifestations. *Lancet* 1:849, 1973.
   DIC occurs in TTP.
8. Jaffe, E. A., Nachman, R. C., and Merskey, C. Thrombotic thrombocytopenic purpura: Coagulation parameters in twelve patients. *Blood* 42:499, 1973.
   Intravascular coagulation thought to be a secondary complication due to the hemolytic process.
9. Clinicopathologic Conference. Lupus erythematosus with severe anemia, selective erythroid hypoplasia and multiple red blood cell isoantibodies. *Am. J. Med.* 44:590, 1968.
   A case of lupus erythematosus associated with the lesions of TTP. TTP has also been observed in Sjögren's syndrome. (See J.A.M.A. *215:757, 1971.)*
10. Watson, C. G., and Cooper, W. M. Thrombotic thrombocytopenic purpura: Concomitant occurrence in husband and wife. *J.A.M.A.* 215:1821, 1971.
    A toxic or infectious cause is suggested.
11. Wallace, D. C., Lovric, A., Clubb, J. S., et al. Thrombotic thrombocytopenic purpura in four siblings. *Am. J. Med.* 58:724, 1975.
    An interaction of genetic and environmental factors may be operative in these patients.
12. Hellman, R. M., Jackson, D. V., and Bass, D. H. Thrombotic thrombocytopenic purpura and hemolytic-uremic syndrome in HLA-identical siblings. *Ann. Intern. Med.* 93:283, 1980.
    Both TTP and hemolytic-uremic syndrome (HUS) appear to be variants of a common disease process.
13. Ponticelli, C., Rivolta, E., Imbasciati, E., et al. Hemolytic uremic syndrome in adults. *Arch. Intern. Med.* 140:353, 1980.
    Recovery does occur.
14. Ahmed, F., Sumalnop, V., Spain, D. M., et al. Thrombohemolytic thrombocytopenic purpura during penicillamine therapy. *Arch. Intern. Med.* 138:1292, 1978.
    Penicillin and its derivatives have been implicated in TTP.
15. Morrison, J., and McMillan, R. Elevated platelet-associated IgG in thrombotic thrombocytopenic purpura. *J.A.M.A.* 238:1944, 1977.
    Elevation of platelet IgG may explain the beneficial effect of splenectomy in some patients.
16. Bayer, A. S., Theofilopoulos, A. N., Eisenberg, R., et al. Thrombotic thrombocytopenic purpura–like syndrome associated with infective endocarditis: A possible immune complex disorder. *J.A.M.A.* 237:408, 1977.
    Immune complexes implicated in the pathogenesis of TTP. (See also Am. J. Clin. Pathol. *67:61, 1977.)*
17. Upshaw, J. D., Jr. Congenital deficiency of a factor in normal plasma that reverses microangiopathic hemolysis and thrombocytopenia. *N. Engl. J. Med.* 298:1350, 1978.

Evidence for a missing plasma factor in a TTP-like syndrome. (See also N. Engl. J. Med. *307:1432, 1982.)*

18. Kitchens, C. S. Studies of a patient with recurring thrombotic thrombocytopenic purpura. *Am. J. Hematol.* 13:259, 1982.
    A fascinating case history. (See also Am. J. Hematol. *17:307, 1984.)*

19. Moake, J. L., Rudy, C. K., Troll, J. H., et al. Unusually large plasma factor VIII:von Willebrand factor multimers in chronic relapsing thrombotic thrombocytopenic purpura. *N. Engl. J. Med.* 307:1432, 1982.
    This is a different syndrome than TTP and probably related to the case cited in reference 18.

20. Shepard, K. V., and Buhouski, R. M. The treatment of thrombotic thrombocytopenic purpura with exchange transfusions, plasma infusions, and plasma exchange. *Semin. Hematol.* 24:178, 1987.
    Plasma exchange is favored.

21. Lichtin, A. E., Schreiber, A. D., Hurwitz, S., et al. Efficacy of intensive plasmapheresis in thrombotic thrombocytopenic purpura. *Arch. Intern. Med.* 147:2122, 1987.
    Early and intensive plasma exchange advocated.

22. Taft, E. G. Thrombotic thrombocytopenic purpura and dose of plasma exchange. *Blood* 54:842, 1979.
    Serum lactic dehydrogenase level correlates with adequacy of plasma exchange and disease severity and provides a guide to the frequency and volume of exchange required.

23. Flaum, M. A., Cuneo, R. A., Appelbaum, F. R., et al. The hemostatic imbalance of plasma-exchange transfusion. *Blood* 54:694, 1979.
    If adequate coagulation factor replacement is not provided, a hemostatic deficit is produced.

24. Walker, B. K., Ballas, S. K., and Martinez, J. Plasma infusion for thrombotic thrombocytopenic purpura during pregnancy. *Arch. Intern. Med.* 140:981, 1980.
    Splenectomy was required to achieve a remission in this patient.

25. Cuttner, J. Thrombotic thrombocytopenic purpura: A ten year experience. *Blood* 56:302, 1980.
    Excellent results achieved with splenectomy, high-dose corticosteroids, and dextran. (For other reports on splenectomy see Am. J. Med. Sci. *277:75, 1979 and* Ann. Surg. *202:318, 1985.)*

26. Zacharski, L. R., Lusted, D., and Glick, J. C. Thrombotic thrombocytopenic purpura in a previously splenectomized patient. *Am. J. Med.* 60:1061, 1976.
    TTP developing after splenectomy for ITP. It may also recur after splenectomy. (See also Br. Med. J. *2:317, 1975.)*

27. Finn, N. G., Wang, J. C., and Hong, K. J. High-dose intravenous γ-immunoglobulin infusion in the treatment of thrombotic thrombocytopenic purpura. *Arch. Intern. Med.* 147:2165, 1987.
    *Based on experimental data (*J. Clin. Invest. *73:548, 1984) this should be effective, but it is still unproved.*

28. Liu, E. T., Linker, C. A., and Shuman, M. A. Management of treatment failures in thrombotic thrombocytopenic purpura. *Am. J. Hematol.* 23:347, 1986.
    Since spontaneous remissions occur, it is difficult to prove what treatment was effective.

29. Brain, M. C., Dacie, J. V., and Hourihane, D. O. B. Microangiopathic haemolytic anaemia: The possible role of vascular lesions in pathogenesis. *Br. J. Haematol.* 8:358, 1962.
    A characteristic blood picture is produced by diseases that affect small vessels.

30. Murgo, A. J. Thrombotic microangiopathies in the cancer patients including those induced by chemotherapeutic agents. *Semin. Hematol.* 24:161, 1987.
    Therapy with agents such as mitomycin C or cyclosporin can produce a syndrome like HUS. (See also Cancer *48:1738 and 2583, 1981, and 55:47, 1985.)*

31. Harkness, D. R., Byrnes, J. J., Lian, E. C.-Y., et al. Hazard of platelet transfusion in thrombotic thrombocytopenic purpura. *J.A.M.A.* 246:1931, 1981.
    Platelet transfusions have no role in the management of TTP.

32. Rosove, M. H., Ho, W. G., and Goldfinger, D. Ineffectiveness of aspirin and dipyridamole in the treatment of thrombotic thrombocytopenic purpura. *Ann. Intern. Med.* 96:27, 1980.
A high incidence of hemorrhagic events was observed.

113. VITAMIN B$_{12}$ DEFICIENCY
Jerry L. Spivak

Man is totally dependent on exogenous sources for the vitamin B$_{12}$ required for metabolic processes. Deficiency of vitamin B$_{12}$ can thus occur with diets devoid of animal protein or from intestinal malabsorption. In addition, an imbalance between supply and demand, as may occur during pregnancy, can produce manifestations of the deficiency state. Lack of vitamin B$_{12}$ results in morphologic and functional changes in epithelial, hematopoietic, and nervous tissue. Except for advanced nervous system changes, all the abnormalities caused by vitamin B$_{12}$ deficiency in the adult can be corrected by microgram quantities of the vitamin administered parenterally. Unfortunately, in spite of the ease with which the deficiency state can be reversed, recognition of vitamin B$_{12}$ lack is too often missed or delayed, resulting in unnecessary morbidity and occasionally death.

The three most common causes of vitamin B$_{12}$ deficiency are gastric and ileal resection and pernicious anemia. Every patient undergoing total gastrectomy and a small percentage of those undergoing partial gastrectomy, particularly for gastric ulcer, develop vitamin B$_{12}$ deficiency in the absence of replacement therapy. If a sufficient length of ileum is resected, vitamin B$_{12}$ deficiency also occurs. The time interval between surgery and the onset of vitamin B$_{12}$ deficiency varies, depending on body stores of the vitamin. Loss of vitamin B$_{12}$ occurs through its excretion in the bile, if the normal absorptive mechanisms are impaired. Pernicious anemia is a syndrome of vitamin B$_{12}$ lack due to the genetically determined development of gastric atrophy with loss of intrinsic factor secretion. The clinical stereotype, an irascible elderly patient with white hair, blue eyes, large ear lobes, and a lemon-tinted skin, represents only the manifestations of the disease in one racial group. It is important to remember that the disease occurs commonly in blacks, and particularly in black females below age 45.

The presenting signs and symptoms of vitamin B$_{12}$ deficiency are nonspecific. Of note, however, is the occurrence of pernicious anemia in females with vitiligo. A decrease in blood pressure in a hypertensive patient may also be a specific clue. Personality changes reversible with vitamin B$_{12}$ therapy occur, but rarely if ever is dementia an early manifestation of the deficiency state. Usually the earliest neurologic signs are paresthesias in the extremities, followed by clumsiness, weakness, and ataxia. Pseudotumor cerebri has been described as a presenting manifestation. Pernicious anemia has been associated with diabetes mellitus, Hashimoto's disease, hypothyroidism, hyperthyroidism, Addison's disease, and hypoparathyroidism. Thus vitamin B$_{12}$ deficiency should be considered when these endocrine disorders are complicated by anemia. Although most patients with classic pernicious anemia are elderly, the disease may present much earlier in patients with adult-onset immunoglobulin deficiency.

The profound changes that occur in red blood cell morphology as a result of vitamin B$_{12}$ lack provide a simple means for recognizing the deficiency state. Unfortunately, errors in interpretation of the peripheral blood smear are too common. Although hypersegmented neutrophils and macroovalocytes (in distinction to the flat macrocyte of liver disease) are characteristic of megaloblastic maturation (due to either vitamin B$_{12}$ or folic acid deficiency), it is important to recognize that there is a hemolytic component to the anemia as well due to the rigidity of the vitamin-deficient red cells. Consequently, red cells of all sizes and shapes are present. It is this *pleomorphic appearance* of the blood smear, with microcytes, fragmented cells, and teardrop forms, as well as macroovalocytes, Howell-Jolly bodies, and hypersegmented neutrophils, that is often misleading but should be diagnostic. Since there is usually a leukoerythroblastic reaction when the hematocrit falls below 30 percent, megaloblastic nucleated red blood cells can also be found in the peripheral blood.

A bone marrow aspirate should be done to confirm the clinical impression. Usually, even in the presence of peripheral pancytopenia, the hypercellular marrow virtually flows out of the needle. A "dry" tap should therefore suggest another diagnosis, such as a hematologic malignancy, which can be confirmed with a bone marrow biopsy. Iron deficiency prevents the expression of megaloblastic maturation, and uremia results in erythroid hypoplasia, but otherwise the characteristic nuclear cytoplasmic asynchrony is seen and giant metamyelocytes and hypersegmented neutrophils will provide a marker for the vitamin deficiency in both conditions. In this regard, it should be noted that blood transfusions do not alter marrow morphology although they may suppress the erythropoietin-mediated erythroid hyperplasia. Establishment of the presence of megaloblastic hematopoiesis does not, however, define its cause nor are serum vitamin B_{12} or red cell folate levels always helpful in this regard. Red cell folate may be falsely low in vitamin B_{12} deficiency while serum vitamin B_{12} levels are falsely low in approximately 50 percent of patients with folic acid deficiency and will rise with folic acid replacement. Falsely low serum vitamin B_{12} levels are also encountered with transcobalamin I deficiency, following administration of certain diagnostic radioisotopes (technetium Tc 99m and gallium citrate 67) or inhalation of nitrous oxide, and occasionally as a consequence of the vitamin assay itself. Falsely normal or high serum vitamin B_{12} levels can occur due to recent parenteral administration of the vitamin, in chronic myelogenous leukemia, with transcobalamin II deficiency, and as an artifact of the vitamin assay. Because of these possibilities for error and because a low value for serum vitamin B_{12} does not establish its cause, a Schilling test should always be performed to determine whether there is malabsorption of the vitamin. Prior therapy with vitamin B_{12} does not interfere with the Schilling test. Achlorhydria and antiparietal cell antibodies are a feature of adult pernicious anemia but are not specific for that disorder and cannot be used as diagnostic tests. Antibodies to intrinsic factor are specific for pernicious anemia but approximately 40 percent of patients with the disorder lack these antibodies.

The patient with profound vitamin B_{12} deficiency needs prompt therapy without the delay required for diagnostic testing. Since the hematologic abnormalities of vitamin B_{12} and folic acid deficiencies are the same, both vitamins should be given. Combination therapy with both vitamins is harmless. It is only when folic acid is given alone that correction of the anemia, followed by progression of neurologic abnormalities, will occur. In this regard, it should be noted that continued therapy with folic acid in a patient with vitamin B_{12} deficiency eventually results in a hypoplastic marrow and hematologic relapse.

1. Carmel, R. Pernicious anemia. *Arch. Intern. Med.* 148:1712, 1988.
   The article emphasizes that the classic laboratory abnormalities may be absent. (See also Arch. Intern. Med. *146:1161, 1986 and* Ann. Intern. Med. *63:951, 1965.)*
2. Carmel, R. Macrocytosis, mild anemia, and delay in the diagnosis of pernicious anemia. *Arch. Intern. Med.* 139:47, 1979.
   Macrocytosis is probably the earliest sign of vitamin B_{12} deficiency. (See also J.A.M.A. *245:1144, 1981.)*
3. Carmel, R. The laboratory diagnosis of megaloblastic anemias. *West. J. Med.* 128:294, 1978.
   An important review of pitfalls and problems.
4. Cooper, B. A., Fehedy, V., and Blanshay, P. Recognition of deficiency of vitamin B_{12} using measurement of serum concentration. *J. Lab. Clin. Med.* 107:447, 1986.
   The reliability of the assay is best at high levels of vitamin B_{12}. (See also Arch. Pathol. Lab. Med. *108:277, 1984.)*
5. Carmel, R. Artifactual radioassay results due to serum contamination by intravenous radioisotope administration: Falsely low serum vitamin B_{12} and folic acid results. *Am. J. Clin. Pathol.* 70:364, 1977.
   Technetium 99m and gallium 67 can interfere with the serum assays for vitamin B_{12} and folic acid.

6. Hitzhusen, J. C., Taplin, M. E., Stephenson, W. P., et al. Vitamin B$_{12}$ levels and age. *Am. J. Clin. Pathol.* 85:32, 1986.
   Vitamin B$_{12}$ levels do not decline with age. For normal differences, see Am. J. Clin. Pathol. *88:195, 1987.*

7. Fairbanks, V. F., Wahner, H. W., and Phyliky, R. L. Tests for pernicious anemia: the "Schilling test." *Mayo Clin. Proc.* 58:541, 1983.
   Only the two-stage test is reliable.

8. Carmel, R., and Johnson, C. S. Racial patterns in pernicious anemia. *N. Engl. J. Med.* 298:647, 1978.
   Black females manifest pernicious anemia at a younger age than white women and also have a much higher incidence of circulating antibody to intrinsic factor. (See also Arch. Intern. Med. *138:388, 1978.)*

9. Chanarin, I., O'Hea, A.-M., Malkowska, V., et al. Megaloblastic anaemia in a vegetarian Hindu community. *Lancet* 2:1168, 1985.
   Some were nutritionally deficient; others had pernicious anemia.

10. Howitz, J., and Schwartz, M. Vitiligo, achlorhydria, and pernicious anemia. *Lancet* 1:1331, 1971.
    Women with vitiligo have an increased incidence of pernicious anemia.

11. Twomey, J. J., Jordan, P. H., Jarrold, T., et al. The syndrome of immunoglobulin deficiency and pernicious anemia. *Am. J. Med.* 47:340, 1969.
    High incidence of pernicious anemia in adult-onset hypogammaglobulinemia.

12. Hughes, W. S., Brooks, F. P., and Conn, H. O. Serum gastrin levels in primary hypogammaglobulinemia and pernicious anemia. *Ann. Intern. Med.* 77:746, 1972.
    A normal gastrin level with pernicious anemia suggests hypogammaglobulinemia.

13. Strickland, R. G. Pernicious anemia and polyendocrine deficiency. *Ann. Intern. Med.* 70:1001, 1969.
    Association of deficiency states characterized by organ-specific antibodies.

14. Lindenbaum, J., Pezzimenti, J. F., Shea, N., et al. Small-intestinal function in vitamin B$_{12}$ deficiency. *Ann. Intern. Med.* 80:326, 1974.
    A significant but reversible impairment of intestinal absorption occurs with vitamin B$_{12}$ deficiency.

15. Schilling, R. F. The role of the pancreas in vitamin B$_{12}$ absorption. *Am. J. Hematol.* 14:197, 1983.
    Brief review.

16. Lindenbaum, J. Aspects of vitamin B$_{12}$ and folate metabolism in malabsorption syndromes. *Am. J. Med.* 67:1037, 1979.
    Detailed review.

17. Hall, C. A. The transport of vitamin B$_{12}$ from food to use within the cells. *J. Lab. Clin. Med.* 94:811, 1979.
    Brief review.

18. Jacob, E., Baker, S. J., and Herbert, V. Vitamin B$_{12}$-binding proteins. *Physiol. Rev.* 60:918, 1980.
    Comprehensive review.

19. Carmel, R. Nutritional vitamin B$_{12}$ deficiency. *Ann. Intern. Med.* 88:647, 1978.
    Food vitamin B$_{12}$ malabsorption suggested as a cause for overt vitamin B$_{12}$ deficiency in vegans. (See also Ann. Intern. Med. *94:57, 1981.)*

20. Marcoullis, G., Parmentier, Y., Nicolas, J.-P., et al. Cobalamin malabsorption due to nondegradation of R proteins in the human intestine. *J. Clin. Invest.* 66:430, 1980.
    Due to impaired secretion of proteolytic enzymes in chronic pancreatitis, the R protein–vitamin B$_{12}$ complex is not degraded, preventing the formation of intrinsic factor–vitamin B$_{12}$ complexes. (See also J. Clin. Invest. *61:47, 1978.)*

21. Katz, M., Lee, S. K., and Cooper, B. A. Vitamin B$_{12}$ malabsorption due to a biologically inert intrinsic factor. *N. Engl. J. Med.* 287:425, 1972.
    Abnormal intrinsic factor capable of binding to vitamin B$_{12}$ but not to ileal receptors.

22. Hakami, N., Neiman, P. E., Canellos, G. P., et al. Neonatal megaloblastic anemia due to inherited transcobalamin II deficiency in two siblings. *N. Engl. J. Med.* 285:1163, 1971.
    The consequences of transcobalamin II deficiency are impaired absorption and utilization of vitamin B$_{12}$. (See also N. Engl. J. Med. *303:1209, 1980.)*

23. Amess, J. A. L., Burman, J. F., Rees, G. M., et al. Megaloblastic haemopoiesis in patients receiving nitrous oxide. *Lancet* 2:339, 1978.
    Nitrous oxide appears to interfere with vitamin B_{12}. (See also Lancet 2:613, 1978.)
24. Victor, M., and Lear, A. A. Subacute combined degeneration of the spinal cord. *Am. J. Med.* 20:896, 1956.
    Problems in the diagnosis of a treatable condition.
25. Johnson, G. E. Reversible orthostatic hypotension of pernicious anemia. *J.A.M.A.* 257:1084, 1987.
    As a corollary, spontaneous remission of hypertension should suggest pernicious anemia.
26. Shorvon, S. D., Carney, M. W. P., Chanarin, I., et al. The neuropsychiatry of megaloblastic anaemia. *Br. Med. J.* 281:1036, 1980.
    Differences between vitamin B_{12} and folic acid deficiency reviewed.
27. Murphy, F., Srivastava, P. C., Varodi, S., et al. Screening of psychiatric patients for hypovitaminosis B_{12}. *Br. Med. J.* 3:559, 1969.
    A low-yield procedure.
28. Lee, C. A., and Fielding, J. Combined dietary vitamin-B_{12} deficiency and beta-thalassemia trait. *Lancet* 2:127, 1975.
    Initially the mean corpuscular volume is normal; with vitamin B_{12} replacement it becomes microcytic.
29. Will, J. J., Mueller, J. F., Brodine, C., et al. Folic acid and vitamin B_{12} in pernicious anemia. *J. Lab. Clin. Med.* 53:22, 1959.
    Therapy with folic acid in pernicious anemia eventually results in a hypoplastic marrow and subacute combined degeneration.
30. Hillman, R. S., Adamson, J., and Burka, E. Characteristics of vitamin B_{12} correction of the abnormal erythropoiesis of pernicious anemia. *Blood* 31:419, 1968.
    Megaloblasts do not change to normoblasts with vitamin B_{12} therapy.
31. Mason, J. D., and Leavell, B. S. The effect of transfusions of erythrocytes on untreated pernicious anemia. *Blood* 11:632, 1956.
    Transfusions do not convert a megaloblastic marrow to normoblastic maturation.
32. Jeffries, G. H., Todd, J. E., and Sleisenger, M. H. The effect of prednisolone on gastric mucosal histology, gastric secretion, and vitamin B_{12} absorption in patients with pernicious anemia. *J. Clin. Invest.* 45:803, 1966.
    Correction with steroids of the gastric mucosal lesion and gastric secretory function.
33. Scott, J. M., Wilson, P., Dinn, J. J., et al. Pathogenesis of subacute combined degeneration: a result of methyl group deficiency. *Lancet* 2:334, 1981.
    An interesting hypothesis.
34. Scott, J. M., and Weir, D. G. The methyl folate trap. *Lancet* 2:337, 1981.
    The most acceptable explanation for the adverse effects of folic acid on vitamin B_{12} deficiency. (See also Blood 66:479, 1985.)
35. Hesp, R., Chanarin, I., and Tait, C. E. Potassium changes in megaloblastic anaemia. *Clin. Sci. Mol. Med.* 49:77, 1975.
    Significant changes in serum potassium with treatment were not observed.
36. de Aizpurua, H. J., Ungar, B., and Toh, B.-H. Autoantibody to the gastrin receptor in pernicious anemia. *N. Engl. J. Med.* 313:479, 1985.
    Another immunologic abnormality in pernicious anemia.
37. Carmel, R., and Spencer, C. A. Clinical and subclinical thyroid disorders associated with pernicious anemia. *Arch. Intern. Med.* 142:1465, 1982.
    Both hypo- and hyperthyroidism can occur.
38. Matchar, D. B., Feussner, J. R., Millington, D. S., et al. Isotope-dilution assay for urinary methylmalonic acid in the diagnosis of vitamin B_{12} deficiency. *Ann. Intern. Med.* 106:707, 1987.
    If available, this would be the most specific assay for vitamin B_{12} deficiency.
39. Lindenbaum, J., Healton, E. B., Savage, D. G., et al. Neuropsychiatric disorders caused by cobalamin deficiency in the absence of anemia or macrocytosis. *N. Engl. J. Med.* 318:1720, 1988.
    Whether this is a rare or common event remains to be established. For a perspective on the problem, see the accompanying editorial on page 1752.

VII. INFECTIOUS DISEASES

114. ACQUIRED IMMUNODEFICIENCY SYNDROME (AIDS)

Steven M. Holland
Thomas C. Quinn

The acquired immunodeficiency syndrome (AIDS) is an immunologic disorder caused by the human immunodeficiency virus (HIV). The clinical spectrum of HIV infection includes an initial acute nonspecific viral infection followed by a prolonged asymptomatic, but infectious, stage which may be associated with immunologic abnormalities such as immune thrombocytopenic purpura, anemia, or lymphadenopathy. After a mean incubation of 8 to 10 years, and with further immunologic impairment, about 50 percent of infected individuals develop AIDS, characterized by disseminated opportunistic infections and neoplasms. It is currently estimated that there are 1 million Americans infected with HIV and that by 1992 there will be 365,000 cases of AIDS in the United States with over 200,000 deaths. Worldwide an estimated 10 million people are infected with HIV. One million people will develop AIDS in 140 countries over the next 2 years.

HIV is a human retrovirus of the lentivirus family. The virus is composed of an mRNA and protein core surrounded by a cell-derived lipid membrane. The viral envelope protein gp120 binds to the CD4 molecule, a marker found in abundance on T4 (helper) lymphocytes and to a lesser extent on monocytes/macrophages. Viral infection of cells occurs through binding of virus at the CD4 receptor, fusion with the cell membrane, uncoating of the viral RNA in the cytoplasm, and reverse transcription of viral RNA into DNA. Virally encoded DNA can exist in integrated or unintegrated forms and characteristically remains clinically dormant for years. In addition to the basic retroviral group antigen (*gag*), envelope (*env*), and polymerase (*pol*) genes, HIV has unique genetic elements. These include a transactivator (*tat*) gene which increases viral transcription, a negative regulatory factor (*nef*) gene which downregulates viral transcription, a regulator of viral expression (*rev*) gene which allows structural gene expression, and a viral infectivity factor (*vif*) gene which enhances cell-free virus infectivity. Another virus, HIV-2, causing a similar clinical syndrome and sharing about 60 percent genetic homology with HIV, has been found in West Africa.

The clinical occurrence of an opportunistic infection correlates directly with a decreasing number of CD4+ (T4+ or helper T) lymphocytes. The precise mechanisms of T4 depletion are unclear, but possibilities include direct viral killing, cell-cell fusion and death, autoimmune destruction, stem cell dysfunction, or the effect of circulating toxins. HIV also depresses T cell and B cell responsiveness to specific antigens, inhibits monocyte/macrophage chemotaxis, phagocytosis, and intracellular killing, and causes hypergammaglobulinemia. Although virus can be found in the CNS, gut, heart, lung, eye, and cervix, the specific cells harboring HIV in these tissues are debated.

Detection of HIV infection is mainly by serologic analysis. An enzyme-linked immunosorbent assay (ELISA) for detection of antibody to HIV uses disrupted infected cells applied to plastic plates to detect antibody to viral components. In the general population, this test has high sensitivity but poor specificity. Therefore, a more specific test used to confirm seroreactivity is the Western blot, which uses separated viral antigens bound to a membrane to detect specific antiviral antibody. The Western blot is considered negative only if no bands are present. Bands against the *gag, env,* and *pol* products are required for a positive blot. Western blots with some but not all of the above bands are considered indeterminate and should be repeated in 3 to 4 months. ELISA tests using recombinant viral antigens should allow for greater specificity. A recently developed ELISA test for viral core antigen p24 can detect viral antigen in the blood and CSF before the emergence of antibody early in disease and after the waning of antibody late in disease. Culture of the virus is possible from blood and CSF. DNA and RNA–based detection systems are able to demonstrate virus in situ and in clinical samples. With use of the polymerase chain reaction, a DNA amplification technique, the HIV genome has been demonstrated in peripheral blood lymphocytes months before the emergence of antibody or antigen.

The modes of transmission are sexual, parenteral, and perinatal. Between 20 and 50 percent of homosexual men studied have been HIV antibody–positive. Practices that cause rectal trauma such as receptive anal intercourse and douching carry a high risk of HIV infection. Heterosexual transmission is the major mode of spread in Africa and the most rapidly increasing mode of spread in the United States. Factors enhancing heterosexual spread include genital ulceration, lack of male circumcision, and sexually transmitted diseases which disrupt genital mucosal integrity. In sex partners of hemophiliacs, 10 to 25 percent are seropositive, and transmission of HIV correlates inversely with T4 cell counts. In contrast, about 50 percent of the sex partners of infected intravenous drug users (IVDU) are seropositive. Among prostitutes in the United States, infection correlates with the use of intravenous drugs; in African prostitutes, infection correlates with genital ulceration and clients from Central Africa.

Parenteral transmission from blood and blood product infusions has been reduced markedly following the introduction of blood screening for HIV in March 1985. Because of the long latency of the disease, however, many cases of AIDS due to transfusion between 1979 and 1985 will continue to evolve. Between 15 and 90 percent of hemophiliacs who received replacement factors during that interval are infected, depending on the severity of their disease and the number of treatments. IVDU accounts for 17 percent of reported cases nationally, but in some cities IVDU-related AIDS is more frequent than homosexually transmitted AIDS.

About 40 to 50 percent of babies born to infected mothers may become infected with HIV. Perinatal transmission occurs both in utero and post partum from exposure during labor and occasionally by breast-feeding. Diagnosis of infection in the newborn is complicated by the presence of transplacentally acquired maternal IgG. IgM detection, culture, or nucleic acid detection must be used during the period of maternal antibody persistence. Alternatively, after 6 to 9 months maternal antibody is lost and endogenous IgG antibody can be measured.

Occupational exposure has led to infection infrequently. Less than 1 percent of needle sticks from seropositive patients has led to seroconversion. This contrasts with the 20 to 30 percent seroconversion rate following hepatitis B needle sticks. Laboratory workers who handled concentrated virus and health care workers who were exposed to infected blood through skin abrasions and mucous membranes have become infected. Despite isolation of virus from saliva and tears, there have been no cases of household or casual spread.

Primary HIV infection is usually unrecognized, but it can present as a mononucleosis-like syndrome with atypical lymphocytosis, aseptic meningitis, encephalitis, or rash. During this period, p24 antigen and viral culture may be positive while standard antibody tests remain negative. Following acute infection, seroconversion usually occurs within 3 to 6 months. Adults may remain entirely asymptomatic for an average of 8 years (range 2–15 years). Children under 5 years old become symptomatic more rapidly. The factors that cause progression to full-blown AIDS may include T cell activation by intercurrent infections. Stimulation of HIV-bearing T cells causes increased viral transcription in vitro. A progressive decline in the number of T4 cells below 200 per microliter is a poor prognostic sign that precedes the development of opportunistic infections (OI). More than 50 percent of patients die within 1 year and 80 percent within 2 years of the diagnosis of AIDS. Those surviving more than 2 years have been homosexual men with Kaposi's sarcoma.

The diagnosis of AIDS is usually made by the detection of specific OI or neoplasms. A prodrome of fever, nonproductive cough, and dyspnea is a common presentation of *Pneumocytis carinii* pneumonia (PCP), the most frequent OI seen in AIDS patients. The chest x-ray usually shows diffuse interstitial infiltrates but may be normal. This is the most common AIDS-defining illness in this country, occurring in 60 percent of patients. A further 25 percent will develop PCP later in the course of their disease. Diagnosis is made by demonstration of organisms in pulmonary secretions or tissue. Sputum induction, when performed and interpreted in an experienced center, is up to 79 percent sensitive. If sputum is negative or unavailable, bronchoalveolar lavage, which has a sensitivity greater than 95 percent, should be performed. High-dose intravenous trimethoprim-sulfamethoxasole or pentamidine is severely limited by adverse drug reactions. Duration of therapy is usually 3 weeks. Short-course corticosteroids show some benefits for patients with severe pulmonary disease. Mortality per episode of PCP is between 20 and 40 percent. In view of the high relapse and mortality rates, prophylactic regimens of trimethoprim-sulfamethoxasole, dapsone, and aerosolized pentamidine are under study.

Other treatable pulmonary pathogens include *Mycobacterium tuberculosis,* cytomegalovirus (CMV), encapsulated bacteria (*Streptococcus pneumoniae, Haemophilus influenzae*), *Cryptococcus neoformans, Histoplasma capsulatum, Coccidioides immitis,* and *Strongyloides stercoralis. Mycobacterium avium-intracellulare* is frequently recovered from pulmonary specimens, but its specific role in disease is unclear. There is no consensus on therapy for this organism in AIDS patients. Kaposi's sarcoma can cause pulmonary infiltration or effusion. It is difficult to diagnose as it requires biopsy, and treatment to date has been disappointing.

Dysphagia or odynophagia suggest esophageal candidiasis, especially when accompanied by oral thrush. Definitive diagnosis requires endoscopy with biopsy showing mucosal invasion by *Candida.* Treatment consists of intravenous amphotericin for severe cases or oral ketoconazole for milder ones. Long-term prophylaxis with an oral antifungal agent is usually required.

Fever, headache, or altered mental status, alone or together, suggest cryptococcal meningitis. This infection occurs in about 9 percent of AIDS patients. Neuroradiologic imaging is usually normal. CSF may be inflammatory or normal, but often shows numerous cryptococci on India Ink preparation. Cryptococcal antigen is almost always present but may be in great excess, giving a prozone phenomenon and false-negative results. Intravenous amphotericin for 4 to 6 weeks with or without flucytosine (5-FC) is the treatment of choice. Without maintenance therapy recurrence is about 50 percent. Many centers currently use weekly intravenous amphotericin prophylaxis for life but new oral azole antifungals such as fluconazole are promising.

Encephalitis due to *Toxoplasma gondii* occurs in about 30 percent of AIDS patients with antibody to *Toxoplasma.* Although fever, headache, and altered mentation may suggest cryptococcal infection, the presence of focal neurologic defects, seizures, or coma strongly suggests toxoplasmosis. Definitive diagnosis requires brain biopsy, but presumptive diagnosis and therapy are made by the finding of multiple, bilateral, hypodense lesions on contrast head computed tomography (CT). Magnetic resonance imaging (MRI) is more sensitive in nonfocal presentations. The presence of a single intracranial lesion is suspicious for lymphoma, abscess, or Kaposi's sarcoma, while nonenhancing hypodense lesions on CT suggest progressive multifocal leukoencephalopathy, a dementing illness caused by a papovavirus. Steroid administration is determined by the extent of cerebral edema. Treatment of toxoplasmic encephalitis consists of pyrimethamine and sulfadiazine for several months. Therapy is complicated by cytopenias and rashes which may force discontinuation. Alternative regimens, often including clindamycin, are unproved. Relapse is quite common with toxoplasmic encephalitis, and therefore lifelong maintenance therapy is desirable.

Persistent oral, genital, or perianal ulceration is often due to herpes simplex infections. When present for more than 1 month, this constitutes an AIDS-defining illness. Diagnosis is confirmed by Tzanck smear, biopsy, or culture. Treatment consists of acyclovir orally or intravenously. As with many infections in AIDS, long-term therapy is often required. Herpes zoster occurs at a higher rate than normal in asymptomatic and symptomatic carriers of HIV. In those that are otherwise well, zoster can be managed palliatively as in uninfected patients.

Severe diarrhea is a common problem in HIV disease. Etiologic agents include cryptosporidia, *Isospora, Giardia,* entamoebae, salmonella, shigella, *campylobacter,* mycobacterium avium intracellulare (MAI), gonorrhea, chlamydia, *Treponema pallidum,* cytomegalovirus (CMV), herpes simplex virus (HSV), HIV, Kaposi's sarcoma, and lymphoma. Evaluation should include stool for culture and examination for leukocytes and parasites. Endoscopic examination is helpful if these are negative. As in other organ systems, infections are often multiple and therefore concurrent infections should be considered. Therapy for most agents is the same as in the normal population. Salmonella, an organism normally killed in macrophages, is poorly cleared in AIDS and may require chronic suppression. Cryptosporidia and *Isospora* are refractory to current therapies.

Kaposi's sarcoma, high-grade B cell lymphoma in a patient with a positive HIV serology, and primary CNS lymphoma are diagnostic of AIDS. Hodgkin's disease, chronic lymphocytic leukemia (CLL), and anal cancer may all be more common in AIDS patients. These neoplasms (with the exception of CLL) are more aggressive and have poorer responses to therapy than in uninfected patients.

Primary neurologic manifestations of HIV include meningitis, encephalitis, myelopathy, demyelinating and inflammatory peripheral neuropathy, and dementia. Psychiatric syndromes and suicide are also quite common in AIDS. Opportunistic infections must be ruled out. There is some response of the demyelinating neuropathy to plasmapheresis and of dementia to azidothymidine. Other primary manifestations of HIV infection include anemia, immune thrombocytopenia, and immune neutropenia.

The mainstay of 1990 antiretroviral therapy is azidothymidine (AZT; zidovudine). This oxythymidine analogue is phosphorylated by cellular enzymes to the triphosphate which causes chain termination of reverse transcribed viral DNA. In patients with AIDS, AZT reduces the frequency and severity of OI, prolongs survival, increases body weight and CD4 number, and improves performance levels. Toxicities include headache, nausea, insomnia, macrocytosis, anemia, and neutropenia. Acute dose reduction can lead to an acute meningoencephalitis. Close monitoring of clinical and hematologic status is necessary. Comprehensive drug treatment protocols are available through the AIDS Treatment Evaluation Units nationwide. Many new drugs, treatment strategies, and vaccines are being evaluated.

1. Sande, M. A., and Volberding, P. A. (eds.). Medical management of AIDS. *Infect. Dis. Clin. North Am.* 2:1988.
   A comprehensive compilation of articles dealing with pathogenesis, epidemiology, transmission, specific clinical syndromes, and therapy.
2. Curran, J. W., Jaffe, H. W., Hardy, A. M., et al. Epidemiology of HIV infection and AIDS in the United States. *Science* 239:610, 1988.
   Thorough, well-referenced review.
3. Piot, P., Plummer, F. A., Mhalu, F. S., et al. AIDS: An international perspective. *Science* 239:573, 1988.
   The spread of HIV in the Third World is predominantly heterosexual and perinatal. Patterns and contributing factors discussed.
4. Fauci, A. S. The human immunodeficiency virus: Infectivity and mechanisms of pathogenesis. *Science* 239:617, 1988.
   Review of cell tropism, latency, and activation of HIV, and mechanisms of T4 depletion.
5. Ho, D. D., Pomerantz, R. J., and Kaplan, J. C. Pathogenesis of infection with human immunodeficiency virus. *N. Engl. J. Med.* 317:278, 1987.
   Excellent, in-depth review of HIV with special emphasis on the role of monocytes and CNS infection.
6. Price, R. W., Brew, B., Sidtis, J., et al. The brain in AIDS: Central nervous system HIV-1 infection and AIDS dementia. *Science* 239:586, 1988.
   AIDS dementia complex, neuropathology, and pathogenesis.
7. Pomerantz, R. J., de la Monte, S. M., Donegan, S. P., et al. Human immunodeficiency virus (HIV) infection of the uterine cervix. *Ann. Intern. Med.* 108:321, 1988.
   Cervical endothelium, monocyte/macrophages, and lymphocyte-like cells are infected with HIV. A mild cervicitis accompanied HIV infection in this group.
8. Pomerantz, R. J., Kuritzkes, D. R., de la Monte, S. M., et al. Infection of the retina by human immunodeficiency virus type 1. *N. Engl. J. Med.* 317:1643, 1987.
   Retinal endothelium and glial components were infected in autopsy specimens.
9. Nelson, J. A., Reynolds-Kohler, C. R., Margaretten, W., et al. Human immunodeficiency virus detected in bowel epithelium from patients with gastrointestinal symptoms. *Lancet* i:259, 1988.
   Intestinal columnar epithelial cells and enterochromaffin cells were infected in biopsy specimens.
10. Weiss, S. H., Goedert, J. J., Sarngadharan, M. G., et al. Screening test for HTLV-III (AIDS agent) antibodies. *J.A.M.A.* 253:221, 1985.
    Sensitivity and specificity of the ELISA are greater than 95%.

11. Loche, M., and Mach, B. Identification of HIV-infected seronegative individuals by a direct diagnostic test based on hybridization to amplified viral DNA. *Lancet* 2:418, 1988.
    By use of the polymerase chain reaction, infection was demonstrated in 5/16 seronegative sex partners of seropositive individuals.
12. Farzadegan, H., Polis, M. A., Wolinsky, S. M., et al. Loss of human immunodeficiency virus type 1 (HIV-1) antibodies with evidence of viral infection in asymptomatic homosexual men: A report from the multi-center AIDS cohort study. *Ann. Intern. Med.* 108:785, 1988.
    Persistent HIV infection demonstrated by polymerase chain reaction after loss of anti-HIV antibody.
13. Quinn, T. C., Mann, J. M., Curran, J. W., et al. AIDS in Africa: An epidemiologic paradigm. *Science* 234:955, 1986.
    HIV is a largely sexually transmitted disease in Africa. Clinical spectrum of disease is different from United States.
14. Simonsen, J. N., Cameron, W., Gakinya, M. N., et al. Human immunodeficiency virus infection among men with sexually transmitted diseases: Experience from a center in Africa. *N. Engl. J. Med.* 319:274, 1988.
    HIV infection was more common in men with intact foreskins or histories of genital ulcer disease.
15. Winkelstein, W., Lyman, D. M., Padian, N., et al. Sexual practices and risk of infection by the human immunodeficiency virus: The San Francisco men's health study. *J.A.M.A.* 257:321, 1987.
    Seropositivity in homosexual men correlated with number of partners, receptive anal intercourse, and douching.
16. Friedland, G. H., Saltzman, B. R., Rogers, M. F., et al. Lack of transmission of HTLV-III/LAV infection to household contacts of patients with AIDS or AIDS-related complex with oral candidiasis. *N. Engl. J. Med.* 314:344, 1986.
    No household transmission of HIV found.
17. Holmberg, S. D., Stewart, J. A., Gerber, A. R., et al. Prior herpes simplex virus type 2 infection as a risk factor for HIV infection. *J.A.M.A.* 259:1048, 1988.
    Acquisition of HSV-2, whether symptomatic or not, correlated with acquiring HIV.
18. Friedland, G. H., and Klein, R. S. Transmission of the human immunodeficiency virus. *N. Engl. J. Med.* 317:1125, 1987.
    Thorough review of how HIV is and is not transmitted.
19. McCray, E., and the Comparative Needle Stick Surveillance Group. Occupational risk of the acquired immunodeficiency syndrome among health care workers. *N. Engl. J. Med.* 314:1127, 1986.
    The rate of seroconversion following mucosal or percutaneous exposure to body fluids of AIDS patients is less than 1%. 40% of these exposures were easily preventable.
20. Centers for Disease Control. Update: Acquired immunodeficiency syndrome and human immunodeficiency virus infection among health-care workers. *M.M.W.R.* 37:229, 1988.
    Risk of acquiring HIV by needle stick is less than 1%. HIV laboratory workers are also at risk.
21. Daul, C. B., deShazo, R. D., and Andes, W. A. Human immunodeficiency virus infection in hemophiliac patients: A three-year prospective evaluation. *Am. J. Med.* 84:801, 1988.
    Decline in lymphocyte function is more prominent than fall in lymphocyte number.
22. Lui, K.-J., Darrow, W. W., and Rutherford, G. W., III. A model-based estimate of the mean incubation period for AIDS in homosexual men. *Science* 240:1333, 1988.
    A mean incubation of 7.8 years is calculated.
23. Rothenberg, R., Woelfel, M., Stoneburner, R., et al. Survival with the acquired immunodeficiency syndrome: Experience with 5833 cases in New York City. *N. Engl. J. Med.* 317:1297, 1987.
    Overall cumulative probability of survival for 1 year < 50%; for 5 years, 15%. White

homosexual men with Kaposi's sarcoma only had cumulative 1 year probability of survival of 80%; black women IVDU, 30%.

24. Polk, B. F., Fox, R., Brookmeyer, R., et al. Predictors of the acquired immunodeficiency syndrome developing in a cohort of seropositive homosexual men. *N. Engl. J. Med.* 316:61, 1987.
    Predictors of AIDS include low T4, increased T8, low HIV titer, high CMV titer, and history of sex with someone who developed AIDS.

25. Goedert, J. J., Biggar, R. J., Melbye, M., et al. Effect of T4 count and cofactors on the incidence of AIDS in homosexual men infected with human immunodeficiency virus. *J.A.M.A.* 257:331, 1987.
    The 3-year risk of AIDS was 40% in those with T4 counts < 300 μl.

26. Curran, J. W., Lawrence, D. N., Jaffe, H., et al. Acquired immunodeficiency syndrome (AIDS) associated with transfusions. *N. Engl. J. Med.* 310:69, 1984.
    Evidence that AIDS is transmitted by blood transfusions.

27. Centers for Disease Control. Revision of the CDC surveillance case definition for acquired immunodeficiency syndrome. *M.M.W.R.* 36:1S, 1987.
    Diagnostic criteria for patients with and without the HIV serology.

28. Glatt, A. E., Chirgwin, K., and Landesman, S. H. Treatment of infections associated with human immunodeficiency virus. *N. Engl. J. Med.* 318:1439, 1988.
    Review of the major treatable infections in people with HIV.

29. Murray, J. F., Felton, C. P., Garay, S. M., et al. Pulmonary complications of the acquired immunodeficiency syndrome. Report of a National Heart, Lung, and Blood Institute Workshop. *N. Engl. J. Med.* 310:1682, 1984.
    Review of the spectrum of pulmonary pathogens encountered in HIV infection.

30. Sattler, F. R., Cowan, R., Nielsen, D. M., et al. Trimethoprim-sulfamethoxazole compared with pentamidine for treatment of *Pneumocytosis carinii* pneumonia in the acquired immunodeficiency syndrome. *Ann. Intern. Med.* 109:280, 1988.
    The authors show that one can continue to treat with either trimethoprim-sulfamethoxasole or pentamidine despite adverse effects by adjusting the dose. The former seemed more effective.

31. Montgomery, A. B., Luce, J. M., Turner, J., et al. Aerosolized pentamidine as sole therapy for *Pneumocystis carinii* pneumonia in patients with acquired immunodeficiency syndrome. *Lancet* 2:480, 1987.
    13/15 (87%) of patients with mild to moderate PCP were treated successfully.

32. McFadden, D. K., Hyland, R. H., Inouye, T., et al. Corticosteroids as adjunctive therapy in treatment of *Pneumocystis carinii* pneumonia in patients with acquired immunodeficiency syndrome. *Lancet* 1:1477, 1987.
    9/10 patients with severe PCP treated with short-course steroids survived.

33. Fischl, M. A., Dickinson, G. M., and La Voie, L. Safety and efficacy of sulfamethoxazole and trimethoprim chemoprophylaxis for *Pneumocystis carinii* pneumonia in AIDS. *J.A.M.A.* 259:1185, 1988.
    800 mg sulfamethoxasole and 160 mg trimethoprim twice a day prevented recurrence of PCP.

34. Meduri, G. U., Stover, D. E., Lee, M., et al. Pulmonary Kaposi's sarcoma in the acquired immune deficiency syndrome: Clinical, radiographic, and pathologic manifestations. *Am. J. Med.* 81:11, 1986.
    Nodular infiltrates and effusions are the most common radiographic signs. Transbronchial biopsy, brushing, or effusion analysis not helpful in diagnosis.

35. Gabuzda, D. H., and Hirsch, M. S. Neurologic manifestations of infection with human immunodeficiency virus: Clinical features and pathogenesis. *Ann. Intern. Med.* 107:383, 1987.
    Review of the neurologic manifestations and infections of HIV.

36. Dismukes, W. E. Cryptococcal meningitis in patients with AIDS. *J. Infect. Dis.* 157:624, 1988.
    Brief review of the clinical and therapeutic approaches to cryptococcal meningitis.

37. Navia, B. A., Petito, C. K., Gold, J. W. M., et al. Cerebral toxoplasmosis complicating the acquired immune deficiency syndrome: Clinical and neuropathologic findings in 27 patients. *Ann. Neurol.* 19:224, 1986.
    Clinical and pathologic aspects.

38. Haverkos, H. W. Assessment of therapy for *Toxoplasma* encephalitis: The TE study group. *Am. J. Med.* 82:907, 1987.
   Median survival from initiation of therapy was 4 months. Clinical relapse 50%.
39. Berger, J. R., Kaszovita, B., Donovan-Post, M. J., et al. Progressive multifocal leukoencephalopathy [PML] associated with human immunodeficiency virus infection: A review of the literature with a report of sixteen cases. *Ann. Intern. Med.* 107:78, 1987.
   Clinical and pathologic description. No effective therapy for PML yet.
40. Smith, P. D., Lane, H. C., Gill, V. J., et al. Intestinal infections in patients with the acquired immunodeficiency syndrome (AIDS): Etiology and response to therapy. *Ann. Intern. Med.* 108:328–333, 1988.
   One or more gastrointestinal pathogens found in 85%.
41. Laughon, B. E., Druckman, D. A., Vernon, A., et al. Prevalence of enteric pathogens in homosexual men with and without acquired immunodeficiency syndrome. *Gastroenterology* 94:984, 1988.
   Gastrointestinal pathogens found in both symptomatic and asymptomatic populations.
42. Knowles, D. M., Chamulak, G. A., Subar, M., et al. Lymphoid neoplasia associated with the acquired immunodeficiency syndrome (AIDS). *Ann. Intern. Med.* 108:744, 1988.
   Non-Hodgkin's lymphoma (NHL), Hodgkin's lymphoma, and CLL found in AIDS patients. Response to therapy and survival worse in NHL and HL.
43. Berman, A., Espinoza, L. R., Diaz, J. D., et al. Rheumatic manifestations of human immunodeficiency virus infection. *Am. J. Med.* 85:59, 1988.
   Arthralgias, oligoarthritis, and Reiter's seen in AIDS.
44. Sreepada Rao, T. K., Friedman, E. A., and Nicastri, A. D. The types of renal disease in the acquired immunodeficiency syndrome. *N. Engl. J. Med.* 316:1062, 1987.
   Focal glomerular sclerosis, nephrotic syndrome seen in AIDS. Irreversible uremia responds very poorly to dialysis.
45. Yarchoan, R., and Broder, S. Development of antiretroviral therapy for the acquired immunodeficiency syndrome and related disorders: A progress report. *N. Engl. J. Med.* 316:557, 1987.
   Mechanism and use of AZT and its analogues.
46. DeVita, V. T., Broder, S., Fauci, A. S., et al. Developmental therapeutics and the acquired immunodeficiency syndrome. *Ann. Intern. Med.* 106:568, 1987.
   Antivirals, immunomodulators, antibiotics, and antifungals described.
47. Fischl, M. A., Richman, D. D., Grieco, M. H., et al. The efficacy of 3'-azido-3'-deoxythymidine (azidothymidine) in the treatment of patients with AIDS and AIDS-related complex: A double-blind placebo-controlled trial. *N. Engl. J. Med.* 317:185, 1987.
   Reduction in frequency and severity of OI. Marked reduction in mortality.
48. Richman, D. D., Fischl, M. A., Grieco, M. H., et al. The toxicity of azidothymidine (AZT) in the treatment of patients with AIDS and AIDS-related complex. *N. Engl. J. Med.* 317:192, 1987.
   Anemia, neutropenia, nausea, myalgia, insomnia, and headache were reported. Multiple transfusions were required.
49. Jackson, G. G., Paul, D. A., Falk, L. A., et al. Human immunodeficiency virus (HIV) antigenemia (p24) in the acquired immunodeficiency syndrome (AIDS) and the effect of treatment with zidovudine (AZT). *Ann. Intern. Med.* 108:175, 1988.
   AZT at 200–250 mg. every 4 hours reduced p24 antigen levels up to 90%.
50. Spivak, J. L., Bender, B. S., and Quinn, T. C. Hematologic abnormalities in the acquired immune deficiency syndrome. *Am. J. Med.* 77:224, 1984.
   Anemia and leukopenia were common as were myelofibrosis, plasmacytosis, lymphoid infiltrates, and maturation abnormalities. Erythropoietin levels are also inappropriately low (J.A.M.A. 261:3104, 1989).
51. Schnittman, S. M., Psallidopoulos, M. C., Lane, H. C., et al. The reservoir for HIV-1 in human peripheral blood is a T cell that maintains expression of CD4. *Science* 245:305, 1989.

Circulating HIV infected cells are CD4+. These constitute about 1 percent of CD4+ cells in patients with AIDS.

52. Ho, D. D., Moudgil, T., Alam, M. Quantitation of human immunodeficiency virus type 1 in the blood of infected persons. *N. Engl. J. Med.* 321:1621, 1989.

HIV titer in plasma and peripheral mononuclear cells increases with progression from asymptomatic to symptomatic HIV infection. Plasma viremia, but not peripheral mononuclear cell viremia, is reduced with AZT treatment.

115. ASEPTIC MENINGITIS
H. Verdain Barnes

Aseptic meningitis is characterized by fever, signs and symptoms of meningeal inflammation, and abnormal but sterile cerebrospinal fluid (CSF). Typically there is a 3- to 4-day history of fever, headache, varying degrees of nuchal rigidity, lethargy often associated with irritability and confusion, and occasionally nausea and vomiting. These signs and symptoms can range from striking to subtle and any one may dominate the clinical picture. Examination of the CSF shows some degree of pleocytosis, normal or increased protein, normal or low sugar, and negative bacterial and fungal stains. The cell count is usually below 1000 per microliter but may rarely be higher. The cell type is variable. In general, late in the course of the illness there is a predominance of mononuclear cells, whereas early in the course a predominance of polymorphonuclear leukocytes is common. The sugar content is typically greater than 40 percent of a simultaneously drawn blood sugar. A variety of conditions can have these general features. They fall into the following major categories: (1) viral meningitis, (2) inadequately treated bacterial meningitis, (3) parameningeal inflammation, (4) spirochete meningitis, (5) tumor metastases, (6) fungal meningitis, and (7) miscellaneous. The vast majority are viral, but the ever-present possibility that one of the other types is involved often leads to diagnostic and therapeutic difficulties.

1. Viral meningitis has some clinically useful, epidemiologic symptoms and features. The most common reported etiologies are the enteroviruses (about 80%) followed by mumps, lymphocytic choriomeningitis, herpes simplex, herpes zoster, and arboviruses. Enterovirus disease usually occurs between June and October, with the peak in August. Men are more frequently affected than women. In most series about 60 percent of the patients are between the ages of 5 and 20 years. Clinically about 10 to 15 percent complain of a sore throat, but exudative pharyngitis is rare. Rhinitis with or without a cough is equally as common. Five to eight percent complain of some type of chest or abdominal pain. A petechial or maculopapular rash may be seen, but is rare. Myalgias and gastroenteritis are variable in frequency. From 10 to 12 percent have one or more of the following serious manifestations of central nervous system dysfunction: grand mal or (rarely) focal seizures, severe lethargy or coma, objective unilateral muscle weakness, blurred optic disks without a clear increase in CSF pressure, sensory defects, and (rarely) oculogyric crisis, choreiform movements, transverse myelitis, or truncal ataxia. For the most part, the entire illness, regardless of severity, lasts less than 2 weeks. Fever initially ranges from 38.3 to 40°C (101–104°F). The fever, headache, stiff neck, and vomiting tend to resolve first. The CSF cell count can range from 10 to 2000 per microliter, with about 30 percent of patients having a count greater than 300. Except for mumps, which is dominated by a mononuclear pleocytosis throughout, the early predominance is neutrophilic in about 70 percent. CSF protein is slightly to modestly elevated in two-thirds of patients. CSF glucose is typically normal. The peripheral white blood cell count may range from less than 6000 to more than 20,000 per microliter. No one clinical finding is diagnostic.

About 50 percent of patients have some complaints during convalescence. These complaints may last weeks to months, but more than 95 percent of patients are totally asymptomatic within a year. The most frequent convalescent complaints are recurrent headache or asymmetric muscle weakness or tightness, which follows the acute episode in 20 to 30 percent. The muscles most frequently involved are the gluteus medius, gastrocnemius-soleus, and abdominal recti.

Coxsackie viruses may cause an aseptic meningitis. The Coxsackie viruses involved are, in order of frequency, group A type 9 and group B types 5, 4, 3, 2, and 1. Other less common viruses include polioviruses types 1 and 3, measles, rubella, chickenpox, hepatitis A and B viruses, and the arthropod-borne viruses. Viral isolation from CSF is definitive. Finally, aseptic meningitis is the most common neurologic manifestation of infectious mononucleosis.

2. Inadequately treated bacterial meningitis can result in an aseptic meningitis picture and needs no further elaboration.

3. The parameningeal inflammations that can produce aseptic meningitis are intracerebral abscess, epidural abscess, thrombosis of the intracranial venous sinuses, and encephalitis.

4. The spirochete infections leptospirosis and acute syphilis can produce the syndrome.

5. A variety of malignancies have been associated with an aseptic meningitis syndrome, the most common ones being the acute leukemias, lymphomas, and Hodgkin's disease. Rare tumors include cavernous hemangiomas, ependymomas, dermoid and hydatid cysts. Metastatic carcinomatous meningitis has been reported with such carcinomas as breast, stomach, lung, and malignant melanoma.

6. The most common fungal cause of aspectic meningitis is cryptococcosis, followed by histoplasmosis, coccidioidomycosis, and blastomycosis. Aspectic meningitis has also been reported with psittacosis, lymphogranuloma, Q fever, Rift Valley fever, Lyme disease, *Mycoplasma pneumoniae*, and *Toxoplasma gondii*.

7. The etiologies in the miscellaneous category of aseptic meningitis are varied. All are rare. They include recurrent benign endothelio-leukocytic meningitis (Mollaret's meningitis), sarcoidosis, Behçet's syndrome, Vogt-Koyanagi-Harada disease, granulomatous angiitis, chronic benign lymphocytic meningitis, parasitic meningitis, systemic lupus erythematosus, and drug-induced meningitis.

Finally, and of particular importance, the CSF findings in early tuberculous meningitis may be indistinguishable from those of viral aseptic meningitis. Consequently any patient with aseptic meningitis must be appropriately evaluated for tuberculosis. In summary, viral aseptic meningitis is a diagnosis of exclusion.

1. Wallgren, A. Acute aseptic meningitis: New infections of central nervous system? *Acta Paediatr.* 4:158, 1925.
   The initial description.
2. Edwards, G. A., and Domm, B. M. Human leptospirosis. *Medicine* 39:117, 1960.
   Meningitis occurs in phase 2 of the disease.
3. Bhandari, Y. S., and Sarkari, N. B. S. Subdural empyema: Review of 37 cases. *J. Neurosurg.* 32:35, 1970.
   Another example of parameningeal infections to be considered.
4. Schwartz, J. H., Canellos, G. P., Young, R. C., et al. Meningeal leukemia in the blastic phase of chronic granulocytic leukemia. *Am. J. Med.* 59:819, 1975.
   Meningeal involvement occurred in about 7% of these patients, but it rarely if ever occurs in the chronic phase.
5. Griffin, J. W., Thompson, R. W., Mitchinson, M. J., et al. Lymphomatous leptomeningitis. *Am. J. Med.* 51:200, 1971.
   The authors found the cytologic examination of the CSF to be useful in making the diagnosis.
6. Gautier-Smith, P. C. Neurological complications of glandular fever. *Brain* 88:323, 1965.
   Aseptic meningitis is the most common CNS manifestation of infectious mononucleosis.
7. Cantu, R. C., and Wright, R. L. Aseptic meningitis syndrome with cauda equina epidermoid tumor. *J. Pediatr.* 73:114, 1968.

8. Harbert, J. C. Aseptic meningitis following isotope cisternography. *J. Nucl. Med.* 13:778, 1972.
   Rare causes of aseptic meningitis are discussed in articles 7, 8.
9. Canoso, J. J., and Cohen, A. S. Aseptic meningitis in systemic lupus erythematosus. *Arthritis Rheum.* 18:369, 1975.
10. Sergent, J. S., Lochshin, M. D., Klempner, M. S., et al. Central nervous system disease in systemic lupus erythematosus. *Am. J. Med.* 58:644, 1975.
    Aseptic meningitis can occur before other manifestations (article 9) or during the course (article 10) of lupus erythematosus.
11. Hodges, G. R., Fass, R. G., and Saslaw, S. Central nervous system disease associated with *Mycoplasma pneumoniae* infection. *Arch. Intern. Med.* 130:277, 1972.
    Another rare cause.
12. Galdi, A. P. Benign recurrent aseptic meningitis (Mollaret's meningitis): Case reports and clinical review. *Arch. Neurol.* 36:657, 1979.
    "Endothelial cells" in the CSF during the first 24 hours of the illness are diagnostic.
13. Gonyea, E. F. The spectrum of primary blastomycotic meningitis: A review of central nervous system blastomycosis. *Ann. Neurol.* 3:26, 1978.
    An excellent review.
14. Fujita, N. K., Reynard, M., Sapico, F. L., et al. Cryptococcal intracerebral mass lesions: The role of computed tomography and nonsurgical management. *Ann. Intern. Med.* 94:382, 1981.
    An interesting finding in cryptococcal meningitis; about 18% have no focal neurologic signs.
15. Ruppert, G. B., and Barth, W. F. Tolmetin-induced aseptic meningitis. *J.A.M.A.* 245:67, 1981.
    Fenoprofen calcium, ibuprofen, and tolmetin sodium are all potentials.
16. Varki, A. P., and Puthuran, P. Value of second lumbar puncture in confirming a diagnosis of aseptic meningitis: A prospective study. *Arch. Neurol.* 36:581, 1979.
    The change from polymorphonuclear neutrophils to mononuclear cells occurred in all their patients within 18 to 48 hours. This author believes they have overstated their case for initially withholding antibiotics. Otherwise a useful article.
17. Salaki, J. S., Louria, D. B., and Chmel, H. Fungal and yeast infections of the central nervous system: A clinical review. *Medicine* 63:108, 1984.
    A comprehensive, well-referenced review.
18. Dougherty, J. M., and Jones, J. Cerebrospinal fluid cultures and analysis. *Ann. Emerg. Med.* 15:317, 1986.
    A useful discussion of acrinidine orange stain, counterimmunoelectrophoresis, agglutination tests, enzyme immunoassay, and bacterial antigen quantitation in the diagnosis of meningitis.
19. Ratzan, K. R. Viral meningitis. *Med. Clin. North Am.* 69:399, 1985.
    A concise review; the enteroviruses are the most common of the reported etiologies.
20. Reik, L., Jr., Burgdorfer, W., and Donaldson, J. O. Neurologic abnormalities in Lyme disease without erythema chronicum migrans. *Am. J. Med.* 81:73, 1986.
    Another cause to keep in mind by an increasingly reported disease.

116. BACTERIAL MENINGITIS

H. Verdain Barnes

Untreated bacterial meningitis is almost invariably fatal. Clinical suspicion, accurate diagnosis, and appropriate antibiotic therapy are paramount in reducing morbidity and mortality. Meningitis can occur at any age, but it is most common in infancy, early childhood, and in old age.

The clinical onset and symptom picture are variable. In about 25 percent the onset is abrupt, with a rapid progression of signs and symptoms. In this setting there are usually no respiratory signs or symptoms. In about 50 percent of patients there is a slow progression of meningeal symptoms over a period of 1 to 7 days. Nearly one-third of the patients have associated upper respiratory tract complaints. In another 20 percent meningeal signs develop rapidly or slowly after a 1- to 3-week upper respiratory tract infection. The remaining patients do not have a characteristic presentation. The most common complaints are, in decreasing order of frequency, fever, confusion, vomiting, headache, stiff neck, and chills. Initially many patients have only one or two of these symptoms. In infants and children the only manifestations may be fever and vomiting. In some adults the only symptoms are fever and confusion. On physical examination about 80 percent have a stiff neck and a Kernig's or Brudzinski's sign; patients without these signs are most often infants, elderly, or markedly obtunded. Approximately 96 percent have some alteration in mental status, ranging from lethargy to deep coma. About 50 percent exhibit other neurologic signs, such as seizures, Babinski's reflex, doll's eye movements, fixed pupils, hemiparesis, anisocoria, nystagmus, or involvement of the fourth, sixth, seventh, or eighth cranial nerves. A petechial rash occurs in about two-thirds of persons with meningococcal meningitis, and rarely in persons with pneumococcal, staphylococcal, streptococcal, and *Haemophilus influenzae* infections. The most common etiologic organisms are *Diplococcus pneumoniae, H. influenzae,* and *Neisseria meningitidis,* which account for over 70 percent of all cases. Other less common organisms are *Staphylococcus aureus, Escherichia coli,* other β-hemolytic streptococci, *Proteus, Pseudomonas,* diphtheroids, *Listeria monocytogenes,* and *Neisseria gonorrhoeae.* In the final analysis, however, any organism is a potential cause. About 4 percent of patients have more than one organism, while, at the opposite end of the spectrum, in up to 10 percent no organism can be identified. In general, meningococcal meningitis is more common in persons under age 30; pneumococcal more common in persons under age 1 and over age 40, and *H. influenzae* tends to predominate in patients age 5 years and under. The other organisms are generally distributed among all ages.

The organism involved may depend on a predisposing factor. For example, in pneumococcal meningitis close to 25 percent of patients are alcoholics and about one-third have accompanying pneumonia or endocarditis. Prior head trauma, otitis media, chronic or acute sinusitis, leukemia, lymphoma, and acquired immunodeficiency syndrome (AIDS) are also relatively commonly associated conditions. In *H. influenzae* meningitis, the most common association is otitis media, followed by upper respiratory tract infection. In adults, meningitis associated with these conditions usually arises in the setting of a congenital communicating anatomic defect, head trauma, a parameningeal focus of infection, or defective immunologic status. Patients with meningococcal meningitis almost invariably have a predisposing upper respiratory tract source of infection. Staphylococcal meningitis is usually associated with prior craniotomy, sinusitis, cranial osteomyelitis, or bacterial endocarditis. Meningitis due to *E. coli* or other gram-negative organisms often has a predisposing factor, such as a craniotomy, laminectomy, spinal anesthesia, or a chronic debilitating disease. Other associated factors include mastoiditis, brain abscess, omphalitis, ophthalmitis, cellulitis, furunculosis, endometritis, malnutrition, and diabetes mellitus. In 10 to 25 percent of all cases no demonstrable predisposing factor is found.

The three crucial elements in diagnosis are the cerebrospinal fluid (CSF), bacterial stain and culture, and blood culture. Lumbar puncture (LP) should not be delayed in patients suspected of having a purulent meningitis unless there is an equal suspicion of a focal lesion, such as a tumor or abscess. In those cases emergency computed tomography (CT) of the head should be performed before the LP. Lumbar puncture in the presence of increased intracranial pressure and a mass lesion increases the potential of irreversible cerebellar or temporal lobe herniation and death. In bacterial meningitis, the CSF cell count is frequently greater than 1000 per microliter, with a definite leukocytosis. However, the count may be as low as 1 per microliter early in the course of the illness. Counts of less than 100 are seen in 5 to 20 percent of all types of pyogenic meningitis. Cell counts of over 50,000 per microliter can be seen, but when present raise the possibility of a ruptured brain abscess. In the majority of patients the CSF sugar level is less than 40 percent of that in a simultaneously drawn blood sample. Low CSF sugar levels may also be seen in mycotic and mumps meningitis, as well as an occasional case of carcinomatous or hypersensitivity reaction meningitis. Hypoglycorrhachia is caused by an inhibition of the glucose carrier transport mechanisms, increased brain utilization of glucose, and increased utilization of glucose by the bacteria and phagocytic cells. The CSF protein is elevated in about 90 percent of patients with pneumococcal and *H. influenzae* and in 80 percent of patients with meningococcal meningitis. Paramen-ingeal foci of infection, some viruses, hypersensitivity meningitis, chemical meningitis, and neoplastic meningitis may mimic the CSF findings of bacterial meningitis. In sum-mary, none of the CSF findings are diagnostic of bacterial meningitis. Recent studies support the usefulness of counterimmunoelectrophoresis (CIE), latex agglutination (LA), enzyme immunoassay, and bacterial antigen quantitation tests in the diagnosis of bacterial meningitis. All, however, can have false-positive and, more importantly, false-negative results. The CIE and LA tests appear to have the greatest utility. These tests, if available, may speed the diagnostic process.

In most series the CSF Gram stain reveals an organism in about 80 percent of pa-tients, with correct identification of the organism ranging from 80 to 90 percent. Acrin-idine orange, which stains bacterial nucleic acids, is sensitive, easy to perform, and has greater sensitivity than the Gram stain. However, it does not provide the same potential for specific organism identification as does the Gram stain. Abnormal CSF specimens that are negative on Gram stain should routinely be stained for acid-fast organisms. Careful CSF cultures on appropriate media are positive in over 90 percent of patients. Of those with negative cultures, many have had some prior antibiotic therapy. Blood cultures are positive in about 50 percent of patients with pneumococcal meningitis, 75 percent of persons with *H. influenzae,* 30 percent of patients with meningococcal or streptococcal meningitis, and 20 percent of patients with staphylococcal meningitis. Up-per respiratory tract cultures grow a predominance of the offending organism in less than one-third of patients.

Mortality is due to a variety of factors; the overall incidence is about 6 to 33 percent depending on the organism. In most series the highest mortality occurs with gram-negative meningitis, followed by pneumococcal and staphylococcal. Recurrent meningi-tis may occur in as many as 4 percent of patients, most frequently in those with head trauma, CSF rhinorrhea, or otorrhea.

1. Swartz, M. N., and Dodge, R. R. Bacterial meningitis: A review of selected aspects. *N. Engl. J. Med.* 272:728, 779, 842, 898, 954, 1003, 1965.
   A well-referenced, comprehensive review.
2. Carpenter, R. R., and Petersdorf, R. G. The clinical spectrum of bacterial meningitis. *Am. J. Med.* 33:262, 1962.
   Three modes of onset characterize bacterial meningitis.
3. Harter, D. H. Preliminary antibiotic therapy in bacterial meningitis. *Arch. Neurol.* 9:343, 1963.
   Negative CSF cultures are twice as frequent in patients who have received antibiotic therapy.
4. Milhorat, T. H., Hammock, M. R., Fenstermacher, J. D., et al. Cerebrospinal fluid production by the choroid plexus and brain. *Science* 173:330, 1971.
5. Davison, H., Hollingsworth, G., and Segal, M. B. The mechanism of cerebrospinal fluid. *Brain* 93:665, 1970.
   Articles 4 and 5 provide a quick symposium on CSF physiology.
6. Cooper, A. J., Beaty, H. N., Oppenheimer, S. I., et al. Studies on pathogenesis of meningitis: VII. Glucose transport and spinal fluid production in experimental pneu-mococcal meningitis. *J. Lab. Clin. Med.* 71:473, 1968.
   Low CSF glucose—one contributing factor is the inhibition of the glucose carrier transport mechanism.
7. Petersdorf, R. G., Swarmer, D. R., and Garcia, M. Studies in pathogenesis of men-ingitis: III. Relationship of phagocytosis to the fall in cerebrospinal fluid sugar in experimental pneumococcal meningitis. *J. Lab. Clin. Med.* 61:745, 1963.
   Low CSF glucose—another contributing factor is increased utilization of glucose by bacteria and phagocytic cells.

8. Menkes, J. H. The causes for low spinal fluid sugar in bacterial meningitis: Another look. *Pediatrics* 44:1, 1969.
   Low CSF glucose—a third contributing factor is an increased brain utilization of glucose.

9. Hand, W. L., and Sanford, J. P. Posttraumatic bacterial meningitis. *Ann. Intern. Med.* 72:869, 1970.
   Always search the history for this possibility. 71% of the cases are pneumococcal.

10. Merselis, J. G., Jr., Sellers, T. F., Johnson, E. J., III, et al. *Hemophilus influenzae* meningitis in adults. *Arch. Intern. Med.* 110:837, 1962.
    Usually associated with CSF rhinorrhea, agammaglobulinemia, diabetes mellitus, or alcoholism.

11. Margaretten, W., and McAdams, A. J. An appraisal of fulminant meningococcemia with reference to the Shwartzman phenomenon. *Am. J. Med.* 25:868, 1958.
    Adrenal hemorrhage was seen in 3.3%.

12. Rahal, J. J., Jr. Treatment of gram-negative bacillary meningitis in adults. *Ann. Intern. Med.* 77:295, 1972.
    Usually associated with chronic systemic disease, invasive central nervous system procedures, or head trauma. Well-referenced for all gram-negative meningitis.

13. Taubin, H. L., and Landsberg, L. Gonococcic meningitis. *N. Engl. J. Med.* 285:504, 1971.
    It is probably more common than realized. Almost all patients have other signs and symptoms of gonorrhea.

14. Soscia, J. L., DiBenedetto, R., and Crocco, J. *Klebsiella pneumoniae* meningitis. *Arch. Intern. Med.* 113:569, 1964.
    Rare; 50% mortality; it is seen most often with diabetes mellitus.

15. Roberts, W. C., and Buchbinder, N. A. Right-sided valvular infective endocarditis. *Am. J. Med.* 53:7, 1972.
    A common tetrad to keep in mind: alcoholism, acute pneumonia, acute meningitis, and infective endocarditis.

16. Smilack, J. D. Group-Y meningococcal disease. *Ann. Intern. Med.* 81:740, 1974.
    Another virulent strain to keep in mind.

17. Hodges, G. R., and Perkins, R. L. Hospital-associated bacterial meningitis. *Am. J. Med. Sci.* 271:335, 1976.
    The most common organisms were Pseudomonas, staphylococcus, *and* streptococcus.

18. Bayer, A. S., Seidel, J. S., Yoshikawa, T. T., et al. Group D enterococcal meningitis. *Arch. Intern. Med.* 136:883, 1976.
    The CSF white count and glucose levels are usually low, and mortality is usually high.

19. Feldman, W. E. Relationship of concentrations of bacteria and bacterial antigen in cerebrospinal fluid to prognosis in patients with bacterial meningitis. *N. Engl. J. Med.* 296:433, 1977.
    The concentration of bacteria in the CSF probably has the best correlation with prognosis.

20. Heerema, M. S., Ein, M. E., Musher, D. M., et al. Anaerobic bacterial meningitis. *Am. J. Med.* 67:219, 1979.
    Beware of anaerobes as the cause in patients with chronic otitis media and mastoiditis, chronic sinusitis and recent craniotomy, or abdominal trauma.

21. Cherubin, C. E., Marr, J. S., Sierra, M. F., et al. *Listeria* and gram-negative bacillary meningitis in New York City, 1972–1979: Frequent causes of meningitis in adults. *Am. J. Med.* 71:199, 1981.
    These two organisms were the fourth and fifth most common causes of meningitis in their institution.

22. Powers, W. J. Cerebrospinal fluid to serum glucose ratios in diabetes mellitus and bacterial meningitis. *Am. J. Med.* 71:217, 1981.
    A ratio of less than 0.31 provided the best differentiation, but only 70.3% of those with meningitis had an abnormally low ratio while 97.2% of the uninfected were above this ratio.

23. Rahal, J. J., and Simberkoff, M. S. Host defense and antimicrobial therapy in adult gram-negative bacillary meningitis. *Ann. Intern. Med.* 96:468, 1982.
    Therapy must be carefully selected when the etiologic bacteria are encapsulated.

24. Kleiman, M., Reynolds, J., and Watts, N. Superiority of acrinidine orange stain versus Gram stain in partially treated bacterial meningitis. *J. Pediatr.* 104:401, 1984.
   An easy-to-do stain with high sensitivity.
25. Kaplan, S. Antigen detection in cerebrospinal fluid: Pros and cons. *Am. J. Med.* 75:109, 1983.
26. Tilton, R., Dias, F., and Ryan, R. Comparative evaluation of three commercial products and counterimmunoelectrophoresis for the detection of antigens in the cerebrospinal fluid. *J. Clin. Microbiol.* 20:231, 1984.
27. Pebble, J., Moxon, E., and Yolken, R. Indirect enzyme-linked immunoabsorbent assay for quantitation of the type-specific antigen of *Haemophilus influenza* B: A preliminary report. *J. Pediatr.* 92:233, 1980.
   These three articles (25–27) discuss CSF testing for specific bacterial antigens.
28. Mayefsky, J. H., and Roghmann, K. J. Determination of leukocytosis in traumatic spinal tap specimens. *Am. J. Med.* 82:1175, 1987.
   An old problem and a method for interpretation.
29. Neu, H. C. Impact of the patient at risk on current and future antimicrobial therapy. *Am. J. Med.* 76(Suppl. 5A):193, 208, 215, 224, 231, 1984.
   These five papers detail patient risk factors and considerations in management.
30. Weber, D. J., Wolfson, J. S., Swartz, M. N., et al. *Pasteurella multocida* infections: Report of 34 cases and review of the literature. *Medicine* 63:133, 1984.
   Seventeen cases of meningitis were identified.
31. Klein, N. C., Dansker, B., and Hirschman, S. Z. Mycobacterial meningitis: Retrospective analysis from 1970 to 1983. *Am. J. Med.* 79:29, 1985.
   An old disease that can present as acute, subacute, or chronic meningitis.
32. Peacock, J. E., Jr., McGinnis, M. R., and Cohen, M. S. Persistent neutrophilic meningitis: Report of four cases and review of the literature. *Medicine* 63:379, 1984.
   Both infectious and noninfectious etiologies were found.
33. Gorse, G. J., Thrupp, L. D., Nudleman, K. L., et al. Bacterial meningitis in the elderly. *Arch. Intern. Med.* 144:1603, 1984.
   Of those over 50 years old, bacterial accounted for 76% and aseptic for 11%.
34. Weinstein, L. Bacterial meningitis: Specific etiologic diagnosis on the basis of distinctive epidemiologic, pathogenetic, and clinical features. *Med. Clin. North Am.* 69:219, 1985.
   The personal experience of an old pro.
35. Bolan, G., and Barza, M. Acute bacterial meningitis in children and adults: A perspective. *Med. Clin. North Am.* 69:231, 1985.
   A concise, up-to-date review.
36. Schlech, W. F., III, Ward, J. I., Band, J. D., et al. Bacterial meningitis in the United States, 1978 through 1981: The national bacterial meningitis surveillance study. *J.A.M.A.* 253:1749, 1985.
   Haemophilus influenzae *was the most common bacterial organism (48.3%) followed by* Neisseria meningitidis *(19.6%) and* Streptococcus pneumoniae *(13.3%).*
37. Quagliarello, V. J., and Scheld, W. M. Review: Recent advances in the pathogenesis and pathophysiology of bacterial meningitis. *Am. J. Med. Sci.* 292:306, 1986.
   A concise current review of pathophysiology and pathogenesis.

117. BACTERIAL OSTEOMYELITIS

H. Verdain Barnes

Osteomyelitis may result from bacteremia or direct extension of a local infection. Acute hematogenous osteomyelitis occurs most frequently in infants, children, and adolescents, in whom more rapid bone growth and turnover are present. The pathophysiology in children and youth is best explained by the anatomy of the metaphyseal area where infection occurs. Nutrient arterioles loop sharply near the epiphysis, where these non-anastomotic branches enter large venous sinusoids. Flow is sluggish in the sinusoids and is ideal for bacterial growth. The infection spreads laterally through the bone cortex to the subperiosteal space. Although the epiphyseal growth plate usually protects the epiphysis, in children under age 1 year the capillaries still penetrate the epiphyseal growth plate, allowing the infection to spread into the epiphysis and often into the joint. A similar situation exists in the adult, whose epiphyseal growth plate has been reabsorbed. In addition, the periosteum in the adult is firmly affixed to the bone, thereby allowing less subperiosteal elevation and abscess formation. Consequently, in the infant, hematogenous osteomyelitis often destroys epiphyses, has a high incidence of associated septic arthritis, and forms a large involucrum, whereas in the child there is primarily cortical destruction and involucrum formation with only infrequent involvement of the adjacent epiphysis or joint. In adults, joint infection is not uncommon and little or no involucrum is formed. In infants and children, long-bone involvement is the rule; in adults, it is far less common. In adults, chronic osteomyelitis results more commonly than in children and infants.

Recent studies show an increasing incidence of hematogenous osteomyelitis in heroin addicts and those over age 50 years, with vertebral involvement becoming more frequent. The general distribution of involvement is as follows: about 35 percent femur, 15 percent tibia, 15 percent vertebrae, 14 percent humerus, 6 percent tarsal bones, 5 percent clavicle, 4 percent pelvis, 2 percent radius, 2 percent fibula, and 2 percent carpal bones. Approximately 13 percent have multifocal involvement.

Acute hematogenous osteomyelitis has an abrupt onset. The disease runs a toxic course in about 56 percent while in the remainder, the course is more indolent. When the onset is abrupt, there is usually an accompanying high fever, chills, headache, local tenderness and suppuration, marked malaise, and occasional nausea and vomiting. These patients seek attention early and are almost invariably diagnosed in less than 21 days of the onset. Combining acute and subacute presentations, local tenderness occurs in about 88 percent of patients, fever in 75 percent, local swelling in 52 percent, limitation of motion in 50 percent, local heat in 32 percent, local erythema in 22 percent, local drainage in 10 percent, and adjacent joint effusion in 8 percent. One-third of patients have a history of preceding blunt trauma to the involved area. Patients who run a subacute course of metaphyseal osteomyelitis with a quiescent subperiosteal accumulation of pus have a so-called Brodie's abscess. With the more indolent course, the constitutional signs and symptoms are less severe, with approximately 25 percent being afebrile. It is not uncommon for these patients to go longer than a month before seeking help. Two groups seem particularly prone to an indolent course—heroin addicts and patients with hemoglobin S-S disease. Patients with recurrent osteomyelitis often have few constitutional signs or symptoms.

The appearance of radiographic evidence of osteomyelitis is delayed by the natural physiochemistry of bone. Periosteal elevation usually begins within the first 10 days but on occasion may be delayed for a year or more. Soft tissue swelling is commonly seen between 11 and 20, but it likewise may be delayed. Lytic lesions are rarely seen within the first 10 days, but in the majority become visible between days 11 and 90. Sclerotic lesions tend to occur between 1 and 20 months.

It should be kept in mind that the radiographic changes of healing are usually delayed compared to the clinical course. In fact, in the early stages, bone changes may progress as the patient improves clinically. Ewing's sarcoma on occasion cannot be differentiated clinically or radiographically from osteomyelitis. Bone biopsy or aspiration should be performed when the diagnosis or pathogen is in doubt. Most patients have white blood cell counts between 10,000 and 16,000 per microliter, with a shift to the left. The erythrocyte sedimentation rate is usually elevated. Anemia is frequently present; hematocrit values decrease an average of 15 percent during the typical hospital course. When treated appropriately, 85 percent of the patients recover fully while the remainder progress to chronic osteomyelitis.

Osteomyelitis may arise as a result of an adjacent infectious process. In 60 percent of cases, the precipitating factor is an open reduction of a fracture. The major nonsurgical factor is soft tissue infection. About 30 percent of the contiguous foci are in the thigh; 21 percent in the calf; 10 percent in the jaw, calvarium, phalanges, and fibula; and the remainder are scattered in other areas of the skeleton. Most cases are diagnosed within 30 days of the onset of the inciting infection. Seventy-five percent of the patients are over age 41 years. Fever, local swelling, and erythema occur in approximately 50 percent. A demonstrable draining sinus is present in about 20 percent. The disease course is often insidiously progressive.

Patients with diabetes or peripheral vascular insufficiency are more likely to develop osteomyelitis of the feet and toes. About 50 percent have associated indolent ulcers, frequently of long standing. Associated cellulitis is common. Radiographically the picture is usually that of mottled lytic lesions. Success with nonamputation therapy is rare.

A wide spectrum of bacteria has been identified in hematogenous osteomyelitis, but *Staphylococcus aureus* continues to be the major organism, occurring in 48 to 80 percent. Next in frequency are the group A streptococci, followed by *Salmonella* and a variety of other organisms. In the heroin addict, fungi and gram-negative organisms are the most common. *Salmonella paratyphi* is the dominant organism in sickle cell patients.

Osteomyelitis due to local invasion from adjacent foci of infection is likewise dominated by the *S. aureus,* occurring in about 60 percent. The gram-negative organisms follow in frequency in most series. About 25 percent of patients have more than one organism. In diabetics and patients with vascular insufficiency, more than one organism is typical, frequently staphylococcus and streptococcus.

The index of suspicion should be high for osteomyelitis when there is an unexplained illness with bone pain, whether it is acute or chronic.

1. Waldvogel, F. A., Medoff, G., and Swartz, M. N. Osteomyelitis: A review of clinical features, therapeutic considerations and unusual aspects. *N. Engl. J. Med.* 282:198, 260, 316, 1970.
   A thorough, well-referenced review.
2. Trueta, J. The three types of acute haematogenous osteomyelitis: A clinical and vascular study. *J. Bone Joint Surg.* [Am.] 41:671, 1959.
   Good pathophysiology discussion relating the varying vascular patterns to the clinical picture.
3. Winters, J. L., and Cohen, I. Acute hematogenous osteomyelitis: A review of 66 cases. *J. Bone Joint Surg.* [Am.] 42:691, 1960.
   85% of patients are children or adolescents. In the past 85% of cases were due to staphylococcus.
4. Harris, N. H., and Kirkaldy-Willis, W. H. Primary subacute pyogenic osteomyelitis. *J. Bone Joint Surg.* [Br.] 47:526, 1965.
   Brodie's abscess may run an indolent course, thus delaying diagnosis.
5. Nance, C. L., Jr., Roberts, W. M., and Miller, G. R. Ewing's sarcoma mimicking osteomyelitis. *South. Med. J.* 60:1044, 1967.
   Occasionally, an exact mimic; if the diagnosis is in doubt, a biopsy is the best approach, although a definitive answer may not result unless the biopsy is deep into the involved area.
6. Holzman, R. S., and Bischko, F. Osteomyelitis in heroin addicts. *Ann. Intern. Med.* 75:693, 1971.
   The course is often indolent, and gram-negative organisms and yeast are frequent offenders.
7. Lee, Y. H., and Kerstein, M. D. Osteomyelitis and septic arthritis: Complication of subclavian venous catheterization. *N. Engl. J. Med.* 285:1179, 1971.
   Beware.
8. Leonard, A., Comty, C. M., and Shapiro, F. L. Osteomyelitis in hemodialysis patients. *Ann. Intern. Med.* 78:651, 1973.
   The ribs and thoracic vertebrae are most commonly involved. Diagnosis is frequently delayed.
9. Engh, C. A., Hughes, J. L., Abrams, R. C., et al. Osteomyelitis in the patient with sickle-cell disease: Diagnosis and management. *J. Bone Joint Surg.* 53:1, 1971.
   Salmonella paratyphi A is the offender in the majority of sickle cell patients.

10. Blumenfeld, R. J., and Skolnid, E. M. Intracranial complications of sinus disease. *Trans. Am. Acad. Ophthalmol. Otolaryngol.* 79:899, 1966.
Next to surgery, sinus disease is the most common cause of osteomyelitis of the calvarium.

11. Brandt, K., Cathcart, E. S., and Cohen, A. S. Clinical analysis of the course and prognosis of 42 patients with amyloidosis. *Am. J. Med.* 44:955, 1968.
Secondary amyloidosis can result from chronic osteomyelitis.

12. Sedlin, E. D., and Fleming, J. L. Epidermoid carcinoma arising in the chronic osteomyelitis foci. *J. Bone Joint Surg. [Am.]* 45:827, 1963.

13. Hejna, W. F. Squamous-cell carcinoma developing in the chronic draining sinuses of osteomyelitis. *Cancer* 18:128, 1965.
Tumors can arise in areas involved with chronic osteomyelitis (articles 12, 13).

14. Sapico, F. L., and Montgomerie, J. Z. Pyogenic vertebral osteomyelitis: Report of nine cases and review of the literature. *Rev. Infect. Dis.* 1:754, 1979.
An excellent review; over 50% had symptoms for longer than 3 months before diagnosis and the ESR was consistently elevated. Staphylococcus was the most common organism.

15. Kahn, F. W., Gornick, C. C., and Tofte, R. W. Primary cutaneous *Nocardia asteroides* infection with dissemination. *Am. J. Med.* 70:859, 1981.
Another cause of osteomyelitis.

16. Sapico, F. L., and Montgomerie, J. Z. Vertebral osteomyelitis in intravenous drug abusers: Report of three cases and review of the literature. *Rev. Infect. Dis.* 2:196, 1980.
Here the most common organism was Pseudomonas species.

17. Gathe, J. C., Jr., Harris, R. L., Garland, B., et al. *Candida* osteomyelitis: Report of five cases and review of the literature. *Am. J. Med.* 82:927, 1987.
Usually associated with disseminated candidiasis, the most common site of infection is the lumbar vertebrae.

18. Schlaeffer, F., Mikolich, D. J., and Mates, S. M. Technetium Tc 99m diphosphonate bone scan: False-normal findings in elderly patients with hematogenous vertebral osteomyelitis. *Arch. Intern. Med.* 147:2024, 1987.
This completes the spectrum of false-negatives in infants, children, and adults.

19. Waldvogel, F. A., and Vasey, H. Osteomyelitis: The past decade. *N. Engl. J. Med.* 303:360, 1980.
An effective review and discussion of changing trends in osteomyelitis.

20. McHenry, M. C., Duchesneau, P. M., Keys, T. M., et al. Vertebral osteomyelitis presenting as spinal compression fracture: Six patients with underlying osteoporosis. *Arch. Intern. Med.* 148:417, 1988.
Another presentation of osteomyelitis which merits attention. An unexplained ESR elevation was a clue.

21. Modic, M. T., Feiglan, D. H., Piraino, D. W., et al. Vertebral osteomyelitis: Assessment using MR. *Radiology* 157:157, 1985.
Magnetic resonance can be useful in diagnosis.

22. Bambergen, D. M., Daus, G. P., and Gerding, D. N. Osteomyelitis in the feet of diabetic patients: Long-term results, prognostic factors, and the role of antimicrobial and surgical therapy. *Am. J. Med.* 83:653, 1987.
A concise review. If there is no gangrene or extensive necrosis, antibiotic therapy may be curative.

23. Weinstein, M. P., Stratton, C. W., Hawley, H. B., et al. Multicenter collaborative evaluation of a standardized serum bactericidal test as a predictor of the therapeutic efficacy in acute and chronic osteomyelitis. *Am. J. Med.* 83:218, 1987.
One of the advantages of high-technology medicine. In acute osteomyelitis the serum bactericidal level should be 1:2 or greater, and in chronic 1:4 or greater, for the best results.

24. Gelfand, M. J., and Silberstein, E. B. Radionuclide imaging: Use for diagnosis of osteomyelitis in children. *J.A.M.A.* 237:245, 1977.
About 53% of patients had scan changes before routine x-ray changes.

118. BACTERIAL PNEUMONIA
Jerry L. Spivak

Bacterial pneumonia continues to be a common cause of morbidity and mortality in the antibiotic era. The most frequent offending pathogen is the pneumococcus, which accounts for over 60 percent of bacterial pneumonias; gram-negative organisms have displaced staphylococci as the most common pulmonary invader seen in hospitals. *Haemophilus* is being recognized as a pulmonary pathogen with increasing frequency as is pneumonia due to *Legionella* species. The latter organisms should be considered particularly when pneumonia is associated with gastrointestinal symptoms. In endemic areas, tularemia should always be considered in the differential diagnosis of pulmonary infiltrates.

Bacterial pneumonias arise either from aspiration of infectious material or seeding of the pulmonary parenchyma during bacteremia. The factors responsible for the initiation of bacterial pneumonia via the respiratory route are unclear. With the exception of viral influenza, no other viral respiratory illness has been consistently found to predispose to bacterial pneumonia. For pneumococcal infection, host factors, such as sickle cell disease, alcoholism, chest trauma, and congestive heart failure, are important. Most patients with gram-negative infections have an underlying illness that impairs host defense mechanisms. Such underlying illnesses include chronic pulmonary and renal disease, diabetes mellitus, hematologic malignancies, and chronic alcoholism. Colonization of the oropharynx with gram-negative organisms is a major factor contributing to gram-negative pneumonias in hospitalized patients. With scrupulous attention to decontamination of ventilatory equipment and to aseptic care of endotracheal tubes and tracheotomies, the incidence of nosocomial pneumonia can be reduced.

Determination of the offending agent in bacterial pneumonia is often difficult, particularly in patients with pneumococcal infections and in patients who have been receiving antimicrobial therapy. In the former, the sputum culture is negative in 45 percent of the patients with positive blood cultures. The use of mouse inoculation improves this figure but in close to 20 percent of cases sputum and blood cultures will still be at variance. This is in part due to improper culture techniques (e.g., the hot loop syndrome, delay in transporting the specimen to the laboratory, and failure to sample more than one area of the sputum, since distribution of organisms in sputum is uneven) as well as to inadequate sputum production. The gram-stained sputum smear is also subject to the dangers of heating the slide or inadequate sampling as well as to observer error (e.g., poor staining, confusion of streptococci, staphylococci, and pneumococci). Consequently, the use of the quellung reaction has been advocated to reduce observer error. The finding of gram-positive organisms in the sputum, of course, does not guarantee that they are the causative agents in the pneumonic process. In patients with chronic disease or prior antibiotic therapy, colonization of the sputum with gram-negative organisms can also cause considerable confusion. If the presence of organisms is associated with neutrophils in the sputum, infection rather than colonization is more likely. The chest x ray can also be misleading if dehydration (*Am. J. Roentgenol.* 148:853, 1987) or altered pulmonary anatomy results in atypical patterns of infiltration instead of the expected lobar or segmental consolidation. Occasionally there is considerable disparity between the chest x ray and the physical findings, particularly in staphylococcal pneumonia. Blood cultures are the best single method of defining the identity of the pathogen, although bacteremia is found in less than one-third of cases. A considerable source of confusion occurs when *Haemophilus* or both *Haemophilus* and pneumococci are found in the sputum. Both agents produce a similar clinical picture and both can cause pneumonia in previously healthy persons, but the antibiotic therapy for each differs. The role of transtracheal aspiration in the diagnosis of pneumonia is controversial but is not usually indicated in community-acquired infections and should only be performed by someone skilled in the technique.

In the absence of complicating factors, the pneumococcus is the most common cause of community-acquired pneumonia, and since penicillin is more effective than ampicillin, it seems best to start therapy with penicillin, to follow the clinical course, and to await culture results. It should be emphasized, however, that community-acquired staphylococci are frequently penicillin-resistant, and alternate therapy should be chosen if staphylococci are a consideration clinically. Ampicillin-resistant strains of *Haemophilus influenzae* are also being recognized, but these respond to third-generation cephalosporins. In a seriously ill patient, particularly an elderly one, treatment with a newer cephalosporin and erythromycin should provide coverage of gram-positive and most gram-negative organisms, including *Legionella,* until the actual invading organism is identified. In uncomplicated pneumococcal pneumonia, defervescence can be expected within 48 to 72 hours. Prolonged fever occurs in some patients and may take more than a week to resolve. Prolonged fever can also be due to multilobular involvement, leukopenia, diabetes mellitus, chronic alcoholism, or a suppurative complication, such as empyema, pericarditis, arthritis, meningitis, peritonitis, or endocarditis. The possibility of a drug reaction, incorrect diagnosis, bronchial obstruction, or superinfection must also be considered. In a small percentage of patients, x-ray resolution takes more than 4 weeks. It has been emphasized in the past and again recently that pneumococcal pneumonia is a virulent illness, with most deaths occurring early in the course of the illness and irrespective of the type of therapy employed. This observation applies to the later stages of the illness as well, and altered mental status should never be attributed to fever or alcoholic withdrawal. It is not uncommon in such instances to find pneumococci in the spinal fluid.

Given the variety of pneumococcal serotypes capable of causing infection and the obligate mortality and substantial morbidity of these infections, the development of a vaccine against the pneumococcus was a welcome advance. The vaccine, which now contains the capsular carbohydrate antigens of the 23 pneumococcal serotypes most frequently identified as causing infections in humans, has not proved to be uniformly effective, particularly in immunosuppressed patients or those at high risk of pneumococcal infection by virtue of an underlying illness. Whether the new "23-valent" vaccine will prove more efficient than its "14-valent" predecessor is unclear, but given the obligate mortality of severe pneumococcal infections, its use is recommended in high-risk groups such as asplenic or human immunodeficiency virus (HIV)–positive individuals and those who have previously had a pneumococcal infection. Such patients should also receive influenza vaccine, and both vaccines can be administered simultaneously without untoward reactions or impairment of antibody formation.

1. Shulman, J. A., Phillips, L. A., and Petersdorf, R. G. Errors and hazards in the diagnosis and treatment of bacterial pneumonias. *Ann. Intern. Med.* 62:41, 1965.
   An important review.
2. Verghese, A., and Berk, S. L. Bacterial pneumonia in the elderly. *Medicine* 62:271, 1983.
   All aspects reviewed.
3. Barrett-Connor, E. The nonvalue of sputum culture in the diagnosis of pneumococcal pneumonia. *Am. Rev. Respir. Dis.* 103:845, 1971.
   Sputum culture failed to grow pneumococci in 45% of cases.
4. Austrian, R. Pneumococcal pneumonia. *Chest* 90:738, 1986.
   Advocates the use of pneumococcal vaccine. (See also Ann. Intern. Med. *108:757, 1988.) For invasive pneumococcal infections, see* Rev. Infect. Dis. *7:133, 1985.*
5. Pratter, M. R., and Irwin, R. S. Transtracheal aspiration: Guidelines for safety. *Chest* 76:518, 1979.
   Guidelines for reducing the risks of the procedure.
6. Bartlett, J. G. Diagnostic accuracy of transtracheal aspiration bacteriologic studies. *Am. Rev. Respir. Dis.* 115:777, 1977.
   Only 1% false-negative and 21% false-positive cultures.
7. Merrill, C. W., Gwaltney, J. M., Jr., Hendley, J. O., et al. Rapid identification of pneumococci: Gram stain vs. Quellung reaction. *N. Engl. J. Med.* 288:510, 1973.
   The quellung reaction improves diagnostic accuracy of the Gram's stain.
8. Ziskind, M. M., Schwarz, M. I., George, R. B., et al. Incomplete consolidation in pneumococcal pneumonia complicating pulmonary emphysema. *Ann. Intern. Med.* 72:835, 1970.
   Distorted architecture results in an atypical x-ray pattern.

9. Austrian, R., and Gold, J. Pneumococcal bacteremia with especial reference to bacteremic pneumococcal pneumonia. *Ann. Intern. Med.* 60:759, 1964.
   Early mortality is uninfluenced by the type of therapy employed. (See also J.A.M.A. 249:1055, 1983 and Chest 83:598, 1983.)
10. Pallares, R., Gudiol, F., Linares, J., et al. Risk factors and response to antibiotic therapy in adults with bacteremic pneumonia caused by penicillin-resistant pneumococci. *N. Engl. J. Med.* 317:18, 1987.
   Previous hospitalization, nosocomial pneumonia, and previous antibiotic therapy were identifiable risk factors. (See also Lancet 1:1142, 1988.)
11. Alvarez, S., Guarderas, J., Shell, C. G., et al. Nosocomial pneumococcal bacteremia. *Arch. Intern. Med.* 146:1509, 1986.
   Use of pneumococcal vaccine advocated in debilitated patients. (See also Am. J. Med. 77:1091, 1984.)
12. Yangco, B. G., and Deresinski, S. C. Necrotizing or cavitating pneumonia due to *Streptococcus pneumoniae*: Report of four cases and review of the literature. *Medicine* 59:449, 1980.
   Cavitation is a rare event in pneumococcal pneumonia and probably due to concomitant anaerobic infection (see Am. Rev. Respir. Dis. 129:317, 1984).
13. Taryle, D. A., Potts, D. E., and Sahn, S. A. The incidence and clinical correlates of parapneumonic effusions in pneumococcal pneumonia. *Chest* 74:170, 1978.
   The incidence of effusions correlates with the duration of the pneumonia before therapy.
14. Jay, S. J., Johanson, W. G., Jr., and Pierce, A. K. The radiographic resolution of *Streptococcus pneumoniae* pneumonia. *N. Engl. J. Med.* 293:798, 1975.
   Slow resolution of radiographic abnormalities in bacteremic pneumococcal pneumonia is common.
15. Brewin, A., Arango, L., Hadley, K., et al. High dose penicillin therapy and pneumococcal pneumonia. *J.A.M.A.* 230:409, 1974.
   If there was any doubt about dosage, this article should settle it. There is no need for more than 1.2 million units of procaine penicillin G per day.
16. Levy, M., Dromer, F., Brion, N., et al. Community-acquired pneumonia. *Chest* 93:43, 1988.
   A Gram stain and chest x ray were the best diagnostic tests. (See also Chest 87:631, 1985.)
17. Boerner, D. F., and Zwadyk, P. The value of the sputum gram's stain in community-acquired pneumonia. *J.A.M.A.* 247:642, 1982.
   The Gram-stained sputum smear remains a valuable diagnostic aid. (See also J.A.M.A. 239:2671, 1978.)
18. Helms, C. M., Viner, J. P., Weisenburger, D. D., et al. Sporadic legionnaires' disease: Clinical observations on 87 nosocomial and community-acquired cases. *Am. J. Med. Sci.* 288:2, 1984.
   Legionella pneumonia has a high mortality rate. (See also Medicine 62:120, 1983 and J.A.M.A. 249:3184, 1983.)
19. Crowe, H. M., and Levitz, R. E. Invasive *Haemophilus influenzae* disease in adults. *Arch. Intern. Med.* 147:241, 1987.
   Most organisms were penicillin-sensitive. (See also Ann. Intern. Med. 99:444, 1983.)
20. Hirschmann, J. V., and Everett, E. D. *Haemophilus influenzae* infections in adults: Report of nine cases and a review of the literature. *Medicine* 58:80, 1979.
   Haemophilus pneumonia in adults is being observed with increasing frequency.
21. Levin, D. C., Schwarz, M. I., Matthay, R. A., et al. Bacteremic *Hemophilus influenzae* pneumonia in adults. *Am. J. Med.* 62:219, 1977.
   Pleural involvement was common; the x-ray pattern was not distinctive, and ampicillin was the most effective drug. (See also Am. J. Med. 64:87, 1978.)
22. Bartlett, J. G., O'Keefe, P., Tally, F. P., et al. Bacteriology of hospital-acquired pneumonia. *Arch. Intern. Med.* 146:868, 1986.
   Gram-negative and anaerobic organisms predominated. (See also Rev. Infect. Dis. 7(Suppl. 3):357 and 371, 1985.)

23. Basiliere, J. L., Bistrong, H. W., and Spence, W. F. Streptococcal pneumonia. *Am. J. Med.* 44:580, 1968.
    High incidence of empyema.
24. Pierce, A. K., and Sanford, J. P. Aerobic gram-negative bacillary pneumonias. *Am. Rev. Respir. Dis.* 110:647, 1974.
    A comprehensive review.
25. Manfredi, F., Daly, W. J., and Behnke, R. H. Clinical observations of acute Friedländer pneumonia. *Ann. Intern. Med.* 58:642, 1963.
    Loss of lung volume with tracheal deviation is an important clue.
26. Tillotson, J. R., and Lerner, A. M. Characteristics of pneumonia caused by *Bacillus proteus. Ann. Intern. Med.* 68:287, 1968.
    Proteus produces lobar involvement.
27. Tillotson, J. R., and Lerner, A. M. Characteristics of nonbacteremic pseudomonas pneumonia. *Ann. Intern. Med.* 68:295, 1968.
    A necrotizing bronchopneumonia.
28. Tillotson, J. R., and Lerner, A. M. Bacteroides pneumonia. *Ann. Intern. Med.* 68:308, 1968.
    Empyema is common.
29. Irwin, R. S., Woelk, W. K., and Coudon, W. C., III. Primary meningococcal pneumonia. *Ann. Intern. Med.* 82:493, 1975.
    An unusual cause of pneumonia in healthy persons. (See also Am. J. Med. *62:661, 1977.)*
30. Miller, R. F., and Bates, J. H. Pleuropulmonary tularemia. *Am. Rev. Respir. Dis.* 99:31, 1969.
    Look for the cutaneous ulcer.
31. Mason, W. L., Ergelsbach, H. T., Little, S. F., et al. Treatment of tularemia, including pulmonary tularemia with gentamicin. *Am. Rev. Respir. Dis.* 121:39, 1980.
    Gentamicin found to be an effective antibiotic for the treatment of tularemia. (See also Arch. Intern. Med. *47:265, 1987.)*
32. Karnad, A., Alvarez, S., and Berk, S. L. Pneumonia caused by gram-negative bacilli. *Am. J. Med.* 79:61, 1985.
    Gram-negative pneumonias have a poor prognosis in spite of improvements in antibiotic therapy. (See also Am. J. Med. *70:664, 1981.)*
33. Polsky, B., Gold, J. W., Whimbey, E., et al. Bacterial pneumonia in patients with the acquired immunodeficiency syndrome. *Ann. Intern. Med.* 104:38, 1986.
    These infections can be fulminant. (See Chest *87:486, 1985.)*
34. Rosenon, E. C., III, Wilson, W. R., and Cocherill, F. R., III. Pulmonary disease in the immunocompromised host. *Mayo Clin. Proc.* 60:473, 610, 1985.
    Comprehensive review. (See also J.A.M.A. *253:1769, 1985 and* Medicine *56:241, 1977.)*
35. Hopkin, J. M., Turney, J. H., Young, J. A., et al. Rapid diagnosis of obscure pneumonia in immunosuppressed renal patients by cytology of alveolar lavage fluid. *Lancet* 2:299, 1983.
    Successful use of bronchoalveolar lavage.
36. Winterbauer, R. H., Bedon, G. A., and Ball, W. A., Jr. Recurrent pneumonia: Predisposing illness and clinical patterns in 158 patients. *Ann. Intern. Med.* 70:689, 1969.
    Bronchography is more productive diagnostically than bronchoscopy in patients with recurrent pneumonia.
37. Edelstein, P. H., and Meyer, R. D. Legionnaires' disease. *Chest* 85:114, 1984.
    Brief review.
38. Muder, R. R., Yu, V. L., and Zuravleff, J. J. Pneumonia due to the Pittsburgh pneumonia agent: New clinical perspective with a review of the literature. *Medicine* 62:120, 1983.
    A cause of pneumonia in debilitated patients.
39. Zuravleff, J. J., Yu, V. L., Shonnard, J. W., et al. Diagnosis of legionnaires' disease. *J.A.M.A.* 250:1981, 1983.
    Discussion of the use of cultures, immunofluorescence, and antibodies for diagnosis.

40. Kirby, B. D., Peck, H., and Meyer, R. D. Radiographic features of legionnaires' disease. *Chest* 76:562, 1979.
    Initially, unilateral involvement is common but a variety of abnormalities can be observed. (See also Radiology *127:577, 1978.)*
41. Bartlett, J. G. Anaerobic bacterial infections of the lung. *Chest* 91:901, 1987.
    State-of-the-art review.
42. MacFarlane, J. T. Treatment of lower respiratory infections. *Lancet* 2:1446, 1987.
    Concise review. (See also Am. J. Med. *80:70, 1986 and* Am. J. Med. *79:25, 1985.)*
43. Donowitz, G. R., and Mandell, G. L. Empiric therapy for pneumonia. *Rev. Infect. Dis.* 5:S40, 1983.
    Fitting the antibiotic to the infection. (See also Am. J. Med. *80:70, 1986.)*
44. Donowitz, G. R., and Mandell, G. L. Drug therapy: Beta-lactam antibiotics. *N. Engl. J. Med.* 318:419 and 490, 1988.
    Comprehensive review.
45. Graham, W. G. B., and Bradley, D. A. Efficacy of chest physiotherapy and intermittent positive-pressure breathing [IPPB] in the resolution of pneumonia. *N. Engl. J. Med.* 299:624, 1978.
    Neither physiotherapy nor IPPB hastened resolution of uncomplicated bacterial or mycoplasmal pneumonia.

119. CANDIDIASIS
Jerry L. Spivak

Candida is a saprophytic, dimorphic fungus commonly found on the mucous membranes or in the gastrointestinal tract. Ordinarily not an invasive organism, under certain conditions it becomes a pathogen for its host, often with a serious or fatal result. Factors predisposing to infection with *Candida* include therapy with multiple antibiotics, corticosteroids, x ray, or immunosuppressive agents; bowel disease or bowel surgery; hematopoietic malignancy; uremia; leukopenia; endocrine insufficiency (diabetes mellitus or the syndrome of ectodermal dysplasia and polyendocrinopathy); prolonged use of intravenous or bladder catheters; hyperalimentation; and defective cellular immunity. *Candida* infection can be localized, as in thrush, intertrigonous infection, or the vaginitis seen in pregnancy or diabetes mellitus; or it can be invasive, producing endocarditis or disseminated tissue infection.

Candida endocarditis can be a consequence of treatment for bacterial endocarditis since the latter requires prolonged periods of intravenous therapy with multiple antibiotics. It is also not uncommon in narcotic addicts who repeatedly inject contaminated material (often mixed with toilet water) intravenously. *Candida* endocarditis occurs most often on previously damaged heart valves and has involved prosthetic valves as well. Clinically, the endocarditis behaves similarly to subacute bacterial endocarditis, except that embolization, particularly to large arteries and the mesentery, is more common. The importance of intravenous catheters in compromising host defenses is seen by the ability of *Candida* species other than *C. albicans* to cause endocarditis when indwelling catheters are employed. Such organisms are not otherwise associated with deep tissue infection.

In contrast to endocarditis, with its constant fungemia, embolic phenomena, and indolent course, disseminated candidiasis is a more fulminant disease but one much harder to document. Dissemination is usually associated with fever, clinical deterioration, and azotemia. The site of dissemination, however, is not usually apparent, although it has become evident that gastrointestinal tract candidiasis frequently precedes disseminated infection. Fungi can pass through the intact intestinal wall, and significant esophageal infection can be present without evidence of oral candidiasis. In disseminated infection the kidneys, heart, and lungs are most frequently affected, but hepatic and splenic involvement can also occur. Blood cultures are often negative, but urine cultures are frequently positive. However, since the patients most susceptible to invasion are also most likely to be colonized with the organisms, it is often difficult to determine the significance of a positive urine or sputum culture. The problem is further complicated by the well-documented occurrence of transient candidemia associated with intravenous catheters.

In an effort to arrive at an accurate diagnosis rapidly and to avoid unnecessary administration of amphotericin B, a number of different serologic tests have been employed but none have proved totally reliable, particularly in immunosuppressed patients. A helpful clue is the finding of *Candida* organisms on a blood smear. Success is most likely if the buffy coat is examined. The presence of mycelial forms in the urine or stool is also suggestive of invasive disease. A careful examination of the retina is important since embolic lesions may occur there. In the appropriate setting, the development of a papular skin rash or polymyalgia or arthralgias should suggest disseminated candidiasis. Biopsy of skin lesions or a tender area of muscle is a useful approach for obtaining evidence of fungal invasion early in its course.

In the final analysis the decision to treat may depend on the clinical status of the patient. In the patient recovering from a bacterial infection in whom blood cultures become positive for *Candida,* removal of all catheters, discontinuation of antibiotics, if possible, and careful observation seem reasonable. On the other hand, in the immunocompromised host who is deteriorating or when large masses of *Candida* appear in the urine, amphotericin B therapy should be initiated.

Since disseminated candidiasis is fulminant but difficult to recognize, it seems prudent to place emphasis on prophylaxis. Avoidance of prolonged use of intravenous or bladder catheters is important, but it is equally important to recognize local *Candida* infections and eradicate them. Particular attention should be paid to gastrointestinal candidiasis, and if this cannot be eradicated with oral fungicides, amphotericin B therapy is indicated.

1. Edwards, J. E., Jr., Lehrer, R. I., Stiehm, E. R., et al. Severe candidal infections. *Ann. Intern. Med.* 89:91, 1978.
   An important review.(See also Medicine *41:307, 1962.)*
2. Harvey, R. L., and Myers, J. P. Nosocomial fungemia in a large community teaching hosptial. *Arch. Intern. Med.* 147:2117, 1987.
   The usual predisposing factors were present. (See also Rev. Infect. Dis. *7:646, 1986.)*
3. Thaler, M., Pastakia, B., Shawker, T. H., et al. Hepatic candidiasis in cancer patients: The evolving picture of the syndrome. *Ann. Intern. Med.* 108:88, 1988.
   A complication being seen with increasing frequency. (See also Am. J. Med. *83:17, 1987,* J. Comput. Assist. Tomogr. *11:795, 1987, and* Radiology *166:417, 1988.)*
4. Taschdjian, C. L., Kozinn, P. J., and Toni, E. F. Opportunistic yeast infections with special reference to candidiasis. *Ann. N. Y. Acad. Sci.* 174:606, 1970.
   Review of the differences between colonization and invasion.
5. Kozinn, P. J., Taschdjian, C. L., Goldberg, P. K., et al. Advances in the diagnosis of renal candidiasis. *J. Urol.* 119:184, 1978.
   A colony count of 10,000–15,000/ml in a catheterized urine specimen is suggested as indicating infection.
6. Sandford, G. R., Merz, W. G., Wingard, J. R., et al. The value of fungal surveillance cultures as predictors of systemic fungal infections. *J. Infect. Dis.* 142:503, 1980.
   The incidence of colonization was high; in the absence of colonization systemic fungal infection rarely occurred.
7. Ellis, C. A., and Spivack, M. L. The significance of candidemia. *Ann. Intern. Med.* 67:511, 1967.
   Removal of intravenous catheters may terminate candidemia.
8. Curry, C. R., and Quie, P. G. Fungal septicemia in patients receiving parenteral hyperalimentation. *N. Engl. J. Med.* 285:1221, 1971.
   Tissue invasion occurs in this group of patients.
9. Bodey, G. P., and Luna, M. Skin lesions associated with disseminated candidiasis. *J.A.M.A.* 229:1466, 1974.
   Macronodular lesions beautifully illustrated. (See also Arch. Intern. Med. *146:385, 1986 and* Am. J. Med. *80:679, 1986.)*

10. Jarowski, C. I., Fialk, M. A., Murray, H. W., et al. Fever, rash and muscle tenderness. *Arch. Intern. Med.* 138:544, 1978.
A diagnostic triad is proposed for disseminated candidiasis. For the importance of early biopsy, see Arch. Intern. Med.*138:429, 1978.*

11. Edwards, J. E., Jr., Foos, R. Y., Montgomerie, J. Z., et al. Ocular manifestations of *Candida* septicemia: Review of seventy-six cases of hematogenous *Candida* endophthalmitis. *Medicine* 53:47, 1974.
A not uncommon complication of Candida *septicemia.*

12. Portnoy, J., Wolf, P. L., Webb, M., et al. *Candida* blastospores and pseudohyphae in blood smears. *N. Engl. J. Med.* 285:1010, 1971.
Buffy coat smears as well as peripheral smears can aid in the diagnosis of Candida *septicemia. (See also* J.A.M.A. *260:2926, 1988.)*

13. Glew, R. H., Buckley, H. R., Rosen, H. M., et al. Serologic tests in the diagnosis of septicemic candidiasis. *Am. J. Med.* 64:586, 1978.
Absence of Candida *precipitins correlates with absence of systemic infection. A positive immunodiffusion precipitin reaction does not always correlate with systemic infection. (See also* J. Infect. Dis. *135:349, 1977.)*

14. Wheeler, R. R., Peacock, J. E., Jr., Cruz, J. M., et al. Esophagitis in the immunocompromised host: Role of esophagoscopy in diagnosis. *Rev. Infect. Dis.* 9:88, 1987.
More than one infectious agent can be present. Candida, *in this situation, may be resistant to ketoconazole. (See* Gastroenterology *90:443, 1986.)*

15. Joshi, S. N., Garvin, P. J., and Sunivoo, Y. C. Candidiasis of the duodenum and jejunum. *Gastroenterology* 80:829, 1981.
Aggressive diagnosis and therapy can be curative.

16. Myerowitz, R. L., Pazin, G. J., and Allen, C. M. Disseminated candidiasis. *Am. J. Clin. Pathol.* 68:29, 1977.
Gastrointestinal involvement thought to be the source for disseminated infection, particularly C. tropicalis. *(See* Am. J. Clin. Path. *85:498, 1986.)*

17. Murray, H. W., Fialk, M. A., and Roberts, R. B. *Candida* arthritis: A manifestation of disseminated candidiasis. *Am. J. Med.* 60:587, 1976.
Transient candidemia is not always benign.

18. Gathe, J. C., Jr., Harris, R. L., Garland, B., et al. *Candida* osteomyelitis. Report of five cases and review of the literature. *Am. J. Med.* 82:927, 1987.
This complication can occur in spite of amphotericin B therapy.

19. Rubenstein, E., Noriega, E. R., Simberkoff, M. S., et al. Fungal endocarditis. *Medicine* 54:331, 1975.
Invading species varies with underlying host pathology.

20. Seelig, M. S., Speth, C. P., Kozinn, P. J., et al. Patterns of *Candida* endocarditis following cardiac surgery. *Prog. Cardiovasc. Dis.* 17:125, 1974.
Serologic testing advocated to detect invasion by Candida *early.*

21. Gomes, J. A. C., Calderon, J., Lajam, F., et al. Echocardiographic detection of fungal vegetations in *Candida parapsilosis* endocarditis. *Am. J. Med.* 61:273, 1976.
A simple test that can aid in the early diagnosis of this disorder.

22. Kraus, W. E., Valenstein, P. N., and Corey, G. R. Purulent pericarditis caused by *Candida*: Report of three cases and identification of high-risk populations as an aid to early diagnosis. *Rev. Infect. Dis.* 10:34, 1988.
A rare and frequently unrecognized complication.

23. Masur, H., Rosen, P. P., and Armstrong, D. Pulmonary disease caused by *Candida* species. *Am. J. Med.* 63:914, 1977.
Candida *pneumonia is uncommon. (See also* AJR *138:645, 1982.)*

24. Tennant, F. S., Remmers, A. R., and Perry, J. E. Primary renal candidiasis. *Arch. Intern. Med.* 122:435, 1968.
A complication associated with diabetes mellitus and renal disease. (See also Lancet *2:1000, 1988 and* J. Urol. *139:1245, 1988.)*

25. Bayer, A. S., Edwards, J. E., Jr., and Seidel, J. S. *Candida* meningitis. *Medicine* 55:477, 1976.
Invasion is by either hematogenous dissemination or direct inoculation.

26. Bayer, A. S., Blumenkrantz, M. J., Montgomerie, J. Z., et al. *Candida* peritonitis. *Am. J. Med.* 61:832, 1976.
    A complication of peritoneal dialysis, gastrointestinal perforation, or surgery.
27. Struijk, D. K., Krediet, R. T., Boeschoten, E. W., et al. Antifungal treatment of *Candida* peritonitis in continuous ambulatory peritoneal dialysis patients. *Am. J. Kidney Dis.* 9:66, 1987.
    Intraperitoneal therapy was effective. (But see also Am. J. Kidney Dis. *8:265, 1986 for catheter persistence.)*
28. Dupont, B., and Drouhet, E. Cutaneous, ocular, and osteoarticular candidiasis in heroin addicts: New clinical and therapeutic aspects in 38 patients. *J. Infect. Dis.* 152:577, 1985.
    Metastatic skin lesions were common.
29. Kenney, F. M., and Holliday, M. A. Hypoparathyroidism, moniliasis, Addison's and Hashimoto's disease. *N. Engl. J. Med.* 271:708, 1971.
    A polyendocrine deficiency state commonly complicated by moniliasis.
30. Dwyer, J. M. Chronic mucocutaneous candidiasis. *Annu. Rev. Med.* 32:491, 1981.
    Comprehensive review of an interesting syndrome; the role of iron deficiency remains unexplained.
31. Kirkpatrick, C. H., and Windhorst, D. B. Mucocutaneous candidiasis and thymoma. *Am. J. Med.* 66:939, 1979.
    Acquired mucocutaneous candidiasis may be a clue to the presence of a thymoma.
32. Petersen, E. A., Alling, D. W., and Kirkpatrick, C. H. Treatment of chronic mucocutaneous candidiasis with ketoconazole. *Ann. Intern. Med.* 93:791, 1980.
    Successful control of skin infection was achieved with oral ketoconazole. For the effectiveness of oral clotrimazole in treating oral candidiasis in these patients see N. Engl. J. Med. *299:1201, 1978.*
33. Wingard, J. R., Merz, W. G., and Saral, R. *Candida tropicalis*: A major pathogen in immunocompromised patients. *Ann. Intern. Med.* 91:539, 1979.
    In this series, colonization with C. albicans *was more frequent but infection with* C. tropicalis *was more common.*
34. Medoff, G., and Kobayashi, G. S. Strategies in the treatment of systemic fungal infections. *N. Engl. J. Med.* 302:145, 1980.
    A useful review of antifungal agents and their use.
35. Young, R. C., Bennett, J. E., and Geelhoed, G. W. Fungemia with compromised host resistance. *Ann. Intern. Med.* 80:605, 1974.
    Guidelines on when to treat and when to withhold antifungal therapy.
36. Bindschalder, D., and Bennett, J. E. Pharmacologic guide to the clinical use of amphotericin B. *J. Infect. Dis.* 120:427, 1969.
    Alternate-day therapy is effective.
37. Medoff, G., Dismukes, W. E., Meade, R. H., III, et al. A new therapeutic approach to *Candida* infections. *Arch. Intern. Med.* 130:241, 1972.
    Low-dose amphotericin B therapy suggested, except in the presence of meningitis or endocarditis.
38. Rubenstein, E., Noriega, E. R., Simberkoff, M. S., et al. Tissue penetration of amphotericin B in *Candida* endocarditis. *Chest* 66:376, 1974.
    Amphotericin B does not always penetrate vegetations well.
39. Douglas, J. B., and Healy, D. K. Nephrotoxic effects of amphotericin B, including renal tubular acidosis. *Am. J. Med.* 46:154, 1969.
    Renal tubular acidosis as a complication of amphotericin B therapy.
40. Panhey, G. A., and Daloviso, J. R. Fungemia caused by *Torulopis glabrata*. *Medicine* 52:395, 1973.
    An opportunistic saprophyte that can cause high fever and hypotension.
41. Platenkamp, G. J., Van Duin, A. M., Porsius, J. C., et al. Diagnosis of invasive candidiasis in patients with and without signs of immune deficiency: A comparison of six detection methods in human serum. *J. Clin. Pathol.* 40:1162, 1987.
    For an overview, see Lancet 2:1373, 1986.
42. Lew, M. A. Diagnosis of systemic *Candida* infections. *Annu. Rev. Med.* 40:87, 1989.
    The laboratory provides only limited assistance.

43. Powderly, W. G., Kobayashi, G. S., Herzig, G. P., et al. Amphotericin B–resistant yeast infection in severely immunocompromised patients. *Am. J. Med.* 84:826, 1988. Candida *infections in immunocompromised hosts are frequently resistant to the usual concentrations of amphotericin B achieved in vivo.*
44. Kirkpatrick, C. H. Host factors in defense against fungal infections. *Am. J. Med.* 77:1, 1984.
    Part of a symposium on candidiasis.

120. FEVER OF UNKNOWN ORIGIN
H. Verdain Barnes

Fever, the ancient hallmark of disease, is not completely understood, and its origin may be obscure. Current evidence suggests that most fevers arise from the release of an endogenous pyrogen or from dysfunction of the hypothalamic thermoregulatory center. A variety of stimuli evoke the release of endogenous pyrogenic substances from granulocytes, monocytes, macrophages, and Kupffer's cells. Release of endogenous pyrogen seems to be the common denominator in illnesses other than pheochromocytoma, thyrotoxic crisis, Addisonian crisis, heat stroke, and noninfectious brain disease. The normal person maintains a temperature within fairly narrow limits. The normal oral temperature ranges from 35.8 to 37.3°C (96.5–99.2°F), with a normal diurnal pattern with a low at about 4 A.M. and a high about 4 P.M. The rectal temperature is 0.3 to 0.5°C (0.5–1°F) higher than the oral temperature. An undiagnosed fever that lasts for 10 or more days qualifies as a *fever of unknown origin (FUO)*.

The FUO demands a careful and complete evaluation. In most series the final diagnostic breakdown is infection (in 30–50%), neoplastic diseases (15–31%), collagen-vascular diseases (10–25%), and undiagnosed (5–39%). The need for meticulous history taking and physical examination in these patients cannot be overemphasized. In the history a careful search should be made for exposures to ill family or friends, animals, birds, drugs, or chemicals. A careful review of the patient's past medical history is needed to establish the exact chronology of any illnesses that might be related to the FUO, such as the slowly unfolding natural history of a collagen-vascular disease. In questioning the patient about the fever, careful probing into any suspected precipitating actions or events may provide the diagnostic clue. The areas that require special emphasis in the physical examination are (1) the entire integument, which should be visualized and palpated, (2) the eyes, particularly the fundi, (3) the mouth, with emphasis on the teeth, gums, tongue, and tonsils, (4) the bones, especially the sternum, (5) the muscles, particularly the trapezius and diaphragm, (6) the navel, (7) the testes, and (8) the rectum. Careful auscultation of the heart, liver, and abdomen is essential. In palpating for lymph nodes, emphasis should be placed on the supraclavicular areas since nodes there are easily accessible to biopsy and have a higher diagnostic yeild than do most other easily accessible nodes. Repeated history taking and daily physical examinations are essential until a diagnosis is made.

The most common infection presenting as an FUO is tuberculosis. In this setting the most common sites are the liver, pericardium, peritoneum, abdominal or hilar lymph nodes, and genitourinary tract. Next in frequency is infective endocarditis, followed closely by a variety of abscesses—subdiaphragmatic, liver, biliary tract, and renal. Almost the entire spectrum of infectious disease has been reported to at times present as an FUO.

A variety of malignant tumors can present as an FUO. The most common are hypernephroma, lymphoma, Hodgkin's disease, and (less frequently) leukemia, hepatoma, and carcinoma of the pancreas, stomach, colon, and bone. In the collagen-vascular disease group, systemic lupus erythematosus, rheumatic fever, giant cell arteritis, and periarteritis nodosa are the most common. In recent years drug fevers have come to the fore. Patients with drug-induced fevers often feel well except for the constitutional symptoms related to the hyperpyrexia itself. Theoretically, any drug can produce a hypersensitivity response and/or fever. Drug fever usually develops early in the course of therapy but may occur after months or years of taking the drug. The miscellaneous FUO categories of note are the inflammatory bowel diseases; thrombophlebitis, particularly pelvic, with or without pulmonary embolization; subacute thyroiditis; familial Mediterranean fever with or without amyloidosis; sarcoidosis; and factitious fever. Factitious fever should be considered when the temperature rises above 40.5°C (105°F) in the absence of heat intoxication or hypothalamic dysfunction when constitutional accompaniments of high fever are absent. Finally, it should be remembered that a low-grade physiologic temperature elevation is often seen with strenuous exercise, hot weather, ovulation, and pregnancy.

In general, the height of the temperature elevation and pattern offer no specific diagnostic help, with the possible exceptions of the double quotidian and Pel-Ebstein patterns. No pattern alone can be said to prove or disprove a diagnosis. Laboratory evaluation must be carefully planned to include chemical, radiographic, and isotope scan studies of suspect organ systems. Blood cultures are essential. Biopsy of skin lesions, easily accessible lymph nodes, and the liver may establish the diagnosis. If all such studies are negative, consideration should be given to an exploratory laparotomy or a clinical therapeutic trial. If the abdomen seems clearly to be the focus of the illness, an exploratory laparotomy is in order. If there is no clue as to the primary focus of the disease and the patient's condition is deteriorating, a therapeutic trial is appropriate. Unless the patient's clinical condition prohibits, the therapeutic trial should be aimed at a specific disease process, and the drugs should be given in adequate doses and continued for a predetermined period of time. An exploratory laparotomy or a therapeutic trial should only be performed if the clinical situation demands.

A fever without evidence of major organ system involvement or focus can be watched. An axiom to keep in mind is that most FUO patients have a common disease presenting in an unusual manner rather than a rare disease.

1. Atkins, E., and Bodel, P. Fever. *N. Engl. J. Med.* 286:27, 1972.
   Still a useful review of fever physiology.
2. Petersdorf, R. G., and Beeson, P. B. Fever of unexplained origin: Report on 100 cases. *Medicine* 40:1, 1961.
   A classic article.
3. Sheon, R. P., and Van Ommen, R. A. Fever of obscure origin: Diagnosis and treatment based on a series of sixty cases. *Am. J. Med.* 34:486, 1963.
   Lymph node, liver, and muscle biopsy are likely to be helpful under the conditions defined.
4. Tumulty, P. A. The patient with fever of undetermined origin: A diagnostic challenge. *Johns Hopkins Med. J.* 120:95, 1967.
   A master clinician offers an approach to the FUO. Should be read by all.
5. Bottiger, L. E., Nordenstam, H. H., and Wester, P. O. Disseminated tuberculosis as a cause of fever of obscure origin. *Lancet* 1:19, 1962.
   Skin tests and chest x rays are often negative in this unconquered disease.
6. Rakatansky, H., and Kirsner, J. B. The gastrointestinal tract: An often forgotten source of prolonged fever. *Arch Intern. Med.* 119:321, 1967.
   A common site of pathology leading to an FUO; therefore, a full gastrointestinal evaluation is essential.
7. Rosenberg, M. Chronic subphrenic abscess. *Lancet* 2:379, 1968.
   A problem to be considered in any patient within a year or two of abdominal surgery.
8. Petersdorf, R. G., and Bennett, I. L., Jr. Factitious fever. *Ann. Intern. Med.* 46:1039, 1957.
   Think of this when the complaints are many and the findings are few.
9. Deller, J. J., and Russell, P. K. An analysis of fevers of unknown origin in American soldiers in Vietnam. *Ann. Intern. Med.* 66:1129, 1967.
   An example of how exposure outside the United States changes the differential diagnosis.

10. Dunn, L. J., and Van Voorhis, L. W. Enigmatic fever and pelvic thrombophlebitis. *N. Engl. J. Med.* 276:265, 1967.
   To be considered in females with known or suspected pelvic disease.
11. Nolan, J. P., and Klatskin, G. The fever of sarcoidosis. *Ann. Intern. Med.* 61:455, 1964.
   Do not count sarcoidosis out; fever was prominent in 41% of this series.
12. Reimann, H. A. Caffeinism: A cause of long-continued, low-grade fever. *J.A.M.A.* 202:1105, 1967.
   Think of simple causes too.
13. Hopkins, B. G., Kan, M., and Mende, C. W. Early ^{67}Ga scintigraphy for the localization of abdominal abscesses. *J. Nucl. Med.* 16:990, 1975.
   This technique correctly identified and localized 18 of 20 surgically proven cases.
14. Murray, H. W., Tuazon, C. U., Guerrero, I. C., et al. Urinary temperature: A clue to early diagnosis of factitious fever. *N. Engl. J. Med.* 296:23, 1977.
   Urine temperature is within 1 to 1.5°C (1.8–2.7°F) of simultaneously taken oral temperatures. A simple technique.
15. Murray, H. W., Mann, J. J., Genecin, A., et al. Fever with dissecting aneurysm of the aorta. *Am. J. Med.* 61:140, 1976.
16. Campbell, E. W., Brantly, R., Harrold, M., et al. Angiomyolipoma presenting as fever of unknown origin. *Am. J. Med.* 57:843, 1974.
   Articles 15, 16 report on rare causes of fever to keep in mind.
17. Esposito, A. L., and Gleckman, R. A. Fever of unknown origin in the elderly. *J. Am. Geriatr. Soc.* 26:498, 1978.
   17% had giant cell arteritis and 11% an intraabdominal abscess.
18. Rothman, D. L., Schwartz, S. I., and Adams, J. T. Diagnostic laparotomy for fever of abdominal pain of unknown origin. *Am. J. Surg.* 133:273, 1977.
   The diagnosis was made in 87% of the FUOs and 82% of the abdominal pain patients.
19. Simon, H. B., and Daniels, G. H. Hormonal hyperthermia. *Am. J. Med.* 66:257, 1979.
   The culprits were hyperthyroidism, acute nonsuppurative thyroiditis, primary and secondary hypoadrenal corticism, and pheochromocytoma.
20. Aduan, R. P., Fauci, A. S., and Dale, D. C. Factitious fever and self induced infection: A report of 32 cases and review of the literature. *Ann. Intern. Med.* 90:230, 1979.
   An excellent article on these two perplexing entities and their associated psychologic problems.
21. Esposito, A. L., and Gleckman, R. A. A diagnostic approach to the adult with fever of unknown origin. *Arch. Intern. Med.* 139:575, 1979.
   A well-referenced review.
22. Levinson, S. L., and Barondess, J. A. Occult dental infection as a cause of fever of obscure origin. *Am. J. Med.* 66:463, 1977.
   Periodontal disease should be looked for early in the evaluation of an FUO.
23. Mackowiak, P. A., and LeMoistre, C. F. Drug fever: A critical appraisal of conventional concepts. *Ann. Intern. Med.* 106:728, 1987.
   There was no characteristic fever pattern, a highly variable lag time from drug institution and fever, and only a few with eosinophilia or skin rash.
24. Bodley, G. P. Fungal infection and fever of unknown origin in neutropenic patients. *Am. J. Med.* 80(Suppl. 5C):112, 1986.
   A special subset of FUO patients which require special considerations.
25. Marantz, P. R., Linzer, M., Feiner, C. J., et al. Inability to predict diagnosis in febrile intravenous drug abusers. *Ann. Intern. Med.* 106:823, 1987.
   Another special and unpredictable subset.
26. Semel, J. D. Complex partial status epilepticus presenting as fever of unknown origin. *Arch. Intern. Med.* 147:1571, 1987.
   Another rare cause to keep in mind.

121. HERPES ZOSTER
Jerry L. Spivak

The viruses of the herpes group—herpes simplex, herpes zoster, varicella, Epstein-Barr, and cytomegalovirus—are morphologically similar, contain a double-stranded DNA core, and share a tendency toward latent infection and subsequent reactivation.

Varicella is the result of the initial infection with the varicella-zoster virus. This contagious illness occurs most often in children and has an incubation period of 11 to 22 days. The major manifestation of the disease is a cutaneous vesicular eruption occurring in crops in a centripetal distribution in association with headache, fever, malaise, and pruritus. Characteristically, due to the asynchronous development of the vesicles, lesions in all stages of development are seen in a single area. Steroids, however, can modify the pleomorphic character of the rash. The disease tends to be more severe in adults. Complications include thrombocytopenia, meningoencephalitis, pneumonitis, and secondary bacterial pneumonia.

Herpes zoster is characterized by the development of grouped vesicles on an erythematous base distributed over an area defined by one or more cutaneous dermatomes. Unlike the seasonal pattern of varicella, herpes zoster appears to occur sporadically and its incidence as well as its severity increases with age. The rash is usually preceded by a prodromal period of pain or paresthesia. This interval between pain and rash is presumably due to the time required for the virus to travel from the dorsal root ganglion to the skin. The duration of the rash is proportional to the period during which the vesicles appear. Usually the rash evolves over a period of 6 days and resolves within 5 weeks. The thoracic and upper lumbar ganglia and the ophthalmic division of the trigeminal nerve are most frequently involved. Regional lymphadenopathy and fever may accompany the rash. Occasionally ganglia at different levels are involved simultaneously. Complications include gangrene of the affected area, corneal ulceration, extraocular muscle paralysis, local muscular weakness, phrenic nerve paralysis, the Ramsay Hunt syndrome, meningoencephalitis, postherpetic neuralgia, dissemination, and pneumonia. Headache may signify the presence of spinal fluid pleocytosis, which is most common in patients with cervical root involvement. Meningoencephalitis usually occurs within 3 weeks of the onset of the rash and is of variable severity. Dissemination can occur in normal persons, usually those with cranial nerve or cervical ganglion involvement, but it is most common in patients with altered cellular immune mechanisms. Pneumonia is a complication of disseminated zoster, but pleurisy can occur without x-ray changes or dissemination of the rash.

While the factors responsible for the development of herpes zoster have not been fully defined, the disorder appears to result from reactivation of endogenous, previously acquired varicella virus. Herpes zoster occurs in otherwise healthy individuals and the incidence increases with age; the highest incidence is in immunosuppressed patients, particularly those with Hodgkin's disease in whom predisposing factors include advanced-stage, splenectomy, and impaired delayed hypersensitivity. Dissemination, which may be associated with poor prognosis, occurs most often in patients with advanced Hodgkin's disease and has been correlated with all the factors mentioned above except splenectomy. Corticosteroids do not appear to predispose to zoster but chemotherapy does. This is true also for patients with neoplasms other than Hodgkin's disease. In contrast to varicella, in which virus disappears from the vesicle fluid within 3 days, in herpes zoster the virus persists even in the presence of circulating antibodies. In addition, dissemination can occur in the presence of serum antibodies. Recent studies indicate that a fall in antibody titer does not occur with age and thus cannot account for the increased incidence of herpes zoster in the elderly. Antibodies appear to play some role, however, since lymphoma patients without antibodies to the virus are more prone to the development of herpes zoster than are those with such antibodies. Cellular immunity appears to have an important role since there is a correlation between dissemination and lack of reactivity to dinitrochlorobenzene. Additionally, the high incidence of herpes zoster in advanced Hodgkin's disease supports this contention as well. Recent studies in cancer patients have suggested that impaired cutaneous interferon production may be responsible for the dissemination of the cutaneous infection.

The skin lesions of disseminated herpes zoster and varicella must be distinguished from those caused by herpes simplex, generalized vaccinia, smallpox, aspergillosis, staphylococcal pyoderma, and rickettsial pox. Multinucleated giant cells with intranuclear inclusions in biopsies or vesicle scrapings are characteristic of the herpesviruses, but serologic testing is required to differentiate the various types.

The mortality of herpes zoster in immunosuppressed patients is less than 10 percent, and the illness is usually self-limited. In children under the age of 15 with a congenital or acquired immunodeficiency state, zoster immune globulin, if administered within 96 hours of exposure to varicella or herpes zoster, will prevent or modify infection by the virus. Zoster immune globulin will not prevent dissemination of localized disease in immunosuppressed individuals nor does it alter the course of cutaneous disseminated zoster in immunosuppressed patients. Interferon also appears to be effective in limiting the extent of herpes zoster in patients with cancer (*N. Engl. J. Med.* 298:981, 1978). While cytosine arabinoside, an inhibitor of DNA synthesis, has not been found to be a useful agent for treating infections due to the varicella-zoster virus, adenine arabinoside (vidarabine) and acycloguanosine (acyclovir) are. Both of these agents, which are not without toxic side effects, are effective in immunosuppressed hosts in reducing new lesion formation and dissemination when initiated early during the course of the infection. Acyclovir is the agent of choice.

1. Straus, S. E., Ostrove, J. M., Inchauspe, G., et al. Varicella-zoster virus infections. *Ann. Intern. Med.* 108:221, 1988.
   An important review.
2. Ragozzino, M. W., Melton, I. J., III, Kurland, L. T., et al. Population-based study of herpes zoster and its sequelae. *Medicine* 61:310, 1982.
   Epidemiology of herpes zoster in the community. (See also J.A.M.A. 164:265, 1957.)
3. Gold, E. Serologic and virus-isolation studies of patients with varicella or herpes-zoster infection. *N. Engl. J. Med.* 274:181, 1966.
   Virus persists in the vesicle fluid longer in herpes zoster than in varicella.
4. Merselis, J. G., Kaye, D., and Hook, E. W. Disseminated herpes zoster. *Arch. Intern. Med.* 113:679, 1964.
   Dissemination usually occurs 2 to 10 days after onset of rash.
5. Gallagher, J. G., and Merigan, T. C. Prolonged herpes-zoster infection associated with immunosuppressive therapy. *Ann. Intern. Med.* 91:842, 1979.
   A consequence of aggressive chemotherapy.
6. Armstrong, R. W., Gurwith, M. J., Waddell, D., et al. Cutaneous interferon production in patients with Hodgkin's disease and other cancers infected with varicella or vaccinea. *N. Engl. J. Med.* 283:1182, 1970.
   Dissemination of herpes zoster correlated with impaired production of cutaneous interferon.
7. Gershon, A. A., and Steinberg, S. P. Antibody responses to varicella-zoster virus and the role of antibody in host defense. *Am. J. Med. Sci.* 282:12, 1981.
   Humoral antibodies have little influence on the development or dissemination of herpes zoster.
8. Gershon, A. A., Steinberg, S. P., Gelb, L., et al. Clinical reinfection with varicella-zoster virus. *J. Infect. Dis.* 149:137, 1984.
   Reinfections are usually mild.
9. Atkinson, K., Meyers, J. D., Storb, R., et al. Varicella-zoster virus infection after marrow transplantation for aplastic anemia or leukemia. *Transplantation* 29:47, 1980.
   Varicella-zoster virus infection occurs with a high incidence within the first 12 months after transplant; the mortality in this series was 8%. (See also J. Infect. Dis. 152:1172, 1985.)
10. Rusthoven, J. J., Ahlgren, P., Elhakim, T., et al. Risk factors for varicella zoster disseminated infection among adult cancer patients with localized zoster. *Cancer* 62:1641, 1988.
    Risk of dissemination increased with Hodgkin's and non-Hodgkin's lymphoma and

head and neck cancer. (See also Arch. Intern. Med. *148:1561, 1988 and* Cancer *56:642, 1985.)*

11. Pek, S., and Gikos, P. W. Pneumonia due to herpes zoster. *Ann. Intern. Med.* 62:350, 1965.
    Pneumonia associated with disseminated herpes zoster.
12. Schlossberg, D., and Littman, M. Varicella pneumonia. *Arch. Intern. Med.* 148:1630, 1988.
    This can be a devastating complication in adults. Acyclovir therapy is recommended.
13. Jemsek, J., Greenberg, S. B., Taber, L., et al. Herpes zoster–associated encephalitis: Clinicopathologic report of 12 cases and review of the literature. *Medicine* 62:81, 1983.
    Most patients were elderly, immunosuppressed, and had cutaneous dissemination. Acquired immunodeficiency syndrome (AIDS) can cause a chronic encephalitis. (See Neurology *38:1150, 1988 and* Ann. Neurol. *19:182, 1986.)*
14. Eidelberg, D., Sotrel, A., Horoupian, D. S., et al. Thrombotic cerebral vasculopathy associated with herpes zoster. *Ann. Neurol.* 19:7, 1986.
    Vasculopathy due to direct viral vessel invasion. (See also Arch. Pathol. Lab. Med. *112:173, 1988.)*
15. Buss, D. H., and Schorjy, M. Herpes virus infection of the esophagus and other visceral organs in adults. *Am. J. Med.* 66:457, 1979.
    Esophageal involvement is often asymptomatic. (See also Radiology *14:611, 1981.)*
16. Shanbrom, E., Miller, S., and Haar, H. Herpes zoster in hematologic neoplasias: Some unusual manifestations. *Ann. Intern. Med.* 53:523, 1960.
    Herpes zoster infection causing the Ramsay Hunt syndrome.
17. Patterson, S. D., Larson, E. B., and Corey, L. Atypical generalized zoster with lymphadenitis mimicking lymphoma. *N. Engl. J. Med.* 302:848, 1980.
    An unusual cause of lymphadenopathy.
18. Jellinek, E. H., and Tulloch, W. S. Herpes zoster with dysfunction of bladder and anus. *Lancet* 2:1219, 1976.
    An unusual and reversible complication.
19. Melbye, M., Grossman, R. J., Goedert, J. J., et al. Risk of AIDS after herpes zoster. *Lancet* 1:728, 1987.
    Herpes zoster can be used as a predictor of AIDS. (See also Am. J. Med. *84:1076, 1988.)*
20. Kalman, C. M., and Laskin, O. L. Herpes zoster and zosteriform herpes simplex virus infections in immunocompetent adults. *Am. J. Med.* 81:775, 1986.
    Zosterlike rashes can be caused by herpes simplex.
21. Brunell, P. A., Ross, A., Miller, L. H., et al. Prevention of varicella by zoster immune globulin. *N. Engl. J. Med.* 280:1191, 1969.
    Herpes zoster immune globulin is effective in preventing chickenpox.
22. Stevens, D. A., and Merigan, T. C. Zoster immune globulin prophylaxis of disseminated zoster in compromised hosts: A randomized trial. *Arch. Intern. Med.* 140:52, 1980.
    Zoster immune globulin does not prevent or modify disseminated disease. (See also J.A.M.A. *239:1877, 1978.)*
23. Varicella-zoster immune globulin for the prevention of chickenpox. *Ann. Intern. Med.* 100:859, 1984.
    Guidelines for the use of varicella-zoster immune globulin.
24. Shepp, D. H., Dandliker, P. S., and Meyers, J. D. Treatment of varicella-zoster virus infection in severely immunocompromised patients. *N. Engl. J. Med.* 314:208, 1986.
    Acyclovir was superior to vidarabine in this controlled study. (See also Am. J. Med. *85:68, 1988.)*
25. Dorsky, D. I., and Crumpacker, C. S. Drugs five years later: Acyclovir. *Ann. Intern. Med.* 107:859, 1987.
    A comprehensive review. (See also Arch. Intern. Med. *144:1241, 1984.)*
26. Winston, D. J., Eron, L. J., Pazin, G., et al. Recombinant interferon alpha-2a for treatment of herpes zoster in immunosuppressed patients with cancer. *Am. J. Med.* 85:147, 1988.
    Interferon can modify the severity of herpes zoster.

27. Watson, P. N., and Evans, R. J. Postherpetic neuralgia. A review. *Arch. Neurol.* 43:836, 1986.
   Amitriptyline may be useful. (See also Ann. Neurol. *20:651, 1986.)*
28. Esmann, V., Geil, J. P., Kroon, S., et al. Prednisolone does not prevent post-herpetic neuralgia. *Lancet* 2:126, 1987.
   Neither acyclovir nor corticosteroids prevent the development of neuralgia.
29. Balfour, H. H. Varicella zoster virus infections in immunocompromised hosts. *Am. J. Med.* 85(Suppl. 2A):68, 1988.
   Part of a symposium on antiviral therapy.

122. INFECTIVE ENDOCARDITIS
H. Verdain Barnes

Infective endocarditis (IE) is a disease with protean manifestations that may be subtle or flagrant. Untreated IE means certain death. The clinical spectrum of the disease continues to change, making diagnosis more and more of a challenge. The most common manifestations are nonspecific, with fatigue, malaise, anorexia, myalgias, sweats, weight loss, and fever leading the list. Fever is present in at least 80 to 95 percent of cases. It is most often low grade. It may be persistent, intermittent, or spiking with or without associated chills or chilliness. Most likely to be afebrile are patients who (1) have received antibiotics within 2 weeks of evaluation, (2) have congestive heart failure or uremia, or (3) are taking antipyretics or are on a short course of steroids. A heart murmur, another classic feature of the disease, is absent in about one-third of patients with left heart endocarditis and in about two-thirds of those with right heart disease. Patients in whom the illness is running an acute course are unlikely to have a heart murmur at the time of presentation. A distinct, clinically recognizable change in a preexistent murmur occurs in less than 20 percent. Splenomegaly occurs in about 50 percent of patients with a subacute course and in about 25 percent of patients with an acute course. The skin manifestations include petechiae (20–40% of patients), Osler's nodes, and subungual splinter hemorrhages (10–15%). None of these manifestations are diagnostic. Petechiae are seen in a variety of other infections; Osler's nodes can also be seen in systemic lupus erythematosus and marantic endocarditis, as well as nonendocarditis *Salmonella* and gonococcal infections; and splinter hemorrhages have been reported to occur in up to 66 percent of normal persons. Clubbing of the nails may occur in up to 50 percent of IE patients.

Embolism, a hallmark of IE, usually occurs after the patient is well into the disease course or after 2 to 3 weeks of effective antibiotic therapy. Some form of embolism occurs in 30 to 40 percent in most series. The most common site in left-sided endocarditis is the spleen and in right-sided endocarditis, the lung. In addition, renal, cerebral, retinal, coronary, and small peripheral arteries are not uncommonly involved. Large artery occlusion is seen almost exclusively in fungal endocarditis.

A definite diagnosis is made by histologic evidence of IE at surgery or autopsy or by a positive culture and/or positive organism stain of a valve, vegetation, or peripheral embolus. Von Reyn et al. (1981) define a highly probable diagnosis as including a persistently positive blood culture plus a new regurgitant murmur or predisposing heart disease or vascular embolic phenomenon, or negative or intermittently positive blood culture plus a fever, a new regurgitant murmur, and vascular embolic phenomenon. Because the bacteremia of infective endocarditis is most often continuous, recent data support the use of at least three blood culture sets if the probability of IE is high and at least four culture sets if the probability of IE is high and the potential organism is a common skin contaminant, the patient has received an antibiotic within the previous 2 weeks, or the suspected organism is difficult to grow. The percentage of patients reported to have culture-negative endocarditis ranges from 5 to 28 percent. The three major reasons for negative cultures in infective endocarditis are (1) administration of antibiotics in the recent past, (2) frequent absence of generalized bacteremia in right-sided endocarditis, and (3) poor culture technique or routine media incapable of supporting the growth of vitamin B_6–dependent *Streptococcus viridans*. Appropriate technique requires culturing for anaerobic as well as aerobic organisms, use of penicillinase when appropriate, use of hypertonic culture media for protoplast growth, use of a media that will support the growth of vitamin B_6–dependent organisms, and observation of cultures for at least 3 weeks. Two recently reported methods to improve the diagnosis of staphylococcal IE are the lysis-centrifugation blood culture technique and an immunoassay for *Staphyloccus epidermidis* IgG antibodies or antigens. The latter appears to be useful in separating IE patients from those with non-IE bacteremia. Two-dimensional echocardiography to identify a vegetation is also a useful diagnostic technique which appears to be particularly useful in the diagnosis of culture-negative IE and in predicting the need for surgical valve replacement based on the size of the vegetation.

The white blood cell count may or may not be elevated or shifted to the left. Toxic granulation is common. The erythrocyte sedimentation rate is elevated in about 90 percent of patients, and a positive latex fixation test approaches the same incidence by 6 weeks in untreated patients. Anemia occurs at some point in 50 to 80 percent of patients. Rapidly progressive anemia is seen most often with gonococcal and staphylococcal infection.

The bacteria responsible for infective endocarditis is changing. In most recent unselected series, *Streptococcus* infections continue to dominate, with an increase in enterococcal and *S. bovis* and a decrease in *S. viridans* infections. Staphylococcal endocarditis has increased, particularly in prosthetic heart valve patients and in heroin addicts, as has gram-negative endocarditis. Fungal endocarditis occurs most often in patients undergoing long-term antibiotic or steroid therapy, in heroin addicts, and in prosthetic heart valve patients. The most frequent aerobic gram-negative organism is *Escherichia coli;* the most common anaerobic organism is *Bacteroides* sp. Although staphylococcal, enterococcal, or gonococcal endocarditis is usually invasive and destructive, it may also run a prolonged and indolent course.

The prognosis in appropriately treated cases depends on the age of the patient, the duration of the illness before treatment, the infecting organism, the presence or absence of associated chronic disease, and the extent of valve damage. In general, the mortality increases with age, apparently because of the increased incidence of other serious underlying diseases. With a subacute course, about 90 percent of patients survive if therapy is initiated within 2 weeks, whereas after a delay of 2 months or more, only about 75 percent survive. With an acute course, even with prompt initiation of antibiotics, the mortality is high. Mortality is highest with staphylococcal, enterococcal, gram-negative, and fungal disease.

Intractable cardiac decompensation is a consequence of extensive valve damage, valve perforation, ruptured chordae tendineae, torn cusps, or marked valve deformity after healing. The major complications of infective endocarditis (other than heart failure) are myocarditis or myocardial abscesses, focal or diffuse immune complex glomerulonephritis with associated renal failure, embolic phenomena, and mycotic aneurysms. Septic embolization may result in brain, lung, joint, liver, and splenic abscesses. Mycotic aneurysms occur due to an occlusion of the vasa vasorum and tend to rupture late in the course of the disease. These aneurysms most often involve the cerebral arteries but can involve the abdominal aorta and splenic and coronary arteries.

The possibility of IE must be considered in patients who have *unexplained* fevers for longer than 2 weeks, anemia, septic arthritis, nephritis, intracranial hemorrhage, meningitis, pleuritis, pneumonitis, optic neuritis, lung abscess, brain abscess, sudden peripheral arterial occlusion, focal costovertebral or left upper quadrant abdominal pain, congestive heart failure, or signs of focal cerebral damage. Patients at an increased risk of developing IE are those with valve deformity (congenital or acquired) such as a bicuspid aortic valve, mitral valve prolapse (particularly males and those with a distinct murmur), degenerative disease of the aortic or mitral valve, rheumatic heart disease, compromised immune status such as patients on therapeutic steroids or with acquired immunodeficiency syndrome (AIDS), and intravenous drug abusers ranging from heroin to cocaine.

1. Lerner, P. I., and Weinstein, L. Infective endocarditis in the antibiotic era. *N. Engl. J. Med.* 274:199, 259, 323, 388, 1966.
   A superb, well-referenced review.
2. Blumenthal, S., Griffiths, S. P., and Morgan, B. C. Bacterial endocarditis in children with heart disease. *Pediatrics* 26:993, 1960.
   Bacterial endocarditis can occur in all varieties of congenital heart disease in adolescents, children, and infants.
3. Cooper, E. S., Cooper, J. W., and Schnabel, T. G., Jr. Pitfalls in the diagnosis of bacterial endocarditis. *Arch. Intern. Med.* 118:55, 1966.
   The pitfalls include prominent unrelated disease, no heart murmur or embolic phenomenon, and lack of familiarity with the protean manifestations and complications of endocarditis.
4. Kilpatrick, Z. M., Greenberg, P. A., and Samford, J. P. Splinter hemorrhages: Their clinical significance. *Arch. Intern. Med.* 115:730, 1965.
   As high as 60% of normal persons have splinter hemorrhages.
5. Alpert, J. S., Krous, H. F., Dalen, J. E., et al. Pathogenesis of Osler's nodes. *Ann. Intern. Med.* 85:471, 1976.
   Most Osler's nodes are due to septic microemboli.
6. Jones, H. R., Jr., Sieker, R. G., and Geraci, J. E. Neurologic manifestations of bacterial endocarditis. *Ann. Intern. Med.* 71:21, 1969.
   60% had a neurologic chief complaint or major component; of those, 50% had cerebrovascular lesions.
7. Perez, G. O., Rothfield, N., and Williams, R. C. Immune-complex nephritis in bacterial endocarditis. *Arch. Intern. Med.* 136:334, 1976.
   IgM and C3 were found in all glomeruli studied.
8. Felner, J. M., and Dowell, V. R., Jr. Anaerobic bacterial endocarditis. *N. Engl. J. Med.* 283:1188, 1970.
   Bacteroides *species are most common.*
9. Nastro, L. J., and Finegold, S. M. Endocarditis due to anaerobic gram-negative bacilli. *Am. J. Med.* 54:482, 1973.
   Major embolization in 67%.
10. Mandell, G. L., Kaye, D., Levison, M. E., et al. Enterococcal endocarditis: An analysis of 38 patients observed at the New York Hospital-Cornell Medical Center. *Arch. Intern. Med.* 125:258, 1970.
    The most common associated conditions were genitourinary tract infection, antecedent childbirth, or abortion.
11. Tumulty, P. A. Management of bacterial endocarditis. *Geriatrics* 22:122, 1967.
    Endocarditis caused by Staphylococcus aureus, Streptococcus fecalis, *or gonococci may run an indolent course.*
12. Rosen, P., and Armstrong, D. Nonbacterial thrombotic endocarditis in patients with malignant neoplastic diseases. *Am. J. Med.* 54:23, 1973.
    A cause of noninfectious endocarditis that must be kept in mind.
13. Wilson, W. R., Jaumin, P. M., Danielson, G. K., et al. Prosthetic valve endocarditis. *Ann. Intern. Med.* 82:751, 1975.
    The most common early postoperative organism was Staphylococcus aureus; *for late onset it was* Streptococcus viridans.
14. Rubinstein, E., Noriega, E. R., Simberkoff, M. S., et al. Fungal endocarditis: Analysis of 24 cases and review of the literature. *Medicine* 54:331, 1975.
    Candida *was most common in narcotic addicts and in patients with long-term intravenous lines or antibiotic therapy, whereas* Aspergillus *was common after cardiovascular surgery.*
15. Vergue, R., Selland, B., Gobel, F. L., et al. Rupture of the spleen in infective endocarditis. *Arch. Intern. Med.* 135:1265, 1975.
16. Pfeifer, J. F., Lipton, M. J., Oury, J. H., et al. Acute coronary embolism complicating bacterial endocarditis: Operative treatment. *Am. J. Cardiol.* 37:920, 1976.
    Two rare but important complications of IE (articles 15 and 16).
17. Von Reyn, C. F., Levy, B. S., Arbeit, R. D., et al. Infective endocarditis: An analysis based on strict case definitions. *Ann. Intern. Med.* 94:505, 1981.

Useful clinical definitions of definite, probable, and possible IE, plus a good review of clinical manifestations.

18. Chun, C. H., Raff, M. J., Contreras, L., et al. Splenic abscess. *Medicine* 59:50, 1980.
    A rare entity, most often resulting from IE.

19. Pesanti, E. L., and Smith, I. M. Infective endocarditis with negative blood cultures: Analysis of 52 cases. *Am. J. Med.* 66:43, 1979.
    An important article that should be read.

20. Kerr, A., Jr., and Tan, J. S. Biopsies of the Janeway lesion of infective endocarditis. *J. Cutan. Pathol.* 6:124, 1979.
    These lesions are from bacterial emboli and local suppuration.

21. Reymann, M. T., Holley, H. P., Jr., and Cobbs, C. G. Persistent bacteremia in staphylococcal endocarditis. *Am. J. Med.* 65:729, 1978.
    Persistent bacteremia usually signifies abscess formation.

22. Weinberg, M. S., Ellis, C. A., and Levy, S. B. Nutritionally deficient streptococcus: Investigation of the hidden culprit in culture-negative endocarditis. *South. Med. J.* 73:1647, 1980.
    An important group of organisms to keep in mind; some are vitamin B_6–dependent.

23. Wilson, W. R. (ed.). Symposium on infective endocarditis. *Mayo Clin. Proc.* 57:3, 81, 145, 1982.
    An up-to-date symposium covering the key aspects of infective endocarditis.

24. Devereux, R. B., Hawkins, I., Kramer-Fox, R., et al. Complications of mitral valve prolapse: Disproportionate occurrence in men and older patients. *Am. J. Med.* 81:751, 1986.
    Men and those with a murmur are at the greatest risk for developing IE.

25. McKinsey, D. S., Ratts, T. E., and Bisno, A. L. Underlying cardiac lesions in adults with infective endocarditis: The changing spectrum. *Am. J. Med.* 82:681, 1987.
    The underlying lesions were mitral valve prolapse (29%), degenerative valve lesions (21%), congenital heart disease (13%), rheumatic heart disease (6%), and the remaining had no identifiable heart lesion.

26. Bayer, A. S., Lam, K., Ginzton, L., et al. *Staphylococcus aureus* bacteremia: Clinical, serologic, and echocardiographic findings in patients with and without endocarditis. *Arch. Intern. Med.* 147:457, 1987.

27. Chambers, H. F., Korzeniowski, O. M., Sande, M. A., et al. *Staphylococcus aureus* endocarditis: Clinical manifestations in addicts and non-addicts. *Medicine* 62:170, 1983.

28. Espersen, F., and Frimodt-Moller, N. *Staphylococcus aureus* endocarditis: A review of 119 cases. *Arch. Intern. Med.* 146:1118, 1986.
    Three key articles (26–28) on staphyloccal IE.

29. Robbins, M. J., Frater, R. W. M., Soeiro, R., et al. Influence of vegetation size on clinical outcome of right-sided infective endocarditis. *Am. J. Med.* 80:165, 1986.

30. Tape, T. G., and Panzer, R. J. Echocardiography, endocarditis, and clinical information bias. *J. Gen. Intern. Med.* 1:300, 1986.

31. Espersen, F., Wheat, J., Bemis, A. T., et al. Solid-phase radioimmunoassay of IgG antibodies to *Staphyloccus epidermidis:* Use in serious coagulase-negative staphyloccal infections. *Arch. Intern. Med.* 147:689, 1987.

32. Aronson, M. D., and Bor, D. H. Blood cultures. *Ann. Intern. Med.* 106:246, 1987.

33. Walker, R. C., Henry, N. K., Washington, J. A., II, et al. Lysis-centrifugation blood culture technique: Clinical impact in *Staphylococcus aureus* bacteremia. *Arch. Intern. Med.* 146:2341, 1986.
    These articles (29–33) discuss the current status of selected diagnostic modalities.

34. Chambers, H. F., Morris, D. L., Tauber, M. G., et al. Cocaine use and the risk for endocarditis in intravenous drug users. *Ann. Intern. Med.* 106:833, 1987.
    Another risk factor to keep in mind.

35. Griffin, M. R., Wilson, W. R., Edwards, W. D., et al. Infective endocarditis. *J.A.M.A.* 254:1199, 1985.
    Total rate from 1970–1981 was 3.9. The 60-day fatality rate is declining.

36. Cantrell, M., and Yoshikawa, T. T. Infective endocarditis in the aging patient. *Gerontology* 30:316, 1984.
    A concise, well-referenced review.

37. Williams, R. C. Jr., and Kirkpatrick, K. Immunofluorescence studies of the cardiac valves in infective endocarditis. *Arch. Intern. Med.* 145:297, 1985.
38. Sullam, P. M., Drake, T. A., and Sande, M. A. Pathogenesis of endocarditis. *Am. J. Med.* 78(Suppl. 6B):110, 1985.
    Two articles (37, 38) updating the pathogenesis of IE.
39. Weinstein, M. P., Stratton, C. W., Ackley, A., et al. Multicenter collaborative evaluation of a standardized serum bactericidal test as a prognostic indicator in infective endocarditis. *Am. J. Med.* 78:262, 1985.
    A peak bactericidal titer of 1:64 and a trough titer of 1:32 or more are recommended for optimal medical therapy.
40. Kaye, D. Prophylaxis for infective endocarditis: An update. *Ann. Intern. Med.* 104:419, 1986.
    Current strategy for prophylaxis.
41. Douglas, A., Moore-Gillon, M., and Eykyn, S. Fever during treatment of infective endocarditis. *Lancet* 1:1341, 1986.
    Usually a bad omen.

123. INFECTIOUS MONONUCLEOSIS
H. Verdain Barnes

Infectious mononucleosis (IM) is a lymphoproliferative disease that may involve any age group although about 60 percent of cases occur in persons between ages 15 and 24 years. The etiologic agent is the Epstein-Barr virus (EBV) of the herpes group. Initially the virus infects the pharyngeal epithelial cells and then spreads to the subepithelial cells and B lymphocytes, all of which have EBV receptors. The result is about 1 percent of B lymphocytes being infected and stimulated to proliferate and secrete immunoglobulins, primarily IgM. Typically, there is an associated activation of the suppressor T cells which inhibit further B cell activation as well as activated T lymphocytes and natural killer cells which appear to be cytotoxic to the EBV-infected B lymphocyte. There are at least two antigens (M and K) located on the EBV nucleus to which antibodies can be generated. K antigen antibodies are typical both with and without M antigen antibodies. Some patients with chronic EBV disease have only M antigen antibodies.

Clinically there are at least four potential components of the disease. The prodromal phase lasts from 3 to 7 days and usually consists of malaise, fever, and a mild pharyngitis or tonsillitis. It is followed by a 4- to 30-day phase of active disease (discussed below). Convalescence, the final phase, may last from 2 weeks to 28 months. Brief recrudescences are not uncommon during this period. During convalescence patients progressively regain their strength and sense of well-being. The final component, "chronic EBV disease," remains controversial. These patients can be divided into a small group with specific lymphoproliferative, hypoplastic, or other immune deficiency disorders and a larger group with what has been termed a "chronic fatigue syndrome." During the prodrome and active disease phases, most series report sore throat in about 85 percent of patients, feverishness and chilliness in 77 percent, malaise in 70 percent, headache in 52 percent, myalgias in 46 percent, daytime and/or nighttime sweats in 18 percent, and cough and chest pain in 2 percent.

The predominant signs of the disease include lymphadenopathy and fever (over 95% of patients), pharyngeal and tonsillar inflammation (in about 90%), splenomegaly (over 50%), hepatomegaly (50%), palatal enanthema (about 42%), periorbital and eyelid edema (36%), tonsillar exudate (33%), jaundice (4%), and rash and neurologic manifestations (2%). The fever is often irregular, with peaks in the 39.4 to 40°C (103–104°F) range. Fever persists for over a week in about 90 percent and longer than 2 weeks in about 50 percent. Fever typically returns during recrudescences and may last as long as a week. In general, the lymphadenopathy is bilateral and nontender. Posterior cervical nodes are the most often involved. Histologically enlarged lymph nodes show follicular hyperplasia with a blurred appearance due to lymphocytic proliferation in the medullary cords. Perivascular aggregates of normal or atypical lymphocytes are common.

Laboratory findings are variable. The white blood cell count may range from leukopenia to marked leukocytosis with 80 percent of patients having white cell counts between 6000 and 15,000 per microliter. Initially there may be a shift to the left of the granulocytes with an ultimate change to a moderate to marked lymphocytosis and a predominance of atypical lymphocytes. This lymphocytosis is primarily due to an increase in the T cell subset of lymphocytes. Atypical lymphocytes usually begin to appear about 2 days into the disease and peak between the seventh and tenth days. On occasion, however, atypical lymphocytes may not appear until the second week of the illness. Atypical lymphocytes frequently constitute over 20 percent of the differential count. It should be noted, however, that atypical lymphocytosis can be seen in diseases other than IM. Anemia is rare. The serum immunoglobulins IgG, IgM, and IgA increase during the disease. IgA and IgM reach a peak in about 7 days, whereas the IgG peak occurs somewhat later. Cold agglutinins and latex fixation tests may be transiently positive. A biologic false-positive VDRL test for syphilis may rarely occur. Liver enzyme elevations are seen in over 70 percent. The diagnosis of IM is confirmed by a rise in the heterophile titer. The heterophile antibody is absorbed by beef but not by guinea pig kidney antigens, whereas in serum sickness the antibody is absorbed by guinea pig kidney. A presumptive diagnosis of current or recent IM can be made if the heterophile titer is 1:160 or greater, with or without a demonstrable rise. More sophisticated and specific serologic testing by an immunofluorescent or an enzyme-linked immunoassay is readily available. Antibody titers to anti-EBNA (latent infection), anti-EA (early replication), or anti-VCA (late replication) are useful in staging the disease. In acute primary IM the anti-EA and IgM anti-VCA titers are high while IgG anti-VAC and anti-EBNA titers are low or absent. In convalescent patients these titer levels are reversed. The latter titers may persist for years. Serologic diagnosis may be atypical in immunosuppressed or deficient patients such as those with acquired immunodeficiency syndrome (AIDS) or X-linked immune deficiency. It is of note that patients with cytomegalovirus (CMV) infectious mononucleosis-like disease show no cross reactivity with the test for antibodies to EBV capsid antigens (IgM-VCA), whereas patients with EBV-IM often cross-react with the anti-CMV (IgM-CMV) test.

Signs and symptoms related to a specific system may rarely dominate the picture. The most common nervous system manifestations are aseptic meningitis or encephalitis. Cranial nerve paralysis, transverse myelitis, anterior horn cell disease, and Guillain-Barré syndrome have been reported. Cardiovascular manifestations include pericarditis, epicarditis, and/or an arteritis. Pulmonary manifestations are uncommon. Pulmonary infiltrates or pleural effusions have been reported, usually in the presence of significant hilar adenopathy. Hepatitis and pancreatitis with or without ascites have been recorded. Some degree of hepatitis is common. Hematologically a severe hemolytic anemia or thrombocytopenia may be seen on a rare occasion. Glomerulitis and orchitis are rare manifestations. Splenic rupture and hemorrhage can be life-threatening but occur in less than 0.5 percent. The most common skin manifestation is a maculopapular erythematous eruption. Urticaria and vesicular lesions may occur, but are rare.

Fortunately, death is rare, but it can occur with complications such as splenic rupture, respiratory paralysis, overwhelming septicemia, hemorrhage from deep tonsillar ulcers, or upper airway obstruction due to edema of the glottis. The most lethal acute complication is the virus-associated hemophagocytic syndrome. Several viruses are known to cause infectious mononucleosis–like illnesses and should be differentiated from true IM. Those reported include CMV, rubella, adenoviruses, hepatitis virus, AIDS, and *toxoplasma gondii*.

1. Bernstein, A. Infectious mononucleosis. *Medicine* 19:85, 1940.
   A classic.
2. Henle, W., and Henle, G. Epstein-Barr virus and infectious mononucleosis. *N. Engl. J. Med.* 288:263, 1973.
   EBV is the culprit.

3. Sawyer, R. N., Evans, A. S., Niederman, J. C., et al. Prospective studies of a group of Yale University freshmen: I. Occurrence of infectious mononucleosis. *J. Infect. Dis.* 123:263, 1971.
   51% of entering freshmen had a positive EBV antibody titer. 13% became positive within 9 months.

4. Allansmith, M., and Bergstresser, P. Sequence of immunoglobulin changes resulting from an attack of infectious mononucleosis. *Am. J. Med.* 44:124, 1968.
   IgM and IgA rise early and IgG later.

5. Kilpatrick, Z. M. Structural and functional abnormalities of liver in infectious mononucleosis. *Arch. Intern. Med.* 117:47, 1966.
   Sinusoidal infiltration by mononuclear cells is commonly seen.

6. Gelb, D., West, M., and Zimmerman, H. J. Serum enzymes in disease: Analysis of factors responsible for elevated values in infectious mononucleosis. *Am. J. Med.* 33:279, 1962.
   AST(SGOT), ALT(SGPT), and alkaline phosphatase are elevated in about 80% of patients.

7. Bernstein, T. C., and Wolff, H. G. Involvement of the nervous system in infectious mononucleosis. *Ann. Intern. Med.* 33:1120, 1950.
   Aseptic meningitis and encephalitis are most common.

8. Eaton, O. M., Stevens, H., and Silver, H. M. Respiratory failure in polyradiculoneuritis associated with infectious mononucleosis. *J.A.M.A.* 194:609, 1965.
   Guillain-Barré syndrome in IM.

9. Fekete, A. M., and Kerpelman, E. J. Acute hemolytic anemia complicating infectious mononucleosis. *J.A.M.A.* 194:1326, 1965.
   Hemolysis is probably autoimmune.

10. McCarthy, J. T., and Hoagland, R. J. Cutaneous manifestations of infectious mononucleosis. *J.A.M.A.* 209:153, 1969.
    The rash is usually erythematous and maculopapular.

11. Wislocki, L. C. Acute pancreatitis in infectious mononucleosis. *N. Engl. J. Med.* 275:322, 1966.
    A rare but important complication.

12. Jondal, M., and Klein, G. Surface markers on human B and T lymphocytes: II. Presence of Epstein-Barr virus receptors on B lymphocytes. *J. Exp. Med.* 138:1365, 1973.
    The EBV attacks only the B lymphocyte.

13. Pattengale, P. K., Smith, R. W., and Perlin, E. Atypical lymphocytes in acute infectious mononucleosis. *N. Engl. J. Med.* 291:1145, 1974.
    The overwhelming majority of atypical lymphocytes are T lymphocytes.

14. Royston, I., Sullivan, J. L., Periman, P. O., et al. Cell-mediated immunity to Epstein-Barr virus transformed lymphoblastoid cells in acute infectious mononucleosis. *N. Engl. J. Med.* 293:1159, 1975.
    Acute phase lymphocytes are cytotoxic against EBV-infected cells.

15. Niederman, J. C., Miller, G., Pearson, H. A., et al. Infectious mononucleosis: Epstein-Barr virus shedding in saliva and the oropharynx. *N. Engl. J. Med.* 294:1355, 1976.
    Kissing can do it.

16. Horwitz, C. A., Henle, W., Henle, G., et al. Heterophile-negative infectious mononucleosis and mononucleosislike illnesses: Laboratory confirmation of 43 cases. *Am. J. Med.* 63:947, 1977.
    CMV accounted for 30 of the cases, 7 had EBV infections, 1 each had rubella and toxoplasmosis, and the remainder were unidentified. EBV patients often cross-reacted in the IgM-CMV test, but the CMV patients did not cross-react with the IgM-VCA test.

17. Carter, J. W., Edson, R. S., and Kennedy, C. C. Infectious mononucleosis in the older patient. *Mayo Clin. Proc.* 53:146, 1978.
    After age 60 the clinical picture is often nonspecific and may mimic chronic lymphocytic leukemia or present as a fever of unknown origin.

18. Tosato, G., Magarth, I., Koski, I., et al. Activation of suppressor T-cells during Epstein-Barr virus-induced infectious mononucleosis. *N. Engl. J. Med.* 301:1133, 1979.
    A unique host defense mechanism in IM.

19. Dagan, R., and Powell, K. R. Postanginal sepsis following infectious mononucleosis. *Arch. Intern. Med.* 147:1581, 1987.
20. Whittingham, S., McNeilage, J., and Mackay, I. R. Primary Sjögren's syndrome after infectious mononucleosis. *Ann. Intern. Med.* 102:490, 1985.
21. Fuhrman, S. A., Gill, R., Horowitz, C. A., et al. Marked hyperbilirubinemia in infectious mononucleosis: Analysis of the laboratory data in seven patients. *Arch. Intern. Med.* 147:850, 1987.
22. Guilleminault, C., and Mondini, S. Mononucleosis and chronic daytime sleepiness: A long term follow-up study. *Arch. Intern. Med.* 146:1333, 1986.
    These articles (19–22) describe some of the ever-increasing number of associations or complications of IM.
23. Sullivan, J. L., Woda, B. A., Herrod, H. G., et al. Epstein-Barr virus associated hemophagocytic syndrome: Virologic and immunopathologic studies. *Blood* 65:1097, 1985.
24. Mroczek, E. C., Weisenburger, D. D., Grierson, H. L., et al. Fatal infectious mononucleosis and virus associated hemophagocytic syndrome. *Arch. Pathol. Lab. Med.* 111:530, 1987.
    A deadly complication (articles 23, 24).
25. Jones, J. F., Ray, G., Minnich, L. L., et al. Evidence for active Epstein-Barr virus infection in patients with persistent unexplained illnesses: Elevated anti-early antigen antibodies. *Ann. Intern. Med.* 102:1, 1985.
26. Straus, S. E., Tosato, G., Armstrong, G., et al. Persisting illness and fatigue in adults with evidence of Epstein-Barr virus infection. *Ann. Intern. Med.* 102:7, 1985.
27. Miller, G., Grogan, E., Fischer, D. K., et al. Antibody responses to two Epstein-Barr virus nuclear antigens defined by gene transfer. *N. Engl. J. Med.* 312:750, 1985.
28. Schooley, R. T., Carey, R. W., Miller, G., et al. Chronic Epstein-Barr virus infection associated with fever and interstitial pneumonitis. *Ann. Intern. Med.* 104:636, 1986.
    Although still controversial, the evidence favors a chronic EBV disease with a myriad of potential manifestations (articles 25–28).
29. Sixbey, J. M., Nedrud, J. C., Raab-Traub, N., et al. Epstein-Barr virus replication in oropharyngeal epithelial cells. *N. Engl. J. Med.* 310:1225, 1984.
    These cells have an EBV receptor.
30. Horwitz, C. A., Henle, W., Henle, G., et al. Clinical and laboratory evaluation of cytomegalovirus-induced mononucleosis in previously healthy individuals. *Medicine* 65:124, 1986.
    A good review of this IM look-alike.
31. Birx, D. L., Redfield, R. R., and Tosato, G. Defective regulation of Epstein-Barr virus infection in patients with acquired immunodeficiency syndrome (AIDS) or AIDS-related disorders. *N. Engl. J. Med.* 314:874, 1986.
    These patients have a marked defect in T cell immunity to EBV as well as large numbers of EBV-infected B cells.

124. LISTERIOSIS
Jerry L. Spivak

Listeria monocytogenes is a gram-positive motile rod, capable of partial hemolysis, that usually grows well on conventional media. Because of its similarity to diphtheroids, it is often mistaken for these organisms; and due to changes in morphology and staining characteristics during growth in culture, it can be confused with *Haemophilus influenzae* as well. *Listeria* is a facultative intracellular parasite, a characteristic it shares with mycobacteria, fungi, *Toxoplasma, Salmonella,* and *Brucella.* It is found in sewage, soil, mammals, fowl, and man, but only rarely has either a source or a portal of entry for a human *Listeria* infection been identified. Since excellent documentation has been obtained recently that contamination of dairy products by the organism was responsible for several epidemics of listeriosis, it is possible that many ostensibly "sporadic" cases of listeriosis may be due to foodborne transmission.

Clinical syndromes caused by *Listeria* include neonatal granulomatosis, bacteremia, endocarditis, conjunctivitis, septic arthritis, peritonitis, and meningitis. Meningitis is the most common of these and is the most severe form of infection in the adult. Rarely a mononucleosis-like syndrome has been observed, and in pregnancy a mild infection may be associated with severe disease in the fetus. Factors predisposing to listeriosis include extremes of age, lymphoreticular neoplasms, diabetes mellitus, chronic alcoholism, pregnancy, hemodialysis, underlying cardiac disease, and therapy with corticosteroids or radiation. Recently, splenectomy has been associated with an increased susceptibility to *Listeria* infection. Furthermore, as might be expected with such an opportunistic organism, listeria infections have been documented in acquired immunodeficiency syndrome (AIDS) patients.

Infection with *Listeria* initially elicits a neutrophilic response followed by an increase in monocytes. Intracellular multiplication of the organism is followed in several days by an increase in monocyte bactericidal activity. This is associated with the development of delayed hypersensitivity to the organism. The ability of macrophages to kill *Listeria* is dependent on the presence of immunocompetent T lymphocytes that are capable of simulating hypersensitivity and resistance to the organism. Humoral factors are unimportant in this regard. Conditions that impair lymphocyte multiplication (and subsequent macrophage activation) increase susceptibility to *Listeria* (as well as to other organisms, such as *Brucella, Salmonella,* and fungi).

Clinically, there is little to distinguish listeriosis from other infections. Most commonly the onset is sudden, with fever as the major manifestation. When meningitis is present, neurologic signs develop quickly, with altered mental consciousness, seizures, fasciculations, ataxia, tremors, and hemiparesis. Bacteremia is usually accompanied by fever or chills. Granulocytosis is not uncommon, and in patients with lymphomas, lymphopenia is the rule. Monocytosis seems to be more characteristic of the rabbit than man. The cerebrospinal fluid findings are variable in terms of cell count and differential, with either neutrophils or mononuclear cells predominating. Cerebrospinal fluid protein content is usually high and the glucose content often normal; low glucose levels are associated with a poor prognosis. The diagnosis of listeriosis will not be missed if the possibility is considered in every situation in which fever develops in an immunosuppressed host. The difficulty in distinguishing *Listeria* meningitis from tuberculous meningitis must also be kept in mind.

Listeria is usually sensitive to penicillin, ampicillin, cephalexin, tetracycline, erythromycin, and chloramphenicol, and resistant to oxacillin, lincomycin, and colistin. Individual strains vary in their susceptibility but usually require more penicillin for a "cidal" effect than do pyogenic gram-positive organisms. Tetracycline has been suggested as the drug of choice because it localizes in the reticuloendothelial system, where the organism is found. Others have advocated the use of ampicillin, but controlled studies have not been done. Clinical reports reveal a tendency of patients to relapse after an initial response to therapy regardless of the agent used. In this regard, it should be recognized that with recovery from meningeal inflammation, antibiotic diffusion into the CSF will diminish, permitting microbial persistence. Thus, the inhibitory activity of both the serum and the CSF must be monitored and therapy prolonged in immunosuppressed patients. It is also apparent that if host defenses are markedly impaired, little can be expected from antibiotics alone.

1. Gellin, B. G., and Broome, C. V. Listeriosis. *J.A.M.A.* 261:1313, 1989.
   State-of-the-art review.
2. Mackaness, G. B. Cellular resistance to infection. *J. Exp. Med.* 116:381, 1962.
   Elegant experiments demonstrating the importance of cellular immunity in the defense against Listeria.
3. Medoff, G., Kurz, L. J., and Weinberg, A. N. Listeriosis in humans: An evaluation. *J. Infect. Dis.* 123:247, 1971.
   Infections can be seen in normal persons.

4. Buckner, L. H., and Schneierson, S. S. Clinical and laboratory aspects of *Listeria monocytogenes* infections. *Am. J. Med.* 45:904, 1968.
   Recommends the use of tetracycline.
5. Louria, D. B., Hensle, T., Armstrong, D., et al. Listeriosis complicating malignant disease. *Ann. Intern. Med.* 67:261, 1967.
   An opportunistic infection in patients with an impaired cellular immune response.
6. Salata, R. A., King, R. E., Gose, F., et al. *Listeria monocytogenes* cerebritis, bacteremia, and cutaneous lesions complicating hairy cell leukemia. *Am. J. Med.* 81:1068, 1986.
   An example of a lymphoma complicated by infection with this organism.
7. Louria, D. B., Blevens, A., and Armstrong, D. *Listeria* infections. *Ann. N.Y. Acad. Sci.* 174:548, 1970.
   Steroid therapy is a predisposing factor.
8. Pollock, S. S., Pollock, T. M., and Harrison, M. J. G. Infection of the central nervous system by *Listeria monocytogenes. Q. J. Med.* 53:331, 1984.
   Cerebritis occurs as well as meningitis. (See also Q. J. Med. 37:281, 1968.)
9. Lavetter, A., Leedom, J. M., Mathies, A. W., et al. Meningitis due to *Listeria monocytogenes. N. Engl. J. Med.* 285:598, 1971.
   Ampicillin therapy recommended.
10. Elson, H. R., Zencka, A. E., and Sketch, M. H. *Listeria monocytogenes* endocarditis. *Arch. Intern. Med.* 124:488, 1969.
    Can be confused in the laboratory with Erysipelothrix, *streptococcus, and diphtheroids.*
11. Johnson, W. D., and Kay, D. Serious infections caused by diphtheroids. *Ann. N.Y. Acad. Sci.* 174:568, 1970.
    Another gram-positive rod with which Listeria *is commonly confused.*
12. Moellering, R. C., Jr., Medoff, G., Leech, I., et al. Antimicrobial synergism against *Listeria monocytogenes. Antimicrob. Agents Chemother.* 1:30, 1972.
    "Cillins" are static, "mycins" are cidal; a combination of penicillin and streptomycin or gentamicin advocated in the high-risk situation.
13. Gantz, N. M., Myerowitz, R. L., Medeiros, A. A., et al. Listeriosis in immunosuppressed patients. *Am. J. Med.* 58:637, 1975.
    Meningitis is not uncommon in renal transplant recipients. (See also Arch. Intern. Med. 137:1395, 1977.)
14. Cherubin, C. E., Marr, J. S., Sierra, M. F., et al. *Listeria* and gram-negative bacillary meningitis in New York City, 1972–1979: Frequent causes of meningitis in adults. *Am. J. Med.* 71:199, 1981.
    Chloramphenicol was found to be inferior to other antibiotics.
15. Neiman, R. E., and Lorber, B. Listeriosis in adults: A changing pattern: Report of eight cases and review of the literature, 1968–1978. *Rev. Infect. Dis.* 2:207, 1980.
    Comprehensive review. (See also Rev. Infect. Dis. 4:665, 1982.)
16. Carvajal, A., and Frederiksen, W. Fatal endocarditis due to *Listeria monocytogenes. Rev. Infect. Dis.* 10:616, 1988.
    Antecedent valvular disease is usually present and systemic emboli are common. (See also Am. J. Med. Sci. 273:319, 1977 and Scand. J. Infect. Dis. 20:359, 1988.)
17. Watson, G. W., Fuller, T. J., Elms, J., et al. *Listeria* cerebritis. *Arch. Intern. Med.* 138:83, 1978.
    Cerebritis with an abnormal brain scan but normal CSF can occur with inadequate therapy; in immunosuppressed patients, antibiotics should be given for 4 to 6 weeks. (See also Arch. Intern. Med. 137:1395, 1977.)
18. Ho, J. L., Shands, K. N., Friedland, G., et al. An outbreak of type 4b *Listeria monocytogenes* infection involving patients from eight Boston hospitals. *Arch. Intern. Med.* 146:520, 1986.
    Suggestion that antacid and H_2 blockers facilitated infections with this organism.
19. Ciesielski, C. A., Hightower, A. W., Parsons, S. K., et al. Listeriosis in the United States: 1980–1982. *Arch. Intern. Med.* 148:1416, 1988.
    Foodborne transmission may be an important factor in infection with this organism.

20. Fleming, D. W., Cochi, S. L., and MacDonald, K. L. Pasteurized milk as a vehicle of infection in an outbreak of listeriosis. *N. Engl. J. Med.* 312:404, 1985.
    Milk products may be an important vector as the organism may survive pasteurization and grow in the cold. (See also N. Engl. J. Med. *312:438, 1985 and 308:203, 1983.)*
21. Mascola, L., Lieb, L., Chiu, J., et al. Listeriosis: An uncommon opportunistic infection in patients with acquired immunodeficiency syndrome. A report of five cases and a review of the literature. *Am. J. Med.* 84:162, 1988.
    This was inevitable. (See also Am. J. Med. *85:737, 1988.)*
22. Mossey, R. T., and Sondheimer, J. Listeriosis in patients with long-term hemodialysis and transfusional iron overload. *Am. J. Med.* 79:397, 1985.
    Another example of immunosuppression complicated by listeriosis.
23. Soto-Hernandez, J. L., Nunley, D., Gutierrez, C. C., et al. *Listeria monocytogenes* peritonitis. *Am. J. Gastroenterol.* 83:180, 1988.
    It is surprising that this does not occur more often.

125. MILIARY TUBERCULOSIS
Jerry L. Spivak

Miliary tuberculosis in the adult most often occurs as a result of late activation of a latent focus of tuberculosis acquired during the hematogenous dissemination of a primary tuberculous infection. The disease seems to have a predilection for older persons and blacks. Predisposing factors include steroid therapy, pregnancy, and hematologic malignancies.

The most common symptoms of miliary tuberculosis—weight loss, anorexia, and fever—are nonspecific and of no help in diagnosis. Symptoms referable to the head, chest, or abdomen are usually the result of tuberculous involvement of the meninges, lungs, or peritoneum. Fever is present in most (80%) but not all patients.

Pulmonary abnormalities are the most common findings on physical examination, and at least 20 percent of patients will have signs of meningitis. Choroidal tubercles are not found frequently, and lymphadenopathy and hepatomegaly occur more often than splenomegaly. A high percentage of patients have an abnormal chest x ray, but the classic miliary pattern is found in only 25 to 65 percent of cases. Liver function tests may reveal abnormalities associated with infiltrative disease (Bromsulphalein retention, alkaline phosphatase elevation). The presence of hyponatremia should suggest the possibility of meningeal disease or adrenal insufficiency. The tuberculin test is positive in up to 80 percent of patients, and in many of the rest serial testing reveals a conversion or a booster effect. Hematologic abnormalities are variable, but anemia is commonly found. The leukocyte count can be high, normal, or low. A low leukocyte count may be a reflection of a concurrent underlying illness, whereas a high count may indicate the presence of meningitis. A leukemoid reaction is not common and should suggest the presence of an underlying disease. Although much has been written about the ability of tuberculous infection to produce either pancytopenia or mimic leukemia, a review of all such cases reveals that most are instances of leukemia or aplastic anemia complicated by tuberculosis. Tuberculosis is not more common in patients with leukemia or myeloproliferative disorders, but when such patients develop tuberculosis, it is likely to be the miliary form. An exception, however, to the statement that tuberculosis rarely causes pancytopenia is provided by disseminated atypical mycobacterial infections. The published reports of this association are convincing.

In the presence of a classic chest x ray, miliary tuberculosis will not be overlooked although sarcoidosis, pneumoconiosis, and histoplasmosis must be considered in the differential diagnosis. When the chest x ray is normal, however, the diagnosis of miliary tuberculosis can be more difficult to establish. This is not an uncommon problem since in many cases the site of dissemination is extrapulmonary, as reflected by the fact that sputum cultures are negative in 50 percent of cases. Liver and lymph node biopsies are helpful procedures, but bone marrow biopsy has a much lower positive yield. Serial x rays are often helpful since the miliary pattern may develop over a period of several weeks. In a small percentage of elderly patients, however, the diagnosis may still not be apparent after careful evaluation. These patients have been designated as having "cryptic" tuberculosis. In some the clinical illness may be acute; in others it is indolent. In order to avoid missing such cases, a trial of chemotherapy has been advised in elderly patients with unexplained fever. When embarking on such a course, the physician must remember that early defervescence does not prove that tuberculosis was the cause of fever, nor does persisting fever prove that tuberculosis is not present. The latter response can be seen with miliary disease.

1. Slavin, R. E., Walsh, T. J., and Pollack, A. D. Late generalized tuberculosis: A clinical pathologic analysis and comparison of 100 cases in the preantibiotic and antibiotic eras. *Medicine* 59:352, 1980.
   An important review emphasizing diagnostic problems and pathophysiology.
2. Nice, C. M. The pathogenesis of tuberculosis. *Dis. Chest* 17:550, 1950.
   An old but excellent review.
3. Munt, P. W. Miliary tuberculosis in the chemotherapy era. *Medicine* 51:139, 1972.
   A thorough clinical review. Hyponatremia was not uncommon.
4. Miliary Tuberculosis. In J. E. Johnson, III (ed.), *Rational Control and Therapy of Tuberculosis.* Gainesville: University of Florida Press, 1970. P. 63.
   Dissemination is usually from an extrapulmonary focus.
5. Grieco, M. H., and Chmel, H. Acute disseminated tuberculosis as a diagnostic problem. *Am. Rev. Respir. Dis.* 109:554, 1974.
   Cutaneous anergy occurring with old age can obscure the diagnosis.
6. Gelb, A. F., Leffler, C., Brewin, A., et al. Miliary tuberculosis. *Am. Rev. Respir. Dis.* 108:1327, 1973.
   Sputum and gastric washings together were diagnostic in 77%.
7. Sahn, S. A., and Neff, T. A. Miliary tuberculosis. *Am. J. Med.* 56:495, 1974.
   Review of all aspects of the disease.
8. Yu, Y. L., Chow, W. H., Humphries, M. J., et al. Cryptic miliary tuberculosis. *Q. J. Med.* 59:421, 1986.
   An underlying illness was common. (See also Lancet 1:650, 1978 and 1:1176, 1979.)
9. Berger, H. W., and Samortin, T. G. Miliary tuberculosis: Diagnostic methods with emphasis on the chest roentgenogram. *Dis. Chest* 58:586, 1970.
   Subtle nature of early miliary lesions is emphasized and follow-up films advised.
10. Massaro, D., Katz, S., and Sacks, M. Choroidal tubercles: A clue to hematogenous tuberculosis. *Ann. Intern. Med.* 60:231, 1964.
    Choroidal tubercles are usually associated with a positive chest x ray.
11. Zysser, R. D., Rau, J. E., Ricketts, R. R., et al. Tuberculous pseudotumors of the liver. *Am. J. Med.* 61:946, 1976.
    An unusual presentation of disseminated tuberculosis.
12. Carr, W. P., Kyle, R. A., and Bowie, E. J. W. Hematologic changes in tuberculosis. *Am. J. Med. Sci.* 248:714, 1964.
    Anemia and leukopenia are not common.
13. Glasser, R. M., Walker, R. I., and Herion, J. C. The significance of hematologic abnormalities in patients with tuberculosis. *Arch. Intern. Med.* 125:691, 1970.
    Pancytopenia in a patient with tuberculosis is usually due to a hematologic disease. (See also Br. J. Haematol. 25:793, 1973 and Postgrad. Med. J. 63:801, 1987.)
14. Katzen, H., and Spagnolo, S. V. Bone marrow necrosis from miliary tuberculosis. *J.A.M.A.* 244:2438, 1980.
    An unusual association. (See also Chest 75:208, 1979.)
15. Bagby, G. C., Jr., and Gilbert, D. N. Suppression of granulopoiesis by T-lymphocytes in two patients with disseminated mycobacterial infection. *Ann. Intern. Med.* 94:478, 1981.
    Possible mechanism for cytopenias associated with tuberculous infection.

16. Goldfine, J. D., Schacter, H., Barclay, W. R., et al. Consumption coagulopathy in miliary tuberculosis. *Ann. Intern. Med.* 71:775, 1969.
   Disseminated intravascular coagulation resulting from extensive tissue necrosis. (See also Chest *73:539, 1978.)*

17. Willcox, P. A., Potgeiter, P. D., Bateman, E. D., et al. Rapid diagnosis of sputum negative miliary tuberculosis using the flexible fibreoptic bronchoscope. *Thorax* 41:681, 1986.
   Biopsy was diagnostic in 73% and by brushings in 57%.

18. Engstrom, P. F., Dewey, G. C., and Barrett, O. W. Disseminated *Mycobacterium kansasii* infection. *Am. J. Med.* 52:533, 1972.
   Pancytopenia may be a feature of atypical tuberculous infections. (See also Arch. Intern. Med. *121:424, 1968.)*

19. Cucin, R. L., Coleman, M., Eckardt, J. J., et al. The diagnosis of miliary tuberculosis: Utility of peripheral blood abnormalities, bone marrow and liver needle biopsy. *J. Chronic Dis.* 26:355, 1973.
   Liver biopsy is superior to bone marrow biopsy: bone marrow biopsy yields are highest when anemia, leukopenia, and monocytosis are present. (See also Am. J. Med. *60:1, 1976.)*

20. Williams, M. H., Jr., Yoo, O. H., and Kane, C. Pulmonary function in miliary tuberculosis. *Am. Rev. Respir. Dis.* 107:858, 1973.
   Impairment of diffusing capacity was the most striking abnormality.

21. Witham, R. R., Johnson, R. H., and Roberts, D. L. Diagnosis of miliary tuberculosis by cerebral computerized tomography: Meningitis or tuberculoma may accompany disseminated tuberculosis. *Arch. Intern. Med.* 139:479, 1979.
   Computed tomography scanning is an excellent screening test.

22. Pasculle, A. W., Kapadia, S. B., and Ho, M. Tuberculous bacillemia, hyperpyrexia, and rapid death. *Arch. Intern. Med.* 140:426, 1980.
   Acute tuberculous sepsis producing hyperpyrexia and the adult respiratory distress syndrome. (See also Chest *73:37, 1978 and* Crit. Care Med. *13:12, 1985.)*

23. Alvarez, S., and McCabe, W. R. Extrapulmonary tuberculosis revisited: A review of experience at Boston City and other hospitals. *Medicine* 63:56, 1984.
   Extrapulmonary tuberculosis is still a significant problem in the elderly.

24. Dutt, A. K., Moers, D., and Stead, W. W. Short-course chemotherapy for extrapulmonary tuberculosis. Nine years' experience. *Ann. Intern. Med.* 104:7, 1986.
   Isoniazid and rifampin for 9 months were effective. (See also Lancet *1:1423, 1986.)*

126. MUCORMYCOSIS

Jerry L. Spivak

The zygomycetes are aerobic saprophytic fungi that reside in soil and decaying matter. They grow rapidly in culture, display broad, nonseptate, branching hyphae, and stain more readily with hematoxylin and eosin than with PAS. In tissue sections they can easily be misconstrued by the uninitiated as artifacts of the preparation process. The size of the hyphae, the wide angle of branching, and the staining characteristics distinguish these fungi from *Aspergillus*. This distinction is important since both fungi cause pulmonary infection and both have a predilection for blood vessel invasion. Under normal circumstances zygomycetes are not pathogenic in man, but in the presence of diabetes mellitus, acidosis from any cause, hematologic malignancies, diarrheal illnesses, burns, malnutrition, renal disease, and therapy with corticosteroids, antibiotics, x ray, and cytotoxic agents, they become invasive. In contrast to infections with other fungi zygomycotic infections are often rapidly progressive.

The taxonomy of the fungi belonging to the class Zygomycetes (Phycomycetes) is complex. The clinically most important fungi belong to families within the order Mucorales and of these, the family Mucoraceae is the most important. Although mucormycosis is the descriptive term applied to infections with these fungi, in addition to *Mucor*, several other genera, including *Rhizopus* and *Absidia*, can cause them.

Invasion can occur by several routes. Superficial infections develop in necrotic areas, most often after a burn injury, but rarely does the infection remain localized. Occasionally a localized superficial infection develops in an otherwise normal area of the skin. Such lesions should always be considered as embolic in origin. Gastrointestinal invasion occurs in the setting of diarrhea or colitis or during the course of a debilitating illness. Infarction, ulceration, and perforation of the bowel occur, and the fungi disseminate to other areas of the body, most notably the lungs. Primary pulmonary involvement is most common in patients with hematologic malignancies. Often the fungal infection is preceded by a bacterial infection. Chest x ray may reveal infiltrates, consolidation, cavitation, fungus balls, or effusions. Hemoptysis and pleurisy also occur. Positive sputum cultures have been obtained, and the fungus has been demonstrated in potassium hydroxide preparations of the sputum. Invasion of blood vessels results in embolization of the fungus to all parts of the body, most often to the brain but also to the kidney, spleen, and liver. Severe jaundice in zygomycotic infection is usually the result of hepatic artery occlusion with liver necrosis. Endocarditis and mycotic aneurysms can develop. Myocardial infarction, hemiplegia, aortic blockade, and peripheral gangrene result from mycotic endocarditis.

The most characteristic syndrome caused by the zygomycetes is rhinocerebral infection. Patients with diabetes mellitus are most prone to this complication. Initial manifestations are usually nondescript. They include fever, neck pain, and pharyngitis. Epistaxis, facial tenderness, ptosis, proptosis, periorbital swelling, loss of vision, ophthalmoplegia, sensory deficits, seizures, and coma follow. Physical examination may reveal crusting or ulceration of the palate or black necrotic debris (infarcted turbinates) in the nasal passages. The change from local symptoms to specific neurologic defects can be rapid. In most cases the issue is further complicated by ketoacidosis. However, it must be emphasized that rhinocerebral zygomycosis can occur in the absence of ketoacidosis. In addition, the illness can be slowly progressive and if limited to the ethmoidal and sphenoidal sinuses, few clinical findings are present to permit an early diagnosis. Although these organisms elicit a marked pyogenic tissue reaction, both fever and leukocytosis can be absent. The pathway of infection is from the pharynx, palate, or nose into the paranasal sinuses, through the cribriform plate into the meninges and brain, and into the orbit via the nasolacrimal duct. Blood vessel invasion results in epistaxis, systemic dissemination, cerebral abscesses, aneurysm formation, and ischemic infarction. Central retinal artery occlusion is common. Extension from the sphenoidal sinus leads to basilar meningitis, and spread from the ophthalmic veins into the cavernous sinus produces abnormalities of the third, fourth, and sixth cranial nerves and the ophthalmic division of the fifth cranial nerve. Depending on the degree of involvement, the cerebrospinal fluid (CSF) can be normal or xanthochromic with evidence of subarachnoid hemorrhage, or it can exhibit an elevated protein level and a neutrophilic leukocytosis. Changes in CSF sugar level are usually obscured by the uncontrolled diabetic state. However, even in the presence of extensive cerebral disease the CSF can be normal, and the fungus has never been isolated from the CSF.

Rhinocerebral zygomycosis is easily overlooked initially, and the patient may be considered to have diabetic ophthalmoplegia, thyroid disease, orbital tumor, Wegener's granulomatosis, nasal pharyngeal carcinoma, intracranial aneurysm, arteriovenous anomaly, or septic cavernous sinus thrombosis. The diagnosis will not be missed if zygomycosis is considered in any diabetic with ophthalmoplegia, sinusitis, sudden blindness, or unilateral exophthalmos. The presence of a bruit should suggest a vascular anomaly, while sparing of vision is more common in septic cavernous sinus thrombosis. Soft tissue x rays may be helpful in revealing thickening of sinus linings and bony destruction; if the infection is deep-seated, tomography is required. Arteriography is an important tool to demonstrate the extent of vascular involvement, and tissue biopsy usually settles the diagnostic issue.

The treatment of rhinocerebral zygomycosis consists of amphotericin B therapy, extensive surgical debridement of the affected bone and tissue with adequate drainage, and correction of the underlying metabolic disorder. Expectant treatment in patients with septic cavernous sinus thrombosis is not unreasonable until culture reports are available.

1. Parfrey, N. A. Improved diagnosis and prognosis of mucormycosis. A clinicopathologic study of 33 cases. *Medicine* 65:113, 1986.
   A comprehensive review. (See also Lancet *1:1362, 1986.)*
2. Bigby, T. D., Serota, M. L., Tierney, L. M., Jr., et al. Clinical spectrum of pulmonary mucormycosis. *Chest* 89:435, 1986.
   In addition, aggressive pneumonia occurs in leukemic patients, endobronchial invasion in diabetics.
3. Gamba, J. L., Woodruff, W. W., Djang, W. T., et al. Craniofacial mucormycosis: Assessment with CT. *Radiology* 160:207, 1986.
   Magnetic resonance imaging (MRI) is also useful in this disorder. (See J. Comput. Assist. Tomogr. *12:744, 1988.)*
4. Price, D. L., Wolpow, E. R., and Richardson, E. P. Intracranial phycomycosis: A clinico-pathological and radiological study. *J. Neurol. Sci.* 14:359, 1971.
   Use of arteriography to demonstrate the extent of infection.
5. Prokop, L. D., and Silva-Hutner, M. Cephalic mucormycosis (phycomycosis). *Arch. Neurol.* 17:379, 1967.
   Skull erosions and carotid occlusion due to mucormycosis.
6. Abramson, E., Wilson, D., and Arky, R. A. Rhinocerebral phycomycosis in association with diabetic ketoacidosis. *Ann. Intern. Med.* 66:735, 1967.
   A thorough review of a classic association.
7. Sandler, R., Tallman, C. F., Keamy, D. G., et al. Successfully treated rhinocerebral phycomycosis in diabetes. *N. Engl. J. Med.* 285:1180, 1971.
   Mucormycosis without ketoacidosis.
8. Erdos, M. S., Butt, K., and Weinstein, L. Mucormycotic endocarditis of the pulmonary valve. *J.A.M.A.* 222:951, 1972.
   Endocarditis complicated by disseminated intravascular coagulation.
9. Murray, H. W. Pulmonary mucormycosis with massive fatal hemoptysis. *Chest* 68:65, 1975.
   Vessel wall erosion terminating in pulmonary hemorrhage.
10. Bartrum, R. J., Jr., Watnick, M., and Herman, P. G. Roentgenographic findings in pulmonary mucormycosis. *Am. J. Roentgenol. Radium Ther. Nucl. Med.* 117:810, 1973.
    Pleural effusion is uncommon, but no roentgenographic finding is characteristic.
11. Medoff, G., and Kobayaski, G. S. Pulmonary mucormycosis. *N. Engl. J. Med.* 286:86, 1972.
    Spores are not sensitive to amphotericin B, but the germinating organism is.
12. Brown, J. F., Jr., Gottlieb, L. S., and McCormick, R. A. Pulmonary and rhinocerebral mucormycosis: Sucessful outcome with amphotericin B and griseofulvin therapy. *Arch. Intern. Med.* 137:936, 1977.
    Recovery in spite of widespread infection.
13. Cohen, M. S., Brook, C. J., Naylor, B., et al. Pulmonary phycomycetoma in a patient with diabetes mellitus. *Am. Rev. Respir. Dis.* 116:519, 1977.
    Postpneumonic phycomycetoma in a diabetic.
14. Connor, B. A., Anderson, R. J., and Smith, J. W. Mucor mediastinitis. *Chest* 75:524, 1979.
    Mucor invasion of the mediastinum, pericardium, and pleura.
15. Wright, R. N., Saxena, A., Robin, A., et al. Pulmonary mucormycosis (phycomycetes) successfully treated by resection. *Ann. Thorac. Surg.* 129:166, 1980.
    Pulmonary resection advocated for localized disease.
16. Windus, D. W., Stokes, T. J., Julian, B. A., et al. Fatal *Rhizopus* infections in hemodialysis patients receiving deferoxamine. *Ann. Intern. Med.* 107:678, 1987.
    Deferoxamine proposed as a precipitating factor. (See also Arch. Ophthal. *106:1089, 1988.)*
17. Parkhurst, G. F., and Vlahides, G. D. Fatal opportunistic fungus disease. *J.A.M.A.* 202:279, 1967.
    Jaundice is a frequent complication of disseminated mucormycosis.

18. Lyon, D. T., Schubert, T. T., Mantra, A. G., et al. Phycomycosis of the gastrointestinal tract. *Am. J. Gastroenterol.* 72:379, 1979.
    Comprehensive review.
19. Meyer, R. D., Kaplan, M. H., Ong, M., et al. Cutaneous lesions in disseminated mucormycosis. *J.A.M.A.* 225:737, 1973.
    Cutaneous vasculitis due to fungal embolization. (See also Lab. Invest. *11:1091, 1962.)*
20. Agger, W. A., and Maki, D. G. Mucormycosis: A complication of critical care. *Arch. Intern. Med.* 138:925, 1978.
    Mucor *is being recognized with increasing frequency as a nosocomial pathogen.*
21. Vainrub, B., Macareno, A., Mandel, S., et al. Wound zygomycosis (mucormycosis) in otherwise healthy adults. *Am. J. Med.* 84:546, 1988.
    Extensive sore contamination of traumatic wounds leading to invasive mucormycosis in nonimmunosuppressed hosts.
22. Gartenberg, G., Bottone, E. T., Keusch, G. T., et al. Hospital-acquired mucormycosis *(Rhizopus rhizopodoformus)* of skin and subcutaneous tissue. *N. Engl. J. Med.* 299:1115, 1978.
    Skin inoculation at the site of a surgical wound from a contaminated bandage can produce disseminated infection. (See also J.A.M.A. *241:1032, 1979.)*
23. Wilson, W. S., Grotta, J. C., Schold, C., et al. Cerebral mucormycosis: An unusual case. *Arch. Neurol.* 36:725, 1979.
    Rhinocerebral infection without prominent clinical findings in a patient taking corticosteroids. (See also Arch. Neurol. *42:578, 1985.)*
24. Meyers, B. R., Wormser, G., Hirschman, S. Z., et al. Rhinocerebral mucormycosis. *Arch. Intern. Med.* 129:557, 1979.
    Facial or orbital pain in the appropriate setting (diabetes, immunosuppression) should suggest mucormycosis.
25. Caraveo, J., Trowbridge, A. A., Amaral, B. W., et al. Bone marrow necrosis associated with a mucor infection. *Am. J. Med.* 62:404, 1977.
    An interesting association.
26. Cuadrado, L. M., Guerrero, A., Garcia Asenjo, J. A., et al. Cerebral mucormycosis in two cases of acquired immunodeficiency syndrome. *Arch. Neurol.* 45:109, 1988.
    This is not at all surprising.
27. Echols, R. M., Selinger, D. S., Hallowell, C., et al. *Rhizopus* osteomyelitis. *Am. J. Med.* 66:141, 1979.
    A rare occurrence in the absence of established infection elsewhere.
28. Woods, K. F., and Hanna, B. J. Brain stem mucormycosis in a narcotic addict with eventual recovery. *Am. J. Med.* 80:126, 1986.
    See also Surg. Neurol. *28:468, 1987 and* Neurology *20:261, 1970.*
29. Battock, D. J., Grausz, H., Bobrowski, M., et al. Alternate-day amphotericin B therapy in the treatment of rhinocerebral phycomycosis. *Ann. Intern. Med.* 68:122, 1968.
    Successful therapy with alternate-day amphotericin B therapy.
30. Lehrer, R. I., Howard, D. H., Sypherd, P. S., et al. Mucormycosis. *Ann. Intern. Med.* 93:93, 1980.
    Review of all aspects of mucormycosis.
31. Washburn, R. G., Kennedy, D. W., Begley, M. G., et al. Chronic fungal sinusitis in apparently normal hosts. *Medicine* 67:231, 1988.
    Other fungi can also cause sinusitis. (See also Medicine *67:77, 1988.)*
32. Ventura, G. J., Kantarjian, H. M., Anaissie, E., et al. Pneumonia with *Cunninghamella* species in patients with hematologic malignancies. A case report and review of the literature. *Cancer* 1:1534, 1986.
    The lung is the target organ for zygomycotic infections in patients with leukemia or lymphoma. (See also Am. J. Med. *81:1065, 1986,* Cancer *58:2717, 1986, and* Ann. Intern. Med. *77:871, 1972.)*

127. PULMONARY TUBERCULOSIS
Jerry L. Spivak

As physicians of an earlier generation were advised to know syphilis, it is not inappropriate to advise today's physicians to know tuberculosis, particularly if their patients are from the inner city. The analogy is suitable not only because tuberculosis has protean manifestations but also because, like syphilis, it too is a latent infection. This latter feature guarantees a reservoir of new cases and a constant source of infection, particularly in areas where poverty, ignorance, overcrowding, and inadequate health care exist (*N. Engl. J. Med.* 315:1570, 1986 and *Public Health Rep.* 101:481, 1986). In addition, the emergence of human immunodeficiency virus (HIV) infection with its attendant profound compromise of the immune system and the increasing prevalence of HIV infection in intravenous drug abusers have provided new hosts for tuberculosis to flourish in. The influx of immigrants from Southeast Asia has also provided another population harboring this infection and, in particular, drug-resistant organisms.

The tuberculin skin test is the simplest test for documenting the presence of tuberculous infection. False-positive reactions can result from passive transfer of sensitivity by blood transfusion or as a nonspecific booster effect following skin testing for atypical organisms. Conditions responsible for false-negatives include testing before the skin reactivity associated with infection develops (2–10 weeks), variation in preparation potency, adsorption of unstabilized test material to glass, viral infection, live viral vaccination, immunosuppressive therapy, Hodgkin's disease, sarcoidosis, uremia, corticosteroids, old age, overwhelming infection, infection with atypical mycobacteria, observer variation, and in some patients the activation of cells that suppress the immune response. Isoniazid usually diminishes but does not abolish the reaction, whereas faulty injection technique may result in the production of erythema without induration. The relationship of a negative skin test to prognosis in patients with active infection depends on the reason for the negative test; it should not be assumed that loss of cutaneous hypersensitivity is inevitably associated with impairment of host immune resistance (cf. *Chest* 136:575, 1987).

In the United States, tuberculosis is usually acquired via the respiratory tract. The initial nidus of infection is generally asymptomatic, with only tuberculin conversion providing evidence that tissue invasion has occurred. In some cases calcification in the area of the initial pneumonitis and lymphadenitis (Ghon complex) provides visual but less specific evidence of the event. Concomitant with the primary infection is hematogenous dissemination, and metastatic foci develop most often in the lung apices, meninges, kidneys, and bone. This localization is presumably due to the high oxygen tensions found in these areas. Although the course of primary tuberculosis is usually silent and progression of metastatic foci is hindered by the development of immunity, in some patients progressive pulmonary or miliary tuberculosis develops. The reason for this is unknown but the phenomenon is not limited to children. Consequently, the recognition of a positive tuberculin test is an important observation since progressive pulmonary tuberculosis can produce extensive destruction of lung parenchyma in a short period of time. In most adults, however, progressive primary disease does not develop, and the subsequent development of pulmonary tuberculosis represents reactivation of a latent focus acquired during the hematogenous dissemination of the primary infection. The factors responsible for activation of the latent pulmonary focus in tuberculin-positive persons are unknown, but predisposing causes include corticosteroid therapy, diabetes mellitus, silicosis, immunosuppressive illnesses, and invasive carcinoma. In any event, the physician must also assume that other less obvious extrapulmonary foci are equally likely to be activated and further hematogenous dissemination can also occur. Evaluation and therapy must be planned with this in mind.

The presence of hyponatremia, an interesting complication of pulmonary tuberculosis, always raises the possibility of an associated pulmonary neoplasm, meningitis, or hypoadrenalism. In most cases none of these are found, and evidence suggests that the hyponatremia is due to inappropriate secretion of antidiuretic hormone (ADH). In some of the reported cases, as well as in some of our own, sudden death has occurred with no lesions apparent outside the lungs at autopsy.

The most promising advance in the management of tuberculosis has been the development of treatment regimens employing isoniazid and rifampin, which yield a high cure rate and low relapse rate with short-term (9 months) therapy. The addition of ethambutol is advised if drug resistance is suspected while susceptibility tests are being conducted. More recently, the efficacy of a 6-month regimen employing isoniazid, rifampin, and pyrazinamide for 2 months, followed by isoniazid and rifampin for 4 months in patients with sensitive organisms, has been established. Pyrazinamide appears to be of particular value because of its effectiveness at an acid pH and against intracellular organisms. Isoniazid toxicity appears to be potentiated by rifampin and this may be a particular problem in "slow acetylators." Isoniazid prophylaxis is recommended for close contact of individuals recently infected with tuberculosis, individuals whose skin test has converted within 2 years, those with a positive skin test under age 35, those with a positive skin test and an abnormal chest x ray, and those with a positive skin test and risk factors such as silicosis, end-stage renal disease, diabetes mellitus, immunosuppressive drug therapy, or the acquired immunodeficiency syndrome (AIDS).

1. Glassroth, J., Robins, A. G., and Snider, D. E., Jr. Tuberculosis in the 1980s. *N. Engl. J. Med.* 302:1441, 1980.
   An important review. (See also the symposium in Arch. Intern. Med. *139:1375, 1979.)*
2. O'Brien, R. J., Geiter, L. J., and Snider, D. E., Jr. The epidemiology of nontuberculous mycobacterial diseases in the United States. *Am. Rev. Respir. Dis.* 135:1007, 1987.
   See also Arch. Intern. Med. *148:953, 1988 and* Am. Rev. Respir. Dis. *119:107, 1979.*
3. Reichman, L. B. Tuberculin skin testing. *Chest* 76S:764S, 1979.
   Useful review. (See also Am. Rev. Respir. Dis. *104:769, 1971.)*
4. Sokal, J. E. Measurement of delayed skin-test responses. *N. Engl. J. Med.* 293:501, 1975.
   Good advice. For the problem of variability see Am. Rev. Respir. Dis. *132:175 and 177, 1985 and* Arch. Intern. Med. *148:2457, 1988.*
5. Holden, M., Dubin, M. R., and Diamond, P. H. Negative intermediate-strength tuberculin sensitivity in active tuberculosis. *N. Engl. J. Med.* 285:1506, 1971.
   Glass adsorption results in loss of potency with nonstabilized preparations, but false-negatives still occur with stabilized purified protein derivative (PPD).
6. Comstock, G. W. False tuberculin test results. *Chest* 68:465s, 1975.
   Part of a symposium on tuberculosis. (See also Am. Rev. Respir. Dis. *95:411, 1967.)*
7. Thompson, N. J., Glassroth, J. L., Snider, D. E., Jr., et al. The booster phenomenon in serial tuberculin testing. *Am. Rev. Respir. Dis.* 119:587, 1979.
   The booster phenomenon is due to remote tuberculous infection or sensitization by an atypical organism with initial loss of reactivity.
8. Reichman, L. B., and O'Day, R. The influence of a history of a previous test on the prevalence and size of reactions to tuberculin. *Am. Rev. Respir. Dis.* 115:737, 1977.
   Tuberculin skin testing is not contraindicated when there is a history of a previous positive reaction.
9. Strumpf, I. J., Tsang, A. Y., and Sayre, J. W. Re-evaluation of sputum staining for the diagnosis of pulmonary tuberculosis. *Am. Rev. Respir. Dis.* 119:599, 1979.
   Reliability of sputum staining reaffirmed. (See also Ann. Intern. Med. *92:512, 1980.)*
10. Hinson, J. M., Jr., Bradsher, R. W., and Bodner, S. J. Gram-stain neutrality of *Mycobacterium tuberculosis*. *Am. Rev. Respir. Dis.* 123:365, 1981.
    M. tuberculosis *is not stained by Gram's stain and appears ghostlike in such preparations.*
11. Schacter, E. N. Tuberculin negative tuberculosis. *Am. Rev. Respir. Dis.* 106:587, 1972.
    Atypical mycobacteria as a cause of pulmonary disease with a negative skin test with intermediate PPD.
12. McMurray, D. N. Mechanisms of anergy in tuberculosis. *Chest* 77:4, 1980.
    Brief review. (See also Am. Rev. Respir. Dis. *123:556, 1981.)*

13. Smith, L. S., Schillaci, R. F., and Sarlin, R. F. Endobronchial tuberculosis. *Chest* 91:644, 1987.
    This is now a complication of the primary infection. (See also Chest *89:727, 1986 and 93:836, 1988.)*
14. Stead, W. W., and Bates, J. H. Evidence of a "silent" bacillemia in primary tuberculosis. *Ann. Intern. Med.* 74:559, 1971.
    Proof of dissemination of organisms at the time of primary infection.
15. Stead, W. W., Kerby, G. R., Schlueter, D. P., et al. The clinical spectrum of primary tuberculosis in adults. *Ann. Intern. Med.* 68:731, 1968.
    Rapid progression with pulmonary disabilities may occur.
16. Stead, W. W. Pathogenesis of a first episode of chronic pulmonary tuberculosis in man: Recrudescence of residuals of the primary infection or exogenous reinfection? *Ann. Rev. Respir. Dis.* 95:729, 1967.
    Chronic pulmonary tuberculosis is the result of reactivation of a latent focus and not of an exogenous reinfection.
17. Woodring, J. H., Vandiviere, H. M., Fried, A. M., et al. Update: The radiographic features of pulmonary tuberculosis. *Am. J. Roentgenol.* 146:497, 1986.
    Comprehensive review. (See also Am. J. Med. *62:31, 1977,* Chest *89:75, 1986, and 94:316, 1988.)*
18. Chang, S. C., Lee, P. Y., and Perng, R. P. Lower lung field tuberculosis. *Chest* 91:230, 1987.
    Tuberculosis can simulate bacterial pneumonia, particularly in diabetics. (See also Chest *65:522, 1974.)*
19. Alvarez, S., Shell, C., and Berk, S. L. Pulmonary tuberculosis in elderly men. *Am. J. Med.* 82:602, 1987.
    Often the diagnosis is not considered. For skin testing in this population, see Chest *92:237, 1987.*
20. Epstein, D. M., Kline, L. R., Albelda, S. M., et al. Tuberculous pleural effusions. *Chest* 91:106, 1987.
    The complication is now being seen in older patients with reactivation tuberculosis.
21. Kent, D. C., and Elliott, R. C. Hilar adenopathy in tuberculosis. *Am. Rev. Respir. Dis.* 96:439, 1967.
    This article must be reviewed with Ann. Intern. Med. *78:65, 1973.*
22. Bowry, S., Chan, C. H., Weiss, H., et al. Hepatic involvement in pulmonary tuberculosis. *Am. Rev. Respir Dis.* 101:941, 1970.
    25% incidence of noncaseating granulomas.
23. Snider, D. The relationship between tuberculosis and silicosis. *Am. Rev. Respir. Dis.* 118:455, 1978.
    Silicosis may predispose to tuberculosis by impairing macrophage function.
24. Byrd, R. B., Fisk, D. E., Roethe, R. A., et al. Tuberculosis in Oriental immigrants: A study in military dependents. *Chest* 76:136, 1979.
    Tuberculosis acquired in the Orient is frequently drug-resistant.
25. Rutsky, E. A., and Rostand, S. G. Mycobacteriosis in patients with chronic renal failure. *Arch. Intern. Med.* 140:57, 1980.
    Patients with chronic renal failure have a high incidence of tuberculosis. (See also Am. J. Med. *68:59, 1980.)*
26. Handwerger, S., Mildvan, D., Senie, R., et al. Tuberculosis and the acquired immunodeficiency syndrome at a New York City hospital: 1978–1985. *Chest* 91:176, 1987.
27. Diagnosis and management of mycobacterial infection and disease in persons with human immunodeficiency virus infection. *Ann. Intern. Med.* 106:254, 1987.
    M. avium-intracellulare is the most common organism for which established therapy is not effective. (See also J. Infect. Dis. *157:863, 1988,* Ann. Intern. Med. *105:184, 1986,* J.A.M.A. *256:362, 1986, and* Radiology *160:77, 1986.)*
28. Klatt, E. C., Jensen, D. F., and Meyer, P. R. Pathology of *Mycobacterium avium-intracellulare* infection in acquired immunodeficiency syndrome. *Hum. Pathol.* 18:709, 1987.
    Typical granulomas are not the rule. (See also Am. J. Clin. Pathol. *85:67, 1986.)*

29. Rohwedder, J. J. Upper respiratory tract tuberculosis. *Ann. Intern. Med.* 80:708, 1974.
    A complication of pulmonary tuberculosis.
30. Moss, J. D., and Knauer, C. M. Tuberculous enteritis. *Gastroenterology* 65:959, 1973.
    A complication that can occur in the setting of active pulmonary tuberculosis.
31. Goodwin, R. A., Nickell, J. A., and Des Prez, R. M. Mediastinal fibrosis complicating healed primary histoplasmosis and tuberculosis. *Medicine* 51:227, 1972.
    An unusual complication of granulomatous infection of lymph nodes.
32. Snider, G. L., and Placik, B. The relationship between pulmonary tuberculosis and bronchogenic carcinoma. *Am. Rev. Respir. Dis.* 99:229, 1969.
    Tuberculosis masking the presence of lung carcinoma.
33. Vorherr, H., Massry, S. G., Fallet, R., et al. Antidiuretic principle in tuberculous lung tissue of a patient with pulmonary tuberculosis and hyponatremia. *Ann. Intern. Med.* 72:383, 1970.
    Further evidence for inappropriate secretion of ADH. (See also Ann. Intern. Med. *70:943, 1969.)*
34. Treatment of tuberculosis and tuberculosis infection in adults and children. *Am. Rev. Respir. Dis.* 134:355, 1986.
    Guidelines for treatment and prophylaxis (see also Am. Rev. Respir. Dis. *133:423, 1986 and 136:1475, 1987).*
35. Selwyn, P. A., Hartel, D., Lewis, V. A., et al. A prospective study of the risk of tuberculosis among intravenous drug users with human immunodeficiency virus infection. *N. Engl. J. Med.* 320:545, 1989.
    Chemoprophylaxis advised when the PPD test is positive in HIV-infected patients.
36. Van Scoy, R. E., and Wilkowshe, C. J. Antituberculosis agents. *Mayo Clin. Proc.* 62:1129, 1987.
    Brief review.
37. Steele, M. A., and Des Prez, R. M. The role of pyrazinamide in tuberculosis chemotherapy. *Chest* 94:845, 1988.
    Review of a useful drug in the first-line treatment of tuberculosis.
38. Barnes, P. F., Leedom, J. M., Chan, L. S., et al. Predictors of short-term prognosis in patients with pulmonary tuberculosis. *J. Infect. Dis.* 158:366, 1988.
    Advanced age, lymphopenia, alcoholism, granulocytosis, and extrapulmonic disease were among the poor prognostic factors.
39. Lee, C. H., Wang, W. J., Lan, R. S., et al. Corticosteroids in the treatment of tuberculous pleurisy. *Chest* 94:1256, 1988.
    Symptoms and effusions cleared more quickly but residual pleural thickening was not affected.
40. Berger, H. W., and Rosenbaum, I. Prolonged fever in patients treated for tuberculosis. *Am. Rev. Respir. Dis.* 97:140, 1968.
    70% of cases defervesce within 3 weeks; miliary or far-advanced pulmonary disease takes longer. (See also Am. Rev. Respir. Dis. *123:20, 1981.)*
41. Mitchell, J. R., Zimmerman, H. J., Iskak, K. G., et al. Isoniazid liver injury: Clinical spectrum, pathology and probable pathogenesis. *Ann. Intern. Med.* 84:181, 1976.
    A problem in patients over age 35. (See also Chest *62:71, 1972.)*
42. Steiner, M., Chaves, A., and Lyons, H. A. Primary drug-resistant tuberculosis. *N. Engl. J. Med.* 283:1353, 1970.
    Importance of determining the sensitivity of the organism to the standard drugs.
43. Smith, D. W. Why not vaccinate against tuberculosis? *Ann. Intern. Med.* 72:419, 1970.
    BCG recommended for high-risk groups.

128. PYOGENIC LIVER ABSCESS
H. Verdain Barnes

Pyogenic liver abscess is rare. Abscess formation typically occurs as a complication of intestinal or biliary tract disease such as ascending cholangitis secondary to biliary or pancreatic carcinoma, choledocholithiasis, pancreatitis, or biliary tract surgery, systemic bacteremia, pylephlebitis, acute appendicitis, infected hepatic cysts, diverticulitis, chronic cholecystitis, chronic pancreatitis, peptic ulcer disease, inflammatory bowel disease, infective endocarditis, penetrating or nonpenetrating abdominal trauma, and local extension from perinephric, subphrenic, or subhepatic abscesses. In most series up to 20 percent are cryptogenic. In recent years a majority have been over age 40. The sex distribution is equal. Most patients have macroscopic abscesses, but a significant number have only microscopic lesions. About 50 percent of the patients have a single abscess, with 50 to 75 percent occurring in the right lobe. When there are multiple abscesses, about two-thirds involve both lobes. In most cases of biliary tract origin the abscesses are multiple. The overall mortality ranges from 25 to 90 percent, depending on the series. Multiple factors influence prognosis. The mortality with multiple abscesses is 4 times greater than with a single abscess. Mortality is higher in old age, when more than one organism is involved, and when the serum albumin is less than 2 gm/dl at the time of diagnosis.

The clinical presentation is variable and often masked by the associated disease. Fever is the most common symptom. No fever pattern predominates. Other common symptoms and approximate percentages include pleuritic or abdominal pain (75%), chills (60%), nausea and vomiting (60%), weight loss (50%), malaise (40%), anorexia (40%), diarrhea (17%), and pruritus (12%). Less frequent symptoms are abdominal distention, hiccups, and dyspnea. The most frequent physical finding is an enlarged liver, seen in about 50 percent. Jaundice and abdominal tenderness occur in 40 to 75 percent; diminished breath sounds or rales, splenomegaly, and an abdominal mass or distention in about 20 percent. Less common findings include a friction rub over the liver, ascites, decreased mentation, and a pleural effusion or rub.

Clinical laboratory tests are not diagnostic. Anemia, leukocytosis, prolonged prothrombin time, elevated erythrocyte sedimentation rate, and elevated levels of direct and/or indirect bilirubin, alkaline phosphatase, aspartate aminotransferase (AST), and alanine aminotransferase (ALT) are common. Serum vitamin B_{12} levels may be increased. The chest x ray is normal in the majority but may show an elevated right hemidiaphragm basilar atelectasis, right pleural effusion, or pneumonitis. The most helpful noninvasive diagnostic technique is the radioisotope scan of the liver. In addition to the anterior, lateral and posterior views should be performed or some defects will be missed. Currently available scanning techniques cannot distinguish a liver abscess from a tumor or congenital cyst. Over 80 percent of the scans are positive in pyogenic liver abscess when the lesion is 1 cm or more in diameter. This is true also of a hepatic angiogram. Most recent series expound the use of needle aspiration for diagnosis. Spread or secondary infection, however, is a potential complication that should be considered. Aspirated fluid should be cultured for aerobic and anaerobic organisms. A Gram's stain should be performed. Cultures from aspirated fluid will be positive in at least 50 percent. Blood cultures are positive in 30 to 40 percent of patients.

The most common causative aerobes, in essentially the descending order of frequency, are *Escherichia coli, Klebsiella, Enterobacter* species, enterococci, *Pseudomonas aeruginosa, Staphylococcus aureus, Proteus* sp., *Serratia marcescens,* and *Alcaligenes* sp. A variety of anaerobic organisms have been isolated; the most common are microaerophilic streptococci, peptococci, *Bacteroides, Fusobacterium, Clostridium,* and *Actinomyces.* Anaerobes may be the only organisms found, accounting for 18 to 45 percent in most recent series. These organisms may well explain the high incidence of sterile liver abscesses reported in the past.

The primary differential diagnosis includes congenital cysts, neoplasm, and amebic abscess. Unless secondarily infected, congenital cysts offer no signs or symptoms. Malignancy often provides other clues to diagnosis, but on occasion can only be ruled out by microscopic examination. Amebic abscesses (described in a separate chapter) have some differentiating characteristics. The brown "anchovy sauce" fluid characteristic of an amebic abscess is helpful if present, but on occasion it may be simulated by a pyogenic abscess. Positive indirect hemagglutination, complement fixation or agar gel diffusion tests for *Entamoeba histolytica,* or demonstration of the organism confirms the diagnosis. For patients with pyogenic liver abscess, therapy consists of correcting the underlying disease, high-dose antibiotics, and, when required, surgical drainage. The median time for defervescence with appropriate antibiotic therapy is about 8 days.

1. Ochsner, A., DeBakey, M., and Murray, S. Pyogenic abscess of the liver. *Am. J. Surg.* 40:292, 1938.
   A classic from the preantibiotic era.
2. Lazarchick, J., DeSouza, N. A., Nichols, D. R., et al. Pyogenic liver abscess. *Mayo Clin. Proc.* 48:349, 1973.
   25% had two or more organisms.
3. Rubin, R. H., Swartz, M. N., and Malt, R. Hepatic abscesses: Changes in clinical, bacteriologic and therapeutic aspects. *Am. J. Med.* 57:601, 1974.
   Two-thirds of patients had macroscopic abscesses. The highest mortality was in patients over age 50 years.
4. Neale, G., Caughey, D. E., Mollin, D. L., et al. Effects of intrahepatic and extrahepatic infection on liver function. *Br. Med. J.* 1:382, 1966.
   Serum vitamin B_{12} levels are increased in intrahepatic infections.
5. Pyrtek, L. J., and Bartus, S. A. Hepatic pyemia. *N. Engl. J. Med.* 272:551, 1965.
   Liver function studies may be normal if the process is localized.
6. Patterson, D. K., Ozeran, R. S., Alantz, G. J., et al. Pyogenic liver abscess due to microaerophilic streptococci. *Ann. Surg.* 165:362, 1967.
   A high percentage of sterile liver abscesses may be due to poor anaerobic culturing.
7. Sabbaj, J., Suller, V. L., and Finegold, S. M. Anaerobic pyogenic liver abscess. *Ann. Intern. Med.* 77:629, 1972.
   45% were anaerobes in this series.
8. Zipser, R. D., Rau, J. E., Ricketts, R. R., et al. Tuberculous pseudotumors of the liver. *Am. J. Med.* 61:946, 1976.
   A rare manifestation of tuberculosis that on scan is compatible with neoplasia or multiple abscesses.
9. Pitt, H. A., and Zuidema, G. D. Factors influencing mortality in the treatment of pyogenic hepatic abscess. *Surg. Gynecol. Obstet.* 140:228, 1975.
   Escherichia coli was the most common organism isolated. Multiple organisms were isolated in 65%, anaerobic abscesses were generally solitary, and ascending cholangitis was the most frequent cause.
10. Cheung, N. K., Malfitan, R. C., Najem, A. Z., et al. Pyogenic liver abscess. *Am. Surg.* 16:272, 1978.
    The most useful diagnostic tests were the radioisotope liver scan and hepatic angiography.
11. Verlenden, W. L., III, and Frey, C. F. Management of liver abscess. *Am. J. Surg.* 140:53, 1980.
    Factors predisposing to multiple liver abscesses were biliary tract diseases, cancer, chemotherapy, steroids, and alcoholism.
12. Liebert, C. W., Jr. Hepatic abscess resulting from asymptomatic diverticulitis of the sigmoid colon. *South. Med. J.* 74:71, 1981.
    Another potential cause of "cryptogenic" liver abscess.
13. Liu, Y.-C., Cheng, D.-L., and Lin, C.-L. *Klebsiella pneumoniae* liver abscess associated with septic endophthalmitis. *Arch. Intern. Med.* 146:1913, 1986.
    A potential complication which often has a tragic outcome.
14. Barnes, P. F., DeCock, K. M., Reynolds, T. N., et al. A comparison of amebic and pyogenic abscess of the liver. *Medicine* 66:472, 1987.
    A retrospective review of 96 cases of amebic and 48 cases of pyogenic abscess. Needle aspiration is recommended for diagnosis.

15. Laud, M. A., Moinuddin, M., and Bisno, A. L. Pyogenic liver abscess: Changing epidemiology and prognosis. *South. Med. J.* 78:1426, 1985.
Now seen more commonly in the elderly without a clear predisposing disease.

129. ROCKY MOUNTAIN SPOTTED FEVER
H. Verdain Barnes

Rocky Mountain spotted fever (RMSF) is caused by *Rickettsia rickettsii.* The tick serves as a reservoir and vector for the disease. *Dermacentor andersoni,* the wood tick, and *Dermacentor variabilis,* the American dog tick, are the primary vectors. The disease is endemic in many areas of the United States. In recent years, most cases have come from Wyoming, Montana, and Colorado in the West and from Virginia, North Carolina, Maryland, Georgia, South Carolina, Pennsylvania, New York, West Virginia, and New Jersey in the East and Southeast. In all areas the number of cases has decreased in recent decades. Almost all cases occur from April through September, the time of maximum tick activity. The organism, once inoculated into man, invades endothelial cells throughout the body. Reproduction occurs primarily in these cells. The result is endothelial proliferation, edema, and perivascular inflammation. Progression of the process results in increased capillary permeability and small vessel occlusion. These vascular manifestations appear to result, at least in part, from the early activation of the fibrinolytic system, platelets, and coagulation pathways.

A history of tick bite can be obtained in about 60 to 80 percent of patients. The incubation period ranges from 2 to 14 days, averaging 2 to 4 days. The onset is abrupt in about 75 percent and gradual but not insidious in the remainder. Virtually all patients have malaise, fever, and a rash at some point during their illness. The fever characteristically spikes in the afternoon into the 40 to 41.1°C (104–106°F) range, declining by 1.7 to 2.8°C (3–5°F) by morning. Some patients, however, have a constant fever in the 38.8 to 39.4°C (102–103°F) range. The erythematous, maculopapular rash is characteristically seen on the wrists, ankles, palms, and soles. The first appearance, however, may be diffuse or localized to the abdomen, arms, or perineum. Within 72 hours of onset the rash typically becomes diffuse and eventually becomes petechial. The rash can appear any time within the first 10 days of the illness, but it is usually present by the third day. The duration of the rash is variable but rarely disappears in less than 4 days. Other common features are a constant intractable headache, mental confusion, generalized myalgias with associated muscle tenderness, nausea, vomiting; and constipation. Less common findings are arthralgia, splenomegaly, hepatomegaly, lymphadenopathy, chills, abdominal pain, photophobia, transient deafness, bilateral orbital pain, periorbital edema, subconjunctival hemorrhage, conjunctivitis, diarrhea, and epistaxis.

About one-third of patients will have one or more complications; the most common are neurologic. Meningismus is the most frequent with a majority having a normal spinal fluid. Patients with nuchal rigidity have a high frequency of associated grand mal seizures. Hemiplegia or ascending paralysis may occur. Other complications include parotitis, interstitial pneumonitis, myocarditis, oliguria, pulmonary edema, hepatitis, and disseminated intravascular coagulation (DIC). Some degree of thrombocytopenia is seen in about 75 percent of patients. Platelet counts of less than 50,000 per microliter may occur. The most common cause of death is a diffuse meningoencephalitis. These complications occur or are most severe from the seventh to the fourteenth days of the illness, which is the time of maximum vascular damage. Consequently patients should be monitored with particular care during this critical period.

Early diagnosis on clinical grounds is often difficult. In one large series from an endemic area, about 38 percent had an initial diagnosis other than RMSF. The diagnoses most often confused are infectious mononucleosis, viral encephalitis, meningococcal aseptic meningitis, and rubella. When these diseases are in the differential diagno so also is RMSF, especially if it is the appropriate season in an endemic area. No consistent or characteristic changes are found in hematologic, urine, or electrolyte determinations. The diagnosis can be confirmed as early as day 4 by demonstrating the organism by skin biopsy and the use of an immunofluorescent staining technique. Later in the course of the disease the diagnosis can be proved by serologic testing. Serologic confirmation cannot be made before day 7 or 8. In general, peak titers are seen from the fifteenth to the thirtieth days. Complement-fixing antibodies in dilutions of 1 : 5 or greater are diagnostic. These 19S antibodies become very low or nonmeasurable within a year. Antibodies demonstrated by the fluorescent technique may remain high for years. The traditional Weil-Felix test for OX-19 agglutinins usually becomes positive in diagnostic titers after the tenth day and falls by the thirtieth day. OX-19 titers must be 1 : 160 or greater to support the diagnosis, and in some patients are never significantly elevated.

Most authors agree that early antibiotic therapy diminishes the incidence of serious complications and death. To initiate antibiotic therapy is of little or no value after the seventh to tenth day of the illness. Therapy should be instituted without delay when the diagnosis is suspected, particularly in an undiagnosed febrile illness occurring between April and September in patients under the age of 20 years living in or having recently visited an endemic area.

1. Harrell, G. T. Rocky Mountain spotted fever. *Medicine* 28:333, 1949.
   A classic review.
2. Vianna, N. J., and Hinman, A. R. Rocky Mountain spotted fever on Long Island. *Am. J. Med.* 51:725, 1971.
   High fever, malaise, and maculopapular rash were seen in all 260 patients.
3. Hand, W. L., Miller, J. B., Reinarz, J. A., et al. Rocky Mountain spotted fever: A vascular disease. *Arch. Intern. Med.* 125:879, 1970.
   Early diagnosis and specific antibiotic therapy reduce the mortality.
4. Mengel, C. E., and Trygstad, C. Thrombocytopenia in Rocky Mountain spotted fever. *J.A.M.A.* 183:886, 1963.
   Thrombocytopenia is commonly seen and can be mild to severe.
5. Trigg, J. W., Jr. Hypofibrinogenemia in Rocky Mountain spotted fever: Report of a case. *N. Engl. J. Med.* 270:1042, 1964.
   Another cause of DIC.
6. Pincoffs, M. C., Guy, E. C., Lister, L. M., et al. Treatment of Rocky Mountain spotted fever with chloromycetin. *Ann. Intern. Med.* 29:656, 1948.
   Sulfa drugs may make the illness worse.
7. Woodward, T. E., Pedersen, C. E., Oster, C. N., et al. Prompt conformation of Rocky Mountain Spotted Fever: Identification of Rickettsiae in skin tissues. *J. Infect. Dis.* 134:297, 1976.
   An important technique to prove the diagnosis of RMSF early in the course of the disease.
8. Walker, D. H., Burday, H. S., Folds, J. D., et al. Laboratory diagnosis of acute Rocky Mountain spotted fever. *South. Med. J.* 73:1443, 1980.
   Test sensitivity during the acute phase of the illness were skin biopsy 70%, proteus OX-19 65%, hemagglutination 19%, proteus OX-2 18%, and complement fixation 0% with overall specificity rates of 100%, 78%, 99%, and 96%, respectively.
9. Middleton, D. B. Rocky Mountain spotted fever: Gastrointestinal and laboratory manifestations. *South. Med. J.* 71:629, 1978.
   Gastrointestinal manifestations were present in 80%. Enzyme elevations included (ALT) in 90%, SGPT (AST) in 83%, SGOT creatine phosphokinase in 76%, and lactic dehydrogenase 65%. Liver function elevations included total bilirubin in 69% (mostly direct) and prothrombin time in 41%.
10. Donohue, J. F. Lower respiratory tract involvement in Rocky Mountain spotted fever. *Arch. Intern. Med.* 140:223, 1980.
    Some degree of lower respiratory involvement occurred in 42%.
11. Yamada, T., Harber, P., Pittit, G. W., et al. Activation of the kallikrein-kinin system in Rocky Mountain spotted fever. *Ann. Intern. Med.* 88:764, 1978.

The kallikrein-kinin system may play a major role in the pathogenesis of the vasculitis, DIC, and shock in this disease.

12. Walker, D. H., and Mattern, W. D. Acute renal failure in Rocky Mountain spotted fever. *Arch. Intern. Med.* 138:443, 1979.
13. Ramphal, R., Kluge, R., Cohen, V., et al. Rocky Mountain spotted fever and jaundice. *Arch. Intern. Med.* 138:260, 1978.
    Two (articles 12 and 13) uncommon, but important complications.
14. Turner, R. C., Chaplinski, T. J., and Adams, H. G. Rocky Mountain spotted fever presenting as thrombocytopenic purpura. *Am. J. Med.* 81:153, 1986.
15. Walker, D. H., Lesensne, H. R., Varma, V. A., et al. Rocky Mountain spotted fever mimicking acute cholecystitis. *Arch. Intern. Med.* 145:2194, 1985.
    Two (articles 14, 15) rare presentations of RMSF.
16. Milunski, M. R., Gallis, H. A., and Fulkerson, W. J. *Staphyloccus aureus* septicemia mimicking fulminant Rocky Mountain spotted fever. *Am. J. Med.* 83:801, 1987.
    An interesting look-alike.
17. Rao, A. K. Schapira, M., Clements, M. L., et al. A prospective study of platelets and plasma proteolytic systems during the early stages of Rocky Mountain spotted fever. *N. Engl. J. Med.* 318:1021, 1988.
18. Randall, M. B., and Walker, D. H. Rocky Mountain spotted fever. *Arch. Pathol. Lab. Med.* 108:963, 1984.
    Two insights into the pathogenesis of RMSF (articles 17, 18).
19. Massey, E. W., Thames, T., Coffey, C. E., et al. Neurologic complications of Rocky Mountain spotted fever. *South. Med. J.* 78:1288, 1985.
    A concise review. Sequalae appear to be rare.
20. Salgo, M. P., Telzak, E. E., Currie, B., et al. A focus of Rocky Mountain spotted fever within New York City. *N. Engl. J. Med.* 318:1345, 1988.
    RMSF can occur without a history of being in an endemic area.

130. SEPTIC (PYOGENIC) ARTHRITIS
H. Verdain Barnes

Pyogenic joint disease is relatively common. The usual mode of bacterial entry into the joint space is hematogenous. Infection, however, can result by the spread of bacteria from an adjacent focus or can be introduced by joint penetration. The latter may be accidental, self-inflicted, or iatrogenic. The joint space and fluid provide an ideal environment for bacterial growth, with the necessary nutrients as well as lower concentrations of antibodies and complement than are found in the plasma. Furthermore, once the inflammatory process begins, bacterial metabolism decreases, thus making it more difficult for antibiotics that require rapid cell metabolism to be effective.

Classically, septic arthritis is acute in onset and involves a single joint. There is a clear predilection for the larger weight-bearing, diseased, or traumatized joints. For instance, acutely septic joints are being recognized more frequently in patients with chronic osteoarthritis, rheumatoid arthritis, and in prosthetic joints, a point to keep in mind when evaluating patients with what appears to be an acute exacerbation of known chronic joint disease or post–prosthetic joint surgery. To overlook this diagnosis can be fatal.

A septic joint is almost invariably warmer than surrounding skin—even frankly hot— tender to palpitation and movement, and most often erythematous. A demonstrable effusion is rarely lacking with superficial joint involvement. The patient may have a low-grade, high persistent, or spiking fever. On rare occasions patients who are uremic, debilitated, or taking steroids are afebrile. A careful search for a bacterial source, such as pneumonia, a furuncle, or a discharge from the urethra or cervix, often reveals the source of the offending organism in the joint.

An important diagnostic procedure is athrocentesis. Joint fluid examination should not be delayed in evaluating these patients. In general, pyogenic joint fluid has the following characteristics: yellow color, turbidity or frank purulence, reduced viscosity, poor or friable mucin clot, 7000 to 250,000 cells per microliter with a predominance of segmented neutrophils, and a synovial fluid to simultaneous blood sugar ratio of less than 0.5. These features, however, are not invariably present, and may not differ from findings typical of a nonpyrogenic inflammatory joint fluid. Consequently, only a carefully done Gram's stain and culture can confirm or exclude the diagnosis. If any amount of fluid is obtained, stain and culture should be given first priority. Blood agar, chocolate agar, thioglycolate broth, Sabouraud's agar, and ATS media or their equivalents should be routinely used. Thayer-Martin medium is good for gonococci, but it does not support growth of many other pathogens of potential importance, such as *Haemophilus* sp. Gonococcal protoplast forms can usually be grown in media of high ionic strength. The joint fluid should have Gram's, Wright's, and acid-fast stains. Standard x ray is frequently not helpful in the acute septic joint, but magnetic resonance imaging may prove useful in selected patients.

The most common organisms found in adolescents and adults are, in order of decreasing frequency, *Neisseria gonorrhoeae, Staphylococcus aureus, Streptococcus pyogenes, Diplococcus pneumoniae, Escherichia coli, Salmonella* sp., *Pseudomonas* sp., *Haemophilus influenzae,* and *Mycobacterium tuberculosis.* In children the order is *Haemophilus, Staphylococcus, Streptococcus, Pneumococcus,* gram-negative organisms, and *Mycobacterium tuberculosis.* A wide variety of other organisms have also been implicated: *Klebsiella, Vibrio fetus, Bacteroides* sp., *Micrococcus tetragenus, Proteus mirabilis, Serratia marcescens, Clostridium welchii, Meningococcus, Brucella,* Shiga's bacillus, *Streptobacillus moniliformis,* anthrax bacillus, diphtheria organisms, *Treponema pallidum, Sporotrichum, Coccidioides immitis, Histoplasma capsulatum, Blastomyces dermatitidis, Cryptococcus, Actinomyces, Nocardia,* and *Candida albicans* to name a few.

Since gonococcal arthritis is increasing in frequency, some additional comments are warranted. The initial presentation is often a migratory polyarthritis, which may localize in more than one joint. Although tenosynovitis and dermatitis may occur it is less frequent than in disseminated gonorrhea without septic arthritis. The majority have temperatures of less than 39.4°C (103°F) and about 10 percent are afebrile. Women predominate over men 4:1 in most series. With appropriate therapy, a clinical response is rarely delayed beyond 72 hours. Recurrent effusion requiring arthrocentesis may occur for a week or more after therapy is initiated.

1. Ward, J. R., and Atcheson, S. G. Infectious arthritis. *Med. Clin. North Am.* 61:313, 1977.
   A good general review.
2. Goldenberg, D. L., and Cohen, A. S. Acute infectious arthritis: A review of patients with nongonococcal joint infections. *Am. J. Med.* 60:369, 1976.
   There is an increase in the incidence of gram-negative organisms and the usefulness of needle joint aspiration in therapy is shown.
3. Goldenberg, D. L., Brandt, K. D., Cathcart, E. S., et al. Acute arthritis caused by gram-negative bacilli: A clinical characterization. *Medicine* 53:197, 1974.
   Joint damage is usually severe and mortality higher than in gram-positive joint infections.
4. Brandt, K. D., Cathcart, E. S., and Cohen, A. S. Gonococcal arthritis: Clinical features correlated with blood, synovial fluid and genitourinary cultures. *Arthritis Rheum.* 17:503, 1974.
   No clinical differences found between the so-called bacteremic and septic joint types of arthritis.
5. Rimoin, D. L., and Wennberg, J. E. Acute septic arthritis complicating chronic rheumatoid arthritis. *J.A.M.A.* 196:617, 1966.
   A pyogenic process superimposed on chronic joint disease is not uncommon.
6. Smith, W. S., and Ward, R. M. Septic arthritis of the hip complicating perforation of abdominal organs. *J.A.M.A.* 195:170, 1966.
   Pyrogenic arthritis can arise from a variety of adjacent infections; here it was an intraabdominal abscess.

7. Rabinowitz, M. S. Pyarthrosis of the knee joint following intra-articular hydrocortisone. *Bull. Hosp. Joint Dis.* 16:158, 1955.
   Just one example of how bacteria can be iatrogenically introduced into the joint.
8. Holmes, K. K., Gutman, L. T., Belding, M. E., et al. Recovery of *Neisseria gonorrhoeae* from "sterile" synovial fluid in gonococcal arthritis. *N. Engl. J. Med.* 284:318, 1971.
   In gas chromatography, L-forms may be recovered by using a hypertonic media.
9. Rice, P. A., and Goldenberg, D. L. Clinical manifestations of disseminated infection caused by *Neisseria gonorrhoeae* are linked to differences in bacterial reactivity of infecting strains. *Ann. Intern. Med.* 95:175, 1981.
   Tenosynovitis and dermatitis are less frequent in those who develop septic arthritis. Those with septic arthritis are more sensitive to the bactericidal activity of normal serum than are those with disseminated disease without a septic joint.
10. Gelberman, R. H., Menon, J., Austerlitz, M. S., et al. Pyogenic arthritis of the shoulder in adults. *J. Bone Joint Surg [Am.]* 62A:550, 1980.
    All had predisposing disorders.
11. Gordon, G., and Kabins, S. A. Pyogenic sacroiliitis. *Am. J. Med.* 69:50, 1980.
    Symptoms are often vague. This entity may be more common than currently appreciated.
12. Doll, N. J., and Jackson, F. N. Acute pseudogout simulating septic arthritis. *J.A.M.A.* 242:1768, 1979.
13. Good, A. E., Hague, J. M., and Kauffmann, C. A. Streptococcal endocarditis initially seen as septic arthritis. *Arch. Intern. Med.* 138:805, 1978.
    Two (articles 12 and 13) rarities.
14. Brook, I., Reza, M. J., Bricknell, K. S., et al. Synovial fluid lactic acid: A diagnostic aid in septic arthritis. *Arthritis Rheum.* 21:774, 1978.
    Lactic acid levels were high in nongonococcal septic arthritis and much lower in nonseptic arthritis and gonococcal septic arthritis.
15. Sharp, J. T., Lidsky, M. D., Duffy, J., et al. Infectious arthritis. *Arch. Intern. Med.* 139:1125, 1979.
    A good review of 120 episodes and a useful list of organisms. Gonorrhea was the most common.
16. Schmid, F. R. (ed). Infectious arthritis. *Clin. Rheum. Dis.* 12:343, 1986.
    This volume discusses Lyme disease, septic arthritis in children, imaging of septic arthritis, therapy, and prosthetic joint infections.
17. Baer, P. A., Tenenbaum, J., Fam, A. G., et al. Coexistent septic and crystal arthritis: Report of four cases and literature review. *J. Rheumatol.* 13:604, 1986.
    A rare but important association.
18. Nakashima, A. K., McCarthy, M. A., Martone, W. J., et al. Epidemic septic arthritis caused by *Serratia marcescens* and associated with a benzalkonium chloride antiseptic. *J. Clin. Microbiol.* 25:104, 1987.
    Another iatrogenic infection to keep in mind.
19. Pischel, K. D., Weisman, M. H., and Cone, R. O. Unique features of group B streptococcal arthritis in adults. *Arch. Intern. Med.* 145:97, 1985.
    Multiple joints can be involved and the infection behave aggressively.
20. Borenstein, D. G., and Simon, G. L. *Haemophilus influenzae* septic arthritis in adults: A report of four cases and a review of the literature. *Medicine* 65:191, 1986.
    Most were monoarticular and the joint fluid is typically purulent and greenish.
21. McGuire, N. M., and Kauffman, C. A. Septic arthritis in the elderly. *J. Am. Geriatr. Soc.* 33:170, 1985.
    A concise review of this disease in the older population.

131. SEXUALLY TRANSMITTED DISEASES
Gina A. Dallabetta
Thomas C. Quinn

The term *sexually transmitted diseases (STDs)* now describes an expanded array of clinical syndromes beyond the classic venereal diseases. This is due to the recognition of new pathogens (human immunodeficiency virus [HIV], *Mobiluncus*), the recognition of the sequelae of STDs (pelvic inflammatory diseases, infertility, neonatal infections), the recognition of the sexual spread of old diseases (hepatitis B, shigellosis, amebiasis), and the association with chronic or fatal diseases (herpes simplex virus, human papilloma virus, acquired immunodeficiency syndrome [AIDS]). In the evaluation of patients at risk for STDs the etiologic diagnosis can often not be readily made at the time of initial visit. Consequently, the most symptomatic individuals will be treated based on history and clinical presentation for the most likely organisms with modification of therapy based on test results. However, treatment of only symptomatic patients will fail to identify many infected individuals; thus, routine screening of those at high risk and evaluation and treatment of sexual contacts of infected persons will identify many asymptomatic individuals.

Urethritis in sexually active men under 40 years of age is most commonly sexually acquired and is either gonococcal or nongonococcal urethritis (NGU). Symptoms of urethritis include dysuria and discharge. The symptoms of NGU tend to be milder and of longer duration as compared to gonococcal urethritis, but clinical presentation is not reliable in their differentiation. Gram-stained smears of urethral discharge with polymorphonuclear neutrophils (PMNs) containing gram-negative diplococci are highly predictive (sensitivity and specificity >95%) for a positive culture for *Neisseria gonorrhoeae*. Smears that show atypical intracellular gram-negative organisms or only extracellular gram-negative diplococci are called equivocal, but are still sufficiently predictive of a positive culture to warrant therapy. The absence of gram-negative intracellular diplococci and greater than 4 PMNs per oil immersion field fulfill the criteria for NGU. The etiologies of NGU include *Chlamydia trachomatis* (30–50%) and *Ureaplasma urealyticum*. Other rare nonbacterial causes include herpes simplex virus, intraurethral warts, and *Trichomonas vaginalis*. Complications of urethritis in men include urethral strictures, epididymitis, and prostatitis.

Lower genital tract infections in women include infections of the cervix, vulva, urinary tract, and vagina. The symptoms produced by these infections overlap and include dysuria, dyspareunia, increased vaginal discharge, and vulvar pruritus. A systematic evaluation of women can differentiate sites of infection, identify etiologic agents, and exclude more serious upper tract disease. Cervicitis is a clinical diagnosis based on the presence of mucopurulent endocervical discharge, the presence of 10 or more PMNs on oil immersion field of a Gram stain of endocervical discharge, friability, and edema of the zone of ectopy. The recognized and suspected etiologies of mucopurulent cervicitis (MPC) include both infectious and noninfectious causes, the most common being *C. trachomatis, N. gonorrhoeae,* herpes simplex virus, human papilloma virus, and *T. vaginalis*. In women with gonococcal cervicitis, endocervical Gram stains will have gram-negative intracellular diplococci 40 to 60 percent of the time. Pelvic inflammatory disease (PID), frequently due to either gonorrhea, chlamydia, and/or anaerobes, is the major complication of cervicitis, which often results in severe long-term sequelae such as infertility, ectopic pregnancy, chronic pelvic pain, and recurrent infection.

Disseminated gonococcal infection (DGI) is a complication of untreated gonococcal infection in both men and women. Patients present with fever, arthritis, or dermatitis. Cultures of blood, joint fluid, and skin lesions as well as cervix or urethra, throat, and rectum should be performed. Hospitalization and parenteral antibiotics are indicated for DGI.

Patients with uncomplicated urogenital gonorrhea should receive therapy for both *N. gonorrhoeae* and *C. trachomatis,* as coinfection with chlamydia occurs in 20 to 50 percent of patients with gonorrhea. While many strains of gonorrhea remain penicillin-sensitive, an increase in both penicillinase-producing *N. gonorrhoeae* (PPNG) and tetracycline-resistant gonorrhea has been noted in selected areas. In women with MPC and men with NGU, where gonorrhea has been ruled out, initial therapy should be directed against chlamydia using either tetracycline or erythromycin. Epididymitis should be treated with therapy for gonorrhea and chlamydia. PID requires prolonged therapy against gonorrhea, chlamydia, facultative gram-negative organisms, and anaerobes.

Vaginitis syndromes include trichomoniasis, candidiasis, and bacterial vaginosis (formerly nonspecific vaginitis or *Gardnerella* vaginitis). Vaginitis syndromes can be differentiated at the time of speculum examination by examination of a wet mount for identification of *T. vaginalis* and clue cells, by examination of a potassium hydroxide preparation for *Candida albicans,* and by identification of clue cells and elevated vaginal pH in bacterial vaginosis. Bacterial vaginosis is a disequilibrium syndrome and is diagnosed with the presence of three of the four criteria: homogeneous gray-white discharge, vaginal pH greater than 4.6, greater than 20 percent clue cells on wet mount, and positive amine odor upon application of KOH to the vaginal fluid.

Genital ulceration with regional lymphadenopathy encompasses another group of organisms other than those causing urethritis and cervicitis. Herpes simplex virus (HSV) and *Treponema pallidum,* the causative agent of syphilis, are the most common causes of genital ulceration in the United States. *Haemophilus ducreyi,* the cause of chancroid, is an uncommon cause of genital ulceration in the United States, but is increasing in certain areas. Granuloma inguinale and lymphogranuloma venereum are rare in the United States, but should be considered in patients who have been in endemic areas. Other causes of genital ulceration include fixed drug eruption, carcinoma, and trauma. The clinical manifestations and symptoms of genital ulcer syndromes are not distinctive enough to permit accurate diagnosis. Nonetheless, definitive diagnosis is important given the wide spectrum of possible pathogens.

Herpes accounts for 30 to 60 percent of ulcerative lesions in STD clinic patients. The incubation period for genital herpes is 3 to 10 days following exposure. Classically, herpes presents as multiple small grouped vesicular lesions, although most patients present after the vesicles have ruptured into ulcerative lesions. In patients with a primary genital herpes infection the ulceration tends to be more extensive with bilateral, coalesced lesions associated with bilateral tender inguinal adenopathy and systemic symptoms such as myalgias, arthralgias, and low-grade fever. A primary outbreak resolves in about 3 weeks. In recurrent episodes the ulcers tend to be fewer in number, shorter in duration, and not associated with systemic symptoms. Laboratory diagnostic tests are extremely important in the diagnosis of herpes, especially in patients without classic lesions. These diagnostic tests include virus culture, detection of viral antigen by immunologic methods, or demonstration of giant cells or intranuclear inclusions by Papanicolaou or Giesma staining. HSV serology can be useful in documenting a primary infection but has little utility in recurrent disease. Because herpes is the most common cause of ulcerative lesions in the United States, an uncommon presentation of herpes is a more likely cause of genital ulceration than other, less frequent causes of ulceration. Acyclovir is an effective therapy for herpes and is useful in primary infections and in severe, recurrent disease.

Syphilis accounts for 12 to 17 percent of genital ulcerative lesions in STD patients in the United States. The initial lesion, a chancre, appears between 7 and 21 days after exposure. Classically, a syphilitic chancre is a single, painless ulcer with firm, indurated edges, a clean base, and with nontender regional lymphadenopathy. Dark-field microscopy of serum exuded from the dermal layer of the lesion is often positive in those patients who have not used antibiotics or topical antibacterial agents. About 30 percent of patients with primary syphilis will be seronegative at the time of initial evaluation and it is therefore advisable to repeat serology 7 days after initial presentation. If primary syphilis goes untreated, patients will manifest signs and symptoms of secondary syphilis in about 6 weeks. These signs and symptoms are protean and include rash, generalized lymphadenopathy, fever, and malaise. In this stage serologic tests are almost invariably reactive, with false-negative reactions due to technical problems or antibody excess (1–2%), termed the *prozone phenomenon*. Other stages of syphilis are identified by serologic testing, history, and lumbar puncture. The neurologic manifestations of syphilis can occur at any stage of the infection.

Homosexual men, because of their sexual practices, are at risk for acute anorectal and enteric infections as well as HIV infection and AIDS. The pathogens associated with the enteric syndromes include the classic STDs (gonorrhea, chlamydia, HSV, and syphilis) as well as traditional enteric organisms (*Entamoeba histolytica, Giardia lambdia, Shigella* sp., *Salmonella* sp., and *Campylobacter* sp.). Since many organisms, all with widely different therapies, have similar presentations a systematic approach to diagnosis and therapy is necessary, including anoscopy, sigmoidoscopy, and cultures.

1. Perine, P., Handsfield, H. H., Holmes, K. K., et al. Epidemiology of sexually transmitted disease. *Annu. Rev. Public Health* 6:85, 1985.
2. Jacobs, N. F., and Kraus, S. S. Gonococcal and non-gonococcal urethritis in men. Clinical and laboratory differentiation. *Ann. Intern. Med.* 82:7, 1975.
   Compares microscopic findings to culture.
3. Stamm, E. W., Koutsky, L. A., Benedetti, J. K., et al. *Chlamydia trachomatis* urethral infections in men: Prevalence, risk factors, and clinical manifestations. *Ann. Intern. Med.* 100:47, 1984.
   A study of the spectrum in disease due to C. trachomatis *in men.*
4. Kristensen, J. K., and Scheibel, J. H. The etiology of acute epididymitis presenting in a venereal disease clinic. *Sex Transm. Dis.* 11:32, 1984.
   The most common etiology is C. trachomatis.
5. Brunham, R. C., Paavonen, J., Stevens, C. E., et al. Mucopurulent cervicitis—The ignored counterpart in women of urethritis. *N. Engl. J. Med.* 311:1, 1984.
   This paper defines the clinical entity of mucopurulent cervicitis and its associated pathogens.
6. Amsel, R., Follen, P. A., Spiegel, C. A., et al. Nonspecific vaginitis. Diagnostic criteria and microbial and epidemiologic associations. *Am. J. Med.* 74:14, 1983.
   Describes the clinical diagnostic criteria.
7. Wasserheit, J. N. Pelvic inflammatory disease and infertility. *Md. State Med. J.* 36:58, 1987.
   A review of etiology, diagnosis, therapy, and complications.
8. Stamm, W. E. Diagnosis of *Chlamydia trachomatis* genitourinary infections. *Ann. Intern. Med.* 108:710, 1988.
   A complete discussion of all aspects of diagnosis.
9. Alexander, E. R., and Harrison, H. R. Role of *Chlamydia trachomatis* in perinatal infection. *Rev. Infect. Dis.* 5:713, 1983.
   A review of perinatal transmission of chlamydia and its effect on pregnancy and the infant.
10. Thompson, S. E., and Washington, A. E. Epidemiology of sexually transmitted *Chlamydia trachomatis* infections. *Epidemiol. Rev.* 5:96, 1983.
    An excellent review of the clinical spectrum of chlamydia and the groups at highest risk.
11. Stamm, W. E, Wagner, K. F., Amsel, R., et al. Causes of the acute urethral syndrome in women. *N. Engl. J. Med.* 310:409, 1980.
    Chlamydia can cause dysuria and culture-negative pyuria in women.
12. Handsfield, H. H., Jasman, L. L., Roberts, P. L., et al. Criteria for selective screening for *Chlamydia trachomatis* infection in women attending family planning clinics. *J.A.M.A.* 255:1930, 1986.
    Identifies criteria for identifying high-risk women for chlamydial infection.
13. Dallabetta, G., Hook, E. W., III. Gonococcal infections. *Infect. Dis. Clin. North Am.* 1:25, 1987.
    Overview of gonococcal pathogenesis, clinical manifestations, and therapy.
14. Centers for Disease Control. Sexually transmitted disease treatment guidelines, 1989. *M.M.W.R.* 38(Suppl. S-8):1, 1989.
    A complete review of recommended therapy for sexually transmitted diseases.
15. Centers for Disease Control. *Chlamydia trachomatis* infections: Policy guidelines for prevention and control. *M.M.W.R.* 34(Suppl. 3s): 53s, 1985.
    Guidelines for diagnosis and therapy.
16. Eisenstein, B. I., and Masi, A. T. Disseminated gonococcal infection (DGI) and gono-

coccal arthritis (GCA): I. Bacteriology, epidemiology, host factors, pathogen factors and pathology. *Semin. Arthritis Rheum.* 10:155, 1981.
A thorough description of the disease.

17. Chapel, T. A., Brown, W. J., Jeffries, C., et al. How reliable is the morphological diagnosis of penile ulcerations? *Sex Transm. Dis.* 4:150, 1987.
Clinical diagnosis of ulcers is often inaccurate.

18. Diaz-Mitoma, F., Bennington, G., Slutchuk, M., et al. Etiology of nonvesicular ulcers in Winnipeg. *Sex Transm. Dis.* 14:35, 1987.
Herpes still a common cause of ulceration.

19. Schmid GP, Sanders, L. L., Blount, J. H., et al. Chancroid in the United States. *J.A.M.A.* 258:3265, 1987.
In the United States chancroid is most common in specific areas with a history of prostitute contact.

20. Corey, L., Adams, H. G., Brown, Z. A., et al. Genital herpes simplex virus infections: Clinical manifestations, course and complications. *Ann. Intern. Med.* 98:958, 1983.

21. Cory, L., and Holmes, K. K. Genital herpes simplex virus infections: Current concepts in diagnosis, therapy and prevention. *Ann. Intern. Med.* 98:973, 1983.
These two papers are a thorough review of the subject.

22. Sparling, F. P. Diagnosis and treatment of syphilis. *N. Engl. J. Med.* 284:642, 1971.
A full discussion of diagnosis, especially serology.

23. Simon, R. P. Neurosyphilis. *Arch. Neurol.* 42:606, 1985.
Discusses full spectrum of the disease which occurs in all stages of syphilis.

24. Berry, R. D., Hooton, T. M., Collier, A. C., et al. Neurologic relapse after benzathine penicillin therapy for secondary syphilis with HIV infection. *N. Engl. J. Med.* 316:1587, 1987.
HIV infection may alter response to therapy of syphilis.

25. Quinn, T. C., Stamm, W. E., Goodell, S. E., et al. The polymicrobial origin of intestinal infections in homosexual men. *N. Engl. J. Med.* 309:576, 1983.
This paper describes the syndromes and associated pathogens in sexually acquired intestinal infections.

26. Howley, P. M. The role of Papilloma Virus in Human Cancer. In V. T. DeVita Jr., S. Hellman, and S. A. Rosenberg (eds.), *Important Advances in Oncology.* Philadelphia: J. B. Lippincott, 1987. P. 55.

27. Kirby, P., and Corey, L. Genital human papillomavirus infections. *Infect. Dis. Clin. North Am.* 1:123, 1987.
These papers (articles 26, 27) give a full overview of the evidence linking HPV to human cancers.

132. STAPHYLOCOCCAL INFECTIONS
Jerry L. Spivak

Colonization by staphylococci is common, but infection, either localized or disseminated, usually occurs only under conditions in which host resistance is impaired. These conditions include viral respiratory tract infections, the presence of foreign bodies (sutures, drains, catheters, shunts), burns, trauma, diabetes mellitus, narcotic addiction, leukopenia, vascular disease, chronic renal failure, and therapy with corticosteroids or broadspectrum antibiotics. Although gram-negative organisms are currently the most frequent cause of opportunistic and nosocomial infections, it is important not to overlook the possibility of staphylococcal invasion since the organism possesses the potential to produce disseminated infection, to attack and destroy normal heart valves, and to cause overwhelming sepsis even in an otherwise healthy host.

Metastatic pulmonary infection is not uncommon as a complication of staphylococcal bacteremia. The progression of the pulmonary lesions can be rapid, with considerable involvement apparent on chest x ray in the absence of any physical findings. The fulminant nature of some staphylococcal infections should not, however, obscure the fact that staphylococcal infection can exhibit considerable latency, occasionally to the extent that the initiating event is no longer evident. This is a feature of staphylococcal infection of bone, and often the first indication of such infection is the development of a paraspinal or epidural abscess. Abscess formation can result in sinus tracts, and in such instances the diagnostic possibilities include tuberculosis and actinomycosis as well as staphylococcal infection.

A particular problem in the management of staphylococcal infection is determination of whether bacteremia represents or has produced endocarditis. The incidence of endocarditis-associated bacteremia is 15 to 25 percent in unselected patients, but in the narcotic addict with a staphylococcal bacteremia or staphylococcal pneumonia, endocarditis should always be considered present. In other situations, persistent bacteremia suggests endocarditis or endarteritis, whereas intermittent bacteremia is usually associated with soft tissue abscesses. In general, endocarditis is usually present when bacteremia is not associated with a definable primary focus of infection, is community-acquired, and metastatic sequelae are present. Serologic studies have been useful in identifying those patients with an endocarditis-associated bacteremia. Echocardiography may also be useful in this regard in patients with community-acquired infection.

Methicillin-resistant staphylococci, which are essentially a hospital-associated phenomenon, are a serious problem mainly in debilitated hosts. A more troublesome problem is the emergence of coagulase-negative staphylococci as a hospital pathogen, of which the commonest species is *Staphylococcus epidermidis,* and multiantibiotic resistance is frequent. These organisms are often the cause of bacteremia in patients with intravenous lines, but other implanted devices (shunts, cardiac, vascular, and joint prostheses) may be involved. Infection of a native cardiac valve usually only occurs when the valve is anatomically abnormal. It is thought that slime production is an important pathogenetic feature of those coagulase-negative strains which infect implanted devices.

In the management of any staphylococcal infection, penicillin resistance should be assumed. However, antibiotic sensitivities should be determined since penicillin is a more effective agent than its semisynthetic analogues. The possibility of methicillin resistance should also be examined. Methicillin-resistant *Staphylococcus aureus* infections are best treated with vancomycin as are those due to multidrug-resistant *S. epidermidis.* Slow resolution of fever and continued bacteremia are not uncommon during the initial phase of antibiotic therapy for staphylococcal infections. Persistence of fever, however, should suggest the possibility of antibiotic resistance or metastatic abscesses for which surgical drainage is necessary. In the case of antibiotic resistance, either a change in antibiotic or addition of a second agent will be necessary. Available evidence suggests that while the duration of bacteremia is reduced in staphylococcal endocarditis with combination therapy, the clinical response is no different than when a single agent is employed initially. Consequently, combination therapy should be reserved for those situations when a single agent has proved ineffective or where the diagnosis is in doubt.

1. Sheagren, J. N. *Staphylococcus aureus:* The persistent pathogen. *N. Engl. J. Med.* 310:1368, 1437, 1984.
   Comprehensive review.
2. Eykyn, S. J. Staphylococcal sepsis. *Lancet* 1:100, 1988.
   Concise review.
3. Brumfitt, W., and Hamilton-Miller, J. Methicillin-resistant *Staphylococcus aureus.* *N. Engl. J. Med.* 320:1188, 1989.
   State-of-the-art review.
4. Martin, M. A., Pfaller, M. A., and Wenzel, R. P. Coagulase-negative staphylococcal bacteremia. *Ann. Intern. Med.* 110:9, 1989.
   This is associated with a significant mortality rate.
5. Bayer, A. S., Lam, K., Ginzton, L., et al. *Staphylococcus aureus* bacteremia. *Arch. Intern. Med.* 147:457, 1987.
   Comparison of patients with and without endocarditis.

6. Chambers, H. F., Karzencowski, C. M., and Saude, M. A. *Staphylococcus aureus* endocarditis. *Medicine* 62:170, 1983.
   Staphylococci are the commonest cause of endocarditis in narcotic addicts where the disease is usually on the tricuspid valve; in nonaddicts, the left side of the heart is involved and congestive failure is more common. (See also Ann. Intern. Med. *109:619, 1988.)*

7. Watanakunakorn, C., and Baird, I. M. *Staphylococcus aureus* bacteremia and endocarditis associated with a removable infected intravenous device. *Am. J. Med.* 63:253, 1977.
   Over 30% of patients in this series developed endocarditis as a consequence of a contaminated intravenous line.

8. Manolis, A. S., and Melita, H. Echocardiographic and clinical correlates in drug addicts with infective endocarditis. Implications of vegetation size. *Arch. Intern. Med.* 148:2461, 1988.
   The tricuspid valve is most frequently involved. (See also Chest *93:247, 1988 and* Am. J. Med. *80:165, 1986.)*

9. Espersen, F., and Frimodt-Mller, N. *Staphylococcus aureus* endocarditis. A review of 119 cases. *Arch. Intern. Med.* 146:1118, 1986.
   A diagnosis which is frequently unsuspected.

10. Caputo, G. M., Archer, G. L., Calderwood, S. B., et al. Native valve endocarditis due to coagulase-negative staphylococci. *Am. J. Med.* 83:619, 1987.
    Preexisting anatomic abnormalities are the rule. (See also Am. J. Clin. Pathol. *87:408, 1987 and* Arch. Intern. Med. *146:119, 1986.)*

11. Hart, R. G., Kagan-Hallet, K., and Joerns, S. E. Mechanisms of intracranial hemorrhage in infective endocarditis. *Stroke* 18:1048, 1987.
    Septic arteritis is more common than mycotic aneurysms.

12. Quale, J. M., Mandel, L. J., Bergasa, N. V., et al. Clinical significance and pathogenesis of hyperbilirubinemia associated with *Staphylococcus aureus* septicemia. *Am. J. Med.* 85:615, 1988.
    Hyperbilirubinemia is often associated with overwhelming sepsis.

13. Jacobson, M. A., Gellermann, H., and Chambers, H. *Staphylococcus aureus* bacteremia and recurrent staphylococcal infection in patients with acquired immunodeficiency syndrome and AIDS-related complex. *Am. J. Med.* 85:172, 1988.
    Human immunodeficiency virus (HIV)–infected patients are at a high risk for staphylococcal bacteremia.

14. Stein, J. M., and Pruett, B. A., Jr. Suppurative thrombophlebitis: A lethal iatrogenic disease. *N. Engl. J. Med.* 282:1452, 1970.
    Advocates surgical excision of the involved vein.

15. Ho, G., Jr., Fue, A. D., and Kaplan, S. R. Septic bursitis in the prepatellar and olecranon bursae. *Ann. Intern. Med.* 89:21, 1978.
    A high incidence of staphylococcal infection was observed in this series. (See also Am. J. Med. *83:661, 1987.)*

16. Levin, M. J., Gardner, P., and Waldvogel, F. A. "Tropical" pyomyositis: An unusual infection due to *Staphylococcus aureus*. *N. Engl. J. Med.* 284:196, 1971.
    The abscesses are deep, signs of inflammation are lacking, and a tropical background is not necessary. (See also Lancet *1:862, 1978 and* J. Clin. Pathol. *39:1116, 1986.)*

17. Fred, H. L., and Harle, T. S. Septic pulmonary embolism. *Dis. Chest* 55:483, 1969.
    Careful evaluation of the chest x ray is important in recognizing this problem.

18. Schlesinger, L. S., Ross, S. C., and Schaberg, D. R. *Staphylococcus aureus* meningitis: a broad-based epidemiologic study. *Medicine* 66:148, 1987.
    Comprehensive review. (See also Am. J. Med. *78:965, 1985.)*

19. Danner, R. L., and Hartman, B. J. Update of spinal epidural abscess: 35 cases and review of the literature. *Rev. Infect. Dis.* 9:265, 1987.
    Staphylococci are the most common cause and the presentation can be subtle.

20. Quarles, L. D., Rutsky, E. A., and Rostand, S. G. *Staphylococcus aureus* bacteremia in patients on chronic hemodialysis. *Am. J. Kidney Dis.* 6:412, 1985.
    Vascular access sites are the usual portal of entry.

21. Eisenberg, E. S., Ambalu, M., Szylagi, G., et al. Colonization of skin and development

of peritonitis due to coagulase-negative staphylococci in patients undergoing peritoneal dialysis. *J. Infect. Dis.* 156:478, 1987.
A not uncommon problem in this population.

22. Neefe, L. I., Tuazon, C. U., Cardella, T. A., et al. Staphylococcal scalded skin syndrome in adults: Case report and review of the literature. *Am. J. Med. Sci.* 277:99, 1979.
The importance of a skin biopsy is emphasized.

23. Elias, P. M., Fritsch, P., and Epstein, E. H. Staphylococcal scalded skin syndrome. *Arch. Dermatol.* 113:207, 1977.
Staphylococcal scalded skin syndrome contrasted with toxic epidermal necrolysis. (See also J.A.M.A. 229:425, 1974.)

24. Davis, J. P., Chesney, P. J., Wand, P. J., et al. Toxic-shock syndrome: Epidemiologic features, recurrence, risk factors, and prevention. *N. Engl. J. Med.* 303:1429, 1980.
A disease of "progress." (See also J.A.M.A. 259:394, 1988.)

25. Rahal, J. J., Jr., MacMahon, H. E., and Weinstein, L. Thrombocytopenia and symmetrical peripheral gangrene associated with staphylococcal and streptococcal bacteremia. *Ann. Intern. Med.* 69:35, 1968.
Disseminated intravascular coagulation with gram-positive cocci.

26. Mandell, G. L. Staphylococcal infection and leukocyte bactericidal defect in a 22-year-old woman. *Arch. Intern. Med.* 130:754, 1972.
Something to consider in an adult with recurrent staphylococcal infections. (See also Lancet 2:880, 1987.)

27. Tu, W. H., Shearn, M. A., and Lee, J. C. Acute diffuse glomerulonephritis in acute staphylococcal endocarditis. *Ann. Intern. Med.* 71:335, 1969.
Reversible immune complex nephritis.

28. Demuth, P. J., Gerding, D. N., and Crossley, K. *Staphylococcus aureus* bacteriuria. *Arch. Intern. Med.* 139:78, 1979.
Staphylococcal urinary infection is usually a consequence of urinary tract manipulation.

29. Lee, B. K., Crossley, K., and Gerding, D. N. The association between *staphylococcus aureus* bacteremia and bacteriuria. *Am. J. Med.* 65:303, 1978.
Bacteriuria frequently occurs during staphylococcal bacteremia and does not signify significant renal involvement or endocarditis.

30. Detecting host response to staphylococcal infection. *Lancet* 1:953, 1986.
Concise review of serologic testing in staphylococcal infections.

31. Tenney, J. H., Moody, M. R., Newman, K. A., et al. Adherent microorganisms on luminal surfaces of long-term intravenous catheters. Importance of *Staphylococcus epidermidis* in patients with cancer. *Arch. Intern. Med.* 146:1949, 1986.
Slime production is an important feature of the infecting organism.

32. Rhinehart, E., Shlaes, D. M., Keys, T. F., et al. Nosocomial clonal dissemination of methicillin-resistant *Staphylococcus aureus*. Elucidation by plasmid analysis. *Arch. Intern. Med.* 147:521, 1987.
Cross-transmission by hospital personnel caused this outbreak. (See also Lancet 2:189, 1985 and Medicine 60:62, 1981.)

33. Sabath, L., Wheeler, N., Laverdiere, M., et al. A new type of penicillin resistance of *Staphylococcus aureus*. *Lancet* 1:443, 1977.
The three forms of penicillin resistance are reviewed.

34. Rajashekaroiah, K. R., Rue, T., Ruo, V. S., et al. Clinical significance of tolerant strains of *Staphylococcus aureus* in patients with endocarditis. *Ann. Intern. Med.* 93:796, 1980.
Tolerance appears to adversely affect the treatment of endocarditis but not other types of bacteremia. (See accompanying editorial on p. 924 for a balanced review of the significance of tolerance.)

35. Abrams, B., Sklaver, A., Hoffman, T., et al. Single or combination therapy of staphylococcal endocarditis in intravenous drug abusers. *Ann. Intern. Med.* 90:789, 1979.
Single-agent therapy was sufficient. (See also Arch. Intern. Med. 139:1090, 1979.)

36. Onorato, I. M., and Axelrod, J. L. Hepatitis from intravenous high-dose oxacillin therapy. *Ann. Intern. Med.* 89:497, 1978.
Hepatitis developed with doses greater than 6 gm/day.

37. Cook, F. V., and Farrar, W. E., Jr. Vancomycin revisited. *Ann. Intern. Med.* 88:813, 1978.
    Review of the pharmacology and clinical usefulness of this drug.
38. Kaplan, M. H., and Tenenbaum, M. J. Staphylococcus aureus: Cellular biology and clinical application. *Am. J. Med.* 72:248, 1982.
    Comprehensive review.
39. Coagulase-negative staphylococci. *Lancet* 1:139, 1981.
    Concise review.
40. Christensen, G. D., Bisno, A. L., Parisi, J. T., et al. Nosocomial septicemia due to multiple antibiotic-resistant *Staphylococcus epidermidis*. *Ann. Intern. Med.* 96:1, 1982.
    A problem usually associated with intravenous catheters.
41. Louria, D. B., Sen, P., Kapila, R., et al. Anterior thigh pain or tenderness. *Arch. Intern. Med.* 145:657, 1985.
    An interesting diagnostic sign of bacteremia.

133. STREPTOCOCCAL INFECTIONS

H. Verdain Barnes

A wide variety of common and uncommon infections are caused by streptococci. Streptococci are currently grouped A through H and K through T on the basis of serologic cell wall properties. The group A β-hemolytic streptococci are by far the most common offenders in man, but groups B, C, D, F, G, H, K, and O and some nongroupable strains have been cultured from active infectious foci and the blood of humans. Of these, the group D strains are often labeled enterococci.

Virulent group A streptococci produce an M surface protein that inhibits leukocyte phagocytosis. The following substances are liberated: erythrogenic toxin (ET), streptolysins O and S, streptokinase, nicotinamide adenine dinucleotidase, deoxyribonuclease (DNase), proteinase, and hyaluronidase. Only ET, of which there are three serologic forms, has proved to have pathogenic significance; it produces malaise, fever, nausea, vomiting, and a scarlatiniform rash. A specific antibody to streptolysin O (ASO) forms in about 80 percent of patients with streptococcal pharyngitis. This antibody appears about the second week, peaks around the fifth postinfection week, and usually remains elevated for months. The antibody to DNase B is commonly produced, and an anti-DNase B titer can on occasion identify patients with remote infections in whom the ASO is not elevated. Infections by other pathogenic streptococcal groups cannot be so identified.

Group A streptococci are the most common cause of bacterial pharyngitis and/or tonsillitis. In addition, they have been reported to cause acute appendicitis, septic arthritis, myositis, brain abscess, acute bronchitis, conjunctivitis, meningitis, otitis media, otitis externa, primary peritonitis, pneumonia, osteomyelitis, impetigo, cellulitis, empyema, and puerperal infections. Group A pneumonia is most often secondary, usually occurring in the setting of measles, influenza, or chronic bronchitis. Primary pneumonias, however, may be seen. The pneumonia is an interstitial bronchopneumonia that spreads rapidly via lymphatic channels to the pleural surface. Consequently, a serosanguineous pleural effusion early in the illness is common. The pleural effusion almost invariably has numerous streptococcal chains on Gram's stain.

Group B streptococci have been identified as producing septicemia, endocarditis, osteomyelitis, pneumonia, empyema, wound infections, puerperal infections, local skin infections, multiple abscesses, peritonitis, urinary tract infection, septic arthritis, neonatal sepsis, and meningitis. About 20 percent in one series show in vitro insensitivity to the 2-unit penicillin G disk test. There is a frequent but unexplained association with diabetes mellitus. Group C streptococci can cause genital tract, skin, and wound infections; endocarditis; pharyngitis; meningitis; tonsillitis; and pneumonia.

Group D infections have increased in frequency over the past few decades. Infections are more common in elderly debilitated patients or patients receiving antibiotics, corticosteroids, or antimetabolites. The following infections have been identified: endocarditis; biliary tract infection; appendicitis; cervicitis; endometritis; pyelophlebitis; septic pelvic thrombophlebitis; urinary tract infection; enterocolitis; cellulitis; wound infection; pneumonia; empyema; meningitis; sinusitis; osteomyelitis; and skin, wound, tuboovarian, liver, and perinephric abscesses. The streptococci of this group are often not sensitive to penicillin alone.

Group F infections have been reported in the upper respiratory tract, brain, meninges, lungs, pleura, and urinary tract. Group G streptococci can cause cellulitis, endocarditis, ascending cholangitis, empyema, pharyngitis, endometritis, pneumonia, osteomyelitis, peritonitis, septicemia, skin infections, and wound abscesses. These infections are often puerperal. The most common infection produced by group H is bacterial endocarditis, but sinusitis and meningitis have also been reported. Group K has been isolated in sinusitis, endocarditis, cholangitis, pneumonitis, empyema, and otitis media. Group O is rare but can produce nasopharyngeal infections and pneumonia. The large group of nongroupable strains is capable of producing most if not all infections cited.

Bacteremia is not infrequent in patients with streptococcal infections. The initial clinical picture in bacteremia is similar for all groups of streptococci in the absence of endocarditis. High fever, shaking chills, anorexia, nausea, vomiting, and mental confusion predominate. The fever may follow any pattern except double quotidian. Hypotension of variable degree is present in almost all patients with sepsis. The white blood cell count usually ranges from 15,000 to 30,000, with a shift to the left and toxic granulations. Patients may have low serum sodium levels, even in the absence of demonstrable renal disease.

The nonsuppurative complications of group A infections include acute rheumatic fever, acute glomerulonephritis, gangrene, purpura fulminans, scleredema, Schönlein-Henoch purpura, and erythema nodosum. Except for purpura fulminans, these complications have not been reported in non–group A streptococcal infections.

1. Wannamaker, L. W., and Matsen, J. M. *Streptococci and Streptococcal Diseases*. New York: Academic Press, 1972.
   A comprehensive discussion of the streptococci.
2. Duma, R. J., Weinberg, A. N., Medrek, T. F., et al. Streptococcal infections. *Medicine* 48:87, 1969.
   A good, well-referenced, general review with emphasis on bacteremia. Serum sodium was often low.
3. Feingold, D. S., Stagg, N. L., and Kunz, L. J. Extrarespiratory streptococcal infections: Importance of the various serologic groups. *N. Engl. J. Med.* 275:356, 1966.
   Group A, C, and G infections mimic one another.
4. Basiliere, J. L., Bistrong, H. W., and Spence, W. F. Streptococcal pneumonia: Recent outbreaks in military recruit populations. *Am. J. Med.* 44:580, 1969.
   Chest pain and empyema were present in 66%. The incidence of positive blood cultures was low.
5. Altemeier, W. A. The bacterial flora of acute, perforated appendicitis with peritonitis. *Ann. Surg.* 107:517, 1938.
6. Salvatierra, O., Jr., Bucklen, W. B., and Morrow, J. W. Perinephric abscesses: A report of 71 cases. *J. Urol.* 98:296, 1967.
7. Swartz, M. N., and Dodge, P. R. Bacterial meningitis. *N. Engl. J. Med.* 272:275, 779, 842, 898, 1965.
   Articles 5–7 point out the place of streptococci in their respective areas of infection.
8. Reinarz, J. A., and Stanford, J. P. Human infections caused by non-group A or D streptococci. *Medicine* 44:81, 1965.
   A review of non-group A infections, past and present.
9. Sanders, V. Bacterial endocarditis due to a group C beta hemolytic streptococcus. *Ann. Intern. Med.* 58:858, 1963.
   A look at group C disease.
10. Rantz, L. A. Streptococcal meningitis. *Ann. Intern. Med.* 16:716, 1942.
    Group F was the culprit.

11. Leirisalo, M., and Laitinen, O. Rheumatic fever in adult patients. *Ann. Clin. Res.* 7:244, 1975.
    A useful review. Yersinia enterocolitica *infections are pointed out as an important acute rheumatic fever look-alike.*
12. Peter, G., and Smith, A. L. Group A streptococcal infections of the skin and pharynx. *N. Engl. J. Med.* 297:311, 365, 1977.
    A concise review covering clinical courses, epidemiologies, and therapy.
13. Lerner, P. I., Gapalakrishna, K. V., Wolinsky, E., et al. Group B streptococcus (*S. agalactiae*) bacteremia in adults: Analysis of 32 cases and review of the literature. *Medicine* 56:457, 1977.
    An opportunistic pathogen especially in the presence of malignancy and diabetes.
14. Mohr, D. N., Feist, D. J., Washington, J. A., II, et al. Meningitis due to group C streptococci in an adult. *Mayo Clin. Proc.* 53:529, 1978.
15. Stevens, D. L., Haburchak, D. R., McNitt, T. R., et al. Group B streptococcal osteomyelitis in adults. *South Med. J.* 71:1450, 1978.
    Two unusual infections by these organisms (articles 14 and 15).
16. Faro, S. Group B beta-hemolytic streptococci and puerperal infections. *Am. J. Obstet. Gynecol.* 139:686, 1981.
17. Ogden, E., and Amstey, M. S. Peurperal infection due to group A beta hemolytic streptococcus. *Obstet. Gynecol.* 52:53, 1978.
    These articles (16 and 17) offer good clinical discussions of group A and B puerperal infections.
18. Murray, H. W., and Roberts, R. B. *Streptococcus bovis* bacteremia and underlying gastrointestinal disease. *Arch. Intern. Med.* 138:1097, 1978.
    Streptococcus bovis *bacteremia may be the presenting manifestation of gastrointestinal malignancy.*
19. DiSciascio, G., and Taranta, A. Rheumatic fever in children. *Am. Heart J.* 99:635, 1980.
    An excellent, up-to-date review.
20. Bayer, A. S., Yoshikawa, T. T., Nolan, F., et al. Non-group D streptococcal meningitis misidentified as enterococcal meningitis: Diagnostic and therapeutic implications of misdiagnosis by screening microbiology. *Arch. Intern. Med.* 138:1645, 1978.
    An important potential error to keep in mind.
21. Murray, H. W., Gross, K. C., Masur, H., et al. Serious infections caused by *Streptococcus milleri.* *Am. J. Med.* 64:759, 1978.
    This species of viridans streptococci can cause abscesses, peritonitis, endocarditis, cholangitis, empyema, and cellulitis.
22. Vartian, C., Lerner, P.I., Shlaes, D. M., et al. Infections due to Lancefield group G streptococci. *Medicine* 64:75, 1985.
    An important nosocomial and opportunistic organism.
23. Gallagher, P. G., and Watanakunakorn, C. Group B streptoccocal bacteremia in a community teaching hospital. *Am. J. Med.* 78:795, 1985.
    About 46% were hospital-acquired. Outside the perinatal setting the mortality was 70%.
24. Adams, E. M., Gudmundsson, S., Yocum, D. E., et al. Streptoccocal myositis. *Arch. Intern. Med.* 145:1020, 1985.
    Another group A infection to keep in mind.
25. Braman, S. S., and Donat, W. E. Explosive pleuritis: Manifestation of group A beta-hemolytic streptococcal infection. *Am. J. Med.* 81:723, 1986.
    Pleuritis in the absence of pneumonia.
26. Decker, M. D., Lavely, G. B., Hutcheson, R. H., Jr., et al. Food-borne streptococcal pharyngitis in a hospital pediatric clinic. *J.A.M.A.* 253:679, 1985.
    The rice dressing appeared to be the culprit.

134. TUBERCULOUS MENINGITIS
Jerry L. Spivak

Tuberculous meningitis arises as a result of direct extension of a localized intracranial caseous focus to involve the meninges or cerebrospinal fluid. Although untreated miliary tuberculosis is commonly complicated by meningeal infection and most patients with meningeal tuberculosis have evidence of tuberculosis elsewhere, the available evidence suggests that tuberculous meningitis does not develop immediately following hematogenous dissemination. Both we and others have seen patients in whom the meningitis developed after head trauma. Whether the trauma was a fortuitous occurrence or facilitated the breakdown of a caseous focus is unclear.

The presenting manifestations of tuberculous meningitis can vary from fever and headache to seizures, focal neurologic signs, or coma. Physical examination usually reveals meningismus, altered mental status, and often cranial nerve palsies. The tuberculin skin test is usually positive, and tuberculous lesions are found on chest x ray in over 60 percent of patients. Findings on spinal fluid examination vary, depending on when the lumbar puncture is performed. Early in the course of the disease, neutrophils can predominate and the sugar content may not be reduced. Typically the spinal fluid protein level is elevated, the glucose concentration reduced, and the cell count increased, with lymphocytes predominating. In some patients the cerebrospinal fluid pressure may be high; such patients are at risk from herniation. In others there is evidence of cerebrospinal fluid blockade, with a marked elevation in protein concentration. Acid-fast bacilli are found on stained spinal fluid smears in 10 to 30 percent of patients, and spinal fluid cultures are positive in approximately 70 percent of patients. Positive cultures from the sputum or other sources are found in over 50 percent.

In the patient with typical findings, particularly with evidence of tuberculosis elsewhere, the diagnosis is not difficult. On the other hand, when the spinal fluid findings are not typical or there is no other evidence of tuberculous infection, the diagnosis may not be easy to establish. A particular problem occurs in patients who have been partially treated for bacterial meningitis or in those with aseptic meningitis. In such cases careful observation with repeated spinal fluid examinations may obviate a long course of unnecessary chemotherapy. On the other hand, in the critically ill patient with evidence of progressive neurologic deterioration, treatment with chemotherapy should not be delayed. Isoniazid (INH) and rifampin are an effective combination with ethambutol being employed initially if drug resistance is suspected, as in Asian or Hispanic immigrants. A four-drug regimen, INH, rifampin, pyrazinamide, and streptomycin, for 2 months, followed by isoniazid and rifampin for 7 months, has also been effective. However, despite excellent chemotherapeutic agents, the morbidity and mortality rates associated with tuberculous meningitis remain high.

Computed axial tomography (CT) is an ideal technique for following the progress of tuberculous meningitis and its response to treatment. With CT scanning, the extent of meningeal involvement and hydrocephalus and the development of tuberculomas can be evaluated. The latter complication is being recognized with increasing frequency in patients with tuberculous meningitis. Tuberculomas do not usually require surgical intervention, but hydrocephalus will require surgical drainage if there is associated neurologic deterioration.

A particular problem in patients with tuberculous meningitis is the development of cerebral edema and herniation. Steroid therapy has been shown to be efficacious in reducing cerebrospinal fluid pressure and the incidence of herniation. Steroids may also be useful in the management of tuberculomas when these are associated with increased intracranial pressure.

Spinal fluid recovery from tuberculous meningitis is slow, and although the glucose level returns to normal within several weeks, elevations of protein and cell count can persist for many months. Fever usually subsides within 4 weeks. Poor prognostic factors include old age, coma, race, and chronic alcoholism. Neurologic sequelae are not uncommon; they include hydrocephalus, organic brain syndrome, hemiplegia, paraplegia, seizures, optic atrophy, and cranial nerve paralysis. Panhypopituitarism has also been documented in younger patients.

1. Ogawa, S. K., Smith, M. A., Brennessel, D. J., et al. Tuberculous meningitis in an urban medical center. *Medicine* 66:317, 1987.
   The mortality rate was high particularly when the disease was at an advanced stage. (See also Med. Clin. North Am. 69:315, 1985.)

2. Klein, N. C., Damsker, B., and Hirschman, S. Z. Mycobacterial meningitis. Retrospective analysis from 1970 to 1983. *Am. J. Med.* 79:29, 1985.
   The clinical presentation is variable, and it is important that chemotherapy be instituted as soon as possible.

3. Anderson, N. E., and Willoughby, E. W. Chronic meningitis without predisposing illness—a review of 83 cases. *Q. J. Med.* 63:283, 1987.
   Tuberculosis was the most common cause.

4. Bishburg, E., Sunderam, G., Reichman, L. B., et al. Central nervous system tuberculosis with the acquired immunodeficiency syndrome [AIDS] and its related complex. *Ann. Intern. Med.* 105:210, 1986.
   Tuberculosis is an important consideration in the AIDS patient with neurologic symptoms.

5. Traub, M., Colchester, A. C., Kingsley, D. P., et al. Tuberculosis of the central nervous system. *Q. J. Med.* 53:81, 1984.
   Advocates avoiding surgery for diagnostic purposes.

6. Stockstill, M. T., and Kauffman, C. A. Comparison of cryptococcal and tuberculous meningitis. *Arch. Neurol.* 40:81, 1983.
   A difficult diagnostic problem.

7. Rich, A. R., and McCordock, H. A. The pathogenesis of tuberculous meningitis. *Bull. Johns Hopkins Hosp.* 52:31, 1933.
   Tuberculous meningitis arises from activation of a latent central nervous system focus, not as a direct result of miliary dissemination.

8. Falk, A. U.S. Veterans Administration Armed Forces Cooperative Study on the Chemotherapy of Tuberculosis: XIII. Tuberculous meningitis in adults with special reference to survival, neurologic residuals and work status. *Am. Rev. Respir. Dis.* 91:823, 1965.
   Organic brain syndrome is the most common severe sequela.

9. Hinman, A. R. Tuberculous meningitis at Cleveland Metropolitan General Hospital 1959 to 1963. *Am. Rev. Respir. Dis.* 95:670, 1967.
   Spinal fluid abnormalities can persist for many weeks after initiation of therapy.

10. Udani, P. M., Parekh, U. C., and Dastur, D. K. Neurological and related syndromes in CNS tuberculosis. *J. Neurol. Sci.* 14:341, 1971.
    A detailed review of neurologic syndromes occurring with tuberculous infection of the central nervous system.

11. Kocen, R. S., and Parsons, M. Neurological complications of tuberculosis: Some unusual manifestations. *Q. J. Med.* 39:31, 1970.
    Early spinal fluid changes can be quite misleading.

12. Phuapradit, P., and Vejjajiva, A. Treatment of tuberculous meningitis: Role of short-course chemotherapy. *Q. J. Med.* 62:249, 1987.
    Four drugs employed for 2 months; then isoniazid and rifampin for 7 months was an effective form of therapy.

13. Clark, W. C., Metcalf, J. C., Jr., Muhlbauer, M. S., et al. *Mycobacterium tuberculosis* meningitis: A report of twelve cases and a literature review. *Neurosurgery* 18:604, 1986.
    An aggressive approach advocated to prevent hydrocephalus. (See also Am. J. Med. 70:895, 1981.)

14. O'Toole, R. D., Thornton, G. F., Mukherjee, M. K., et al. Dexamethasone in tuberculous meningitis: Relationship of cerebrospinal fluid effects to therapeutic efficacy. *Ann. Intern. Med.* 70:39, 1969.
    Use of steroids to control cerebral edema.

15. Kingsley, D. P., Hendrickse, W. A., Kendall, B. E., et al. Tuberculous meningitis: Role

of CT in management and prognosis. *J. Neurol. Neurosurg. Psychiatry* 50:30, 1987.
Abnormalities detected by CT scanning may already be too advanced for surgical correction.

16. Sherman, B. M., Gorden, P., and DiChirio, G. Post-meningitic selective hypopituitarism with suprasellar calcification. *Arch. Intern. Med.* 128:600, 1971.
A complication of tuberculous meningitis.

17. Haas, E. J., Madhavan, T., Quinn, E. L., et al. Tuberculous meningitis in an urban general hospital. *Arch. Intern. Med.* 137:1518, 1977.
Delays in diagnosis were frequent in this series.

18. Whitener, D. R. Tuberculous brain abscess. *Arch. Neurol.* 35:148, 1978.
A rare form of CNS tuberculosis that presents clinically like a pyogenic abscess. (See also J. Neurology 232:118, 1985.)

19. Kennedy, D. H., and Fallon, R. J. Tuberculous meningitis. *J.A.M.A.* 241:264, 1979.
Early institution of therapy is important in reducing neurologic sequelae.

20. Daniel, T. M. New approaches to the rapid diagnosis of tuberculous meningitis. *J. Infect. Dis.* 155:599, 1987.
Review of the available tests for diagnosis using CSF. There is as yet no proven test.

135. TUBERCULOUS PERICARDITIS
Jerry L. Spivak

Tuberculous pericarditis accounts for approximately 10 percent of cases of pericarditis for which a cause can be established. It is an uncommon complication of tuberculosis, and it occurs predominantly in black men. The pericarditis is rarely a primary form of tuberculosis but results from direct extension of infection in mediastinal nodes or less commonly as a consequence of hematogenous miliary dissemination. The release of caseous material containing tuberculoprotein into the pericardial sac produces an exudative inflammatory reaction with an accumulation of fluid. The latter is encouraged by poor drainage due to involvement of the mediastinal lymph nodes.

Clinically, the illness can develop acutely with symptoms indistinguishable from those of acute viral pericarditis or myocardial infarction. More commonly the onset is insidious, with progressive dyspnea, nonproductive cough, weight loss, edema, and abdominal distention. Physical examination reveals fever, tachycardia, cardiomegaly, neck vein distention, edema, hepatomegaly, and often ascites. Downward displacement of the left lobe of the liver has been described frequently enough to suggest that it is a reliable sign of pericardial effusion. A pericardial friction rub is heard in approximately 50 percent of patients, and the incidence increases after pericardial fluid is removed. Pleural effusion or friction rubs are not uncommon, and frequently signs of consolidation at the left base are present due to compression of lung by the distended pericardium. As is characteristic of tuberculous infection in general, the patient can appear well in spite of an elevated temperature and in many cases the white cell count is not elevated. ECG abnormalities depend on the stage of the disease, with low voltage and inverted T waves being the most common findings. The volume and characteristics of the pericardial fluid also depend on the stage of the illness; most often a serosanguineous fluid is obtained, with a high specific gravity, elevated protein content, and increase in mononuclear cells. Only rarely are tubercle bacilli found on staining, and positive cultures are obtained in only 50 percent of patients.

In the absence of demonstrable tubercle bacilli or a known focus of tuberculosis elsewhere, the diagnosis of tuberculous pericarditis can be difficult to establish. The disease must be distinguished from other illnesses causing acute or chronic pericarditis, particularly acute rheumatic fever, fungal infection, carcinomatosis, and collagen-vascular disease. Insufflation of air into the pericardial sac after removal of fluid is often helpful because it provides definition of the pericardial wall and heart size. A thickened pericardium and a normal heart size effectively exclude myocardiopathy or rheumatic fever as the cause of the problem. Exclusion of viral or nonspecific pericarditis may be more difficult. Pericardial biopsy is often not helpful, revealing only nonspecific inflammation. This is not surprising since tubercles may be few and widely scattered.

Given the characteristic clinical picture, a positive tuberculin skin test, and the absence of another treatable cause of the pericarditis, institution of antituberculous therapy is indicated. If left untreated, tuberculous pericarditis pursues a relentless course, with death due to myocardial failure or to the development of other tuberculous complications. In the pretreatment era, patients with negative pericardial fluid cultures appeared to fare better, even though they too often developed other manifestations of tuberculosis. Contrary to common doctrine, the incidence of pericardial calcification is low.

The treatment of tuberculous pericarditis does not end with the institution of chemotherapy. The immediate threat to life in these patients is pericardial tamponade. Chemotherapy does not reverse lesions already present, nor is the effect of drugs quick enough to prevent continued fluid accumulation. Chemotherapy appears to be most effective in patients who are treated early in the course of the illness. In such patients steroids may also hasten resolution of the inflammatory process. Controlled studies indicate that corticosteroid therapy reduces mortality, rapid pericardial fluid accumulation, and the need for repeated pericardiocentesis, but not the risk of constrictive pericarditis. In patients with signs of tamponade or continued elevation of the venous pressure despite removal of pericardial fluid, neither chemotherapy nor steroids should be relied on and pericardiectomy should be performed. Open drainage or internal windows are equally unsatisfactory owing to rapid obstruction of both routes of drainage and the risk of pyogenic superinfection with open drainage. Adjunctive therapy with digitalis is helpful owing to the tendency toward myocardial dilatation after pericardial stripping and to the frequency of atrial arrhythmias. However, myocardial sensitivity to digitalis is also increased and ventricular arrhythmias can be precipitated.

1. Harvey, A. M., and Whitehall, M. R. Tuberculous pericarditis. *Medicine* 16:45, 1937.
   A classic description of this disease before the advent of chemotherapy.
2. Schwartz, M. J., Nay, H. R., and Fitzpatrick, H. F. Pericardial biopsy. *Arch. Intern. Med.* 112:917, 1963.
   Pericardial biopsy often fails to provide a definitive diagnosis.
3. Strang, J. I. G., Gibson, D. G., Mitchison, D. A., et al. Controlled clinical trial of complete open surgical drainage and of prednisolone in treatment of tuberculous pericardial effusion in Transkei. *Lancet* 2:759, 1988.
   Prednisone reduced mortality and fluid accumulation but not constrictive pericarditis.
4. Ortbals, D. W., and Avioli, L. V. Tuberculous pericarditis. *Arch. Intern. Med.* 139:231, 1979.
   A useful review.
5. Sagrista-Sauleda, J., Permanyer-Miralda, G., and Soler-Soler, J. Tuberculous pericarditis: Ten year experience with a prospective protocol for diagnosis and treatment. *J. Am. Coll. Cardiol.* 11:724, 1988.
   The clinical presentation is variable but tamponade is common.
6. Larrieu, A. J., Tyers, F. O., Williams, E. H., et al. Recent experience with tuberculous pericarditis. *Ann. Thorac. Surg.* 29:464, 1980.
   Early surgical intervention recommended if the response to chemotherapy is not prompt.
7. Quale, J. M., Lipschik, G. Y., and Heurich, A. E. Management of tuberculous pericarditis. *Ann. Thorac. Surg.* 43:653, 1987.
   Pericardiectomy is advocated if thickening is associated with a major effusion.
8. Knoll, S. M., and Slovin, A. J. Tuberculosis in uremic pericarditis. *Chest* 66:205, 1974.
   The possibility of tuberculosis as a cause of pericarditis should always be considered.

136. TUBERCULOUS PERITONITIS
Jerry L. Spivak

Tuberculous peritonitis usually occurs as a result of activation of a latent focus of tuberculosis in the peritoneal cavity. Rarely the infection is due to contiguous spread from an intestinal ulcer or urogenital lesion or hematogenous dissemination from a tuberculous focus outside the abdominal cavity. As in the case of tuberculous pericarditis, this extrapulmonary manifestation of tuberculosis is more common in blacks. Its predominance in women has not been explained, but it does not appear to be due to differences in the anatomy of the male and female urogenital tracts.

The presenting manifestations of tuberculous peritonitis include fever (which may be intermittent and associated with chills), weight loss, abdominal pain, and abdominal enlargement. The onset is usually insidious, but it can be acute if a large amount of caseous material is released into the peritoneal cavity. Diarrhea occurs in a small percentage of cases; it is usually due to involvement of the bowel by adhesions and inflammatory masses rather than to intrinsic mucosal disease. The most common physical findings are fever, ascites, abdominal tenderness, and an abdominal mass. The mass is due either to a matted omentum, which can mimic an enlarged liver, or to adherent loops of bowel. The classic "doughy abdomen" appears to be much more common in textbooks than in actual practice. In a small number of patients, pleural effusions or lymphadenopathy is present.

With the exception of the tuberculin skin test, laboratory data provide little evidence as to the nature of the underlying process. Most patients are not anemic and the white cell count is usually less than 10,000 per microliter. Parenchymal pulmonary lesions are found in less than 10 percent of cases. Barium contrast studies of the intestines may reveal abnormalities in luminal size and motility, but most of these defects are due to extramural inflammation and adhesions. Liver function tests are usually normal unless there is an underlying parenchymal disease, such as cirrhosis or, rarely, tuberculous hepatitis. In keeping with this, liver biopsy is not a helpful diagnostic procedure. The ascitic fluid can be clear, serosanguineous, or frankly hemorrhagic. The protein content is usually greater than 3 gm/dl, and the leukocyte count more than 250 cells per microliter with more than 75 percent being lymphocytes. However, documented cases of tuberculous peritonitis have occurred in which the ascitic fluid contained fewer than 250 cells per microliter and a protein concentration of less than 2.5 gm/dl. Rarely are tubercle bacilli seen in the ascitic fluid, and in up to 50 percent of cases ascitic fluid cultures for tuberculosis are negative although there is evidence to suggest that the culture results may depend on the volume of the fluid cultured. Occasionally a false-positive cytopathology result is obtained. Positive cultures for tuberculosis may be obtained from other body fluids or tissue, but this is not proof that the intraabdominal disorder is due to the same process. The diagnosis is best established by demonstration of caseous granulomas in peritoneal tissue obtained at laparotomy, peritoneoscopy, or by blind peritoneal biopsy.

Due to the nonspecific presentation, physical findings, and laboratory data, tuberculous peritonitis can be easily confused with many other diseases. These include Meigs' syndrome, pancreatic ascites, inflammatory bowel diseases, carcinomatosis, intraabdominal lymphoma, cirrhosis, hepatoma, congestive heart failure, and myxedema. Since the mortality in untreated patients is over 50 percent, it is important to recognize the presence of tuberculous peritonitis. This can be done only if a high level of suspicion is maintained in evaluating patients with exudative ascites (and those with transudative ascites who are not progressing satisfactorily). A particular problem in this regard occurs in patients with cirrhosis, who are particularly prone to develop intraabdominal processes that cause pain and fever. These include pancreatitis, peptic ulcer with perforation, spontaneous bacterial peritonitis, acute alcoholic hepatitis, hepatoma, and pyelonephritis with renal papillary necrosis. In addition, cirrhotics have a high incidence of tuberculous peritonitis. A transudative fluid with a protein content less than 2 gm/dl and a predominance of neutrophils suggests bacterial peritonitis, but if the diagnosis is in doubt, tissue should always be obtained to evaluate the possibility of tuberculous peritonitis.

Tuberculous peritonitis is only one manifestation of a sytemic disease, and as such it should be treated with triple-drug chemotherapy. Some investigators have recommended the use of steroids to abort the possibility of late fibrotic complications such as adhesions; others have found steroids to be unnecessary, and the question has not been resolved.

1. Bastani, B., Shariatzadeh, R., and Dehdashti, F. Tuberculous peritonitis—report of 30 cases and review of the literature. *Q. J. Med.* 56:549, 1985.
   Fever, abdominal pain, swelling, and weight loss were prominent.
2. Jakubowski, A., Elwood, R. K., and Enarson, D. A. Clinical features of abdominal tuberculosis. *J. Infect. Dis.* 158:687, 1988.
   Peritonitis is the most common form. (See also Am. J. Gastroenterol. *67:324, 1977 and* Surg. Gynecol. Obstet. *167:167, 1988.)*
3. Burack, W. R., and Hollister, R. M. Tuberculous peritonitis. *Am. J. Med.* 28:510, 1960.
   Pitfalls in the diagnosis of a treatable disease.
4. Hyman, S., Villa, F., Alvarez, S., et al. The enigma of tuberculous peritonitis. *Gastroenterology* 42:1, 1967.
   Tuberculous peritonitis is easily confused with other causes of ascites.
5. Johnston, F. F., and Sanford, J. P. Tuberculous peritonitis. *Ann. Intern. Med.* 54:1125, 1961.
   The occurrence of chills should not be taken to exclude tuberculous infection.
6. Sochocky, S. Tuberculous peritonitis. *Am. Rev. Respir. Dis.* 95:398, 1967.
   A review of the disease as it occurred in a tuberculosis sanatorium.
7. Gonnella, J. S., and Hudson, E. K. Clinical patterns of tuberculous peritonitis. *Arch. Intern. Med.* 117:164, 1966.
   Liver biopsy is not a helpful diagnostic procedure.
8. Levine, H. Needle biopsy diagnosis of tuberculous peritonitis. *Am. Rev. Respir. Dis.* 97:889, 1968.
   High yield of involved tissue obtained with peritoneal needle biopsy.
9. Berner, C., Fred, H. C., Riggs, S., et al. Diagnostic probabilities in patients with conspicuous ascites. *Arch. Intern. Med.* 113:687, 1964.
   Think of tuberculosis when the cause of ascites is not readily apparent.
10. Mauk, P. M., Schwartz, J. T., Lowe, J. E., et al. Diagnosis and course of nephrogenic ascites. *Arch. Intern. Med.* 148:1577, 1988.
    Tuberculosis must always be considered.
11. Borhanmanesh, F., Hekmat, K., Vaezzadeh, K., et al. Tuberculous peritonitis. *Ann. Intern. Med.* 76:567, 1972.
    The use of steroids was found to be unnecessary. For the opposite view, see N. Engl. J. Med. *281:1091, 1969.*
12. Klimach, O. E., and Ormerod, L. P. Gastrointestinal tuberculosis: A retrospective review of 109 cases in a district general hospital. *Q. J. Med.* 56:569, 1985.
    This can mimic chronic inflammatory bowel disease. (See also Am. J. Med. *27:509, 1959.)*
13. Wolfe, J. H. N., Behn, A. R., and Jackson, B. T. Tuberculous peritonitis and role of diagnostic laparoscopy. *Lancet* 1:852, 1979.
    The classic "doughy" abdomen was not observed; laparoscopy is advocated for rapid diagnosis.
14. Sherman, S., Rohwedder, J. J., Ravikrishnan, K. P., et al. Tuberculous enteritis and peritonitis: Report of 36 general hospital cases. *Arch. Intern. Med.* 140:506, 1980.
    The diagnosis of tuberculous enteritis was usually made unexpectedly at surgery. (See also Am. J. Surg. *31:55, 1988.)*
15. Schulze, H., Warner, H. A., and Murray, D. Intestinal tuberculosis: Experience at a Canadian teaching institution. *Am. J. Med.* 63:735, 1977.
    Only 3 of 13 patients had active pulmonary disease.

16. Essop, A. R., Posen, J. A., Hodkinson, J. H., et al. Tuberculosis hepatitis: A clinical review of 96 cases. *Q. J. Med.* 53:465, 1984.
   An uncommon but serious illness.
17. Voigt, M. D., Trey, C., Lombard, C., et al. Diagnostic value of ascites adenosine deaminase in tuberculous peritonitis. *Lancet* 1:751, 1989.
   The usefulness of this test remains to be established.

137. VIRAL, MYCOPLASMAL, AND CHLAMYDIAL PNEUMONIA
Jerry L. Spivak

Nonbacterial pneumonia can be either a localized, benign, self-limited infection or a diffuse pulmonic process resulting in considerable morbidity and mortality. The former is usually seen with rhinovirus, adenovirus, influenza virus, and parainfluenza virus, as well as with mycoplasmal infections, whereas the latter is characteristic of varicella-zoster and cytomegalovirus pneumonia. Occasionally, a localized pneumonic process becomes widespread or the viral infection is complicated by secondary bacterial pneumonia. These complications can occur in normal persons but are most likely to occur in patients with underlying cardiopulmonary disorders or during pregnancy.

Clinically, most patients with viral or mycoplasmal pneumonia present with a history of fever, rhinorrhea, pharyngitis or otitis, headache, cough, myalgias, and substernal or occasionally pleuritic chest pain. Rarely chills are experienced. On physical examination cervical adenopathy may be found, as well as pharyngitis or myringitis. Skin rashes usually occur late in the course of the infection. Auscultation of the chest reveals localized rales, wheezing, and diminished breath sounds. In some patients, a friction rub or evidence of pleural fluid will be found. Chest x ray usually reveals a localized reticular or nodular segmental infiltrate, most often in a lower lobe; hilar adenopathy may be present, and diffuse interstitial involvement can occur. Involvement of more than one lobe has been described, and the appearance of new infiltrates during the course of the illness is not uncommon. Pleural effusions can be demonstrated in at least 20 percent of patients if lateral decubitus views are employed. The fluid is usually an exudate. Sputum is usually minimal and clear, but can be purulent. Lymphopenia and neutrophilia with either a normal or elevated leukocyte count are usual, although the neutrophilia declines during the course of the illness. Transient elevations of serum transaminase levels may occur and myoglobinuria is being reported with increasing frequency. In most patients with localized disease, fever resolves within 5 to 7 days and x-ray resolution occurs within 2 weeks, although the course can be more prolonged, particularly with mycoplasmal infections, and occasionally febrile relapses occur.

When confronted with the patient who has a fever and a localized pulmonary infiltrate, the physician must decide whether he is dealing with a bacterial infection, viral infection, pulmonary infarction, tuberculosis, collagen-vascular disease, or aspiration. It is obvious that a shaking chill, purulent sputum, pleurisy, exudative pleural effusion, neutrophilia, or a friction rub cannot be used as evidence in favor of a bacterial process and that negative sputum or blood cultures cannot be used as evidence against one. The problem is further compounded by the fact that patients with viral pneumonias can develop pulmonary infarction as part of the illness. A negative tuberculin skin test is also without value since this reaction can be suppressed during a viral infection. Serologic studies are useful but only in retrospect. Signs of consolidation and an elevated erythrocyte sedimention rate are two findings that do support a bacterial etiology, but in the end the decision to treat or observe is usually based on clinical assessment of the patient. Knowledge of a current viral epidemic is helpful in this regard.

In the patient with diffuse pulmonary involvement, diagnostic considerations include pulmonary edema, tuberculosis, aspiration, acute interstitial fibrosis (Hamman-Rich syndrome), desquamative interstitial pneumonia, pulmonary alveolar proteinosis, allergic pneumonitis, sarcoidosis, lymphangitic carcinomatosis, pulmonary hemorrhage, and, in patients with impaired cellular immunity or receiving immunosuppressive drugs, *Pneumocystis carinii*, aspergillosis, cryptococcosis, or *Pseudomonas* infection. Needle biopsy of the lung may be helpful in this situation. A complicating feature in patients with viral pneumonia and diffuse pulmonary involvement is the development of disseminated intravascular coagulation (DIC) and viral invasion of many organs besides the lungs.

A major advance in the therapy of viral infections has been the development of agents such as acyclovir, which is active against herpes simplex and varicella-zoster, and ganciclovir, which is effective against cytomegalovirus. Both agents have been employed in the treatment of pneumonia caused by these viruses, but the extent to which they will be effective is still unknown.

1. Mansel, J. K., Rosenow, E. C., III, Smith, T. F., et al. *Mycoplasma pneumoniae* pneumonia. *Chest* 95:639, 1989.
   Comprehensive clinical review. For pathology, see Arch. Pathol. Lab. Med. *110:34, 1986.*
2. Tew, J., Calenoff, L., and Berlin, B. S. Bacterial or nonbacterial pneumonia: Accuracy of radiographic diagnosis. *Radiology* 124:607, 1977.
   The distinction between a bacterial, mycoplasmal, or viral pneumonia on chest x ray is often difficult. (See also Am. Rev. Respir. Dis. *96:1144, 1967.)*
3. Douglas, R. G., Alford, R. H., Cote, T. R., et al. The leukocyte response during viral respiratory illness in man. *Ann. Intern. Med.* 64:521, 1966.
   Clinical infection is usually associated with an initial neutrophilic leukocytosis.
4. George, R. B., and Mogabgab, W. J. Atypical pneumonia in young men with rhinovirus infections. *Ann. Intern. Med.* 71:1073, 1969.
   A neutrophilic leukocytosis is often seen.
5. Bryant, R. E., and Rhoades, E. R. Clinical features of adenoviral pneumonia in Air Force recruits. *Am. Rev. Respir. Dis.* 96:717, 1967.
   Anterior cervical adenopathy may be a helpful clue.
6. Dudding, B. A., Wagner, S. C., Zeller, J. A., et al. Fatal pneumonia associated with adenovirus type 7 in three military trainees. *N. Engl. J. Med.* 286:1289, 1972.
   Viral pneumonia complicated by DIC.
7. Louria, D. B., Blumenfeld, H. L., Ellis, J. T., et al. Studies on influenza in the pandemic of 1957–1958: II. Pulmonary complications of influenza. *J. Clin. Invest.* 38:213, 1959.
   A classic review.
8. Kaye, D., Rosenbluth, M., Hook, E. W., et al. Endemic influenza: II. The nature of the disease in the post-pandemic period. *Am. Rev. Respir. Dis.* 85:9, 1962.
   Severe pulmonary complications usually occur in patients with cardiovascular disease.
9. Tashiro, M., Ciborowski, P., Klenk, H. D., et al. Role of staphylococcus protease in the development of influenza. *Nature* 325:536, 1987.
   Activation of influenza virus by staphylococci.
10. Triebwasser, J. H., Harris, R. E., Bryant, R. E., et al. Varicella pneumonia: Report of seven cases and a review of the literature. *Medicine* 46:409, 1967.
    Diffuse nodular infiltrate occasionally accompanied by effusion and pleurisy.
11. Schlossberg, D., and Littman, M. Varicella pneumonia. *Arch. Intern. Med.* 148:1630, 1988.
    Favorable results with acyclovir. See Thorax *43:627, 1988 for the converse.*
12. Finucane, K., Colebatch, H. J. H., Robertson, M. R., et al. The mechanism of respiratory failure in a patient with viral (varicella) pneumonia. *Am. Rev. Respir. Dis.* 101:949, 1970.
    Decreased compliance, alveolar collapse, and intrapulmonic shunting.
13. Hall, W. J., Douglas, R. G., Jr., Hyde, R. W., et al. Pulmonary mechanics after uncomplicated influenza A infection. *Am. Rev. Respir. Dis.* 113:141, 1976.
    Pulmonary dysfunction persists after the acute infection has subsided.
14. Zaroukian, M. H., Kashyap, G. H., and Wentworth, B. B. Respiratory syncytial virus

infection: A cause of respiratory distress syndrome and pneumonia in adults. *Am. J. Med. Sci.* 295:218, 1988.
This infection can be fatal. (See Arch. Intern. Med. *147:791, 1987.)*

15. Ferstenfeld, J. E., Schlueter, D. P., Rytel, M. W., et al. Recognition and treatment of adult respiratory distress syndrome secondary to viral interstitial pneumonia. *Am. J. Med.* 58:709, 1975.
A difficult therapeutic problem.

16. Glick, N., Levin, S., and Nelson, K. Recurrent pulmonary infarction in adult chicken pox pneumonia. *J.A.M.A.* 222:173, 1972.
An unusual complication.

17. Klemola, E., Stenstrom, R., and von Essen, R. Pneumonia as a clinical manifestation of cytomegalovirus infection in previously healthy adults. *Scand. J. Infect. Dis.* 4:7, 1972.
Atypical lymphocytosis and a negative heterophile test.

18. Meyers, J. D., Flourney, N., and Thomas, E. D. Risk factors for cytomegalovirus infection after human marrow transplantation. *J. Infect. Dis.* 153:478, 1986.
Cytomegalovirus pneumonia was common and lethal.

19. Wallace, J. M., and Hannah, J. Cytomegalovirus pneumonitis in patients with AIDS. *Chest* 92:198, 1987.
CMV alone can cause severe lung damage and disseminated infection.

20. Springmeyer, S. C., Hackman, R. C., Holle, R., et al. Use of bronchoalveolar lavage to diagnose acute diffuse pneumonia in the immunocompromised host. *J. Infect. Dis.* 154:604, 1986.
This approach was more effective than needle biopsy. (See also Ann. Intern. Med. *104:476, 1986.)*

21. Frank, I., and Friedman, H. M. Progress in the treatment of cytomegalovirus pneumonia. *Ann. Intern. Med.* 109:769, 1988.
Concise review.

22. Olson, R. W., and Hodges, G. R. Measles pneumonia. *J.A.M.A.* 232:363, 1975.
A high incidence of bacterial superinfection, particularly with sero group Y Neisseria, *was observed.*

23. Martin, D. B., Weiner, L. B., Nieburg, P. I., et al. Atypical measles in adolescents and young adults. *Ann. Intern. Med.* 90:877, 1979.
Atypical presentation attributed to previous measles vaccination. (See also Ann. Intern. Med. *90:882, 1976.) The pulmonary manifestations are diverse and a large population of young adults is at risk.*

24. Marrie, T. J., Grayston, J. T., Wang, S. P., et al. Pneumonia associated with the TWAR strain of chlamydia. *Ann. Intern. Med.* 106:507, 1987.
A newly appreciated cause of pneumonia.

25. Grayston, J. T. *Chlamydia pneumoniae,* strain TWAR. *Chest* 95:664, 1989.
Comprehensive review.

26. Ellenbogen, C., Graybill, J. R., Silva, J., Jr., et al. Bacterial pneumonia complicating adenoviral pneumonia. *Am. J. Med.* 56:169, 1974.
Antibiotic prophylaxis does not prevent the development of secondary bacterial pneumonia.

27. Josselson, J., Pula, T., and Sadler, J. H. Acute rhabdomyolysis associated with an echovirus 9 infection. *Arch. Intern. Med.* 140:1671, 1980.
Viral infections can produce rhabdomyolysis and even renal failure. This article lists the reported cases.

28. Little, J. W., Hall, W. J., Douglas, R. G., et al. Amantadine effect on peripheral airways abnormalities in influenza. *Ann. Intern. Med.* 85:177, 1976.
Amantadine promoted resolution of pulmonary dysfunction in patients with uncomplicated influenza A infection. (See also Med. Lett. Drugs Ther. *20:25, 1978.)*

29. Murray, H. W., Masur, H., Senterfit, L. B., et al. The protean manifestations of *Mycoplasma pneumoniae* infection in adults. *Am. J. Med.* 58:229, 1975.
A detailed review. (See also J. Infect. Dis. *123:74, 1971.)*

30. Teisch, J. A., Shapiro, L., and Walzer, R. A. Vesiculopustular eruption with mycoplasma infection. *J.A.M.A.* 211:1694, 1970.

Skin rash, characteristically an erythema multiforme, is not uncommon in myco-
plasma infections.

31. Fine, N. L., Smith, L. R., and Sheedy, P. F. Frequency of pleural effusions in mycoplasma and viral pneumonias. *N. Engl. J. Med.* 283:790, 1970.
   Pleural effusion was present in 20% of cases.

32. Sands, M. J., Satz, J. E., Turner, W. E., et al. Pericarditis and perimyocarditis associated with active mycoplasma pneumoniae infection. *Ann. Intern. Med.* 86:544,
1977.
   Myocardial and pericardial involvement occurring with mycoplasmal pneumonia.

33. Koletsky, R. J., and Weinstein, A. J. Fulminant *Mycoplasma pneumoniae* infection.
Am. Rev. Respir. Dis. 122:491, 1980.
   Overwhelming infection occurs but is uncommon.

34. Longstreth, G. F., and Edgington, T. S. Clinical and immunologic features of transient cold agglutinin hemolytic anemia. *Am. J. Med.* 54:514, 1973.
   A complication of mycoplasma infection.

35. Smith, C. B., Freidewald, W. T., and Chanock, R. M. Shedding of *Mycoplasma pneumoniae* after tetracycline and erythromycin therapy. *N. Engl. J. Med.* 276:1172,
1967.
   Organisms persist in the sputum during and after treatment.

36. Byron, N. P., Walls, J., and Mair, H. J. Fulminant psittacosis. *Lancet* 1:353, 1979.
   The clinical features in these patients were similar to legionnaires' disease.

37. Marrie, T. J., Schlech, W. F., III, Williams, J. C., et al. Q fever pneumonia associated
with exposure to wild rabbits. *Lancet* 22:427, 1986.
   This can be confused with tularemia.

38. Hughes, W. T. *Pneumocystis carinii* pneumonitis. *Chest* 85:810, 1984.
   Another frequent cause of pneumonia in immunosuppressed patients.

VIII. DISEASES OF THE KIDNEY

138. ACUTE RENAL FAILURE
Alan Watson
Luis F. Gimenez

Acute renal failure may be defined as a sudden reduction of renal function with the retention of nitrogenous waste normally excreted by the kidneys.

Acute renal failure (ARF) is traditionally characterized according to its cause as prerenal, intrinsic renal, and postrenal. Prerenal ARF is characterized by diminished renal perfusion resulting from a reduction in blood volume, be it effective (e.g., cardiac failure) or absolute (e.g., hemorrhage, dehydration, or fluid sequestration). Disease processes causing intrinsic acute renal failure are classified according to the primary site of injury for example, glomerulus (glomerulonephritis), tubule (acute tubular necrosis), interstitial tissue (interstitial nephritis), or blood vessels (thrombotic thrombocytopenic purpura, hemolytic uremic syndrome). The most common type of intrinsic ARF encountered in clinical practice is acute tubular necrosis, which may be ischemic or nephrotoxic in origin or the result of a pigment-induced (myoglobin, hemoglobin) injury. Postrenal ARF is caused by disease states resulting in obstruction to urine flow.

A careful history and physical examination will, in many cases, provide a reliable guide as to whether ARF is intrinsic or due to prerenal or postrenal causes. Particular attention should be paid to the hydration status of the patient by examining for poor skin turgor and the presence of orthostatic hypotension. Because of the recent recognition that nonoliguric ARF is more common than previously recognized, assessment of urine flow rates, for example, oliguria (<400ml/24 hours) is no longer regarded as helpful in excluding the presence of ARF. Total anuria should, however, alert one to consider the possibility of bilateral cortical necrosis, vascular occlusion, rapidly progressive glomerulonephritis, or complete mechanical obstruction to urine outflow. Analysis of the urine sediment is also helpful. In prerenal and postrenal disease states, a normal sediment is usual. Red cell casts suggest glomerular disease whereas eosinophiliuria suggests allergic interstitial nephritis, and tubular epithelial cells, cellular casts, and debris are commonly seen in acute tubular necrosis.

Biochemical analysis of the urine is increasingly used in differentiating prerenal ARF from acute tubular necrosis. The various parameters commonly measured include urine osmolality, urine sodium, and the calculated fractional excretion of sodium. Typical values for prerenal ARF would be urine osmolality greater than 500 mOsm/kg, urine sodium less than 10 mEq/liter, and fractional excretion of sodium less than 1 percent; for acute tubular necrosis: less than 350 mOsm/kg, greater than 20 mEq/liter, and greater than 1%, respectively. It should be remembered, however, that these studies are reflective of the integrity of tubular function and as such the pattern of prerenal disease may be seen in acute renal failure due to glomerulonephritis and early obstructive uropathy. Radiologic evaluation of the kidneys and the urinary tract is a necessary undertaking in all patients with ARF to rule out the possibility of obstructive uropathy. Sonography is the most commonly used method and has simplified greatly the assessment of the patency of the urinary tract. On occasion, where the proposed sequence of diagnostic steps fails to identify the cause of ARF, a renal biopsy may prove useful, particularly if there is a history suggesting a multisystem disease process or ingestion of pharmacologic agents known to be associated with tubulointerstitial nephritis.

The management of the patient with ARF in whom reversible factors (e.g., dehydration, obstruction) have been excluded is largely directed at the many potential complications associated with this condition. Electrolytes need to be followed on a daily basis, monitoring for the development of hyponatremia, hyperkalemia, or metabolic acidosis. Restriction of free water and dietary reduction of potassium (40 mEq/day), sodium (2 gm/day), and protein (40 gm/day) should be instituted at an early stage. Serious hyperkalemia necessitates more aggressive management with glucose and insulin, sodium bicarbonate, or calcium gluconate if necessary. These maneuvers, of course, merely antagonize the effects of hyperkalemia or redistribute potassium between cellular and extracellular compartments and are temporary measures. Cation exchange resins (sodium polystyrene sulfonate [Kayexalate]) or dialysis are necessary for actual removal of potassium from the body. Metabolic acidosis and hyperphosphatemia are common findings in ARF and are treatable with alkali supplements and phosphate-binding antacids respectively.

Sepsis and bleeding remain major causes of mortality in ARF. Intravenous catheters should be used only where necessary, for example, for parenteral nutrition. Urinary catheters should be avoided. Since leukocytosis is a feature of ARF per se and fever may be suppressed by uremia, extreme vigilance for the development of sepsis is mandatory. Prophylactic antibiotic therapy, however, should not be used. The hemorrhagic tendency of uremia is well recognized and most frequently involves the mucosal surface of the gastrointestinal tract. Usually clinical bleeding is minimal but on occasion can be life-threatening. Some authorities recommend the regular use of either antacids or cimetidine on a long-term basis to avoid a gastrointestinal hemorrhage.

Desmopressin (DDAVP) in the dose of 0.3 to 0.4 µg/kg given in 20 ml of saline over 20 minutes, or cryoprecipitate (10 units), have proved useful in stopping hemorrhage or when an invasive procedure is planned.

Aggressive use of dialysis therapy is widely used in the management of ARF. Proponents argue that complications such as bleeding are avoided and that volume status is easily controlled allowing for uninterrupted parenteral nutrition and a better state of overall health. There is, however, no hard evidence that mortality per se is reduced by the institution of early dialysis. Absolute indications for dialysis include volume overload, progressive hyperkalemia, acidosis, or a blood urea nitrogen level greater than 100 mg/dl. Hemodialysis and peritoneal dialysis have respective advantages and disadvantages. Hemodialysis is rapidly effective but predisposes to the disequilibrium syndrome, requires creation of a vascular access, and may be hazardous to the patient with cardiovascular instability. Peritoneal dialysis provides a more gentle exchange but necessitates insertion of a peritoneal catheter, immobilizing the patient, and predisposes to infection, hyperglycemia, and hypoalbuminemia.

In the setting of oliguric ARF, due to acute tubular necrosis, an increasing urine output may herald recovery of overall renal function. This is known as the diuretic or polyuric phase of acute tubular necrosis, and during this phase attention should be directed to replacement of electrolytes, including sodium, potassium, and magnesium, which can be lost in the urine in large quantities in this stage. It is important to realize that during this apparent recovery phase, the glomerular filtration rate may remain depressed for a variable period of time and aggressive therapy as outlined above should be continued.

The majority of individuals with ARF are on drug therapy of various sorts. Attention therefore should be given to whether a particular drug is normally excreted by the kidney, and if so the dosage should be modified appropriately. Further dose adjustments are necessary when dialysis is required.

1. Luke, R. G. Diagnostic possibilities in acute renal failure. *Geriatrics* 31:92, 1976.
   A good review of a diagnostic approach to the individual with acute renal failure.
2. Appel, G. D., and Neu, H. C. The nephrotoxicity of antimicrobial agents. *N. Engl. J. Med.* 296:663, 772, 784, 1977.
   A classic review of mechanisms of nephrotoxicity of antimicrobial agents.
3. Bennett, W. N., Singer, I., Golper, T., et al. Guidelines for drug therapy in renal failure. *Ann. Intern. Med.* 86:754, 1977.
   This comprehensive review provides guidelines for drug usage in patients with renal insufficiency. Nephrotoxicity or adverse effects in patients with renal disease are described and adjustments for dialysis suggested.
4. van Ypersele de Strihou, C. Acute oliguric interstitial nephritis. *Kidney Int.* 16:751, 1979.
   This presentation deals with several aspects of clinical and experimental acute interstitial nephritis.
5. Espanel, C. H., and Gregory, A. W. Differential diagnosis of acute renal failure. *Clin. Nephol.* 13:73, 1980.
   A review of the clinical approach to unraveling the pathophysiology underlying the individual with ARF.
6. Linton, A. L., Clark, W. F., Driger, A. A., et al. Acute interstitial nephritis due to drugs. *Ann. Intern. Med.* 93:735, 1980.

This report highlights the fact that acute interstitial nephritis due to drugs commonly presents as ARF. It reviews the types of drugs commonly involved, and the potential immunologic mechanisms underlying the renal damage. Various diagnostic approaches are also reviewed.

7. Nolph, K. D., Miller, F., Rubin, J., et al. New directions in peritoneal dialysis concepts and applications. *Kidney Int.* 18:111, 1980.
   A review of recent advances in peritoneal dialysis.

8. Harkonen S., and Kjellstrand, C. Contrast nephropathy. *Am. J. Nephrol.* 1:69, 1981.
   A review of contrast-dye–induced renal injury, an increasing cause of hospital-acquired acute renal insufficiency.

9. McPhaul, J. I. Acute glomerular disease presenting as acute renal failure. *Semin. Nephrol.* 1:21, 1981.
   This report emphasizes the fact that acute glomerular disease can result in acute renal insufficiency and must be considered in the differential diagnosis of any such patient.

10. Feinstein, E. I., Blumenkrantz, M. J., Healy, M., et al. Clinical and metabolic responses to acute renal failure. *Medicine* 60:124, 1981.
    This study examines various metabolic problems that occur in the setting of ARF and highlights the multiple derangements that can occur during uremia.

11. Watson, A. J. S., and Keogh, J. A. B. Effect of 1-deamino-8-arginine vasporessin in the prolonged bleeding time of chronic renal failure. *Nephron* 32:49, 1982.
    This is the original description of desmopressin as a treatment of the hemorrhagic diathesis of renal insufficiency and provides a review and rationale for the use of this agent.

12. Rota, S., Mougenot, B., and Baudouin, B. Multiple myeloma in severe renal failure: A clinical pathologic study of outcome and prognosis in 34 patients. *Medicine* 66:126, 1982.
    This study reevaluates the outcome, precipitating conditions, and prognostic factors of renal failure in multiple myeloma and identifies a high rate of renal failure reversibility. Statistical analysis of potential prognostic factors is undertaken and the discussion provides a good review of ARF associated with this neoplastic process.

13. Hou, S. H., Bushinskey, D. A., Wish, J. A., et al. Hospital acquired renal insufficiency: A prospective study. *Am. J. Med.* 74:243, 1983.
    The iatrogenic factors (e.g., antibiotic, contrast agents) accounted for 55% of hospital-acquired acute renal failure.

14. Kurokawa, K. Acute renal failure and rhabdomyolysis. *Kidney Int.* 23:888, 1983.
    A good review of the available hemodialysis techniques and the complications that occur during such treatments. Myoglobinuria renal failure is characterized by refractory hypertension and severe hyperkalemia, hyperphosphatemia, and hypocalcemia.

15. Mustonen, J., Pasternak, A., and Helin, A. Renal biopsy in acute renal failure. *Am. J. Nephrol.* 4:27, 1984.
    Renal biopsy proved valuable in settling the diagnosis, determining the prognosis, and planning the treatment of acute intrinsic renal failure.

16. Garella, S., and Mapraraes, R. A. Renal effect of prostaglandins in clinical adverse effects of non-steroidal anti-inflammatory agents. *Medicine* 63:165, 1984.
    This is an excellent review of all the various nephrotoxic effects that nonsteroidal anti-inflammatory drugs may exert through their ability to inhibit cyclooxygenase activity.

17. Rasmussen, H. H., Pitt, E. A., Ibold, L. S., et al. Prediction of outcome in acute renal failure by discriminant analysis of clinical variables. *Arch. Intern. Med.* 145:2015, 1985.
    The poor outcome of renal failure can be predicted in a considerable proportion of patients by a weighted evaluation of clinical variables.

18. Dixon, B. S., and Anderson, B. J. Non-oliguric renal failure. *Am. J. Kidney Dis.* 2:71, 1985.
    This report highlights the fact that although oliguria has long been considered a cardinal feature of ARF, the majority of cases with ARF now occur in the setting of well-maintained urine output. It also emphasizes the fact that the nonoliguric state

may occur in the setting of pre- and postrenal azotemia as well as in acute tubular necrosis.

19. Pru, C., and Kjellstrand, C. Urinary indices and chemistries in the differential diagnosis of pre-renal failure and acute tubular necrosis. *Semin. Nephrol.* 5:224, 1985.
This is an excellent review of the various diagnostic tests used in ARF ranging from urine specific gravity and osmolality to free water clearance and renal failure index. The value of these tests in differentiating acute tubular necrosis from prerenal azotemia is emphasized.

20. Watson, A. J., and Whelton, A. Therapeutic manipulations in uremic bleeding. *J. Clin. Pharmacol.* 25:305, 1985.
A thorough review of the pathophysiology of the hemorrhagic diathesis of renal insufficiency and potential new treatments.

21. Cronin, R. E. Drug therapy in the management of acute renal failure. *Am. J. Med. Sci.* 292:112, 1986.
This report reviews the experimental data utilizing pharmacologic intervention in ARF and comes to the conclusion that apart from mannitol and/or loop diuretics, very little is of benefit.

22. Myers, B. D., and Moran, M. S. Hemodynamically mediated acute renal failure. *N. Engl. J. Med.* 314:97, 1986.
A good review of the pathophysiologic role of renal blood flow in ARF.

23. Corwin, H. L., and Bonaventure, J. V. Acute renal failure. *Med. Clin. North Am.* 70:1037, 1986.
A very thorough review of etiology, pathophysiology, and clinical features of ARF.

24. Shusterman, N., Strom, B. L., Murray, T. G., et al. Risk factors and outcome of hospital-acquired acute renal failure. *Am. J. Med.* 83:65, 1987.
An often fatal illness precipitated by volume depletion, aminoglycosides, contrast dyes, and septic shock.

139. HYPERNEPHROMA
H. Verdain Barnes

Renal cell carcinoma, because of its protean presentations, is appropriately called the internist's tumor. Hypernephroma is the most frequent renal malignancy. It occurs 3 times more often in men than in women, with a peak incidence after age 50 years. Metastases often occur early by hematogenous or lymphatic routes or by direct invasion.

The classic triad of gross hematuria, flank pain, and palpable mass is uncommon. In most series, gross hematuria occurs in only about 18 percent of patients, while flank pain and palpable masses occur in 15 to 42 percent and 37 to 63 percent, respectively. Most often the tumor presents as a systemic or hormone syndrome. The various presentations are: (1) Fever of unknown origin—the fever is usually high-spiking and intermittent and may or may not be associated with weight loss or fatigue. (2) Hypercalcemia is most often associated with the production of a parathyroid hormone–like substance by the tumor and therefore with a low normal or low serum phosphorus level. (3) Peripheral neuropathy or myopathy can be seen. The neurologic process is usually a polyneuropathy, often presenting with progressive weakness or dysesthesias. (4) Secondary amyloidosis has been reported. (5) Refractory anemia, which is most often normochromic, normocytic, frequently associated with an elevated erythrocyte sedimentation rate, can be seen. (6) Polycythemia, a secondary erythrocytosis, is due to the production of erythropoietin by the tumor. (7) Congestive heart failure is usually high output failure secondary to an arteriovenous fistula of the involved kidney. (8) Cushing's syndrome, hyperadrenocorticism, is caused by the production of an ACTH-like substance by the tumor. (9) Nonmetastatic liver dysfunction may include an elevated alkaline phosphatase, increased thymol turbidity, Bromsulphalein (BSP) retention, increased alpha-2 globulin level, decreased prothrombin time, and/or decreased serum albumin level. (10) Vascular syndromes include thrombophlebitis (in about 15% of patients), inferior vena cava obstruction (in up to 6%), and varicocele (in 1–3%). (11) Finally, the initial presentation may be in association with Lindau-von Hippel disease or as a metastatic lesion to the lung, liver, or brain with or without associated organ dysfunction.

A renal mass can be most confidently excluded by contrast computerized tomographic (CT) scan or magnetic resonance. Cyst aspiration for cytology guided by ultrasound or CT is an important adjunct. If intravenous pyelography is used, nephrotomograms should be included for optimal evaluation. In certain patients selective renal arteriography is useful but is less often needed today. Hypernephroma, if present, can be demonstrated in virtually all patients by an effective combination of these diagnostic methods.

1. Kiely, J. Hypernephroma: The internist's tumor. *Med. Clin. North Am.* 50:1067, 1966.
   A good, short general review of the protean presentations of hypernephroma.
2. Cronin, R. S., Kaehny, W. D., Miller, P. D., et al. Renal cell carcinoma: Unusual systemic manifestations. *Medicine* 55:291, 1976.
   The best complete, and well-referenced study available—an important article.
3. Berger, A. L. Systemic manifestations of hypernephroma: A review of 273 cases. *Am. J. Med.* 22:791, 1957.
4. Clarke, B. G., and Goade, W. J., Jr. Fever and anemia in renal cancer. *N. Engl. J. Med.* 254:107, 1956.
   Articles 3 and 4 show a 3:1 sex ratio (male-female); increasing incidence after age 50; 2–5% of patients presented with fever as a chief complaint; 28% have a fever sometime during the course of their disease, and 25% have an anemia.
5. Utz, D. C., Warren, M. M., Gregg, J. A., et al. Reversible hepatic dysfunction associated with hypernephroma. *Mayo Clin. Proc.* 45:161, 1970.
   A detailed discussion of the nonmetastatic liver dysfunction seen in 40% of this series.
6. Rubin, P. Cancer of the urogenital tract-kidney: Locally advanced and metastatic renal adenocarcinoma. *J.A.M.A.* 204:604, 1968.
   Summarizes pathogenesis, basis of hormonal therapy, reasons for nephrectomy, regression of hypernephroma, and pelvis as opposed to cortical tumors.
7. Zusman, R. M., Snider, J. J., Cline, A., et al. Antihypertensive function of renal cell carcinoma: Evidence for prostaglandin A–secreting tumor. *N. Engl. J. Med.* 290:843, 1974.
8. Marcus, R. M., and Grayzel, A. I. A lupus antibody syndrome associated with hypernephroma. *Arthritis Rheum.* 22:1396, 1979.
   What more can this tumor do? (Articles 7 and 8).
9. Clayman, R. V., Williams, R. D., and Frawley, E. E. Current concepts in cancer: Pursuit of the renal mass. *N. Engl. J. Med.* 300:72, 1979.
   An approach to diagnosis with an emphasis on cost considerations.
10. Dawson, N. A., Barr, C. F., and Alving, B. M. Acquired dysfibrinogenemia: Paraneoplastic syndrome in renal cell carcinoma. *Am. J. Med.* 78:682, 1985.
    Another manifestation of hypernephroma.
11. Yamamoto, I., Kitamura, N., Aoki, J., et al. Circulating 1,25-dihydroxyvitamin D concentrations in patients with renal cell carcinoma–associated hypercalcemia are rarely suppressed. *J. Clin. Endocrinol. Metab.* 64:175, 1987.
    Only 11% had low levels while 87% of hypercalcemic patients with bony metastases from other malignancies had low levels.

140. NEPHROLITHIASIS
Mohammad G. Saklayen

Renal stone disease, or nephrolithiasis, affects 1 to 2 percent of the population, the highest incidence being in young males. Sixty to seventy percent of all kidney stones are composed of calcium oxalate. Most of the other stones are composed of calcium phosphate, uric acid, or struvite. Cystine, triamterene, and adenine stones are rare. Precipitation of crystals out of a urine supersaturated with the stone-forming elements is the primary event in the pathogenesis of renal stones. In addition to supersaturation, lack of certain organic and inorganic crystal growth inhibitors and the presence of a favorable nidus enhance the growth of stone.

Idiopathic hypercalciuria is the most common metabolic abnormality leading to calcium stone formation. Hypercalciuria secondary to primary hyperparathyroidism, distal renal tubular acidosis, sarcoidosis, milk-alkali syndrome, medullary sponge kidney, Paget's disease, malignancy, immobilization, vitamin D intoxication, etc., can lead to calcium stone formation also. Primary oxaluria, or more commonly, secondary oxaluria due to steatorrhea, is frequently the cause of recurrent calcium oxalate stone. Hyperuricosuria with or without gout favors the formation of either uric acid or calcium stones. Struvite stone is almost always due to recurrent urinary tract infection by urease-producing bacteria. The rare hereditary disorder homozygous cystinuria causes cystine stone.

The stone usually starts to form on the tip of the papillae of the kidney and except for microscopic or gross hematuria may lie silent in the pelvicaliceal system until it starts to move downstream with the urine. If the stone is quite small, it can pass without much pain, but more often than not it gets lodged in a narrow point in the ureter causing severe, sometimes unbearable, colicky pain. Ureteral stone may also present as asymptomatic hydronephrosis causing renal failure. Struvite stones and occasionally cystine and uric acid stones grow to fill up the whole pelvicaliceal system, giving rise to the staghorn calculi. Untreated staghorn calculus can cause complete destruction of the kidney. Urinary tract infection is always present with struvite stone, but it can be present with other types of stones also.

With the exception of uric acid stones, all renal stones are radiopaque, and plain x ray of the kidney-ureter-bladder area is often adequate to show their presence within the urinary tract. Urinalysis usually reveals the presence of red cells in the urine. The presence of leukocytes and bacteria in the urine usually indicates associated urinary tract infection.

For the etiologic diagnosis of renal stone disease, in addition to routine urinalysis and urine culture, measurement of calcium and uric acid in the serum and 24-hour urine are the most useful and cost-effective initial investigations. If these tests fail to establish the etiology, more elaborate tests may be necessary. X-ray diffraction study to determine the composition of the stone can help in the investigation. In recurrent stone diseases, measurement of oxalate, citrate, or cystine in 24-hour urine and the ammonium chloride loading test to assess urinary acidification are often necessary to pinpoint the etiology.

Most cases of nephrolithiasis are self-limited. Half of the patients presenting with the first episode of stone will not have a recurrence. Of the remaining half, most will have two or more episodes of stones in their lifetime. A small subgroup will have frequent recurrences, sometimes one or two episodes per month. Metabolic workup is cost-effective in these recurrent patients. Thiazide diuretics, allopurinol, neutral phosphates, and potassium citrate are some of the drugs commonly used in the prevention of renal stones. The choice of agent will depend on the underlying pathophysiology in the individual patient. Penicillamine is used in the treatment of cystine stone. Struvite stones are very difficult to treat and need removal of stone as well as continued antibiotic treatment to keep the urine sterile. The use of ultrasonic radiation to break down stone has been the notable recent development in the treatment of renal stone disease. Lithotripsy, percutaneous as well as extracorporeal, has reduced the need for extensive surgical procedures.

1. Smith, L. H., ed. Symposium on stones. *Am. J. Med.* 45:649, 1968.
2. Gill, W. B. Urolithiasis update: Biophysical and radiologic advances enhance anti-stone therapy. *Am. J. Kidney Dis.* 1:66, 1981.
   Articles 1 and 2 are good reviews of the subject.
3. Melick, R. A., and Henneman, P. H. Clinical and laboratory studies of 207 consecutive patients in a kidney-stone clinic. *N. Engl. J. Med.* 259:307, 1958.
4. Marsahl, V., and White, R. H., and Saintonge, M. C. The natural history of renal and ureteric calculi. *Br. J. Urology.* 47:117, 1975.
5. Coe, F. L., Keck, J., and Norton, E. R. The natural history of calcium urolithiasis. *J.A.M.A.* 238:1519, 1977.
   Articles 3–5 detail the natural history of the disease. Renal stones tend to recur in the majority of patients, most within 2 years. Incidence of the disease is higher in males and has increased in the last two decades.
6. Herring, L. C. Observation on the analysis of ten thousand urinary calculi. *J. Urol.* 88:545, 1962.
7. Prien, E. L. Crystallographic analysis of urinary calculi: A 23-year survey study. *J. Urol.* 89:917, 1963.
   The two studies (articles 7, 8) report on the analysis of 35,000 stones. X-ray diffraction is the best way to study stone composition. Calcium oxalate and phosphate were the predominant stone types (80%).
8. Prien, E. L., and Prien, E. L., Jr. Composition and structure of urinary stone. *Am. J. Med.* 45:654, 1968.
   Detailed review of the subject.
9. Roth, C. S., Bowyer, B. A., and Berquist, T. H. Utility of the plain abdominal radiograph for diagnosing ureteral calculi. *Ann. Emerg. Med.* 14:311, 1985.
10. Zangerle, K. F., Iserson, K. V., and Bjellard, J. C. Usefulness of abdominal flat plate radiographs in patients with suspected ureteral calculi. *Ann. Emerg. Med.* 14:316, 1985.
    Sensitivity and specificity of plain abdominal radiographs in detecting ureteral calculi were 62% and 67%, respectively, in contrast to traditional belief in 90% sensitivity and specificity.
11. Vermeulen, C. W., and Lyon, E. S. Mechanism of genesis and growth of calculi. *Am. J. Med.* 45:684, 1968.
12. Boyee, W. H. Organic matrix of human urinary concretions. *Am. J. Med.* 45:673, 1968.
    Articles 11 and 12 are good reviews of the basic physicochemical changes in urine that lead to kidney stone formation.
13. Howard, J. E., and Thomas, W. C. Control of crystallization in urine. *Am. J. Med.* 45:693, 1968.
    Citrate, pyrophosphate, and some ill-defined peptides present in urine are inhibitors of calcium stone formation. Other inhibitors are discussed.
14. Pak, C. Y. Physiological basis for absorptive and renal hypercalciuria. *Am. J. Physiol.* 237:F415, 1979.
    Review of the pathogenetic mechanism of idiopathic hypercalciuria—the single most common metabolic abnormality leading to kidney stone.
15. Robertson, W. G., and Peacock, M. The cause of idiopathic calcium stone disease: Hypercalciuria or hyperoxaluria. *Nephron* 26:105, 1980.
    Only 10% of all hypercalciurics develop calcium stones. Other factors, like the presence of a mild degree of hyperoxaluria, may be important. See also reference 17.
16. Parks, J. H., and Coe, F. L. A urinary calcium citrate index for the evaluation of nephrolithiasis. *Kidney Int.* 30:85, 1986.
    Underscores the importance of low citrate levels in urine in the pathogenesis of calcium stone.
17. Pak, C. Y., and Fuller, C. Idopathic hypocitruric calcium-oxalate nephrolithiasis successfully treated with potassium citrate. *Ann. Intern. Med.* 104:33, 1986.
    Correction of hypocitruria with oral supplementation by potassium citrate was effective in preventing recurrence in 90% of these patients.

18. Parks, J. H., Coe, F. L., and Farus, M. Hyperparathyroidism in nephrolithiasis. *Arch. Intern. Med.* 140:1479, 1980.
    Incidence of primary hyperparathyroidism among kidney stone patients was about 5%. Many of these patients had only mild (10.15–10.95 mg/dl) and intermittent hypercalcemia.
19. Derrick, F. C., Jr. Renal calculi in association with hyperparathyroidism: A changing entity. *J. Urol.* 127:226, 1982.
    Much lower incidence (0.2%) observed in this study. The reason could be a less rigorous search for hyperparathyroidism. Since hypercalcemia is often mild and intermittent, the diagnosis of hyperparathyroidism can be easily missed.
20. Kimbrough, J. C., and Denslow, J. C. Urinary tract calculi in recumbent patient. *J. Urol.* 61:837, 1949.
21. Cockett, A. T., Beechler, C. C., and Roberts, J. E. Astronautic urolithiasis: A potential hazard during prolonged weightlessness in space travel. *J. Urol.* 88:542, 1962.
    Articles 20 and 21 underscore the importance of immobilization as a factor in hypercalciuria and kidney stone formation.
22. Albright, F., Consolazio, W. V, and Coombs, F. S. Metabolic studies and therapy in a case of nephrocalcinosis with rickets and dwarfism. *Bull. Johns Hopkins Hosp.* 66:7, 1940.
23. Buckalew, V. M., Purvis, M. L., and Shulman, M. G. Hereditary renal tubular acidosis. *Medicine* 53:229, 1974.
    Two classic studies on distal-type renal tubular acidosis. Nephrocalcinosis is quite common in this entity.
24. Sage, M. R., Lawson, A. D., and Marshall, V. R. Medullary sponge kidney and urolithiasis. *Clin. Radiol.* 33:435, 1982.
    Medullary sponge kidney is associated with tubular abnormality, including renal hypercalciuria, and often leads to urolithiasis. Authors cite 17% incidence of this disease in renal stone patients.
25. Gregory, J. G., Park, K. Y., and Schoenberg, H. W. Oxalate stone disease after intestinal resection. *J. Urol.* 117:631, 1977.
    Of 543 patients with jejunoileal bypass, 65 patients developed renal stones. Most had recurrent stones.
26. Dobbins, J. W., and Bender, H. J. Importance of the colon in enteric hyperoxaluria. *N. Engl. J. Med.* 296:298, 1977.
    Oxalate is absorbed in the colon. Bypassing the colon in ileum corrects hyperoxaluria due to ileal dysfunction.
27. Gregory, J. G. Hyperoxaluria and stone disease in the gastrointestinal bypass patient. *Urol. Clin. North Am.* 8:331, 1981.
    Good review of this interesting iatrogenic cause of kidney stones.
28. Hatch, M., Mulgrew, S., and Bourke, E. Effect of megadoses of ascorbic acid on serum and urinary oxalate. *Eur. Urol.* 6:166, 1980.
    Using megadoses of vitamin C is not without hazard. One known side effect is the risk of developing kidney stone.
29. Williams, H. E., and Smith, L. H. Disorders of oxalate metabolism. *Am. J. Med.* 45:715, 1968.
    State-of-the-art review of the biochemistry of oxalate metabolism, and the mechanism of primary and secondary hyperoxaluria, and their management.
30. Gutman, A. B. Uric acid nephrolithiasis. *Am. J. Med.* 45:756, 1968.
    Extensive review of the prevalence, pathogenesis, and management of uric acid stone. Well-referenced with illustrative cases.
31. Pak, C. Y., Waters, O., and Arnold, L. Mechanism for calcium urolithiasis among patients with hyperuricosuria. *J. Clin. Invest.* 59:426, 1977.
32. Millman, S., Strauss, A. C., and Parks, J. H. Pathogenesis and clinical course of mixed calcium oxalate and uric acid nephrolithiasis. *Kidney Int.* 22:366, 1982.
    These articles (31, 32) discuss the mechanism, incidence, and management of calcium stones in hyperuricosuric patients.
33. Crawhall, J. C., and Watts, R. W. Cystinuria. *Am. J. Med.* 45:736, 1968.
    An extensive review of the genetics, biochemistry, clinical, and therapeutic aspects of this inherited metabolic disorder.

34. Seegmiller, J. E. Xanthine stone formation. *Am. J. Med.* 45:780, 1968.
    Review of a rare but interesting type of kidney stone.
35. Gault, M. H., Simmonds, H. A., and Snedden, W. Urolithiasis due to 2.8-dihydroxy-adenine in an adult. *N. Engl. J. Med.* 305:1570, 1981.
    Yet another abnormality of purine metabolism leading to a rare kind of kidney stone.
36. Ettinger, B., Oldroyd, N. O., and Sorgel, F. Triamterene nephrolithiasis. *J.A.M.A.* 244:2443, 1980.
    Triamterene, a frequently prescribed drug in hypertension therapy, has been implicated as causing a new kind of stone. The incidence, however, is rare.
37. Chute, R., and Suby, H. I. Prevalence and importance of urea-splitting bacterial infections of the urinary tract in the formation of calculi. *J. Urol.* 44:590, 1943.
    One of the very early reports showing the importance of urea-splitting bacterial infection, e.g., proteus, in the genesis of struvite stone.
38. Singh, M., Chapman, R., and Tresidder, G. C. The fate of the un-operated stag-horn calculus. *Br. J. Urol.* 45:581, 1973.
    Expectant treatment of these patients led either to subsequent nephrectomy or progressive renal failure and death.
39. Nimoy, N. J., and Stamey, T. A. Surgical, bacteriological, and biochemical management of infection stones. *J.A.M.A.* 215:1470, 1971.
40. Resnick, M. I. Evaluation and management of infection stones: *Urol. Clin. North Am.* 8:265, 1981.
    These articles (39, 40) summarize the management of one of the most difficult kinds of kidney stone.
41. Pak, C. Y., Britton, F., and Peterson, R. Ambulatory evaluation of nephrolithiasis. *Am. J. Med.* 69:19, 1980.
    Diagnostic metabolic workup of kidney stone disease in ambulatory clinic setting well outlined.
42. Smith, C. L. When should the stone patient be evaluated? Early evaluation of single stone formation. *Med. Clin. North Am.* 68:455, 1984.
43. Erickson, S. B. When should the stone patient be evaluated? Limited evaluation of single stone formation. *Med. Clin. North Am.* 68:461, 1984.
    Limited evaluation and fluid diet therapy as initial approach is cost-effective. Extensive workup reserved for multiple recurrences.
44. Segura, J. W., Patterson, D. E., and Leroy A. J. Percutaneous removal of kidney stones: review of 1000 cases. *J. Urol.* 134:1077, 1985.
    Percutaneous lithotripsy is relatively easy to do and has a high success rate (88–98%) and few complications (3%).
45. Newman, R. C., Bezirdjian, L., and Steinbook, G. Complications of extracorporeal shock wave lithotripsy: Prevention and treatment. *Semin. Urol.* 4:170, 1986.
    Complications of this new modality are rare but include ureteral obstruction, flank pain, hematoma, cardiac dysrhythmia, upper extremity paresis, and burn.
46. Health and Public Policy Committee, American College of Physicians. Lithotripsy. *Ann. Intern. Med.* 103:626, 1985.
    Review of the status of these newer modes of surgical therapy for kidney stones with recommendations when to use.
47. Yendt, E. R., and Cohanim, M. Prevention of calcium stones with thiazides. *Kidney Int.* 13:397, 1978.
    354 patients were treated with a success rate of 90%. A detailed review by a pioneer in the field.
48. Coe, F. L. Prevention of kidney stones. *Am. J. Med.* 71:514, 1981.
    Brief summary of medical management of recurrent stones by a well-known specialist in the field.

141. NEPHROTIC SYNDROME
H. Verdain Barnes

The nephrotic syndrome is characterized by the presence of (1) proteinuria (3.5 gm/24 hours or greater), (2) hypoalbuminemia (3 gm/dl or less), and (3) lipiduria, including free fat, oval fat bodies, and/or fatty casts in the urine. Hypercholesterolemia with a cholesterol level of 300 mg/dl or greater is frequently present. Edema is present in 80 percent of adults and 98 percent of children. The chief complaint is generally that of edema, which is usually insidious in onset but may occur abruptly. The edema is usually bilateral, involving the lower extremities, hands, and periorbital areas, but it may be unilateral or localized to one of these areas or to the scrotum or abdominal wall. Anasarca occurs in some younger patients, who may collect fluid weight equal to or greater than 50 percent of their dry body weight. Ascites, pleural effusion, pericardial effusion, and hydroarthrosis are not uncommon. Pharyngeal and epiglottal swelling may precipitate respiratory emergencies.

Other clinical features of the syndrome, excluding those accompanying the underlying disease, are (1) a retinal sheen and light reflex, predominantly on the nasal side of the disk, (2) Muehrcke lines (paired white lines on the fingernails), (3) growth retardation in children and adolescents, and (4) eruptive xanthomas in patients with marked hyperlipidemia. Infection, particularly of the urinary tract, is common, regardless of the therapy used. Approximately 20 percent of patients have positive urine cultures at some time during the course of their illness. Septic peritonitis can occur; it is most often due to pneumococci. The classic nephrotic "crisis" is uncommon, but it can present a diagnostic and therapeutic dilemma. The features are prostration, behavior changes, abdominal pain, vomiting, obstipation, and fever. In the majority no underlying cause is documented, whereas in others there may be an associated staphylococcal enterocolitis or an enteritis produced by other bacteria or fungi. Some patients have been found at laparotomy to have localized edema of Treitz's ligament, which may be an underlying cause of this symptom constellation. Another complication of nephrotic syndrome is thromboembolism in up to 28 percent of patients. A variety of coagulation abnormalities have been reported including decreased antithrombin III levels; increased or decreased levels of the vitamin K–dependent factors II, VII, IX, and X; increased protein C and S antigen levels, but decreased protein S activity; and increased levels of plasma fibrinopeptide and B beta 15–42. Consequently, some nephrotic syndrome patients exhibit a hypercoagulable state which may result in venous or arterial thrombosis. In one recent series almost 50 percent had documentable renal vein thrombosis, although it appeared to have little demonstrable effect on the course of the disease or outcome. Other sites of thrombosis, particularly when accompanied by embolism, may result in significant clinical outcomes.

The known causes of the nephrotic syndrome are numerous but they bear enumeration. Most common is a variety of primary glomerular diseases. These include (1) minimal change disease, (2) idiopathic membranous glomerulonephritis, (3) acute, subacute, or chronic proliferative glomerulonephritis, (4) focal segmented glomerulosclerosis, and (5) lobular glomerulonephritis. Collagen-vascular causes include systemic lupus erythematosus, periarteritis nodosa, Goodpasture's disease, dermatomyositis, erythema multiforme, progressive systemic sclerosis, and giant-cell arteritis. In addition, nephrotic syndrome has been associated with Hodgkin's disease; multiple myeloma; chronic lymphocytic leukemia; clonal T cell leukemia; non-Hodgkin's lymphomas; carcinoid, bronchogenic, gastric, colon, pharyngeal, mouth, breast, prostrate, and ovarian carcinomas; Waldenström's macroglobulinemia; melanoma; nephroblastoma; carotid body and colon tumors; sickle cell anemia; spherocytosis; diabetic glomerulosclerosis; pheochromocytoma; myxedema (acquired and familial); amyloidosis; renal artery stenosis; acute and chronic renal vein thrombosis; pulmonary artery thrombosis; inferior vena cava obstruction; constrictive pericarditis; tricuspid insufficiency; congestive heart failure; infectious endocarditis; hereditofamilial nephritis; pregnancy; malignant mesothelioma; primary hyperparathyroidism; massive obesity; renal transplantation; intravenous heroin abuse; and the ingestion of trimethadione (Tridione), paramethadione, probenecid, lithium, tolbutamide, fenoprofen, naproxen, and penicillamine. Nephrotoxins, such as the mercurial diuretics, mercury, bismuth, and gold, may produce the nephrotic syndrome. The other major associations include a variety of allergens and infectious agents. The allergens reported are bee stings, snake bites, wool, poison oak, poison ivy, and a variety of pollens. The infectious associations are secondary syphilis, schistosomiasis, plasmodium malaria, tuberculosis, herpes zoster, typhus, and cytomegalovirus disease.

The common feature of these diverse causes is glomerular damage resulting in increased permeability. The type of glomerular lesion varies from minimal histologic change in the glomerulus to proliferation of the mesangial, endothelial, and parietal epithelial cells and basement membrane to marked thickening of the capillary walls in the absence of hypocellularity to a combination of proliferative and membranous changes. Immunohistologically there is rarely if ever IgG or C3 deposition detectable on the glomerular basement membrane or capillary walls in minimal change disease, whereas in the other histologic variations, deposition of these immunoglobulins is usually found.

The edema which develops in nephrotic syndrome is probably multifactorial and may differ from patient to patient. The classic pathophysiologic explanation based on decreased vascular volume due to a low level of albumin appears to be operative in most patients, particularly children. In this setting the hypovolemia results in a rise in circulating levels of plasma renin activity, catecholamines, aldosterone, and vasopressin in an effort to increase vascular volume. In other patients these levels are essentially normal, in which setting there may be an intrarenal defect which triggers glomerular vasoconstriction. Other, as yet undefined, mechanisms may also be operative. Diagnosis of the syndrome is usually made easily on clinical and routine chemical and urine evaluations. Specific analysis of urinary protein may be of diagnostic and prognostic help. Selective proteinuria is asociated with minimal glomerular change disease, while unselective proteinuria is associated with the other types. Minimal change disease usually responds to steroids. A histologic diagnosis may help direct therapy and define prognosis. A closed-needle biopsy of the kidney is a safe, reliable procedure when carefully performed by an experienced nephrologist. The specimen should be evaluated by light microscopy with both hematoxylin and eosin and PAS stains and by immunohistochemical techniques. However, one recent decision analysis study concludes that a renal biopsy is rarely required in managing adult patients with nephrotic syndrome.

Minimal change disease with no immunochemical deposition and selective proteinuria offers the best prognosis, while the other varieties have a poorer prognosis, particularly in the presence of any of the following features: (1) nephrotic syndrome of greater than 6 months' duration, (2) hypertension, (3) azotemia, (4) relatively low serum cholesterol level, and (5) significant hematuria.

1. Earley, L. E., and Forland, M. Nephrotic Syndrome. In L. E. Earley and C. W. Gottschalk (eds.), *Strauss and Welt's Diseases of the Kidney* (3rd ed.). Boston: Little, Brown, 1979.
   An excellent, well-referenced review of all aspects of the syndrome.
2. Muehrcke, R. C. The finger-nails in chronic hypoalbuminemia: A new physical sign. *Br. Med. J.* 1:1327, 1956.
   A helpful clinical sign that may help date the onset of the syndrome.
3. Newmark, S. R., Anderson, C. F., Donadio, J. V., et al. Lipoprotein profiles in adult nephrotics. *Mayo Clin. Proc.* 50:359, 1975.
   The most common lipoprotein types were IIa, IIb, and V.
4. Hopper, J. J., Ryan, P., Lee, J. C., et al. Lipoid nephrosis in 31 adults: Renal biopsy study by light, electron, and fluorescent microscopy with experience in treatment. *Medicine* 49:321, 1970.
5. McIntosh, R. M., Ting, B., Kaufman, D., et al. Immunohistology in renal disease: Diagnostic, prognostic, therapeutic, and etiologic value and limitations. *Q. J. Med.* 40:385, 1971.
   Articles 4 and 5 provide a comprehensive review of the histologic evaluation of renal tissue in the nephrotic syndrome.
6. Herdman, R. C., Pickering, R. J., Michael, A. F., et al. Chronic glomuerulonephritis associated with low serum complement activity. *Medicine* 49:207, 1970.
   An interesting entity that has diagnostic as well as prognostic significance.

7. Farr, L. E., and MacFayden, D. A. Hypoamino-acidemia in children with nephrotic crisis. *Am. J. Dis. Child.* 59:782, 1940.
   Nephrotic crisis—an important and interesting phenomenon.
8. Gerber, M. A., and Paronetto, F. IgE in glomeruli of patients with nephrotic syndrome. *Lancet* 1:1097, 1971.
   IgE seen along capillary walls in a segmental linear pattern in 80% with minimal change disease.
9. Jenis, E. H., Teichman, S., Briggs, W. A., et al. Focal segmental glomerulosclerosis. *Am. J. Med.* 57:695, 1974.
10. Cheigh, J.-S., Stenzel, K. H., Susin, M., et al. Kidney transplant nephrotic syndrome. *Am. J. Med.* 57:730, 1974.
11. Conser, W. G., Wagonfeld, J. B., Spargo, B. H., et al. Glomerular deposition of tumor antigen in membranous nephropathy associated with colonic carcinoma. *Am. J. Med.* 57:962, 1974.
12. Gagliano, R. G., Costanzi, J. J., Beathard, G. A., et al. The nephrotic syndrome associated with neoplasia: An unusual paraneoplastic syndrome. *Am. J. Med.* 60:1026, 1976.
13. Alexander, F., and Atkins, E. L. Familial renal amyloidosis: Case reports, literature review and classification. *Am. J. Med.* 59:121, 1975.
14. Falcao, H. A., and Gould, D. B. Immune complex nephropathy in schistosomiasis. *Ann. Intern. Med.* 83:148, 1975.
15. Moorthy, A. V., Zimmerman, S. W., and Burkholder, P. M. Nephrotic syndrome in Hodgkin's disease: Evidence for pathogenesis alternative to immune complex deposition. *Am. J. Med.* 61:471, 1976.
16. Martelo, O. J., Schultz, D. R., Pardo, V., et al. Immunologically-mediated renal disease in Waldenström's macroglobulinemia. *Am. J. Med.* 58:567, 1975.
17. O'Regan, S., Fong, J. S. C., de Chadarevian, J.-P., et al. Treponemal antigens in congenital and acquired syphilitic nephritis. *Ann. Intern. Med.* 85:325, 1976.
18. Weisinger, J. R., Kempson, R. L., Eldridge, F. L., et al. The nephrotic syndrome: A complication of massive obesity. *Ann. Intern. Med.* 81:440, 1974.
19. Humpherys, S. R., Holley, K. E., Smith, L. H., et al. Mesenteric angiofollicular lymphoid hyperplasia (lymphoid hamartoma) with nephrotic syndrome. *Mayo Clin. Proc.* 50:317, 1975.
20. Palma, A., Sanchez-Palencia, A., Armas, J. R., et al. Progressive systemic sclerosis and nephrotic syndrome. *Arch. Intern. Med.* 141:520, 1981.
21. Cade, R., Spooner, G., Juncos, L., et al. Chronic renal vein thrombosis. *Am. J. Med.* 63:387, 1977.
22. Wakashin, M., Wakashin, Y., Iesato, K., et al. Association of gastric cancer and nephrotic syndrome: An immunologic study in three patients. *Gastroenterology* 78:749, 1980.
23. DePace, N. L., Elquezabal, A., and Hardenburg, H. C. Pulmonary carcinoid tumor associated with nephrotic syndrome. *Arch. Intern. Med.* 140:552, 1980.
24. Bennett, W. M., Plamp, C., and Porter, G. A. Drug-related syndromes in clinical nephrology. *Ann. Intern. Med.* 87:582, 1977.
25. Richman, A. V., Masco, H. L., Rifkin, S. I., et al. Minimal-change disease and the nephrotic syndrome associated with lithium therapy. *Ann. Intern. Med.* 92:70, 1980.
26. Brezin, J. H., Katz, S. M., Schwartz, A. B., et al. Reversible renal failure and nephrotic syndrome associated with nonsteroidal antiinflammatory drugs. *N. Engl. J. Med.* 301:1271, 1979.
27. Kumar, A., and Shapiro, A. P. Proteinuria and nephrotic syndrome induced by renin in patients with renal artery stenosis. *Arch. Intern. Med.* 140:1631, 1980.
   Articles 9–27 detail an array of causes and pathogeneses for nephrotic syndrome.
28. Anderson, D. C., York, T. L., Rose, G., et al. Assessment of serum factor B, serum opsonins, granulocyte chemotaxis and infection in nephrotic syndrome of children. *J. Infect. Dis.* 140:1, 1979.
   Decreased serum chemotaxis and factor B may be responsible for the increased susceptibility to infection.

29. Kauffmann, R. H., Veltkamp, J. T., Tilburg, N. H. V., et al. Acquired antithrombin III deficiency and thrombosis in the nephrotic syndrome. *Am. J. Med.* 65:607, 1978.

30. Saito, H., Goodnough, L. T., Makker, S. P., et al. Urinary excretion of Hageman factor (factor XII) and the presence of nonfunctional Hageman factor in the nephrotic syndrome. *Am. J. Med.* 70:531, 1981.
    Articles 29, 30 discuss clotting system changes and their potential relation to hypercoagulability in nephrotic syndrome.

31. Lowenstein, J., Schacht, R. G., and Baldwin, D. S. Renal failure in minimal change nephrotic syndrome. *Am. J. Med.* 70:227, 1981.
    In this setting the renal failure often responds to diuresis and may be related to intrarenal edema.

32. Idelson, B. A., Smithline, N., Smith, G. W., et al. Prognosis in steroid-treated idiopathic nephrotic syndrome in adults: Analysis of major predictive factors after ten-year follow-up. *Arch. Intern. Med.* 137:891, 1977.
    A useful discussion of prognosis.

33. Nolasco, F., Cameron, J. S., Heywood, E. F., et al. Adult-onset minimal change nephrotic syndrome: A long-term follow-up. *Kidney Int.* 29:1215, 1986.
    The response to steroids is slower than in children, but age was not a factor in the response to therapy.

34. Orman, S. V., Schechter, G. P., Whang-Peng, J., et al. Nephrotic syndrome associated with a clonal T-cell leukemia of large granular lymphocytes with cytotoxic function. *Arch. Intern. Med.* 146:1827, 1986.

35. Stuart, K., Fallon, B. G., and Cardi, M. A. Development of the nephrotic syndrome in a patient with prostatic cancer. *Am. J. Med.* 80:295, 1986.

36. Seney, F. D., Jr., Federgreen, W. R., Stein, H., et al. A review of nephrotic syndrome associated with chronic lymphocytic leukemia. *Arch. Intern. Med.* 146:137, 1986.

37. Fellner, S. K., and Spargo, B. H. Nephrotic syndrome from hypercalcemia in a patient with primary hyperparathyroidism. *Am. J. Med.* 83:355, 1987.

38. Schroeter, N. J., Rushing, D. A., Parker, J. P., et al. Minimal-change nephrotic syndrome associated with malignant mesothelioma. *Arch. Intern. Med.* 146:1834, 1986.
    Articles 34–38 report additional causes to keep in mind.

39. Vigano-D'Angelo, S., D'Angelo, A., Kaufman, C. E., Jr., et al. Protein S deficiency occurs in the nephrotic syndrome. *Ann. Intern. Med.* 107:42, 1987.

40. Tomura, S., Oono, Y., Kuriyama, R., et al. Plasma concentrations of fibrinopeptide A and fibrinopeptide Bβ 15–42 glomerulonephritis and the nephrotic syndrome. *Arch. Intern. Med.* 145:1033, 1985.

41. Wagoner, R. D., Stanson, A. W., Holley, K. E., et al. Renal vein thrombosis in idiopathic membranous glomerulopathy and nephrotic syndrome: Incidence and significance. *Kidney Int.* 23:368, 1983.
    Clotting system abnormalities (articles 39, 40) and a potential outcome (article 41).

42. Roscher, W., and Tulassay, T. Hormonal regulation of water metabolism in children with nephrotic syndrome. *Kidney Int.* 32:583, 1987.

43. Brown, E. A., Markandu, N., Sagnella, G. A., et al. Sodium retention in nephrotic syndrome is due to an intrarenal defect: Evidence from steroid-induced remission. *Nephron* 39:290, 1985.
    Potential mechanisms for the edema in nephrotic syndrome (articles 42, 43).

44. Levey, A. S., Lau, J., Pauker, S. G., et al. Idiopathic nephrotic syndrome: Puncturing the biopsy myth. *Ann. Intern. Med.* 107:697, 1987.
    These authors conclude from decision analysis that renal biopsy is rarely needed to direct patient management.

45. Mitas, J. A., II. Exogenous protein as a cause of nephrotic-range proteinuria. *Am. J. Med.* 79:115, 1985.
    Factitous proteinuria (3.2 gm/24 hours) documented by immunoelectrophoresis.

46. Beaman, M., Howie, A. J., Hardwicke, J., et al. The glomerular tip lesion: A steroid responsive nephrotic syndrome. *Clin. Nephrol.* 27:217, 1987.
    A rare cause of nephrotic syndrome with a good prognosis.

142. POSTSTREPTOCOCCAL GLOMERULONEPHRITIS
H. Verdain Barnes

Acute glomerulonephritis is not an uncommon complication of β-hemolytic streptococcal infection. The most common streptococcal types involved, in order of frequency, are types 12, 14, 49, and 1. The incidence ranges up to 25 percent of those infected, depending on the type of infection. Most often, the antecedent infection involves the pharynx, ears, or skin. With some streptococcal types, particularly type 49, there is a higher incidence of glomerulonephritis with skin than with pharyngeal infections. Acute poststreptococcal glomerulonephritis (APSG) can occur at any age. The peak incidence in children is between the ages of 3 and 7 years while in the adult the average age is in the mid-thirties. Men show about a 2:1 predominance over women.

The classic clinical presentation is well-known and need not be described; however, some comments about variations in the clinical picture are warranted. First, the time from acute infection to the onset of clinical APSG may be as short as 2 days or as long as 56 days, compared to the average of about 10 days. As many as 20 percent have a latent period of less than 1 week. In general, the latent period for exacerbations of chronic poststreptococcal glomerulonephritis is between 1 and 4 days; however, it may be as long as 14 days. Second, overt manifestations may be lacking or may be dominated by nonrenal symptoms. Some patients have no clinical signs or symptoms except for an abnormal urine sediment. On the other hand, a rare patient has a typical clinical presentation, but a normal urine at the time of first evaluation. Weakness may be the dominant symptom and the last to disappear; in fact, it may persist for several months after the urine and other manifestations have returned to normal. In the over-50 age group, unexplained acute pulmonary edema or dyspnea and orthopnea should raise the question of APSG. Abdominal complaints, such as nausea with or without vomiting, constipation, or diarrhea, may dominate the clinical picture, focusing the physician's attention away from the kidney. Moderate degrees of fluid retention may not result in easily demonstrable edema. In this instance, its presence may be fully realized only after diuresis has occurred. Third, hypertension, when present, is characteristically mild, but APSG must enter the differential diagnosis of any encephalopathy associated with hypertension, particularly in younger patients, whose mild hypertension may represent a marked elevation above their normal blood pressure. Finally, hematuria, the most common single manifestation of this disease, may persist for months. Gross hematuria can persist for more than 30 days, particularly in patients with exacerbations of chronic poststreptococcal disease.

The glomerular disease in APSG is probably related to the deposition of antigen-antibody complexes within the glomerulus. Granular glomerular deposits of IgG, anti-IgG, and C3 have been demonstrated. Histologically, acute inflammation is seen about equally in all glomeruli. The capillary tufts are enlarged, and the lumen is obstructed to varying degrees. Both the epithelial and mesangial cells are increased in number, whereas the tubules and interstitium show little or no change. These pathologic changes typically result in changes in renal function. There is a decrease in glomerular filtration rate despite a normal or increased renal blood flow. Tubular reabsorption is decreased, as is renal oxygen consumption. The urine on gross inspection may be clear, smoky, or reddish-brown. Urinary protein usually ranges from 1 to 4 gm/24 hours but on rare occasions may be as high as 15 gm/day. Some hyaline, granular, white cell, or red cell casts may be seen, and on occasion they approach 20 per high-power field. Red cell casts can almost always be found with a diligent search. White cell casts, though more typical of pyelonephritis, may be seen in any acute inflammatory response in the kidney, including APSG, lupus nephritis, and anaphylactoid purpura. Finally, on occasion oval fat bodies are seen.

A variety of renal disorders may at some point in their course be clinically indistinguishable from APSG. First, there are those entities that may confuse the picture on the basis of the initial clinical course and urinary findings. These include acute exacerbations of chronic glomerulonephritis, focal glomerulonephritis, and malignant hypertension. Second are the diseases in which the urine findings may be similar or identical to those in APSG. These include anaphylactoid purpura, Wegener's granulomatosis, polyarteritis nodosa, Goodpasture's disease, rapidly progressive glomerulonephritis, acute tubular necrosis, hereditary nephritis, lipoid nephrosis, bacterial endocarditis, febrile proteinuria, and exercise proteinuria or hematuria.

1. McCluskey, R. T., and Klassen, J. Immunologically-mediated glomerular, tubular, and interstitial renal disease. *N. Engl. J. Med.* 288:564, 1973.
   Most glomerular diseases appear to be immunologically mediated.
2. Churg, J., and Girshman, E. Ultrastructure of immune deposits in renal glomeruli. *Ann. Intern. Med.* 76:479, 1972.
   A good study in immunopathology.
3. Nissenson, A. R., Baraff, L. J., Fine, R. N., et al. Poststreptococcal acute glomerulonephritis: Fact and controversy. *Ann. Intern. Med.* 91:76, 1979.
   An up-to-date review. C3 levels are usually low, occasionally normal.
4. Freedman, P., Meister, H. P., Lee, H. W. J., et al. The renal response to streptococcal infection. *Medicine* 49:433, 1970.
   A study of the renal pathology and subsequent acute glomerulonephritis.
5. Sagel, I., Treser, G., Ty, A., et al. Occurrence and nature of glomerular lesions after group A streptococci infections in children. *Ann. Intern. Med.* 79:492, 1973.
   CH_{50} and/or urine sediment abnormalities were seen in 21% after an acute group A streptococcal infection.
6. Bernstein, S. H., and Stillerman, M. A study of the association of group A streptococci with acute glomerulonephritis. *Ann. Intern. Med.* 52:1026, 1960.
   Types 12 and 14 were most common.
7. Dunn, M. J. Acute glomerulonephritis with normal results from urinalyses. *J.A.M.A.* 201:933, 1967.
   Beware.
8. Sapir, D. G., Yardley, J. H., and Walker, W. G. Acute glomerulonephritis in older patients. *Johns Hopkins Med. J.* 123:145, 1968.
   Dyspnea and orthopnea may dominate the clinical picture.
9. Leonard, C. D., Nagle, R. B., Striker, G. E., et al. Acute glomerulonephritis with prolonged oliguria. *Ann. Intern. Med.* 73:703, 1970.
   Oliguria may last as long as 39 days before renal function begins to return.
10. Anthony, B. F., Kaplan, E. L., Wanamaker, L. W., et al. Attack rates of acute nephritis after type 49 streptococcal infection of the skin and of the respiratory tract. *J. Clin. Invest.* 48:1697, 1969.
    23.8% with skin infection developed APSG as compared to 4.5% with throat infection.
11. Dodge, W. F., Spargo, B. H., Travis, L. B., et al. Poststreptococcal glomerulonephritis. *N. Engl. J. Med.* 286:273, 1972.
    A switch to an orthostatic pattern of proteinuria may indicate a better prognosis.
12. Hinglais, N., Garcia-Torres, R., and Kleinknecht, D. Long-term prognosis in acute glomerulonephritis. *Am. J. Med.* 56:52, 1974.
    Early clinical and pathologic features may have predictive value.
13. Lewy, J. E., Salinas-Madgigal, L., Herdson, P. B., et al. Clinico-pathologic correlations in acute poststreptococcal glomerulonephritis. *Medicine* 50:435, 1971.
    An excellent, well-referenced review.
14. Baldwin, D. S., Gluch, M. C., Schacht, R. G., et al. The long-term course of poststreptococcal glomerulonephritis. *Ann. Intern. Med.* 80:342, 1974.
    Follow-up from 2–15 years revealed long-term proteinuria, hypertension, or reduced glomerular filtration rate in 50% of these authors' 115 patients.
15. Schacht, R. G., Gluch, M. C., Gallow, G. R., et al. Progression to uremia after remission of acute poststreptococcal glomerulonephritis. *N. Engl. J. Med.* 295:977, 1976.
    Six patients had renal function return essentially to normal. Then over a period of from 2 to 12 years increasing renal failure developed, with increasing glomerular sclerosis without proliferative or fibrohyaline changes.
16. Rodriguez-Iturbe, B., Rabideau, D., Garcia, R., et al. Characterization of the glomer-

ular antibody in acute poststreptococcal glomerulonephritis. *Ann. Intern. Med.* 92:478, 1980.
No streptococcal enzymes or proteins were found in the kidney—just IgG and anti-IgG.

17. Sanjad, S., Tolaymat, A., Whitworth, J., et al. Acute glomerulonephritis in children: A review of 153 cases. *South. Med. J.* 70:1202, 1977.
    Impetigo was the major association and APSG continues to appear to be self-limiting in children.

18. Lien, J. W. K., Mathew, T. H., and Meadows, R. Acute poststreptococcal glomerulonephritis in adults: A long term study. *Q. J. Med.* 48:99, 1979.
    In this series the majority had a good prognosis.

19. DeBeukelear, M. M., and Yound, G. F. Subarachnoid hemorrhage complicating acute poststreptococcal glomerulonephritis. *Arch. Neurol.* 35:473, 1978.
    A rarity to keep in mind if the patient has meningeal signs or symptoms.

20. Smith, M. C., Cooke, J. H., Zimmerman, D. M., et al. Asymptomatic glomerulonephritis after nonstreptococcal upper respiratory infections. *Ann. Intern. Med.* 91:697, 1979.
    Some common viruses can do it.

21. Gibney, R., Reineck, J., Bannayan, G. A., et al. Renal lesions in acute rheumatic fever. *Ann. Intern. Med.* 94:322, 1981.
    The renal lesions were variable and may be more common than previously thought.

22. Vogl, W., Renke, M., Mayer-Eichberger, D., et al. Long-term prognosis for endocapillary glomerulonephritis of poststreptococcal type in children and adults. *Nephron* 44:58, 1986.
    In this series, only 2% progressed to chronic renal failure. The prognosis was poorer in those with an initial nephrotic syndrome.

23. Ferrario, F., Kowilsky, O., and Morel-Maroger, L. Acute endocapillary glomerulonephritis in adults: A histologic and clinical comparison between patients with and without initial acute renal failure. *Clin. Nephrol.* 19:17, 1983.
    The disease in adults is well characterized by clinical presentation.

24. Rodriguez-Iturbe, B. Epidemic poststreptococcal glomerulonephritis. *Kidney Int.* 25:129, 1984.
    Children recover more rapidly than adults.

25. Ben-Dov, I., Berry, E. M., and Kopolovic, J. Poststreptococcal nephritis and acute rheumatic fever in two adults. *Arch. Intern. Med.* 145:338, 1985.
    Although rare, this coexistence can occur in both children and adults.

143. PYELONEPHRITIS
Kim Goldenberg

Pyelonephritis is an inflammation of the renal parenchyma and pelvis. Pyelonephritis and tubulointerstitial (or interstitial) kidney disease produce the same pathologic changes. However, pyelonephritis commonly refers to upper urinary tract infection and interstitial kidney disease to a chemical, physical, or immunologic insult to the kidney. In acute disease, the distinction between these terms, based on the etiology, that is, infection versus other factors, is usually possible. In chronic disease, however, an etiology is often not found. The exact incidences of acute and chronic pyelonephritis are unknown. Pregnancy, associated with bacteriuria, results in an increased incidence of acute pyelonephritis. This predisposition to pyelonephritis that is seen in pregnancy results in part from diminished ureteral tone and peristalsis, and incompetence of the vesicoureteral valves. Autopsy studies suggest that chronic pyelonephritis, exclusive of diabetes and obstructive uropathy, is present in less than 1 percent of the population. Diabetics and hypertensives have a greater incidence of pyelonephritis.

The possibility that chronic pyelonephritis has been caused by repeated episodes of acute pyelonephritis is suggested by a history of recurrent urinary tract infections, an underlying renal defect such as vesicoureteral reflux, asymmetric renal atrophy, and pathologic involvement of the pelvicaliceal system (which is not usually discernible by needle biopsy). Acute pyelonephritis may develop by an ascending, hematogenous, or lymphatic spread of a microbial agent. The ascending route is most common. The normal urinary tract is void of organisms except for the distal urethra which is colonized with species of viridan streptococcus, *Staphylococcus epidermidis,* diphtheroids, lactobacillis, *Gardenerella vaginalis,* and anaerobes. These organisms rarely cause infection. The great majority of infections are due to gram-negative coliforms, mostly *Escherichia coli,* which colonize the introitus, periurethral skin, and migrate to the distal urethra.

In susceptible individuals, bacteria enter the bladder by transurethral migration and, in a minority, enter the kidney via the ureters. Predisposing factors that favor ascending infection include a short urethra, for example, in women; incompetent vesicoureteral valves that allow urinary reflux; urethral instrumentation, especially in diabetics; incomplete bladder emptying that allows residual urine and growth for bacteria; and foreign bodies such as calculi that may act as a nidus for infection. *Proteus mirabilis,* a common coliform, produces urease which decomposes urea to ammonia and carbon dioxide. The resulting alkaline urine favors the formation of struvite (magnesium ammonium phosphate) stones. *Klebsiella pneumoniae* may also favor stone formation by producing extracellular polysaccharides and mucin. *Proteus, Klebsiella-Enterobacter, Pseudomonas, Streptococcus faecalis,* and *Staphylococcus* species are more commonly acquired in the hospital where instrumentation and antibiotic-resistant isolates are likely. However, gram-positive bacteria rarely cause pyelonephritis that is acquired outside of the hospital.

Hematogenous spread of infection is rare and may occur because of virulent organisms in the blood, that is, due to *Staphylococcus aureus* endocarditis or with an anatomic abnormality of the kidney. *Mycobacterium tuberculosis,* which can disseminate from foci in the lung or lymph nodes, may be clinically silent except for a urine which contains white and red cells without bacteria. Lymphatic spread of infection is seen in animals other than humans.

Irrespective of the route of infection, acute pyelonephritis produces an inflammatory response in the interstitium of the medulla and cortex consisting of increased polymorphonuclear cells, tubule necrosis, and abscesses on the cortex surface. Antibodies may protect against the occurrence of pyelonephritis by inhibiting the adherence of organisms to uroepithelial cells and by binding to specific structural and fimbrial antigens. The medulla is usually more damaged than the cortex, which is due, in part, to the decreased phagocytosis and leukocyte mobilization that occurs in the relative hypertonic medulla. Chronic pyelonephritis, if active, shows foci of inflammation with lymphocytes, plasma cells, and fibrosis. Tubules may be dilated and contain leukocyte and colloid casts with eosinophilic material. Remnants of tubules may resemble thyroid follicles, so-called thyroidization. Glomeruli are not usually affected until late in the disease course.

The clinical manifestations of acute pyelonephritis are variable. In a review of 185 hospitalized patients, with an initial diagnosis of acute pyelonephritis, only about half had explicit clinical and laboratory criteria for making this diagnosis. Clinical manifestations may consist of classic upper urinary tract symptoms (flank pain and fever $\geq 101°F$ [$38.3°C$]) and/or lower tract symptoms (dysuria, frequency, urgency, and suprapubic pain). Nausea, vomiting, diarrhea, or constipation may be seen with both. Shaking chills suggest bacteremia. In the elderly and in patients with indwelling urinary catheters, fever and pain may be minimal or absent. Physical examination often reveals tenderness in the flank or costovertebral angle but tenderness in the epigastric or upper abdominal areas is also seen. Chronic pyelonephritis may present with the symptoms of an acute event, with fever, malaise, and weight loss, or without symptoms.

A diagnostic evaluation of pyelonephritis requires an examination of a clean-voided, midstream urine specimen. The majority of patients show greater than 10 leukocytes (centrifuged) per high-power field, and usually grow a single pathogen in urine culture, unless complicating factors such as renal calculi or anatomic defects are present. White cell casts are suggestive of, but are neither sensitive nor specific for, pyelonephritis.

Bacteria may not be seen if the count is less than 30,000 per milliliter or if caused by tuberculosis (sterile pyuria). Culture from a midstream voided urine is considered positive if the colony count is 100,000 per milliliter or more or between 10,000 and 100,000 on two determinations. Blood culture is positive in up to 40 percent of patients and the number of positives increase with age, especially in elderly females. Positive blood cultures or non–*E. coli* infections suggest renal calculi or genitourinary tract abnormalities. Localization of urinary infection to the upper tracts may be helped by antibody-coated bacteria testing with a fluorescein-labeled anti–human globulin. However, this test is usually not practical because of a 15 percent false-negative rate where 10 to 14 days are required for an adequate antibody response. False-positive rates are also 15 percent due to prostatitis, stones, and neoplasms and tissue invasion and contamination by yeast and pseudomonads from the vagina which may fluoresce.

Gallium 67 may localize infection to the kidney but is expensive. It gives results that are comparable to the more invasive technique, ureteral catheterization. Acute pyelonephritis in a male or female is rare and therefore requires further evaluation for anatomic abnormalities and residual urine by an intravenous pyelogram (IVP) and voiding cystourethrogram. An IVP in chronic pyelonephritis may be normal in the early stages of the disease if no anatomic abnormality exists. Renal biopsy may also be normal owing to the focal nature at this stage. Later in the disease course an IVP reveals bilateral and often asymmetric atrophy, irregular borders, caliceal dilatation and blunting, and cortical scarring. Prognosis is generally good with fluctuations in renal function that relate to episodes of dehydration, infection, or obstruction. Hypertension is not usually present in the early stages of chronic pyelonephritis. Surgical correction of obstruction and antimicrobial treatment of infections may prevent disease progression and deterioration in renal function.

Acute pyelonephritis rarely progresses to chronic pyelonephritis, unless the patient is obstructed or immunocompromised (i.e., diabetes mellitus). Severe complications of acute pyelonephritis, more often seen in this group of predisposed patients, include renal abscess, perinephric abscess, and renal papillary necrosis. Renal abscess may result from pyelonephritis in two-thirds of cases and from hematogenous spread in the remaining one-third, that is, due to *Staphylococcus aureus*. A perinephric abscess usually results from the rupture of an intrarenal abscess and most patients have a concomitant renal calculus or diabetes mellitus. An abscess should be suspected in patients with acute pyelonephritis who do not respond to antibiotic therapy. An intrarenal abscess requires an IVP, ultrasound, or computed tomography (CT) for diagnosis, and a perinephric abscess the last two. Treatment for the abscess is usually surgery as well as antimicrobial therapy. Renal papillary necrosis, like the renal abscess, is more common in diabetics as well as in patients with sickle cell anemia, obstruction, and phenacetin analgesic abuse. Clinical manifestations include the intensification of acute pyelonephritis that should be especially suspected in elderly diabetic patients with renal insufficiency.

1. Cunningham, F. G., Lucas, M. J., and Hankins, G. D. Pulmonary injury complicating antipartum pyelonephritis. *Am. J. Obstet. Gynecol.* 156:797, 1987.
   These women had an increased incidence of multisystem derangement, but no predictable risk factors at admission.
2. Fierer, J. Acute pyelonephritis. *Urol. Clin. North Am.* 14:251, 1987.
   Summary of microbial and host factors, as well as limitations in distinguishing upper and lower urinary tract infections.
3. Claes, H., Vereecken, R., Oyen, R., et al. Xanthogranulomatous pyelonephritis with emphasis on computerized tomography scan. Retrospective study of 20 cases and literature review. *Urology* 29:389, 1987.
   A rare but potentially fatal disease if not diagnosed. Diagnosis is suggested by resistant urinary tract infection, perinephric abscess, and a nonfunctioning kidney.
4. Jacobson, S. H. P-fimbriated *Escherichia coli* in adults with renal scarring and pyelonephritis. *Acta. Med. Scand. (Suppl.)* 713:1, 1986.
   In patients with renal scarring, a higher availability of P-fimbriae receptor on their uroepithelial cells correlated with renal failure.

5. Grover, S. A., Komaroff, A. L., Weisberg, M., et al. The characteristics and hospital course of patients admitted with presumed acute pyelonephritis. *J. Gen. Intern. Med.* 2:5, 1987.
   Presenting clinical features have limited specificity and a midstream urine culture is not highly sensitive.

6. Jacobson, S., Carstensen, A., Kallenius, G., et al. Fluoresence-activated cell analysis of P-fimbriae receptor accessibility on uroepithelial cells of patients with renal scarring. *Eur. J. Clin. Microbiol.* 5:649, 1986.
   P-fimbriae receptor determination may eventually help detect groups at risk for recurrent urinary tract infection.

7. Gilstrap, L. G., Hankins, G. D., Snyder, R. R., et al. Acute pyelonephritis in pregnancy. *Compr. Ther.* 12:38, 1986.
   Bacteriuria in pregnancy should be detected and eradicated to prevent pyelonephritis.

8. Roberts, J. A. Pyelonephritis, cortical abscess, and perinephric abscess. *Urol. Clin. North Am.* 13:637, 1986.
   Diabetes, immunosuppression, stone formation, and obstruction predispose a patient to renal abscess, perinephric abscess, and pyelonephrosis.

9. Weinstein, T., Zevin, D., Gafter, U., et al. Acute renal failure in a solitary kidney due to bacterial pyelonephritis. *J. Urol.* 136:1290, 1986.
   Patients with a single functioning kidney are at increased risk of renal dysfunction after an episode of pyelonephritis.

10. Roberts, J. A., Suarezn, G. M., Kaack, B., et al. Host-parasite relationships in acute pyelonephritis. *Am. J. Kidney Dis.* 8:139, 1986.
    P-fimbriated strains of E. coli and receptor availability are both necessary to the pathogenesis of pyelonephritis.

11. Hida, M., Tasaka, T., Kitamura, M., et al. Autopsy findings in chronic pyelonephritis patients under dialysis—collected from the Annuals of Pathologic Autopsy Cases in Japan. *Tokai. J. Exp. Clin. Med.* 10:551, 1985.
    The incidence of tuberculosis was high in patients with chronic pyelonephritis who were receiving dialysis.

12. Owen, J. P., Ramos, J. M., Keir, M. J., et al. Urographic findings in adults with chronic pyelonephritis. *Clin. Radiol.* 36:81, 1985.
    Severity of renal function is associated with renal scarring and proteinuria.

13. Andriole, V. T. The role of Tamm-Horsfall protein in the pathogenesis of reflux nephropathy in chronic pyelonephritis. *Yale J. Biol. Med.* 58:91, 1985.
    Tamm-Horsfall protein may elicit an autoimmune response that is pathogenic for chronic pyelonephritis in patients with vesicoureteral reflux.

14. Gleckman, R. A. Diagnosing a common kidney infection of the elderly inpatient. *Geriatrics* 40:87, 1985.
    Pathologic pyuria in the elderly may be missed because of infection that is not directly accessible to the collecting system, obstruction distal to the site of the infection, and the prior use of diuretics and antimicrobials.

15. OHanley, T., Low, D., Romero, I., et al. Gal-Gal binding and hemolysin phenotypes and genotypes associated with uropathogenic *Escherichia coli*. *N. Engl. J. Med.* 313:414, 1985.
    Potential for a vaccine against pyelonephritis is supported by the fact that nucleotide sequences in heterologous strains of bacteria share homology in the shared regions of the genome.

16. Kunin, C. M. Does kidney infection cause renal failure? *Annu. Rev. Med.* 36:165, 1985.
    Urinary tract infection rarely causes impairment in renal function in the absence of predisposing factors. These factors may go unheralded until an acute episode of pyelonephritis.

17. Herrmann, B., and Burman, L. G. Pathogenesis of *Escherichia coli* cystitis and pyelonephritis: Apparent lack of significance of the bacterial motility and chemotaxis towards human urine. *Infection* 13:4, 1985.
    Bacterial motility does not appear to be a virulent factor in urinary tract infection.

18. OHanley, P., Lark, D., Falkow, S., et al. Molecular basis of *Escherichia coli* coloni-

zation of the upper urinary tract in BALB/c mice. Gal-Gal pili immunization prevents *Escherichia coli* pyelonephritis in the BALB/c mouse model of human pyelonephritis. *J. Clin. Invest.* 75:347, 1985.
Animal model for the potential prevention of pyelonephritis by the use of an immunogen.

19. Gleckman, R., Bradley, P., Roth, R., et al. Therapy of symptomatic pyelonephritis in women. *J. Urol.* 133:176, 1985.
A 10-day course of therapy in uncomplicated pyelonephritis is as effective as a 21-day extended course.

20. Gleckman, R. A., Bradley, P. J., Roth, R. N., et al. Bacteremic urosepsis: A phenomenon unique to elderly women. *J. Urol.* 133:174, 1985.
In elderly women with nonobstructive pyelonephritis, bacteremia is more common than in young women.

21. Bankoff, M. S., Sarno, R. C., and Mitcheson, H. D. Computed tomography differentiation of pyelonephritis and renal infarction. *J. Comput. Assist. Tomogr.* 8:239, 1984.
Acute renal infarction can mimic acute pyelonephritis in clinical presentation and may be distinguished with computed tomography.

22. Faro, S., Pastorek, J. G., Plauche, W. C., et al. Short course parenteral antibiotic therapy for pyelonephritis in pregnancy. *South. Med. J.* 77:455, 1984.
Women who have pyelonephritis in pregnancy are at high risk for subsequent infection and may benefit from short-term parenteral antibiotic therapy followed by long-term oral suppressive therapy.

23. Thomas, V. L., and Forland, M. Antibody coated bacteria in urinary tract infections. *Kidney Int.* 21:1, 1982.
Although the predictive value of a positive or negative test result for antibody-coated bacteria is over 80%, discrepancy has resulted from lack of standardization.

24. Merritt, J. L., and Keys, T. F. Limitations of the antibody-coated bacteria test in patients with neurogenic bladders. *J.A.M.A.* 247:1723, 1982.
Catheterized paraplegics have high false-positive and false-negative results with antibody-coated testing.

25. Kessler, W. O., Gittes, R. F., Hurwitz, S. R., et al. Gallium-67 scans in the diagnosis of pyelonephritis. *West. J. Med.* 121:91, 1974.
The site of urinary tract infection may be helped in questionable clinical cases with gallium-67.

26. Mayrer, A. R., Miniter, P., and Andriole, V. T. Immunopathogenesis of chronic pyelonephritis. *Am. J. Med.* 75 (Suppl. 1B), 59, 1983.
Description of histologic changes in pyelonephritis resulting from renal injury and radiologic scanning.

144. RENAL ARTERY OCCLUSION
Jerry L. Spivak

Occlusion of the renal artery by embolus or thrombus is not often recognized clinically. The symptoms are nonspecific; if the opposite kidney is uninvolved, and if renal function is not markedly impaired, attention is usually directed to the more evident damage of associated cerebral or peripheral vascular thromboembolic events. Several large retrospective studies have indicated that the incidence of renal infarction in autopsy cases is 1.5 percent, of which only 0.1 percent were recognized before death. In approximately 50 percent of patients, the infarction was bilateral, but the whole kidney was involved in less than 5 percent. The left kidney was more commonly affected, and emboli were frequently found in other organs, such as the spleen and brain.

Renal artery embolization tends to occur in certain clinical settings. These include congestive heart failure, atrial fibrillation, rheumatic heart disease, arteriosclerotic peripheral vascular disease, endocarditis, intracardiac tumors, and prosthetic cardiac valves. Prosthetic cardiac valves are a frequent cause of clinically recognized renal embolization and the increased use of valvular prostheses suggests that renal artery embolization may become a more common clinical problem in the future. Rarely, in patients with multiple pulmonary emboli or intraventricular septal defects, paradoxical emboli may lodge in the kidney. In older patients, surgical manipulation of the aorta or aortography may result in renal artery occlusion with atheromatous emboli. Thrombotic occlusion of the aorta may also extend to involve the renal arteries.

As indicated in retrospective studies, most renal infarcts are silent, including total infarction of the kidney by arterial embolic occlusion. When symptoms are present, they usually consist of nausea, vomiting, and abdominal pain that is often diffuse but may be localized to the upper quadrants or even the chest. Temperature elevation, if present, is usually mild. Flank pain and gross hematuria are more likely to be seen with renal stones, trauma, infection, renal vein thrombosis, carcinoma, dissecting aneurysm, or polyarteritis nodosa. Leukocytosis is usual; proteinuria and microscopic hematuria may be seen in 30 to 50 percent of cases, but hemoglobinuria due to release of pigment from infarcted tissue is a more important clue. Elevation of blood pressure is not invariable, but the diagnosis of thromboembolic occlusion of the renal artery should always be considered when hypertension appears de novo or when there is acceleration of preexisting hypertension. Hypertension is also an indicator that renal blood flow persists in the affected kidney. In one such case, anuria was precipitated by antihypertensive therapy.

Serum enzyme determinations may be helpful in establishing the diagnosis. With renal infarction, the level of serum lactic dehydrogenase (LDH) rises three- to sevenfold within 3 days. Changes in the level of LDH are less marked or absent with renal ischemia. The increase in LDH may be followed by increases in serum aspartate aminotransferase (AST) and alkaline phosphatase levels. Changes in renal function may be present even if only one kidney is involved; when there is bilateral renal involvement or only one kidney is present, oliguria or anuria is the rule. Since intravenous pyelography can result in further deterioration of renal function, isotope scanning is the appropriate diagnostic procedure for evaluation of renal artery embolism. Retrograde pyelography should be used to exclude obstructive uropathy when anuria occurs. Arteriography, of course, provides precise definition of the process.

Therapy for embolic infarction of the kidneys usually is directed toward the underlying disease process responsible for the embolus. The cardinal features of renal embolic disease are recurrence and bilateral involvement. In many reported cases, major involvement of one kidney was followed within months by involvement of the other. Since embolic infarction is often silent, documentation of such an event in one kidney should lead to the careful evaluation of the function of the other kidney. Experimentally, occlusion of the renal artery for more than 3 hours results in tubular necrosis, but the glomeruli are spared. This is in part due to the presence of collateral circulation from the lumbar and iliac vessels to the capsule and peripheral areas of the kidney. A rim of viable cortical tissue is often seen in infarcted kidneys. Collateral vessels are not, however, sufficient to preserve the kidney unless occlusion of the renal artery is incomplete or gradual. It is, of course, important to remember that renal tissue can survive at blood pressures below that required for urine formation. Numerous clinical reports attest to the fact that anuria, even of prolonged duration, is not proof of irreversible tissue damage. In some of the cases, occlusion of the renal artery was not complete, even though arteriographic studies failed to demonstrate renal perfusion. Thrombolytic therapy or anticoagulation may be the treatment of choice in patients with embolic or thrombotic occlusion vessels, even when there is deterioration of renal function. In such cases, dialysis can be employed to support the patient until there is recovery from the thromboembolic episode. In view of the underlying diseases associated with renal artery thromboembolism, many patients are unsuitable candidates for surgery. Given the relative resistance of the kidney to ischemic damage and a demonstration that anticoagulation and supportive therapy are sufficient to achieve restoration of adequate renal function, a conservative approach to the management of renal artery occlusion seems appropriate. When renal artery occlusion, either complete or segmental, produces hypertension or when an infarcted area becomes the site of persistent infection, surgery is indicated. Surgery should also be considered in patients who fail to respond to conservative therapy. Prolonged ischemia or lack of kidney function is not a contraindication to surgery. Reversal of the hypertension and improvement in renal function is usually the rule in patients with angiographic evidence of distal and collateral circulation.

1. Schoenbaum, S., Goldbran, M. A., and Siegelman, S. S. Renal arterial embolization. *Angiology* 22:332, 1971.
   Be aware of renal artery embolism when making a diagnosis of pyelonephritis in a patient with rheumatic heart disease and atrial fibrillation.
2. Sakati, I. A., Devine, P. C., Devine, C. J., et al. Serum lactic dehydrogenase in acute renal infarction and ischemia. *N. Engl. J. Med.* 278:721, 1968.
   Marked elevation of serum LDH occurs 2–4 days following renal infarction.
3. Gault, M. H., and Steiner, G. Serum and urinary enzyme activity after renal infarction. *Can. Med. Asoc. J.* 93:1101, 1965.
   Elevations of AST and alkaline phosphatase follow the rise in LDH.
4. Thomas, T. V., Faulconer, H. J., and Lansing, A. M. Management of embolic occlusion of the renal arteries. *Surgery* 65:576, 1969.
   Recurrent renal embolization with recovery after 2 days of anuria.
5. Patel, H. D., and Harris, J. Isolated metachronous renal artery emboli. *Surgery* 79:37, 1976.
   A review of successfully treated cases.
6. Schramek, A., Hashmonai, C. C., and Better, O. S. Survival following late renal embolectomy in a patient with a single functioning kidney. *J. Urol.* 109:342, 1973.
   Flank pain and anuria were the presenting manifestations. (See also Urology 31:66, 1988.)
7. Smith, H. T., Shapiro, F. L., and Messner, R. P. Anuria secondary to renovascular disease. *J.A.M.A.* 204:176, 1968.
   Thrombotic occlusion of the aorta and renal artery with recovery after 4 days of anuria. (See also J.A.M.A. 187:540, 1964.)
8. Perkins, R. P., Jacobsen, D. S., Feder, F. P., et al. Return of renal function after late embolectomy. *N. Engl. J. Med.* 276:1194, 1967.
   Return of function after 39 days of anuria.
9. Duncan, D. A., and Dexter, R. N. Anuria secondary to bilateral renal artery embolism. *N. Engl. J. Med.* 266:971, 1962.
   Occurrence of spasm in uninvolved segments of renal vasculature.
10. Baird, R. J., Yendt, E. R., and Firor, W. B. Anuria due to acute occlusion of the artery to a solitary kidney. *N. Engl. J. Med.* 272:1012, 1965.
    Importance of collateral flow in saving a kidney after renal artery thrombosis.
11. Mundth, E. D., Shine, K., and Austen, W. G. Correction of malignant hypertension and return of renal function following late renal artery embolectomy. *Am. J. Med.* 46:985, 1969.
    Criteria for potential viability of an ischemic kidney.
12. Kassirer, J. Atheroembolic renal disease. *N. Engl. J. Med.* 280:812, 1969.
    A cause of renal failure in the elderly.
13. Hamilton, P. B., Phillips, R. A., and Heller, A. Duration of renal ischemia required to produce uremia. *Am. J. Physiol.* 152:517, 1948.
    Four hours of experimental renal ischemia causes tubular necrosis but spares the glomeruli.
14. Kaiser, T. F., and Ross, R. R. Total infarction of the kidneys from bilateral arterial emboli. *J. Urol.* 66:500, 1954.
    The natural history of the untreated disease.
15. Gill, J. J., and Dammin, G. J. Paradoxical embolism with renal failure caused by occlusion of the renal arteries. *Am. J. Med.* 25:780, 1958.
    An unusual source of renal embolization.
16. Dobrzinsky, S. J., Voegeli, E., Grant, H. A., et al. Spontaneous reestablishment of renal function after complete occlusion of a renal artery. *Arch. Intern. Med.* 128:266, 1971.
    Gradual occlusion of the renal artery, permitting the development of adequate collateral circulation. Stenosis can have the same effect.

17. Libertino, J. A., Zinman, L., Breslin, J., et al. Renal artery revascularization: Restoration of renal function. *J.A.M.A.* 244:1340, 1980.
    Hypertension and reduced renal function due to renal artery occlusion were corrected by surgery. (See also J. Urol. 124:184, 1980.)
18. Nicholas, G. G., and DeMuth, Jr., W. E. Treatment of renal artery embolism. *Arch. Surg.* 119:278, 1984.
    Surgery is reserved for patients not responding to streptokinase or angioplasty.
19. Lessman, R. K., Johnson, S. F., Coburn, J. W., et al. Renal artery embolism. *Ann. Intern. Med.* 89:477, 1978.
    A favorable response was obtained with anticoagulation and expectant dialysis. (See also Br. Med. J. 4:587, 1969.)
20. Pineo, G. F., Thorndyke, W. C., and Steed, B. L. Spontaneous renal artery thrombosis: Successful lysis with streptokinase. *J. Urol.* 138:1223, 1987.
    Successful use of localized thrombolytic therapy.
21. Cosby, R. L., Miller, P. D., and Schrier, R. W. Traumatic renal artery thrombosis. *Am. J. Med.* 81:890, 1986.
    Spontaneous recovery occurred. (See also J. Trauma 26:941, 1986.)
22. Ouriel, K., Andrus, C. H., Ricotta, J. J., et al. Acute renal artery occlusion: When is revascularization justified. *J. Vasc. Surg.* 5:348, 1987.
    The prognosis varies with the cause of the occlusion. Trauma or embolus carries a worse prognosis than thrombosis.

145. RENAL TUBULAR ACIDOSIS
Alan Watson

The kidneys have an integral role in the maintenance of acid-base homeostasis. Under normal circumstances, the proximal tubule reclaims 85 to 90 percent of bicarbonate that has been filtered by the glomeruli. The distal nephron is capable of reabsorbing any remaining bicarbonate, and, through its ability to form ammonium and titratable acid, determines the net acid excretion of the urine (net acid excretion = titratable acid + ammonium − urine bicarbonate). Renal tubular acidosis (RTA) refers to a group of disorders which impair the kidney's handling of bicarbonate and its ability to acidify the urine normally.

Three major types are recognized in clinical practice: (1) distal RTA [type I] is characterized by reduced net acid excretion and an absolute inability to acidify the urine, (2) proximal RTA [type II], where there is abnormal leakage of bicarbonate from the proximal tubule, and (3) hyperkalemic RTA [type IV], where, in contrast to types I and II, there is a tendency toward hyperkalemia in association with the metabolic acidosis. (A type III RTA has also been described and usually represents a combination of types I and II but is not included in most classifications of RTA.)

The characteristic feature of type I RTA (also known as classic RTA) is an inability to acidify the urine. Pathophysiologically, it is a heterogeneous entity characterized by a secretory defect, backleak gradient defect, and impairment of normal electrical augmentation of hydrogen ion secretion by the distal nephron. There is diminished titratable acid and ammonium excretion and a mild degree of bicarbonaturia, that is, net acid excretion is diminished. A hyperchloremic metabolic acidosis results which is not associated with a high anion gap. In addition, bicarbonaturia promotes kaliuresis resulting in hypokalemia which, on occasion, can be severe. Hypercalciuria is also a common feature of distal RTA and is a direct effect of metabolic acidosis per se. In the presence of an alkaline urine, a high urinary calcium concentration leads to precipitation of calcium phosphate salts resulting in nephrocalcinosis and nephrolithiasis. Osteomalacia is an additional feature of abnormal calcium metabolism seen in children with type I RTA.

The traditional test used to assess urinary acidification is the ammonium chloride loading test. Ammonium chloride [0.1 gm/kg] is given after an overnight fast. Serial urine pH measurements and serum HCO_3 are made. Under normal circumstances, the urine pH will fall to less than 5.5 during the ensuing 4 to 6 hours as a metabolic acidosis develops. If the urine pH fails to fall to less than 5.5, this suggests an abnormal acidification mechanism. Two practical factors should be remembered with regard to this test: (1) a pH meter should always be used, and (2) the presence of a urinary tract infection with a urea-splitting organisms renders the urine pH an unreliable index of acid excretion. Measurement of the ammonium excretion rate and the urine PCO_2 after bicarbonate administration are also helpful tests.

The causes of type I RTA may be broadly classified as primary or secondary; there are genetic forms in both categories. The vast majority of cases are secondary to a variety of autoimmune or tubulointerstitial diseases: common examples include nephrocalcinosis, renal transplant rejection, Sjögren's syndrome, and systemic lupus erythematosus. Type I RTA can also occur as a result of lithium or amphotericin B toxicity or intoxication by toluene or glue. The treatment of type I renal tubular acidosis is the administration of alkali in amounts sufficient to buffer the amount of endogenous acid normally generated [1–3 mEq/kg/day]; children may require higher doses. Whereas one of the classic features of type I RTA is the presence of metabolic acidosis, there are patients who do not manifest a low bicarbonate and yet on testing will demonstrate an inability to acidify the urine: this variant of type I RTA is termed *incomplete distal renal tubular acidosis.*

In type II RTA [proximal RTA], the capacity of the proximal tubule to reclaim bicarbonate is diminished, allowing a large quantity of bicarbonate to reach the distal tubule. Unfortunately, the capacity of the distal nephron to handle bicarbonate is limited, and as a result significant amounts of bicarbonate may be lost in the urine [usually >15% of the filtered load of bicarbonate when serum bicarbonate is in the normal range]. Net loss of bicarbonate leads to a hyperchloremic metabolic acidosis [chloride reabsorption is stimulated by concomitant extracellular volume contraction], with a normal anion gap.

With progressive acidosis, plasma bicarbonate falls and filtered bicarbonate is reduced below the reabsorption threshold of the proximal tubule. Thus the amount leaking out of the proximal tubule diminishes, and at this stage the distal nephron may be able to maximally acidify the urine. Therefore the diagnosis of type II RTA is best established by measuring the fractional excretion of bicarbonate [when serum bicarbonate is in the normal range]. Tests of distal acidification, for example, with ammonium chloride, are not as helpful since this mechanism remains intact.

There are many conditions which can lead to proximal RTA. It may occur as a primary disorder or secondary to a variety of clinical conditions. Examples of such predisposing conditions include amyloidosis, multiple myeloma, renal transplantation, and Wilson's disease. Carbonic anhydrase inhibitors, for example, acetazolamide, can produce a chemical form of proximal RTA. On occasion other proximal tubular defects may coexist, for example, aminoaciduria, phosphaturia, and glycosuria. This is known as Fanconi's syndrome, and because of continued loss of these substances, may become clinically manifest as osteomalacia or malnutrition. As an isolated defect, type II RTA is associated with variable degrees of hypokalemia due to urinary losses of potassium. Nephrolithiasis and bone disease are not observed generally, however. Treatment is with bicarbonate or an equivalent base [citrate mixtures], in a dose calculated to compensate for the degree of bicarbonaturia. As a result, a patient may have to ingest between 20 and 30 mEq/kg/day of alkali. Thiazides have proved useful in diminishing bicarbonate requirements by stimulating extracellular volume contraction and promoting proximal tubular bicarbonate reabsorption. Potassium replacement may also be required, particularly if thiazide diuretics are being used.

Type IV RTA is characterized by decreased net acid excretion but may be differentiated from types I and II RTA by the presence of hyperkalemia and a decreased urinary potassium excretion. The basic defect lies in a disturbance of the renin-angiotensin aldosterone mechanism resulting in underproduction of the mineralocorticoid or in tubular unresponsiveness to the steroid hormone. Since aldosterone is a physiologic stimulator of potassium and hydrogen secretion by the distal nephron, the ability to acidify the urine and excrete potassium is retarded in its absence. An additional important mechanism whereby hyperchloremic acidosis develops in this setting is through suppression of ammonium production by hyperkalemia. Specialized tests indicate a retained ability to acidify the urine in most patients, although net acid excretion is subnormal. There are three pathophysiologic types of type IV RTA: (1) primary aldosterone deficiency (e.g., Addison's disease), (2) hyporeninemic hypoaldosteronism (e.g., diabetes mellitus), (3) decreased renal responsiveness to aldosterone (e.g., interstitial renal disease or pseudohypoaldosteronism). By measuring plasma renin activity, urinary aldosterone, and urinary salt excretion, these subtypes can usually be distinguished. Treatment consists of mineralocorticoid [fludrocortisone]: supraphysiologic doses may often be greater than 0.1 mg/day. Occasionally, a loop diuretic is used to enhance potassium excretion which will improve ammoniagenesis and ameliorate the degree of acidosis.

In summary, the diagnosis of RTA should be suspected in the setting of a hyperchloremic metabolic acidosis [normal anion gap] where the urine is inappropriately alkaline. Concomitant hyperkalemia suggests type IV RTA. Hypokalemia favors a diagnosis of types I and II RTA, which may be further differentiated by testing the kidney's ability to acidify the urine and by determining the fractional excretory rate of bicarbonate. Subsequent investigation should be directed at identification of the etiology of the tubular disorder and in particular to determine whether it is primary or secondary to some other disease process.

1. Sebastian, A., Schambelan, M., Lindenfelt, S., et al. Amelioration of metabolic acidosis with fludrocortisone therapy in hyporeninemic hypoaldosteronism. *N. Engl. J. Med.* 297:576, 1977.
   The rationale for the use of mineralocorticoid therapy in type IV RTA.
2. Gennari, F. J., and Cohen, J. J. Renal tubular acidosis. *Ann. Rev. Med.* 29:521, 1978.
   A concise review of proximal and distal forms of RTA.
3. Aruda, J. A. L., and Kurtzman, N. A. Mechanisms and classifications of deranged distal urinary acidification. *Am. J. Physiol.* 239:F515, 1980.
   This is a detailed review of distal tubular function and RTA and provides a classification of distal acidification defects.
4. Phelps, K. R., Liberman, R. L., Oh, M. S., et al. Pathophysiology of the syndrome of hyporeninemic hypoaldosteronism. *Metabolism* 29:186, 1980.
   A good discussion of the underlying pathophysiology of type IV RTA.
5. McSherry, E. Renal tubular acidosis in childhood. *Kidney Int.* 20:799, 1981.
   A nephrology forum discussing RTA in childhood with emphasis on proximal forms of the disease.
6. Morris, R. C. Renal tubular acidosis. *N. Engl. J. Med.* 304:418, 1981.
   A thorough review of RTA with the pathophysiology and treatment of RTA.
7. Steinbaugh, B. J., Schloeder, F. X., Goldstein, N. B., et al. The pathogenesis of distal renal tubular acidosis. *Kidney Int.* 19:1, 1981.
   A comprehensive discussion of the pathogenesis of distal acidification defects.
8. Battle, D. Delta urine pCO_2 rather than U-B pCO_2 as an index of distal acidification. *Semin. Nephrol.* 2:189, 1982.
   A thorough discussion of the use of specialized tests such as urine PCO_2 in the assessment of the kidney's acidification ability.
9. Brenner, R. J., Spring, D. B., Sebastian, A., et al. Incidence of radiographically evident bone disease, nephrocalcinosis and nephrolithiasis in various types of renal tubular acidosis. *N. Engl. J. Med.* 307:217, 1982.
   A discussion of the bone disease and altered calcium metabolism in the different types of RTA.
10. Donckerwolcke, R. A. Diagnosis and treatment of renal tubular disorders in childhood. *Pediatr. Clin. North Am.* 29:895, 1982.
    Classification and discussion of the types of RTA seen in children.
11. Sebastian, A., Hulter, H., Kurtz, I., et al. Disorders of distal nephron function. *Am. J. Med.* 72:289, 1982.

A review of abnormalities of distal nephron function which includes a good discussion of distal nephron defects.

12. Battle, D. Renal tubular acidosis. *Med. Clin. North Am.* 67:859, 1983.
    A thorough review of RTA.
13. Koeppen, B. M., and Steinmetz, P. R. Basic mechanisms of urine acidification. *Med. Clin. North Am.* 67:753, 1983.
    A good discussion of the kidney's acidification mechanisms.
14. Kurtzman, M. A. Acquired distal renal tubular acidosis. *Kidney Int.* 24:807, 1983.
    This article reviews experimental defects in urinary acidification as they correlate with the clinical forms of distal tubular acidosis.
15. Cannon, R. J. Discussion. In R. J. Glassock and E. I. Feinstein: Metabolic acidosis in a young woman. *Am. J. Nephrol.* 4:59, 1984.
    A clinical example of acquired RTA.
16. Chan, J. C. N., and Alon, U. Tubular disorders of acid-base and phosphate metabolism. *Nephron* 40:257, 1985.
    A good discussion on a variety of tubular disorders including proximal and distal RTA.
17. Halperin, M. L., Goldstein, M. B., Richardson, R. M. A., et al. Distal renal tubular acidosis: A pathophysiological approach. *Am. J. Nephrol.* 5:1, 1985.
    A clinical approach to distal RTA.

IX. DISEASES OF THE LUNG

146. ASPIRATION PNEUMONIA
Jerry L. Spivak

Aspiration of liquid or particulate matter into the bronchial tree is a potential hazard in many clinical situations, and can result in serious complications or death. Since therapy for pulmonary aspiration is limited, prevention and/or early recognition are of paramount importance, and it is important to be aware of those situations in which aspiration is likely to occur. They include drug or alcohol intoxication, anesthesia, the postictal state, coma from any cause, neuromuscular disorders affecting the swallowing mechanism, gastric or esophageal obstruction, esophageal diverticula, drowning, and violent activity, such as a convulsion or cardiac resuscitation. The syndrome may be an occult event (as with the inhalation of oily nose drops, the nocturnal regurgitation of esophageal achalasia, or following overly vigorous abdominal palpation in the comatose or anesthetized patient) or a dramatic event, with the sudden onset of cyanosis and respiratory distress.

Unless the aspiration is witnessed, the diagnosis may be difficult to establish. In the acute situation, radiologic findings are indistinguishable from those of pulmonary edema or bronchopneumonia; chronic aspiration pneumonitis can masquerade as "refractory" pneumonia with negative sputum cultures. The segmental nature of the process and location in a dependent area of the lung, usually the right lower lobe, are important clues in distinguishing aspiration from a primary bacterial pneumonitis. In chronic cases, pulmonary fibrosis, bronchiectasis, or a pulmonary nodule can be found. The type of pulmonary lesion is dependent on the quality and quantity of material aspirated. Aspiration of small amounts of oral contents may result in a putrid lung abscess, whereas a larger volume causes widespread bronchial obstruction, atelectasis, and respiratory distress. The destructive effect of gastric contents is proportional to their volume and pH. Tube feeding with a pH above 5 causes embarrassment by respiratory obstruction, whereas fluid with a pH less than 2.5 causes necrosis of pulmonary tissue. When the lung is burned by acid, there is a rapid exudation of serum into the alveoli, with neutralization of the pH within 15 minutes. Hypovolemia and hypotension ensue, and pulmonary compliance decreases. Hydrocarbon aspiration also causes a necrotizing pneumonitis.

The initial therapy for pulmonary aspiration involves establishment of an airway, oxygenation, and support of the blood volume. Bronchoscopy is indicated for the removal of particulate matter and relief of atelectasis. Bronchial lavage has no value since aspirated fluid is rapidly transported to the alveoli and neutralized, and pulmonary damage by acid or kerosene is instantaneous. In addition, bronchial lavage may result in further reduction in pulmonary compliance. Steroids have no role in treatment of aspiration pneumonia. Administration of steroids to patients with aspiration pneumonia increases the incidence of infection and bleeding and does not lessen mortality. Patients with acute respiratory insufficiency are susceptible to the development of hemorrhagic gastritis and steroids might accelerate this process. In addition, they obscure the signs of infection as well as impair host responses to bacterial invasion.

Administration of antibiotics prophylactically for pulmonary aspiration is also not advisable. Prophylactic administration of antibiotics does not improve survival in patients with aspiration pneumonia. Initial pulmonary injury following aspiration is not due to bacteria, and antibiotics should be withheld until definite evidence of bacterial infection is obtained. Blind antibiotic treatment may only select out resistant nosocomial organisms. If hypoxia is observed, continuous positive pressure ventilation (CPPV) may be beneficial, and there are experimental data suggesting that CPPV may reduce the degree of tissue injury occurring with acid aspiration. The use of CPPV, of course, requires scrupulous attention to the maintenance of the blood volume. The usefulness of osmotically active agents such as albumin to counteract extravasation of fluid into the pulmonary alveoli has not been established clinically. Recently, administration of antacids or cimetidine preoperatively has been advocated for the prophylaxis of aspiration associated with general anesthesia. Antacids, because they add volume and particulate matter to the gastric fluid, are not recommended for prophylaxis. The use of an

H2 receptor antagonist such as cimetidine appears more logical since gastric pH can be increased and there may also be a decrease in gastric volume.

The best therapy is prevention. Comatose patients should be positioned on their side, with the head slightly dependent. Nasogastric tubes should not be passed in the comatose patient without prior tracheal intubation. Hyperinflation of a tracheal tube cuff may result in esophageal obstruction or a tracheoesophageal fistula. Tube feeding should be given in small amounts and only when there is evidence of adequate gastric emptying. Even gastrotomy feeding has been associated with aspiration. The physician must also be aware that any narcotic antagonist, even naloxone, can precipitate vomiting and that control of the airway is the first step in managing a narcotic overdose. The patient with diabetic ketoacidosis should be evaluated for gastric atony and the patient receiving inhalation therapy checked for gastric distention. Patients with neuromuscular disorders are also at risk. Ileus demands the use of gastric suction. With proper precautions a catastrophic event can be avoided.

1. Gardner, A. M. N. Aspiration of food and vomit. *Q. J. Med.* 27:227, 1958.
   A humorous, historical, and experimental study.
2. Ribaudo, C. A., and Grace, W. J. Pulmonary aspiration. *Am. J. Med.* 50:413, 1971.
   A comprehensive review of aspiration of liquids, solids, and gases.
3. Huxley, E. J., Viroslav, J., Gray, W. R., et al. Pharyngeal aspiration in normal adults and patients with depressed consciousness. *Am. J. Med.* 64:564, 1978.
   Aspiration occurs in normal individuals during sleep.
4. Atkinson, W. J. Posture of the unconscious patient. *Lancet* 1:404, 1970.
   Keep the head slightly dependent to prevent aspiration.
5. Bernard, G. R., Luce, J. M., Sprung, C. L., et al. High-dose corticosteroids in patients with the adult respiratory distress syndrome [ARDS]. *N. Engl. J. Med.* 317:1565, 1987.
   Corticosteroids were not beneficial in ARDS whether due to aspiration or other causes.
6. Wolfe, J. E., Bone, R. C., and Ruth, W. E. Effects of corticosteroids in the treatment of patients with gastric aspiration. *Am. J. Med.* 63:719, 1977.
   Infection and bleeding were more frequent with steroid therapy; the mortality was not affected.
7. Kumar, A., Falke, K. J., Geffin, B., et al. CPPV in acute respiratory failure. *N. Engl. J. Med.* 283:1430, 1970.
   Effect of CPPV on cardiopulmonary mechanics.
8. Cameron, J. L., Mitchell, W. H., and Zuidema, G. D. Aspiration pneumonia. *Arch. Surg.* 106:49, 1973.
   Mortality is proportional to the number of lobes involved.
9. Cameron, J. L., Reynolds, J., and Zuidema, G. D. Aspiration in patients with tracheostomies. *Surg. Gynecol. Obstet.* 136:68, 1973.
   High incidence of aspiration with cuffed tracheostomy tubes, but no aspiration was found with oral endotracheal tubes.
10. Eller, W. C., and Haughen, R. K. Food asphyxiation: Restaurant rescue. *N. Engl. J. Med.* 289:81, 1973.
    A reversible catastrophe that is usually mismanaged.
11. Bartlett, J. G., Gorbach, S. L., and Finegold, S. M. The bacteriology of aspiration pneumonia. *Am. J. Med.* 56:202, 1974.
    Anaerobic organisms predominate.
12. McCormick, P. W. Immediate care after aspiration of vomit. *Anaesthesia* 30:658, 1975.
    Good advice.
13. Lorber, B., and Swenson, R. M. Bacteriology of aspiration pneumonia. *Ann. Intern. Med.* 81:329, 1974.
    The bacteriology of community- and hospital-acquired pneumonia was found to differ.
14. Bartlett, J. G., and Gorbach, S. L. The triple threat of aspiration pneumonia. *Chest* 68:560, 1975.
    Antibiotics should be withheld until there is evidence of infection.

15. Bartlett, J. G., and Gorbach, S. L. Treatment of aspiration pneumonia and primary lung abscess. *J.A.M.A.* 234:935, 1975.
    Penicillin G alone is effective in treating aspiration pneumonia, but with a hospital-acquired infection the possible presence of gram-negative organisms or a resistant staphylococcus must be considered.

16. Wynne, J. W., and Modell, J. H. Respiratory aspiration of stomach contents. *Ann. Intern. Med.* 87:466, 1977.
    A critical review of the problem. Little justification was found for the use of corticosteroids, bronchial lavage, or prophylactic antibiotics.

17. Schwartz, D. J., Wynne, J. W., Gibbs, C. P., et al. The pulmonary consequences of aspiration of gastric contents at pH values greater than 2.5. *Am. Rev. Respir. Dis.* 121:119, 1980.
    pH alone is not the only determinant of pulmonary injury. (See also Arch Surg. *116:46, 1981.)*

18. Wynne, J. W., DeMarco, F. J., and Hood, I. Physiological effects of corticosteroids in foodstuff aspiration. *Arch. Surg.* 116:46, 1981.
    Steroids were not found to be beneficial.

19. Stewardson, R. H., and Nyhus, L. M. Pulmonary aspiration. *Arch. Surg.* 112:1192, 1977.
    Neither steroids, antibiotics, nor lavage is advocated; positive pressure ventilation is beneficial if hypoxia is present.

20. Bynum, L. J., and Pierce, A. K. Pulmonary aspiration of gastric contents. *Am. Rev. Respir. Dis.* 114:1129, 1976.
    The routine use of antibiotics does not prevent the subsequent development of infection.

21. Murray, H. W. Antimicrobial therapy in pulmonary aspiration. *Am. J. Med.* 66:188, 1979.
    Prophylactic antibiotics are not recommended.

22. Hughes, R. L., Freilich, R. A., Bytell, D. E., et al. Aspiration and occult esophageal disorders. *Chest* 80:489, 1981.
    Role of esophageal disturbances in pulmonary aspiration.

23. Wolkove, N., Kreisman, H., Cohen, C., et al. Occult foreign-body aspiration in adults. *J.A.M.A.* 248:1350, 1982.
    An interesting reminder.

24. Schmidt-Nowara, W. W., Samet, J. M., and Rosario, P. A. Early and late pulmonary complications of botulism. *Arch. Intern. Med.* 143:451, 1983.
    Pulmonary aspiration is one complication.

25. Coombs, D. W. Aspiration pneumonia prophylaxis. *Anesth. Analg.* 62:1055, 1983.
    Review of the role of cimetidine for prophylaxis (see also Lancet *1:465, 1980).*

26. Whittington, R. M., Robinson, J. S., and Thompson, J. M. Fatal aspiration (Mendelson's) syndrome despite antacids and cricoid pressure. *Lancet* 2:228, 1979.
    Antacids are not a substitute for emptying the stomach.

27. Landay, M. J., Christensen, E. E., and Bynum, L. J. Pulmonary manifestations of acute aspiration of gastric contents. *AJR* 131:587, 1978.
    No pattern is characteristic or prognostic; progressive changes after several days suggest the development of infection, embolism, or ARDS.

147. EMPYEMA

Jerry L. Spivak

Infection in the pleural space can result from extension of an underlying pulmonary infection; drainage from an infected paravertebral lymph node; sepsis; esophageal perforation; extension of a subdiaphragmatic or submaxillary space abscess; or contamination following spontaneous pneumothorax, surgery, thoracentesis, or penetration by a foreign body. Pulmonary infections associated with empyema include bacterial pneumonia, particularly when due to streptococci; staphylococci; *Escherichia coli; Bacteroides;* bronchiectasis; septic infarction; and putrid lung abscess. Actinomycosis is an unusual cause of empyema that should be considered if there is a history of aspiration or if cutaneous abscesses appear. In patients without underlying disease, staphylococcus is the most common infecting organism, whereas in those with underlying illnesses or prior therapy with antibiotics, gram-negative organisms equal or exceed staphylococci in occurrence. Infection with multiple organisms is not uncommon after surgery or when there is a bronchopleural fistula, extension of a subdiaphragmatic infection, or penetration by a foreign body. Empyema in patients receiving steroids has generally been caused by staphylococci or other gram-positive organisms. In patients with lymphoreticular neoplasms, an unusual organism such as salmonella or *Listeria* may be the infecting agent.

The characteristics of the pleural fluid depend on when the thoracentesis is performed, the underlying illness, and whether or not antibiotic therapy has been initiated. Initially, the pleural fluid is an exudate that is usually easy to aspirate. Within a week the pus becomes more viscous and a fibrin layer develops over the pleural surfaces, resulting in loculation of fluid and restriction of the lung. Eventually with fibroblastic activity there is organization of the fibrin membrane into a thick restraining peel. If left unattended, the pus often tracks to the surface or ruptures into a bronchus (empyema necessitatis). The association of pericarditis with pneumococcal empyema suggests that contiguous spread to the pericardium also occurs.

There is usually nothing on physical examination to distinguish an empyema from an uninfected pleural effusion. In patients with rheumatoid arthritis, evaluation is further complicated by the occurrence of a low pleural fluid glucose, a pH less than 7.20, and a high protein content in the absence of infection. Steroids can mask the presence of an empyema, and in some debilitated patients neither fever nor leukocytosis is present. This emphasizes the importance of examining and culturing (both aerobically and anaerobically) every pleural effusion. With prior antibiotic therapy, organisms may not be cultured but the pleural fluid cell count may still be increased.

The treatment of empyema includes both antibiotics and drainage. There has been no controlled study to support the efficacy of high-dose antibiotics, but the poor diffusion of drugs into the pleural space supports this approach. If the fluid is easily aspirated, drainage by thoracentesis is often adequate. However, in the presence of a large accumulation of fluid, a pleural fluid pH less than 7.30, and rapid reaccumulation of the fluid, loculation, or thick pus, closed drainage by a chest tube is necessary since repeated attempts at thoracentesis only result in loculation and allow further organization to occur. With closed drainage, if fever has not resolved within 4 to 6 days or if the lung has not reexpanded, open drainage or decortication will be necessary. The use of enzymes to debride the fibrin exudate has been suggested by several authors, but there is no proof that enzymes aid in resolution of empyema and they are not without side effects. Even today, empyema still carries a high mortality. Adequate drainage is the cornerstone of effective therapy in empyema, and enzymatic debridement should not be used as a substitute.

1. Sahn, S. A. The pleura. *Am. Rev. Respir. Dis.* 138:184, 1988.
   If you have time to read only one reference, this is it.
2. Lemmer, J. H., Botham, M. J., and Orringer, M. B. Modern management of adult thoracic empyema. *J. Thorac. Cardiovasc. Surg.* 90:849, 1985.
   Aggressive management including rib resection advocated particularly for postoperative empyemas and in immunocompromised patients. (See also Chest *93:901, 1988.)*
3. Grant, D. R., and Finley, R. J. Empyema: Analysis of treatment techniques. *Can. J. Surg.* 28:449, 1985.
   Empyema still causes a high mortality. (See also Scand. J. Thorac. Cardiovasc. Surg. *18:85, 1984.)*
4. Andrews, N. C., Parker, E. F., and Shaw, R. R., et al. Management of non-tuberculous empyema. *Am. Rev. Respir. Dis.* 85:935, 1967.
   An excellent summary of the natural history of empyema.

5. Vianna, N. J. Nontuberculous bacterial empyema in patients with and without underlying diseases. *J.A.M.A.* 215:69, 1971.
   Frequent occurrence of gram-negative empyema in debilitated patients.
6. Snider, G. L., and Saleh, S. S. Empyema of the thorax in adults: Review of 105 cases. *Dis. Chest* 54:410, 1968.
   Concise presentation of pathophysiology and management of empyema.
7. Jones, F. C., and Blodgett, R. C. Empyema in rheumatoid pleuropulmonary disease. *Ann. Intern. Med.* 74:665, 1971.
   Increased incidence of empyema in rheumatoid arthritis.
8. Sahn, S. A., Lakshminarayan, S., and Char, D. C. Silent empyema in patients receiving corticosteroids. *Am. Rev. Respir. Dis.* 107:873, 1973.
   Emphasizes the importance of tapping every pleural effusion.
9. Marks, M. I., and Eickhoff, T. C. Empyema necessitatis. *Am. Rev. Respir. Dis.* 101:759, 1970.
   If left untreated, empyema often drains externally.
10. Harvey, J. C., Cantrell, J. R., and Fisher, A. M. Actinomycosis: Its recognition and treatment. *Ann. Intern. Med.* 46:868, 1957.
    An unusual cause of empyema.
11. Boyer, A. S., Nelson, S. C., Galpin, J. E., et al. Necrotizing pneumonia and empyema due to *Clostridium perfringes. Am. J. Med.* 59:851, 1975.
    This organism can be seeded into the pleural cavity by thoracentesis.
12. Bartlett, J. G., and Finegold, S. M. Anaerobic infections of the lung and pleural space. *Am. Rev. Respir. Dis.* 110:56, 1974.
    A comprehensive review.
13. Sahn, S. A., Reller, L. B., Taryle, D. A., et al. The contribution of leukocytes and bacteria to the low pH of empyema fluid. *Am. Rev. Respir. Dis.* 128:811, 1983.
    Both contribute to the low pH. (The pleural membrane may also; see J. Lab. Clin. Med. 93:1041, 1979.)
14. Light, R. W., Girard, W. M., Jenkinson, S. G., et al. Parapneumonic effusions. *Am. J. Med.* 69:507, 1980.
    If the pleural fluid pH is greater than 7.2, loculation and the need for drainage are unlikely. (See also Chest 79:714, 1981.)
15. Schacter, E. N., Kreisman, H., and Putman, C. Diagnostic problems in suppurative lung disease. *Arch. Intern. Med.* 136:167, 1976.
    Differentiation between abscess and empyema. (See also AJR 141:163, 1983. Computed tomography (CT) is useful here.)
16. Baber, C. E., Hedlund, L. W., Oddson, T. A., et al. Differentiating empyema and peripheral pulmonary abscesses. *Radiology* 135:755, 1980.
    Use of CT scanning to distinguish between abscess and empyema.
17. Silverman, S. G., Mueller, P. R., Saini, S., et al. Thoracic empyema: Management with image-guided catheter drainage. *Radiology* 169:5, 1988.
    The adequacy of drainage, not the method, is the most important principle.
18. Mavroridis, C., Symmonds, J. B., Minagi, H., et al. Improved survival in management of empyema thoracis. *J. Thorac. Cardiovasc. Surg.* 82:49, 1981.
    The type of organism did not correlate with the severity of the empyema or the need for surgical drainage.
19. Sullivan, K. M., O'Toole, R. D., Fisher, R. H., et al. Anaerobic empyema thoracis. *Arch. Intern. Med.* 131:521, 1973.
    Loculation is characteristic and thoracentesis may be misleading.
20. Fishman, N. H., and Ellertson, D. G. Early pleural decortication for thoracic empyema in immunosuppressed patients. *J. Thorac. Cardiovasc. Surg.* 74:537, 1977.
    Early decortication recommended in immunosuppressed patients.
21. Reeder, G. S., and Gracey, D. R. Aspiration of intrathoracic abscess. *J.A.M.A.* 240:1156, 1978.
    Drainage of an empyema into the bronchial tree can cause acute respiratory failure.
22. Petty, B. G., and Smith, C. R. The syndrome of inappropriate secretion of antidiuretic hormone associated with anaerobic empyema. *Am. Rev. Respir. Dis.* 115:685, 1977.

(See also Chest *72:796, 1977.) Another example of antidiuretic hormone secretion associated with a pulmonary disorder.*

23. MacMillan, J. C., Milstein, S. H., and Samson, P. C. Clinical spectrum of septic pulmonary embolism and infarction. *J. Thorac. Cardiovasc. Surg.* 75:670, 1978.
    The incidence of empyema was 30%.

24. Varkey, B., Rose, H. D., Kutty, C. P. K., et al. Empyema thoracis during a ten-year period. *Arch. Intern. Med.* 141:1771, 1981.
    Anaerobic organisms were responsible in 39% of cases.

25. Valero, V., Senior, J., and Watanakunakorn, C. Liver abscess complicating Crohn's disease presenting as thoracic empyema. *Am. J. Med.* 79:659, 1985.
    An interesting clinical presentation.

26. Neild, J. E., Eykyn, S. J., and Phillips, I. Lung abscess and empyema. *Q. J. Med.* 57:875, 1985.
    Penicillin-resistant organisms were common.

148. INTERSTITIAL LUNG DISEASE
Charles B. Payne, Jr.

There are many causes of diseases of the interstitium of the lung. The etiology is known for only 30 percent of the entire spectrum of diseases. Numerous illnesses of variable prognosis are included in this category. The pneumoconioses, such as silicosis, coal worker's pneumoconiosis, and asbestosis, are members of this group. The lung manifestations of sarcoidosis are also a form of interstitial lung disease but will be discussed separately. Lymphangitic spread of neoplasms to the lung involves the interstitium but is also excluded from this discussion. Hypersensitivity pneumonitis, familial interstitial lung disease, interstitial disease associated with collagen-vascular disease, postinfectious interstitial disease, and interstitial lung disease of unknown etiology will be briefly discussed.

Terminology varies. The British use "cryptogenic fibrosing alveolitis" to describe the most common type of idiopathic interstitial lung disease. Nomenclature derived from descriptive pathology would call this "usual interstitial pneumonitis" (UIP), or use "desquamative interstitial pneumonitis" (DIP) and "lymphocytic interstitial pneumonitis" (LIP) depending on the major cell type seen on microscopic examination of biopsy specimens. We will call the most common type of idiopathic interstitial lung disease *diffuse interstitial lung disease (DILD)*. The term *Hamman-Rich syndrome* should be reserved for the type of rapidly progressive, fatal cases of DILD described by Hamman and Rich.

The pathogenetic mechanism involves an inflammatory reaction which is generally referred to as an "alveolitis," although the vasculature, lymphatics, small airways, and connective tissue of the lung parenchyma are involved. In various types of interstitial disease the initial insult to the lung may be infectious, genetically mediated, allergic, or secondary to the effects of an inhalant. The lung may be involved in a general immune response such as in sarcoidosis or in collagen-vascular disease. In DILD, the initial insult is unknown. The inflammatory reaction involves the alveolar spaces with destruction or dedifferentiation of the alveolar type I lining cells. Desquamation of these cells, together with debris, may fill alveolar spaces.

An inflammatory infiltrate, primarily of polymorphonuclear leukocytes in DILD, involves the pulmonary capillary endothelium, the ground substance, and connective tissue of the interstitium and small airways. Mediators of inflammation such as lymphokines, leukocyte chemotactic factors, macrophage inhibitory factor, and others are produced. The inflammatory process and repair occur simultaneously at varying stages throughout the lung. This inflammatory and repair process may resolve or continue to be active. The active cellular components vary with the disease process so that bronchial lavage studies show sarcoidosis to produce a fluid rich in lymphocytes, while in DILD polymorphonuclear leukocytes predominate.

During attempts at repair, abnormal fibrosis and collagen deposition occur in the parenchyma leading to altered lung mechanics and gas transport. The lung becomes "stiffer" (decreased compliance), increasing the work of breathing and stimulating nerve receptors in the lung which are responsible for the sensation of dyspnea. Airflow obstruction is usually not seen. Distortion of the lung architecture reduces the surface area available for gas exchange so that the diffusing capacity (DLCO) is reduced. Ventilation-perfusion mismatching is responsible for the majority of hypoxemia seen although a true diffusion abnormality is difficult to exclude. During the inexorable course of fibrosis, significant true shunting may occur in the lung.

Common presentations in most interstitial lung diseases involve complaints of exertional dyspnea, nonproductive and chronic cough, with clubbing of the digits which occurs in up to 60 percent of published series. Weight loss may occur. In interstitial disease accompanying systemic illnesses, the complaints may be those of the systemic illness, such as rheumatoid arthritis, lupus erythematosus, or polyarteritis nodosa.

Physical examination shows tachypnea. Central cyanosis may be present. In addition to digital clubbing, characteristic auscultatory findings include fine crackles called "Velcro" or "cellophane" crackles. Pleural effusions may occur in some interstitial diseases. Examination of the heart frequently reveals an accentuated second heart sound at the pulmonic area with a right ventricular lift or heave. With progression of the disease, other signs of pulmonary hypertension and cor pulmonale, such as hepatomegaly and peripheral edema, occur.

The chest x ray may be normal or show patterns varying from a ground-glass appearance to nodular, reticular, or reticulonodular diffuse infiltrates. Full-blown honeycombing is usually a late manifestation. Although each disease may have suggestive radiologic features, definitive diagnoses cannot be made solely by x ray. Lung biopsy is required either by thoracotomy or transbronchial biopsy with sufficient tissue being obtained to minimize sampling error since the disease process is heterogeneous. Bronchoalveolar lavage is frequently performed for various reasons and may offer confirmatory evidence in diagnosis. It has a larger role in measuring disease activity and as an investigational tool.

Specific blood tests are not available. A variety of immunologically based tests may be abnormal such as the rheumatoid factor and DNA antibody determinations. These may be nonspecific in many cases.

Therapy is based on interrupting or suppressing the inflammatory process. Determination of disease activity is vital because of evidence that treatment is most effective before fibrosis is irreversible. Gallium lung scans are positive during the inflammatory phase with serial scanning suggested as a means of following treatment. Serial measurements of the diffusing capacity and alveolar-arterial oxygen gradient [$P(A-a)O_2$] may be performed. Recently serial magnetic resonance imaging (MRI) studies have been reported to be as effective as other methods of determining activity and do not use ionizing radiation. Serial lung biopsies have also been used. The prognosis of DILD is quite unpredictable, ranging from fulminant, progressive fatal disease to survival of up to 15 years from the time of diagnosis. Interstitial lung disease patients are also at an increased risk of developing adenocarcinomas of the lung.

At this time, the mainstay of therapy is the corticosteroids. These are normally begun in suppressive doses, then tapered to maintenance levels based on clinical response and the studies described above. Other immunosuppressive regimens, alone or in combination with steroids, include cyclophosphamide, azathioprine, chlorambucil, methotrexate, vincristine, and vinblastine. Antimalarials are under evaluation. Small patient numbers in treatment protocols, the lack of established measures of disease activity, and a variable prognosis limit attempts to define therapy. Neither lavage, gallium scanning, nor MRI has been used long enough to know how well the results correlate with prolonged patient survival.

1. Fulmer, J. D. An introduction to the interstitial lung diseases. *Clin. Chest Med.* 3:457, 1982.

...cellent overview classifying interstitial lung diseases, with an excellent bibli-
..graphy of both clinical and research value.

2. Hance, A. J., and Crystal, R. G. The Connective Tissue of Lung. In *Lung Disease: State of the Art 1975–1976.* New York: American Thoracic Society, 1977. P. 219.
   A necessary introduction to any more recent study of the connective tissue of the lung with information on models of pulmonary fibrosis.

3. Hamman, L., and Rich, A. R. Acute diffuse interstitial fibrosis of the lungs. *Bull. Johns Hopkins Hosp.* 74:177, 1944.
   After an initial report in 1935, this paper defined idiopathic pulmonary fibrosis and directed attention to the condition.

4. Fraser, R. G. The radiology of interstitial lung disease. *Clin. Chest Med.* 3:475, 1982.
   Succinct and authoritative descriptions of the radiologic appearances of interstitial lung disease.

5. Snider, G. L. Interstitial pulmonary fibrosis. *Chest* 89:115, 1986.
   Reviews animal models of lung injury other than that caused by inhalation of partic- ulate matter producing fibrosis.

6. Liebow, A. A., and Carrington, C. B. Alveolar Diseases: The Interstitial Pneumonias. In M. Simon (ed.), *Frontiers of Pulmonary Radiology.* New York: Grune & Stratton, Inc., 1967. P. 214.
   Thorough pathologic review by these pioneers from whom sprang the descriptive ter- minology.

7. Flint, A. The interstitial lung diseases: A pathologist's view. *Clin. Chest Med.* 3:491, 1982.
   A modern review of terminology, anatomic basis of pathologic diagnosis, methods of lung biopsy, and need for clinician and pathologist cooperation.

8. Rosenberg, D. M. Inherited forms of interstitial lung disease. *Clin. Chest Med.* 3:635, 1982.
   A short but well-referenced review of various familial forms of interstitial lung dis- ease.

9. Chapman, J. R., Charles, P. J., Venables, P. J. W., et al. Definition and clinical relevance of antibodies to nuclear ribonucleoprotein and other nuclear antigens in patients with cryptogenic fibrosing alveolitis. *Am. Rev. Respir. Dis.* 130:439, 1984.
   British experience relating antinuclear antibody titers in interstitial lung disease to specific connective tissue diseases showing the nonspecificity of these antibodies.

10. Davis, W. B., and Crystal, R. G. Chronic interstitial Lung Disease. In D. H. Simmons (ed.), *Current Pulmonology,* New York. John Wiley, 1984. Vol. 5.
    A thorough review of the scope of chronic interstitial diseases including 668 references from recognized authorities.

11. Winterbauer, R. H., and Hammar, S. P. Sarcoidosis and Idiopathic Pulmonary Fibro- sis: A Review of Recent Events. In D. H. Simmons (ed.), *Current Pulmonology.* Chi- cago: Year Book Medical Publishers, 1986. Vol. 7, p. 117.
    Well-conceived comparisons and contrasts between sarcoidosis and idiopathic pul- monary fibrosis with excellent illustrations and advice on management.

12. Fulmer, J. D. Bronchoalveolar lavage (editorial). *Am. Rev. Respir. Dis.* 126:961, 1982.
    Little has changed since 1982 to establish lavage as an essential procedure in inter- stitial lung diseases although acquired immunodeficiency syndrome (AIDS) may be changing this.

13. Turner-Warwick, M., and Haslam, P. L. The value of serial bronchoalveolar lavages in assessing the clinical progress of patients with cryptogenic fibrosing alveolitis. *Am. Rev. Respir. Dis.* 135:26, 1987.
    Information from the Brompton Hospital with early suggestions that serial bron- choalveolar lavage may be valuable, but calling for more studies.

14. Haslam, P. L., Dewar, A., Butchers, P., et al. Mast cells, atypical lymphocytes, and neutrophils in bronchoalveolar lavage in extrinsic allergic alveolitis. *Am. Rev. Res- pir. Dis.* 135:35, 1987.
    Hypersensitivity pneumonitis cell populations show the mast cell involved in the in- flammatory response as well as lymphocytes.

15. Carrington, C. B., and Liebow, A. A. Lymphocytic interstitial pneumonia (abstract). *Am. J. Pathol.* 48:36, 1966.
   The initial description of LIP.

16. Yoshizawa, Y., Ohdama, S., Ideda, A., et al. Lymphoid interstitial pneumonia associated with depressed cellular immunity and polyclonal gammopathy. *Am. Rev. Respir. Dis.* 130:507, 1984.
   Although Young and others have shown association of LIP with monoclonal and polyclonal gammopathy, this recent report shows decreased circulating T cell activity.

17. Grieco, M. H., and Chinoy-Archarya, P. Lymphocytic interstitial pneumonia associated with the acquired immune deficiency syndrome. *Am. Rev. Respir. Dis.* 131:952, 1985.
   This and the paper by Solal-Celigny and associates in the same issue establish the link between LIP and AIDS.

18. Kornstein, M. J., Pietra, G. G., Hoxie, J. A., et al. The pathology and treatment of interstitial pneumonitis in two infants with AIDS. *Am. Rev. Respir. Dis.* 133:1196, 1986.
   An LIP-like pathologic picture in 12- and 18-month-old infants with AIDS.

19. Tenholder, M. F., Russell, M. D., Knight, E., et al. Orthodeoxia: A new finding in interstitial fibrosis. *Am. Rev. Respir. Dis.* 136:170, 1987.
   Arterial desaturation worsened while upright and improved by recumbency in this neat clinical report.

20. McFadden, R. G., Carr, T. J., and Wood, T. E. Proton magnetic resonance imaging to stage activity of interstitial lung disease. *Chest* 92:31, 1987.
   Although costly, the authors show convincing illustrations that the greater the disease activity, the greater the intensity of MRI of the lung.

21. Meyer, C. E., and Liebow, A. A. Relationship of interstitial pneumonia, honeycombing and atypical epithelial proliferation to cancer of the lung. *Cancer* 18:322, 1965.
   Report of the now well-known relationship of lung cancer to chronic interstitial pulmonary fibrosis.

22. Rudd, R. M., Haslam, P. L., and Turner-Warwick, M. Cryptogenic fibrosing alveolitis: Relationships of pulmonary physiology and bronchoalveolar lavage to response to treatment and prognosis. *Am. Rev. Respir. Dis.* 124:1, 1981.
   Correlates physiologic and lavage data with the ability to predict response to treatment and mentions some treatment regimens.

23. Marchlinsky, F. F., Gansler, T. S., Waxman, H. L., et al. Amiodarone pulmonary toxicity. *Ann. Intern. Med.* 97:839, 1982.
   A reminder that a multitude of drugs, some old, some new, such as amiodarone, produce interstitial lung diseases.

149. MEDIASTINAL MASSES

H. Verdain Barnes

Mediastinal masses are diagnostically perplexing regardless of the patient's age. Although the majority of patients present with cardiac or pulmonary signs or symptoms, about 14 percent are asymptomatic and have the mass discovered on a routine chest x ray. The area of the mediastinum in which the mass is located provides a general guideline for differential diagnosis. The superior mediastinum is the area bounded by the manubrium anteriorly and the third and fifth thoracic vertebrae posteriorly. This area is further divided into anterior and posterior. Masses in the anterior superior area are most often of thymic, thyroid, or parathyroid origin, whereas those in the posterior area are most often of neurogenic origin. Other types of masses in the superior mediastinum include aneurysms, bronchogenic cysts, cystic hygromas, lymphomas, metastatic carcinomas, myxomas, and mesotheliomas.

...or mediastinum is the area anterior to the heart from the inferior border of ...erior mediastinum to the diaphragm. The most common masses in this area are ... dermoid cysts, teratomas, and lymph nodes involved by lymphomas, Hodgkin's disease, tuberculosis, sarcoid, or histoplasmosis. Other types include aortic aneurysms, abscesses, hematomas, Morgagni's hernias, lipomas, epicardial fat pads, fibromas, lymphangiomas, hemangiomas, sarcomas, thymomas, goiters, and parathyroid adenomas and carcinomas.

The posterior mediastinum is the area between the vertebral column and lungs from the inferior border of the superior mediastinum to the diaphragm. By far the most common masses in this area are tumors of neurogenic origin. Other masses common to this area include sarcomas, lymphomas, myxomas, enterogenous cysts, hiatal hernias, pancreatic pseudocysts, esophageal diverticula, tumors, meningoceles, hematomas, loculated pleural effusion, thoracic duct cysts, aortic aneurysms, extramedullary hemopoiesis, and paravertebral abscesses.

The middle mediastinum is that area bounded by the inferior border of the superior mediastinum to the diaphragm and from the posterior border of the anterior mediastinum to the anterior border of the posterior compartment. The most common masses in this area are those arising from lymph nodes or lung parenchyma. The causes are primarily lymphomas, Hodgkin's disease, primary lung malignancies, metastatic malignancies, tuberculosis, and sarcoid. Other less common causes include various vascular anomalies, bronchogenic cysts, pericardial cysts, lipomas, abscesses, hiatus hernias, hematomas, and lymph node involvement by erythema nodosum, infectious mononucleosis, and fungi.

In most series about 18 percent of the masses occur in the superior mediastinum and 82 percent in the anterior, middle, and posterior segments. Of the primary neoplasms and cysts of the mediastinum, the most common ones are the neurogenic tumors, followed by thymomas and the various cysts. Of the neurogenic tumors the most common ones are ganglioneuromas, neurinomas, and neurofibromas. Thymomas are usually benign, but about 25 percent are malignant. The most common cysts are bronchogenic, dermoid, or unclassifiable. Undifferentiated primary carcinoma of the mediastinum is not uncommon. The other types of mediastinal masses are relatively rare.

The clinical features are, for the most part, nonspecific, but the majority of patients are to some degree symptomatic. Nonspecific chest pain is the most common complaint, occurring in 33 percent of patients with benign lesions and in over 50 percent of those with a malignancy. Cough is present in about 50 percent of those with malignancy and 20 percent of those with benign processes. Weight loss, dysphagia, and hoarseness are far more common in the group with malignant lesions, whereas dyspnea and hemoptysis occur with about equal frequency in benign and malignant disease. In the patients with metastases to the mediastinum, the most common primary tumors outside the chest are renal, breast, colon, rectum, cervix, thyroid, and uterus. The physical findings in patients with mediastinal masses are variable; however, many exhibit cardiac findings. In as many as 8 percent of patients, the initial diagnosis is intrinsic cardiovascular disease. Computed tomography (CT) is the most effective noninvasive initial diagnostic method for essentially all mediastinal masses or suspected masses regardless of the type or location. In patients with cardiac findings, angiography is also a useful diagnostic tool. In patients suspected of having a thyroid cause, a radioiodine scan can offer differential help; however, since many substernal goiters are not functional, the study is helpful only if the results are positive. Biopsy of a palpable supraclavicular lymph node will often provide a specific diagnosis. In the final analysis, however, most of these patients require fine-needle aspiration biopsy of the lesion, mediastinoscopy, or thoracotomy for a definitive diagnosis.

1. Sabiston, D. C., and Scott, H. W. Primary neoplasms and cysts of the mediastinum. *Ann. Surg.* 136:777, 1952.
   An excellent general review of the subject.
2. Drash, E. C., and Hyer, H. J. Mesothelial mediastinal cysts. *J. Thorac. Surg.* 19:755, 1950.
3. Rusby, N. L. Dermoid cysts and teratoma of the mediastinum. *J. Thorac. Surg.* 13:169, 1944.

4. Olenek, J. L., and Tandatnick, J. W. Congenital mediastinal cysts of foregut origin. *Am. J. Dis. Child.* 71:466, 1946.

5. Stewart, F. W., and Copeland, M. M. Neurogenic sarcoma. *Am. J. Cancer* 15:1235, 1931.

6. Stout, A. P. Ganglioneuroma of the sympathetic nervous system. *Surg. Gynecol. Obstet.* 84:101, 1947.

7. Wakeley, C. P. G., and Mulvany, J. H. Intrathoracic goiter. *Surg. Gynecol. Obstet.* 70:702, 1940.

8. Dyer, N. H. Cystic teratomas and thymic cysts: A review. *Thorax* 22:408, 1967.

9. Cheng, T. O. Aneurysm of a nonpatent ductus arteriosus: An unusual cause of mediastinal mass. *Dis. Chest* 55:497, 1969.

10. Cheng, T. O. Pseudocoarctation of the aorta: An important consideration in the differential diagnosis of superior mediastinal mass. *Am. J. Med.* 49:551, 1970.

11. Weidmann, P., Rutishauser, W., and Siegenthaler, W. Mediastinal pseudocyst of the pancreas. *Am. J. Med.* 46:454, 1969.

12. Bodman, S. F., and Condemi, J. J. Mediastinal widening in iatrogenic Cushing's syndrome. *Ann. Intern. Med.* 67:399, 1967.

13. Grelier, J. M., and Hardin, J. G. Synovial cyst of sternoclavicular joint as mediastinal mass. *Ann. Intern. Med.* 83:525, 1975.

14. DeCosta, J. L., Loh, Y. S., and Hanam, E. Extramedullary hemopoiesis with multiple tumor-simulating mediastinal masses in hemoglobin E–thalassemia disease. *Chest* 65:210, 1974.

15. Enquist, R. W., Torney, D. C., Jenis, E. H., et al. Malignant chemodectoma of the superior mediastinum with elevated urinary homovanillic acid. *Chest* 66:209, 1974.

16. Feldman, L., and Kricun, M. E. Malignant melanoma presenting as a mediastinal mass. *J.A.M.A.* 241:396, 1979.

17. Olson, J. L., and Salyer, W. R. Mediastinal paragangliomas (aortic body tumor): A report of four cases and a review of the literature. *Cancer* 41:2405, 1978.

18. Shub, C., Parkin, T. W., and Lie, J. T. An unusual mediastinal lipoma simulating cardiomegaly. *Mayo Clin. Proc.* 54:60, 1979.

19. Osnosa, K. L., and Harrell, D. D. Isolated mediastinal mass in primary amyloidosis. *Chest* 78:786, 1980.

20. Arbona, G. L., Lloyd, T. V., and Lucas, J. Mediastinal extramedullary plasmacytoma. *South. Med. J.* 73:670, 1980.

21. Siddorn, J. A., and Worsornu, L. Dilation of the azygos vein simulating a mediastinal tumor. *Thorax* 34:117, 1979.
    Articles 20, 21 detail a variety of etiologies.

22. Oldham, H. N., and Sabiston, D. C. Primary tumors and cysts of the mediastinum. *Arch. Surg.* 96:71, 1968.
    8% of these patients with mediastinal masses were incorrectly diagnosed as having primary cardiovascular disease.

23. Goodwin, R. A., Nickell, J. A., Des Proz, R. M. Mediastinal fibrosis complicating healed primary histoplasmosis and tuberculosis. *Medicine* 51:227, 1972.
    Symptom complexes include superior vena caval obstruction, bronchial stenosis, and obstruction of pulmonary arteries or veins.

24. Rimon, D., Cohen, L., and Rosenfield, J. Thrombosed giant left atrium mimicking a mediastinal tumor. *Chest* 71:406, 1977.
    Two problems mimicking mediastinal masses; the first (article 23) is not rare.

25. Davidson, K. G., Walbaum, P. R., and McCormack, J. M. Intrathoracic neural tumors. *Thorax* 33:359, 1978.

26. Adam, A., and Hochholzer, L. Ganglioneuroblastoma of the posterior mediastinum. *Cancer* 47:373, 1981.
    Two (articles 25 and 26) good reviews of neurogenic tumors of the mediastinum.

27. Akwari, O. E., Payne, W. S., Onofrio, B. M., et al. Dumbbell neurogenic tumors of the mediastinum. *Mayo Clin. Proc.* 53:353, 1978.
    About 10% had tumors that extended through an intervertebral foramen.

28. Bower, R. J., and Kiesewetter, W. B. Mediastinal masses in infants and children. *Arch. Surg.* 112:1003, 1977.

About half are malignant neurogenic or lymphoid tumors, the former more common in those age 4 years or less and the latter in those over that age.

29. Homer, M. J., Wechsler, R. J., and Carter, B. L. Mediastinal lipomatosis: Computed tomography confirmation of a normal variant. *Radiology* 128:657, 1978.
    Fat has a characteristic density on CT allowing a confident diagnosis.
30. Lichtenstein, A. K., Levine, A., Taylor, C. R., et al. Primary mediastinal lymphoma in adults. *Am. J. Med.* 68:509, 1980.
    The most common type is diffuse poorly differentiated lymphoma with convoluted morphology usually with disseminated disease.
31. Devkota, J. Mediastinal tumors and pseudotumors: Evaluation by computerized tomography. *South. Med. J.* 78:393, 1985.
    CT proved superior to other imaging techniques for precise location and general differentiation.
32. Weisbrod, G. L. Percutaneous fine-needle aspiration biopsy of the mediastinum. *Clin. Chest Med.* 8:27, 1987.
33. Pedersen, O. M., Aasen, T. B., and Gulsvik, A. Fine needle aspiration biopsy of mediastinal and peripheral pulmonary masses guided by real-time sonography. *Chest* 89:504, 1986.
    A useful diagnostic technique (article 32) and a refinement (article 33).
34. Eagle, K. A., Quertermous, T., Kritzer, G. A., et al. Spectrum of conditions initially suggesting acute aortic dissection but with negative aortograms. *Am. J. Cardiol.* 57:322, 1986.
    In this series 7% had a mediastinal mass rather than a dissection.

150. PLEURAL EFFUSION

H. Verdain Barnes

Excess fluid in the pleural cavity has diagnostic and therapeutic implications. Normally there is a small volume of serous fluid in the pleural cavity that serves as a lubricant between the visceral and parietal pleura. In normal homeostasis the quantity of pleural fluid is controlled by a combination of hydrostatic, colloid osmotic, and pleural pressure in accord with Starling's equation. Normally, pleural fluid is produced by the parietal pleura and absorbed by the visceral pleura. Fluid and low-molecular-weight substances are absorbed by the visceral pleural capillaries, and larger substances primarily by the lymphatics. This dynamic equilibrium can be altered in the direction of pleural fluid accumulation by any process with (1) increases in hydrostatic pressure in the systemic and/or pulmonary capillaries, (2) decreases in intravascular oncotic pressure, (3) increases in the amount of negative pleural pressure, (4) an impediment to lymphatic drainage, or (5) increases in capillary permeability.

The presence of a large pleural effusion is easily documented on physical examination, but small or loculated effusions may escape detection. The symptoms associated with an effusion per se may range from none to pleuritic pain to marked dyspnea and respiratory distress. Respiratory distress is most often present when fluid is accumulating rapidly, is large in amount, or is superimposed on already compromised pulmonary function. The chest x ray is a simple method of documenting a pleural effusion. For radiographs to clearly define a pleural effusion, at least 25 to 30 ml of fluid must be present; however, with special projections and horizontal x-ray beams, as little as 10 to 15 ml can be identified in about 10 percent of normal persons. Consequently, small amounts of pleural effusion may not be pathologically significant. The earliest radiographic signs are blunting of the costophrenic angle on the anteroposterior view and loss of a clear definition of the diaphragm posteriorly on the lateral view. When there is doubt, a lateral decubitus film typically shows a layering of the fluid along the dependent chest wall unless there is loculation. Larger accumulations of fluid offer less of a problem in radiologic diagnosis unless loculated between the lung and diaphragm, in a major or minor fissure, or along the lateral wall of the chest. On routine views, fluid in the last two areas may resemble tumor opacities within the lung—so-called pseudotumor. Loculated effusions or empyema can often be unequivocally diagnosed and accurately followed using sonography, a useful, noninvasive diagnostic technique.

Once a pleural effusion is demonstrated, in most clinical situations a thoracentesis should be performed. The main purposes are to obtain fluid for characterization and to potentially relieve associated respiratory distress. Thoracentesis is a benign procedure when carefully performed in a patient given atropine to avoid the effects of possible reflex vagal stimulation when the pleural cavity is entered. Pneumothorax and hemothorax are rare complications of the procedure, as are intravascular collapse and unilateral pulmonary edema after the withdrawal of large quantities of fluid.

Once obtained, the evaluation of the fluid should be designed to gather the information that will have the greatest impact on resolving the question of etiology. In most clinical settings a description of the gross character of the fluid, anaerobic and aerobic bacterial as well as fungal cultures, total protein or lactic acid dehydrogenase (LDH) levels, Gram's and acid-fast stains, white and red blood cell counts, and cytology are indicated. Depending on the differential diagnosis being considered, one or more of the following may be useful: a fluid pH anaerobically collected, glucose, amylase, carcinoembryonic antigen (CEA), antinuclear antibody (ANA), rheumatoid factor, LE preparation, complement, eosinophil count, lysozyme level, WBC differential, orosomucoid level, cholesterol level, total neutral fat level, or needle biopsy of the parietal pleura.

Classification of an effusion as an exudate or transudate will often help focus the differential diagnosis. The protein content of the fluid is probably the single most helpful determination; a protein level of greater than 3 gm/dl is indicative of an exudate. However, if only this criterion is used, approximately 10 percent of the exudates and 15 percent of the transudates will be misclassified. Accuracy is significantly enhanced by using the following criteria for an exudate: (1) a pleural fluid–serum protein ratio over 0.5 and (2) a pleural fluid–serum LDH ratio over 0.6. The differential diagnosis of an exudate includes such neoplasms as carcinoma of the bronchus, breast, ovary, pancreas, uterus, stomach, liver, kidney, adrenal, testes, larynx, and thyroid; lymphomas and leukemias; and bacterial, fungal, and viral infections. The most common infection is tuberculosis, followed closely by other bacterial infections and less commonly by mycoplasmal and viral pneumonia. The effusions associated with trauma, pulmonary embolization, pancreatitis, postmyocardial infarction syndrome, rheumatoid disease, infectious hepatitis, sarcoidosis, uremia, rheumatic fever, postcardiotomy syndrome, polyarteritis, scleroderma, uremia, Wegener's granulomatosis, rheumatoid arthritis, systemic lupus erythematosus, asbestosis, and pleural mesothelioma are typically exudates, except for the last three, which are about equally as often transudates. A low protein content or transudate is typical in congestive heart failure, cirrhosis, hypothyroidism, Meigs' syndrome, and nephrotic syndrome.

An anaerobically collected pleural fluid pH of less than 7.3 is seen in patients with empyema and esophageal rupture, in about 67 percent with tuberculosis, in about 64 percent with collagen-vascular disease, in about 25 percent with malignancy, and in about 20 percent with hemothorax. In parapneumonic effusions a pH less than 7.0 and/or glucose less than 40 mg/dl indicates need for closed-tube drainage. A pleural fluid mesothelial cell count of less than 1 percent suggests tuberculosis. False-positive or equivocal cytologic studies may rarely occur with nonmalignant inflammatory processes. When total neutral fat is greater than 400 mg/dl, chylothorax can be diagnosed, a finding seen most often with lymphomas, solid tumors, nephrotic syndrome, cirrhosis, and occasionally rheumatoid arthritis. Pleural fluid amylase content may be greater than blood amylase in pancreatitis, carcinoma of the lung, bacterial pneumonias, and esophageal rupture. A rheumatoid factor titer of 1:160 or greater can be seen in rheumatoid arthritis, bacterial pneumonia, tuberculosis, and carcinoma. Grossly bloody fluid is most often seen in malignancy, trauma, pulmonary embolus, and tuberculosis as well as after repeated thoracenteses. The differential cell count may on occasion help to differentiate acute from chronic inflammation. A high eosinophil count may be seen in a variety of situations including repeat thoracentesis, but is usually associated with a benign process.

1. Green, R. A., and Johnston, R. F. Introduction to Pleural Disease. In G. L. Baum (ed.), *Textbook of Pulmonary Diseases* (2nd ed.). Boston: Little, Brown, 1974. P. 941.
   A good review of pleural physiology and pathophysiology.
2. Leuallen, E. C., and Carr, D. T. Pleural effusion: A statistical study of 436 patients. *N. Engl. J. Med.* 252:79, 1955.
   Of these 436 patients with pleural effusion, 52% had tumors.
3. Ungerleider, J. T. The diagnostic significance of pleural effusion. *Dis. Chest* 32:83, 1957.
   Tuberculosis is a common cause of unilateral "idiopathic pleural effusion."
4. Rao, N. V., Jones, P. O., Greenberg, S. D., et al. Needle biopsy of parietal pleura in 124 cases. *Arch. Intern. Med.* 115:34, 1965.
   The article points out the benign nature of needle biopsy of the pleura in the diagnosis of pleural effusions. A positive histologic diagnosis can be made in approximately 70%.
5. Light, R. W., MacGregor, I., Luchsinger, P. C., et al. Pleural effusions: The diagnostic separation of transudates and exudates. *Ann. Intern. Med.* 77:507, 1972.
   Only a rare misclassification of an effusion as an exudate or transudate is made when these authors' criteria are used.
6. Light, R. W., and Ball, W. C. Glucose and amylase in pleural effusions. *J.A.M.A.* 225:257, 1973.
   Glucose levels were of little use, and the lack of specificity of elevated amylase levels is documented.
7. Dye, R. A., and Laforet, E. G. Esophageal rupture: Diagnosis by pleural fluid pH. *Chest* 66:454, 1974.
   The pH was less than 5.
8. Light, R. W., Erozan, Y. S., and Ball, W. C. Cells in pleural fluid: Their value in differential diagnosis. *Arch. Intern. Med.* 132:854, 1973.
   The red cell and white cell counts are of limited help in the differential diagnosis, but the presence of less than 1% mesothelial cells is a helpful finding.
9. Feagler, J. R., Sorenson, G. D., Rosenfeld, M. G., et al. Rheumatoid pleural effusion. *Arch. Pathol.* 92:257, 1971.
   An exhaustive characterization of the pleural fluid in this disease and demonstration of inclusions in the polymorphonuclear leukocytes.
10. Roy, P. H., Carr, D. T., and Payne, W. S. The problem of chylothorax. *Mayo Clin. Proc.* 42:457, 1967.
    The most common causes of chylothorax are trauma to the thoracic duct and lymphoma.
11. Gaensler, E. A., and Kaplan, A. I. Asbestos pleural effusion. *Ann. Intern. Med.* 74:178, 1971.
    Pleural effusion can be seen in asbestosis with or without an associated mesothelioma.
12. Sandweiss, D. A., Hanson, J. C., Gosnik, B. B., et al. Ultrasound in diagnosis, localization, and treatment of loculated pleural empyema. *Ann. Intern. Med.* 82:50, 1975.
    An important, noninvasive diagnostic tool.
13. Vladutiu, A. O., Brason, F. W., and Adler, R. H. Differential diagnosis of pleural effusions: Clinical usefulness of cell marker quantitation. *Chest* 79:297, 1981.
    CEA and orosomucoid levels had an 86% sensitivity in diagnosing malignant pleural effusion.
14. Hirsch, A., Ruffie, P., Nebut, M., et al. Pleural effusion: Laboratory tests in 300 cases. *Thorax* 34:106, 1979.
    The most common causes were cancer in 39%, tuberculosis in 17.6%, and bacterial infection in 12.6%.
15. Light, R. W., Girard, W. M., Jenkinson, S. G., et al. Parapneumonic effusions. *Am. J. Med.* 69:507, 1980.

A pleural fluid pH of <7.0 and/or glucose <40 mg/dl requires immediate closed-chest tube drainage.

16. Kutty, C. P. D., and Varkey, B. "Contarini's condition": Bilateral pleural effusions with markedly different characteristics. *Chest* 74:679, 1978.
    Worth keeping in mind in the immunosuppressed patient. This patient had staphylococcal empyema on the left and a lymphocytic effusion on the right.

17. Horn, B. R., and Byrd, R. B. Simulation of pleural disease by disk space infection. *Chest* 74:575, 1978.

18. Myers, T. J., Cole, S. R., and Pastuszak, W. T. Angioimmunoblastic lymphadenopathy: Pleural-pulmonary disease. *Cancer* 40:266, 1978.

19. Singer, J. A., Kaplan, M. M., and Katz, R. L. Cirrhotic pleural effusion in the absence of ascites. *Gastroenterology* 73:575, 1977.
    Three (articles 17–19) causes of pleural effusion.

20. Chernow, B., and Sahn, S. A. Carcinomatous involvement of the pleura: An analysis of 96 patients. *Am. J. Med.* 63:695, 1977.
    The most common primary tumors were lung, breast, ovary, and stomach in descending order. The pleural effusion was the basis for first diagnosis in 46% and the mean survival was only 3.1 months after diagnosis.

21. Good, J. T., Jr., Taryle, D. A., Maulitz, R. M., et al. The diagnostic value of pleural fluid pH. *Chest* 78:55, 1980.
    A value <7.3 was seen in all patients with empyema or esophageal rupture, tuberculosis (67%), collagen-vascular disease (64%), malignancy (25%), and hemothorax (20%).

22. Light, R. W., Jenkinson, S. G., Minh, V. D., et al. Observations on pleural fluid pressures as fluid is withdrawn during thoracentesis. *Am. Rev. Respir. Dis.* 121:799, 1980.
    The authors recommend termination of fluid withdrawal when the pleural pressure falls below −20 cm of water, perhaps an important guide to how much to take off at one time.

23. Adelman, M., Albelda, S. M., Gottlieb, J., et al. Diagnostic utility of pleural fluid eosinophilia. *Am. J. Med.* 77:915, 1984.
    Most cases were benign process. May help differentiate between exudate and transudate.

24. Chetty, K. G. Transudative pleural effusions. *Clin. Chest Med.* 6:49, 1985.
    Typical causes are discussed ranging from congestive heart failure to hypothyroidism to a misplaced subclavian catheter.

25. Katner, H. P., Treen, B., Pankey, G. A., et al. Pleural effusion and anicteric hepatitis associated with cat-scratch disease. *Chest* 89:302, 1986.

26. Brown, S. E., and Light, R. W. Pleural effusion associated with pulmonary embolism. *Clin. Chest Med.* 6:77, 1985.
    Two (articles 25, 26) rare causes of effusion.

27. Hernando, H. R. V., Jimenez, J. F. M., Juncal, L. D., et al. Meaning and diagnostic value of determining the lysozyme level of pleural fluid. *Chest* 91:342, 1987.

28. Hamm, H., Brohan, U., Bohmer, R., et al. Cholesterol in pleural effusions: A diagnostic aid. *Chest* 92:296, 1987.
    Two (articles 27, 28) potential adjuncts in diagnosis.

29. Irani, D. R., Underwood, R. D., Johnson, E. H., et al. Malignant pleural effusions: A clinical cytopathologic study. *Arch. Intern. Med.* 147:1133, 1987.

30. Sahn, S. A., and Good, J. T., Jr. Pleural fluid pH in malignant effusions: Diagnostic, prognostic and therapeutic implications. *Ann. Intern. Med.* 108:345, 1988.

31. Prakash, U. B. S., and Reiman, H. M. Comparison of needle biopsy with cytologic analysis for the evaluation of pleural effusion: Analysis of 414 cases. *Mayo Clin. Proc.* 60:158, 1985.
    Three articles (29–31) providing current data on the diagnostic evaluation of a potentially malignant effusion.

32. Epstein, D. M., Kline, L. R., Albelda, S. M., et al. Tuberculous pleural effusions. *Chest* 91:106, 1987.
    A concise review; only 62% had pleural fluid lymphocytosis. All fluids were exudates and 15% had a glucose of less than 30 mg/dl.

33. Himelman, R. B., and Callen, P. W. The prognostic value of loculation in parapneumonic pleural effusions. *Chest* 90:852, 1986.
    Loculation correlated with the fluid being an exudate.
34. Good, J. T., Jr., King, T. E., Antony, V. B., et al. Lupus pleuritis: Clinical features and pleural fluid characteristics with special reference to pleural fluid antinuclear antibodies. *Chest* 84:714, 1983.
    The ANA may be helpful in diagnosis.
35. Estenne, M., Yernault, J.-C., Troyer, A. D. Mechanism of relief of dyspnea after thoracentesis in patients with large pleural effusions. *Am. J. Med.* 74:813, 1983.
    Relief is probably primarily due to a decrease in the size of the thoracic cage rather than changes in other pulmonary function parameters.

151. PRIMARY LUNG ABSCESS
Jerry L. Spivak

Primary lung abscess, which is caused by a bronchial embolus of aspirated material, cannot be distinguished on a plain chest x ray from cavitary lung lesions produced by carcinoma, tuberculosis, fungi, sarcoidosis, septic pulmonary infarction, Hodgkin's disease, Wegener's granulomatosis, rheumatoid nodules, amebiasis, staphylococcus, pneumonococcus, streptococcus, *Klebsiella, Pseudomonas,* or tularemia. Physicochemical changes in cancerous or caseating tissue can stimulate cavitation with bronchial communication when neither is present, and benign lung cysts containing fluid can also mimic a lung abscess. Primary lung abscesses are usually found in the bronchopulmonary segments that are most dependent in the supine position, namely, the posterior segments of the upper lobes and superior segments of the lower lobes, most often on the right side. In the upright position, aspiration usually produces abscesses in the basilar segments of the lower lobes. The presence of oral sepsis, alcoholism, epilepsy, sinus disease, esophageal disorders, or a history of unconsciousness from any cause suggests that a cavitary pulmonary lesion is an abscess. The absence of a predisposing cause or an atypical location should suggest another etiology for the cavitation such as a carcinoma or septic embolism. The presence of weight loss, pleural effusion, or hilar adenopathy will not differentiate an abscess from a cavitating carcinoma. It should also be noted that in the narcotic addict, pulmonary cavitation is more often due to septic embolization than to aspiration of infected material.

Sputum is generally an unsatisfactory source for routine bacteriologic studies, but transtracheal aspirates are useful if there are no contraindications to the procedure. Blood cultures are rarely positive in anaerobic lung infections; pleural fluid cultures may prove useful if there is empyema, and transthoracic needle aspiration or fiberoptic bronchoscopy are other options. The last-named is probably best reserved for situations in which the possibility of a cavitating neoplasm exists. Sinus x rays and esophageal studies may also be useful in the diagnostic evaluation. Anaerobic bacteria generally predominate in culture material and the infection is usually polymicrobial. In approximately 15 percent of cases, penicillin-resistant strains are present. The complications of a primary lung abscess include sepsis, hemorrhage, metastatic infection (such as a brain abscess), bronchopleural fistula, bronchiectasis, intrapulmonic aspiration, and empyema.

Although lung abscesses have been observed to heal spontaneously, in the usual situation both antibiotics and drainage are required for adequate healing and to avoid the complications listed above. Historically, penicillin has been the drug of choice in the treatment of primary lung abscess but there is no agreement as to the amount of penicillin that should be employed. Furthermore, recent studies indicate that clindamycin is more effective than penicillin, as might be expected in view of the bacteriologic data. Metronidazole alone is not an effective agent in the treatment of primary lung abscess but can be combined with penicillin.

The healing of a lung abscess with medical therapy is dependent on the duration of symptoms before treatment. If the cavity has been present for longer than 12 weeks, the chances of its closure are poor. For this reason, the addition of a second antibiotic has been advocated to avoid the possibility of a primary treatment failure when penicillin is used alone. In certain situations, such as a hospital-acquired lung abscess from which enteric bacilli have been recovered, addition of an aminoglycoside to the treatment regimen seems reasonable. Other factors affecting healing include cavity size (cavities greater than 8 cm may not close) and associated underlying illnesses. With therapy, fever should subside within 12 days; cavity closure usually begins by 2 weeks, but healing may take 6 months and sometimes longer. Antibiotic therapy should be continued for at least 6 weeks. Cavities that persist with a size greater than 2 cm can give rise to complications, such as recurrent infection and hemorrhage. Surgery is recommended for situations in which a carcinoma cannot be ruled out or in which there is a significant complication, such as persistent bronchial obstruction, hemoptysis, bronchopleural fistula, or bronchiectasis.

1. Bartlett, J. G. Anaerobic bacterial infections of the lung. *Chest* 91:901, 1987.
   Good advice, clearly stated.
2. Barnett, T. B., and Herring, C. L. Lung abscess. *Arch. Intern. Med.* 127:217, 1971.
   Duration of symptoms and cavity size are important determinants of therapeutic success.
3. Perlman, L. V., Lerner, E., and D'Esopo, N. Clinical classification and analysis of 97 cases of lung abscess. *Am. Rev. Respir. Dis.* 99:390, 1969.
   Prognosis is related to the illness that caused the aspiration.
4. Laforet, E. G., and Laforet, M. T. Non-tuberculouis cavitary disease of the lung. *Dis. Chest* 31:665, 1957.
   Catalogues the causes of pulmonary cavitation.
5. LeMay, M., and Piro, A. J. Cavitary pulmonary metastases. *Ann. Intern. Med.* 62:59, 1965.
   Pseudocavitation with carcinoma.
6. Mayock, R. L., Dillon, R. F., and Stead, W. W. Roentgenographic simulation of cavitation by caseous material in lung lesions. *Am. Rev. Tuberc.* 71:529, 1955.
   Solid or liquid caseation can appear radiolucent on x ray.
7. Senecal, J. L., Antoine, P., and Beliveau, C. *Legionella pneumophila* lung abscess in a patient with systemic lupus erythematosus. *Am. J. Med. Sci.* 293:309, 1987.
   Abscess formation appears common in immunocompromised patients. (See also J. Infect. 11:51, 1985 and J.A.M.A. 241:597, 1979.)
8. Pohlson, E. C., McNamara, J. J., Char, C., et al. Lung abscess: A changing pattern of the disease. *Am. J. Surg.* 150:97, 1985.
   Clinical review. (See also Ann. Surg. 197:775, 1983.)
9. Wallace, R. J., Jr., Cohen, A., Awe, R. J., et al. Carcinomatous lung abscess: Diagnosis by bronchoscopy and cytopathology. *J.A.M.A.* 242:521, 1979.
   Cytology was an effective method of identification of a carcinomatous lung abscess; if doubt exists tissue should be obtained for diagnosis.
10. Webb, W. R., and Gamsu, G. Cavitary pulmonary nodules with systemic lupus erythematosus [SLE]: Differential diagnosis. *AJR* 136:27, 1981.
    Pulmonary cavitation in SLE is usually due to infection.
11. Fahey, P. J., Utell, M. J., and Hyde, R. W. Spontaneous lysis of mycetomas after acute cavitating lung disease. *Am. Rev. Respir. Dis.* 123:336, 1981.
    Fungi do not usually colonize an acute lung abscess.
12. Stark, D. D., Federle, M. P., Goodman, P. C., et al. Differentiating lung abscess and empyema. *Am. J. Roentgenol.* 141:163, 1983.
    Computed tomography appears more useful than conventional radiography. (See also Radiology 135:755, 1980.)
13. Bartlett, J. G., Gorbach, S. L., Tally, F. P., et al. Bacteriology and treatment of primary lung abscess. *Am. Rev. Respir. Dis.* 109:510, 1974.
    Anaerobes were obtained in 24 of 26 patients by transtracheal aspiration; mixed aerobic and anaerobic infections occurred in 10 patients.
14. Levison, M. E., Mangura, C. T., Lorber, B., et al. Clindamycin compared with peni-

cillin for the treatment of anaerobic lung abscess. *Ann. Intern. Med.* 98:466, 1983.
Clindamycin was more effective than penicillin in this study.

15. Neild, J. E., Eykyn, S. J., and Phillips, I. Lung abscess and empyema. *Q. J. Med.* 57:875, 1985.
    Penicillin-resistant organisms were common.

16. Kirby, B. D., George, W. L., Sutter, V. C., et al. Gram-negative anaerobic bacilli: Their role in infection and patterns of susceptibility to antimicrobial agents: I. Little-known bacteroides species. *Rev. Infect. Dis.* 2:914, 1980.
    A high percentage of penicillin-resistant bacteroides species were recovered.

17. Schweppe, H., Knowles, J. H., and Kane, L. Lung abscess. *N. Engl. J. Med.* 265:1039, 1961.
    With good bronchial drainage, 2.4 million units of parenteral procaine penicillin per day produced resolution.

18. Louria, D. B., and Brayton, R. G. The efficacy of penicillin regimens. *J.A.M.A.* 186:987, 1963.
    Advocates the use of the smallest amount of a single antibiotic to avoid superinfection.

19. Saunders, C. V., Hanna, B. J., and Lewis, A. C. Metronidazole in the treatment of anaerobic infections. *Am. Rev. Respir. Dis.* 120:337, 1979.
    Treatment failures were frequent; metronidazole is not recommended for treatment of lung abscess.

20. Rumbaugh, J. F., and Prior, J. A. Lung abscess: A review of forty-one cases. *Ann. Intern. Med.* 55:223, 1961.
    Lung abscesses associated with bronchiectasis respond poorly to medical therapy.

21. Weiss, W. Cavity behavior in acute primary nonspecific lung abscess. *Am. Rev. Respir. Dis.* 108:1273, 1973.
    Most cavities resolve within 3 months of initiation of therapy.

22. Block, A. J., Wagley, P. F., and Fisher, A. M. A reevaluation of the indications for surgery. *Johns Hopkins Med. J.* 125:19, 1969.
    Surgery is reserved for clinical deterioration or suspicion of carcinoma, not delayed closure.

23. Parker, L. A., Melton, J. W., Delany, D. J., et al. Percutaneous small bore catheter drainage in the management of lung abscesses. *Chest* 92:213, 1987.
    An alternative approach to surgery. (See also Am. Rev. Respir. Dis. 136:174, 1987 and J. Thorac. Cardiovasc. Surg. 87:308, 1984.)

24. Thoms, N. W., Wilson, R. F., Puro, H. E., et al. Life-threatening hemoptysis in primary lung abscess. *Am. Thorac. Surg.* 14:347, 1972.
    Reopacification of the abscess cavity suggests bleeding and is an indication for surgery.

25. Reeder, G. S., and Gracey, D. R. Aspiration of intrathoracic abscess: Resultant acute ventilatory failure. *J.A.M.A.* 240:1156, 1978.
    Adequate drainage should prevent this complication.

26. Libby, L. S., King, T. E., LaForce, M., et al. Pulmonary cavitation following pulmonary infarction. *Medicine* 64:342, 1985.
    Something to consider in evaluating a pulmonary cavity.

27. Pohlson, E. C., McNamara, J. J., Char, C., et al. Lung abscess: A changing pattern of the disease. *Am. J. Surg.* 150:97, 1985.
    Clinical review (see also Ann. Surg. 197:775, 1983).

152. PULMONARY NODULES

Jerry L. Spivak

The discovery of a pulmonary nodule or nodules in an asymptomatic patient presents an interesting but difficult diagnostic problem. In large series, 40 percent of such lesions are neoplastic (35% primary, 5% metastatic), 40 percent are granulomas, and the rest are of varying origins, including lipomas, arteriovenous fistulas, adenomas, hamartomas, hematomas, hemangiomas, mesotheliomas, neurofibromas, lipoid granulomas, rheumatoid nodules, arteritis, poorly resolving pneumonias, interlobar effusions, and bronchopulmonary sequestration.

Usually, neither the history nor the physical examination is of help in identifying the etiology of a pulmonary nodule. Skin tests and serologic studies, whether positive or negative, do not further define the type of lesion. The usual lack of bronchial communication means that sputum cultures are often negative and sputum cytologies are positive in only 20 percent of carcinomatous lesions. Previous chest x rays provide the most valuable information, since they provide documentation of the age of the lesion, its progression, or the lack of it. The smallest lesion resolvable by the eye on the plain x ray is the 3-mm miliary granuloma. Carcinomatous lesions are not usually seen until they reach 1 cm in diameter. This is because tumors grow irregularly, not concentrically, and their margins are poorly defined. Granulomas grow at a rate of approximately 2 mm per year. Tumors double in size between 20 and 450 days. Growth in carcinomatous lesions is manifested by a visible increase in density before there is a visible increase in size. Concentric or diffuse central calcifications are specific indicators that the lesion is benign; umbilication or notching of the margins suggests malignancy. Failure of a lesion to progress in serial x rays over a 2-year period also suggests a benign etiology.

In the patient with an isolated pulmonary nodule with no signs or symptoms or lesions elsewhere, an extensive tumor search will usually be fruitless. For diagnostic purposes, the pulmonary nodule should be approached directly. As mentioned above, previous chest x rays should always be obtained. If these are not available, or the nature of the lesion remains uncertain, computed tomography (CT) should be employed to assess the pulmonary nodule.

An appropriately performed CT densitometry evaluation can identify approximately 50 percent of the lesions that are benign. For the rest, depending on the circumstances, either fiberoptic bronchoscopy, transthoracic needle aspiration, or thoracotomy will be required to obtain a definitive diagnosis, generally in that sequence. It should be emphasized, however, that a definitive diagnosis of benign lesions is difficult to establish by needle aspiration biopsy because of the physical characteristics of these lesions, and that on an actuarial basis, the difference in life expectancy with intervention as opposed to observation is not always substantial.

1. Inouye, S. K., and Sox, H. C., Jr. Standard and computed tomography in the evaluation of neoplasms of the chest. *Ann. Intern. Med.* 105:906, 1986.
   A superb analysis of the utilization of tomography for pulmonary lesions.
2. Khouri, N. F., Meziane, M. A., Zerhouni, E. A., et al. The solitary pulmonary nodule. Assessment, diagnosis, and management. *Chest* 91:128, 1987.
   Concise review.
3. Cummings, S. R., Lillington, G. A., and Richard, R. J. Estimating the probability of malignancy in solitary pulmonary nodules. *Am. Rev. Respir. Dis.* 134:449, 1986.
   A method for estimating the likelihood of a malignant nodule.
4. Cummings, S. R., Lillington, G. A., and Richard, R. J. Managing solitary pulmonary nodules. *Am. Rev. Respir. Dis.* 134:453, 1986.
   When probability analysis was employed, life expectancy rates were not greatly different for surgery, biopsy, or observation.
5. Zerhouni, E. A., Stitik, F. P., Siegelman, S. S., et al. CT of the pulmonary nodule: a cooperative study. *Radiology* 160:319, 1986.
   Role of CT scanning in diagnosis defined.
6. Levine, M. S., Weiss, J. M., Harrell, J. H., et al. Transthoracic needle aspiration biopsy following negative fiberoptic bronchoscopy in solitary pulmonary nodules. *Chest* 93:1152, 1988.
   Needle aspiration biopsy is useful when bronchoscopy is negative. (See also Chest *93:1254, 1988.)*
7. Coultas, D. B., Samet, J. M., Wiggins, C. L., et al. Clinical features of a population-

based series of patients with lung cancer presenting with a solitary nodule. *Am. Rev. Respir. Dis.* 133:302, 1986.
Forty-nine percent 5-year survival with stage I disease following surgery.

8. Casey, J. J., Stempel, B. G., Scanlon, E. F., et al. The solitary pulmonary nodule in the patient with breast cancer. *Surgery* 96:801, 1984.
Solitary pulmonary nodules in patients with cancer are often due to a second primary tumor. (See also Cancer *33:414, 1974.)*

9. Lillington, G. A. The solitary pulmonary nodule: 1974. *Am. Rev. Respir. Dis.* 110:699, 1974.
Mediastinoscopy may be helpful in determining the resectability of malignant nodules.

10. Trunk, G., Gracey, D. R., and Byrd, R. B. The management and evaluation of the solitary pulmonary nodule. *Chest* 66:236, 1974.
Conservative management is advised for the patient under age 35 since the risk of cancer is 1 in 100.

11. Goldmeier, E. Limits of visibility of bronchogenic carcinoma. *Am. Rev. Dis.* 91:232, 1965.
Carcinomatous lesions less than 1 cm in diameter are not visible.

12. Garland, L. H., Coulson, W., and Wallin, E. The rate of growth and apparent duration of untreated primary bronchial carcinoma. *Cancer* 16:694, 1963.
The average doubling time is 4.2 months for squamous carcinoma and 7.3 months for adenocarcinoma.

13. Garland, L. H. The rate of growth and natural duration of primary bronchial cancer. *Am. J. Roentgenol. Radium Ther. Nucl. Med.* 96:604, 1966.
Squamous carcinoma takes approximately 8 years to reach 2 cm; adenocarcinoma takes 16 years.

14. Theros, E. G. Varying manifestations of peripheral pulmonary neoplasms: A radiologic-pathologic correlative study. *AJR* 128:893, 1977.
40% of peripheral lesions were adenocarcinomas; 11% were carcinoid tumors.

15. Poe, R. H., and Tobin, R. E. Sensitivity and specificity of needle biopsy in lung malignancy. *Am. Rev. Respir. Dis.* 122:725, 1980.
Needle biopsy is a reliable and safe technique. (See also Cancer *43:1533, 1979 and* Chest *80:300, 1981.)*

16. Alazraki, N. P., Ranisdell, J. W., Taylor, A., et al. Reliability of gallium scan chest radiography compared to mediastinoscopy for evaluating mediastinal spread in lung cancer. *Am. Rev. Respir. Dis.* 117:415, 1978.
High correlation found between gallium uptake and the presence of tumor.

17. Chui, C. L., and Sickels, W. Common bony densities simulating disease in the chest. *J.A.M.A.* 234:1171, 1975.
Well-illustrated examples of osseous abnormalities simulating nodular lesions.

18. Goodwin, R. A., and Snell, J. D. The enlarging histoplasmoma. *Am. Rev. Respir. Dis.* 100:1, 1969.
A growing lesion that is easily mistaken for a neoplasm.

19. Gribetz, A. R., Damsker, B., Bottone, E. J., et al. Solitary pulmonary nodules due to nontuberculous mycobacterial infection. *Am. J. Med.* 70:39, 1981.
Solitary granulomatous nodules containing acid-fast bacilli are frequently due to atypical mycobacteria.

20. Herman, P. G., Hillman, B., Pinkus, G., et al. Unusual noninfectious granulomas of the lung. *Radiology* 121:287, 1976.
Interesting examples of nodular pulmonary lesions.

21. Yale, A. M., and Kleitsch, W. P. Solitary pulmonary nodule due to phycomycosis (mucormycosis). *Chest* 62:752, 1972.
Pulmonary infarction presenting as a solitary nodule.

22. Spear, H. C., Daughtry, D. C., Chesney, J. G., et al. Solitary pulmonary lesion due to *Dirofilaria. N. Engl. J. Med.* 278:832, 1968.
An unusual cause of a solitary nodule.

23. Mittman, C., and Bruderman, I. Lung cancer: To operate or not. *Am. Rev. Respir. Dis.* 116:477, 1977.
Excellent review.

24. Wallace, J. M., and Deutsch, A. L. Flexible fiberoptic bronchoscopy and percutaneous needle lung aspiration for evaluating the solitary pulmonary nodule. *Chest* 81:665, 1982.
   Fiberoptic bronchoscopy and needle aspiration complement each other in the diagnosis of malignant nodules. (See also Chest 81:662, 1982.)
25. Westcott, J. L. Percutaneous transthoracic needle biopsy. *Radiology* 169:593, 1988.
   State-of-the-art review.

153. RIGHT MIDDLE LOBE SYNDROME

H. Verdain Barnes

Acute or chronic atelectasis of the right middle lobe is a relatively common x-ray finding. The predilection for this lobe relates to a number of unique anatomic features. First, the main stem bronchus is unusually long and branches distally into the medial and lateral divisions. Second, the caliber of the main right middle lobe bronchus is small in comparison to other bronchi. Third, there is usually an acute angle of takeoff of the right middle lobe bronchus. These three factors result in an increased opportunity for bronchial plugging and pooling of secretions. Fourth, the right middle lobe bronchus is usually surrounded by a collar of lymph nodes that drain almost the entire right lung and some segments of the left lung. These lymph nodes, if inflamed or enlarged, can encroach on the bronchus, causing partial or complete obstruction. Erosion into the bronchus may occur and result in hemoptysis. Obstruction, regardless of its origin, usually occurs about 1 cm into the bronchus. Finally, the right middle lobe is anatomically isolated, totally or in part, from the upper and lower lobes. Consequently there is little or no collateral ventilation through the interalveolar pores of Kohn. Collateral aeration from contiguous alveoli normally protects against atelectasis in the presence of pneumonia and bronchitis and provides propulsion for coughing. In its absence, the middle lobe is prone to poor clearing of secretions, chronic infection, and bronchiectasis.

Patients with this syndrome may go for months or years without signs or symptoms. More commonly they present with the nonspecific symptoms of easy fatigue, malaise, and weight loss. The specific pulmonary complaints are (1) a dry hacking cough productive of little or no sputum (in over 90%), (2) a history of recurrent pneumonia (in about 75%), (3) a dull or pulling pleuritic chest pain confined to the right middle lobe area (in 50%), (4) hemoptysis of minimal to moderate amounts (in about 40%), and (5) on occasion, localized wheezing.

The diagnosis of the syndrome is made by x ray. The right lateral chest view is crucial. There is a triangular or quadrilateral opacified area that may only be seen on the lateral view. An associated finding is depression of the horizontal fissure. Hilar adenopathy with or without calcification is commonly seen. Unless carefully studied, the opacified area may be mislabeled as an interlobar effusion or a prominent right heart border with an elevated right diaphragm. Diagnosis of the underlying cause requires sputum stains and cultures for bacteria, tuberculosis, and fungi; fiberoptic bronchoscopy; biopsy; culture, and washings for cytology; and bronchograms to demonstrate bronchial occlusion or bronchiectasis. If these procedures are inconclusive and the clinical circumstances demand a diagnosis, surgery is warranted. In most series the diagnosis is made by bronchoscopy and bronchography in about two-thirds of patients.

In recent years, the most common causes of right middle lobe syndrome are benign inflammatory disease (about 47%), neoplasia (about 24%), bronchiectasis (about 15%), and tuberculosis (about 9%). The most common neoplasm is squamous cell carcinoma of the lung. Carcinoma is far more frequent in men than in women, whereas the incidence of bronchial adenomas is about equal. Bronchoglandular fistulas and scarring are not uncommon. The most frequent miscellaneous causes are acute bronchitis and bacterial and aspiration pneumonia. Other less common causes include sarcoidosis, coccidioidomycosis, histoplasmosis, foreign body, chronic abscess with organizing pneumonitis, lipoid pneumonia, metastatic carcinoma of the breast and colon/rectum, malignant melanoma, congenital bronchial stenosis, and congenital lung cysts. The most frequent organisms isolated from primary or secondary pneumonias are *Mycobacterium tuberculosis*, streptococci, pneumococci, and staphylococci.

Surgery should be considered if malignancy is suspected, if atelectasis persists despite medical therapy, or if significant hemoptysis occurs.

1. Graham, E. A., Burford, T. H., and Mayer, J. H. Middle lobe syndrome. *Postgrad. Med.* 4:29, 1948.
   The syndrome was first labeled in this article.
2. Hampton, A. O., and King, D. S. Middle lobe of right lung: Its roentgen appearance in health and disease. *Am. J. Roentgenol.* 35:721, 1936.
   A classic.
3. Lindskog, G. E., and Spear, H. C. Middle-lobe syndrome. *N. Engl. J. Med.* 253:489, 1955.
   Reports a variety of causes, including lipoid pneumonia.
4. Culiner, M. M. The right middle lobe syndrome; a non-obstructive complex. *Dis. Chest* 50:57, 1966.
   Bronchial obstruction was found to be rare, and the lack of collateral ventilation was the most common pathogenic mechanism.
5. Simecek, C. Middle lobe syndrome. *Respiration* 27:100, 1970.
   249 cases reported; 53 of the 125 men had carcinoma.
6. Wagner, R. B., and Johnston, M. R. Middle lobe syndrome. *Ann. Thorac. Surg.* 35:679, 1983.
   In this review of 933 patients, benign inflammatory disease was the most common etiology.
7. Ludmerer, K. M., and Kissane, J. M. (eds.). Right middle lobe syndrome progressing to death in a 77-year-old woman. *Am. J. Med.* 82:471, 1987.
   A concise discussion of aspiration, but the patient had tuberculosis.

154. SPONTANEOUS PNEUMOTHORAX
H. Verdain Barnes

Spontaneous pneumothorax must be considered in any patient complaining of a sudden onset of chest pain, dyspnea, or cough in the absence of an obvious cause. The bimodal incidence peaks of this disorder are from 20 to 40 and 50 to 60 years of age. Men predominate in all age groups. On occasion the onset of symptoms is insidious, but less than 1 percent are completely asymptomatic. About 20 percent of patients have a history of physical exertion prior to or coinciding with the onset of symptoms.

Clinically the chest pain is usually pleuritic and over the affected side. To some degree, dyspnea is almost invariably present, and cyanosis is not uncommon, particularly in the elderly. The classic physical findings of decreased breath sounds, decreased vocal and tactile fremitus, hyperresonance over the involved area, and mediastinal shift to the opposite side are often absent when the pneumothorax is less than 50 percent. The findings in pneumothorax can be indistinguishable from those of emphysema. When the diagnosis is suspected, a chest x ray should be obtained. It is important to get both an inspiratory and an expiratory film. The expiratory x ray helps in locating a small pneumothorax since lung collapse is better demonstrated during full expiration. The typical x-ray findings can be mimicked to a significant degree by large acquired or congenital thin-walled cysts, large thin-walled pneumatoceles, diaphragmatic hernias, subphrenic abscesses containing air, and large emphysematous bullae. These possibilities should, therefore, be considered in the differential diagnosis.

Most authors agree that spontaneous rupture of a subpleural bleb or bulla is probably the most common cause of spontaneous pneumothorax as compared to three to five decades ago, when active tuberculosis was the most common etiology. A number of other diseases have been reported to cause spontaneous pneumothorax. They include emphysema, chronic bronchitis, asthma, interstitial pneumonias, organizing pulmonary infarcts, sarcoidosis, diffuse interstitial fibrosis, pneumoconiosis, carcinoma of the lung, scleroderma, Marfan's syndrome, Osler-Weber-Rendu disease, tuberous sclerosis, histiocytosis, acute lymphoblastic leukemia, childhood dermatomyositis, idiopathic pulmonary hemosiderosis, alveolar proteinosis, histoplasmosis, coccidioidomycosis, endometriosis, *Pneumocystis carinii,* and acute bacterial pneumonias, particularly staphylococcal pneumonia. The incidence of left and right pneumothorax is about equal in all conditions, except Hamman-Rich syndrome, in which the left side predominates. About 2.5 percent of patients have simultaneous bilateral pneumothorax. An increasingly common cause of pneumothorax is iatrogenic following subclavian vein catheterization. This is usually an immediate complication, but can become clinically apparent hours or days after the procedure. The patients at highest risk are those on positive pressure respiratory support or who are trapping air.

The clinical course is variable. Some patients present in respiratory failure, with cyanosis and hypotension. Fortunately this presentation is rare. When it does occur, it is more likely to be in older patients with chronic obstructive pulmonary disease and in infants with acute pneumonia. The other dangerous complications are tension pneumothorax (in 10–19% of patients), hemothorax (in 1–7%), and (rarely) air embolism. The mortality in the presence of these complications may be as high as 33 percent. The degree of pneumothorax is variable, but it exceeds 50 percent in two-thirds of diagnosed cases. In patients treated conservatively without thoracotomy, the recurrence rate is about 52 percent after the first attack, 62 percent after the second attack, and 83 percent after the third.

Pathophysiologically the escape of air into the pleural cavity increases the negative intrapleural pressure to atmospheric levels or higher if the pneumothorax is over 50 percent. This usually leads to a mediastinal shift to the unaffected side. The result is a compromise of function in the unaffected side. As a result mediastinal tamponade may occur, with decreased filling of the right heart and a subsequent decrease in cardiac output. Air in the intrapleural space clears itself in time, provided the leak into the area stops. The absorption rate averages about 1.25 percent per day. Consequently, about 4 weeks is required for the resolution of an uncomplicated 35 percent pneumothorax. Recovery time can be substantially reduced by the removal of the air by needle or tube. When the pneumothorax exceeds 15 percent, evacuation of the air by one of these methods is important.

1. Kjaergaard, H. Spontaneous pneumothorax in the apparently healthy. *Acta Med. Scand. (Suppl.)* 43:1, 1932.
   The first study establishing tuberculosis as the primary cause.
2. Ruckley, C. V., and McCormack, R. J. M. The management of spontaneous pneumothorax. *Thorax* 21:139, 1966.
   A good review of the clinical features of spontaneous pneumothorax.
3. Dines, D. E., Clagett, O. T., and Good, C. A. Nontuberculous pulmonary parenchymal conditions predisposing to spontaneous pneumothorax. *J. Thorac. Cardiovasc. Surg.* 53:726, 1967.
   A number of diseases are reviewed in which spontaneous pneumothorax occurs.
4. Dines, D. E., Clagett, O. T., and Payne, W. S. Spontaneous pneumothorax in emphysema. *Mayo Clin. Proc.* 45:481, 1970.
   A good review of the disease in older patients with emphysema. Ten of 57 patients died. Massive gastrointestinal hemorrhage from acute stress ulcers complicated three of these deaths.
5. Mayo, P., Long, G. A., and McElvein, E. B. Diagnosis and treatment of spontaneous pneumothorax in patients aged 40 and over. *J. Ky. Med. Assoc.* 66:967, 1968.
   An expiratory chest x ray highlights the collapsed lung better than the routine inspiratory film.
6. Rottenberg, L. A., and Golden, R. Spontaneous pneumothorax: A study of 105 cases. *Radiology* 53:157, 1949.
   Tension pneumothorax is a complication in 10–19% of patients.

7. Gobbel, W. G., Rhea, W. G., Jr., Nelson, I. A., et al. Spontaneous pneumothorax. *J. Thorac. Cardiovasc. Surg.* 46:331, 1963.
   The recurrence rate is 52% after the first spontaneous pneumothorax, 62% after the second, and 83% after the third.

8. Norris, R. M., Jones, J. G., and Bishop, J. M. Respiratory gas exchange in patients with spontaneous pneumothorax. *Thorax* 3:427, 1968.
   A good discussion of respiratory dysfunction in this entity. In general, the greater the pneumothorax, the larger the arteriovenous shunt and the lower the arterial oxygen tension.

9. Kircher, L. T., and Swartzel, R. L. Spontaneous pneumothorax and its treatment. *J.A.M.A.* 155:24, 1954.
   The absorption rate per day is approximately 1.25%.

10. Shearin, R. P., Hepper, N. G. G., and Payne, W. S. Recurrent spontaneous pneumothorax concurrent with menses. *Mayo Clin. Proc.* 49:98, 1974.
    Pleural or diaphragmatic endometriosis was found in about 25% and diaphragmatic defects in about 19%; the remainder remain enigmatic.

11. Glauser, F. L., and Bartlett, R. H. Pneumo-peritoneum in association with pneumothorax. *Chest* 66:536, 1974.
    A rare but important association to recognize. The precipitating circumstances are discussed.

12. Lake, K. B., Rumsfeld, J., and Van Dyke, J. Infraclavicular subclavian catheterization: Another caution. *Chest* 64:475, 1974.
    Pneumothorax is the most frequent complication of this procedure.

13. Steier, M., Ching, N., Roberts, E. B., et al. Pneumothorax complicating continuous ventilatory support. *J. Thorac. Cardiovasc. Surg.* 67:17, 1974.
    38% of 544 cases were iatrogenic and 28% were spontaneous. The incidence of iatrogenic pneumothorax increased dramatically over an 8-year period; pneumothorax from other causes did not.

14. Singsen, B. H., Tedford, J. C., Platzker, A. C. G., et al. Spontaneous pneumothorax: A complication of juvenile dermatomyositis. *J. Pediatr.* 92:771, 1978.

15. Geltner, D., Friendman, G., Naparstek, E., et al. Acute lymphoblastic leukemia. *Arch. Intern. Med.* 138:292, 1978.

16. Najafi, J. A., and Guzman, L. G. Spontaneous pneumothorax in labor. *Am. J. Obstet. Gynecol.* 129:463, 1977.
    Three (articles 14–16) rare associations.

17. Yeung, K. Y., and Bonnet, J. D. Bronchogenic carcinoma presenting as spontaneous pneumothorax. *Cancer* 39:2286, 1977.
    The pneumothorax preceded the diagnosis of squamous cell carcinoma by 6 months.

18. Ohata, M., and Suzuki, H. Pathogenesis of spontaneous pneumothorax. *Chest* 77:771, 1980.
    The pleural mesothelial cells appear to play a role in Reid type 1 bulla, which the authors believe may leak at certain pressures without rupture.

19. Sivak, S. L. Late appearance of pneumothorax after subclavian venipuncture. *Am. J. Med.* 80:323, 1986.
    The clinical manifestations may not appear for up to 4 days post procedure.

20. Joe, L., Gordin, F., and Parker, R. H. Spontaneous pneumothorax with *Pneumocystis carinii* infection. *Arch. Intern. Med.* 146:1816, 1986.
    Another cause in a patient with the acquired immunodeficiency syndrome.

21. Shashy, S. S., Jones, B. C., and Kitchens, C. S. Spontaneous pneumothorax in a patient with Osler-Weber-Rendu disease. *South. Med. J.* 78:1393, 1985.
    A rare cause of pneumothorax.

22. Hall, J. R., Pyeritz, R. E., Dudgeon, D. L., et al. Pneumothorax in the Marfan syndrome: Prevalence and therapy. *Ann. Thorac. Surg.* 37:500, 1984.
    These authors found a prevalence of 4.4% in 249 patients.

23. Kernodle, D. S., Di Raimondo, C. R., and Fulkerson, W. J. Re-expansion pulmonary edema after pneumothorax. *South. Med. J.* 77:318, 1984.
    A rare complication.

X. MISCELLANEOUS DISORDERS

155. DEMENTIA
David W. Buchholz

Dementia is global deterioration of cognitive function despite clear consciousness. It differs from mental retardation, in which intellectual impairment is chronic and stable, and from delirium, in which consciousness is clouded. In addition, delirium tends to be more acute and reversible than dementia, since delirium is usually caused by a temporary metabolic, toxic, vascular, or traumatic insult to the brain.

Dementia is a symptom complex with many causes, and the symptoms are behavioral alterations consequent to cognitive dysfunction. Patients with mild dementia often recognize their early behavioral changes, but patient self-insight is lost as dementia progresses. Diagnosis is complicated by difficulty in distinguishing the early symptoms of dementia from the normal, mild, age-related decline of cognition, especially memory. This benign, senescent memory loss does not interfere with occupational or social performance. Conversely, demented patients suffering from short-term memory loss tend to routinely forget locations of objects left around the home, purposes of shopping trips, and directions for automotive travel. Eventually, long-term memory also suffers, and patients forget names of close acquaintances and locations of rooms within their homes.

Language, calculation, visuospatial orientation, problem solving, abstract thinking, and judgment all deteriorate in dementia, sometimes even before memory. Demented patients become withdrawn and disinterested, and some are suspicious, irritable, and hostile. They require increasing assistance with formerly independent, self-motivated activities, and, if left unsupervised, demented patients are liable to become lost, have motor vehicle mishaps, and cause household accidents such as kitchen fires. Commonly, unrecognized demented patients with stable, supportive home environments become recognized as a result of hospitalization or some other perturbation of normal routines that causes them to decompensate.

Well over half of cases of dementia are of Alzheimer's type (DAT). It is estimated that 2 to 3 million elderly persons in the United States alone have DAT. There is no meaningful distinction based on age of onset of DAT, and consequently the terms "senile" and "presenile" dementia have become outmoded. In the absence of specific cerebral biopsy findings, the antemortem diagnosis of DAT is always tentative and one of exclusion. The major morphologic changes of DAT include cortical atrophy, loss of large neurons, neurofibrillary tangles, and neuritic plaques. Neurofibrillary tangles are abnormal neurons filled with paired helical filaments, and neuritic plaques are clusters of degenerating nerve terminals containing amyloid protein. All of these changes are found in normal aged brains, but the extent and distribution of the changes are highly characteristic in DAT brains. A fascinating clue to the cause of DAT is the presence of DAT-like clinical and neuropathologic abnormalities in patients with Down's syndrome (trisomy 21) who live at least 40 years. There is therefore speculation that overabundance and neuronal accumulation of a gene product of chromosome 21 is a major factor in DAT. Some cases of DAT appear to have autosomal dominant inheritance with age-dependent onset, and the concordance of monozygotic twins for DAT is about fivefold that of dizygotic twins. Nonetheless, toxic, infective, and traumatic factors may also play roles in the pathogenesis of DAT.

Biochemically, the predominant neurotransmitter disturbance in DAT is a cholinergic deficit, and there is a strong correlation between degree of dementia and cerebral loss of choline acetyltransferase, the enzymatic source of acetylcholine. The finding of preserved cholinergic receptor function in DAT has raised the as yet unfulfilled hope of cholinergic substitution therapy for DAT. Trials of choline and lecithin, the precursors of acetylcholine, have failed. Efforts using physostigmine, which blocks acetylcholinesterase and thereby increases available acetylcholine, have yielded partial benefit in some patients, but physostigmine has many disadvantages as a routine therapeutic agent. Studies of other approaches to cholinergic replacement or enhancement are ongoing, but abnormalities in somatostatinergic and noradrenergic systems in at least some patients with DAT should temper optimism about a strictly cholinergic treatment strategy for DAT.

After DAT, the other major cause of true dementia is multiinfarct dementia (MID). It is not simply the presence of either large vessel disease (atherosclerosis) or small vessel disease (hypertensive lipohyalinosis, vasculitis) that causes dementia; it is the consequent volume and distribution of cerebral infarctions that causes MID. The diagnosis of MID has long been controversial and should be reserved for cases with compelling strokelike clinical features and radiographic evidence. The controversy has been renewed by recent discussions of Binswanger's disease, a condition of periventricular demyelination and multiple microinfarctions in the setting of chronic hypertensive small vessel disease, which high-resolution cranial imaging data suggest may be a more common cause of dementia and gait disorder in the elderly than previously suspected. The primary treatment of MID is prevention of stroke, and alleged cerebral vasodilators do not appear therapeutic for this or any other form of dementia.

Another controversial but less common cause of dementia is normal-pressure hydrocephalus (NPH), a form of communicating hydrocephalus in which intracranial pressure (ICP) is normal most of the time but rises too high for too long during the ICP rise normally accompanying rapid eye movement (REM) sleep. The cause is thought to be impaired cerebrospinal fluid (CSF) resorption, probably as a result of chronic subarachnoid inflammation due to, for example, prior subarachnoid hemorrhage or meningitis. The syndrome of NPH is classically defined as a triad of dementia, gait apraxia, and urinary incontinence, all thought to result from compromise of periventricular white matter tracts consequent to ventricular expansion. Extrapyramidal features such as Parkinsonism are also common in NPH. The diagnosis is often suspected on radiographic grounds, usually cranial computed tomography (CT) scan evidence of enlargement of the ventricles much greater than the cortical sulci and fissures. Diagnostic efforts should include CSF examination to measure ICP and to exclude chronic meningitis, and CSF can be obtained at the time of radionuclide cisternography to look for abnormal accumulation of tracer within the ventricles indicating impaired CSF resorption. Cranial magnetic resonance imaging (MRI) may show transependymal CSF leakage in NPH, and prolonged ICP monitoring may reveal abnormal ICP rises during REM sleep. Serial lumbar punctures in true, reversible NPH should be followed by at least transient measurable improvement in mentation and gait. The definitive treatment of NPH is ventricular decompression via surgical shunting of CSF, but results are often disappointing and sometimes deleterious unless treated patients have a clear-cut predisposing cause for NPH, a relatively brief history of NPH symptoms dominated by gait disorder, and a thorough, positive diagnostic evaluation.

Alcohol abuse causes dementia in many ways, including recurrent head trauma, coagulopathy leading to subdural hematomas, vitamin deficiencies such as thiamine (Korsakoff's syndrome) and niacin (pellagra), and direct neurotoxicity. Abstinence and vitamin replacement may achieve partial recovery. Other neurotoxins such as lead, arsenic, mercury, and illicit, abused substances can lead to dementia. Prescription medication can readily produce reversible dementia, especially agents such as anticholinergics, centrally acting antihypertensives, sedative hypnotics, and narcotic analgesics. Correctable metabolic causes of dementia include hypothyroidism, vitamin B_{12} deficiency, uremia, and hepatic insufficiency. A variety of cerebral and meningeal infections, some of which are treatable, can result in dementia. The list contains neurosyphilis, Lyme disease, fungal and parasitic infections, Creutzfeldt-Jakob disease, and human immunodeficiency virus (HIV) infection. Intracranial mass lesions such as neoplasm (especially frontal meningioma or glioma), subdural hematoma, and high-pressure hydrocephalus can yield dementia and may respond well to surgical treatment. Dementia is often associated with neurodegenerative diseases such as Parkinson's disease, progressive supranuclear palsy, and Huntington's disease as well as multiple sclerosis and a variety of rare metabolic, enzymatic, and storage disorders involving the brain.

The most common source of treatable "dementia" is depression causing "pseudodementia." Depressed elderly patients often have apathy, psychomotor retardation, deficient attention and concentration, and forgetfulness. Mood disturbance may be denied, and these depressed patients therefore seem demented, although they tend to complain much more of their cognitive loss than do truly demented patients. The diagnostic dilemma of dementia vs. pseudodementia is confounded by the high frequency of reactive depression complicating true dementia, especially in the early stages when patient self-insight is preserved. Since depression is a treatable illness, it behooves the clinician to keep it high in the differential diagnosis of dementia, and often an empiric trial of antidepressant medication is worthwhile.

Routine blood studies for dementia should consist of CBC, chemistry panel, thyroid screening, vitamin B_{12} level, and fluorescent treponemal antibody assay (FTA). (Rapid plasma reagin [RPR] is falsely negative for late syphilis in up to one-third of cases.) In some instances it is appropriate to include screening for heavy metal toxicity, abused substances, vasculitis, and HIV and Lyme disease antibodies. Head imaging, either CT or MRI, is essential to look for evidence of multiple infarctions, hydrocephalus, and mass lesions. CSF examination is needed to evaluate positive serum syphilis serology, suspected chronic meningitis, and apparent NPH. Electroencephalography (EEG) in dementia is usually normal or nonspecifically (slowed) and therefore unhelpful but can show diagnostic features of Creutzfeldt-Jakob disease. At minimum, an abbreviated standardized test such as the Mini-Mental State Examination should be performed at baseline and as part of serial follow-up, and more extensive, formal cognitive testing is highly advisable. Such testing can confirm the presence of dementia (as opposed to benign forgetfulness of the elderly), can determine a pattern of cognitive impairment pointing to a specific cause of dementia, and can help sort out the relative contributions of dementia and depression. In a similar vein, psychiatric evaluation may be helpful.

The management of dementia depends on its cause; of course, any treatable underlying disease should be corrected. General medical issues such as maximizing visual and auditory acuity should not be overlooked. Medications should be kept as simple as possible, and unnecessary psychoactive medications should be specifically avoided. The opportunity for abuse of alcohol and illicit drugs should be eliminated. Tricyclic antidepressant therapy such as nortriptyline may be helpful but may also cause undesirable anticholinergic and sedative side effects, and therefore dosage should start low and be increased very slowly. Neuroleptics such as haloperidol in low dosage may assist in controlling nocturnal agitation. The tendency to "sundowning" may be further reduced by keeping demented patients active during the day, avoiding naps, and thereby increasing nocturnal sleep need. Potentially injurious activities such as cooking and driving should be restricted. Psychological and resource counseling is often helpful to families, especially those keeping demented patients at home. Inevitably the care needs of demented patients grow, and institutionalization often becomes a necessity.

1. Gurland, B., and Toner, J. Differentiating Dementia from Nondementia Conditions. In R. Mayeux, and W. G. Rosen (eds.), *The Dementias.* New York: Raven Press, 1983. P. 1.
   Is the forgetful elderly patient demented or simply elderly?
2. Jenkyn, L. R., Reeves, A. G., Warren T., et al. Neurologic signs in senescence. *Arch. Neurol.* 42:1154, 1985.
   More on differentiation between normality and abnormality with aging.
3. Tomlinson, B. E., Blessed, G., and Roth, M. Observations on the brains of nondemented old people. *J. Neurol. Sci.* 7:331, 1968.
   This and the following companion reference are landmark neuropathologic studies.
4. Tomlinson, B. E., Blessed, G. and Roth M. Observations on the brains of demented old people. *J Neurol. Sci.* 11:205, 1970.
5. Folstein, M., Folstein, S., and McHugh, P. R. Mini-Mental State: a practical method for grading the cognitive state of patients for the clinician. *J. Psychiat. Res.* 12:189, 1975.
   The original publication of the most widely used cognitive screening test.
6. Katzman, R. Alzheimer's disease. *N. Engl. J. Med.* 314:964, 1986.
   An outstanding review.
7. McKhann, G., Drachman, D., Folstein, M., et al. Clinical diagnosis of Alzheimer's disease: Report of the NINCDS-ADRDA Work Group under the auspices of Department of Health and Human Services Task Force on Alzheimer's Disease. *Neurology* 34:939, 1984.
   The current diagnostic criteria for DAT.
8. Tierney, M. C., Fisher, R. H., Lewis, A. J., et al. The NINCDS-ADRDA Work Group

criteria for the clinical diagnosis of probable Alzheimer's disease: A clinicopathologic study of 57 cases. *Neurology* 38:359, 1988.
Neuropathologic assessment of the clinical criteria for the diagnosis of DAT.

9. Morris, J. C., and Fulling, K. Early Alzheimer's disease. *Arch. Neurol.* 45:345, 1988.
A look at the initial stages of DAT.

10. Mesulam, M. M. Slowly progressive aphasia without generalized dementia. *Ann. Neurol.* 11:592, 1982.
DAT may begin as a remarkably focal progressive cognitive deficit, such as aphasia, or perhaps this is a different disease.

11. Mayeux, R., Stern, Y., and Spanton, S. Heterogeneity in dementia of the Alzheimer type: Evidence of subgroups. *Neurology* 35:453, 1985.
Either DAT has very variable manifestations or we are lumping together multiple different diseases under the label DAT.

12. Jorm, A. F. Subtypes of Alzheimer's dementia: A conceptual analysis and critical review. *Psychol. Med.* 15:543, 1985.
More on the variety of what we call DAT.

13. Martin, A., Brouwers, P., Lalonde, F., et al. Towards a behavioral typology of Alzheimer's patients. *J. Clin. Exp. Neuropsychol.* 8:594, 1986.
An effort to clinically distinguish DAT variants.

14. Berg, L., Danziger, W. L., Storandt, M., et al. Predictive features in mild senile dementia of the Alzheimer type. *Neurology* 34:563, 1984.
An effort to prognosticate in cases of DAT.

15. Coyle, J. T., Price, D. L., and Delong, M. R. Alzheimer's disease: A disorder of cortical cholinergic innervation. *Science* 219:1184, 1983.
A statement of the essential biochemical defect in DAT.

16. Whitehouse, P. J., Price, D. L., Clark, A. W., et al. Alzheimer's disease: Evidence for selective loss of cholinergic neurons in the nucleus basalis. *Ann. Neurol.* 10:122, 1981.
Some researchers believe that the generalized cortical cholinergic deficit in DAT is a consequence of neuronal depletion in a small subcortical region, the nucleus basalis, that provides diffuse cholinergic input to the cortex.

17. Perry, E., Tomlinson, B., Blessed, G., et al. Correlation of cholinergic abnormalities with senile plaques and mental test scores in senile dementia. *Br. Med. J.* 2:2457, 1978.
Degree of dementia, extent of neuropathology as measured by senile (neuritic) plaques, and cholinergic deficit positively correlate in DAT.

18. Iacono, R. P., and Sandyk, R. Noncholinergic mechanisms in Alzheimer's disease. *Ann. Neurol.* 21:311, 1987.
There are multiple neurochemical disturbances in at least some patients with DAT, not simply cholinergic deficiency.

19. Mace, N. L., and Rabins, P. V. *The 36 Hour Day: A Family Guide to Caring for Persons with Alzheimer's Disease.* Baltimore: Johns Hopkins Press, 1981.
The definitive resource for families of patients with DAT.

20. Whitehouse, P. J. The concept of subcortical and cortical dementia: Another look. *Ann. Neurol.* 19:1, 1986.
A critical reappraisal of this dubious distinction between types of dementias.

21. Cummings, J. L., Miller, B., Hill, M. A., et al. Neuropsychiatric aspects of multi-infarct dementia and dementia of the Alzheimer's type. *Arch. Neurol.* 44:389, 1987.
A look at the clinical similarities and differences between the two leading causes of dementia.

22. Brust, J. C. M. Dementia and Cerebrovascular Disease. In R. Mayeux, and W. G. Rosen (eds.), *The Dementias.* New York: Raven Press, 1983. P. 131.
Not all vascular dementia is alike.

23. O'Brien, M. D. Vascular dementia is underdiagnosed. *Arch. Neurol.* 45:797, 1988.
I doubt it, but this article thoroughly examines the diagnostic difficulties that perpetuate this controversy.

24. Brust, J. C. M. Vascular dementia is overdiagnosed. *Arch. Neurol.* 45:799, 1988.
The other point of view (see above), thoughtfully presented.

25. Caplan, R. R., and Schoene, W. C. Clinical features of subcortical arteriosclerotic encephalopathy (Binswanger's disease). *Neurology* 28:1206, 1978.
   A good description of the full-blown version of this syndrome that we now realize may be much more common in milder forms.
26. Kinkel, W. R., Jacobs, L., and Plachini, I. Subcortical arteriosclerotic encephalopathy (Binswanger's disease): Computed tomographic, nuclear magnetic resonance, and clinical correlations. *Arch. Neurol.* 42:951, 1985.
   A newer look at Binswanger's disease with the help of MRI.
27. Katzman, R. Normal-pressure Hydrocephalus. In C. E. Wells (ed.), *Dementia* (2nd ed.). Philadelphia: F. A. Davis, 1977. P. 69.
   Much remains to be understood about NPH; the final word has yet to be written.
28. Haase, G. R. Diseases Presenting as Dementia. In C. E. Wells (ed.), *Dementia* (2nd ed.). Philadelphia F. A. Davis, 1977. P. 27.
   Exhaustive review of causes of dementia other than DAT and MID.
29. Wells, C. Pseudodementia. *Am. J. Psychiatry* 136:895, 1979.
   A clinical analysis of dementia-like behavior attributable to depression.

156. MEDICAL COMPLICATIONS OF ALCOHOLISM
Jerry L. Spivak

PORTER: *. . . drink, sir, is a great provoker of three things.*
MACDUFF: *What three things does drink especially provoke?*
PORTER: *Marry, sir, nose-painting, sleep, and urine. Lechery, sir, it provokes and it unprovokes; it provokes the desire, but it takes away the performance. . . .*
                                                                         (Macbeth II, i)

Custom, convenience, variety, and legality have made alcohol society's mood-altering drug of choice. Alcohol is a toxin, a by-product of microbial metabolism. It provides calories but no nourishment; it produces relaxation but impairs judgment; it stimulates fatty acid synthesis but blocks gluconeogenesis; it promotes the detoxification of some drugs but increases the toxicity of others. Directly or indirectly, alcohol has been demonstrated to be toxic for every organ in the body. The most common complications of excess alcohol intake are alterations in mental status and physical coordination. If sufficient alcohol is ingested, coma, followed by death, may ensue. The body cannot excrete alcohol efficiently by either the lungs or the kidney, and the liver bears the responsibility for its metabolism. Oxidation of alcohol by the liver is carried out by the alcohol dehydrogenase system and the microsomal ethanol-oxidizing system. These metabolic pathways are saturated at low concentrations of the drug, and consequently alcohol is metabolized at a constant rate that is independent of the blood alcohol level. The rate of metabolism of alcohol is, however, enhanced by constant drinking.

The mood alterations provoked by alcohol are equally balanced by the mood alterations that occur with abstinence. There is a spectrum of symptoms associated with withdrawal from alcohol. Cessation of drinking results in tremulousness, confusion, agitation, disorientation, nausea, vomiting, and insomnia. Coarse tremor and hallucinations may ensue, with peak frequency within the first 24 hours of withdrawal. In spite of the hallucinations, the sensorium is usually otherwise clear. Seizures may occur within the first 48 hours, followed within 72 to 96 hours by delirium tremens, a state of psychic, somatic, and autonomic overactivity that has the potential to be fatal. The severity of withdrawal symptoms is proportional to the duration of drinking. The first clue that a withdrawal syndrome is pending may come on morning rounds. If, when greeting one patient, the patient in the next bed responds, delirium tremens is imminent (Entman's sign).

The clinical features of delirium tremens include fever, tachycardia, hallucinations, agitation, diaphoresis, disorientation, tremulousness, incontinence, and dehydration. Therapy should be directed at correcting or preventing hypovolemia, sedating the patient, and preventing him from being harmful to himself or others. Alcoholics are, of course, prone to traumatic, infectious, and metabolic complications that can coexist with and be obscured by the withdrawal reaction. These must be carefully searched for.

Alcohol itself has not proved to be an effective agent for either prevention or correction of delirium tremens. Phenothiazines also have no place in therapy since they provoke seizures and can produce hypotension. Drugs that share cross-tolerance with alcohol, such as paraldehyde or the benzodiazepines, can prevent withdrawal reactions and act as effective sedatives during withdrawal. The benzodiazepines appear to be more effective than paraldehyde and less toxic. Beta blockers will also ameliorate withdrawal symptoms.

Chronic alcoholism produces damage in many organs. The liver is most commonly affected since it is responsible for metabolizing the drug. Even in the presence of adequate nutrition, prolonged alcohol ingestion results in liver damage. Within the liver, alcohol blocks gluconeogenesis, stimulates fatty acid synthesis and lactate production, and damages mitochondria, in part through its metabolite acetaldehyde. The clinical results of these effects are hypoglycemia, hyperlipidemia, lactic acidosis, hyperuricemia, and acute alcoholic hepatitis with global impairment of liver function. Continued alcohol consumption leads, of course, to cirrhosis with portal hypertension.

Alcohol attacks other areas of the gastrointestinal tract as well, provoking vomiting (a prerequisite for the Mallory-Weiss syndrome), gastritis, peptic ulceration, pancreatitis, and malabsorption of vitamins B_{12}, thiamine, B_6, and possibly folic acid. Other metabolic effects include hypomagnesemia, hypophosphatemia, metabolic alkalosis, ketoacidosis, dehydration, hyperosmolality, glucose intolerance, and impairment of protein synthesis. While acute intoxication impairs the metabolism of anticoagulants, anticonvulsants, hypnotics, and oral hypoglycemic agents, chronic alcoholism results in the enhanced metabolism of warfarin (Coumadin), phenytoin, isoniazid, phenobarbital, tolbutamide and testosterone. As a corollary, drugs such as disulfiram, chlorpropamide, and tolbutamide can potentiate the side effects of alcohol by impairing its metabolism.

The hematologic effects of alcohol include suppression of erythropoiesis, granulopoiesis, and thrombopoiesis, with hyperferremia and vacuolization of early erythroid and myeloid precursors. Alcohol also impairs folic acid metabolism and facilitates the development of ringed sideroblasts. In addition to impairing granulocyte and platelet production, alcohol impairs the function of these cells, thus placing the patients at a greater risk from infection or bleeding.

Cardiac toxicity from alcohol may derive directly from its effects on the myocardium or indirectly from the associated complication of thiamine deficiency. The severity of alcoholic cardiomyopathy is directly proportional to the duration of symptoms.

Musculoskeletal complications of alcohol include acute myopathy and myoglobinuria with a biochemical defect resembling that of McArdle's syndrome. In some patients, a chronic myopathy has been described. Osteoporosis and osteonecrosis of the hip may occur, the latter presumably due to fat embolization.

Alcohol attacks the nervous system in many ways, most of which are not understood. The consequences of excessive intake and of abstinence have been described above. Other syndromes include cerebellar degeneration, central pontine myelinolysis, and peripheral neuropathy. Alcoholics may ingest other toxins, such as methanol and ethylene glycol, or use sedatives or hypnotics whose effects may be potentiated by the alcohol. In addition, concomitant thiamine deficiency (Wernicke-Korsakoff syndrome), niacin deficiency, or ascorbic acid deficiency can contribute to the neurologic abnormalities. Since alcoholics are prone to seizures and loss of consciousness, head trauma and subdural hematoma must be considered in an alcoholic with a neurologic disorder. Once liver disease is advanced, hepatic encephalopathy may complicate the picture. Clearly, alcohol is a formidable agent and it continues to maintain its role as a major public health problem.

1. Sellers, E. M., and Kalant, H. Alcohol intoxication and withdrawal. *N. Engl. J. Med.* 294:757, 1976.
   An important review.

2. Smuckler, E. A. Alcoholic drink: Its production and effects. *Fed. Proc.* 34:2038, 1975.
   Interesting facts discussed in a wry manner.
3. Eckardt, M. J., Harford, T. C., Kaelber, C. T., et al. Health hazards associated with alcohol consumption. *J.A.M.A.* 246:648, 1981.
   Comprehensive review. (See also Johns Hopkins Med. J. *141:235 and 273, 1977).*
4. Mendelson, J. H., and Mello, N. K. Biologic concomitants of alcoholism. *N. Engl. J. Med.* 301:912, 1979.
   Review of the antecedents and consequences of alcohol abuse.
5. Seixas, F. Alcohol and its drug interactions. *Ann. Intern. Med.* 83:86, 1975.
   A brief review.
6. Lieber, C. S. Alcohol, protein metabolism, and liver injury. *Gastroenterology* 79:373, 1980.
   Discussion of the toxic effects of ethanol and acetaldehyde.
7. Van Thiel, D. H., Lipsitz, H. D., Porter, L. E., et al. Gastrointestinal and hepatic manifestations of chronic alcoholism. *Gastroenterology* 81:594, 1981.
   Thorough review. (For further discussion of alcoholic hepatitis, see Gastroenterology *74:276, 1978.)*
8. Orrego, H., Blake, J. E., Blendis, L. M., et al. Long-term treatment of alcoholic liver disease with propylthiouracil. *N. Engl. J. Med.* 317:1421, 1987.
   This was not effective if ethanol intake was high.
9. Victor, M. The role of hypomagnesemia and respiratory alkalosis in the genesis of alcohol-withdrawal symptoms. *Ann. N.Y. Acad. Sci.* 215:235, 1973.
   Hyperexcitability of the nervous system thought to be due to both hypomagnesemia and respiratory alkalosis. (See Lancet *2:549, 1978.)*
10. Ng, S. K., Hauser, A., Brust, J. C. M., et al. Alcohol consumption and withdrawal in new-onset seizures. *N. Engl. J. Med.* 319:666, 1988.
    New-onset seizures were found to be related to the quantity of ethanol consumed rather than ethanol withdrawal. (See also N. Engl. J. Med. *319:715, 1988.)*
11. Thompson, W. L. Management of alcohol withdrawal syndromes. *Arch. Intern. Med.* 138:278, 1978.
    Diazepam recommended for control of withdrawal.
12. Kraus, M. L., Gottlieb, L. D., Horowitz, R. I., et al. Randomized clinical trial of atenolol in patients with alcohol withdrawal. *N. Engl. J. Med.* 313:905, 1985.
    Beta blockade ameliorated withdrawal symptoms. (See also N. Engl. J. Med. *313:951, 1985.)*
13. Madison, L. L., Lochner, A., and Wulff, J. Ethanol-induced hypoglycemia: II. Mechanism of suppression of hepatic gluconeogenesis. *Diabetes* 16:252, 1967.
    Altered NADH/NAD ratio is thought to underlie the hypoglycemic effect of alcohol.
14. Miller, P. D., Heinz, R. E., and Waterhouse, C. Treatment of alcoholic acidosis. *Arch. Intern. Med.* 138:67, 1978.
    Intravenous glucose recommended as the most effective treatment for alcoholic ketoacidosis.
15. Robinson, A. G., and Loeb, J. N. Ethanol ingestion: Commonest cause of elevated plasma osmolality? *N. Engl. J. Med.* 284:1253, 1971.
    Ethanol can markedly raise the plasma osmolality.
16. Green, P. H. R., and Fall, A. R. Drugs, alcohol and malabsorption. *Am. J. Med.* 67:1066, 1979.
    Effects of alcohol on absorption reviewed.
17. Herbert, V., and Colman, N. Introduction: The multifactorial causes of hematologic problems seen with alcoholism. *Semin. Hematol.* 17:83, 1980.
    Part of a symposium devoted to the hematologic complications of alcohol.
18. Savage, D., and Lindenbaum, J. Anemia in alcoholics. *Medicine* 65:332, 1986.
    An excellent algorithim is provided for the evaluation of anemia. (For the mechanism of anemia, see N. Engl. J. Med. *307:845, 1982.)*
19. Smith, F. E., and Palmer, D. L. Alcoholism, infection, and altered host defenses. *J. Chronic Dis.* 29:35, 1976.
    Alcohol impairs lung clearance mechanisms, granulocyte function, and reticuloendothelial system.
20. Heinemann, H. O. Alcohol and the lung. *Am. J. Med.* 63:81, 1977.

Most effects of alcohol on the lung are indirect. (See also Am. Rev. Respir. Dis. 123:16, and Am. J. Med. 71:240, 1981.)

21. Demakis, J. G., Proskey, A., Rahimtoola, S. H., et al. The natural course of alcoholic cardiomyopathy. *Ann. Intern. Med.* 80:293, 1974.
   The longer the duration of symptoms, the poorer the prognosis. (See also Lancet 2:653, 1981.)

22. Ettinger, P. O., Wu, C. F., DeLo Cruz, C., Jr. Arrhythmias and the "holiday heart": Alcohol associated cardiac rhythm disorders. *Am. Heart J.* 95:555, 1978.
   Atrial fibrillation was the most common arrhythmia. (See also N. Engl. J. Med. 301:1049 and 1060, 1979 and Ann. Intern. Med. 98:135, 1983.)

23. Bleich, H. L., and Moore, M. J. Alcoholic myopathy in heart and skeletal muscle. *N. Engl. J. Med.* 301:28, 1979.
   Ethanol is a muscle toxin. (See also the references in the chapter on myoglobinuria.)

24. Rubenstein, A. E., and Wainapel, S. F. Acute hypokalemic myopathy in alcoholism: A clinical entity. *Arch. Neurol.* 34:553, 1977.
   Hypokalemia suggested as a cause of alcohol-induced myopathy. (See also J.A.M.A. 242:1648, 1979.)

25. Poser, C. M. Demyelination in the central nervous system in chronic alcoholism: Central pontine myelinolysis and Marchiafava-Bignami disease. *Ann. N.Y. Acad. Sci.* 215:373, 1973.
   Uncommon neurologic disorders associated with alcoholism.

26. Lee, K., Hardt, F., Moller, L., et al. Alcohol-induced brain damage and liver damage in young males. *Lancet* 2:759, 1979.
   Intellectual impairment is the earliest complication of alcoholism. (See also Science 200:1076, 1978.)

27. Serdaru, M., Hausser-Hauw, C., Laplane, D., et al. The clinical spectrum of alcoholic pellagra encephalopathy. A retrospective analysis of 22 cases studied pathologically. *Brain* 111:829, 1988.
   Pellagra is often unrecognized due to the presence of other vitamin deficiencies. Therefore, vitamin replacement should always include niacin.

28. Wallis, W. E., Willoughby, E., and Baker, P. Coma in the Wernicke-Korsakoff syndrome. *Lancet* 2:400, 1978.
   Thiamine deficiency should always be considered when coma is complicated by hypothermia.

29. Behse, F., and Buchthal, F. Alcoholic neuropathy: Clinical, electrophysiological, and biopsy findings. *Ann. Neurol.* 2:95, 1977.
   Alcohol is directly toxic to peripheral nerves. (See also Lancet 2:1053, 1980.)

30. Feussner, J. R., Linfors, E. W., Blessing, C. L., et al. Computed tomography brain scanning in alcohol withdrawal seizures. *Ann. Intern. Med.* 94:519, 1981.
   Computed tomography scanning is indicated when focal neurologic deficits are observed.

31. Ryback, R. S., Eckardt, M. J., and Pautler, C. P. Clinical relationships between serum phosphorus and other blood chemistry values in alcoholics. *Arch. Intern. Med.* 140:673, 1980.
   Low serum phosphate levels may be predictive of rhabdomyolysis. (See also Arch. Intern. Med. 140:613, 1980 and Am. J. Med. 72:489, 1982.)

32. Laine, L., and Weinstein, W. M. Histology of alcoholic hemorrhagic "gastritis": an evaluation. *Gastroenterology* 94:1254, 1988.
   Edema and subepithelial hemorrhage without significant inflammation.

33. Fuller, R. K., and Roth, H. P. Disulfiram for the treatment of alcoholism. *Ann. Intern. Med.* 90:901, 1979.
   The implied potential toxicity of disulfiram is sufficient to cause abstinence in patients willing to take it.

34. McCoy, H. G., Cipolle, R. J., Ehlers, S. M., et al. Severe methanol poisoning. *Am. J. Med.* 67:804, 1979.
   Hemodialysis and inhibition of methanol metabolism by ethanol are recommended. Peritoneal dialysis is much less effective. (See also Am. J. Med. 64:749, 1978 and Medicine [Baltimore] 60:373, 1981.)

35. Asheley, M. J., Olin, J. S., le Riche, W. H., et al. Skid row alcoholism. *Arch. Intern. Med.* 136:272, 1976.
   A detailed assessment of the derelict.
36. Blass, J. P., and Gibson, G. E. Abnormality of a thiamine-requiring enzyme in patients with Wernicke-Korsakoff syndrome. *N. Engl. J. Med.* 297:1367, 1977.
   Patients who develop Wernicke's encephalopathy may have a genetic predisposition to thiamine deficiency.
37. Clark, W. D. Alcoholism: Blocks to diagnosis and treatment. *Am. J. Med.* 71:275, 1981.
   An important review. (See also Ann. Intern. Med. *77:249, 1972.)*

157. MEDICAL COMPLICATIONS OF OPIATE AND COCAINE ABUSE
Jerry L. Spivak

Self-abuse in the form of opiate addiction results in a formidable array of medical problems. They can be classified into four categories: infectious, allergic, embolic, and toxic. Infectious complications include local abscesses, tetanus, pneumonia, bacterial and fungal endocarditis, septic pulmonary embolization with abscess and empyema formation, mycotic aneurysms, osteomyelitis, septic phlebitis, acquired immunodeficiency syndrome (AIDS), malaria, syphilis, and viral hepatitis. The infectious complication most threatening to life is endocarditis. Any addict with septicemia, empyema, embolic phenomena, osteomyelitis, or a acute lung abscess must be considered to have endocarditis or endarteritis. Septic embolization from right-sided valvular lesions can be very subtle, and the regions where the lung is adjacent to the diaphragm must be carefully examined on chest x ray for nodules or small cavities. In contrast to the chronic alcoholic, who also has frequent episodes of altered consciousness, in the narcotic addict putrid lung abscesses are uncommon. This is probably due to the lack of an adverse effect of opiates on bacterial defense mechanisms. Consequently, in the addict a lung abscess is almost always due to a septic pulmonary embolus. In recent years, shared needles have also become a dominant mechanism for the transmission of human immunodeficiency virus (HIV), leading not only to dissemination of this lethal virus but also to a whole new spectrum of infections and systemic complications in heroin addicts, as a consequence of AIDS.

Repeated subcutaneous injections of the sclerosing agents used to "cut" heroin result in lymphatic obstruction, brawny nonpitting edema, and grotesque swelling of the involved extremities. In such areas deep-seated abscesses are easily overlooked. Erythema and fluctuation may be lacking, and considerable muscle mass can be destroyed without evident weakness. Soft tissue x rays are useful in revealing gas formation, and needle aspiration can be used to locate pus.

Allergic phenomena occur as a consequence of repeated injections of foreign or contaminated matter. Constant antigenic stimulation results in elevated IgM levels and biologic false-positive serologic reactions. A relationship between these findings and the occurrence of necrotizing angiitis or the nephrotic syndrome with IgM and complement deposition in the kidney in narcotic addicts has not been established. A report of necrotizing angiitis in a drug abuser in association with hepatitis B antigen indicates that immune complex disease is responsible for some cases of arteritis in this group of patients.

Nonseptic embolic phenomena are the result of inadvertent intravenous injections of talc or cotton wool along with the narcotic agent. These materials produce interstitial granuloma and eventually pulmonary fibrosis and pulmonary hypertension. Diffusing capacity and compliance are decreased. Hilar adenopathy may be seen, and in early cases pulmonary function is usually reduced out of proportion to the radiologic findings. Talc and other foreign material can also embolize to the eyes.

Toxic effects of narcotic abuse include quinine ambylopia and hemolytic anemia, and less well-defined problems, such as hypothermia, rhabdomyolysis and myoglobinuria, transverse myelitis, and polyneuritis.

The greatest threat to life is from drug overdose. In this situation it must be remembered that the drug abuser does not usually limit himself to one agent, and the comatose addict should be evaluated no differently from any other patient in coma. Attention should be directed initially to maintenance of a patent airway, respiration, circulation, and blood glucose, regardless of the size of the patient's pupils or those of his friends. The availability of the narcotic antagonist naloxone has removed the danger of respiratory depression if coma is due to an opiate. However, naloxone causes emesis and should not be administered to a patient in coma unless the airway is secure. When heroin is in short supply, methadone is often employed as a substitute. This drug has a long duration of action, often lasting 48 hours. If naloxone is relied on in a methadone overdose, repeated administration may be necessary to prevent relapse. It should also be remembered that excessive doses of naloxone can lead to withdrawal symptoms in addicted individuals.

A common complication of opiate overdose is pulmonary edema. This can occur with oral ingestion or inhalation of opiates as well as by intravenous injection and with methadone as well as heroin. The presence of lung edema may be recognized early in the course of the overdose or can occur up to 24 hours later. The edema is not due to cardiac failure or drug allergy. Hypoxia, opiate-induced antidiuretic hormone secretion, and a central neurogenic effect probably all play a role. Naloxone has no effect on opiate-induced pulmonary edema.

In recent years, cocaine has supplanted heroin as the most widely used illicit drug. Although initially considered benign and nonaddicting, cocaine use is not only addictive but can have lethal consequences, often of a sudden and unexpected nature. These include acute myocardial infarction in the absence of preexisting coronary artery disease, cardiac arrhythmias, aortic rupture, cerebrovascular complications such as subarachnoid hemorrhage, stroke, seizures, vasculitis and transient ischemic attacks, hyperthermia, rhabdomyolysis, myoglobinuria, and renal failure in addition to the dysphoric agitation of the acute intoxication. Other complications include myocarditis, pulmonary infiltrates and fibrosis, hepatitis, intestinal ischemia, nasal septum perforation, abruptio placentae, spontaneous abortion, and abnormalities of the fetus. These complications are not restricted to a particular route of administration, a particular quantity of the drug, or a particular age group. While the mechanisms for the toxic effects of cocaine are not completely understood, many are related to its stimulation of adrenergic pathways; others are undoubtedly related to its effects on membrane depolarization.

1. Sapira, J. D. The narcotic addict as a medical patient. *Am. J. Med.* 45:555, 1968.
   An excellent detailed review of the effects of addiction on each organ or tissue of the body.
2. Louria, D. B., Hensle, T., and Rose, J. The major medical complications of heroin addiction. *Ann. Intern. Med.* 67:1, 1967.
   Clinical problems encountered in 96 heroin users.
3. Fultz, J. M., Jr., and Senay, E. C. Guidelines for the management of hospitalized narcotic addicts. *Ann. Intern. Med.* 82:815, 1975.
   Good advice.
4. Garriot, J. C., and Sturner, W. Q. Morphine concentrations and survival periods in acute heroin fatalities. *N. Engl. J. Med.* 289:1276, 1973.
   Sudden death is the result of a drug effect, not hypersensitivity.
5. Steinberg, A. D., and Karliner, J. A. The clinical spectrum of heroin pulmonary edema. *Arch. Intern. Med.* 122:122, 1968.
   A common complication of heroin intoxication that may occasionally have a delayed onset.
6. Katz, S., Aberman, A., Frand, U., et al. Heroin pulmonary edema. *Am. Rev. Respir. Dis.* 106:472, 1972.
   High protein content of the edema fluid suggests capillary damage. (See also Chest 73:471, 1978.)

7. Arnett, E. N., Battle, W. E., Russo, J. V., et al. Intravenous injection of talc-containing drugs intended for oral use. *Am. J. Med.* 60:711, 1976.
   Pulmonary hypertension as a complication. (See also Chest *77:277, 1980.)*
8. Peter Paré, J. A., Fraser, R. G., Hogg, J. C., et al. Pulmonary 'mainline' granulomatosis: Talcosis of intravenous methadone abuse. *Medicine* 58:229, 1979.
   Irreversible pulmonary disease due to granuloma formation and fibrosis. (See also Am. J. Med. *68:231, 1980.)*
9. Atlee, W. E., Jr., Talc and cornstarch emboli in the eyes of drug abusers. *J.A.M.A.* 219:49, 1972.
   Methylphenidate (Ritalin) retinopathy.
10. Reisberg, B. E. Infective endocarditis in the narcotic addict. *Prog. Cardiovasc. Dis.* 22:193, 1979.
    Comprehensive review. (See also Medicine *62:173, 1983,* and Arch. Intern. Med. *148:2461, 1988.)*
11. Miller, D. J., Kleber, H., and Bloomer, J. R. Chronic hepatitis associated with drugs: Significance of hepatitis B virus. *Yale J. Biol. Med.* 52:135, 1979.
    Chronic active hepatitis in narcotic addicts is usually due to hepatitis B infection.
12. Gelb, A. M., Mildvan, D., and Stenger, R. J. The spectrum and causes of liver disease in narcotic addicts. *Am. J. Gastroenterology* 67:314, 1977.
    Alcoholic cirrhosis was common.
13. Sapico, F. L., and Montgomerie, J. Z. Vertebral osteomyelitis in intravenous drug abusers: Report of three cases and review of the literature *Rev. Infect. Dis.* 2:196, 1980.
    Gram-negative organisms predominated; cervical spine involvement was common.
14. Forlenza, S., Axelrod, J. L., and Grieco, M. H. Pott's disease in heroin addicts. *J.A.M.A.* 241:379, 1979.
    Tuberculous osteomyelitis in narcotic addicts is a more acute illness than nontuberculous infectious osteomyelitis.
15. Cherubin, C. E. Infectious disease problems of narcotic addicts. *Arch. Intern. Med.* 128:309, 1971.
    Sudden death is not unusual in addicts stricken with tetanus.
16. Brown, S. M., Stimmel, B., Taub, R. N. Immunologic dysfunction in heroin addicts. *Arch. Intern. Med.* 134:1001, 1974.
    Hyperglobulinemia, biologic false-positives, positive latex fixation, and impaired response to phytohemagglutinin.
17. Geller, S. A., and Stimmel, B. Diagnostic confusion from lymphatic lesions in heroin addicts. *Ann. Intern. Med.* 78:703, 1973.
    Lymphadenopathy in the addict is not always secondary to drug abuse.
18. Sreepada, T. C., Nicastri, A. D., and Friedman, E. A. Renal consequences of narcotic abuse. *Adv. Nephrol.* 7:261, 1978.
    Myoglobinuria, renal failure, necrotizing angiitis, proliferative glomerulonephritis secondary to septicemia, and focal glomerulosclerosis. (See also Am. J. Med. *68:42, 1980.)*
19. Scholes, J., Derosena, R., Appel, G. B., et al. Amyloidosis in chronic heroin addicts with the nephrotic syndrome. *Ann. Intern. Med.* 91:26, 1979.
    A complication associated with long-standing narcotic abuse.
20. Heffernon, J. J., Smith, W. R., Berk, J. E., et al. Hyperamylasemia in heroin addicts. *Am. J. Gastroenterol.* 66:17, 1976.
    The hyperamylasemia is not of pancreatic origin.
21. Crane, L. R., Levine, D. P., Zervos, M. J., et al. Bacteremia in narcotic addicts at the Detroit Medical Center. I. Microbiology, epidemiology, risk factors, and empiric therapy. *Rev. Infect. Dis.* 8:364, 1986.
    The staphylococcus was the most common organism and frequently methicillin-resistant.
22. Dupont, B., and Drouhet, E. Cutaneous, ocular, and osteoarticular candidiasis in heroin addicts: New clinical and therapeutic aspects in 38 patients. *J. Infect. Dis.* 152:577, 1985.
    A new Candida *syndrome in heroin abusers. (See also* Br. Med. J. *292:1096, 1986.)*

23. Miro, J. M., Brancos, M. A., Abello, R., et al. Costochondral involvement in systemic candidiasis in heroin addicts: Clinical, scintigraphic, and histologic features in 26 patients. *Arthritis Rheum.* 31:793, 1988.
    An uncommon complication. (See also Ann. Thorac. Surg. *41:89, 1986.)*
24. Kasantikul, V., Shuangshoti, S., and Taecholarn, C. Primary phycomycosis of the brain in heroin addicts. *Surg. Neurol.* 28:468, 1987.
    An unusual presentation for phycomycotic infection.
25. Haskell, L. P., Glicklich, D., and Senitzer, D. HLA associations in heroin-associated nephropathy. *Am. J. Kidney Dis.* 12:45, 1988.
    A genetic predisposition is postulated.
26. Schreiber, S. N., Leibowitz, M. R., Bernstein, L. H., et al. Limb compression and renal impairment (crush syndrome) complicating narcotic overdose. *N. Engl. J. Med.* 284:368, 1971.
    An important cause of myoglobinuria, acute renal failure, and neurologic damage.
27. Challenor, Y. B., Richter, R. W., Bruun, B., et al. Nontraumatic plexitis and heroin addiction. *J.A.M.A.* 225:958, 1973.
    Another unexplained complication.
28. Pearson, J., Richter, R. W., Baden, M. M., et al. Transverse myelopathy as an illustration of the neurologic and neuropathologic features of heroin addiction. *Hum. Pathol.* 3:107, 1972.
    Part of a symposium on narcotic abuse.
29. Duffy, J., Lidsky, M. D., Sharp, J. T., et al. Polyarthritis, polyarteritis, and hepatitis B. *Medicine* 55:19, 1976.
    Immune complex disease causing either transient polyarthritis or systemic arteritis with multiorgan involvement.
30. Tennant, F. S., Jr. Complications of propoxyphene abuse. *Arch. Intern. Med.* 132:191, 1973.
    Pulmonary edema, respiratory arrest, and death.
31. Glauser, F. L., Smith, W. R., Caldwell, A., et al. Etchlorvynol (Placidyl)-induced pulmonary edema. *Ann. Intern. Med.* 84:46, 1976.
    A nonnarcotic agent causing lung congestion after intravenous administration.
32. Anderson, R. J., Garza, H. R., Garriott, J. C., et al. Intravenous propylhexedrine (Benzedrex) abuse and sudden death. *Am. J. Med.* 67:15, 1979.
    Propylhexedrine abuse appears to produce a predisposition to fatal arrhythmias.
33. Streicher, H. Z., Gabow, P. A., Moss, A. H., et al. Syndromes of toluene sniffing in adults. *Ann. Intern. Med.* 94:758, 1981.
    Muscle weakness and rhabdomyolysis are consequences of this type of drug abuse.
34. Martin, W. R. Naloxone. *Ann. Intern. Med.* 85:765, 1976.
    A thorough review.
35. Kaufman, R. E., and Levy, S. B. Overdose treatment. *J.A.M.A.* 227:411, 1974.
    How addicts treat themselves.
36. Khantzian, E. J., and McKenna, G. J. Acute toxic and withdrawal reactions associated with drug use and abuse. *Ann. Intern. Med.* 90:361, 1979.
    An excellent review.
37. Creglar, L. L., and Mark, H. Medical complications of cocaine abuse. *N. Engl. J. Med.* 315:1495, 1986.
    A comprehensive review.
38. Gawin, F. H., and Ellinwood, E. H., Jr. Cocaine and other stimulants: Actions, abuse and treatment. *N. Engl. J. Med.* 318:1173, 1988.
39. Isner, J. M., Estes, N. A., Thompson, P. D., et al. Acute cardiac events temporally related to cocaine abuse. *N. Engl. J. Med.* 315:1438, 1986.
    Neither the dose nor the route of administration is important. (See also Am. Heart. J. *115:1068, 1988,* Arch. Pathol. Lab. Med. *112:225, 1988, and* Ann. Intern. Med. *107:13, 1987.)*
40. Roth, D., Alarcon, F. J., Fernandez, J. A., et al. Acute rhabdomyolysis associated with cocaine intoxication. *N. Engl. J. Med.* 319:673, 1988.
    Myoglobinuria, hyperthermia, disseminated intravascular coagulation, renal failure, and hepatic dysfunction due to cocaine intoxication. (See also Ann. Intern. Med. *109:335, 1988.)*

41. Mody, C. K., Miller, B. L., McIntyre, H. B., et al. Neurologic complications of cocaine abuse. *Neurology* 38:1189, 1988.
    A variety of complications related to vascular insufficiency have been observed. (See also Neurology *37:1849, 1987 and* J.A.M.A. *258:2104, 1987.)*
42. Chasnoff, I. J., Burns, W. J., Schnoll, S. H., et al. Cocaine use in pregnancy. *N. Engl. J. Med.* 313:666, 1985.
    Adverse effects occur in both the mother and the fetus.
43. Schwartz, R. H. Urine testing in the detection of drugs of abuse. *Arch. Intern. Med.* 148:2407, 1988.
    A comprehensive review.
44. Frishmein, W. H., Karpenos, A., and Molloy, T. J. Cocaine-induced coronary artery disease: Recognition and treatment. *Med. Clin. North Am.* 73:475, 1989.
    A useful review.
45. Rubin, R. B., and Neugarten, J. Cocaine-induced rhabdomyolysis masquerading as myocardial ischemia. *Am. J. Med.* 86:551, 1989.
    Not all cocaine-associated chest pain is myocardial in origin.
46. Lange, R. A., Cigarroa, R. G., Yancy, Jr., C. W., et al. Cocaine-induced coronary-artery vasoconstriction. *N. Engl. J. Med.* 321:1557, 1989.
    A possible mechanism for cocaine-associated myocardial toxicity (see also the accompanying editorial on p. 1604).

158. MYASTHENIC SYNDROME (EATON-LAMBERT SYNDROME)
H. Verdain Barnes

The myasthenic syndrome (Eaton-Lambert syndrome) is a rare disorder that is often associated with malignancy. The patient typically presents with weakness and easy fatigue of the proximal muscles. The pelvic girdle and thighs are almost invariably involved; arm and shoulder girdle complaints are unusual. About 50 percent of patients complain of dry mouth, myalgias, peripheral paresthesias, and impotence. One-third have mild difficulty in swallowing, and 20 percent complain of hoarseness and slurred speech. Transient ptosis, diplopia, and blurred vision have occasionally been reported as have cholinergic autonomic defects of pupillary constriction, sweating, lacrimation, and salivation. The mildness and rarity of ocular and bulbar signs and symptoms are distinctly different from myasthenia gravis, with which the syndrome may be confused. The findings on the physical examination may be completely normal, except for a demonstrable delay in the development of maximum voluntary muscle contraction, as, for example, in the grip. In the majority of patients, however, the deep tendon reflexes, particularly the patellar and Achilles, are weak or absent. Muscle wasting is uncommon and, if present, is not prominent.

Men predominate over women 4 : 1 after age 40 years. About 70 percent of patients in most series have a demonstrable malignancy at the time of presentation or are subsequently found to have one. In the reported series, about 75 percent of the malignancies have been small cell bronchogenic carcinomas. Large cell and squamous cell carcinoma of the lung are next in frequency, followed by rare instances of association with lymphosarcoma; reticulum cell sarcoma; rectal, renal, gastric, and basal cell carcinoma; malignant thymoma; leukemia; rheumatoid arthritis; thyrotoxicosis; sarcoidosis; and combined hypothyroidism and pernicious anemia. The duration of symptoms prior to presentation ranges from weeks to years. Those who have subsequently had tumors demonstrated have gone as long as 2.5 years before the tumor was discovered. Many of the 30 percent who have not shown tumors have now been followed for over 10 years without an explanation for the syndrome. An occasional patient develops amytrophic lateral sclerosis.

The serum potassium, sodium, magnesium, creatinine kinase, and aspartate aminotransferase levels are normal. The hemogram and levels of serum thyroxine and urinary hydroxysteroids and ketosteroids are normal. The cerebrospinal fluid is unremarkable. Muscle biopsy is not distinctive and is frequently normal. The electromyogram (EMG), however, is diagnostic. In rested muscle there is a marked depression of neuromuscular transmission after a single submaximal stimulus, and a marked facilitation of the response during repetitive stimulation at rates greater than 10 per second. This characteristic pattern is seen in all muscles stimulated, not just those in symptomatic areas. Myasthenia gravis shows essentially the opposite EMG findings.

Patients with the Eaton-Lambert syndrome show little or no response to neostigmine. Both this syndrome and myasthenia gravis patients are exquisitely sensitive to tubocurarine. The defect in neuromuscular transmission is due to the small number of acetylcholine quanta being released from the motor nerve terminal in response to the nerve impulse. This dysfunction in some patients appears to involve the cholinergic autonomic system as well as the neuromuscular junction of skeletal muscle. A similar defect is seen with hypermagnesemia and botulinus toxin. The acetylcholine quanta packets at the neuromuscular junction are normal in size but diminished in number. This has been reproduced in vitro using lung cancer tissue from a syndrome patient suggesting that the tumor contained a causative substance(s). The sensitivity of the muscle and endplate receptors is normal. In myasthenia gravis, there is a decrease in the packet size rather than packet number.

Tumor therapy provides improvement in about one-third, with an occasional patient becoming symptom-free with no demonstrable defect in neuromuscular transmission. Guanidine has been used effectively for treatment since it increases the quantity of acetylcholine released from the nerve endings by a single nerve impulse.

1. Lambert, E. H., and Eaton, L. M. Electromyography and electric stimulation of nerves in diseases of motor unit. *J.A.M.A.* 163:1117, 1957.
   A classic description of the syndrome.
2. Lambert, E. H., and Rooke, E. D. *The Remote Effects of Cancer on the Nervous System.* New York: Grune & Stratton, Inc., 1965.
   Most patients have small cell bronchogenic carcinoma.
3. Lambert, E. H. Defects of neuromuscular transmission in syndromes other than myasthenia gravis. *Ann. N.Y. Acad. Sci.* 135:367, 1966.
   The pathologic differences between the Eaton-Lambert syndrome and myasthenia gravis.
4. Wise, R. P. A myasthenic syndrome complicating bronchial carcinoma. *Anaesthesia* 17:488, 1962.
   Myalgias may be prominent.
5. Elmquist, D., and Lambert, E. H. Detailed analysis of neuromuscular transmission in a patient with myasthenic syndrome: Sometimes associated with bronchogenic carcinoma. *Mayo Clin. Proc.* 43:689, 1968.
   The characteristic EMG findings are described in detail.
6. Gutmann, L., Crosby, T. W., Takamori, M., et al. The Eaton-Lambert syndrome and autoimmune disorders. *Am. J. Med.* 53:354, 1972.
   An interesting association with thyroiditis and pernicious anemia.
7. Vroom, F. Q., and Engel, W. K. Nonneoplastic, steroid-responsive Lambert-Eaton myasthenic syndrome. *Neurology* 19:281, 1969.
   Maybe autoimmunity plays a role.
8. Mulder, D. W., Lambert, E. H., and Eaton, L. M. Myasthenic syndrome in patients with amyotrophic lateral sclerosis. *Neurology* 9:627, 1971.
   Another association to keep in mind.
9. Lambert, E. H., and Elmquist, D. Quantal components of end-plate potentials in the myasthenic syndrome. *Ann. N.Y. Acad. Sci.* 181:183, 1971.
   An updated evaluation of the underlying pathophysiology.
10. Rubenstein, A. E., Horowitz, S. H., and Bender, A. N. Cholinergic dysautonomia and Eaton-Lambert syndrome. *Neurology* 29:720, 1979.
    A carefully studied patient with evidence of nicotinic and muscarinic autonomic dysfunction.

11. Lauritzen, M., Smith, T., Fischer-Hansen, B., et al. Eaton-Lambert syndrome and malignant thymoma. *Neurology* 30:634, 1980.
    Another association with references to others.
12. Ishikawa, K., Engelhardt, J. E., Fujisawa, T., et al. A neuromuscular transmission block produced by a cancer tissue extract derived from a patient with the myasthenic syndrome. *Neurology* 27:140, 1977.
    A clear in vitro demonstration of decreased acetylcholine release produced by a substance(s) in the tumor extract.
13. Kalter, S., Dhingra, H. M., and Farha, P. Primary therapy for small cell lung cancer reversing the Eaton-Lambert syndrome. *South. Med. J.* 78:197, 1985.
    EMG findings reverted to normal after successful radio- and chemotherapy.

159. MYOGLOBINURIA

Jerry L. Spivak

Excretion of pigmented urine can be due to such diverse conditions as intravascular hemolysis; porphyria; biliary tract obstruction; parenchymal liver disease; alkaptonuria; ingestion of phenazopyridine (Pyridium), phenacetin, or phenolphthalein; an unstable hemoglobin; melanoma; and myoglobinuria. Myoglobinuria, once thought to be rare, has been recognized with increasing frequency in recent years. Myoglobin is a muscle heme compound with an affinity for oxygen greater than that of hemoglobin and less than that of cytochrome oxidase. It functions as an oxygen storage protein and also facilitates the transport of oxygen for intracellular metabolic processes. The concentration of myoglobin is highest in muscles involved in strong repetitive and sustained contractions. Myoglobin is released into the circulation when muscle is injured, but the insult producing myoglobinemia and myoglobinuria may not be associated with any histologic changes. The molecular weight of myoglobin is 17,000; in contrast to hemoglobin, it is not bound by haptoglobin (but may bind to hemopexin) and is excreted in the urine at concentrations (15–20 mg/dl) below that required to discolor plasma.

Myoglobinuria may be caused by a variety of conditions. In some instances the disorder is hereditary, with no fixed age of onset. The myoglobinuria may occur spontaneously, or it may be precipitated by infection or exercise. In many patients the muscle disorder resulting in myoglobinuria is unknown, but in some, the biochemical defect has been identified. In McArdle's syndrome, there is a deficiency of muscle phosphorylase and affected individuals are incapable of utilizing muscle glycogen for energy. There is easy fatigability, weakness, pain, and muscle cramps with exercise. These patients may also exhibit a "second-wind" phenomenon and have an increased exercise tolerance after resting. Attacks may be associated with omission of a meal before exercise, and exercise testing has resulted in a decrease in blood glucose. It has thus been suggested that seizures occurring in some of the patients with McArdle's syndrome may be the result of hypoglycemia. Although symptoms are usually present in childhood, several cases have been described in which the onset occurred in the fifth decade.

Deficiency of muscle carnitine palmityl transferase is another hereditary disorder producing muscle weakness and myoglobinuria in which the biochemical defect has been identified. Affected individuals develop myoglobinuria with exercise particularly in cold weather, after fasting, and if their diet is rich in fat. They do not exhibit a second-wind phenomenon. As in the case of McArdle's syndrome, the onset of symptoms may not occur until after age 20. Other hereditary enzymatic defects causing myoglobinuria with exertion include phosphofructokinase deficiency, which, like McArdle's syndrome, may be expressed late in life and, in addition, is associated with compensated hemolysis, phosphoglycerate kinase deficiency, phosphoglycerate mutase deficiency, and lactic dehydrogenase (LDH) deficiency.

Ischemia can produce myoglobinuria. This may be the result of compression such as in the anterior tibial syndrome or acute arterial occlusion due to embolism or thrombosis or even vena cava ligation. With sudden arterial occlusion, there is an acute onset of pain followed by extreme stiffness of the involved extremity and myoglobinuria. Massive, brawny edema occurs after 12 hours; it will not be confused with deep venous thrombosis if the urine is examined for myoglobin.

Myoglobinuria associated with carbon monoxide poisoning, heroin or cocaine intoxication, barbiturate overdose, or hypothermia may be the result of muscle ischemia due to the intoxicant, or prolonged compression of muscle due to the immobility of the comatose patient. The latter is a variant of the "crush syndrome," in which the patient's own weight produces the damage. Muscle injury occurring in this fashion may be easily overlooked since the patient is not able to communicate. All comatose patients should be examined carefully for swelling of muscle groups, which may require fasciotomy for decompression. Localized erythema or blisters on an extremity are helpful clues to the presence of prior "crush injury." Acute rhabdomyolysis due to cocaine intoxication is notable for a high incidence of renal failure, severe hepatic dysfunction, and intravascular coagulation (DIC).

Alcohol abuse can result in muscle pain and weakness, myoglobinuria, and a biochemical defect resembling that of McArdle's syndrome. The defect is reversible, but patients with a chronic myopathy due to alcohol have been described. Hypophosphatemia may be in part responsible for the myoglobinuria associated with alcohol abuse. Hypokalemia can produce muscle necrosis and myoglobinuria. This has been observed in renal tubular acidosis, excessive licorice ingestion, and with administration of amphotericin B. Myoglobinuria occurring in heat stroke has also been postulated to be due to potassium depletion. There have also been an increasing number of reports of myoglobinuria associated with viral infections. In some patients acute renal failure has occurred. The viruses implicated include influenza, echovirus 9, Epstein-Barr virus, and herpes simplex. Legionnaires' bacillus and *Francisella tularensis* can also damage skeletal muscle and cause myoglobinuria. Of particular interest are cases of myoglobinuria occurring with exertion in previously healthy persons. Using immunologic techniques, myoglobin can often be demonstrated in the urine following strenuous exercise, but few people develop gross myoglobinuria. Characteristically, exercise-induced myoglobinuria occurs after vigorous activity in an unconditioned person. Such persons, however, with conditioning can return to the same level of activity without problems. Myoglobinuria can also be precipitated by hyperpyrexia due to heat exposure, drug reactions (neuroleptic malignant syndrome), anesthetic agents (malignant hyperthermia), thyroid storm, hyperosmolarity, and methanol or strychnine intoxication. High-dose corticosteroid therapy has also been associated with myoglobinuria.

Recognition of myoglobinuria is important because of the major complications associated with it. They include fascial compression syndromes, respiratory insufficiency, and acute renal failure. The possibility of myoglobinuria should be considered in the appropriate clinical setting, particularly when a pigmented, benzidine-positive, red cell–free urine is excreted and plasma color is normal. It should be noted, however, that in some cases the urine is not grossly discolored. Absolute identification of myoglobin requires spectroscopic, electrophoretic, or immunologic analysis. In some instances, excretion of myoglobin has been delayed for over 24 hours after the onset of muscle pain or tenderness. Severe muscle injury may be accompanied by azotemia, acidosis, oliguria, and hyperkalemia. These metabolic abnormalities should be avoided since they may potentiate myoglobin-induced renal damage. The use of mannitol may be required to maintain urine flow. Hypercalcemia occurring during the diuretic phase is a peculiar feature of renal failure associated with myoglobinuria. The mechanism for this is unknown; presumably it reflects a release of calcium previously deposited in damaged muscle.

1. Gabow, P. A., Kaehny, W. D., and Kelleher, S. P. The spectrum of rhabdomyolysis. *Medicine* 61:141, 1982.
   Comprehensive review. (See also Annu. Rev. Med. *33:435, 1982.)*
2. Grossman, R. A., Hamilton, R. W., Morse, B. M., et al. Nontraumatic rhabdomyolysis and acute renal failure. *N. Engl. J. Med.* 291:807, 1974.

Hypocalcemia followed by hypercalcemia was not uncommon, and visible myoglobinuria was not always present.

3. Koffler, A., Friedler, R. M., and Massry, S. G. Acute renal failure due to nontraumatic rhabdomyolysis. *Ann. Intern. Med.* 85:23, 1976.
   Dehydration and profound hyperuricemia were observed.
4. Akmal, M., Goldstein, D. A., Telfer, N., et al. Resolution of muscle calcification in rhabdomyolysis and acute renal failure. *Ann. Intern. Med.* 89:928, 1978.
   Muscle calcium deposits occur during oliguria and resolve with recovery of renal function.
5. Fowler, W. M., Jr., Chowdhury, S. R., Pearson, C. M., et al. Changes in serum enzyme levels after exercise in trained and untrained subjects. *J. Appl. Physiol.* 17:943, 1962.
   Serum levels of muscle enzymes (LDH, AST, ALT, malic dehydrogenase, aldolase) rise with strenuous exercise.
6. Ritter, W. S., Stone, M. J., and Willison, J. T. Reduction in exertional myoglobinemia after physical conditioning. *Arch. Intern. Med.* 139:644, 1979.
   Muscle myoglobin release with exertion can be reduced by prior conditioning. (See also Arch. Intern. Med. 133:233, 1974.)
7. Perkoff, G. T., Hardy, P., and Velez-Garcia, E. Reversible acute muscular syndrome in chronic alcoholism. *N. Engl. J. Med.* 274:1277, 1966.
   An acquired disorder resembling McArdle's syndrome.
8. Richter, R. W., Challenor, Y. B., Pearson, J., et al. Acute myoglobinuria associated with heroin addiction. *J.A.M.A.* 216:1172, 1971.
   A toxic effect not necessarily associated with coma or intravenous administration of heroin.
9. Schiff, H. B., MacSearrough, E. T. M., and Kallmeyer, J. C. Myoglobinuria, rhabdomyolysis and marathon running. *Q. J. Med.* 47:463, 1978.
   57% of marathon participants had myoglobinemia; less than 15% had myoglobinuria.
10. Kendrich, W. C., Hall, A. R., and Knochel, J. P. Rhabdomyolysis and shock after intravenous amphetamine administration. *Ann. Intern. Med.* 86:381, 1977.
    Aggressive volume replacement was required to compensate for fluid loss into necrotic muscle.
11. Cogen, F. C., Rigg, G., Simmons, J. L., et al. Phencyclidine-associated acute rhabdomyolysis. *Ann. Intern. Med.* 88:210, 1978.
    Patients with phencyclidine (PCP) intoxication are at risk of rhabdomyolysis and renal failure. (See Arch. Intern. Med. 140:568, 1980 and Am. J. Nephrol. 1:91, 1981.)
12. Haimovici, H. Arterial embolism, myoglobinuria, and renal tubular necrosis. *Arch. Surg.* 100:639, 1970.
    Myoglobinuria 12 hours after the arterial occlusion.
13. Dominic, J. A., Koch, M., Guthrie, G. P., et al. Primary aldosteronism presenting as myoglobinuric acute renal failure. *Arch. Intern. Med.* 138:1433, 1978.
    Potassium depletion from any cause can produce myoglobinuria. (See also J.A.M.A. 220:967, 1972, 241:2294, 1979, and N. Engl. J. Med. 274:602, 1966.)
14. Grunfeld, J. P., Ganeval, D., Chanard, J., et al. Acute renal failure in McArdle's disease. *N. Engl. J. Med.* 286:1237, 1972.
    Myoglobinuria, renal failure, and hypercalcemia. (See Am. J. Med. 48:693, 1970 for a review of McArdle's disease.)
15. Reza, M. J., Kor, N. C., Pearson, C. M., et al. Recurrent myoglobinuria due to muscle carnitine palmityl transferase deficiency. *Ann. Intern. Med.* 88:610, 1978.
    A low-fat diet and avoidance of strenuous exertion reduce the frequency of myoglobinuria in this disorder.
16. Vora, S., Davidson, M., Seaman, C., et al. Heterogeneity of the molecular lesions in inherited phosphofructokinase deficiency. *J. Clin. Invest.* 72:1995, 1983.
    Review of the metabolic basis for this disorder.
17. Spivak, J. L., and Conti, C. R. Post-seizure myoglobinuria. *Johns Hopkins Med. J.* 124:18, 1969.
    An unusual form of exercise-induced myoglobinuria.

18. Kopyt, N., Myers, A. R., Mandel, S., et al. Recurrent rhabdomyolysis as a manifestation of alcoholic myopathy. *Arch. Intern. Med.* 144:821, 1984.
19. Simon, N. M., Rovner, R. N., and Berlin, B. S. Acute myoglobinuria associated with type A$_2$ (Hong Kong) influenza. *J.A.M.A.* 212:1704, 1970.
    Viral infection precipitating myoglobinuria in a susceptible host. (See also Ann. Intern. Med. *80:359, 362, 1974 and for herpes viruses, see* Arch. Intern. Med. *138:422, 1978.)*
20. Posner, M. R., Caudill, M. A., Brass, R., et al. Legionnaires' disease associated with rhabdomyolysis and myoglobinuria. *Arch. Intern. Med.* 140:848, 1980.
    The clinical spectrum of legionnaires' disease continues to expand. (See also Chest *84:633, 1983.)*
21. Kaiser, A. B., Rieves, D., Price, A. H., et al. Tularemia and rhabdomyolysis. *J.A.M.A.* 252:241, 1985.
22. Bennett, W. R., and Huston, D. P. Rhabdomyolysis in thyroid storm. *Am. J. Med.* 77:733, 1984.
    An unusual cause of myoglobinuria.
23. Britt, C. W., Jr., Light, R. R., Peters, B. H., et al. Rhabdomyolysis during treatment with epsilon-aminocaproic acid [EACA] *Arch. Neurol.* 37:187, 1980.
    EACA is a muscle toxin.
24. Williams, T. J., O'Hehir, R. E., Czarny, D., et al. Acute myopathy in severe acute asthma treated with intravenously administered corticosteroids. *Am. Rev. Respir. Dis.* 137:460, 1988.
    A potential complication of high-dose corticosteroid therapy.
25. Roth D., Alarcon, F. J., Fernandez, J. A., et al. Acute rhabdomyolysis associated with cocaine intoxication. *N. Engl. J. Med.* 319:673, 1988.
    Acute renal failure, hepatic dysfunction, and DIC were common. (See also Ann. Intern. Med. *109:335, 1988.)*
26. Gibb, W. R. G., and Lees, A. J. The neuroleptic malignant syndrome—a review. *Q. J. Med.* 56:421, 1985.
    Myoglobinuria, respiratory and renal failure may occur. (See also Arch. Intern. Med. *142:601, 1982.)*
27. Shields, R. W., Jr., Root, K. E., Jr., and Wilbourn, A. J. Compartment syndromes and compression neuropathies in coma. *Neurology* 36:1370, 1986.
    A palpable pulse does not exclude tissue damage due to compression.
28. Knochel, J. P., and Schlein, E. M. On the mechanism of rhabdomyolysis in potassium depletion. *J. Clin. Invest.* 51:1750, 1972.
    Local increases in potassium concentration promote arteriolar dilatation and improve muscle blood flow.
29. Knochel, J. P., Barcenas, C., Cotton, J. R., et al. Hypophosphatemia and rhabdomyolysis. *J. Clin. Invest.* 62:1240, 1978.
    Role of phosphorus deficiency in rhabdomyolysis examined experimentally. (See also J.A.M.A. *239:643, 1978.)*
30. Eneas, J. F., Schoenfeld, P. Y., and Humphreys, M. H. The effect of infusion of mannitol-sodium bicarbonate on the clinical course of myoglobinuria. *Arch. Intern. Med.* 139:801, 1979.
    Some but not all patients respond to mannitol with an improvement in renal function.
31. Liach, F., Felsenfeld, A. J., and Haussler, M. R. Pathophysiology of altered calcium metabolism in rhabdomyolysis-induced acute renal failure. *N. Engl. J. Med.* 305:117, 1981.
    It is suggested that hypercalcemia during the oliguric phase is due to increased synthesis of vitamin D. (See also the accompanying editorial on p. 161.)
32. Ward, M. M. Factors predictive of acute renal failure in rhabdomyolysis. *Arch. Intern. Med.* 148:1553, 1988.
    An interesting approach.

160. PARANEOPLASTIC SYNDROMES
Martin D. Abeloff

The clinical effects of cancer can be divided from a pathophysiologic standpoint into two major categories: direct and indirect manifestations. The direct effects are those resulting from mass lesions which result in organ dysfunction. Examples are superior vena caval syndrome and spinal cord compression. *Paraneoplastic syndrome* is a generic term used to describe those indirect manifestations which are a consequence of production of hormones, growth factors by the tumor, or immunologic interactions induced by the tumor.

The most frequently recognized paraneoplastic syndromes are endocrine, neurologic, dermatologic, hematologic, and renal. However, these syndromes can involve virtually all organ systems and occur in approximately 10 to 15 percent of patients with cancer. Systemic manifestations of cancer such as cachexia can also be considered paraneoplastic.

Although paraneoplastic syndromes are sometimes regarded as medical oddities, they are important to clinicians for the following reasons. First, these complexes of signs and symptoms can be the initial clue to the presence of an underlying neoplasm. The Eaton-Lambert syndrome is a rare myasthenic syndrome which presents in the majority of cases as an early finding in patients with small cell carcinoma of the lung. This syndrome is characterized by weakness of the proximal muscles, dry mouth, myalgias, peripheral paresthesias, and impotence. The mildness and rarity of ocular and bulbar signs and symptoms are distinctly different from myasthenia gravis with which the syndrome may be confused. Another clinical difference from myasthenia gravis is the weakness or absence of the deep tendon reflexes, particularly the patellar or Achilles, in Eaton-Lambert syndrome. The electromyogram findings are diagnostic and opposite to those found in myasthenia gravis. In rested muscle, there is a marked depression of neuromuscular transmission after a single submaximal stimulus, and a marked facilitation of the response during repetitive stimulation at rates greater than 10 per second. Tumor therapy produces improvement in about one-third of the cases.

Second, paraneoplastic syndromes can be a marker of the activity of a specific cancer and thus can herald remission or recurrence. The syndrome of inappropriate antidiuretic hormone secretion (SIADH) is one of the most common endocrine paraneoplastic syndromes and is frequently associated with bronchogenic cancer, particularly small cell carcinoma of the lung. SIADH occurs at the time of diagnosis in approximately 10 percent of patients with small cell carcinoma and in an additional 15 percent at the time of tumor relapse or progression. The characteristic features of SIADH are (1) hyponatremia associated with serum hypoosmolality and urinary osmolality in excess of serum, (2) continued urinary excretion of sodium, (3) absence of cardiac, thyroid, renal, and adrenal dysfunction. In many patients with cancer, SIADH is mild and does not result in symptomatology. In responsive neoplasms such as small cell lung cancer and lymphoma, the treatment of the underlying disease results in correction of the hyponatremia. However, fluid restriction or specific pharmacologic intervention such as demeclocycline are also frequently necessary.

Third, clinical effects of the paraneoplastic syndrome can be confused with the direct effects of cancer or toxic effects of cancer therapy. The development of peripheral neuropathy in a patient with cancer can represent an indirect effect of the tumor or can result from commonly used therapeutic agents such as vincristine and cisplatin. Likewise, thrombocytopenia in conjunction with a microangiopathic hemolytic anemia and renal dysfunction can be a paraneoplastic manifestation (hemolytic uremic syndrome) of a variety of cancers but also has been associated with a particular cytotoxic agent, mitomycin C.

Finally, the paraneoplastic symptoms can be as serious and difficult to deal with as the cancer itself. The metabolic and physical consequences of the ectopic ACTH syndrome, that is, hyperglycemia, hypokalemia, and muscle weakness, can represent the dominant symptomatology in a patient with lung cancer. Neurologic paraneoplastic syndromes such as limbic encephalopathy, cortical cerebellar degeneration, and multifocal leukoencephalopathy can be the primary causes of death in patients with underlying tumors. The optimal therapeutic approach to these syndromes is definitive treatment of the underlying neoplasm. However, pharmacologic interventions directed at specific aspects of the paraneoplastic syndrome are frequently required for those patients in whom the antitumor therapy has not been successful in alleviating the consequences of the paraneoplastic process.

1. Abeloff, M. D., Paraneoplastic syndromes: A window on the biology of cancer. *N. Engl. J. Med.* 317:1598, 1987.
   Discussion of paraneoplastic syndromes as clues to biologic behavior of tumors.
2. deBustros, A., and Baylin, S. B. Hormone production by tumours; biological and clinical aspects. *Clin. Endocrinol. Metab.* 14:221, 1987.
   Excellent review with emphasis on biologic aspects.
3. Ellis, D. L., Kafka, S. P., Chow, J. C., et al. Melanoma, growth factors, acanthosis nigricans, the sign of Leser-Trélat, and multiple acrochordons; a possible role for alpha-transforming growth factor in cutaneous paraneoplastic syndromes. *N. Engl. J. Med.* 317:1581, 1987.
   New insight into the potential role of growth factors in paraneoplastic syndromes.
4. Grunwald, G. B., Kornguth, S. E., Towfighi, J., et al. Autoimmune basis for visual paraneoplastic syndrome in patients with small cell lung carcinoma. Retinal immune deposits and ablation of retinal ganglion cells. *Cancer* 60:780, 1987.
   Immunologic basis for retinal complications of malignancy.
5. Hasling, C., Charles, P., and Mosekilde, L. Etidronate disodium in the management of malignancy-related hypercalcemia. *Am. J. Med.* 82:51, 1987.
   Treatment of common paraneoplastic manifestation.
6. Ihde, D. C. Paraneoplastic syndromes. *Hosp. Pract.* 22:105, 1987.
   Excellent review emphasizing pathophysiology.
7. Ishikawa, K., Engelhardt, J. E., Fujisawa, T., et al. A neuromuscular transmission block produced by a cancer tissue extract derived from a patient with the myasthenic syndrome. *Neurology* 30:634, 1980.
   A clear in vitro demonstration of decreased acetylcholine release produced by a substance(s) in the tumor extract.
8. Lambert, E. H., and Eaton, L. M. Electromyography and electric stimulation of nerves in diseases of motor unit. *J.A.M.A.* 163:1117, 1957.
   A classic description of the syndrome.
9. Lambert, E. H., and Rooke, E. D. *The Remote Effects of Cancer on the Nervous System.* New York: Grune & Stratton, 1965.
   Most patients have small cell bronchogenic carcinoma.
10. Lambert, E. H. Defects of neuromuscular transmission in syndromes other than myasthenia gravis. *Ann. N.Y. Acad. Sci.* 135:367, 1966.
    The pathologic differences between the Eaton-Lambert syndrome and myasthenia gravis.
11. Lauritzen, M., Smith, T., Fischer-Hansen, B., et al. Eaton-Lambert syndrome and malignant thymoma. *Neurology* 30:634, 1980.
    Another association with references to others.
12. Markman, M. Response of paraneoplastic syndromes to antineoplastic therapy. *West. J. Med.* 144:580, 1986.
    Discussion of the limitations of antineoplastic therapy in alleviating paraneoplastic syndromes.
13. McLean, D. I. Cutaneous paraneoplastic syndromes. *Arch. Dermatol.* 122:765, 1986.
    Visible clues to underlying cancer.
14. Moertel, C. G. Karnofsky Memorial Lecture. An odyssey in the land of small tumors. *J. Clin. Oncol.* 5:1502, 1987.
    Progress in treatment of endocrine tumors.
15. Trump, D. L. Ectopic Hormone Syndromes. In M. D. Abeloff (ed.), *Complications of Cancer: Diagnosis and Management.* Baltimore: Johns Hopkins University Press, 1979. P. 211.
    Thorough discussion of endocrine paraneoplastic syndromes.

16. Tsukamoto, T., Yoshie, O., Tada, K., et al. Anti-Purkinje cell antibody producing B-cell lines from a patient with paraneoplastic cerebellar degeneration. *Arch. Neurol.* 44:833, 1987.
Immunologic mechanism of cerebellar degeneration in patients with cancer.

161. SARCOIDOSIS
Jerry L. Spivak

Sarcoidosis is a systemic illness of unknown cause characterized by the presence of a noncaseating, granulomatous inflammatory reaction. The principal tissues involved are, in order of frequency, the lungs, mediastinal lymph nodes, peripheral lymph nodes, skin, eyes, liver, spleen, bone, salivary and lacrimal glands, joints, heart, skeletal muscle, central nervous system, and kidneys. Cutaneous anergy with respect to reactions involving delayed hypersensitivity is also common in sarcoidosis, but humoral antibody production is not impaired. Furthermore, in the presence of a tuberculous infection, patients with sarcoidosis are capable of developing a positive tuberculin reaction.

In accordance with the systemic nature of sarcoidosis, its clinical manifestations are protean. The disease is not uncommonly discovered on routine chest x ray in an asymptomatic individual. Bilateral hilar adenopathy (stage I), a combination of hilar adenopathy and pulmonary infiltration (stage II), or pulmonary infiltration (stage III) alone may be seen. Much evidence has been accumulated to support the contention that bilateral hilar adenopathy in the absence of symptoms or in the presence of erythema nodosum and uveitis represents sarcoidosis and not an infectious or neoplastic process. The disease can also present in a more symptomatic form, with cutaneous, ocular, or glandular involvement, cranial nerve paralysis, meningitis, polyarthritis or fever, chills, and organomegaly.

The diagnosis of sarcoidosis is based on the characteristics of the clinical manifestations, the presence of noncaseating granulomas on tissue biopsy, and exclusion of other known causes of granulomatous inflammatory reactions. These include tuberculosis, mycotic infections, syphilis, Hodgkin's disease, berylliosis, brucellosis, Q fever, histiocytosis, tularemia, biliary cirrhosis, drug reactions (sulfonamides, phenylbutazone), leprosy, Wegener's granulomatosis, allergic alveolitis, pulmonary vasculitis, and local sarcoidal reactions in lymph nodes draining the locus of a solid tumor. The presence of noncaseating granulomas in liver or peripheral or scalene lymph nodes does not constitute absolute evidence of sarcoidosis since these may occur in the presence of active pulmonary tuberculosis. Furthermore, the presence of noncaseating granulomas in intrathoracic lymph nodes does not exclude metastatic carcinoma as a cause of parenchymal pulmonary lesions. Lung biopsy provides more certain evidence of the pathologic process, but the frequency of positive lung biopsies in sarcoidosis declines with time. Hyperuricemia, hypercalcemia, hyperglobulinemia, elevated rheumatoid factor levels, and false-positive serologic reactions are all found in patients with sarcoidosis and add to the difficulty of the diagnostic process. Antimitochondrial antibody levels can be used to distinguish sarcoidosis from primary biliary cirrhosis. The level of angiotensin-converting enzyme (ACE) is elevated in the serum of patients with sarcoidosis and has been proposed as a diagnostic test for the disorder. Unfortunately, serum ACE appears to parallel the increased macrophage activity associated with granulomatous inflammation and is elevated in other disorders causing granuloma formation such as miliary tuberculosis and silicosis. Measurement of serum ACE appears to be of most value in following the course of sarcoidosis and its response to treatment.

The course of sarcoidosis is highly variable. Most patients with erythema nodosum (Lofgren's syndrome) as an initial manifestation do well, as do those with asymptomatic hilar adenopathy. However, this is not always the case, nor does extensive pulmonary infiltration inevitably imply a poor prognosis. Complications of sarcoidosis include central nervous system damage with neurologic and endocrine abnormalities, bullous and cavitary pulmonary disease as well as pulmonary fibrosis, mycetomas, myocardial sarcoid with conduction system defects and sudden death, hypercalcemia, nephropathy, hepatic insufficiency with portal hypertension, and progressive ocular disease.

Corticosteroids have been the major therapeutic agent used in the treatment of sarcoidosis, although chloroquine has been effective in controlling cutaneous disease and hypercalcemia. Steroid therapy is indicated for active cardiac, ocular, central nervous system and hepatic disease, symptomatic pulmonary disease, severe constitutional symptoms, and hypercalcemia. At the present time, bronchoalveolar lavage and gallium scanning appear not to be more useful than conventional x-ray studies and pulmonary function tests for monitoring disease activity.

1. Johns, C. J., Scott, P. P., and Schonfeld, S. A. Sarcoidosis. *Annu. Rev. Med.* 40:353, 1989.
   Comprehensive review. (See also Arch. Intern. Med. 31:213, 1986.)
2. Hillerdal, G., Nou, K., Osterman, K., et al. Sarcoidosis: Epidemiology and prognosis. *Am. Rev. Respir. Dis.* 130:29, 1984.
   Natural history of sarcoidosis in a Scandinavian population.
3. Foti, P. R., and Moser, K. M. Laboratory guides to scalene node or liver biopsy in suspected sarcoidosis. *Am. Rev. Respir. Dis.* 99:610, 1969.
   Scalene node biopsy is positive more often than liver biopsy.
4. Gilman, M. J., and Wang, K. P. Transbronchial lung biopsy in sarcoidosis: An approach to determine the optimal number of biopsies. *Am. Rev. Respir. Dis.* 122:721, 1980.
   Four biopsies were found to be sufficient to obtain a tissue diagnosis.
5. Poe, R. H., Israel, R. H., Utell, M. J., et al. Probability of a positive transbronchial lung biopsy result in sarcoidosis. *Arch. Intern. Med.* 139:761, 1979.
   The chest x ray best predicted the likelihood of a positive biopsy.
6. Solomon, D. A., Horn, B. R., Byrd, R. B., et al. The diagnosis of sarcoidosis by conjunctival biopsy. *Chest* 74:271, 1978.
   Examination by slit lamp is required to detect conjunctival lesions; biopsies are most often positive in black patients.
7. Nessan, V. J., and Jacoway, J. R. Biopsy of minor salivary glands in the diagnosis of sarcoidosis. *N. Engl. J. Med.* 301:922, 1979.
   A higher yield procedure than skin or conjunctival biopsy but not as high as transbronchial lung biopsy or liver biopsy.
8. Kent, D. C., Houk, V. N., Elliott, R. C., et al. The definitive evaluation of sarcoidosis. *Am. Rev. Respir. Dis.* 101:721, 1970.
   Open-lung biopsy advocated when the results of other diagnostic procedures are equivocal.
9. Winterbauer, R. H., Belic, N., and Moores, K. D. A clinical interpretation of bilateral hilar adenopathy. *Ann. Intern. Med.* 78:65, 1973.
   Bilateral hilar adenopathy in asymptomatic patients with no other physical findings or with erythema nodosum or uveitis was found to be due exclusively to sarcoidosis.
10. Sharma, O. P. Cutaneous sarcoidosis: Clinical features and management. *Chest* 61:320, 1972.
    Chronic skin lesions associated with bone and eye lesions. (See also Arch. Dermatol. 123:1531, 1987 and Br. J. Dermatol. 112:315, 1985.)
11. Maddrey, W. C., Johns, C. J., Boitnott, J. K., et al. Sarcoidosis and chronic hepatic disease: A clinical and pathologic study of 20 patients. *Medicine* 49:375, 1970.
    A spectrum of liver abnormalities is found, including portal hypertension and cholestatic jaundice. (See also Am. J. Med. 83:977, 1987 and Sarcoidosis 2:38, 1985 for the association of biliary cirrhosis and sarcoidosis.)
12. Romer, F. K. Renal manifestations and abnormal calcium metabolism in sarcoidosis. *Q. J. Med.* 49:233, 1980.
    Hypercalcemia was the most common cause of renal failure in this study. (See also Arch. Intern. Med. 139:1183, 1979.)
13. Neville, E., Carstairs, L. S., and James, D. G. Sarcoidosis of bone. *Q. J. Med.* 46:215, 1977.

44. Trump, D. L., Ettinger, D. S., Feldman, M., et al. Sarcoidosis and sarcoid-like lesions. *Arch. Intern. Med.* 141:37, 1981.
    Sarcoidosis-like lesions developing in conjunction with radiotherapy or chemotherapy. (See also Cancer Treat. Rev. *13:147, 1986.)*
45. Simon, H. B., and Wolff, S. M. Granulomatous hepatitis and prolonged fever of unknown origin: A study of 13 patients. *Medicine* 52:1, 1973.
    A problem in differential diagnosis. (See also Ann. Intern. Med. *79:669, 1973 and* Sarcoidosis *3:30, 1986.)*
46. Thomas, P. D., and Hunninghake, G. W. Current concepts of the pathogenesis of sarcoidosis. *Am. Rev. Respir. Dis.* 135:747, 1987.
    Many clues but still no solution.

INDEX

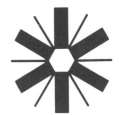
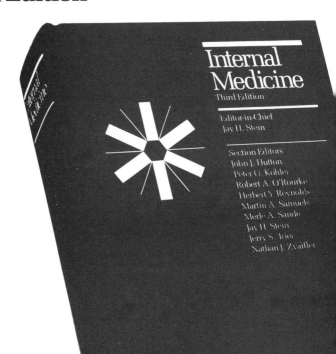

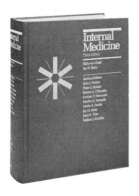
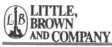

More titles in the *Little, Brown* **Spiral**® *Manual Series*